Amino Acids
Biochemistry and Nutrition

Second Edition

Amino Acids
Biochemistry and Nutrition

Second Edition

Guoyao Wu
Texas A&M University
College Station, Texas, USA

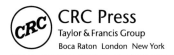

CRC Press
Taylor & Francis Group
Boca Raton London New York

CRC Press is an imprint of the
Taylor & Francis Group, an **informa** business

Second edition published 2022
by CRC Press
6000 Broken Sound Parkway NW, Suite 300, Boca Raton, FL 33487-2742

and by CRC Press
2 Park Square, Milton Park, Abingdon, Oxon, OX14 4RN

© 2022 Taylor & Francis Group, LLC

First edition published by CRC Press 2013

CRC Press is an imprint of Taylor & Francis Group, LLC

Library of Congress Cataloging-in-Publication Data
Names: Wu, Guoyao, 1962- author.
Title: Amino acids : biochemistry and nutrition / Guoyao Wu.
Description: 2nd edition. | Boca Raton : CRC Press, 2021. |
Includes bibliographical references and index. | Summary: "Following its
predecessor, the second edition of Amino Acids: Biochemistry and
Nutrition presents exhaustive coverage of amino acids in the nutrition,
metabolism and health of humans and other animals. Substantially
revised, expanded and updated to reflect scientific advances, this book
introduces the basic principles of amino acid biochemistry and
nutrition, while highlighting the current knowledge of the field and its
future possibilities. The book begins with the basic chemical concepts
of amnio acids, peptides and proteins, and their digestion and
absorption. Subsequent chapters cover cell-, tissue-, and
species-specific synthesis and catabolism of amino acids and related
bioactive metabolites, and the use of isotopes to study amino acids
metabolism in cells and the body. The book details protein turnover,
physiological functions of amino acids, as well as both the regulation
and inborn errors of amino acid metabolism. The book concludes with a
presentation on human and animal dietary requirements of amino acids and
evaluates dietary protein quality"— Provided by publisher.
Identifiers: LCCN 2021011176 (print) | LCCN 2021011177 (ebook) |
ISBN 9780367552787 (hardback) | ISBN 9781032030890 (paperback) |
ISBN 9781003092742 (ebook)
Subjects: MESH: Amino Acids
Classification: LCC QP551 (print) | LCC QP551 (ebook) | NLM QU 60 | DDC
572/.65—dc23
LC record available at https://lccn.loc.gov/2021011176
LC ebook record available at https://lccn.loc.gov/2021011177

ISBN: 9780367552787 (hbk)
ISBN: 9781032030890 (pbk)
ISBN: 9781003092742 (ebk)

Typeset in Times
by codeMantra

Contents

Preface... xxiii
Acknowledgments... xxv
Author xxvii

Chapter 1 Discovery and Chemistry of Amino Acids..1

1.1 Definition and Nomenclature of AAs...3
    1.1.1 Definition of AAs 3
    1.1.2 Definition of Imino Acids...5
    1.1.3 Isomers of AAs...5
        1.1.3.1 L- and D-AAs 5
        1.1.3.2 *R*- and *S*-AAs 9
        1.1.3.3 *cis*- and *trans*-AAs 11
    1.1.4 Proteinogenic and Non-Proteinogenic AAs 12
    1.1.5 Free AAs and Peptide (or Protein)-Bound AAs 12
1.2 Discovery of AAs 16
    1.2.1 L-AAs and Glycine.. 16
    1.2.2 β- and γ-AAs with Physiological Significance 27
    1.2.3 D-AAs...28
        1.2.3.1 Presence of D-AAs in Plant- and Animal-Sourced Foods 28
        1.2.3.2 Presence of D-AAs in the Animal Kingdom...29
        1.2.3.3 Presence of D-AAs in Microbes 30
    1.2.4 Other AAs...31
        1.2.4.1 Other AAs in the Animal Kingdom 31
        1.2.4.2 Other AAs in Spoiled Animal Products..33
        1.2.4.3 Other AAs in Plants..33
        1.2.4.4 Other AAs in Microbes 34
        1.2.4.5 Other AAs in Processed Foods...35
1.3 Chemical Properties of AAs...35
    1.3.1 Physical Appearance, Fluorescence, and Melting Points of Crystalline AAs 35
    1.3.2 Tastes of Crystalline AAs...35
    1.3.3 Solubility of AAs in Water and Organic Solvents..37
    1.3.4 The Zwitterionic Form of AAs...38
    1.3.5 Chemical Stability of AAs 42
        1.3.5.1 Stability of Crystalline AAs 42
        1.3.5.2 Stability of Free AAs in Water and Buffered Solutions at <0°C
              and ≤40°C..42
        1.3.5.3 Stability of Free AAs in Water at High Temperatures 43
        1.3.5.4 Stability of Free AAs in Water under High Pressure and
              High Temperatures..43
        1.3.5.5 Stability of Free AAs in Strong Acid and Alkaline Solutions at ≤25°C.....43
        1.3.5.6 Stability of Free AAs in Strong Acid and Alkaline Solutions at
              High Temperatures..43
    1.3.6 Chemical Reactions of AAs 44
        1.3.6.1 Chemical Reactions of the Amino Group in α-AAs 44
        1.3.6.2 Chemical Reactions of the Carboxyl Group in α-AAs...........................48
        1.3.6.3 Chemical Reactions of the Side Chain in α-AAs 48

    1.3.6.4 Chemical Reactions Involving Both the Amino and Carboxyl
        Groups of α-AAs...49
  1.3.7 Proteins...53
    1.3.7.1 Determination of Protein Concentration 53
    1.3.7.2 Proteins versus Peptides...54
1.4 Summary 59
References...61

Chapter 2 Protein Digestion and Absorption of Peptides and Amino Acids............................67

2.1 Classification and Content of Protein in Diets...69
  2.1.1 Classification of Protein...69
  2.1.2 Protein Content of Foods of Animal and Plant Origin...........................71
2.2 Definitions of Digestion and Absorption...72
  2.2.1 Digestion...72
  2.2.2 Absorption 75
2.3 Protein Digestion and Absorption of Peptides and AAs in Monogastric Animals...............76
  2.3.1 Historical Perspective of Protein Digestion and Absorption..................76
  2.3.2 Digestion of Dietary Protein in the Gastrointestinal Tract....................76
  2.3.3 Developmental Changes in Intestinal Digestion and Absorption...........79
  2.3.4 Determination of Protein Digestibility 81
  2.3.5 Absorption of Free AAs and Small Peptides by the Small Intestine 88
    2.3.5.1 Transport of Free AAs via Transmembrane Transporters..........88
    2.3.5.2 Transport of AAs via the γ-Glutamyl Cycle 88
    2.3.5.3 Transport of Small Peptides by the Small Intestine 92
  2.3.6 Net Balance of AAs Across the Small Intestine in Monogastric Animals 94
  2.3.7 Extensive Recycling of Nitrogen in the Intestine of Monogastric Animals...............96
2.4 Protein Digestion and the Absorption of Peptides and AAs in Ruminants.........................99
  2.4.1 Nutritional Significance of Protein Digestion in Ruminants...................99
  2.4.2 Digestion of Dietary Protein in the Gastrointestinal Tract....................100
  2.4.3 Digestion of Nucleic Acids in the Rumen and Other Parts of
    the Gastrointestinal Tract 103
  2.4.4 Absorption of Free AAs and Small Peptides by the Small Intestine 105
  2.4.5 Nitrogen Recycling in Ruminants and Its Nutritional Implications........105
  2.4.6 Protecting High-Quality Protein and Crystalline AAs from Rumen
    Degradation...106
    2.4.6.1 Heating..106
    2.4.6.2 Chemical Treatment..107
    2.4.6.3 Polyphenolic Phytochemicals 107
    2.4.6.4 Physical Encapsulation of Proteins or AAs 108
    2.4.6.5 Inhibition of AA Degradation..108
  2.4.7 Degradation of Toxic AAs by Ruminal Microbes................................109
2.5 Summary 109
References... 110

Chapter 3 Synthesis of Amino Acids.. 117

3.1 Synthesis of Amino Acids in Tissues and Cells of Humans and Other Animals 118
  3.1.1 Overall View of Amino Acid Synthesis 118
  3.1.2 Cell-, Tissue-, and Species-Specific Synthesis of Amino Acids in
    Humans and Other Animals... 118
    3.1.2.1 Synthesis of AAs in the Liver.. 125

3.1.2.2   Synthesis of Amino Acids in Skeletal Muscle, Heart, Brain, Lungs,
and White Adipose Tissue 125
3.1.2.3   Synthesis of Amino Acids in the Small Intestine 127
3.1.2.4   Synthesis of Amino Acids in the Kidneys 127
3.1.2.5   Synthesis of Amino Acids in Endothelial Cells, Smooth Muscle Cells,
Macrophages, and Lymphocytes 127
3.1.2.6   Synthesis of Amino Acids in Sense Organs 128
3.1.2.7   Synthesis of Amino Acids in Placentae, Mammary Glands,
Ovaries, and Testes 128
3.1.3   Amino Acid Synthesis and Homeostasis in Humans and Other Animals 128
3.1.4   Alterations in the Rates of Amino Acid Synthesis in Disease 131
3.2   General Pathways for the Synthesis of Amino Acids in Animal Cells 132
3.2.1   Overall Pathways for the Synthesis of Amino Acids in Animal Cells 132
3.2.2   Historical Perspectives of Amino Acid Transamination 133
3.3   Specific Pathways for the Synthesis of Amino Acids in Humans and Other Animals 133
3.3.1   Synthesis of Alanine, Glutamine, and Glutamate in Animal Cells 133
3.3.2   Synthesis of Arginine, Citrulline, and Ornithine in Animal Cells 136
3.3.3   Synthesis of Aspartate and Asparagine in Animal Cells 138
3.3.4   Synthesis of Cysteine and Taurine in Animal Cells 138
3.3.5   Synthesis of Homoarginine from Arginine and Lysine in Animal Cells 140
3.3.6   Synthesis of Glycine and Serine in Animal Cells 140
3.3.7   Synthesis of Methylarginines in Animal Cells 146
3.3.8   Synthesis of Proline and Hydroxyproline in Animal Cells 148
3.3.9   Synthesis of Tyrosine in Animal Cells 150
3.3.10 Formation of β-Alanine in Animal Cells 150
3.3.11 Synthesis of Unique Sulfur-Containing Amino Acids in Felidae
Species and Other Animals 151
3.3.12 Synthesis of N-Acetylated Amino Acids in Animal Cells 153
3.3.13 Synthesis of Phosphoryl Amino Acids in Animal Cells 154
3.4   Pathways for the Synthesis of Amino Acids in Microorganisms 154
3.4.1   Overall Pathways for the Synthesis of Amino Acids in Microorganisms 155
3.4.2   Pathways for the Synthesis of AASAs in Microorganisms 156
3.4.2.1   Synthesis of Glutamate and Glutamine 156
3.4.2.2   Synthesis of Arginine 158
3.4.2.3   Synthesis of Aspartate and Asparagine 159
3.4.2.4   Synthesis of Cysteine and Tyrosine 159
3.4.3   Pathways for the Synthesis of Essential Amino Acids in Microorganisms 160
3.4.4   Synthesis of N-Acetylated Amino Acids in Microorganisms 161
3.4.5   Pathways for the Synthesis of 2,6-Diaminopimelic Acid and
2-Aminoethylphosphonate 163
3.4.6   Pathways for the Synthesis of Phosphoryl Amino Acids in Microorganisms 164
3.5   Synthesis of D-AAs from L-AAs in Animal Cells and Microorganisms 164
3.5.1   Human and Other Animals 164
3.5.2   Microorganisms 166
3.5.2.1   Amino Acid Racemases 166
3.5.2.2   Amino Acid Epimerases 167
3.6   Conversion of D-AAs into L-AAs in Animal Cells and Microorganisms 167
3.6.1   Humans and Other Animals 167
3.6.2   Microorganisms 168
3.7   Conversion of α-Ketoacids into L-AAs in Animal Cells and Microorganisms 169
3.8   Summary 170
References 172

Chapter 4   Degradation of Amino Acids 181

4.1   General Characteristics of AA Degradation in Animal Cells... 181
    4.1.1   Overall View of AA Catabolism 181
    4.1.2   Catabolic Pathways of AAs and Their Major Metabolites...................................... 182
    4.1.3   Energetic Efficiencies of AA Catabolism.. 186
    4.1.4   Cell-, Tissue-, and Species-Specific Degradation of AAs................................ 190
    4.1.5   Age-Dependent Changes in AA Catabolism.. 192
    4.1.6   Half-Lives of AAs in the Blood Plasma of Humans and Other Animals 194
    4.1.7   Alterations in the Rates and Patterns of AA Catabolism in Disease 197
4.2   Pathways for the Degradation of AAs in Animal Cells 198
    4.2.1   Historical Perspectives 198
    4.2.2   Catabolism of Alanine, Aspartate, Asparagine, Glutamate, and Glutamine 198
        4.2.2.1   Enzyme-Catalyzed Reactions for the Initiation of Glutamine,
                  Glutamate, Aspartate, and Alanine Catabolism 199
        4.2.2.2   Kidney- and Liver-Type Glutaminases 202
        4.2.2.3   Asparaginase..203
    4.2.3   Catabolism of Arginine, Citrulline, and Ornithine 205
        4.2.3.1   Multiple Enzymes for the Initiation of Arginine Catabolism....................205
        4.2.3.2   Arginases 207
        4.2.3.3   NO Synthases...207
        4.2.3.4   The Arginine Paradox for NO Synthesis..209
        4.2.3.5   Arginine Decarboxylase 211
        4.2.3.6   Syntheses of Polyamines and Creatine from Arginine.......................... 211
    4.2.4   Catabolism of BCAAs 211
        4.2.4.1   BCAA Transaminases 212
        4.2.4.2   BCKA Dehydrogenase.. 214
        4.2.4.3   KIC Dioxygenase 214
        4.2.4.4   Other Enzymes for the Degradation of BCKAs.................................... 215
        4.2.4.5   Nutritional and Physiological Regulation of BCAA Catabolism 216
    4.2.5   Catabolism of Glycine and Serine 217
        4.2.5.1   The Glycine Cleavage System (GCS) 217
        4.2.5.2   Serine Hydroxymethyltransferase (SHMT)....................................... 217
        4.2.5.3   Glycine N-Methyltransferase (GNMT)... 219
        4.2.5.4   Other Enzymes for the Degradation of Serine 219
    4.2.6   Catabolism of Histidine...220
    4.2.7   Catabolism of Lysine 221
        4.2.7.1   Lysine Degradation via Saccharopine and Pipecolate Pathways............. 221
        4.2.7.2   Decarboxylation of Lysine to Cadaverine by ODC in Animal Cells 222
    4.2.8   Catabolism of Phenylalanine and Tyrosine 223
    4.2.9   Catabolism of Proline, 4-Hydroxyproline, and 3-Hydroxyproline..........................225
        4.2.9.1   Proline Oxidase, 4-Hydroxyproline Oxidase, and
                  3-Hydroxyproline Oxidase 226
        4.2.9.2   Metabolism of P5C 226
        4.2.9.3   The "Arginine-Proline Cycle" between Mother and Neonate 227
    4.2.10 Catabolism of Sulfur-Containing AAs...227
        4.2.10.1 Transsulfuration Pathway for Methionine Catabolism............................228
        4.2.10.2 Catabolism of Cysteine to Taurine, H_2S, SO_2, and Sulfate 229
        4.2.10.3 Transamination Pathway for Methionine Catabolism 230
        4.2.10.4 Catabolism of Taurine in Animal Cells.. 231
        4.2.10.5 Catabolism of Taurine in Intestinal Bacteria................................. 231

4.2.11 Catabolism of Threonine..231
4.2.12 Catabolism of Tryptophan...234
      4.2.12.1 The Kynurenine Pathway..234
      4.2.12.2 The Serotonin Pathway...236
      4.2.12.3 The Transamination Pathway 237
4.2.13 Catabolism of Selenocysteine in Animals.......................................237
4.2.14 Catabolism of N-Acetylated AAs in Humans and Other Animals 237
4.3 Catabolism of D-AAs in Animal Cells...238
   4.3.1 D-AA Transporters in Animal Cells..238
   4.3.2 Enzymes for Initiating D-AA Catabolism in Animal Cells.................238
4.4 Catabolism of L-AAs and D-AAs in Microorganisms 239
   4.4.1 L-AA Catabolism in Microbes..239
   4.4.2 D-AA Catabolism in Microbes..241
   4.4.3 Metabolites from the Catabolism of L- and D-AAs in Microbes 241
   4.4.4 Differences in AA Catabolism between Bacteria and Animals............242
4.5 Summary 244
References..245

Chapter 5   Synthesis and Catabolism of Special Substances from Amino Acids.....................255

5.1 Production of Dipeptides Consisting of Histidine or Its Methylated Derivatives................255
   5.1.1 History of Research on Carnosine and Related Dipeptides in Animal Tissues.......255
   5.1.2 Synthesis of Carnosine and Related Dipeptides.............................260
   5.1.3 Regulation of Carnosine Synthesis in Skeletal Muscle 261
      5.1.3.1 Availability of Substrates...261
      5.1.3.2 Age, Sex, Muscle Fiber Type, and Physical Activity.....................262
   5.1.4 Regulation of Anserine Synthesis in the Skeletal Muscle of Nonprimates.............262
   5.1.5 Catabolism of Carnosine and Related Dipeptides.........................263
      5.1.5.1 Carnosinase..263
      5.1.5.2 Anserinase 263
   5.1.6 Species-Specific Tissue Distribution of Carnosine, Anserine, and Balenine...........263
      5.1.6.1 Carnosine 263
      5.1.6.2 Anserine in Nonprimates..264
      5.1.6.3 Balenine 265
5.2 Synthesis and Degradation of GSH...265
   5.2.1 History of GSH Research...265
   5.2.2 Concentrations of GSH in Physiological Fluids and Tissues of
      Humans and Other Animals..265
   5.2.3 GSH Synthesis...266
   5.2.4 Regulation of GSH Synthesis 266
   5.2.5 Transport and Degradation of GSH..268
5.3 Production of Gly-Pro-4-Hydroxyproline 268
   5.3.1 Abundance of Gly-Pro-4-Hydroxyproline in the Milk and Plasma.........................268
   5.3.2 Utilization of Gly-Pro-4-Hydroxyproline by Animals.........................269
5.4 Endogenous and Food-Derived Oligopeptides Consisting of 3–20 or More AA Residues 270
   5.4.1 Endogenous Synthesis of Opioid Peptides in Humans and Other Animals............270
   5.4.2 Bioactive Peptides in Protein Hydrolysates for Improving Human
      Nutrition and Health..271
   5.4.3 Bioactive Peptides in Protein Hydrolysates for Improving Animal
      Nutrition and Health..275
5.5 Synthesis and Catabolism of Polyamines 276

5.5.1   History of Polyamine Research 276
5.5.2   Polyamine Synthesis 277
    5.5.2.1   Pathways of Polyamine Synthesis 277
    5.5.2.2   Regulation of Polyamine Synthesis 279
5.5.3   Polyamine Degradation 279
    5.5.3.1   Diamine Oxidase and Polyamine Oxidase 279
    5.5.3.2   Spermidine/Spermine N^1-Acetyltransferase and
              N^1-Acetylpolyamine Oxidase 281
5.6   Synthesis and Utilization of Creatine 281
5.6.1   History of Creatine Research 281
5.6.2   Creatine Synthesis Through Interorgan Cooperation 281
5.6.3   Regulation of Creatine Synthesis 283
    5.6.3.1   Expression of Arginine: Glycine Amidinotransferase 283
    5.6.3.2   Availability of Substrates 283
5.6.4   Metabolism of Creatine and the Urinary Excretion of Creatinine 284
5.6.5   Tissue Distribution of Creatine 285
5.7   Synthesis and Catabolism of L-Carnitine 285
5.7.1   History of Carnitine Research 285
5.7.2   Carnitine Synthesis Through Interorgan Cooperation in Humans and
    Other Animals 286
5.7.3   Contribution of Diet and Endogenous Synthesis to Carnitine in Humans
    and Other Animals 287
5.7.4   Regulation of Carnitine Synthesis in Humans and Other Animals 288
5.7.5   Catabolism of Carnitine in Humans and Other Animals 288
5.8   Synthesis and Catabolism of Purine and Pyrimidine Nucleotides 290
5.8.1   History of Purine and Pyrimidine Research 290
5.8.2   Purine and Pyrimidine Bases in Nucleotides 291
5.8.3   Synthesis of Purine Nucleotides 292
5.8.4   Synthesis of Pyrimidine Nucleotides 293
5.8.5   Catabolism of Purines and Pyrimidines 295
5.9   Heme Synthesis and Catabolism 296
5.9.1   History of Heme Research 296
5.9.2   Pathways of Heme Synthesis in Animal Cells 298
5.9.3   Regulation of Heme Synthesis in Animal Cells 298
    5.9.3.1   Regulation of Heme Synthesis in Hepatocytes 298
    5.9.3.2   Regulation of Heme Synthesis in Erythroid Cells 300
5.9.4   Catabolism of Heme in Animal Cells 301
5.10   Synthesis and Catabolism of Histamine 303
5.10.1   Synthesis of Histamine 303
5.10.2   Catabolism of Histamine 303
5.11   Synthesis and Catabolism of Catecholamines, Thyroid Hormones, and Melanin 304
5.11.1   Synthesis and Catabolism of Catecholamines 304
5.11.2   Synthesis and Catabolism of Thyroid Hormones 306
5.11.3   Synthesis of Melanin 306
5.11.4   Elimination and Catabolism of Melanin 309
5.12   Synthesis and Catabolism of Serotonin and Melatonin 310
5.12.1   Synthesis of Serotonin and Melatonin 310
5.12.2   Catabolism of Serotonin and Melatonin 310
5.13   Synthesis and Catabolism of D-Glucosamine and Glycosaminoglycans 311
5.13.1   Historical Perspectives 311
5.13.2   Synthesis and Catabolism of D-Glucosamine 311

            5.13.2.1 Synthesis of D-Glucosamine 311
            5.13.2.2 Catabolism of Glucosamine-6-Phosphate 312
      5.13.3 Synthesis and Catabolism of Glycosaminoglycans 312
            5.13.3.1 Synthesis of Glycosaminoglycans 312
            5.13.3.2 Catabolism of Glycosaminoglycans 315
5.14 Synthesis and Catabolism of Choline 317
      5.14.1 History of Choline Research 317
      5.14.2 Synthesis of Choline in Humans and Other Animals 317
            5.14.2.1 Synthesis of Choline in Humans 317
            5.14.2.2 Synthesis of Choline in Farm and Laboratory Animals 318
      5.14.3 Catabolism of Choline in Animal Cells and in Microbes 318
            5.14.3.1 Catabolism of Choline in Cells of Humans and Other Animals 318
            5.14.3.2 Catabolism of Choline in Microbes 319
5.15 Synthesis and Catabolism of Formate 319
      5.15.1 Historic Perspectives 319
      5.15.2 Synthesis and Catabolism of Formate in Animals 320
            5.15.2.1 Synthesis of Formate in Humans and Other Animals 320
            5.15.2.2 Catabolism of Formate in Humans and Other Animals 321
      5.15.3 Synthesis and Catabolism of Formate in Microbes 321
5.16 Conjugation Products for Urinary Excretion 321
      5.16.1 Formation of Hippurate from Glycine 321
      5.16.2 Species-Specific Formation of Phenylacetylglutamine from
              Phenylalanine and Glutamine 322
5.17 Summary 323
References 323

Chapter 6   Synthesis of Urea and Uric Acid 333

6.1 Ammonia Production and Toxicity in Humans and Other Animals 333
      6.1.1 Historical Observations on the Production of Ammonia by Humans and
             Other Animals 333
      6.1.2 Removal of Ammonia in Humans and Other Animals under
             Physiological Conditions 334
      6.1.3 Normal and Abnormal Concentrations of Ammonia in Humans and
             Other Animals 335
      6.1.4 Toxicity of Ammonia to Humans and Other Animals 337
      6.1.5 Biochemical Mechanisms Responsible for Ammonia Toxicity to the
             Nervous System 338
      6.1.6 Treatment of Hyperammonemia 339
6.2 Urea Production in Mammals 339
      6.2.1 Historical Perspectives 339
      6.2.2 The Hepatic Urea Cycle in Mammals 340
            6.2.2.1 Discovery of the Urea Cycle 340
            6.2.2.2 Characteristics of the Urea Cycle 340
            6.2.2.3 Coupling of the Urea Cycle with Gluconeogenesis in the Liver 344
      6.2.3 Synthesis of Urea from Ammonia in the Extrahepatic Cells of Mammals 345
      6.2.4 Calculation of Urea Production by Mammals 346
      6.2.5 Nutritional and Metabolic Implications of Urea Synthesis in Mammals 347
      6.2.6 Regulation of the Urea Cycle in Mammals 348
      6.2.7 Energy Requirement of Ureagenesis in Mammals 349
      6.2.8 Urea Recycling in Ruminants 352

            6.2.9   Excretion of Urea by the Kidneys..353
                     6.2.9.1   Excretion of Urea in the Urine...353
                     6.2.9.2   Important Roles of Renal Transporters of Urea in Its Urinary Excretion ... 354
                     6.2.9.3   Regulation of the Expression of Renal Urea Transporters 356
            6.2.10   Urea Synthesis from Ammonia in Certain Teleost Fish and in the Elasmobranchs... 356
    6.3   Uric Acid Synthesis 357
            6.3.1   Historical Perspectives 357
            6.3.2   Chemistry of Uric Acid 358
            6.3.3   Conversion of Ammonia and Bicarbonate to Purine Nucleosides 358
            6.3.4   Uric Acid Synthesis from Purine Nucleosides 358
            6.3.5   Regulation of Uric Acid Synthesis 360
            6.3.6   Energy Requirement for Uric Acid Synthesis from Ammonia 361
                     6.3.6.1   Energy Required for the Synthesis of Uric Acid from Ammonia
                               via Adenosine..361
                     6.3.6.2   Energy Required for the Synthesis of Uric Acid from Ammonia
                               via Guanosine 362
                     6.3.6.3   Energy Required for the Overall Synthesis of Uric Acid from Ammonia... 364
            6.3.7   Nutritional and Metabolic Significance of Uric Acid Synthesis 364
            6.3.8   Species-Specific Degradation of Uric Acid to Allantoin, Allantoic Acid,
                     Urea, and Glyoxylate 364
            6.3.9   Oxidation of Uric Acid by Reactive Oxygen and Nitrogen Species into Allantoin ...365
            6.3.10   Excretion of Uric Acid by the Kidneys..366
    6.4   Comparisons between Uric Acid and Urea Syntheses 367
            6.4.1   Similarities between Urea and Uric Acid Syntheses.....................................367
            6.4.2   Differences between Urea and Uric Acid Syntheses.....................................367
    6.5   Summary 368
    References..368

    Chapter 7   Use of Isotopes for Studying Amino Acid Metabolism 375

    7.1   Basic Concepts About Isotopes 375
            7.1.1   What Are Isotopes? 375
            7.1.2   Decay of Radioisotopes 377
            7.1.3   Expression of Radioactive and Stable Isotopes 379
            7.1.4   Tracer and Tracee 381
            7.1.5   Concepts of Specific Radioactivity and Isotopic Enrichment 381
                     7.1.5.1   SR of Radioactive Isotopes 382
                     7.1.5.2   Isotopic Enrichment of Stable Isotopes 383
            7.1.6   Significance of SR and IE of a Tracer 385
                     7.1.6.1   Calculations of Rates of Nutrient Metabolism *In Vitro* and *In Vivo*
                               Using Radioisotopes 386
                     7.1.6.2   Calculations of Rates of Nutrient Metabolism *In Vitro* and
                               In Vivo Using Stable Isotopes 388
                     7.1.6.3   Assessments of Product-Precursor Relationships in Metabolism
                               Using Radioactive or Stable Tracers......................................392
            7.1.7   Why Are Isotopes Used in Metabolic Research? 392
                     7.1.7.1   Tracing Metabolic Pathways...392
                     7.1.7.2   High Sensitivity of Detection of Tracers 394
    7.2   Interpretation of Data from Isotope Experiments 394
            7.2.1   Changes in the SR or IE of the Intracellular Labeled Precursor Pool.....................395
                     7.2.1.1   Increased Dilution of Labeled Isotopes in Cells...........................395

7.2.1.2 Decreased Dilution of Labeled Isotopes in Cells 396
7.2.2 Isotope Randomization 396
7.2.3 Isotope Exchange 397
7.2.4 Isotope Recycling 398
7.2.5 Isotopic Non-Steady State 400
7.3 Potential Pitfalls of Isotopic Studies 401
7.4 Summary 403
References 404

Chapter 8 Protein Synthesis 407

8.1 Historical Perspectives of the Protein Synthesis Pathway 407
8.2 Biochemical Pathways of Protein Synthesis in the Cytoplasm of Animal Cells 408
8.2.1 Overall View of Protein Synthesis in the Cytoplasm of Animal Cells 408
8.2.2 Gene Transcription in Animal Cells 409
8.2.3 Initiation of mRNA Translation into Protein in Animal Cells 411
8.2.3.1 Dissociation of Inactive Free 80S Ribosomes into 40s and 60S Subunits 412
8.2.3.2 *Formation of the 43S Preinitiation Complex* 414
8.2.3.3 Formation of the 48S Initiation Complex 414
8.2.3.4 Formation of the Translationally Active 80S Initiation Complex 415
8.2.4 Peptide Elongation in Animal Cells 416
8.2.4.1 Activation of an AA to Form Its Aminoacyl-tRNA 416
8.2.4.2 Addition of an Incoming AA to A tRNA-Bound AA on the 80S Ribosome 416
8.2.4.3 Transfer and Binding of an Incoming Aminoacyl-tRNA to the A Site 416
8.2.4.4 Peptide Bond Formation 417
8.2.4.5 Translocation of the Newly Formed Peptidyl-tRNA 418
8.2.5 Termination of Peptide Chain Elongation 418
8.2.6 Incorporation of L-Selenocysteine (A Special AA) into Selenoproteins 419
8.2.6.1 Historical Perspectives of Research on L-Selenocysteine 419
8.2.6.2 Formation of Selenocysteine and Its Incorporation into Selenoproteins ... 419
8.2.7 Processing and Export of Newly Synthesized Proteins 420
8.2.7.1 Posttranslational Modifications of Newly Synthesized Proteins 420
8.2.7.2 Export of Certain Processed Proteins Synthesized in the Cytosol of Animal Cells into the Extracellular Space 424
8.3 The Biochemical Pathway of Protein Synthesis in the Mitochondria of Animal Cells 424
8.4 Biochemical Pathways of Protein Synthesis in the Cytosol of Prokaryotes 426
8.4.1 Protein Synthesis in the Cytosol of Prokaryotes 426
8.4.2 Major Differences in Protein Synthesis between Prokaryotes and Eukaryotes 426
8.4.2.1 Gene Transcription 426
8.4.2.2 Initiation of mRNA Translation into Protein 427
8.4.2.3 Peptide Elongation and Termination 427
8.4.3 Incorporation of L-Pyrrolysine (A Special AA) into Proteins of Certain Prokaryotes 428
8.5 Biochemical Characteristics and Significance of Protein Synthesis 429
8.5.1 Energy Requirement 429
8.5.2 Physiological Significance of Protein Synthesis 430
8.5.2.1 Physiological Functions of Proteins 430
8.5.2.2 Regulation of Protein Concentrations and Animal Growth 430
8.5.2.3 Production and Replacement of Cells 431
8.5.2.4 Wound Healing and Recovery from Injury 431

                8.5.2.5   Immune Responses and Health..432
8.6   Measurements of Protein Synthesis...432
        8.6.1   Measurement of Protein Synthesis *In Vitro*.......................................432
                8.6.1.1   General Considerations...432
                8.6.1.2   *In Vitro* Preparations..433
                8.6.1.3   Choosing A Labeled AA Tracer 433
                8.6.1.4   Measuring the Rate of Protein Synthesis *In Vitro* 434
        8.6.2   Measurement of Protein Synthesis *In Vivo*.......................................435
                8.6.2.1   General Considerations...435
                8.6.2.2   General Terminologies Used in Measuring Protein Turnover *In Vivo* 436
                8.6.2.3   Pulse Labeling of Proteins by the Single Administration of a
                            Labeled AA...437
                8.6.2.4   Flooding Dose Technique...438
                8.6.2.5   Continuous Infusion of a Tracer AA 440
                8.6.2.6   Leucine Oxidation Method...442
                8.6.2.7   Use of ^2H_2O to Determine Protein Synthesis in Tissues 445
        8.6.3   Rates of Whole-Body and Tissue-Specific Protein Synthesis in
                Humans and Other Animals..448
8.7   Summary 451
References...453

Chapter 9   Intracellular and Extracellular Degradation of Body Proteins 461

9.1   Historic Perspectives of Intracellular Protein Degradation..............................461
9.2   Proteases and Peptidases for Intracellular Protein Degradation 463
        9.2.1   Classification by Reaction Type...463
                9.2.1.1   Exopeptidases (Aminopeptidases and Carboxypeptidases)................464
                9.2.1.2   Endopeptidases (Proteinases) 464
        9.2.2   Classification by Catalytic Site..464
        9.2.3   Classification by Evolutionary Relationship..467
9.3   Intracellular Proteolytic Pathways..467
        9.3.1   The Lysosomal Proteolytic Pathway 467
                9.3.1.1   Entry of Cytosolic Proteins into the Lysosomes via
                            Endocytosis and Autophagy 467
                9.3.1.2   Proteases in the Lysosomes 468
                9.3.1.3   Proteins Degraded by the Lysosomal Proteolytic System........468
        9.3.2   The Nonlysosomal Proteolytic Pathway..470
                9.3.2.1   Overview of the Nonlysosomal Proteolytic System 470
                9.3.2.2   The Ca^{2+}-Dependent Proteolytic System (Calpain System) 470
                9.3.2.3   Caspases..470
                9.3.2.4   The ATP-Dependent and Ubiquitin-Independent Proteolytic System 470
                9.3.2.5   The ATP- and Ubiquitin-Dependent Proteolytic (Proteasome) System.... 471
                9.3.2.6   Proteins Degraded by the Nonlysosomal Proteolytic System 474
9.4   Characteristics and Physiological Significance of Intracellular Protein Degradation 474
        9.4.1   Biological Half-Lives of Proteins 474
        9.4.2   ATP Requirement for Intracellular Protein Turnover..............................477
        9.4.3   Physiological Significance of Intracellular Protein Degradation 477
9.5   Measurements of Intracellular Protein Degradation 479
        9.5.1   Measurement of Intracellular Protein Degradation *In Vitro* 479
                9.5.1.1   General Considerations...479

9.5.1.2 Tracer and Nontracer Methods for Measuring Protein
Degradation *In Vitro* 481
9.5.2 Measurement of Intracellular Protein Degradation *In Vivo* 483
9.5.2.1 General Considerations..483
9.5.2.2 Pulse Labeling of Proteins by the Single Administration of
A Labeled AA 484
9.5.2.3 The Leucine Oxidation Method...485
9.5.2.4 Urinary Excretion of 3-Methylhistidine 485
9.6 Degradation of Extracellular Proteins in Tissues...487
9.6.1 Degradation of Extracellular Matrix Proteins in Tissues..487
9.6.1.1 Extracellular Matrix Proteins 487
9.6.1.2 Degradation of Extracellular Matrix Proteins via
Proteases and Peptidases 487
9.6.2 Degradation of Proteins in the Plasma of Blood 489
9.6.2.1 Proteins in the Plasma of Blood..489
9.6.2.2 Extracellular Degradation of Plasma Proteins by Proteases in the
Blood and the Interstitial Space of Tissues...............................490
9.6.3 Measurement of Extracellular Protein Degradation...491
9.7 Rates of Whole-Body and Tissue-Specific Protein Degradation in Humans and
Other Animals 491
9.8 Summary 492
References..493

Chapter 10 Regulation of Amino Acid Metabolism..499

10.1 Basic Concepts in Metabolism 501
10.1.1 Chemical Reactions 501
10.1.2 Laws of Thermodynamics as Applied to Amino Acid Metabolism.........................501
10.1.2.1 The First Law of Thermodynamics 502
10.1.2.2 The Second Law of Thermodynamics.......................................503
10.1.2.3 The Concept of Free Energy Unifies the First and Second
Laws of Thermodynamics 503
10.1.3 The Concept of Equilibrium in Biochemical Reactions............................504
10.1.4 Near-Equilibrium (Reversible) and Non-Equilibrium (Irreversible) Reactions 505
10.1.5 Enzymes in Biochemical Reactions 506
10.1.5.1 Enzymes as Biological Catalysts 506
10.1.5.2 Reversible Inhibition of Enzymes 506
10.1.5.3 Irreversible Inhibition of Enzymes 508
10.1.6 Intracellular Compartment of Metabolic Pathways..................................508
10.1.7 Metabolic Design Principles...508
10.2 Regulation of Amino Acid Metabolism 509
10.2.1 Allosteric Regulation..510
10.2.2 Reversible Phosphorylation and Dephosphorylation of Protein 510
10.2.3 Concentrations of Substrates and Cofactors 511
10.2.4 Concentrations of Activators and Inhibitors...513
10.2.5 Signal Transduction 514
10.2.5.1 Binding of Extracellular Ligands to the Plasma Membrane....................515
10.2.5.2 Generation of Intracellular Second Messengers 516
10.2.5.3 Covalent Modifications of Target Proteins 516
10.2.5.4 Termination of Signaling Cascades 516
10.2.6 Changes in Cell Volume 517

10.2.7   Other Mechanisms for the Regulation of Enzyme Activity 518
10.3   Effects of Nutritional and Physiological Factors on Amino Acid Metabolism.................... 518
       10.3.1   AA Synthesis 518
                10.3.1.1   Arginine Synthesis 518
                10.3.1.2   Glutamine Synthesis 519
       10.3.2   AA Catabolism 520
                10.3.2.1   Arginine Catabolism 520
                10.3.2.2   Glutamine Catabolism 522
       10.3.3   Intracellular Protein Turnover 522
                10.3.3.1   Mechanistic Target of Rapamycin Cell Signaling (Mechanistic
                           Target of Rapamycin Cell Signaling Complexes 1 and 2).....................522
                10.3.3.2   Factors That Affect Intracellular Protein Turnover.............................525
       10.3.4   Blood Flow as a Regulator of Amino Acid Metabolism *In Vivo*............................527
10.4   Summary 530
References.. 530

Chapter 11   Physiological Functions and Nutritional Supplementation of Amino Acids 537

11.1   Roles of AAs in Protein and Small-Peptide Syntheses 537
       11.1.1   Protein Synthesis 537
       11.1.2   Small-Peptide Synthesis 542
11.2   Roles of AAs in the Synthesis of Nonpeptide Molecules and Other Metabolites................ 542
       11.2.1   Synthesis of Nonpeptide Molecules... 542
       11.2.2   Gaseous Signaling via Nitric Oxide, Carbon Monoxide, and Hydrogen Sulfide 543
                11.2.2.1   Chemical Properties of AA-Derived Gases 543
                11.2.2.2   Functions of Nitric Oxide 544
                11.2.2.3   Functions of Carbon Monoxide 546
                11.2.2.4   Functions of Hydrogen Sulfide 547
       11.2.3   Roles of Select AAs 548
                11.2.3.1   Arginine 548
                11.2.3.2   Glutamine 550
                11.2.3.3   Glutamate... 552
                11.2.3.4   Glycine... 554
                11.2.3.5   Proline.. 555
                11.2.3.6   Tryptophan... 556
       11.2.4   Roles of Select Nitrogenous Products of AAs...557
                11.2.4.1   Functions of Polyamines.. 557
                11.2.4.2   Functions of Creatine... 559
                11.2.4.3   Functions of Glutathione 561
                11.2.4.4   Functions of Purine and Pyrimidine Nucleotides 564
                11.2.4.5   Functions of Taurine 564
                11.2.4.6   Functions of Histamine.. 565
                11.2.4.7   Functions of Melanin... 568
                11.2.4.8   Functions of Melatonin.. 568
                11.2.4.9   Functions of Carnosine and Related Dipeptides....................... 568
                11.2.4.10 Functions of 4-Hydroxyproline 569
                11.2.4.11 Functions of Glucosamine 570
                11.2.4.12 AAs and Their metabolites as Natural Ligands and Activators of
                           Aryl Hydrocarbon Receptors 571
       11.2.5   Functions of AAs in Sensing.. 571
       11.2.6   Functions of D-AAs.. 572

          11.2.6.1 Functions of D-Alanine 572
          11.2.6.2 Functions of D-Aspartate.. 573
          11.2.6.3 Functions of D-Serine.. 573
11.3 Regulatory Roles of AAs in Food Intake, Nutrient Metabolism, and Gene Expression...... 573
     11.3.1 Regulatory Roles of AAs in Food Intake 573
     11.3.2 Regulatory Roles of AAs in Nutrient Metabolism 574
     11.3.3 Regulatory Roles of AAs in Gene Expression and Cell Signaling......... 577
          11.3.3.1 Regulatory Roles of AAs in Gene Expression.................... 577
          11.3.3.2 Regulatory Roles of AAs in Epigenetics 579
          11.3.3.3 Regulatory Roles for AAs in Cell Signaling 581
11.4 Roles for AAs in the Immune Response 583
     11.4.1 Immune Systems in Animals 584
          11.4.1.1 Immune Systems in Mammals and Birds 584
          11.4.1.2 Immune Systems in Fish and Crustaceans 585
          11.4.1.3 Intestinal Immunity and Health in Animals................. 586
          11.4.1.4 Assessments of Immune Function in Animals 586
     11.4.2 Protein Malnutrition and Compromised Immunity....................... 587
          11.4.2.1 Arginine.. 587
          11.4.2.2 Glutamine 588
          11.4.2.3 Glutamate.. 589
          11.4.2.4 Glycine 590
          11.4.2.5 Tryptophan... 590
     11.4.3 Unifying Mechanisms Responsible for the Roles of AAs in Immunity................. 591
11.5 Use of AAs in Human Nutrition and Health, and in Cell Culture 592
     11.5.1 Use of AAs in Medical and Pharmaceutical Therapy 592
     11.5.2 Use of AAs as Dietary Supplements 594
          11.5.2.1 Definition 594
          11.5.2.2 Use of AAs in Human Nutrition................................ 594
          11.5.2.3 Use of AAs in Animal Nutrition and Production 595
     11.5.3 Use of AAs or Their Derivatives as Food Additives 596
          11.5.3.1 AAs as Food Additives 596
          11.5.3.2 Mechanisms for AA-Induced Sensing in the Gastrointestinal Tract........ 596
     11.5.4 Use of AAs in Cosmetic and Toiletry Products........................ 599
     11.5.5 Use of AAs in Cell Culture 599
11.6 Efficacy and Safety of Dietary AA Supplementation............................. 600
     11.6.1 Efficacy of AA Supplementation....................................... 600
     11.6.2 Safety of AA Supplementation 600
          11.6.2.1 Imbalances and Antagonisms among AAs.................... 600
          11.6.2.2 Arginine as an Example for the Safety of AA Supplementation.............. 602
          11.6.2.3 Glutamine as an Example for the Safety of AA Supplementation 603
          11.6.2.4 Glutamate as an Example for the Safety of AA Supplementation............ 604
11.7 Summary 606
References.. 607

Chapter 12 Inborn Errors of Amino Acid Metabolism 623

12.1 Roles of Chromosomes in Genetic Inheritance and Gene Mutations 624
     12.1.1 Autosomal Dominant or Autosomal Recessive Inheritance................. 625
     12.1.2 X-Linked Dominant or Recessive Inheritance 625
12.2 Inherited Diseases Resulting from Abnormal Amino Acid Metabolism............. 625
     12.2.1 All or Most Amino Acids 626

12.2.1.1 Fanconi Syndrome 626
12.2.1.2 Galactosemia 630
12.2.1.3 Wilson's Disease 630
12.2.2 Asparagine and Aspartate 630
12.2.2.1 Asparagine Synthetase Deficiency 630
12.2.2.2 Dicarboxylic Aminoaciduria 631
12.2.3 Basic Amino Acids 631
12.2.3.1 Lysinuric Protein Intolerance 631
12.2.3.2 Hyperornithinemia 631
12.2.4 Branched-Chain Amino Acids 632
12.2.4.1 Maple Syrup Urine Disease 632
12.2.4.2 Isovaleric Acidemia 632
12.2.4.3 Methylbutyric Acidemia 632
12.2.5 Carnitine 632
12.2.5.1 Primary Carnitine Deficiency 632
12.2.5.2 Trimethyllysine Dioxygenase Deficiency 633
12.2.6 Creatine 633
12.2.6.1 Arginine: Glycine Amidinotransferase Deficiency 633
12.2.6.2 Guanidinoacetate Methyltransferase Deficiency 633
12.2.6.3 The X-Linked Creatine Transporter Deficiency 633
12.2.7 Glutamate 633
12.2.7.1 Gamma Aminobutyric Acid Transaminase Deficiency 633
12.2.7.2 Hyperinsulinism and Hyperammonemia Syndrome 634
12.2.7.3 Pyrroline-5-Carbocylate Synthase Deficiency 634
12.2.8 Glutamine 634
12.2.8.1 Glutamine Synthetase Deficiency 634
12.2.8.2 Phosphate-Activated Glutaminase Deficiency 635
12.2.9 Glutathione 635
12.2.9.1 γ-Glutamyl-Cysteine Synthetase Deficiency 635
12.2.9.2 Glutathione Synthetase Deficiency 635
12.2.9.3 5-Oxoprolinuria 635
12.2.10 Glycine 636
12.2.10.1 Dimethylglycine Dehydrogenase Deficiency 636
12.2.10.2 Glycine Encephalopathy 636
12.2.10.3 Glycinemia 636
12.2.10.4 Glycinuria 636
12.2.10.5 Sarcosinemia 637
12.2.10.6 Sideroblastic Anemia 637
12.2.11 Heme Synthesis and Catabolism Disorders 637
12.2.11.1 Dubin–Johnson Syndrome (Conjugated Hyperbilirubinemia) .. 637
12.2.11.2 Gilbert's Syndrome or Crigler–Najjar Syndrome 637
12.2.11.3 Protoporphyria 638
12.2.12 Histidine 639
12.2.12.1 Histidinemia 639
12.2.12.2 Mastocytosis 639
12.2.12.3 Tay–Sachs Disease 639
12.2.12.4 Urocanic Aciduria 639
12.2.13 Phenylalanine and Tyrosine 640
12.2.13.1 Albinism 640
12.2.13.2 Ocular Albinism, Type 1 641
12.2.13.3 Alkaptonuria (Black Urine Disease) 641

12.2.13.4 Aromatic L-Amino Acid Decarboxylase Deficiency 641
12.2.13.5 Hypertyrosinemia 641
12.2.13.6 Hypothyroidism 643
12.2.13.7 Phenylketonuria 644
12.2.13.8 Pheochromocytoma 645
12.2.14 Proline and 4-Hydroxyproline 645
12.2.14.1 Hyperhydroxyprolinemia 645
12.2.14.2 Hyperprolinemia 645
12.2.14.3 Iminoglycinuria 647
12.2.14.4 Prolidase (Imidodipeptidase) Deficiency 647
12.2.15 Purines 648
12.2.15.1 Adenine Phosphoribosyltransferase Deficiency 648
12.2.15.2 Adenosine Deaminase Deficiency 648
12.2.15.3 Adenylosuccinate Lyase Deficiency 648
12.2.15.4 Gout 649
12.2.15.5 Lesch–Nyhan Syndrome 649
12.2.15.6 Myoadenylate Deaminase Deficiency 649
12.2.15.7 Purine Nucleoside Phosphorylase Deficiency 650
12.2.15.8 Xanthinuria 650
12.2.16 Pyrimidines 650
12.2.16.1 β-Aminoisobutyric Aciduria 650
12.2.16.2 Familial Pyrimidinemia 650
12.2.16.3 Hyper-β-Alaninemia 651
12.2.16.4 Orotic Aciduria 651
12.2.17 Serine 651
12.2.17.1 Hypophosphatasia 651
12.2.17.2 Phosphoglycerate Dehydrogenase Deficiency 651
12.2.18 Sulfur-Containing Amino Acids 652
12.2.18.1 Cystathioninuria 652
12.2.18.2 Cystinosis 652
12.2.18.3 Cystinuria 652
12.2.18.4 Homocyst(e)inuria 653
12.2.18.5 Hypermethioninemia 653
12.2.18.6 Glycine N-Methyltransferase Deficiency 654
12.2.18.7 S-Adenosylhomocysteine Hydrolase Deficiency 654
12.2.19 Tryptophan 654
12.2.19.1 Carcinoid Syndrome 654
12.2.19.2 Hartnup Disease 655
12.2.19.3 Aromatic L-Amino Acid Decarboxylase Deficiency 655
12.2.20 The Urea Cycle Defects 655
12.2.20.1 N-Acetylglutamate Synthase Deficiency 656
12.2.20.2 Argininosuccinic Aciduria 656
12.2.20.3 Carbamoyl Phosphate Synthetase I Deficiency 657
12.2.20.4 Hyperargininemia 657
12.2.20.5 Hypercitrullinemia 657
12.2.20.6 Hyperornithinemia 658
12.2.20.7 Hyperornithinemia–Hyperammonemia–Homocitrullinuria Syndrome . 658
12.2.21 Other Organic Acidurias 658
12.2.21.1 Glutaric Acidemia 658
12.2.21.2 Hyperoxaluria 658
12.2.21.3 α-Ketoadipic Acidemia 659

        12.2.21.4 Methylmalonic Acidemia...659
        12.2.21.5 Propionic Acidemia...659
    12.2.22 Polyamines...659
        12.2.22.1 Spermine Synthase Deficiency...660
        12.2.22.2 Elevation of Spermine in the Mucopolysaccharidoses.........................661
12.3 General Considerations for the Treatment of Inborn Errors of Amino Acid Metabolism...661
12.4 Summary 664
References..665

Chapter 13 Dietary Requirements of Amino Acids 671

13.1 Historical Perspectives of Dietary AA Requirements...673
    13.1.1 An Overall View..673
    13.1.2 Studies of Laboratory Animals 673
    13.1.3 Human Studies..675
    13.1.4 Studies of Farm Animals...676
    13.1.5 Dietary Requirements of Humans and Other Animals for AASAs
            (NEAAs *plus* CEAAs)..678
    13.1.6 Functional AAs in Nutrition 681
    13.1.7 Moving Beyond the "Ideal Protein" Concept...683
    13.1.8 Formulating Low-Protein Diets Based on Optimum Ratios of All
            Proteinogenic AAs...683
13.2 Methods for the Determination of Dietary AA Requirements...684
    13.2.1 Nitrogen Balance Studies 685
        13.2.1.1   Measurement of Nitrogen Balances under Various Nutritional and
                    Physiological Conditions 685
        13.2.1.2   Advantages and Limitations of Nitrogen Balance Studies....................689
    13.2.2 The Factorial Method...690
    13.2.3 Dose–Response Feeding Trials...692
    13.2.4 Tracer Methods 693
        13.2.4.1   General Considerations of AA Oxidation Methods for Estimating
                    Dietary AA Requirements 693
        13.2.4.2   The Direct AA Oxidation Method...694
        13.2.4.3   The Indicator AA Oxidation Method 695
        13.2.4.4   Advantages and Disadvantages of Tracer Studies for Estimating
                    Dietary AA Requirements 697
    13.2.5 Substantial Differences in Current Estimated Dietary EAA and Protein
            Requirements by Humans or Other Animals 698
    13.2.6 Potential Use of "-Omics" Technologies to Estimate Dietary AA Requirements ..699
        13.2.6.1   Nutrigenomics...699
        13.2.6.2   Proteomics..700
        13.2.6.3   Metabolomics..701
13.3 Optimum Ratios of AASAs in Diets for Humans and Other Animals 701
13.4 Assessment of Dietary Protein Quality 708
    13.4.1 Chemical Methods...709
        13.4.1.1   AA Analysis 709
        13.4.1.2   AA Score (Chemical Score)...712
        13.4.1.3   EAA Index 713
        13.4.1.4   Dye-Binding Techniques...715
        13.4.1.5   Mutual AA Ratios 715
    13.4.2 Animal Feeding Experiments 716

13.4.2.1 Overall Considerations 716
13.4.2.2 Biological Value... 716
13.4.2.3 Protein Efficiency Ratio.. 716
13.4.2.4 Net Protein Ratio 717
13.4.2.5 Net Protein Utilization.. 718
13.4.2.6 Nitrogen Growth Index 718
13.4.2.7 Relative Nitrogen Utilization.. 718
13.4.2.8 Whole-Body Composition and Lean Tissue Mass.............. 718
13.4.2.9 PDCAAS.. 719
13.4.2.10 DIAAS 721
13.4.3 Metabolic Indicators in Animals.. 722
13.4.3.1 Concentrations of Free AAs in the Plasma or Serum 722
13.4.3.2 Concentrations of Proteins in the Plasma or Serum 722
13.4.3.3 Concentrations of Urea and Ammonia in the Plasma or
         Serum and Urine... 723
13.4.3.4 Enzyme Activities.. 723
13.4.3.5 Whole-Body Protein Turnover....................................... 723
13.4.3.6 Flux of EAAs and Certain AASAs in the Plasma................. 724
13.4.4 Methods Using Microorganisms and Lower Animals 724
13.5 Impacts of AA Nutrition on Human Health 724
13.5.1 General Considerations.. 724
13.5.2 Sarcopenia in Humans during Aging 726
13.5.3 Healthy Humans with Minimum Physical Activity 727
13.5.3.1 The Current RDA of Protein... 727
13.5.3.2 Functional Needs of Humans for Dietary AAs to Maximize Muscle
         Protein Synthesis and Mass 727
13.5.3.3 Suboptimal Values of the Current Protein RDA for Humans and the
         Nutritional Significance of a Higher RDA for Adult Humans........ 727
13.5.3.4 Higher Recommended Protein Requirements for Adult Humans.......... 728
13.5.4 Healthy Humans with Moderate or Intense Physical Activity 728
13.5.4.1 Benefits of Dietary Protein Plus Adequate Exercise on the Protein
         Synthesis and Mass of Skeletal Muscle............................. 728
13.5.4.2 Negative Protein Balance during Moderate or Intense Exercise 728
13.5.4.3 Importance of Adequate Protein Intake to Prevent Muscle Loss
         after Exercise 729
13.5.4.4 Amount and Timing of Dietary Protein to Maximally
         Enhance Skeletal Muscle Protein Synthesis after Exercise 730
13.5.4.5 New Recommended Requirements for Dietary Protein in
         Humans with Moderate or Intense Exercise 731
13.5.5 Obese Humans on a Weight-Reducing Program 731
13.5.6 Distribution of Daily Protein Intake or the Frequency of Meals............. 732
13.5.7 Sources of Dietary AAs.. 732
13.5.7.1 Plant- vs Animal-Sourced Proteins................................. 732
13.5.7.2 Diets Based Solely or Primarily on Plant-Sourced Foods 734
13.5.7.3 Differential Effects of Different Animal Proteins on
         Protein Accretion in the Body 735
13.5.8 Protein Intake and AA Deficiency in Humans 736
13.5.8.1 Global Protein Intake by Adult Humans........................... 736
13.5.8.2 Global Scope and Consequences of Protein Deficiencies 736
13.5.8.3 Means to Prevent AA Deficiency in Humans 737

13.5.8.4   Restriction of Dietary AAs or Protein for Medical
                          Therapy and Longevity 737
        13.5.9   Safe (Tolerable) Upper Limits of Dietary Protein Intake by Humans 739
                13.5.9.1   Healthy Infants and Children 739
                13.5.9.2   Healthy Adult Humans 740
        13.5.10 Concerns over Adverse Effects of High Protein Intake on Human Health 741
                13.5.10.1 General Considerations 741
                13.5.10.2 Definition of and General Concern over High Protein Intake 741
                13.5.10.3 Digestive, Cardiovascular, and Renal Functions 742
                13.5.10.4 Bone Mass and Integrity 743
                13.5.10.5 Cancers 744
                13.5.10.6 Type 1 and Type 2 Diabetes Mellitus 744
13.6 Summary 746
References 747

Index 761

Preface

Since the first edition of this book was published by CRC Press in 2013, the author has received constructive suggestions from readers for expanding the coverage of amino acids (AAs) in the nutrition, metabolism, and health of humans, as well as aquatic and companion animals. This content has now been incorporated into the second edition of this book. The structure of the first edition of "*Amino Acids: Biochemistry and Nutrition*", which has been well appreciated by its readers for the logical flow of the complex knowledge of the subject matter from the basic to the applied, has been retained in the current edition. However, all chapters have been substantially revised, expanded, and updated to reflect significant advances through research over the past eight years. This book presents a comprehensive coverage of these scientific developments, providing a useful reference for students and researchers in both biomedicine and agriculture, and the public.

Specific additions to the new edition include the following: (1) the nutrition and metabolism of AAs and proteins in humans (e.g., infants and young and elderly adults, as well as patients with diabetes and cancers), including the roles of animal- and plant-sourced proteins, vegetarian diets, and dietary supplementation with AAs, protein, and creatine in their growth, health (e.g., sarcopenia, immunity, and longevity), sport nutrition, and exercise performance; (2) the nutrition and metabolism of AAs and proteins in aquatic (e.g., fish and shrimp) and companion (e.g., zoo and domestic pet) animals; (3) recent developments in functional AAs as applied to the health and productivity of humans and other animals; (4) dietary requirements of humans and other animals for biosynthesizable (traditionally classified "nutritionally nonessential") AAs, and of companion animals (e.g., cats and dogs) for all proteinogenic AAs and taurine; (5) new sources of dietary proteins in the nutrition of humans (e.g., insect proteins and algae) and farm animals (e.g., algae meal and fishmeal alternatives); (6) the formulation of cost-effective and environmentally sustainable low-protein diets for livestock, poultry, fish, and shrimp; (7) proteinogenic (protein-creating; e.g., L-selenocysteine and L-pyrrolysine) and non-proteinogenic (e.g., L-homoarginine, L-phosphoarginine, and gizzerosine) AAs; (8) AA metabolism via non-canonical pathways, such as syntheses of polyamines and glycine in animals; (9) the methods and concerns over the current evaluation of dietary protein quality using the protein digestibility-corrected AA score (PDCAAS) and digestible indispensable AA score (DIAAS) systems; (10) the roles of AAs in the prevention and treatment of metabolic (e.g., hypertension, liver dysfunction, obesity, and diabetes) and infectious (e.g., bacterial and viral) diseases, as well as intestinal and reproductive disorders; (11) the safety of dietary AA and protein intakes in humans and other animals; and (12) heated debate over potential contributions of high protein intake to the development of diseases in humans, such as cardiovascular disorders, bone integrity, type 1 and type 2 diabetes mellitus, and cancers.

Biochemistry and nutrition of AAs is an interesting, dynamic, and challenging subject in biological sciences. It spans an immense range from chemistry, metabolism, and physiology to reproduction, immunology, pathology, and cell biology. Since Alton Meister published his two volumes of the monograph "*Biochemistry of The Amino Acids*" in 1965, this field has developed rapidly over the past 56 years. Important technical and conceptual advances include the following: (1) the analysis of AAs by high-performance liquid chromatography and mass spectrometry; (2) isotopic measurements of the synthesis and degradation of proteins and AAs in cells, tissues, and the whole body; (3) the interorgan metabolism of AAs involving the liver, skeletal muscle, small intestine, kidneys, and brain; (4) AAs in cell signaling and the regulation of gene expression; (5) mechanisms for lysosomal proteolysis via autophagy, as well as nonlysosomal proteolysis by ATP- and ubiquitin-dependent proteasomes; (6) the molecular and cellular regulation of intracellular protein turnover and AA metabolism; (7) measurements of true ileal digestibilities of AAs in humans and other animals; (8) the molecular cloning of cell-specific transporters for AAs and small peptides; (9) the development of the ideal protein concept and its revision to optimum ratios of all proteinogenic AAs; (10) dietary requirements of humans and other animals for AASAs (AAs that are synthesizable *de novo* in animal cells); (11) the new nutritional concept of functional AAs in humans and other animals; and (12) the safety and NOAELs (no observed adverse effect levels) for supplemental AAs. Comprehensive and systematic coverage of these new scientific developments in a well-organized book will benefit researchers, students in biomedical and agricultural disciplines, policy makers, and the public to improve both human and animal health, as well as the nutritional value of foods.

The second edition of "*Amino Acids: Biochemistry and Nutrition*" includes 13 chapters. The book begins with the discoveries and basic chemical concepts of AAs, peptides, and proteins. It then advances to protein digestion in the gastrointestinal tract and the absorption of small peptides and individual free AAs in the small intestine. This chapter is followed by a detailed coverage of cell- and tissue-specific synthesis and catabolism of AAs, as well as related nitrogenous substances (including nitric oxide, polyamines, glutathione, creatine, taurine, urea, and uric acid) and hydrogen sulfide in humans and other animals. After the use of isotopes in studying AA metabolism is introduced in Chapter 7, the book continues with intracellular protein turnover, the extracellular degradation of body proteins, the short-term (e.g., via protein phosphorylation) and long-term (e.g., via gene expression, epigenetic modifications, and protein synthesis) regulation of AA metabolism, physiological functions of AAs, and inborn errors of AA metabolism. Finally, the text ends with dietary requirements of AAs/protein by humans and other animals, including the evaluation of dietary protein quality, the roles and safety of dietary AA/protein intake in human physical performance and health, as well as myths and misconceptions over and evidence-based AA/protein nutrition.

While the classical concepts and principles of AA biochemistry and nutrition are emphasized throughout the book, every effort has been made to include the most recent progress in this ever-expanding field so that readers in various biological disciplines can integrate AA biochemistry with nutrition, health, and disease in mammals, birds, and other animal species. At the end of each chapter, selected references provide readers with both comprehensive reviews of the chosen topics and original experimental data on which modern concepts in AA biochemistry and nutrition are based. Reading the scientific literature is essential for a thorough understanding of the history of the field and also provides "food" for creative thinking and for rigorous development as a productive scientist. In the Index section, a list of keywords, phrases, and abbreviations is provided to help readers quickly find information presented in all the chapters.

This book owes its origin to the lecture notes of a graduate course ANSC/NUTR 613 "Protein Metabolism" the author has taught at Texas A&M University for the past 30 years. Its conception was motivated largely by the lack of a suitable textbook for teaching such an advanced course for students majoring in animal science, biochemistry, biomedical engineering, biology, human medicine, kinesiology, veterinary medicine, nutrition, physiology, toxicology, reproductive biology, and other related disciplines. Besides its use as a textbook, all of the chapters provide useful references to general and specific knowledge on AA biochemistry and nutrition for researchers in both biomedicine and agriculture (including animal science, food science, nutrition, and plant breeding).

The sciences of AA biochemistry and nutrition have been built on the shoulders of many giants and pioneers worldwide. Their seminal contributions to the field have made this book possible. The author must apologize to those whose published works are not cited in the text due to limited space. Sincere thanks are also extended to the author's past and current students for their constructive comments on the "Protein Metabolism" course and stimulating discussions in classes, and to other readers of the first edition of this book for their helpful suggestions to further improve its content.

Acknowledgments

The second edition of "*Amino Acids: Biochemistry and Nutrition*" was initiated at the kind invitation of Ms. Randy L. Brehm, a senior editor at CRC Press, and was completed with the patience and guidance of its editorial staff (including Dr. Julia Tanner). The author would like to thank his research assistants Mr. Sudath Dahanayaka and Mr. Neil D. Wu for drawing chemical structures and metabolic pathways of amino acids, Dr. Gregory A. Johnson for illustrating enterocytes of the small intestine, his graduate students (Mr. Kyler R. Gilbreath, Mr. Wenliang He, Ms. Cassandra M. Herring, Dr. Xinyu Li, and Ms. Erin A. Posey) for helpful comments on some chapters, Ms. Marie Lamarche for assistance in studies of immunocyte metabolism, and staff at CodeMantra for their professional typesetting of the entire manuscript. Sincere thanks also go to the following accomplished scientists who critically reviewed various chapters of this book and provided constructive suggestions for improvement:

Prof. Vickie E. Baracos, Ph.D., Faculty of Medicine, University of Alberta, Edmonton, Canada;

Prof. Fuller W. Bazer, Ph.D., Department of Animal Science, Texas A&M University, College Station, TX;

Prof. Werner G. Bergen, Ph.D., Department of Animal Science, Auburn University, Auburn, AL;

Prof. John T. Brosnan, D.Phil., Department of Biochemistry, Memorial University of Newfoundland, St. John's, Canada;

Prof. Margaret E. Brosnan, Ph.D., Department of Biochemistry, Memorial University of Newfoundland, St. John's, Canada;

Prof. Sergio Burgos, Ph.D., Department of Animal Science, McGill University, Quebec, Canada;

Prof. Teresa A. Davis, Ph.D., Department of Pediatrics, Baylor College of Medicine, Houston, TX;

Prof. Jeffrey L. Firkins, Ph.D., Department of Animal Science, Ohio State University, Columbia, OH;

Prof. Catherine J. Field, Ph.D., Faculty of Medicine, University of Alberta, Edmonton, Canada;

Prof. Nick E. Flynn, Ph.D., Department of Chemistry and Physics, West Texas A&M University, Canyon, TX;

Prof. Shaodong Guo, Ph.D., Department of Nutrition, Texas A&M University, College Station, TX;

Prof. Gert Lubec, M.D., Neuroscience Laboratory, Paracelsus Medical University, Salzburg, Austria;

Prof. Errol B. Marliss, M.D., Department of Medicine, McGill University, Montreal, Canada;

Prof. James C. Matthews, Ph.D., Department of Animal Science, University of Kentucky, Lexington, KY;

Prof. Cynthia J. Meininger, Ph.D., Department of Medical Physiology, Texas A&M University, College Station, TX;

Prof. Paul J. Moughan, Ph.D., Riddet Institute, Massey University, Palmerston North, New Zealand;

Prof. J. Marc Rhoads, M.D., Department of Pediatrics, The University of Texas Medical School at Houston, Houston, TX;

Prof. Steven E. Riechman, Ph.D., Departments of Health and Kinesiology, Texas A&M University, College Station, TX;

Prof. Yuxiang Sun, M.D., Ph.D., Department of Nutrition, Texas A&M University, College Station, TX;

Prof. James R. Thompson, Ph.D., Animal Science Program, University of British Columbia, Vancouver, Canada;

Prof. Malcolm Watford, D.Phil., Department of Nutritional Sciences, Rutgers University, New Brunswick, NJ;

Prof. Timothy J. Wester, Ph.D., College of Science, Massey University, Palmerston North, New Zealand.

The author is appreciative of the important contributions of his former and current graduate students, postdoctoral fellows, visiting scholars, research assistants, and undergraduate workers to the conduct of experiments and valuable discussions. The author is also grateful to his graduate advisors Prof. Sheng Yang and Dr. James R. Thompson, as well as postdoctoral mentors Dr. Errol B. Marliss and Dr. John T. Brosnan for rigorous training in amino acid biochemistry and nutrition, as well as their enthusiastic support and inspiration for a lifelong pursuit of this discipline. Productive and enjoyable collaborations with colleagues at Texas A&M University (particularly Drs. Fuller W. Bazer, Robert C. Burghardt, James Cai, Raymond J. Carroll, Michael F. Criscitiello, H. Russell Cross, Kathrin A. Dunlap, Delbert M. Gatlin III, Shaodong Guo, Gregory A. Johnson, Darrell A. Knabe, Jessica L. Leatherwood, Bani K. Mallick, Cynthia J. Meininger, Annie E. Newell-Fugate, Jayanth Ramadoss, Tapasree R. Sarkar, M. Carey Satterfield, Jeffrey W. Savell, Stephen B. Smith, Heewon Seo, Thomas E. Spencer, Yuxiang Sun, Jeffery K. Tomberlin, Shannon E. Washburn, Tryon A. Wickersham, and Renyi Zhang) and at other institutions over the past 30 years (particularly Drs. David H. Baker, Makoto Bannai, Douglas G. Burrin, Zhaolai Dai, Teresa A. Davis, Douglas G. Burrin, Francesca Falco, Susan K. Fried, Elisha Gootwine, Yongqing Hou, Andy C. Hu, Sung Woo Kim, Jessica L. Leatherwood, Defa Li, Ju Li, Peng Li, Yuying Liu, Gert Lubec, Catherine J. McNeal, Shalene H. McNeill, Sidney M. Morris Jr., Tomonori Nochi, Penelope Perkins-Veazie, James M. Phang, Wilson G. Pond, Peter J. Reeds, J. Marc Rhoads, Ana San Gabriel, R. Andrew Shanely, Sue A. Shapses, Izuru Shinzato, Carmen D. Tekwe, Masaaki Toyomizu, Binggen Wang, Fenglai Wang, Junjun Wang, Xiaolong Wang, Malcolm Watford, Zhenlong Wu, Yulong Yin, Shixuan Zheng, Weiyun Zhu, and Roger S. Zoh) are gratefully acknowledged. Furthermore, the author thanks Dr. Peng Li at North American Renderers Association (Alexandria, VA, USA) for helpful discussions on amino acid nutrition in various animal species and new promising sources of protein ingredients to improve animal growth, development, and health.

The author is indebted to Dr. G. Cliff Lamb (Head, Department of Animal Science) and Dr. Patrick J. Stover (Dean, College of Agriculture and Life Sciences) for their support of research and teaching at Texas A&M University. In addition, the timely assistance of helpful librarians at the Texas A&M University's Medical Sciences Library in obtaining research articles to write this book is gratefully appreciated. Work in the author's laboratory is currently supported, in part, by grants from the National Institutes of Health (USA), the United States Department of Agriculture, and the American Quarter Horse Foundation, as well as funds from Texas A&M AgriLife Research (Hatch Project) and Texas A&M University. Such funding support has greatly helped to advance the field of amino acid biochemistry and nutrition.

Special thanks are extended to thousands of scientists who have made great contributions to our understanding of amino acid biochemistry and nutrition over the past century. The author has enjoyed reading their papers and learned a great deal of knowledge from their published works. Finally, I thank my family for their patience and support during the writing of the entire manuscript, as well as Jennifer M. Wu and my graduate students for proofreading all chapters of this book.

Guoyao Wu, Ph.D.
April 2021
College Station, Texas, USA

Author

Dr. Guoyao Wu is a University Distinguished Professor, University Faculty Fellow, and Texas A&M AgriLife Research Senior Faculty Fellow at Texas A&M University. He received a B.S. in Animal Science from South China Agricultural University in Guangzhou, China (1978–1982); an M.S. in Animal Nutrition from China Agricultural University in Beijing, China (1982–1984); and an M.Sc. (1984–1986) and Ph.D. (1986–1989) in Animal Biochemistry from the University of Alberta in Edmonton, Canada. Dr. Wu completed his postdoctoral training in diabetes, nutrition, and biochemistry at McGill University Faculty of Medicine in Montreal, Canada (1989–1991), and Memorial University of Newfoundland Faculty of Medicine in St. John's, Canada (1991). He joined the Texas A&M University faculty in October 1991. Dr. Wu's sabbatical leave was to study human obesity at the University of Maryland School of Medicine in Baltimore, USA (2005).

Dr. Wu has taught graduate (Experimental Nutrition, General Animal Nutrition, Protein Metabolism, and Nutritional Biochemistry) and undergraduate (Problems in Animal Science, Nutrition, and Biochemistry) courses at Texas A&M University over the past 30 years. He has given numerous lectures at other institutions in the United States, Canada, Mexico, Brazil, Europe, and Asia. His research focuses on the biochemistry, nutrition, and physiology of amino acids (AAs) and related nutrients in animals at genetic, molecular, cellular, and whole-body levels. His research interests include (1) functions of AAs in gene expression (including epigenetics) and cell signaling; (2) mechanisms that regulate the intracellular synthesis and catabolism of proteins and AAs; (3) hormonal and nutritional regulation of homeostasis of metabolic fuels; (4) biology and pathobiology of nitric oxide and polyamines; (5) key roles of AAs in preventing metabolic diseases (including diabetes, obesity, and intrauterine growth restriction) and associated cardiovascular complications; (6) essential roles of AAs in the survival, growth, and development of embryos, fetuses, and neonates; (7) dietary requirements of AAs and proteins in the life cycle; and (8) animal models (e.g., pigs, rats, and sheep) for studying human metabolic diseases.

Dr. Wu has published more than 660 papers in peer-reviewed journals, including *Advances in Nutrition, Alcohol, Amino Acids, American Journal of Physiology, Annals of New York Academy of Sciences, Animal Reproduction, Annual Review of Animal Biosciences, Annual Review of Nutrition, Antioxidants & Redox Signaling, Biochemical Journal, Bioessays, Biology of Reproduction, Biometrics, British Journal of Nutrition, Cancer Research, Cell Death & Disease, Clinical and Experimental Immunology, Comparative Biochemistry and Physiology, Diabetes, Diabetologia, Endocrinology, Experimental Biology and Medicine, FASEB Journal, Food & Function, Frontiers in Bioscience, Frontiers in Immunology, Frontiers in Microbiology, Gut, International Journal of Biochemistry, International Journal of Molecular Sciences, Journal of Animal Science, Journal of Animal Science and Biotechnology, Journal of Agricultural and Food Chemistry, Journal of Biological Chemistry, Journal of Chromatography, Journal of Gerontology, Journal of Nutrition, Journal of Nutritional Biochemistry, Journal of Pediatrics, Journal of Physiology (London), Livestock Science, Methods in Molecular Biology, Molecular and Cellular Endocrinology, Molecular Nutrition & Food Research, Molecular Reproduction and Development, Placenta, Proceedings of National Academy of Science USA, Reproduction, Reproductive Toxicology, Scientific Reports, Theriogenology*, and *Trends in Pharmacological Sciences*, and 90 chapters in books. Dr. Wu's work has been extensively cited in Google Scholar over 65,000 times, with an H-index of 126. Three of his papers have each been cited more than 2,900 times. He was a Most Cited Author and a Most Influential Scientific Mind (2014–2020) in the Web of Science (Clarivate Analytics) and was among the 10 most cited scientists in the field of agricultural sciences (2016) worldwide. Dr. Wu edited 6 books related to animal science, human nutrition, and amino acid metabolism for Elsevier and Springer-Nature.

Dr. Wu has received numerous prestigious awards from China, Canada, and the United States, which include China National Scholarship for Graduate Studies Abroad (1984), the University of Alberta Andrew Stewart Graduate Prize (1989), Medical Research Council of Canada Postdoctoral Fellowship (1989), American Heart Association Established Investigator Award (1998), Texas A&M AgriLife Faculty Fellow (2001), Texas A&M University Faculty Fellow (2002), Nonruminant Nutrition Research Award from the American Society of Animal Science (2004), Texas A&M Agriculture Program Vice Chancellor's Award for Excellence in Team (2006) and Individual (2008) Research and in Diversity (2011), Texas A&M University Distinguished Research Achievement Award (2008), Texas A&M AgriLife Research Senior Faculty Fellow Award (2008), FASS–AFIA New Frontiers in Animal Nutrition Research Award from the Federation of Animal Science Societies and American Feed Industry Association (2009), the Samburu Collaboration Award from the International Association of Giraffe Care Professionals (2010), Distinguished Scientist of Sigma Xi Honor Society–Texas A&M University Chapter (2013), and the Morrison Award from American Society of Animal Science (2018).

Dr. Wu is a member and an elected Fellow of the American Association for the Advancement of Science, as well as a member of the American Heart Association, American Society of Animal Science, American Society of Nutrition, and Society for the Study of Reproduction. He has served on Editorial Advisory Boards for *Biochemical Journal* (1993–2005), *Journal of Animal Science and Biotechnology* (2010–present), *Journal of Nutrition* (1997–2003), and *Journal of Nutritional Biochemistry* (2006–present), as well as an Editor and a Consulting Editor of *Amino Acids* (2008–present), an Editor of *Journal of Amino Acids* (2008–2017), Editor-in-Chief of *SpringerPlus–Amino Acids Collections* (2012–2017), a managing Editor (2009–2016) and an Editor (2017–present) of *Frontiers in Bioscience*, and an Editor for four volumes of papers on AAs and animal nutrition in *Advances in Experimental Medicine and Biology* (2018–present).

1 Discovery and Chemistry of Amino Acids

Amino acids (AAs) are present in humans and other animals (including amphibians, cat, cattle, chickens, dogs, fish, goats, insects, mice, pigs, rats, reptiles, sheep, and shrimp), as well as plants (including corn, flowers, rice, soybean, and wheat), microorganisms (including bacteria, fungi, parasites, protozoa, and viruses), and the environment (including the soil, rivers, and oceans). There is a rich history of chemical, biochemical, nutritional, and physiological studies of these organic molecules (Braconnot 1820; Brosnan 2001; Neinast et al. 2019; Vauquelin and Robiquet 1806; Vickery and Schmidt 1931; Watford 2000). This field was pioneered predominantly by European chemists in the 19th century. Over the past 220 years, AA research has been greatly advanced by biochemists, nutritionists, medical professionals, other life scientists, and food scientists worldwide. Specifically, the first discovery of an AA, asparagine, in nature by two French chemists, L.N. Vauquelin and P.J. Robiquet, occurred in 1806, whereas glycine was the first AA isolated from a protein (i.e., gelatin) by hydrolysis with sulfuric acid in 1820 by the French chemist H. Braconnot. Usage of the term *amino acid* in the English language started in 1898. More than 25 years later, in 1925, threonine was discovered as the last addition to the list of 20 canonical AAs required for protein biosynthesis in humans and other animals that are known as proteinogenic (protein-creating) AAs (Table 1.1). The identification of threonine in casein by W.C. Rose in 1935 made it possible to prepare purified diets for feeding humans and other animals. By 1950 and 1983, approximately 200 and 500 natural AAs (AAs present in animals, plants, and microorganisms) had been reported, respectively (Wagner and Musso 1983). Discovery of selenocysteine in 1973 as a rare AA found only in selenoproteins (Stadtman 1996) and of pyrrolysine in 2002 as a rare AA in the Archaea methylamine methyltransferase (Hao et al. 2002; Srinivasan et al. 2002) expanded the list of AAs present in certain unique proteins (Stadtman 1996). It is now known that more than 700 AAs exist in nature. In contrast to other macronutrients (e.g., the carbohydrates and fatty acids), AAs serve as the substrates for the synthesis of proteins, polypeptides, and other biologically active nitrogenous molecules.

The common or trivial names of AAs were derived from (1) the history of their discoveries; (2) their characteristics, including appearance (e.g., arginine and leucine), taste (e.g., glycine), and chemical structure (hydroxyproline, isoleucine, lysine, methionine, proline, and threonine); (3) their sources of isolation (e.g., asparagine, citrulline, cysteine, glutamate, serine, tryptophan, tyrosine, and valine); or (4) the precursors of their chemical syntheses (e.g., the production of alanine and phenylalanine through the Strecker method involving the reaction of an aldehyde with ammonium chloride in the presence of potassium cyanide). Because of variations in their side chains (e.g., carbon numbers, structure, and chemical groups), AAs have remarkably different chemical and biochemical properties as well as nutritional and physiological functions (Agostinelli 2020; Beaumont and Blachier 2020; Closs et al. 2006; Suryawan et al. 2020; Watford 2003; Yang et al. 2020). To appreciate the historical development of AA biochemistry and nutrition, to understand the basis for the different roles of AAs and their interactive networks in the body, and to help stimulate future research in this ever-growing field, this chapter highlights the discoveries, nomenclatures, chemical properties, and analyses of AAs.

TABLE 1.1

Discoveries of Natural Amino Acids

Amino Acids	Year	Source	Scientist(s)
		(1) Neutral Amino Acids	
L-Alanine	1888	Silk fibroin	T. Weyl
β-Alanine	1911	Beef muscle	W. Gulewitsch
γ-Aminobutyrate	1949	Potato tuber	F.C. Steward, J.F. Thompson, and C.E. Dent
β-Aminoisobutyrate	1951	Human urine	Crumpler, H.R., C.E. Dent, H. Harris, and R.G. Westall
L-Asparagine	1806	Asparagus juice	L.N. Vauquelin and P.J. Robiquet
	1932	Edestin	M. Damodaran
L-Citrulline	1930	Watermelon juice	M. Wada
L-Cysteine	1884	Cystine	E. Baumann
L-Cystine	1899	Horn	K.A.H. Mörner
L-Glutamine	1883	Beet juice	E. Schulze and E. Bosshard
	1932	Gliadin	M. Damodaran, G. Jaaback, and A.C. Chibnall
Glycine	1820	Gelatin	H. Braconnot
L-4-Hydroxyproline	1902	Gelatin	E. Fischer
L-Isoleucine	1904	Sugar beet molasses	F. Ehrlich
L-Leucine	1819	Cheese	J.L. Proust
L-Methionine	1922	Casein	J.H. Mueller
L-Phenylalanine	1881	Lupine sprouts	E. Schulze and J. Barbieri
L-Proline	1901	Casein	E. Fischer
L-Serine	1865	Silk gelatin	E. Cramer
Taurine	1827	Ox bile	F. Tiedermann and L. Gmelin
L-Threonine	1925	Oat protein	S.B. Schryver and H.W. Buston
	1925	Teozein	R.A. Gortner and W.F. Hoffmann
	1935	Casein	W.C. Rose
L-Tryptophan	1901	Casein	F.G. Hopkins and S.W. Cole
L-Tyrosine	1846	Crude casein	J. von Liebig
	1849	Casein hydrolysate	F. Bopp
3,5-Diiodotyrosine	1896	Skeleton of coral	E. Drechsel
3,5,3′-Triiodotyrosine	1953	Thyroid tissue	J. Gross and R. Pitt-Rivers
Thyroxine	1915	Thyroid tissue	E.C. Kendall
L-Valine	1856	Animal tissues	E. von Gorup-Besanez
	1879	Albumin	P. Schützenberger
		(2) Basic Amino Acids	
L-Arginine	1886	Lupine seedling extracts	E. Schulze and E. Steiger
	1895	Horn protein	S.G. Hedin
L-Homoarginine	1962	Plants	E.A. Bell
L-Histidine	1896	Sturine protein	A. Kossel
	1896	Various proteins	S.G. Hedin
L-5-Hydroxylysine	1925	Fish gelatin	S.B. Schryver, H.W. Buston, and D.H. Mukherjee
L-Lysine	1889	Casein	E. Drechsel
L-Ornithine	1877	Hen urine	M. Jaffé
L-Pyrrolysine	2002	Archaea (microbes)	J.R. Krzycki and M.K. Chan

(Continued)

TABLE 1.1 (*Continued*)
Discoveries of Natural Amino Acids

Amino Acids	Year	Source	Scientist(s)
		(3) Acidic Amino Acids	
Aminomalonic acid	1984	*Escherichia coli* and HAP	Van Buskirk and colleagues
L-Aspartic acid	1827	Marshmallow extracts	A. Plisson
	1868	Conglutin, legumin	H. Ritthausen
L-Glutamic acid	1866	Gliadin	H. Ritthausen
L-Phosphoarginine	1928	Freshwater crabs	O.F. Meyerhof and K. Lohmann
L-Selenocysteine	1973	Clostridia (anaerobes)	T.C. Stadtman

Source: Greenstein, J.P. and M. Winitz. 1961. *Chemistry of Amino Acids*. John Wiley, New York; and Meister, A. 1965. *Biochemistry of Amino Acids*. Academic Press, New York.

Note: HAP, human atherosclerotic plaque.

1.1 DEFINITION AND NOMENCLATURE OF AAs

1.1.1 DEFINITION OF AAs

AAs are defined as organic substances that contain both amino ($-NH_2$) and acid groups. An acid group in a natural AA can be the carboxyl ($-COOH$; e.g., alanine), sulfonic acid ($-SO_3H$; e.g., taurine), phosphoric acid ($-PO_4H_2$; e.g., phosphoethanolamine), or phosphonic acid ($-PO_3H_2$; e.g., 2-aminoethylphosphonate) group. Some AAs (e.g., phosphoarginine and phosphoserine) possess two different acid groups (e.g., both phosphoric acid and carboxyl groups). AAs are readily ionizable in an aqueous solution. The different carbon atoms of AAs are named in sequence according to the Greek alphabet. If the amino group is linked to the α-carbon (the carbon adjacent to the primary acid group), the AA is designated as an α-AA. The hydrogen atom that is attached to the α-carbon is called the α-hydrogen. Likewise, if the amino group is linked to the β-, γ-, δ-, or ε-carbon, the AA is designated a β-, γ-, δ-, or ε-AA, respectively. Examples of natural α-, ß-, γ-, δ-, or ε-AAs are alanine, β-alanine, γ-aminobutyric acid (GABA), 5-aminovaleric acid, and 6-aminocaproic acid, respectively. Note that aspartate and glutamate have a β- and γ-carboxyl group, respectively; asparagine and glutamine have an amide group at the end of the side chain; and ornithine and lysine have a γ- and ε-amino group, respectively; all of these AAs possess an α-amino group. In addition, arginine has a positively charged guanidino group and citrulline has a neutral ureido group, but these two AAs interconvert via different reactions in humans and other animals, as well as plants and microbes. Thus, some AAs within organisms contain two carboxyl groups, several AAs contain two amino groups, and other AAs contain uncharged side chains. However, despite these variations, all AAs must have a primary amino group ($-NH_2$). Different AAs have different chemical properties (Table 1.2). All proteinogenic AAs are α-AAs.

α-Amino acid   β-Amino acid   γ-Amino acid

(R = side chain)   (R = side chain)   (R = side chain)

TABLE 1.2

Molecular Weights, Number of Nitrogen (N) Atoms, N Content, and Chemical Properties of Amino Acids

Amino Acids	MW (Dalton)	Number of N Atoms	N Content (%)	MP (°C)	Solub[a] in H_2O	pK_1[b]	pK_2[c]	pK_3[d]	pI
(1) Neutral Amino Acids									
L-Alanine ($C_3H_7NO_2$)	89.09	1	15.72	297	16.5	2.35	9.87	–	6.11
β-Alanine ($C_3H_7NO_2$)	89.09	1	15.72	197	82.8	3.55	10.24	–	6.90
γ-Aminobutyrate ($C_4H_9NO_2$)	103.12	1	13.58	202	107.3	4.03	10.56	–	7.30
β-Aminoisobutyrate ($C_4H_9NO_2$)	103.12	1	13.58	176	56.7	4.17	10.32	–	7.25
L-Asparagine ($C_4H_8N_2O_3$)	132.12	2	21.20	236	2.20	2.02	8.80	–	5.41
L-Citrulline ($C_6H_{13}N_3O_3$)	175.19	3	23.99	222	15.2	2.43	9.41	–	5.92
L-Cysteine ($C_3H_7NO_2S$)	121.16	1	11.56	178	17.4	1.96[e]	8.18[e]	10.28[e]	5.07[e]
L-Cystine ($C_6H_{12}N_2O_4S_2$)	240.30	2	11.66	261	0.011	<1.0[f]	8.02[f]	–	5.06[f]
						2.10[f]	8.71[f]	–	
L-DOPA ($C_9H_{11}NO_4$)	197.19	1	7.10	277	0.39	2.32	8.72	9.70	5.52
L-Glu-Na (MSG; $C_5H_8NO_4Na$)	169.11	1	8.28	232	73.9	–	9.47	4.07	6.77
L-Glutamine ($C_5H_{10}N_2O_3$)	146.14	2	19.17	185	4.81[e]	2.17	9.13	–	5.65
Glycine ($C_2H_5NO_2$)	75.07	1	18.66	290	25.0	2.35	9.78	–	6.07
L-4-Hydroxyproline ($C_5H_9NO_3$)	131.13	1	10.68	270	36.1	1.92	9.73	–	5.83
L-Isoleucine ($C_6H_{13}NO_2$)	131.17	1	10.68	284	4.12	2.36	9.68	–	6.02
L-Leucine ($C_6H_{13}NO_2$)	131.17	1	10.68	337	2.19	2.33	9.75	–	6.04
L-Methionine ($C_5H_{11}NO_2S$)	149.21	1	9.39	283	5.06	2.28	9.21	–	5.74
L-Phenylalanine ($C_9H_{11}NO_2$)	165.19	1	8.48	284	2.96	2.20	9.31	–	5.76
L-Proline ($C_5H_9NO_2$)	115.13	1	12.17	222	162.3	1.99	10.6	–	6.30
L-Serine ($C_3H_7NO_3$)	105.09	1	13.33	228	41.3	2.21	9.15	–	5.68
Taurine ($C_2H_7NO_3S$)	125.15	1	11.19	328	10.5	1.50	8.74	–	5.12
L-Threonine ($C_4H_9NO_3$)	119.12	1	11.76	253	9.54	2.15	9.12	–	5.64
L-Tryptophan ($C_{11}H_{12}N_2O_2$)	204.22	2	13.72	282	1.14	2.38	9.39	–	5.89
L-Tyrosine ($C_9H_{11}NO_3$)	181.19	1	7.73	344	0.045	2.20	9.11	10.07	5.66
L-Valine ($C_5H_{11}NO_2$)	117.15	1	11.96	315	5.82	2.29	9.72	–	6.01
(2) Basic Amino Acids									
L-Arginine ($C_6H_{14}N_4O_2$)	174.20	4	32.16	238	18.6	2.17	9.04	12.48	10.76
L-Histidine ($C_6H_9N_3O_2$)	155.15	3	27.08	277	4.19	1.80	9.33	6.04	7.69
L-Homoarginine ($C_7H_{16}N_4O_2$)	188.23	4	29.77	208	0.158	2.49	9.00	12.30	10.65
L-Lysine ($C_6H_{14}N_2O_2$)	146.19	2	19.16	224	78.2[g]	2.18	8.95	10.53	9.74
L-Ornithine ($C_5H_{12}N_2O_2$)	132.16	2	21.20	231[h]	54.5[h]	1.94	8.65	10.76	9.71
L-Pyrrolysine ($C_{12}H_{21}N_3O_3$)	255.31	3	16.46	–	–	–	–	–	–
(3) Acidic Amino Acids									
Aminomalonic acid ($C_3H_5NO_4$)	119.08	1	11.76	243	12.6	1.80	8.50	1.80	1.80
L-Aspartic acid ($C_4H_7NO_4$)	133.10	1	10.52	270	0.45	1.88	9.60	3.65	2.77

(Continued)

TABLE 1.2 (*Continued*)

Molecular Weights, Number of Nitrogen (N) Atoms, N Content, and Chemical Properties of Amino Acids

Amino Acids	MW (Dalton)	Number of N Atoms	N Content (%)	MP (°C)	Solub[a] in H₂O	pK₁[b]	pK₂[c]	pK₃[d]	pI
L-Glutamic acid (C₅H₉NO₄)	147.13	1	9.52	249	0.86	2.19	9.67	4.25	3.22
L-Phosphoarginine (C₆H₁₅N₄O₅P)	254.18	4	22.04	178	2.70	2.02	9.60	Values[i]	<1.98
L-Selenocysteine (C₃H₇NO₂Se)	167.06	1	8.38	145	32.5	2.50	9.50	5.20	3.90

Source: Greenstein, J.P. and M. Winitz. 1961. *Chemistry of Amino Acids*. John Wiley, New York; Meister, A. 1965. *Biochemistry of Amino Acids*. Academic Press, New York; Ennor et al. 1956. *Biochem. J.* 62:358–361; Besant et al. 2009. *Curr. Protein Peptide Sci.* 10:536–550; and https://pubchem.ncbi.nlm.nih.gov. The classification of amino acids as neutral, basic, and acidic amino acids is based on their net charges at neutral pH; neutral AAs have no net charge, basic AAs have a net positive charge, and acidic AAs have a net negative charge.

a   Solubility (Solub); g/100 mL of water at 25°C unless otherwise indicated.

b pK_a for α-COOH (SO₃H for taurine), namely pK_1, at 25°C unless otherwise indicated.

c pK_a for α-NH₃⁺, namely pK₂, at 25°C unless otherwise indicated.

d pK_a for the ionized group in the side chain, namely pK₃, at 25°C unless otherwise indicated.

e   Determined at 30°C.

f   Determined at 35°C.

g   L-Lysine-H₂O.

h   L-Ornithine-HCl.

i   The pK_a values of the first H and the second H of the phosphoric acid moiety are <1.96 and 4.5, respectively. The pK_a value of the side-chain guanidino is 11.2.

Note: L-DOPA, 3,4-dihydroxy-L-phenylalanine (3-hydroxy-L-tyrosine); MP, melting point; MSG, monosodium glutamate (the sodium salt of glutamic acid); MW, molecular weight.

1.1.2   DEFINITION OF IMINO ACIDS

Imino acids are defined as organic substances that contain both secondary α-amino (α-imino) group (–NH) and acid groups. Proline and 4-hydroxyproline belong to this class of molecules. Because proline is a substrate for protein synthesis like other α-AAs and because hydroxyproline is the post-translational metabolite of proline within organisms, proline and hydroxyproline are loosely referred to as α-AAs in biochemistry and nutrition. Hydroxyproline occurs as both 4-hydroxyproline (the major form) and 3-hydroxyproline (the minor form) in animals, with the ratio of 4-hydroxyproline to 3-hydroxyproline being approximately 100:1. The hydroxyprolines have both structural and physiological functions in the body (Li and Wu 2018).

1.1.3   ISOMERS OF AAS

1.1.3.1   L- and D-AAs

The ability of an aqueous solution of a natural AA to exhibit optical activity and rotate plane-polarized light was first observed by L. Pasteur in 1851. The absolute configuration of an AA (L- or D-isomers as first introduced by Emil Fischer in 1908) is arbitrarily defined with reference to L- and D-glyceraldehyde (Figure 1.1). Fischer projections, which are commonly used to represent AAs, are abbreviated structural forms that convey valuable stereochemical information about them in the absence of their three-dimensional representations.

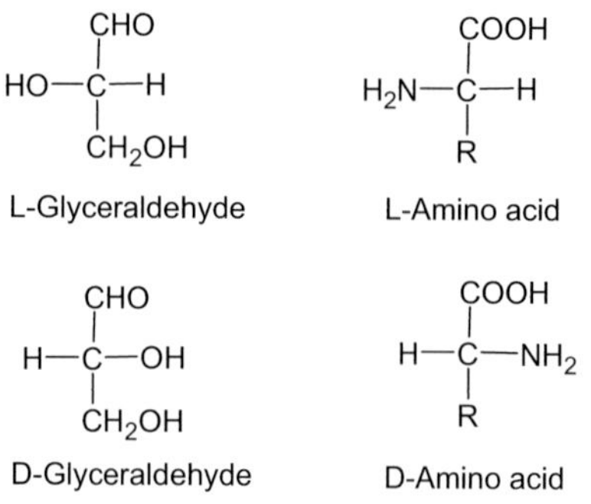

CHO
HO—C—H
CH$_2$OH

L-Glyceraldehyde

COOH
H$_2$N—C—H
R

L-Amino acid

CHO
H—C—OH
CH$_2$OH

D-Glyceraldehyde

COOH
H—C—NH$_2$
R

D-Amino acid

FIGURE 1.1 Fisher projections for configurations of amino acids relative to L- and D-glyceraldehydes. The general structure of an amino acid in its non-ionized form is shown.

Except for glycine (the simplest AA in nature with a single hydrogen side chain), all proteinogenic AAs can have both D- and L-isomers (Bischoff and Schlüter 2012). That is, when a beam of plane-polarized light is passed through the solution of an optical isomer, the light will be rotated either to the right or to the left. Because each asymmetric carbon can have two possible configurations, an AA with n asymmetric carbons has 2^n different possible stereoisomers and 2^{n-1} enantiomeric pairs (non-superimposable mirror images). For example, the β-carbon atom in isoleucine and threonine is also asymmetric; therefore, these two AAs can possibly exist in four optical isomeric forms. Like glycine, some non-proteinogenic AAs, such as GABA, β-alanine, taurine (which are all physiological metabolites in humans and other animals), and aminomalonic acid (which is known to be present in humans and microbes), have no optical activity or D- and L-isomers.

The chemical structures of proteinogenic L-AAs and glycine in humans and other animals at neutral pH are illustrated in Figure 1.2. L-AAs are the predominant physiological isomers of AAs found in nature. However, D-AAs also exist in animals, bacteria, yeast, plants, and foods. L-AAs are generally the most abundant physiological isomers and account for > 99.9% of the total AAs in animals.

The nomenclature of an AA with more than one asymmetric carbon includes an allo-form. Namely, if the β- or γ-carbon configuration in an AA is opposite to the configuration of the α-carbon, this AA is said to have an allo-form. For example, a synthetic L-threonine whose β-carbon has a configuration opposite to that of the α-carbon is called L-allo-threonine. L-Threonine and L-allo-threonine are called diastereomers, and the relationship between the two AAs is diastereomerism (Figure 1.3).

Optical isomerism of organic molecules has traditionally been described as dextrorotatory (right, "+", or *d*) or levorotatory (left, "−", or *l*), depending on the direction of optical rotation. Because measurement conditions can affect the angle of optical rotation, the terms "dextrorotatory" and "levorotatory" have been abandoned. In chemistry, the specific rotation of an AA is measured by a polarimeter under certain experimental conditions, such as solvent, solute concentration, temperature, and the pH of the aqueous solution (Hayashi et al. 1966). Values of the specific rotation of AAs are given in Table 1.3, which are useful for their identification and the assessment of their optical purity. The D and L-configurations for an organic substance may not necessarily determine the rotation of plane-polarized light. For example, the naturally occurring form of fructose is the D (−) isomer (D-configuration with a levorotatory optical activity). When equal amounts of D- and L-AAs (e.g., DL-methionine) are present, the resulting mixture has no optical activity.

The chemical configuration of AAs is not changed in their crystalline form. Standard conditions for acid (6 M HCl at 110°C for 24 h under nitrogen gas), alkaline (4.2 M NaOH plus 1% thiodiglycol, antioxidant, at 105°C for 20 h), or enzymatic hydrolysis of proteins do not affect the configuration of the preexisting isomer of AAs in peptides. However, L- or D-AAs may lose their optical activity (known as racemization) in stronger acid or stronger alkaline solutions at higher temperature (e.g., >110°C) (Greenstein and Winitz 1961). To date, D-AAs are often analyzed by high-performance liquid chromatography on a chiral or ligand column, or using pre-column derivatization with reagents that convert the enantiomers to diastereomers to improve their chromatographic resolution (Miyoshi et al. 2012).

Name	Symbol	Structural formula at neutral pH

With aliphatic side chains

Name	Symbol	Structural formula at neutral pH
Glycine	Gly [G]	$H-\underset{\underset{NH_3^+}{\vert}}{\overset{\overset{H}{\vert}}{C}}-COO^-$
Alanine	Ala [A]	$H_3C-\underset{\underset{NH_3^+}{\vert}}{CH}-COO^-$
Valine	Val [V]	$\underset{H_3C}{\overset{H_3C}{>}}CH-\underset{\underset{NH_3^+}{\vert}}{CH}-COO^-$
Leucine	Leu [L]	$\underset{H_3C}{\overset{H_3C}{>}}CH-CH_2-\underset{\underset{NH_3^+}{\vert}}{CH}-COO^-$
Isoleucine	Ile [I]	$\underset{H_3C}{\overset{H_3C-CH_2}{>}}CH-\underset{\underset{NH_3^+}{\vert}}{CH}-COO^-$

With side chains containing hydroxylic (OH) groups

Name	Symbol	Structural formula at neutral pH
Serine	Ser [S]	$H_2\underset{\underset{OH}{\vert}}{C}-\underset{\underset{NH_3^+}{\vert}}{CH}-COO^-$
Threonine	Thr [T]	$H_3C-\underset{\underset{OH}{\vert}}{CH}-\underset{\underset{NH_3^+}{\vert}}{CH}-COO^-$
Tyrosine	Tyr [Y]	See aromatic amino acids

With side chains containing sulfur atoms

Name	Symbol	Structural formula at neutral pH
Cysteine	Cys [C]	$HS-CH_2-\underset{\underset{NH_3^+}{\vert}}{CH}-COO^-$
Methionine	Met [M]	$H_3C-S-CH_2-CH_2-\underset{\underset{NH_3^+}{\vert}}{CH}-COO^-$

With side chains containing acidic groups

Name	Symbol	Structural formula at neutral pH
Aspartate	Asp [D]	$^-OOC-CH_2-\underset{\underset{NH_3^+}{\vert}}{CH}-COO^-$
Glutamate	Glu [E]	$^-OOC-CH_2-CH_2-\underset{\underset{NH_3^+}{\vert}}{CH}-COO^-$

FIGURE 1.2 Chemical structures of proteinogenic amino acids in humans and other animals at neutral pH. These amino acids also occur in viruses, bacteria, archaea, and algae. Except for selenocysteine (a rare, special peptide-bound amino acid in selenoproteins), the 20 canonical proteinogenic amino acids are present in yeast and higher plants.

(*Continued*)

Name	Symbol	Structural formula at neutral pH

With side chains containing amide groups

| Asparagine | Asn [N] | $H_2N-\underset{O}{\overset{\parallel}{C}}-CH_2-\underset{\overset{+}{N}H_3}{\overset{\mid}{C}H}-COO^-$ |
| Glutamine | Gln [Q] | $H_2N-\underset{O}{\overset{\parallel}{C}}-CH_2-CH_2-\underset{\overset{+}{N}H_3}{\overset{\mid}{C}H}-COO^-$ |

With side chains containing basic groups

Arginine	Arg [R]	$HN-CH_2-CH_2-CH_2-\underset{\overset{+}{N}H_3}{\overset{\mid}{C}H}-COO^-$
Lysine	Lys [K]	
Histidine	His [H]	

With side chains containing aromatic rings

Phenylalanine	Phe [F]	
Tyrosine	Tyr [Y]	
Tryptophan	Trp [W]	

With side chain containing seleno group

| Selenocysteine | Sec [U] | $HSe-CH_2-\underset{\overset{+}{N}H_3}{\overset{\mid}{C}H}-COO^-$ |

With side chain containing imino group

| Proline | Pro [P] | |

FIGURE 1.2 (*CONTINUED*)   Chemical structures of proteinogenic amino acids in humans and other animals at neutral pH. These amino acids also occur in viruses, bacteria, archaea, and algae. Except for selenocysteine (a rare, special peptide-bound amino acid in selenoproteins), the 20 canonical proteinogenic amino acids are present in yeast and higher plants. Note that arginine has a guanidino group.

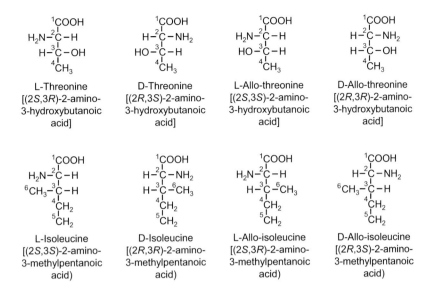

FIGURE 1.3 The *R/S* configurations of L-threonine, D-threonine, L-isoleucine, and D-isoleucine. If two diastereomers have a different configuration in the β- or γ-carbon, they are designated with the prefix "allo". Note that d*iastereomers* are stereoisomers with two or more stereocenters that are not mirror images of one another and are non-superimposable on one another.

1.1.3.2   *R*- and *S*-AAs

To better distinguish some naturally occurring and synthetic AAs (e.g., threonine, isoleucine, and hydroxyproline) with more than one chirality center, the *R/S* nomenclature is used to name their absolute configurations, where *R* is *rectus* (right) and *S* is *sinister* (left) in Latin. This nomenclature system does not involve a reference molecule such as glyceraldehyde, but is based on the prioritized spatial arrangement of the four different groups that are attached to the chirality center, namely 1 = the group with the highest atomic number, 2 = the group with the second highest atomic number, 3 = the group with the third highest atomic number, and 4 = the group with the lowest atomic number. To determine whether the chirality center is in the *R* or *S* configuration, one needs to first prioritize all four of the groups connected to the chirality center based on their atomic numbers (i.e., a higher atomic number takes precedence over a lower atomic number). Then, the molecule is rotated so that the fourth (the lowest) priority group points away from you (a dashed line). If the sequence for the first three priority groups 1-2-3 is clockwise, the designation is *R*. If the sequence for the first three priority groups (1-2-3) is counterclockwise, the designation is *S*. The *R/S* system has no fixed relation to the (+; dextrorotatory form)/(−; levorotary form) system. An *R* isomer can be either dextro-rotatory or levorotatory, depending on its exact substituents. In the *R/S* system, naturally occurring AAs are mostly in the *S* configuration for the first chiral center like a carbohydrate. The *R/S* configurations of L-threonine, D-threonine, L-isoleucine, and D-isoleucine are illustrated in Figure 1.3.

TABLE 1.3
Specific Rotation of Amino Acids (AAs) in Aqueous Solutions

Amino Acids	$[\alpha]_{20}^{D}$		Concentration of AA (%; g/100 ml)	Solvent	Temperature (°C)
	Range[a]	Mean			
(1) Neutral Amino Acids					
L-Alanine	+14.3° to +15.2°	+14.7°	10	6 M HCl	20
L-Alanine	–	+15.5°	10	2 M HCl	20
L-Alanine	+13.7° to +15.1°	+14.4°	10	6 M HCl	25
L-Asparagine	+34.3° to +36.5°	+35.4°	10	6 M HCl	20
L-Citrulline	+24.5° to +26.8°	+25.8°	8	6 M HCl	20
L-Cysteine	+8.3° to +9.5°	+8.9°	8	1 M HCl	20
L-Cysteine	–	+6.5°	2	5 M HCl	25
L-Cysteine-HCl·H$_2$O	+6.1° to +7.8°	+7.0°	8	1 M HCl	20
L-Cystine	−215° to −225°	−220°	2	1 M HCl	20
L-DOPA	−11.5° to −13.0°	−12.3°	5	1 M HCl	20
L-Glutamine	+6.3° to +7.3°	+6.5°	4	Water	20
L-4-Hydroxyproline	−74.0° to −77.0°	−75.1°	4	Water	20
L-Isoleucine	+39.5° to +41.5°	+40.7°	4	6 M HCl	20
L-Leucine	+14.9° to +16.0°	+15.1°	4	6 M HCl	20
L-Methionine	+23.0° to +24.0°	+23.5°	2	6 M HCl	20
L-Methionine	–	+24.2°	8	4–6 M HCl	20
L-Phenylalanine	−33.5° to −35.0°	−34.3°	2	Water	20
L-Proline	−84.5° to −86.0°	−84.8°	4	Water	20
L-Serine	+14.4° to +15.5°	+15.0°	10	2 M HCl	20
L-Threonine	−27.6° to −29.0°	−28.5°	6	Water	20
L-Tryptophan	−30.5° to −32.5°	−31.5°	1	Water	Warm[b]
L-Tyrosine	−11.3° to −12.1°	−12.0°	5	1 M HCl	20
L-Valine	+27.6° to +28.7°	+28.0°	8	6 M HCl	20
(2) Basic Amino Acids and Their HCl Salts					
L-Arginine	+26.9° to +27.9°	+27.4°	8	6 M HCl	20
L-Arginine-HCl	+22.1° to +22.9°	+22.5°	8	6 M HCl	20
L-Histidine	+12.0° to +12.4°	+12.2°	11	6 M HCl	20
L-Histidine·HCl·H$_2$O	+8.9° to +9.5°	+9.3°	11	6 M HCl	20
L-Homoarginine	+12.0° to +16.0°	+14.0°	2	1 M HCl	20
L-Homoarginine·HCl	+16.0° to +20.0°	+18.0°	8	6 M HCl	20
L-Homoarginine·HCl	–	+18.0°	1	1 M HCl	20
L-Lysine·HCl	+20.8° to +21.5°	+21.2°	8	6 M HCl	20
L-Ornithine·HCl	+23.0° to +25.0°	+24.0°	4	6 M HCl	20
(3) Acidic Amino Acids and Their Hydrochloride or Sodium Salts					
L-Aspartic acid	+24.8° to +25.8°	+25.3°	8	6 M HCl	20
L-Aspartic acid	–	+26.2°	10	2–3 M HCl	20
L-Glutamic acid	+31.5° to +32.4°	+32.0°	10	2 M HCl	20
L-Glutamic acid·HCl	+25.2° to +25.8°	+25.5°	10	2 M HCl	20
L-Glu-Na (MSG)	+24.8° to +25.3°	+25.1°	10	2 M HCl	20
L-Glu-Na (MSG)	+24.2° to +25.5°	+24.9°	8	1 M HCl	25
L-Selenocystine	Unknown	−28.0°	1	1 M NaOH	20

Source: Hayashi et al. 1996. *Agric. Biol. Chem.* 30:1221–1237; Ajinomoto® 2003. *Ajinomoto's Amino Acid Handbook.* Tokyo, Japan; and https://pubchem.ncbi.nlm.nih.gov.

[a] The value refers to the angle to which the AA causes the polarized light to rotate under certain experimental conditions such as temperature, wavelength, concentration, and pH.

[b] The water was warmed for the dissolution of tryptophan.

The collagen and plasma of animals contain 4-hydroxy-L-proline (4-hydroxy-L-pyrrolidine-2-carboxylic acid) and 3-hydroxy-L-proline (3-hydroxy-L-pyrrolidine-2-carboxylic acid), with their ratio being approximately 100:1. According to the *R/S* nomenclature system, the physiological isoform of 4-hydroxyproline in collagen and its enzymatic hydrolysates is L-4-hydroxyproline, and the physiological isoform of 3-hydroxyproline is L-3-hydroxyproline.

1.1.3.3 *cis*- and *trans*-AAs

If an organic compound contains a double bond and the double bond cannot rotate, or if an organic compound (e.g., 4-hydroxyproline) with ≥2 functional groups being attached to its carbons has a ring structure where the rotation of bonds is restricted, *cis* and *trans* isomers occur in such a molecule (Figure 1.4). When the two functional groups of a diastereomer (also called diastereo-isomer) are oriented in the same direction, the diastereomer is referred to as *cis*, such as *cis*-4-hydroxy-L-proline [*cis*-(2S,4S)-4-hydroxyproline]. By contrast, when the two functional groups of a diastereomer are oriented in opposite directions, the diastereomer is referred to as *trans*, such as *trans*-4-hydroxy-proline [*trans*-(2S,4R)-4-hydroxy-proline]. The physiological isoform of 4-hydroxyproline in animal collagen and its enzymatic hydrolysates is *trans*-4-hydroxy-L-proline, and that of 3-hydroxy-L-proline is *trans*-3-hydroxy-L-proline [*trans*-(2S,3S)-3-hydroxyproline] (Li and Wu 2018). However, the acid hydrolysis of collagen at high temperatures (e.g., 110°C) yields a small amount of 4-hydroxyproline and 3-hydroxyproline in the *cis* isoform. *cis*-4-Hydroxy-L-proline [*cis*-(2S,4S)-4-hydroxyproline] and *cis*-3-hydroxy-L-proline [(2S,3R)-3-hydroxyproline] have been identified in certain bacteria and fungi, and the microbes may also contain *trans*-4-hydroxy-D-proline [*trans*-(2S, 4S)-4-hydroxyproline] and *cis*-4-hydroxy-D-proline [*cis*-(2R,4R)-4-hydroxy-proline] (Hara and Kino 2009; Watanabe et al. 2017). Note that the *cis/trans* nomenclature is not the same as the *R/S* nomenclature. In the following molecules, the solid hard line and the dash line denote that the functional group points toward and away from the viewer, respectively.

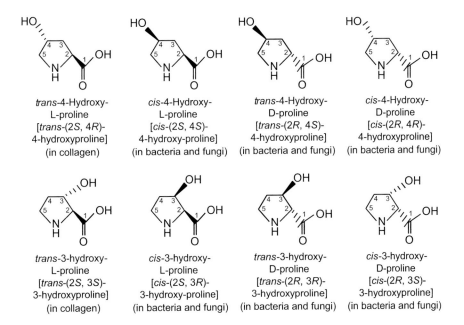

trans-4-Hydroxy-
L-proline
[*trans*-(2S, 4R)-
4-hydroxyproline]
(in collagen)

cis-4-Hydroxy-
L-proline
[*cis*-(2S, 4S)-
4-hydroxy-proline]
(in bacteria and fungi)

trans-4-Hydroxy-
D-proline
[*trans*-(2R, 4S)-
4-hydroxyproline]
(in bacteria and fungi)

cis-4-Hydroxy-
D-proline
[*cis*-(2R, 4R)-
4-hydroxyproline]
(in bacteria and fungi)

trans-3-hydroxy-
L-proline
[*trans*-(2S, 3S)-
3-hydroxyproline]
(in collagen)

cis-3-hydroxy-
L-proline
[*cis*-(2S, 3R)-
3-hydroxy-proline]
(in bacteria and fungi)

trans-3-hydroxy-
D-proline
[*trans*-(2R, 3R)-
3-hydroxyproline]
(in bacteria and fungi)

cis-3-hydroxy-
D-proline
[*cis*-(2R, 3S)-
3-hydroxyproline]
(in bacteria and fungi)

FIGURE 1.4 The *trans* and *cis* configurations of 4-hydroxy-L-proline and 4-hydroxy-D-proline, as well as 3-hydroxy-L-proline and 3-hydroxy-D-proline. The physiological isoform of 4-hydroxyproline and 3-hydroxy-proline in animal collagen and its enzymatic hydrolysates is *trans*-4-hydroxy-L-proline and *trans*-3-hydroxy-L-proline. *trans*-4-Hydroxy-L-proline and *trans*-3-hydroxy-L-proline, as well as their D-isomers, occur in microbes. Note that the *cis/trans* nomenclature is not the same as the *R/S* nomenclature.

1.1.4 PROTEINOGENIC AND NON-PROTEINOGENIC AAS

The AAs that are incorporated into proteins during mRNA translation are called proteinogenic AAs. There are 22 genetically encoded (proteinogenic) AAs in nature. Twenty-one of them (including selenocysteine; Figure 1.2) occur in humans and other animals, as well as viruses, bacteria, archaea, and algae (e.g., *Chlamydomonas reinhardtii*, a single-cell green alga) (Fu et al. 2002; Stadtman 1996). Pyrrolysine is another proteinogenic AA in some proteins of certain methanogenic archaea and bacteria. Twenty of them, namely those in Figure 1.2 excluding selenocysteine, are directly encoded for protein synthesis by the universal genetic code of all organisms (i.e., both eukaryotes and prokaryotes) and, therefore, are called canonical proteinogenic AAs. By contrast, selenocysteine and pyrrolysine are incorporated into proteins through unique mechanisms involving the UGA and UAG stop codons, respectively (Chapter 8), and, therefore, are referred to as non-canonical proteinogenic AAs. Yeast and higher plants contain the 20 canonical proteinogenic AAs (Wu 2018) but no selenocysteine or pyrrolysine (Lu and Holmgren 2008; Wong et al. 2012). The AAs that are not the building blocks of proteins are known as non-proteinogenic AAs (e.g., taurine, 4-hydroxyproline, 3-methylhistidine, β-alanine, citrulline, ornithine, and homocysteine). Some non-proteinogenic AAs occur in certain proteins due to posttranslational modifications.

According to the International Union of Biochemistry and Molecular Biology, a three-letter abbreviation can be used to designate a proteinogenic AA, with one capital letter followed by two lowercase letters, such as Glu for glutamate, Gln for glutamine, and Arg for arginine (Figure 1.2). A one-letter abbreviation is used to represent an AA in protein or polypeptide sequences, such as E, Q, and R for glutamate, glutamine, and arginine, respectively (Figure 1.2).

Based on the foregoing definitions, not all AAs present in polypeptides are classified as proteinogenic AAs. This is because some of the AA residues in polypeptides are formed during posttranslational events. An example is 4-hydroxyproline, which is generated from proline by peptidyl proline hydroxylase after a protein is synthesized. Other examples of the formation of new AA residues in polypeptides due to posttranslational modifications include citrulline and asymmetric dimethylarginine from arginine; 1-methylhistidine and 3-methylhistidine from histidine (primarily in actin and myosin); hydroxyserine and hydroxythreonine from serine and threonine, respectively; hydroxytyrosine and nitrosylated tyrosine from tyrosine; and acetylated lysine, hydroxylysine, and methylated lysine from lysine (Chapter 8).

1.1.5 FREE AAS AND PEPTIDE (OR PROTEIN)-BOUND AAS

Free AAs are defined as those AAs that are not covalently bound in dipeptides, oligopeptides, or polypeptides. Peptide (or protein)-bound AAs are those AAs that are linked in peptides or proteins via peptide bonds. Selenocysteine can be considered to be a special protein-bound AA found in selenoproteins, because it is derived from serine and selenium at the translational step of protein synthesis (Chapter 8). A free pool of selenocysteine does not exist in animals because its high reactivity with many electrophiles (e.g., H^+, NO^+, Zn^{2+}, nitroalkene derivatives of fatty acids, and unsaturated carbonyls) would lead to cellular damage. When two AAs form a peptide bond in protein, one molecule of water is lost. Strictly speaking, proteins contain AA residues (AAs without one molecule of water) but not intact AAs. Thus, 100 g of protein contains 100 g of AA residues but not 100 g of AAs, whereas the complete hydrolysis of 100 g of protein yields more than 100 g of free, intact AAs (e.g., 100 g of protein in pork meat provides 118 g of AAs after its enzymatic hydrolysis). This fundamental principle should be borne in mind when analyzing AA composition in proteins (including those in tissues, cells, human foods, and animal-sourced protein feedstuffs), as well as designing and interpreting nutritional studies involving dietary supplementation with protein and a mixture of AAs.

The composition of peptide bond-linked AAs can vary greatly among different proteins, but is largely similar among different mammalian and avian species (He et al. 2021; Zhang et al. 2021). On the gram or molar basis, glycine is the most abundant AA in the whole body and collagen proteins of animals, followed by proline, glutamate, and arginine in descending order; and the content of leucine and alanine in the whole body and all tissues is similar to that of arginine (Table 1.4). When data on peptide-bound AAs in protein and true protein content in the body are presented, it is very important to indicate how the results are calculated (e.g., based on the molecular weights of either intact AAs or AA residues) and expressed (e.g., g of AA residue/100 g of true protein or g of intact AA/100 g of intact AAs), as indicated for AA content in 6-month-old pigs. This potential problem can be avoided by using the unit of mol rather than g for peptide-bound AAs, but g is commonly used in feeding. Unclear data calculation and expression can cause unintended troubles in both research and nutritional practice.

TABLE 1.4

Composition of Amino Acids (AAs) in the Carcasses of 6-Month-Old Pigs[a]

Amino Acid	Total AA in the Body/kg of BW[b]			AA in Protein			
	g of Intact AAs[c]	g of AA Residues[d]	mmol of AA	mg of Intact AA/g of intact AAs[c]	mg of AA Residue/g of True Protein[d]	μmol of AA/g of True Protein	mg of AA Residue/g of BW[d]
Ala	7.59	6.06	85.19	63.7	59.9	843	5.99
Arg	7.72	6.92	44.32	65.4	69.1	442	6.90
Asn	4.01	3.46	30.35	34.0	34.6	303	3.46
Asp	4.84	4.19	36.36	40.7	41.5	361	4.16
Asp + Asn	8.85	7.65	66.71	74.7	78.1	664	7.62
Cys	1.47	1.25	12.13	12.4	12.4	120	1.24
Gln	6.23	5.46	42.63	48.6	50.2	393	5.04
Glu	9.66	8.48	65.66	80.7	83.5	646	8.34
Glu + Gln	15.89	13.94	108.29	129.3	133.7	1,039	13.38
Gly	15.76	11.98	209.94	132.5	118.8	2,082	11.88
His	2.33	2.06	15.02	19.5	20.3	148	2.03
Ile	3.96	3.42	30.19	33.5	34.1	301	3.41
Leu	7.66	6.61	58.4	64.9	66.0	583	6.60
Lys	6.78	5.95	46.38	57.4	59.3	463	5.94
Met	2.08	1.83	13.94	17.5	18.2	139	1.82
Phe	3.82	3.40	23.12	32.3	33.9	230	3.39
Pro	11.56	9.75	100.41	96.8	96.2	991	9.63
OH-Pro	5.78	4.99	44.06	49.0	49.8	440	4.98
Pro + OH-Pro	17.34	14.74	144.47	145.8	146.0	1,431	14.61
Ser	4.95	4.10	47.10	41.9	40.9	470	4.09
Thr	3.96	3.36	33.24	33.3	33.3	329	3.33
Trp	1.23	1.12	6.79	10.4	11.2	60	1.12
Tyr	3.03	2.73	16.72	25.5	27.1	166	2.71
Val	4.74	4.01	40.38	40.1	40.0	403	4.00
Total	119.2	101.1	1,002.3	1,000	1,000	9,913	100.0

[a] The carcasses of barrows (6-month-old castrated male pigs; 110 kg of body weight) without hooves, heads, leg bones, gastrointestinal contents, and blood were analyzed for AAs, as described by Wu et al. (1999). The content of true protein in the body is 10.0% (g/g).

[b] Sum of peptide- and protein-bound AAs as well as free AAs. Calculations for peptide- and protein-bound AAs were based on the molecular weights of intact AAs.

[c] Calculations for peptide- and protein-bound AAs were based on the molecular weights of intact AAs. 100 g of intact AAs is equivalent to 84.86 g protein.

[d] Calculations were based on the molecular weights of AA residues (molecular weights of an intact AA − 18).

Note: BW, body weight.

Interestingly, the composition of many AAs in the whole body of juvenile carnivorous fish (e.g., hybrid-striped bass and largemouth bass) and shrimp (Li et al. 2021a, b) differs appreciably from that in young pigs (Zhang et al. 2021) and chickens (He et al. 2021). Available evidence shows that the concentrations of individual free AAs can differ markedly among cells, tissues, and species. For example, concentrations of free glutamine are 0.5 and 1 mM in the plasma of healthy humans and chickens, respectively, and are 20–25 and 1.5–15 mM in their skeletal muscles, respectively. Values for human plasma and skeletal muscle are shown in Table 1.5. Intramuscular concentrations of free AAs are also influenced by the type of muscle fiber [e.g., 1.5 and 14 mM glutamine in chicken breast (predominantly glycolytic fiber) and leg muscle (mainly oxidative fiber), respectively]. Also,

TABLE 1.5

Concentrations of Free Amino Acids (Means) in the Plasma (or Serum), Skeletal Muscle, Red Blood Cells, Cerebrospinal Fluid (CSF), and Urine of Healthy Adult Humans

AA	Plasma[a] (µM) Men (20–36 years)	Plasma[a] (µM) Women (20–35 years)	Skeletal Muscle[a] (mM) Men (20–36 years)	Skeletal Muscle[a] (mM) Women (20–35 years)	Red Blood Cells[a] (µM)	CSF[b] (µM)	Serum[c] (µM) Men (23–50 years)	Serum[c] (µM) Women (29–53 years)	Urine[c] (µM) Men (23–50 years)	Urine[c] (µM) Women (29–53 years)
Ala	347	388	2.51	3.58	419	23.2	368	307	215	185
Arg	82	72	0.51	0.95	258	18.3	103	90	98	64
Asp	10	18	1.18	2.45	–	0.6	14	17	49	33
Asn	63	64	0.57	0.46	155	5.4	45	38	72	68
Cys[d]	–	–	–	–	–	0.1	101	95	44	49
Glu	34	43	3.93	5.15	446	11.3	91	75	22	18
Gln	696	637	18.5	20.9	758	444	634	580	340	312
Gly	258	332	1.18	2.33	544	4.7	212	226	794	877
His	77	114	0.44	0.58	120	11.9	78	71	674	539
Ile	62	69	0.09	0.11	71	3.9	74	59	11	9.2
Leu	121	159	0.17	0.22	137	10.1	137	112	28	22
Phe	63	68	0.06	0.10	62	6.5	65	57	43	40
Lys	166	223	0.88	1.63	177	21.7	199	180	155	176
Met	32	29	0.05	0.05	20	1.9	43	35	27	26
Pro	192	233	1.04	1.47	–	–	246	230	114	106
Ser	120	188	1.45	1.42	211	24.5	89	89	186	157
Thr	130	209	0.81	1.06	157	27.7	131	114	176	158
Trp	–	–	–	–	–	–	84	72	89	70
Tyr	60	85	0.06	0.15	82	6.4	82	72	126	97
Val	206	264	0.39	0.30	248	15	251	198	61	48
β-Ala	–	–	–	–	–	–	7.8	5.6	67	45
Cit	40	36	0.05	0.13	47	1.5	29	24	22	11
Orn	97	115	0.40	0.44	271	3.7	69	58	47	35
Tau	84	108	15.3	24.0	196	6.8	210	212	880	285

[a] Healthy young adults (Alteheld et al. 2004). The skeletal muscle was quadriceps femoris muscle.

[b] Healthy adult humans (Neveux et al. 2004). The concentration of total free cysteine (cysteine + ½ cystine) in plasma was 52 µM.

[c] Healthy overweight or obese persons (McNeal et al. 2018).

[d] Total cysteine (cysteine + ½ cystine). "1/2 cystine" denotes that 1 mol cystine is composed of 2 mol cysteine.

Note: Cit, citrulline; FAA, free amino acids; Hyp, 4-hydroxyproline; ND, not detectable (below the limit of detection); Orn, ornithine; PAA, peptide-bound amino acids; TAA, total amino acids; Tau, taurine; "–", data are not available.

concentrations of free glycine are approximately 0.25 and 1 mM in the plasma of healthy humans and pigs, respectively. Interestingly, glycine, rather than glutamine, is the most abundant free AA in the plasma of postnatal ungulate mammals studied (e.g., pigs, cattle, and sheep). Furthermore, concentrations of arginine, glutamine, citrulline, and serine can be as high as 1, 25, 10, and 20 mM, respectively, in ovine allantoic fluid during gestation, whereas values for the corresponding AAs in porcine allantoic fluid are 6, 2.5, 0.1, and 0.2 mM, respectively. These differences in concentrations of free AAs reflect tissue and species differences in AA metabolism.

The ratio of total free AAs to total peptide-bound AAs in the whole body and most tissues (e.g., skeletal muscle, liver, and small intestine) is approximately 1:30 (g:g), meaning that total free AAs represent ~3% of total AAs (free plus peptide-bound) in humans and other animals. However, a ratio of some individual free AAs to the same peptide-bound AAs can be greater than 1:10 or lower than 0.1:100 (g:g). For example, in human skeletal muscle, the ratio of free glutamine to peptide-bound glutamine is approximately 2:10 (g:g), whereas the ratio of free tryptophan to peptide-bound tryptophan is only 0.06:100 (g:g).

Free AAs and their metabolites are widely present in animals (Figures 1.2, 1.5, and 1.6). Many of them (e.g., GABA, citrulline, ornithine, β-alanine, putrescine, spermidine, and spermine) commonly occur in plants and microorganisms. Taurine is present in animals but absent from plants or microorganisms. Some free AAs in plants [e.g., L-theanine (N-ethyl-L-glutamine; an analogue of L-glutamine) in teas and citrulline in watermelon] are beneficial for animal health, whereas others [e.g., β-cyanoalanine, djenkolic acid (two cysteine radicals connected by a methylene group), and mimosine (chemically similar to tyrosine)] are toxic to mammals (Figure 1.7). Note that L-theanine has been recognized by the U.S. Food and Drug Administration (FDA) as a GRAS (Generally Recognized as Safe) dietary supplement. Also, synthetic N-ethyl-L-glutamine (marketed as Suntheanine®) is now readily available in health food stores in the United States.

In most food ingredients of plant (Table 1.6) and animal (Table 1.7) origin, approximately 97%–98% of total AAs are present in proteins and polypeptides, whereas only small amounts (2%–3% of total AAs) occur in a free form. However, some free AAs represent significant amounts of total AAs in certain animal- and plant-sourced foods. For example, free glutamate and glutamine (1 and 4 mM,

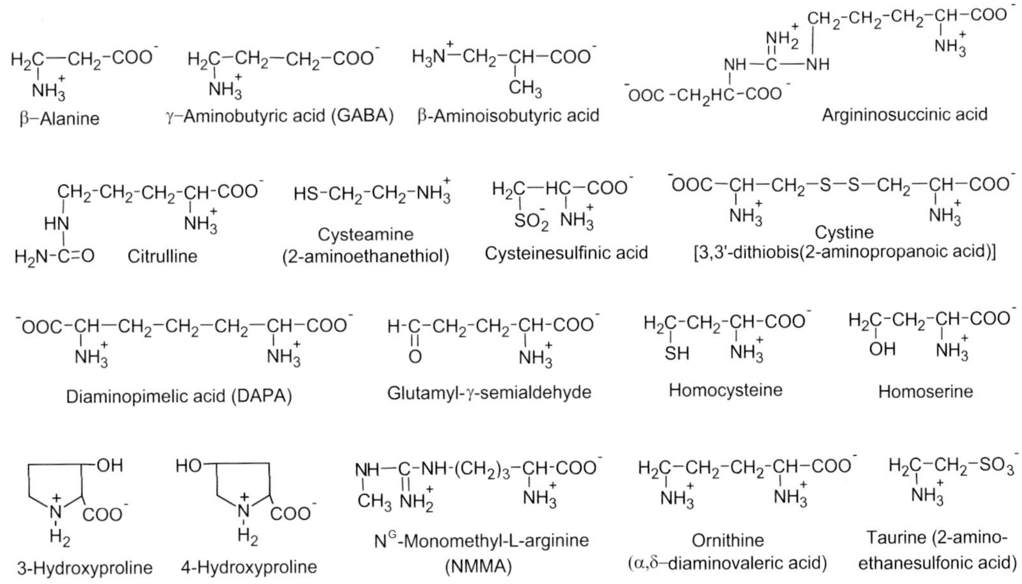

FIGURE 1.5 Chemical structures of non-proteinogenic amino acids in animals at neutral pH. These substances occur in physiological fluids of animals, and some of them are also present in microorganisms and plants. Taurine is present only in animals as a free amino acid. Note that citrulline has a ureido group.

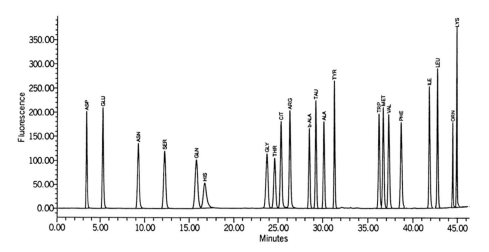

FIGURE 1.6 Analysis of primary amino acids (AAs) as their *o*-phthaldialdehyde (OPA) derivatives using high-performance liquid chromatography (HPLC). The concentration of each AA standard used for the HPLC analysis is 10 μM. Before loading into the HPLC autosampler, the glass vial for AA standards contains 0.1 mL of 1.2% benzoic acid (an antimicrobial; prepared in saturated potassium borate), 0.1 mL of the 10 μM AA standard solution, and 1.4 mL of HPLC-grade water. The vial is then vortexed for 10 s. An aliquot (15 μL) of this solution is programed to mix with 15 μL of the 30 mM OPA reagent for 1 min in an autosampler. The resultant AA-OPA derivatives are separated by HPLC columns, followed by fluorescence detection at an excitation wavelength of 340 nm and an emission wavelength of 455 nm. (Reprinted from Wu, G. and C.J. Meininger. *Methods Enzymol.* 440:177–189, 2008, with permission from Elsevier.)

respectively) account for approximately 2.5% and 10% of total glutamate and glutamine (free plus peptide-bound), respectively, in sow's milk on day 29 of lactation (Table 1.8). Similar results regarding the relatively high abundance of free glutamate and glutamate have been reported for human milk. Also, the concentration of free taurine in human and porcine milk can be as high as 0.35 and 1.5 mM, respectively (Table 1.8). In both humans (Agostoni et al. 2000; Baldeón et al. 2014) and sows (Wu and Knabe 1994; Wu et al. 2011), the concentrations of free glutamate and glutamine in milk increase gradually during the lactation until the mature lactation stage. These milk-borne AAs play an important role in the growth and development of the neonatal small intestine (Hou and Wu 2018; Wu et al. 2011) and may also protect infants against neonatal inflammation, infections, and allergies (van Sadelhoff et al. 2020). In addition, free AAs represent 34.4% and 28.5% of total AAs in potatoes and sweet potatoes, respectively (Hou et al. 2019).

Some free AAs are particularly abundant in plant-sourced foods. For example, free glycine accounts for 26.2% and 21.5% of total free AAs in peanuts and pistachio nuts, respectively; free asparagine represents 32.3%, 17.5%, and 19.4% of total free AAs in potatoes, sweet potatoes, and white rice, respectively; and free glutamine constitutes 13.1% and 25.5% of total free AAs in corn grains and potatoes, respectively. Free glutamine constitutes 10.2%, 2.7%, 11.2%, and 5.8% of total glutamine in beef loin, chicken breast, chicken gastrocnemius, and pig gastrocnemius muscles, respectively. Free AAs contribute to the flavor of foods and are of nutritional significance in humans and other animals.

1.2 DISCOVERY OF AAs

1.2.1 L-AAs and Glycine

L-Alanine (α-aminopropionic acid) was the first AA to be obtained through chemical synthesis before its presence as a component of protein was recognized. Specifically, alanine was first synthesized from acetaldehyde, KCN, and NH₄Cl by Adolph Strecker in 1850. In 1875, P. Schutzenberger and A. Bourgeois hydrolyzed silk proteins with barium hydroxide in an autoclave at 150°C–200°C

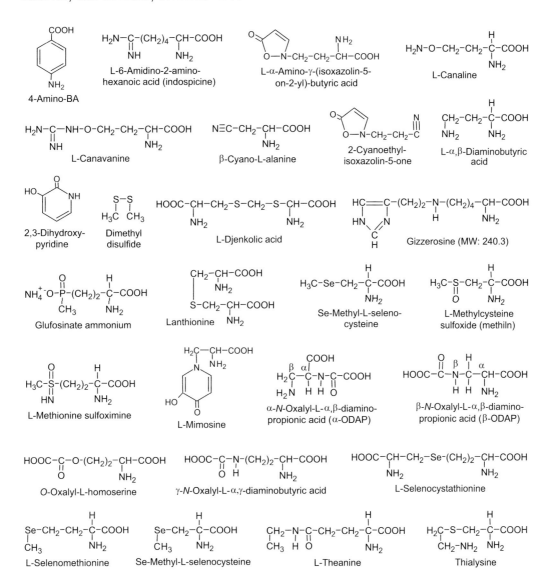

FIGURE 1.7 Chemical structures of non-proteinogenic amino acids in certain plants and of gizzerosine in fishmeal and synthetic glufosinate ammonium in the nonionized form. These substances are generally absent from live animals. Gizzerosine (a toxic amino acid) is formed from histamine and L-lysine in fishmeal at elevated temperatures (e.g., 130°C for 4 h). β-Cyano-L-alanine and glufosinate (an analogue of glutamate) occur naturally in microorganisms. Canavanine present in certain plants is structurally similar to arginine, whereas djenkolic acid present in certain plants is structurally similar to cystine, mimosine to tyrosine, and theanine to glutamine. BA, benzoic acid.

and reported that the fractional crystallization of the resulting hydrolysate contained 30% alanine and 70% other AAs. However, none of these products were rigidly identified. In 1888, T. Weyl isolated alanine from the hydrolytic cleavage products of silk fibroin as its particularly abundant constituent. The structure and configuration of alanine were established in 1901 by its conversion to lactic acid through chemical deamination.

Aminomalonic acid (2-aminopropanedioic acid; an amino dicarboxylic) was chemically synthesized by A. Baeyer in 1864. Despite a lack of experimental evidence, in 1914, F. Knoop suggested that this AA might be a physiological metabolite of protein metabolism in animals. Aminomalonic

TABLE 1.6

Content of Free Amino Acids (FAAs) and Peptide-Bound Amino Acids (PAAs) in Plant-Sourced Foods

AA	Corn Grain		Peanut		Pistachio Nut		Potato		Soybean		Sweet Potato		Wheat Flour		White Rice	
	FAA	PAA	FAA	PAA	FAA	PAA	FAA	PAA	FAA	PAA	FAA	PAA	FAA	PAA	FAA	PAA
Ala	224	7.74	344	12.1	746	10.6	243	2.58	146	22.7	1,342	3.46	70.4	5.35	33.8	4.55
Arg	37.8	4.30	781	34.7	722	23.1	2,058	3.10	1,819	35.4	467	2.61	84.6	7.12	35.5	7.25
Asp	151	4.59	128	14.0	269	9.62	2,017	2.04	240	37.1	1,803	1.53	256	3.33	21.0	4.25
Asn	114	3.77	154	19.6	112	10.1	10,095	9.15	435	24.1	3,686	8.28	237	4.23	93.7	4.51
Cys[a]	32.6	2.14	28.5	4.12	26.0	3.54	387	0.75	40.2	7.73	220	1.41	14.7	3.02	5.48	1.62
Glu	410	6.72	572	28.0	833	17.6	112	0.89	601	52.0	2,250	3.21	165	2.64	65.7	7.32
Gln	429	11.4	8.30	28.9	39.5	26.9	7,957	8.36	15.2	43.0	603	1.59	88.2	45.4	10.3	7.95
Gly	193	4.24	1,082	17.9	1,019	10.7	108	2.63	48.5	24.0	401	3.12	24.7	6.28	7.02	3.95
His	40.2	2.64	35.8	6.94	36.6	5.27	965	0.74	217	12.5	183	0.99	14.8	3.53	8.20	2.19
Hyp	ND	0.04	ND	0.79	ND	0.59	ND	0.08	ND	0.78	ND	0.05	ND	0.43	ND	0.04
Ile	119	3.73	88.0	10.7	77.9	10.1	731	2.46	32.3	23.9	671	2.64	14.3	4.91	8.28	3.73
Leu	225	12.5	136	18.0	116	16.7	514	4.21	50.7	39.9	813	4.07	52.6	9.95	40.5	7.22
Lys	84.3	2.77	83.8	9.90	82.5	11.8	492	4.64	86.2	32.6	297	3.32	28.8	3.62	6.37	2.32
Met	35.7	2.23	34.0	3.39	35.5	3.76	483	1.05	34.2	6.39	274	0.95	11.2	2.47	5.85	2.02
Phe	72.5	5.11	164	14.7	103	11.4	824	3.10	56.2	25.6	1,319	3.51	15.9	7.51	7.47	4.39
Pro	280	11.0	60.7	16.4	56.4	12.8	689	2.33	109	28.3	1,246	1.40	78.3	23.2	43.8	5.36
Ser	233	4.82	96.0	14.3	95.8	13.9	679	2.88	62.7	30.0	1,946	2.60	42.7	6.86	34.2	4.05
Thr	197	3.38	89.7	8.04	129	7.01	399	2.79	24.3	20.9	1,485	2.26	16.8	4.07	10.3	3.01
Trp	20.2	0.73	24.0	2.70	23.0	2.60	322	0.69	34.6	6.99	193	0.29	5.73	1.70	4.61	1.12
Tyr	146	4.66	80.5	10.9	78.3	5.24	619	1.73	38.7	18.4	632	2.36	20.6	3.84	15.2	2.36
Val	162	4.90	108	12.6	91.1	13.1	1,463	3.58	39.1	24.6	1,103	3.36	26.1	6.22	19.8	5.17
β-Ala	9.92	–	16.7	–	23.3	–	46.0	–	69.3	–	12.2	–	3.99	–	2.38	–
Cit	28.5	–	12.9	–	17.6	–	18.7	–	22.3	–	12.7	–	2.30	–	1.68	–
Orn	19.2	–	8.10	–	11.8	–	91.8	–	9.08	–	21.7	–	6.79	–	0.83	–
Total[b]	3,266	103.5	4,137	288.8	4,745	226.4	31,314	59.8	4,231	516.5	20,981	53.0	1,282	155.6	482	84.4
Total[c]	88.5	–	–	248.3	–	194.7	–	51.3	–	444.0	–	45.3	–	133.8	–	72.5

Source: Hou et al. 2019. *Amino Acids* 51:1153–1165. Values (the means) for free AAs and peptide-bound are expressed as μg/g of dry matter and mg/g of dry matter, respectively.

[a] Total cysteine (cysteine + ½ cystine). "½ cystine" denotes that 1 mol cystine is composed of 2 mol cysteine.

[b] The molecular weights of intact amino acids were used to calculate the amount of peptide-bound amino acids.

[c] The molecular weights of amino acid residues (i.e., the molecular weights of intact amino acids − 18) were used to calculate the amount of peptide-bound amino acids. Total peptide-bound amino acids represent true proteins plus peptides in foods.

Note: Cit, citrulline; Hyp, 4-hydroxyproline; Orn, ornithine.

TABLE 1.7

Content of Free Amino Acids (FAAs) and Peptide-Bound Amino Acids (PAAs), and the Percentages of FAAs as Total AAs, in the Skeletal Muscle of Domestic Animals

AA	Beef Loin Muscle			Chicken Breast Muscle			Chicken GM Muscle			Pig GM Muscle		
	FAA	PAA	PFT (%)	FAA	PAA	PFT (%)	FAA	PAA	PFT (%)	FAA	PAA	PFT (%)
Ala	1,258	44.1	2.77	608	46.4	1.29	1,764	46.7	3.64	496	48.9	1.00
Arg	170	52.2	0.33	354	55.6	0.63	357	55.4	0.64	114	56.4	0.20
Asp	65	41.0	0.16	335	42.6	0.78	346	42.7	0.80	67	42.7	0.16
Asn	206	33.2	0.62	236	34.8	0.67	546	34.6	1.55	68	34.2	0.20
Cys[a]	362	10.7	3.27	112	11.4	0.97	118	11.7	1.00	41	12.5	0.33
Glu	801	74.0	10.7	1,069	73.7	1.43	1,804	74.6	2.36	902	74.3	1.20
Gln	5,069	44.8	10.2	1,211	43.6	2.70	5,590	44.3	11.2	2,678	43.5	5.80
Gly	456	33.2	1.35	555	33.9	1.61	1,183	34.7	3.30	765	30.0	2.49
His	338	31.4	1.06	334	27.1	1.22	353	27.0	1.29	132	25.1	0.52
Hyp	73	1.70	4.12	25	1.92	1.29	26	2.01	1.28	24	2.60	0.92
Ile	236	40.9	0.57	66	42.5	0.16	64	42.4	0.15	41	42.6	0.10
Leu	398	66.2	0.60	130	67.9	0.19	184	68.1	0.27	63	66.1	0.10
Lys	349	71.7	0.48	235	63.0	0.37	241	62.8	0.38	81	60.7	0.13
Met	180	25.2	0.71	68	24.2	0.28	66	24.0	0.27	38	23.2	0.16
Phe	352	33.2	1.05	205	35.8	0.57	215	35.6	0.60	70	40.2	0.17
Pro	535	32.4	1.62	524	33.0	1.56	141	33.9	0.41	846	32.1	2.57
Ser	365	35.0	1.03	374	36.6	1.01	1,485	35.8	3.98	107	34.8	0.31
Thr	389	36.5	1.05	415	37.6	1.09	434	38.3	1.12	175	39.0	0.45
Trp	67	9.95	0.67	58	10.5	0.55	59	10.5	0.56	43	10.9	0.39
Tyr	244	29.8	0.81	164	31.1	0.53	152	30.9	0.49	86	30.7	0.28
Val	278	47.2	0.59	127	48.3	0.26	43	48.4	0.89	59	48.0	0.12
β-Ala	712	–	–	722	–	–	926	–	–	267	–	–
Cit	63	–	–	11	–	–	11	–	–	69	–	–
Orn	195	–	–	22	–	–	24	–	–	42	–	–
Tau	2,920	–	–	11,773	–	–	7,296	–	–	4,818	–	–
Total[b]	16,088	795	1.98	19,732	802	2.40	23,426	805	2.83	12,090	798	1.49
Total[c]	–	684	–	–	690	–	693	–	–	688	–	–

Source: Wu et al. 2016. *J. Anim. Sci.* 94:2603–2613 for the skeletal muscle of cattle; He et al. 2021. *Adv. Exp. Med. Biol.* 1285:109–131, for 42-day-old broiler chickens; and Zhang et al. 2021. *Adv. Exp. Med. Biol.* 1285:81–107, for 42-day-old pigs. Values (the means) for free AAs and peptide-bound AAs are expressed as μg/g of dry matter and mg/g of dry matter, respectively.

[a] Total cysteine (cysteine + ½ cystine). "1/2 cystine" denotes that 1 mol cystine is composed of 2 mol cysteine.

[b] The molecular weights of intact amino acids were used to calculate the amount of peptide-bound amino acids.

[c] The molecular weights of amino acid residues (i.e., the molecular weights of intact amino acids – 18) were used to calculate the amount of peptide-bound amino acids. Total peptide-bound amino acids represent true proteins plus peptides in foods.

Note: Cit, citrulline; GM, gastrocnemius; Hyp, 4-hydroxyproline; Orn, ornithine; PFT, percentages of FAAs in total AAs (i.e., 100 × FAAs/total AAs); Tau, taurine; "–", data are not available.

acid decarboxylase, which decarboxylates aminomalonic acid to glycine, was identified in silkworm glands in 1956 and in the rat liver and microbes in 1963. However, the natural presence of the enzyme substrate had not been reported, although it was found to be a structural unit in *arcamine* [a dipeptide, hypotauryl-aminomalonate (a fish attractant)] and malonomycin (an antibiotic of bacterial origin) in the 1970s. This is possibly because free aminomalonic acid is chemically unstable at neutral pH (undergoing spontaneous decarboxylation to glycine at a slow rate) and its concentration is exceedingly low. In

TABLE 1.8
Concentrations of Free, Peptide-Bound, and Total Amino Acids in Human, Bovine, and Porcine Whole Milk

AA	Human Whole Milk			Cow's Whole Milk			Sow's Whole Milk[a]		
	FAA (μM)	PAA[b] (mM)	TAA (mM)	FAA (μM)	PAA[b] (mM)	TAA (mM)	FAA (μM)	PAA (mM)	TAA (mM)
Ala	237[c]–273[d]	4.24	4.49[e]	20[f]	12.1	12.1[e]	742	17.1	17.6
Arg	9[d]–13[f]	2.06	2.07[e]	14[g]	6.56	6.57[e]	71	10.6	10.7
Asp	27[c]–56[d]	3.33	3.37[e]	6[f]	9.15	9.16[e]	490	17.3	17.8
Asn	7[h]	3.09	3.10[e]	trace	8.55	8.55[e]	236	16.2	16.4
Cys[i]	22[d]–12[f]	0.82	0.84[e]	3[f]	1.26	1.26[e]	432	2.92	3.35
Glu	1,246[c]–1,203[d]	5.87	7.09[e]	44[f]	25.2	25.2[e]	1,156	32.7	33.9
Gln	560[c]–612[d]	5.23	5.82c	28[f]	22.2	22.2[e]	3,425	29.2	32.6
Gly	117[c]–132[d]	2.81	2.93[e]	249[f]	7.81	8.06[e]	1,518	18.2	19.7
His	21[c]–20[d]	1.46	1.48[e]	5[f]	5.20	5.20[e]	547	4.39	4.94
Hyp	17	1.01	1.03	28	3.64	3.67	54	6.23	6.28
Ile	23[c]– 30[f]	4.04	4.05[e]	8[f]	12.1	12.1[e]	25	10.4	10.4
Leu	39[c]–55[f]	7.91	7.94[e]	8[f]	25.4	25.4[e]	56	29.0	29.1
Lys	35[c]–68[f]	4.84	4.86[e]	30[f]	19.8	19.8[e]	71	33.6	33.7
Met	5[d]–10[f]	1.08	1.08[e]	trace	5.86	5.86[e]	24	6.13	6.15
Phe	18[c]–20[f]	2.23	2.24[e]	24[f]	10.2	10.2[e]	40	9.20	9.24
Pro	35[c]–26[d]	8.23	8.26[e]	38[f]	29.2	29.2[e]	122	48.2	48.3
Ser	296[c]–126[d]	5.60	5.81[e]	12[f]	17.9	17.9[e]	473	16.0	16.5
Thr	99[c]–73[d]	3.61	3.70[e]	13[f]	11.9	11.9[e]	486	11.3	11.8
Trp	ND	–	0.99[j]	21[f]	2.10	2.10[k]	20	2.72	2.74
Tyr	10[d]–25[f]	2.50	2.54[e]	1[f]	8.73	8.73[e]	78	10.6	10.7
Val	57[c]–46[d]	4.31	4.36[e]	16[f]	14.9	14.9[e]	146	13.9	14.0
β-Ala	–	0.00	–	–	0.00	–	46	0.00	0.046
Cit	39[f]	0.00	0.039	5[f]	0.00	0.005	54	0.00	0.054
Orn	19[f]	0.00	0.019	11[f]	0.00	0.011	63	0.00	0.063
Tau	285[c]–357[d]	0.00	0.32	57[f]	0.00	0.057	1,521	0.00	1.52

[a] Mean values for the mature milk (day 29 of lactation) of 10 sows fed a diet containing 18.4% crude protein (Wu et al. 2011).

[b] Estimated values based on the reported data on the concentrations of free and total amino acids in the mature milk of women and cows.

[c] Mean values for the lactation of women at 3 months after giving term births (Agostoni et al. 2000).

[d] Mean values for the mature milk of women giving term births (Baldeón et al. 2014).

[e] Mean values for the mature milk of women and cows (Davis et al. 1994). Human and cow's whole mature milk contain 10 and 33.6 g amino acids/L, respectively. The total amounts of peptide-bound glutamate plus glutamine in human and cow's milk were 11.1 and 47.4 mM, respectively. The total amounts of peptide-bound aspartate plus asparagine in human and cow's milk were 6.42 and 17.7 mM, respectively. The ratios of glutamate to glutamine in the proteins of the mature milk of women and cows are 1.122:1.000 and 1.135:1.000, respectively, as analyzed by an enzymatic method (Li and Wu 2020). The ratios of aspartate to asparagine in the proteins of the mature milk of women and cows are 1.076:1.000 and 1.070:1.000, respectively, as analyzed by an enzymatic method (Li and Wu 2020).

[f] Mean values for the lactation of women and cows at 2 months after giving births (Ghadimi and Pecora 1963).

[g] Mean values for the mid-lactation of cows (Rassin et al. 1978).

[h] Mean values for the lactation of women at 1 month after giving births (Nishikawa et al. 1984).

[i] Total cysteine (cysteine + ½ cystine). "1/2 cystine" denotes that 1 mol cystine is composed of 2 mol cysteine.

[j] Mean values for the lactation of women at 4 months after giving births (Zhang et al. 2013).

[k] Mean value for the mature milk of women (Heine 1994).

Note: Cit, citrulline; FAA, free amino acids; Hyp, 4-hydroxyproline; ND, not detectable (below the limit of detection); Orn, ornithine; PAA, peptide-bound amino acids; TAA, total amino acids; Tau, taurine; "–", data are not available.

the early 1980s, aminomalonic acid was first identified to be a natural AA in proteins of *Escherichia coli* and the human atherosclerotic plaque after they were hydrolyzed under alkaline conditions (2 M KOH, 110°C, and 24 h; Van Buskirk et al. 1984). This AA is not formed from any of the 20 major AAs during the hydrolysis procedure. The hydrolysates of *Escherichia coli* and human atherosclerotic plaque proteins contain 0.3 and 0.2 aminomalonic acid residues per 1,000 AA residues, respectively (Copley et al. 1992; Van Buskirk et al. 1984). Possible sources of aminomalonic acid in proteins may be errors in protein synthesis, oxidative damage to AA residues in proteins, and the posttranslational carboxylation of glycine residues in proteins. Free aminomalonic acid also exists in human fecal microbes, and its concentration increases after endurance exercise (Zhao et al. 2018). The biological functions of this AA are largely unknown, but it may impart the calcium binding property of proteins like the carboxylation of glutamate in blood-clotting factor proteins. There is also evidence that aminomalonic acid, as an

$$HOOC-CH-COOH \quad \text{Aminomalonic acid } (C_3H_5O_4N; MW = 119.08)$$
$$|$$
$$NH_2$$

analogue of aspartic acid, is a potent inhibitor of mammalian and microbial asparagine synthetases.

L-Arginine (2-amino-5-guanidinovaleric acid) was first isolated in 1886 by E. Schulze and E. Steiger from extracts of etiolated lupine seedlings as a basic substance. In 1895, S.G. Hedin isolated arginine from the hydrolysate of horn protein as a silver nitrate precipitate. One year later, A. Kossel found that arginine is an abundant AA in the basic proteins from fish sperm. The structure of arginine was established through (1) alkaline hydrolysis to yield stoichiometrically ornithine and urea in 1897 (E. Schulze and E. Winterstein), (2) arginase-catalyzed hydrolysis to yield ornithine and urea in 1904 (A. Kossel), and (3) chemical synthesis from benzoylornithine in 1910 (S.P.L. Sörensen). In 1924, A. Kossel discovered that arginine forms a highly insoluble and beautifully crystalline compound with 2,4-dinitro-α-naphthol-7-sulfonic acid. Endogenous synthesis of arginine by mammals was deduced in the classic nutrition studies of W.C. Rose and his colleagues in 1930. The discovery of the urea cycle (ornithine cycle) by H.A. Krebs and K. Henseleit in 1932 revealed a key role for arginine in metabolic pathways. In 1988, arginine was found to be the nitrogenous precursor of nitric oxide (NO) in animal cells. NO is a vasodilator, as well as a cytotoxic molecule for microorganisms and tumor cells.

L-Asparagine (α-aminosuccinamic acid) was first isolated from asparagus juice by the French chemists L.N. Vauquelin and P.J. Robiquet in 1806. However, due to technical difficulties in the analysis of peptide-bound asparagine (i.e., the conversion of asparagine to aspartate under both acid and alkaline hydrolysis conditions), a key role for asparagine in nutrition was not recognized for over a century after its initial discovery. Fortunately, based on the enzymatic hydrolysis of edestin (a globular legumin protein in hemp seeds) by pepsin, trypsin, and dipeptidases, the occurrence of asparagine in protein was finally reported by M. Damodaran in 1932.

L-Aspartate (α-aminosuccinic acid) was first obtained by A. Plisson and É.O. Henry in 1827 from the alkaline hydrolysis of marshmallow root-derived asparagine in the presence of boiling lead hydroxide. The composition of aspartate was proposed by A. Plisson in 1830 and firmly established by A.F. Boutron-Charlard and T.J. Pelouze in 1833. In 1838, J. von Liebig obtained aspartate by hydrolyzing asparagine with potassium hydroxide. The first chemical synthesis of aspartate was accomplished by V. Dessaignes in 1850 by heating the ammonium salts of malic, maleic, and fumaric acids at 160°C–200°C. The presence of aspartate in plant and animal proteins was first identified in 1868 and 1869, respectively. Derivatives of aspartate such as N-acetyl-L-aspartate and phosphoaspartate are present in animal tissues (including the brain, liver, kidneys, and muscles).

L-Citrulline (α-amino-δ-carbamidovaleric acid) was originally isolated by M. Wada from watermelon (the Latin word for *citrullus*) juice as an abundant free AA in 1930. Two years later, H.A. Krebs proposed that citrulline is an intermediate of the hepatic urea cycle. H.G. Windmueller and A.E. Spaeth discovered the release of citrulline from the rat small intestine in 1975. This seminal work revolutionized the field of AA biochemistry and nutrition. In 2003, G. Wu and colleagues found that ovine allantoic fluid contains an extremely high concentration of citrulline during early gestation (approximately 10 mM on day 60; Kwon et al. 2003), which is similar to the concentration in watermelon juice. This AA is an effective substrate for arginine synthesis in mammals and birds, as well as possibly fish and crustaceans. Interestingly, some arginine residues in certain proteins can be enzymatically deiminated to form citrulline residues. Circulating autoantibodies specific for citrullinated peptides and proteins are useful markers for the diagnosis of rheumatoid arthritis.

L-Cysteine (α-amino-β-mercaptopropionic acid) was named after cystine which was discovered in 1810 by W.H. Wollaston as a component of a bladder calculus ("kystis" in the Greek for bladder). The name "cysteine" was coined by J.J. Berzelius in 1832. A.E. Baudrimont and F.J. Malaguti reported in 1837 that cystine contains sulfur. In 1884, E. Baumann discovered that cysteine was the product of cystine reduction. Subsequently, in 1899 it was found that cystine was a major constituent of horn protein. This observation raised the possibility that cysteine was utilized for polypeptide synthesis in animals. The structures of cystine and cysteine were established by chemical synthesis in 1903 and 1904. Cysteine is an abundant AA in hairs and wools.

L-Glutamate (α-aminoglutaric acid) was first isolated by K.H. Ritthausen from wheat gluten (gliadin) hydrolysate in 1866. Seven years later, H. Hlasiwetz and J. Habermann obtained glutamate from casein, the first protein of animal origin shown to contain this AA. Glutamate was synthesized chemically from levulinic acid by Ludwig Wolff in 1890. Monosodium glutamate (MSG; L-glutamic acid in the form of its monosodium salt) was discovered by the Japanese chemist K. Ikeda in 1907 as the substance in kombu broth (a Japanese type of seaweed) that gave the fifth basic taste he coined "*umami*" that is distinct from the other four tastes (bitter, salty, sour, and sweet) known at that time. Glutamic acid stimulates specific receptors in taste buds to induce a "savory" or "meaty" flavor. It is an abundant free AA in the milk of mammals (such as humans, cows, and pigs) and the intracellular fluid of animal tissues, as well as an abundant AA in both animal (e.g., milk and muscle) and plant (e.g., soybean and corn) proteins. Two glutamate derivatives (*N*-acetylglutamate and phosphoglutamate) are present in animals.

L-Glutamine (α-aminoglutaramic acid) was first obtained as a free AA from sugar beet juice by E. Schulze and E. Bosshard in 1883. E. Fischer recognized in 1904 that glutamine is a major source of the ammonia produced upon acid hydrolysis of proteins. After much effort to refine laboratory procedures, glutamine was eventually isolated from the enzymatic hydrolysates of gliadin by M. Damodaran and coworkers in 1932. One year later, this AA was first synthesized chemically from carbobenzoxy-L-glutamic acid anhydride by M. Bergmann, L. Zervas, and L. Salzmann. In 1935, H.A. Krebs reported that glutamine is synthesized from glutamate ammonia and hydrolyzed into its precursors in animal tissues. In the 1940s through the 1960s, glutamine was not considered to be a nutrient needed in diets for animals, and received little attention in classic nutrition textbooks. In 1965, E.M. Neptune discovered that small-intestinal (ileal) preparations from various animal species (guinea pigs, hamster, monkeys, rabbits, and rats) have high rates of glutamine oxidation. This began a new era of biochemical and nutritional research on glutamine in humans and other animals. Glutamine is an abundant free AA in the plasma, brain, and skeletal muscle of mammals (such as humans, cows, and pigs) and birds, as well as the milk and fetal fluids of mammals.

Glycine (aminoacetic acid), the simplest AA in nature, was isolated from the acid hydrolysates of gelatin by the French chemist H. Braconnot in 1820. He found that glycine was as sweet as glucose. In 1838, G.J. Mulder reported that glycine could also be obtained from gelatin and meat using alkaline hydrolysis with potassium hydroxide. In 1845, V. Dessaignes identified glycine as a component of hippuric acid. The correct composition of glycine was determined independently in 1846 by three chemists: E.N. Horsford, A. Laurent, and G.J. Mulder. The structure of glycine was established by A.T. Cahours in 1857, and 1 year later, it was synthesized chemically from ammonia and monochloroacetic acid. Of note, in 2009, scientists of the National Aeronautics and Space Administration discovered the presence of glycine on a comet (an icy, small solar system body), suggesting its formation in space. Glycine accounts for about one-third of all AA residues in collagen proteins, which represent approximately 29%–35% (g:g) of total proteins in postnatal animals (including humans). Glycine is the most abundant free AA in the plasma of some postnatal animals (e.g., pigs, sheep, and cattle) and the most abundant AA in the whole-body proteins of humans and other terrestrial animals.

L-Histidine (α-amino-β-imidazolepropionic acid) was first isolated from acid hydrolysates of sturine protein by A. Kossel in 1896. This finding was published in the *Proceedings of the Prussian Academy of Science* on April 9, 1896. One month later, on May 11, 1896, Editors of *Zeitschrift für physiologische Chemie* received a manuscript from S.G. Hedin, who reported the isolation of histidine from various proteins using a superior method. The simultaneous discovery of histidine by the two different groups is truly remarkable. The structure of histidine, which possesses an imidazole ring, was elucidated by H. Pauly in 1904 and confirmed through chemical synthesis from diaminoacetone by F.L. Pyman in 1911. Two American biochemists, L. Baumann and T. Ingvaldsen, identified histidine as a component of carnosine (an abundant dipeptide in skeletal muscle) in 1918. Histidine is an abundant AA in hemoglobin (the major protein in red blood cells) and is an unusually abundant free AA in the plasma and whole body of some fish (e.g., largemouth bass).

L-Homoarginine [(2*S*)-2-amino-6-(diaminomethylideneamino)hexanoic acid], a structural homologue of L-arginine, was first chemically synthesized from L-lysine and cyanamide by H. Steib in 1926, and subsequently identified by E.A. Bell in 1962 as a naturally occurring substance in plants. Alkaline hydrolysis of L-homoarginine at 105°C yields L-lysine and urea. Compared with L-arginine, L-homoarginine has an additional $-CH_2$ group on its main carbon chain. Synthesis of L-homoarginine by rats and humans was discovered by W.L. Ryan and I.C. Wells in 1964, with the liver and kidneys being the major sites of synthesis. The concentration of L-homoarginine in the urine of adult humans is 0.1–0.48 mg/mL (Ryan and Wells 1964). In animals, L-arginine:glycine amidinotransferase may play a role in synthesizing L-homoarginine from L-arginine and L-lysine. Concentrations of L-homoarginine in the plasma are relatively low (approximately 2–3 μM) in healthy humans, pigs, and rats, and may increase up to 20 μM in hyperargininemic patients. Intracellular concentrations of L-homoarginine in the brain, kidney, and liver of 35-day-old pigs are 2, 95, and 110 μM, respectively (Hou et al. 2015). Physiological concentrations of L-homoarginine may be beneficial for normal cardiovascular and neurological functions.

trans-4-Hydroxy-L-proline (L-4-hydroxypyrrolidine-2-carboxylic acid; the physiological isomer of 4-hydroxy-L-proline in animals) was originally produced from the acid hydrolysates of gelatin by E. Fischer in 1902 soon after his discovery of L-proline. A racemic mixture of 4-hydroxy-L-proline was first synthesized chemically from epichlorhydrin and sodium malonic ester by H. Leuchs in 1905. Subsequently, *trans*-4-hydroxy-L-proline was found to be an abundant constituent of collagen and elastin. Studies in the 1960s revealed that *trans*-4-hydroxy-L-proline is derived from the post-translational hydroxylation of L-proline in proteins (primarily collagen) in the presence of oxygen, ascorbic acid, α-ketoglutarate, and Fe^{2+}, but is not a substrate for protein synthesis. Plants contain much less *trans*-4-hydroxy-L-proline than animals. This AA is a precursor for glycine synthesis and a potent antioxidant in animal tissues, but covalently conjugates polysaccharides to form glycoproteins in plants. In the medicinal industry, *trans*-4-hydroxy-L-proline is a useful precursor for the chemical synthesis of cosmetic and pharmaceutical products (Remuzon 1996).

L-Isoleucine (α-amino-β-methylvaleric acid) was one of the three branched-chain AAs (BCAAs) abundant in both plant proteins and most animal proteins but was the last BCAA to be discovered. Specifically, it was first isolated from sugar beet molasses by the German chemist F. Ehrlich in 1904 and chemically synthesized from D-amyl alcohol by two French chemists, L. Bouveault and R. Locquin, in 1905. In the following years, this AA was obtained from a pancreatic digest of fibrin and from acid hydrolysates of wheat gluten, egg albumin, and beef muscle. F. Ehrlich reported in 1907 that isoleucine had the same chemical composition as leucine but different physicochemical properties (e.g., melting point, optical activity, and solubility). The structure of isoleucine was established through its degradation to amylamine and chemical synthesis from D-isovaleraldehyde by F. Ehrlich in 1908.

L-Leucine (α-aminoisocaproic acid) was the first BCAA to be obtained from cheese by the French chemist J.L. Proust in 1819. One year later, H. Braconnot isolated leucine from acid hydrolysates of skeletal muscle and wool. The term "leucine" was coined by H. Braconnot to indicate the white crystalline substance that was separated from the acid hydrolysates of protein upon the addition of alcohol. In 1839, G.J. Mulder reported that leucine could also be obtained by the alkaline hydrolysis of proteins. A. Laurent and C. Gerhardt correctly determined the composition of leucine in 1848. Its structure was established through chemical synthesis from isovaleraldehyde by E. Schulze in 1891. Among the three BCAAs, leucine is usually the most abundant BCAA in both plant and animal proteins. This AA activates the mechanistic target of rapamycin (MTOR) cell signaling pathway to initiate protein synthesis in animal cells.

L-Lysine (α,ε-diaminocaproic acid) was discovered by E. Drechsel in 1889 as an alkaline substance in casein hydrolysates. In 1891, M.A. Siegfried, a member of E. Drechsel's laboratory, identified lysine as a component in the hydrolysates of other proteins, including conglutin, glutenfibrin, and egg albumin. In the same year, the composition of lysine was determined by E. Drechsel and the term "lysine" was coined by E. Fischer to indicate the release of urea from this new substance upon alkaline hydrolysis by barium hydroxide. The structure of lysine was proposed by A. Ellinger in 1899 and established through chemical synthesis from γ-cyanopropylmalonic ester by E. Fischer and F. Weigert in 1902. Crystalline lysine was first prepared by two American chemists, H.B. Vickery and C.S. Leavenworth, in 1928.

L-Methionine (α-amino-γ-methylthiobutyric acid) was discovered by the American chemist J.H. Mueller in 1922 as a substance in an acid hydrolysate of casein during his studies to define growth factors for hemolytic streptococcus. One year later, the composition of methionine as a sulfur-containing AA was proposed by J.H. Mueller after developing an improved method to obtain a large amount of this substance from casein. Meanwhile, he successfully isolated methionine from other sources of proteins, including egg albumin, edestin, and wool. Likewise, in 1925, S. Odake obtained methionine from yeast extracts and coined this name. The structure of methionine was established through chemical synthesis from β-methylthiolpropaldehyde by two British chemists, G. Barger and F.P. Coyne, in 1928. Commercial synthesis of DL-methionine at Degussa Corporation was achieved by W. Schwarze, H. Wagner, and H. Schulz in 1946. This AA is often added to the plant-based diets for nonruminants (e.g., swine and poultry) in the unprotected form and to those for ruminants (e.g., lactating cows and sheep) in a rumen-protected form.

L-Ornithine (α,δ-diaminovaleric acid) was discovered by M. Jaffé in 1877 as a hydrolysis product of ornithuric acid in the urine of hens fed benzoic acid. The structure of ornithine was established through chemical synthesis from phthalimidopropylmalonic ester by E. Fischer in 1901. Subsequently, ornithine was identified by A. Kossel in 1904 as a product of arginine hydrolysis by arginase. In 1932, H.A. Krebs found that ornithine served as a catalyst to stimulate the conversion of ammonia into urea in liver slices and proposed the urea (ornithine) cycle involving ornithine as an intermediate for urea synthesis in mammals. Ornithine is an immediate precursor of polyamines, which are essential for animal growth and development, but an excess of ornithine can result in retinal damage.

L-Phenylalanine (α-amino-β-phenylpropionic acid) was first obtained from yellow etiolated lupine sprouts by E. Schulze and J. Barbieri in 1879. Two years later, these authors isolated phenylalanine from hydrolysates of plant proteins (e.g., those from lupine seedlings) and correctly determined its composition. In 1882, E. Erlenmeyer and A. Lipp reported the first chemical synthesis of phenylalanine from phenylacetaldehyde, hydrocyanic acid, and ammonia. Following its synthesis by E. Schulze and A. Barbieri in 1883, the structure of the phenylalanine that they had originally isolated from lupine sprouts was finally established. This advance was highly significant in the late 19th century, as it meant that another aromatic AA (after tyrosine) had been discovered in nature. In 1934, the Norwegian doctor I.A. Følling discovered an inborn metabolic disorder called phenylketonuria that was shown in 1947 to result from the impaired catabolism of phenylalanine. This AA is a precursor of neurotransmitters and plays an essential role in neurological function. Of particular note, P.S. Buck, who wrote the tragic story *The Child Who Never Grew: A Memoir* about her daughter's experience with phenylketonuria, became the first American woman to win the Nobel Prize for literature in 1938.

L-Phosphoarginine, also known as L-arginine phosphate or 2S-2-amino-5-{[amino-(phosphonoamino)methylidene]amino}-pentanoic acid, was first isolated from the muscle of freshwater crabs by Meyerhof and Lohmann (1928). It is a major phosphagen in marine invertebrates, such as shrimp and crabs (Nimura and Sato 1982; Rockstein 1971). The concentrations of

L-phosphoarginine in the skeletal muscles of some crustacean species (e.g., crayfish) have been reported to be 83–106 mM (Ennor et al. 1956; Marcus and Morrison 1964). This AA is generated from L-arginine and ATP by arginine kinase, which also reversibly catalyzes the hydrolysis of L-phosphoarginine into L-arginine and inorganic phosphate under favorable conditions. L-Phosphoarginine is usually extracted from tissues with perchloric acid (e.g., 1.5 M) or trichloroacetic acid (e.g., 9%) and can be hydrolyzed into L-arginine and inorganic phosphate in the presence of hot acids (e.g., 0.2 M trichloroacetic acid in boiling water for 1 min) (Ennor et al. 1956; Morrison et al. 1957). L-Phosphoarginine is stable in an alkaline solution (e.g., pH 9.8) for 6 h at 23°C and for 1 min in boiling water, but decomposes when heated in a strong alkaline solution (Nimura and Sato 1983). The nucleophilic attack on the guanidino group of L-homoarginine by a strong base may generate L-citrulline and phosphoramidate (Besant et al. 2009).

L-Proline (pyrrolidine-2-carboxylic acid) derived its name from pyrrolidine (a constituent component of the molecule) and was the second AA to be obtained through chemical synthesis before its discovery as a component of protein in nature. Specifically, proline was originally synthesized chemically from α,δ-dibromopropylmalonic ester by R.M. Willstätter in 1900. One year later, without the knowledge of R.M. Willstätter's published results, E. Fischer discovered proline as a component of casein's acid hydrolysates and established its structure through chemical synthesis from phthalimide propylmalonic ester. Thereafter, E. Fischer obtained proline from a tryptic digest of casein, the alkaline hydrolysates of casein, and an enzymatic digest of gliadin in 1901, 1902, and 1911, respectively, to rule out the possibility that the ring structure of the proline molecule could result from an artifact during the processes of acid hydrolysis and AA esterification. Subsequently, proline and hydroxyproline were found to constitute about 21.4% of all AA residues in collagens, the extracellular proteins that comprise approximately 35% of body proteins in adults. Proline is an abundant AA in the whole body of animals.

L-Pyrrolysine (Pyl: N^6-{[(2R,3R)-3-methyl-3,4-dihydro-2H-pyrrol-2-yl]carbonyl}-L-lysine; $C_{12}H_{21}N_3O_3$) is the 22nd genetically encoded AA in select proteins (e.g., methylamine methyltransferase) of certain methanogenic archaea and bacteria and is the most recent addition to the list of AAs in proteins (Hao et al. 2002; Srinivasan et al. 2002). This rare AA consists of a (4R,5R)-4-methyl-5-carboxypyrroline ring linked to the ε-nitrogen of L-lysine. L-Pyrrolysine is not present in humans and other animals. L-Pyrrolysine is derived from two molecules of L-lysine during the translation of the mRNA and is not created by posttranslational modifications of proteins. Free L-pyrrolysine is a substrate for protein synthesis in those microbes. The discovery of L-pyrrolysine in nature prompted research on its chemical synthesis from (1) (4R,5R)-4-methylpyrroline-5-carboxylic acid and lysine or (2) N-(tert-butylphenylmethylidene)glycine tert-butyl ester and methyl crotonate (Wong et al. 2012).

L-Pyrrolysine (Pyl, O)

L-Selenocysteine (Sec; 2-amino-3-selanylpropanoic acid; $C_3H_7NO_2Se$) is the 21st genetically encoded AA in certain proteins of both prokaryotes and eukaryotes and is not created by posttranslational modifications of proteins. This AA has a structure similar to that of cysteine, with a selenium atom replacing the sulfur atom of cysteine to form a selenol group that is deprotonated at physiological pH. L-Selenocysteine is not a canonical precursor for protein synthesis in known organisms, but rather is generated in animals, bacteria, archaea, and algae under the guidance of a genetic code during the translation of mRNA on ribosomes (Chapter 8). Among the analyzed proteins, only selenoproteins have been found to contain selenocysteine. Selenocysteine is not universal in all organisms.

L-Serine (α-amino-β-hydroxypropionic acid) was isolated from a hydrolysate of silk protein (named sericine) by the German chemist E. Cramer in 1865. This author also correctly determined the composition of serine and found it to be similar to alanine. In 1901, E. Fischer and A. Skita obtained serine from the acid hydrolysates of silk. The structure of serine was established through chemical synthesis from glycolic aldehyde and cyanohydrin by E. Fischer and F.H. Leuchs in 1902. Serine was identified in human sweat by G. Embden and H. Tachau in 1910 and isolated from extracts of green alfalfa leaves by H.B. Vickery in 1925. In 1931, Floyd S. Daft and R.D. Coghill reported that serine was highly unstable when heated in a strongly alkaline solution. This finding paved a way to optimize AA analysis in protein. Serine abundantly accounts for ~9% and 32% of total AAs in whole egg proteins and silkworm sericin, respectively. The occurrence of serine as a phosphate ester (i.e., phosphoserine) in acid hydrolysates of proteins (e.g., casein) was reported by F.A. Lipmann and P.A. Levene in 1932, which laid the foundation for the future discovery of protein phosphorylation in cells.

L-Threonine (α-amino-β-hydroxybutyric acid) was the last proteinogenic AA to be discovered. It was first isolated from oat protein by S.B. Schryver and H.W. Buston and also from teozein (a protein in a plant called teosinte) by R.A. Gortner and W.F. Hoffmann in 1925. Ten years later, W.C. Rose and coworkers identified threonine as a component of the acid hydrolysates of casein. This finding made it possible to prepare purified or semi-purified diets containing crystalline AAs for nutritional research. The structure of threonine was established through chemical synthesis by H.E. Carter in 1935. The occurrence of threonine as a phosphate ester in proteins, reported for the first time in 1952, is a result of posttranslational protein phosphorylation. Threonine is a major AA in certain proteins. For example, threonine constitutes as much as 30% of the AA content of intestinal mucins (Combet et al. 2000), 12%–14% of the AA content of 4E-binding protein-1 (an important translational initiation pathway; Combet et al. 2000), and 8.4% of the AA content of the plasma γ-globulin (Cannon 1945).

L-Tryptophan (α-amino-β-3-indolepropionic acid) was obtained from a pancreatic digest of casein by F.G. Hopkins and S.W. Cole in 1901. Two years later, these authors determined the composition of tryptophan and A. Ellinger reported that tryptophan was the precursor of indole in the intestine. In 1906, F.G. Hopkins prepared a tryptophan-free diet using acid hydrolysates of casein and found that dietary tryptophan is required for animal growth. After much discussion among the contemporary chemists, the structure of tryptophan was finally established through the chemical synthesis of DL-tryptophan from β-indolealdehyde by A. Ellinger and C. Flamand in 1907. Note that about 50 years before the discovery of tryptophan, some of its metabolites were identified in animals, including kynurenic acid in dog urine that was first reported by the German chemist J. von Liebig in 1853.

L-Tyrosine [α-amino-β-(p-hydroxyphenyl)propionic acid] was discovered in a crude casein preparation by J. von Liebig in 1846. One year later, he obtained the same substance from fibrin and serum albumin preparations and named it "tyrosine". In 1848, W. de La Rue correctly determined the composition of tyrosine as $C_9H_{11}NO_3$. This AA was isolated in 1849, for the first time, from an acid hydrolysate of casein by F. Bopp. In 1861, C. Bödeker identified that a large amount of homogentisic acid was formed from tyrosine in the urine of patients with alkaptonuria. The structure of tyrosine was established through chemical synthesis from p-aminophenylalanine by E. Erlenmeyer and A. Lipp in 1883. This AA is a precursor of neurotransmitters and melanin, and therefore plays an essential role in neurological function and skin pigmentation.

L-Valine (α-aminoisovaleric acid) was the second BCAA to be discovered. It was first isolated from extracts of animal tissues (liver, pancreas, spleen, thymus, and thyroid) by E. von Gorup-Besanez in 1856. Valine was obtained from an acid hydrolysate of albumin by P. Schützenberger in 1879, and then from a pancreatic protein hydrolysate by E. Fischer in 1901. The structure of valine was established through chemical synthesis by E. Fischer in 1906. In the same year, E. Fischer named α-aminoisovaleric acid as "valine". Valine is usually the second most abundant BCAA in animal and plant proteins.

1.2.2 β- AND γ-AAS WITH PHYSIOLOGICAL SIGNIFICANCE

β-Alanine (β-aminopropionic acid; also known as 3-aminopropanoic acid) was first synthesized by W.H. Heintz in 1870, only 20 years after the chemical synthesis of α-alanine. In 1911, the Russian biochemist W. Gulewitsch discovered that β-alanine is a component of carnosine (β-alanyl-L-histidine) in beef muscle. In subsequent years, two additional β-alanine-containing peptides (anserine and balenine) were discovered in the skeletal muscle and in the brain in a species-dependent manner. The concentrations of β-alanine are low in the plasma of humans and other monogastric animals (e.g., rats and pigs; 1–5 μM) and are greater in the plasma of chickens (~60 μM) and ruminants (e.g., cattle and sheep; 12–20 μM; Gilbreath et al. 2019). By contrast, free β-alanine is much more abundant in skeletal muscles of mammals and birds [e.g., ~0.5 mM in the vastus lateralis muscle of men (Varanoske et al. 2017); 3.5 mM in chicken gastrocnemius muscle (He et al. 2021)].

γ-Aminobutyric acid (γ-aminobutyrate in the ionized form) was first synthesized by K. Schotten in 1883. In 1949, F.C. Steward, J.F. Thompson, and C.E. Dent discovered that GABA is a constituent of the potato tuber. Using paper chromatography for AA analysis, the work of E. Roberts and S. Frankel in 1950 revealed that GABA is a free AA and is formed from L-glutamate in the brain of mice. These authors also reported the presence of GABA in the brains of humans and other animals (rats, rabbits, guinea pigs, and frogs). Subsequent investigations identified that GABA was a product of L-glutamate decarboxylation by glutamate decarboxylase in bacteria, animals, fungi, and plants. GABA is now known to be the principal inhibitory neurotransmitter in the brain and a major inhibitory neurotransmitter in the spinal cord. The concentrations of GABA are low in the plasma (0.5–3 μM) and non-neurological tissues of humans and other animals (e.g., rats, pigs, and chickens; 2–50 μM) but are highly abundant in the brain of mammals and birds (~3.5 mM in rats; He and Wu 2020).

β-Aminoisobutyric acid (3-amino-2-methylpropanoic or 3-aminoisobutanoic acid; β-aminoisobutyrate in the ionized form) is a physiological metabolite in humans and other animals. In 1951, it was originally discovered by H.R. Crumpler and colleagues to occur in the urine of healthy humans. This substance has two physiological enantiomers in biological systems: R-β-aminoisobutyrate (D-β-aminoisobutyrate) and S-β-aminoisobutyrate (L-β-aminoisobutyrate). R-β-aminoisobutyrate and S-β-aminoisobutyrate are the normal metabolites of pyrimidines (cytosine, uracil, and thymine) and L-valine, respectively, in mammals, birds, fish, and crustaceans. These two substances are interconvertible through the vitamin B_6-dependent stereo-isomerization reaction. The concentrations of R-β-aminoisobutyrate and S-β-aminoisobutyrate in the plasma and urine are relatively low (0.5–2 μM), but increase during exercise. The ratios of R-β-aminoisobutyrate to S-β-aminoisobutyrate depend on the activities of purine and L-valine catabolism in the body, as well as the racemase activity. Recent studies suggest that β-aminoisobutyrate may induce browning of white fat and stimulate hepatic β-oxidation (Roberts et al. 2014), but whether the effect of S-β-aminoisobutyrate is more potent than that of R-β-aminoisobutyrate is unknown.

Taurine (2-aminoethanesulfonic acid) contains an α-sulfonic acid group ($-SO_3H$) and a β-amino group and, therefore, is a β-AA. It was the first sulfur-containing AA to be discovered in nature. Specifically, in 1827, two Austrian scientists, F. Tiedermann and L. Gmelin, isolated taurine from bile acids of the ox, *Bos taurus*. The term "taurine" was coined by H. Demarcay in 1838, in reference to the original substance isolated from "taurus" (meaning bull in Latin). In the same year, two French chemists, J.B. Dumas and E. Pelouze, determined the composition of taurine, but both of them overlooked its sulfur atom, thereby incorrectly giving it the formula $C_2H_7NO_5$. In 1846, another Austrian chemist, J. Redtenbacher, recognized the presence of sulfur in the taurine molecule and correctly identified its formula to be $C_2H_7NO_3S$. The structure of taurine was established through chemical synthesis from ethylene dibromide, potassium thiocyanate, and ammonia by H. Kolbe in 1862. By the 1910s, taurine was known to be widely distributed in the animal kingdom and to be present in relatively high concentrations in all mammalian and avian tissues, including the blood, intestine, liver, skeletal muscle, heart, brain, kidneys, and retina. A 70-kg person has ~70 g taurine (Huxtable 1992). Concentrations of taurine in mammalian and avian cells range from 5 to 60 mM, depending on species and cell type (Wright et al. 1986). Human skeletal muscle, heart, retina, and placenta contain 15–20, 28–40, 20–35, and 20–35 mM taurine, respectively. Because of its large mass [e.g., accounting for 45% of body weight in healthy, non-obese adults], skeletal muscle is the major site (about 70%) of taurine storage in the 70-kg adult. Taurine is abundant in the milk of mammals (e.g., 0.4 mM in humans, 0.8 mM in mice, and 2.8 mM in cats) as a physiologically essential nutrient for infants and children (Sturman 1993). This AA is also highly abundant in fish and crustaceans. Interestingly, taurine is the most abundant free AA in the plasma or serum of some species of fish (e.g., about 1 mM in hybrid striped bass and largemouth bass; Li et al. 2021a), in comparison with its concentrations in the human plasma or serum (0.1–0.2 mM; Table 1.5).

1.2.3 D-AAs

Chemists in the 19th century had known that D-AAs could be obtained from chemical synthesis. Although the occurrence of D-AAs in animals and higher plants had been occasionally reported since 1884, the presence of D-AAs in nature was first definitively recognized in 1927, when an AA metabolite (octopine) derived from L-arginine and D-alanine was discovered in octopus. Furthermore, two American chemists, W.A. Jacobs and L.C. Craig, reported the presence of D-proline in ergotinine [a tripeptide alkaloid isolated from ergot (a group of fungi)] in 1935. Thereafter, relatively large amounts of some D-AAs were isolated from both bacteria and fungi (Berg 1953). This work led to the recognition that (1) D-alanine, D-aspartate, and D-glutamate are essential components of peptidoglycans in bacterial cell walls and (2) antibiotics or their metabolites contain a relatively high content of D-AAs [e.g., D-leucine and D-valine from gramicidin, D-phenylalanine from tyrocidine, and D-β-thiol-valine from D-penicillamine (a metabolite of penicillins)]. The presence of D-AAs in animal tissues and processed foods was demonstrated in the 1950s (Berg 1953). The discovery of D-AAs in natural proteins and the physiological fluids of animals, microbes, and plants marks the beginning of an important chapter in AA biochemistry and physiology.

$(C_9H_{18}N_4O_4;\ MW = 246.26\ Da)$

Octopine (an amino acid metabolite derived from L-arginine and D-alanine in the octopus)

1.2.3.1 Presence of D-AAs in Plant- and Animal-Sourced Foods

D-AAs (including D-alanine, D-aspartate, D-glutamate, D-proline, D-serine, and D-tryptophan) are widespread in plants as a result of uptake from the soil and de novo synthesis (Grishin et al. 2019). Interestingly, D-alanine is the most prevalent D-AA in higher plants and aquatic animals (Abe et al. 2005). In addition to its free form, N-malonyl-D-alanine and L-glutamyl-D-alanine (sources of D-alanine) are present in pea seedlings. Likewise, many D-AAs occur in animals (see below). Of particular note, free D-AAs represent approximately 2% of total free AAs in unprocessed cow's milk, and it is likely that the D-AAs are derived primarily from microbial activity in the digestive tract of ruminants (Friedman 1999a). Thus, natural plant (e.g., wheat flour, rice, corn, and soybean) and animal products (e.g., milk, cheese, meat, and eggs) contain some D-AAs (Grishin et al. 2019; Nagata 1999). Furthermore, processing food at high temperatures (e.g., >100°C) can result in the formation of both free and peptide-bound D-AAs in a time- and pH-dependent manner (Friedman 1999a). The rates of racemization of different L-AA residues to their respective D-isomers in a food protein can vary, but the relative rates for the same D-AAs in different proteins are similar under the same conditions. For example, alkali-treated food proteins contain a significant amount of D-alanine, D-aspartate, D-glutamate, D-leucine, D-phenylalanine, D-proline, and D-valine (Masters and Friedman 1979). The ratio of each of these D-AAs to the corresponding L-AAs in untreated casein, lactalbumin, soy protein, and wheat gluten is only 0.02-0.03 but increases substantially (e.g., up to 0.45 for D-aspartate:L-aspartate ratio in soy proteins) in response to alkaline treatment with 0.1 N NaOH at 65°C for 3 h. Subsequent studies have shown the presence of other D-AAs (including D-asparagine, D-serine, and D-threonine) in other processed foods. Racemization of AAs in proteins as well as the formation of D-peptide bonds and the cross-linked AAs (e.g., lanthionine and lysinoalanine) may impair digestibility and nutritional value.

1.2.3.2 Presence of D-AAs in the Animal Kingdom

To date, a significant amount of D-arginine and D-proline has not been reported in animal cells. However, some D-AAs have been reported to be present in both free and peptide-bound forms in the animal kingdom. In mammals and birds, D-AAs account for < 0.02% of total AAs in the body. However, D-AAs can exceed 1% of total AAs in certain marine shellfish (Abe et al. 2005). To date, D-alanine, D-aspartate, and D-serine in the free form have been found in mammalian (e.g., rat and mouse), avian (e.g., chicken and pigeon), and invertebrate (e.g., insect and aquatic crustacean) tissues, as well as in physiological fluids (e.g., the plasma and saliva), with concentrations varying greatly among tissues and animal species (Grishin et al. 2020; Ota et al. 2014). Of note, D-glutamate has been identified in the rat brain (Mangas et al. 2007) and neurons (Covenas et al. 2017), although it is not as abundant as D-aspartate (Patel et al. 2017; Weatherly et al. 2017). Some free D-AAs may be erroneously incorporated into proteins and polypeptides in animal cells through the action of aminoacyl-tRNA synthetase, which will result in metabolic disorders. D-AAs may play an important role in health and disease states (e.g., retinal, neurological, and kidney disorders) of humans and other animals (Kimura et al. 2020). In support of this view, physiological concentrations of D-aspartate and D-serine are likely crucial for neurological development and function, but an excess of D-serine may contribute to neurodegenerative disorders, including amyotrophic lateral sclerosis (Yoshimura and Goto 2008). Furthermore, the concentrations of D-serine, D-aspartate, D-asparagine, and D-threonine in the proteins of human cataract lenses are substantially greater than those in the proteins of age-matched normal lenses (Hooi and Truscott 2011).

D-Alanine is not synthesized in mammalian cells due to the lack of D-alanine racemase, but insects and certain aquatic animals possess this enzyme for D-alanine formation (Yoshimura and Goto 2008). Because of the synthesis by gastrointestinal microorganisms and possibly intake from plant-based rodent diets, free D-alanine is present in the pancreas (e.g., ~400 μM in rat islets of Langerhans), the pituitary gland (e.g., 13 μM in the rat anterior/intermediate pituitary tissue), and peripheral tissues (Ota et al. 2014). Furthermore, a relatively large amount of D-alanine is found in the urine of mice, which is of primarily bacterial, but not dietary, origin. Finally, D-alanine is present in insects at relatively low concentrations but is highly abundant in certain crustaceans, mollusks, and other aquatic animals. For example, aquatic crustaceans and some bivalve mollusks contain up to 100 mM D-alanine in tissues (e.g., 70 mM in the siphon of the otter clam shell), depending on species (Abe et al. 2005). In these aquatic animals studied, free D-alanine represents up to 80% of total free alanine (L-alanine plus D-alanine), as reported for the mantle muscle of the otter clam shell.

D-Aspartate was discovered in the brain of cephalopods (*Octopus vulgaris*) by A. D'Aniello and A. Guiditta in 1977 and found in the brain and peripheral organs of rodents and man by D.S. Dunlop and colleagues in 1986. In all brain areas of rats at all stages of life, D-aspartate is exclusively restricted to the neuronal population and localized in both the cytoplasm and fiber tracts. Interestingly, free D-aspartate occurs in substantial amounts in the brain at the embryonic phase and during the first few days of postnatal life but greatly decreases in adulthood. The concentration of D-aspartate in the human frontal cortex at gestational week 14 exceeds that of L-aspartate (D-aspartate = 0.36 μmol/g; L-aspartate = 0.21 μmol/g) and then dramatically declines after birth (Hashimoto et al. 1993). In adult mice, concentrations of D-aspartate are approximately 50 μM in the striatum, cortex, cerebellum, and olfactory bulbs and approximately 200 μM in the hippocampus. In addition to nervous tissues, D-aspartate is present in endocrine glands (e.g., pancreas, pineal, adrenal, and pituitary), reproductive organs (e.g., testes, ovaries, and placentae), organs of the immune system (e.g., spleen and thymus), heart, and physiological fluids (e.g., the plasma and saliva) in mammals (Errico et al. 2012). There is a rapid decline in neuronal D-aspartate concentrations, such that D-aspartate in the brain of rats decreases substantially at 1 week after birth and almost disappears by 1 month of age (Schell et al. 1997). Furthermore, results of recent studies indicate that D-aspartate is widespread in both nervous and endocrine tissues in birds and marine invertebrates. There is also evidence that the mammalian brain expresses D-aspartate racemase (Kim et al. 2010).

D-Serine was initially identified in the mammalian brain by T. Nishikawa, A. Hashimoto, and coworkers in 1992. This AA is present in protoplasmic astrocytes and neurons of the forebrain regions where its concentrations remain relatively high throughout postnatal life. The levels of D-serine in the rodent brain can be as much as one-third of L-serine levels. There is evidence that mammalian brain expresses D-serine racemase (Wolosker et al. 1999). Besides the nervous tissues, D-serine is present in the peripheral tissues (e.g., blood, heart, pancreas, spleen, liver, kidney, testis, epididymis, lung, skeletal muscle, and retina) of mice. Similarly, D-serine has been detected in the plasma, brain, and urine of humans and in the brain and kidney of chickens. Besides mammals and birds, D-serine occurs in microorganisms, certain insects (e.g., silkworms), aquatic animals, and other invertebrates (Wolosker et al. 1999; Yoshimura and Esak 2003). Interestingly, in certain species of insects, D-serine accounts for <1% and about 5%–50% of total serine in larvae and pupae, respectively (Nishikawa 2011).

Kreil (1997) summarized evidence for D-AA-containing peptides produced by animals, which include (1) opioid peptides (consisting of a D-alanine or D-methionine residue; first reported in the early 1980s) and antimicrobial peptides (containing a D-alanine residue) from amphibian skin, (2) neuropeptides from snail ganglia (fulicin; consisting of a D-asparagine residue), (3) a hyperglycemic hormone (consisting of D-phenylalanine) from crustaceans, and (4) a constituent of a protein (containing D-serine) from the venom of the funnel-web spider *Agelenopsis aperta*. Peptide bonds formed from D-AAs are resistant to attacks by proteases.

The sources of D-AAs in animals are as follows: (1) diet; (2) the posttranslational action of peptidyl D-AA racemases on peptide-bound L-AAs in proteins; and (3) synthesis of D-AAs from free L-AAs by specific racemases. Racemization of D-AAs to form L-AAs may occur in both gastrointestinal microorganisms and animals [e.g., mammals, birds, freshwater and marine invertebrates (e.g., snails, crayfish, and lobster), insects, and worms]. As indicated previously, the expression of D-AA racemases is cell-, tissue-, and species-specific (Grishin et al. 2020; Kimura et al. 2020).

1.2.3.3 Presence of D-AAs in Microbes

Microbes are capable of synthesizing free D-AAs from free L-AAs and, therefore, contain a relatively high content of D-AAs (up to millimolar levels in some cell cultures; Radkov and Moe 2014), as noted previously. In these cells, D-AAs can be linked via peptide bonds by enzymes that are not part of the mRNA translation machinery to form small peptides. Furthermore, the presence of D-AAs in microbial proteins and polypeptides results from the posttranslational racemization (or isomerization) by peptidyl D-AA racemase. For example, D-aspartic acid, D-glutamic acid, D-alanine, and D-proline exist in bacterial cell wall peptidoglycans. Interestingly, proline racemase is expressed in the unicellular eukaryotic parasite *Trypanosoma cruzi* to convert L-proline into D-proline (Chamond et al. 2005). F. Lipmann and coworkers reported in 1941 that D-AAs account for 20% and 45%, respectively, of total AAs in tyrocidine and gramicidin (peptide antibiotics produced by an aerobic spore-forming organism, *Bacillus brevis*). It is possible that a tRNA is erroneously charged with a D-AA to generate a D-aminoacyl-tRNA, which erroneously enters the ribosomal AA-tRNA binding (A) site for protein synthesis in microorganisms, including bacteria (Grishin et al. 2020). Peptides that are rich in D-AAs not only have a structural function but also provide bacteria and other microbes as well as parasites with a unique ability to resist degradation by the host's proteases and peptidase. Disruption of D-AA synthesis in microbes can lead to cell death. Thus, enzymes (e.g., D-AA racemases) may be the promising targets for the development of antimicrobials (Radkov and Moe 2014).

1.2.4 OTHER AAS

1.2.4.1 Other AAs in the Animal Kingdom

In addition to the AAs noted previously, animals also contain other non-proteinogenic AAs as either normal metabolites or diet-derived substances. Some of them have important physiological significance, but some may be toxic and passed along a food chain via farm animal intermediates. Some hormones (e.g., thyroid hormones) and L-DOPA [3,4-dihydroxy-L-phenylalanine (3-hydroxy-L-tyrosine), a precursor of catecholamine neurotransmitters] are derivatives of AAs and are also AAs. Other AAs include (1) 3-hydroxyproline, which was first isolated from bovine tendon collagen in 1961 and whose content is relatively high in basement membrane collagen; (2) desmosine, which is a derivative of four separate lysine residues in collagen and the fibrous protein elastin to stabilize its structure; (3) 5-hydroxylysine, which occurs in the fibrous protein collagen of connective tissues; (4) palythine [a mycosporine-like metabolite with strong UV radiation-absorbing properties that is present in some marine invertebrates (e.g., corals and sea hares); Solano 2020]; (5) N-acetyl-L-histidine, which is particularly abundant in the lens of fish, such as the Atlantic salmon, rainbow trout, and skipjack tuna, up to 32 mM (Togashi et al. 1998), and occurs at low concentrations in the heart and brain of fish, mammals, amphibians, and reptiles (O'Dowd et al. 1988, 1990; Yamada and Furuichi 1990); (6) N-acetyl-π-methylhistidine, which occurs in the brain, heart, and skeletal muscle of mammals (O'Dowd et al. 1992), as well as some tissues [e.g., the brain (up to 2.3 mM) and stomach of fish (up to 0.55 mM)] of fish (e.g., the skipjack tuna; Togashi et al. 1998); and (7) N-acetyl-aspartate (discovered by H.H. discovered in 1956), which is highly abundant in the brain of mammals (including humans, cows, cats, and rats), fish, and reptiles (Baslow 1997), as well as its dipeptide (N-acetyl-aspartyl-glutamate). The N-acetylated AAs are distributed in a species- and tissue-specific manner and may serve as either neurotransmitters in the central nervous system or osmolytes in the lens of the eyes. Abnormal changes in these AAs may contribute to neurological dysfunction in mammals or cataract in fish (e.g., Atlantic salmon and rainbow trout). The concentrations of N-acetyl-L-histidine, N-acetyl-aspartate, and N-acetyl-π-methylhistidine in the brain and eye lens of select animals are summarized in Table 1.9.

Desmosine ($C_{24}H_{40}N_5O_8$; MW = 526.61 Da)   Palythine ($C_{10}H_{16}N_2O_5$; MW = 244.24 Da)

Trace amounts of free and peptide (e.g., type I and II collagen)-bound homocitrulline are found in humans, which induce the production of autoantibodies that may be useful indicators of the onset of rheumatoid arthritis. In addition, N-methyllysine occurs in myosin (a contractile protein of muscle), whereas 3-methyl-histidine is present in the actin and myosin proteins of skeletal, smooth, and cardiac muscles. γ-Carboxyglutamate is a functional component of the blood-clotting protein prothrombin and some other proteins that bind Ca^{2+}. Furthermore, proteins, blood, and urine of humans and animals contain N^G-monomethylarginine, asymmetric dimethylarginine, and symmetric dimethylarginine, which are products of the posttranslational methylation of arginine residues

TABLE 1.9

Concentrations of N-Acetyl-Aspartate, N-Acetyl-L-Histidine, and N-Acetyl-π-Methylhistidine in the Brain and in the Eye Lens of Humans and Other Animals[a]

Animal	N-Acetyl-Aspartate	N-Acetyl-L-Histidine	N-Acetyl-π-Methylhistidine[b]
Brain			
Humans	5.50	Not detected	Not detected
Mouse	5.90	0.0	–
Rat	5.60	0.30	–
Chick	5.25	0.0	–
Turtle	1.04 (0.88–1.2)	2.08	–
Frog	0.14	2.94	–
Bony fish	3.95 (0.80–5.33)	5.88	–
Sharks	6.89 (5.85–7.93)	0.0	–
Skipjack tuna (fish)	–	0.046	1.61
Perch (fish)	–	6.70	0.0
White croaker (fish)	–	0.48	0.03
Bigeye tuna (fish)	–	1.88	0.14
Japanese barracuda (fish)	–	1.43	0.0
Atlantic salmon	Not detected	Detected	0.0
Coho salmon (fish)	–	0.12	0.014
Rainbow trout (fish)	–	3.11	0.0
Japanese char (fish)	–	2.23	0.024
Japanese eel (fish)	–	4.65	0.038
Conger eel (fish)	–	2.19	0.0
Goldfish (fish)	2.17	5.80	0.0
Lens of the Eyes			
Carp	–	8.4[c]	0.0
Skipjack tuna (fish)	–	22.6	0.0
Perch (fish)	–	4.70	0.014
White croaker (fish)	–	2.83	0.048
Bigeye tuna (fish)	–	11.4	0.045
Japanese barracuda (fish)	–	3.44	0.0
Atlantic salmon	–	1.6–5.7	0.0
Coho salmon (fish)	–	1.68	0.045
Rainbow trout (fish)	–	3.15	0.040
Japanese char (fish)	–	4.85	0.055
Japanese eel (fish)	–	1.98	0.022
Conger eel (fish)	–	1.17	0.0

Source: Baslow, M.H. 1997. *J. Neurochem.* 68:1335–1344; Baslow, M.H. and D.N. Guilfoyle. 2015. *Biomolecules* 5:635–646; Tallan, T.T., S. Moore, and W.H. Stein. 1956. *J. Biol. Chem.* 219:257–264; and Togashi, M., E. Okuma, and H. Abe. 1998. *Fish. Sci.* 64:174–175

[a] Values are expressed as μmol/g of fresh tissue.

[b] An N-acetylated derivative of 1-methylhistidine.

[c] Calculated on the basis of the assumption that the tissue contains 70%.

in proteins. Urinary excretion of free methylarginines is a useful noninvasive indicator of renal and cardiovascular functions.

Mammals synthesize *N*-acetyl-glutamate in the hepatocytes of the liver and the enterocytes of the small intestine as an activator of arginine synthesis (Chapter 3). In addition, humans and other animals also contain relatively small amounts of *N*-acetylated AAs (e.g., *N*-acetylasparagine, *N*-acetylaspartate, *N*-acetylcysteine, *N*-acetylglutamine, *N*-acetylhistidine, *N*-acetylleucine, *N*-acetyllysine, *N*-acetylornithine, *N*-acetylserine, *N*-acetyltaurine, and *N*-acetylthreonine) in a tissue-dependent manner; they are all the metabolites of intestinal microbes (Liu et al. 2019). These substances are either synthesized from the corresponding free AAs or the products of the *N*-acetylation of proteins (e.g., N^ε-acetylated lysine in histones; de Ruijter et al. 2003). Furthermore, all animal cells generate carbamoyl aspartate as an intermediate in the pathway of pyrimidine synthesis.

Free and protein-bound methionine undergoes *S*-oxidation of methionine by reactive oxygen species, including peroxynitrite, hypochlorite, hydrogen peroxide, and singlet oxygen, to generate methionine sulfoxide (a toxic substance). The latter is normally present at low concentrations in the plasma of healthy humans and other animals due to the action of methionine sulfoxide reductase, but at much higher levels in individuals with hypermethioninemia characterized by hepatotoxicity and growth depression. Methionine sulfoxide also occurs in patients with Alzheimer's disease and is associated with the self-assembly of amyloid β-protein into *toxic* oligomers and fibrillar polymers.

Venomous animals (e.g., snakes, spiders, scorpions, toads, frogs, and ants) contain non-proteinogenic AAs and AA metabolites [e.g., suberoyl arginine, bufalin-3-*O*-succinate-arginine, bufalin-3-*O*-pimelate-arginine acylpolyamines, octopamine (an analogue of norepinephrine and an inhibitor of monoamine oxidase), and *N'*-*N'*-dimethyl-serotonin (bufotenin)] for use as poisons and venoms to attack other animals (Klupczynska et al. 2018). Finally, marine sponges (sessile animals that primarily live in salt water) and cyclopeptide antibiotics (e.g., telomycin) have both (2*S*,3*S*) and (2*S*,3*R*) 3-hydroxyproline.

1.2.4.2 Other AAs in Spoiled Animal Products

Gizzerosine (2-amino-9(4-imidazolyl)-7-azanonanoic acid) is formed from histamine and L-lysine in fishmeal during prolonged storage at elevated temperatures (e.g., 130°C for 4 h; Masumura et al. 1985). This compound is highly toxic to animals, as its presence in diets at the very low level of 2.2 ppm results in severe gizzard erosion in chicks within a week after consumption (Okazaki et al. 1983). In addition, free and protein-bound methionine in foods, particularly methionine-rich animal-sourced foods, may become oxidized to form methionine sulfoxide during product processing and prolonged storage at high temperatures. Animal products contaminated with microbes contain non-proteinogenic L-AAs (including L-homoarginine, L-homoserine, L-homocitrulline, and *N*-acetyl-AAs), D-AAs (e.g., D-alanine, D-aspartate, D-glutamate, and D-serine), and non-AA metabolites (e.g., agmatine, indole, p-cresol, phenol, and excessive polyamines).

1.2.4.3 Other AAs in Plants

Besides the AAs listed in Figure 1.7, plants also contain many non-proteinogenic AAs (Nunn et al. 2010). For example, homoserine is an important substrate for methionine synthesis in plants. 5-Hydroxylysine occurs in plant cell wall proteins. By contrast, L-α,γ-diaminobutyric acid (an analogue of L-ornithine) occurs in many plants, including *Polygonatum multiflorum*, *L. latifolius*, *L. sylvestris*, and *Acacia angustissima*. Of note, this AA induces ammonia toxicity and subsequent neurotoxicity in animals (including sheep, cattle, and rats) by inhibiting ornithine carbamoyltransferase in the liver and small intestine. Similarly, ruminants (e.g., cattle) that consume a large amount of *Brassica oleracea var. acephala* (marrowstem kale) containing L-methylcysteine sulfoxide develop hemolytic anemia because it is metabolized by ruminal microbes to dimethyl disulfide (an active hemolytic factor). Furthermore, some palatable leguminous forage plants contain indospicine (L-2-amino-6-amidinohexanoic acid), which is a hepatotoxin for animals, including ruminants.

α-*N*-Oxalyl-α,β-diamino propionic acid (α-ODAP) and β-*N*-oxalyl-α,β-diamino propionic acid (β-ODAP) are found in certain plants (e.g., *Lathyrus* species) and their seeds (e.g., legume *L. sativus*, a grass pea). As analogues of glutamate, α-ODAP and β-ODAP are neurotoxins. Interestingly, the concentrations of α-ODAP and β-ODAP in plants are increased in response to drought. In humans, consumption of β-ODAP results in neurolathyrism (a motor-neuron disease). Serious outbreaks of this disease among affected populations in the Middle East, China, Ethiopia, and the Indian sub-continent usually coincide with periods of famine when *Lathyrus* seeds are a major food due to the limited supply of other food sources (Nunn et al. 2010).

Furthermore, alfalfa and lentils contain canavanine (L-2-amino-4-guanidinooxy-butanoic acid, an analogue of L-arginine and a toxic substance) and homoarginine (also an analogue of L-arginine; an uncompetitive inhibitor of liver and bone alkaline phosphatases and a toxic substance at high concentrations), respectively. In animals, canavanine is hydrolyzed by arginase to canaline (L-2-amino-4-aminoxybutanoic acid), which is highly toxic to insects, but little is known of its toxicological activity in higher animals. Likewise, mimosine (β-[N-(3-hydroxy-4-pyridone)]-L-2- aminopropanoic acid) is present in high concentrations in the leaves and seeds of *Leucaena leucocephala* and toxic to animals particularly ruminants.

L-Methionine sulfoximine occurs naturally in three species of the Connaraceae family (*Cnestis polyphylla*, *C. glabra*, and *Rourea orientalis*). This substance inhibits glutamine synthetase and γ-glutamylcysteine synthetase (an enzyme of the γ-glutamyl cycle). Likewise, plants, particularly those grown in selenium-rich soil, have relatively high levels of selenocysteine, selenocystine, and selenomethionine, which are all toxic to humans and other animals.

Finally, seaweeds (e.g., *Chondria armata*) and pennate phytoplanktonic diatom (e.g., *Pseudonitzschia pungens*) contain domoic acid [3-carboxymethyl-4-(5-carboxy-1-methylhexa-1,3-dienyl)-L-proline (an analogue of glutamate)], which is toxic to the gastrointestinal and neurological systems in humans and many other animal species. Of note, the presence of domoic acid in mussels that have been fed with seaweeds containing this substance can cause gastrointestinal and neurological illness among individuals who consume these shellfish (Wright et al. 1989).

1.2.4.4 Other AAs in Microbes

Microbes produce many AAs. One of them is glufosinate [(*RS*)-2-amino-4-(hydroxy(methyl)phosphonoyl)butanoic acid; an analogue of glutamate], which is a naturally occurring broad-spectrum herbicide produced by several species of *Streptomyces* soil bacteria. It inhibits glutamine synthetase by binding to its active glutamate site. Glufosinate-treated plants die due to a buildup of ammonia in the lumen of thylakoids inside chloroplasts, leading to the uncoupling of photophosphorylation and, therefore, the excessive production of reactive oxygen species that cause lipid peroxidation and membrane destruction (Donn and Köcher 2012). A commercial product of glufosinate is glufosinate ammonium, which was first brought to market in 1984 and is now widely used globally for weed control on farms with a variety of crops (e.g., soybeans, corn, canola, and cotton).

Another microbial metabolite is 2,6-diaminopimelic acid (also known as L,L-α-ε-diaminopimelate, DAPA). It was discovered in bacteria by E. Work in 1949. DAPA is an intermediate in the metabolic pathway for lysine synthesis and present in the peptide component of peptidoglycans in the cell wall of Gram-negative bacteria. The content of DAPA in the ruminal bacteria of sheep and cattle is 0.865 and 0.872 g/100 g of bacterial protein, respectively (Gilbreath et al. 2021). DAPA is used as a marker for bacterial protein in the study of protein nutrition in ruminants and may also have implications for research on colonic AA metabolism and colon cancer in humans.

cis-4-Hydroxy-L-proline [*cis*-(2*S*,4*S*)-4-hydroxyproline, an imino acid], which is a stereoisomer of *trans*-L-4-hydroxyproline, is enzymatically synthesized from the 4-position hydroxylation of free L-proline by L-proline cis-4-hydroxylase in certain organisms (Hara and Kino 2009). As an analogue of L-proline, *cis*-4-hydroxy-L-proline inhibits collagen synthesis in animals and has been tested as an anticancer drug. Interestingly, *cis*-4-hydroxy-L-proline is present in the toxic cyclic peptides from *Amanita* mushrooms (fungi). Thus, not all mushrooms are edible and proper caution should be exercised before consuming unknown fungi.

As noted previously, microorganisms synthesize many different *N*-acetylated AAs. These modified AAs can be formed from free AAs by *N*-acetyl-AA synthetase (e.g., *N*-acetylarginine synthetase). In addition, *N*-acetyltransferases catalyze the posttranslational *N*-acetylation of AA residues in protein, and proteolysis results in the generation of *N*-acetylated AAs (de Ruijter et al. 2003). These AAs are excreted in the feces and urine of humans and other animals.

1.2.4.5 Other AAs in Processed Foods

During the cooking of starchy food with oil at high temperatures, asparagine condenses with carbohydrate (e.g., glucose or fructose) via the Maillard reaction to form *N*-glycosyl-L-asparagine. Upon pyrolysis (the thermal decomposition of materials at elevated temperatures in an inert atmosphere), *N*-glycosyl-L-asparagine is cleaved to produce acrylamine and an Amadori product with *N*-substituted succinimide (Pruser and Flynn 2011). In Greek, "*pyro*" and "*lysis*" mean "fire" and "separating", respectively. Because free asparagine is highly abundant in potato, frying this food contributes to the formation of acrylamide, which has been classified by the International Agency for Research on Cancer as a probable carcinogen.

D-Glucose + L-Asparagine → (Maillard reaction, High Temperature (> 100 °C)) → *N*-Glycosyl-L-asparagine → (Pyrolysis) → Amadori product with *N*-substituted succinimide; Acrylamide (C_3H_5NO; MW, 71.08 Da)

1.3 CHEMICAL PROPERTIES OF AAs

Knowledge of the chemical properties of AAs in water, physiological fluids, and organic solvents is crucial for the preparation of AA solutions for cell culture, nutritional support, and medical therapy. Such information can also guide the practice of processing, storing, and analyzing biological samples. In addition, the chemical properties of AAs can be utilized to develop new delicious and healthy foods for consumption by humans and other animals.

1.3.1 Physical Appearance, Fluorescence, and Melting Points of Crystalline AAs

AA crystals are generally white. Three AAs, phenylalanine, tyrosine, and tryptophan, are naturally fluorescent, with different maximum excitation (Ex) and emission (Em) wavelengths (Yang et al. 2015). Tryptophan (Ex 280 nm, Em 348 nm) is much more fluorescent than phenylalanine (Ex 260 nm, Em 280 nm) or tyrosine (Ex 275 nm, Em 304 nm). All of crystalline α-AAs, except for glutamine, cysteine, phosphoarginine, and selenocysteine, have a high melting point of over 200°C. Glutamine, cysteine, and phosphoarginine have melting points of 185°C, 178°C, and 145°C, respectively. At or above their melting points, AAs decompose spontaneously. The hydrochlorides of L-arginine (L-arginine-HCl), L-lysine (L-lysine-HCl), and L-ornithine (L-ornithine-HCl) have melting points of 235°C, 236°C, and 231°C, respectively (Table 1.2). Interestingly, the melting points of L-arginine and L-arginine-HCl are nearly identical.

1.3.2 Tastes of Crystalline AAs

The taste of AAs results from their interactions with specific receptors [guanine nucleotide-binding protein (G protein)-coupled receptors] on the tongue (San Gabriel et al. 2009; Fernstrom et al. 2012). Different AAs have different structures, and therefore confer different tastes. Generally speaking, small AAs [except for small sulfur AAs (taurine and cysteine) and β-alanine] confer sweet taste, whereas most of the large L-AAs have bitter tastes (Wu 2020a). For example, glycine has a sweet taste, whereas L-alanine, L-citrulline, L-proline, L-serine, and L-threonine have a slightly sweet taste (Kawai et al. 2012). L-Arginine base has a characteristic bitter and unpleasant taste by itself, but in a mixture with citric acid in drinking water, it is palatable. L-Isoleucine, L-lysine, and L-phenylalanine have a slightly bitter taste. β-Alanine, L-cystine, L-methionine, and L-tyrosine are flat (lacking taste), whereas L-cysteine, L-histidine, L-leucine, L-ornithine, and L-tryptophan have a flat-to-bitter taste. Of particular note, L-glutamate [e.g., monosodium glutamate and monopotassium glutamate (an alternative to monosodium glutamate)] and glutamic acid have a "meaty" umami taste (San Gabriel et al. 2009). By contrast, D-glutamate is almost tasteless, and D-cystine is flat. Unlike most L-AAs as well as D-glutamate and D-cystine, many D-AAs are sweet substances (Table 1.10).

Interestingly, some AAs have complex tastes. For example, L-aspartate has a sour taste with a slight umami flavor, L-valine has a bitter taste after an initial slightly sweet flavor, and L-histidine-HCl has a slightly bitter taste after an initial sour flavor. In addition, the taste of basic AAs is altered by their hydrochloride salts (San Gabriel et al. 2009), such that L-arginine-HCl, L-lysine-HCl, and L-ornithine-HCl, which are manufactured by neutralizing the bases with HCl, have a mild but very characteristic taste.

Note that different individuals may have a different tasting response to the same AA. Furthermore, the taste of an AA may differ among animal species. For example, pigs and rats tolerate crystalline L-arginine (in either the base or HCl form) very well, when supplemented into their pellet diets. However, humans are very sensitive to the unpleasant taste of the L-arginine base and would not consume any unencapsulated crystalline L-arginine or its solution. Thus, when L-arginine-HCl (with a slight characteristic taste) is orally administered to humans, it is usually dissolved in a lemon-based or flavored solution to induce palatability.

TABLE 1.10
Tastes of Free Amino Acids as Perceived by Humans

Taste	Amino Acids
Sweet	L-Alanine[a], γ-aminobutyrate, L-citrulline[a], glycine, L-4-hydroxyproline[a], L-proline[a], L-serine[a], L-threonine[a]
	D-Alanine; D-asparagine, D-glutamine, D-histidine, D-isoleucine, D-leucine, D-methionine, D-phenylalanine, D-serine, D-threonine, D-tryptophan, D-tyrosine, D-valine
Sour	L-Aspartate (with a slight umami flavor), L-cysteine-HCl, L-glutamic acid-HCl
	D-Aspartate[b], D-aspartic acid, D-cysteine, D-glutamic acid, D-histidine-HCl[b]
Bitter	L-Arginine (a characteristically unpleasant taste), L-glutamate monoammonium, L-isoleucine[c], L-phenylalanine[c], L-lysine[c], L-histidine-HCl[c] (slightly bitter after an initial sour taste), L-valine (bitter after an initial slightly sweet taste)
	D-Arginine, D-cysteine, D-4-hydroxyproline, D-lysine, D-lysine-HCl, D-proline
Umami[d]	L-Glutamate (e.g., L-monosodium glutamate and monopotassium glutamate), glutamic acid
Flat[e]	β-Alanine, L-cystine, L-methionine, L-tyrosine, D-cystine
	L-Asparagine (flat to slightly sweet), L-glutamine (flat to slightly sweet and meaty), D-glutamate (almost tasteless), taurine (flat to very slightly sour)
Flat to SB	L-Cysteine, L-histidine, L-leucine, L-ornithine, L-tryptophan
SCT	L-Arginine-HCl, L-lysine, L-ornithine-HCl

[a] Slightly sweet.
[b] Complex with sour and slightly bitter tastes.
[c] Slightly bitter.
[d] Meaty, broth-like, or savory taste.
[e] Flat (lacking tastiness or flavor; tasteless) to slightly bitter.
Note: SB, slightly bitter; SCT, slight characteristic tastes, with each of these three amino acids having different characteristic tastes.

1.3.3 Solubility of AAs in Water and Organic Solvents

All AAs are soluble in water at room temperature (e.g., 20°C–25°C). Leucine, isoleucine, valine, phenylalanine, tryptophan, methionine, tyrosine, and cysteine are among the most hydrophobic AAs. All AAs (except for cystine) are soluble in Krebs bicarbonate buffer (pH 7.4 at 25°C) at concentrations that are at least ten times greater than those found in the plasma of animal blood. The solubility of α-AAs in water varies with their side chains, with proline and cystine being the most and least soluble, respectively (Table 1.2). The solubility of β-alanine and γ-aminobutyrate in water is higher than that of lysine. Salts affect the solubility of AAs in water, but such an effect depends on their structures (Table 1.11). The very low solubility of cystine and tyrosine in water presents a challenge in their intravenous administration to humans and other animals directly or through total parenteral nutrition. This problem can be mitigated through the use of N-acetyl-cysteine and N-acetyl-tyrosine, which are readily soluble in water and are effective precursors of cysteine and tyrosine in animals.

The solubility of AAs generally increases in acidic or alkaline solutions and with elevated temperatures. The pH of a solution affects the solubility of AAs by influencing their dissociation into ionic forms. For example, compared with a range of pH 3–8.5, a pH lower than 3 or higher than 8.5 can increase the solubility of asparagine and glutamine, as well as tyrosine, aspartic acid, and glutamic

TABLE 1.11
Effects of Salts on the Solubility of Amino Acids in Water

Amino Acids	Salts	Change in Solubility in Water[a]
Glycine	5 mM $BaCl_2$	↑ 21.1%
	5 mM $CaCl_2$	↑ 23.6%
	10 mM $CaCl_2$	↑ 39.5%
	10 mM NaCl	↑ 3.9%
	10 mM LiCl	↑ 8.0%
	10 mM KCl	↑ 1.0%
	20 mM KCl	↓ 34.5%
	10 mM $NaNO_3$	↑ 12.2%
	10 mM KNO_3	↑ 5.9%
	20 mM KNO_3	↓ 4.7%
L-Aspartic acid	5 mM $BaCl_2$	↑ 68.3%
	5 mM $CaCl_2$	↑ 51.9%
	10 mM $CaCl_2$	↑ 51.9%
	5 mM NaCl	↑ 28.8%
	5 mM LiCl	↑ 16.1%
	5 mM KCl	↑ 31.7%
	10 mM KCl	↑ 31.7%
	10 mM KNO_3	↑ 54.4%
L-Glutamic acid	20 mM NaCl	↑ 31.0%
	20 mM LiCl	↑ 5.7%
	20 mM KCl	↑ 31.2%
	20 mM KNO_3	↑ 80.1%
L-Leucine	5 mM $BaCl_2$	↑ 15.4%
	5 mM $CaCl_2$	↑ 17.6%
	20 mM NaCl	↓ 33.4%
	20 mM LiCl	↓ 9.4%
	20 mM KCl	↓ 34.5%

Source: Greenstein, J.P. and M. Winitz. 1961. *Chemistry of Amino Acids.* John Wiley, New York.

[a] Compared with the absence of salt.

Note: ↑, increase; ↓, decrease.

acid in an aqueous solution. With the exception of proline and hydroxyproline, AAs are generally insoluble in organic solvents (e.g., absolute ethanol). Because of their pyrrole ring structures, proline and hydroxyproline are fairly soluble in absolute ethanol (approximately 1.6 g/100 mL at 20°C).

The hydrochloride salts of AAs (both neutral and basic) are generally more soluble in water than the corresponding free AAs. Most of the AA hydrochlorides are highly soluble in absolute ethanol, because HCl is readily soluble in both ethanol and water. The hydrochloride salts of basic AAs (e.g., arginine, lysine, and ornithine) are often used because of their neutralization in water and in physiological solution. The sodium salts of most AAs dissolve more readily in water and are more ethanol-soluble than the corresponding free AAs.

1.3.4 THE ZWITTERIONIC FORM OF AAS

Because the amino and acidic groups have opposite electrical charges, an AA (an amphoteric electrolyte) acts as a base or an acid by accepting or supplying a hydrogen ion, respectively. Thus, all AAs form intramolecular salts both in the crystalline state and in an aqueous solution. This structure, in which a molecule has both positive and negative electrical charges, is known as a dipolar ion or zwitterion (ionizable). The term "Zwitterion" is derived from the German word for "double" (zwitter) and the word "ion". Uncharged (non-dissociated) forms of AAs almost do not exist. For example, the ratio of charged dipolar (ionized α-amino and α-carboxyl groups) to uncharged forms of L-aspartic acid in an aqueous solution is approximately 28,000:1 at pH 7.0 (Greenstein and Winitz 1961). Similarly, the proportion of charged dipolar (ionized α-amino and α-carboxyl groups) to uncharged forms of L-lysine in an aqueous solution is approximately 320,000:1 at pH 7.0 (Greenstein and Winitz 1961). In an aqueous solution, the ionizable groups of AAs interact with water through ionic interactions, hydrogen bonds, and van der Waals interactions. Note that the simple non-ionized forms of AAs appear in some sections of this book.

$$
\overset{\text{R}}{\underset{\text{H}}{\overset{|}{\underset{|}{\text{H}_3\overset{+}{\text{N}}-\text{C}_\alpha-\text{COO}^-}}}}
$$

The zwitterionic (ionized) form of an AA

In an aqueous solution, the carboxyl and amino groups of an AA dissociate in a pH-dependent manner and, therefore, have their respective dissociation constants (pK_a). The pK_a is the negative log of the acid dissociation constant (K_a) and a measure of the tendency of a group to lose a proton (H^+) or the strength of an acid. A lower pK_a value indicates a stronger acid. Namely, the acid dissociates to a greater extent in water to give up its proton (H^+).

$$
K_1 = \frac{[H_3\overset{+}{N}CHRCOO^-][H^+]}{[H_3\overset{+}{N}CHRCOOH]} \qquad K_2 = \frac{[H_2NCHRCOO^-][H^+]}{[H_3\overset{+}{N}CHRCOO^-]}
$$

The relationship between the pH of an aqueous solution and the pK_a for an acid or an ionizable group is mathematically represented by the following Henderson–Hasselbalch equation:

$$HA = A^- + H^+; \quad pH = pK_a + \log\frac{[A^-]}{[HA]}; \quad pK_a = pH - \log\frac{[A^-]}{[HA]}$$

In this equation, HA is an acid or a protonated form, and A^- is a conjugate base or a deprotonated form. AAs contain more than one ionizable group. The protonated and corresponding deprotonated forms of their groups are shown in Table 1.12. The ratio of $[A^-]$ (e.g., the acid or an ionizable group in a protonated form) to $[HA]$ (e.g., the base or an ionizable group in a deprotonated form) can be calculated with the use of the Henderson–Hasselbalch equation (Table 1.13). When the pH of an aqueous solution is equal to pK_a, the ionizable group is 50% protonated and 50% deprotonated.

The dissociation constants for the acid, amino, and side-chain groups are termed pK_1 (pK_a for the carboxyl group), pK_2 (pK_a for the amino group), and pK_3 (pK_a for the side-chain functional group), respectively. Note that at a neutral pH, the side-chain functional groups of cysteine and tyrosine (with the pK_a values of 10.28 and 10.07, respectively) are essentially not ionized. By contrast, the *seleno group of selenocysteine has the pK_a of 5.2 and therefore exists in a deprotonated state at* neutral pH. Likewise, the side-chain carboxyl group of glutamic acid has the pK_a of 4.25 and gives up its proton at neutral pH. Some AAs, such as phosphoarginine, may have more than one ionizable group in their side chains. The pH of an aqueous solution at which an AA has no net electrical charge is called the isoelectric point (pI). When an AA is dissolved in pure water until the solution is saturated, the pH of this solution will approach the pI value of the AA.

The pI values of AAs in solutions are based on the dissociation constants for their acid, amino, and side-chain groups. For an AA without an ionizable side chain, $pI = (pK_{a1} + pK_{a2})/2$.

Examples for alanine and citrulline are as follows:

$$\text{For alanine, } pI = (2.35 + 9.87)/2 = 6.11$$

$$\text{For citrulline, } pI = (2.43 + 9.41)/2 = 5.92$$

For an AA with an ionizable side chain, pI = the average of the pK_a values of the two most similar acid groups. Examples for acid groups are (1) –COOH, – SO_3H, –PO_4H_2, –SH and –SeH that have no electrical charge in their protonated form and (2) –NH_3^+, –NH_2^+, and –NH^+ that are positively charged

TABLE 1.12

Protonated and Deprotonated Forms of Ionizable Groups in Amino Acids (AAs)

Functional Group	Chemical Formula	Protonated Form Proximate pK_a Values for Proteinogenic AAs	Deprotonated Form
Carboxyl	–COOH	1.8–2.4	–COO⁻
Amino	–NH_3^+	8.7–10.6	–NH_2
Sulfuric acid	–SO_3H	2.2	–SO_3^-
Side-Chain Group			
Guanidino	–NH_2^+	12.5 (e.g., arginine)	=NH
Active N	–NH^+	6.0 (e.g., histidine)	=N
Phenolic hydroxyl	–OH	10 (e.g., tyrosine)	–O⁻
Thiol	–SH	10 (e.g., cysteine)	–S⁻
Seleno	–SeH	5.2 (e.g., selenocysteine)	–Se⁻

TABLE 1.13

Proportions of an Ionizable Group of Amino Acids (AAs) in the Protonated and Deprotonated Forms in Aqueous Solutions at Different pH[a]

Condition	Difference between the pH of an Aqueous Solution and the pK_a of an Ionizable Group of an AA $(pH - pK_a)$	Log $[A^-]/$ $[HA]$	$[A^-]/[HA]$	Percent (%) of the Ionizable Group in the Deprotonated Form (A^-) $X = (100 \times [A^-])/([A^-] + [HA])$	Percent (%) of the Ionizable Group in the Protonated Form (HA) $Y = 100 - X$
$pH = pK_a$	0 (e.g., pH = 4; pK_a = 4)	0	1	50.00 [i.e., 1/(1 +1) = 0.5]	50.00
$pH < pK_a$	−1 (e.g., pH = 3; pK_a = 4)	−1	0.1	9.09 [i.e., 0.1/(0.1 + 1) = 0.0909]	90.91
$pH < pK_a$	−2 (e.g., pH = 2; pK_a = 4)	−2	0.01	0.99 [i.e., 0.01/ (0.01 + 1) = 0.0099]	99.01
$pH < pK_a$	−3 (e.g., pH = 1; pK_a = 4)	−3	0.001	0.10 [i.e., 0.001/ (0.001 + 1) = 0.001]	99.90
$pH > pK_a$	1 (e.g., pH = 5; pK_a = 4)	1	10	90.91 [i.e., 10/(10 + 1) = 0.9091]	9.09
$pH > pK_a$	2 (e.g., pH = 6; pK_a = 4)	2	100	99.01 [i.e., 100/ (100 + 1) = 0.9901]	0.99
$pH > pK_a$	3 (e.g., pH = 7; pK_a = 4)	3	1,000	99.90 [i.e., 1,000/ (1,000 + 1) = 0.9990]	0.10

[a] The ratio of $[A^-]$ (the concentration of a conjugate base) to [HA] (the concentration of an acid) can be calculated with the use of the Henderson–Hasselbalch equation: $pH = pK_a + \log [A^-]/[HA]$. $\log [A^-]/[HA] = pH - pK_a$. A conjugated base is formed from an acid after the removal of its proton.

Note: $[A^-]$, the deprotonated form (e.g., $-COO^-$; NH_2) of an amino acid (also known as a conjugate base); [HA], the protonated form (e.g., $-COOH$; NH_3^+) of an amino acid.

in their protonated state. In the case of aspartic acid, the two similar acids are the α-carboxyl group and the side-chain carboxyl group. For arginine, the two similar acids are the α-amino group and the guanidinium species on the side chain.

Examples for aspartic acid and arginine are as follows:

$$\text{For aspartic acid, pI} = (1.88 + 3.65)/2 = 2.77$$

$$\text{For arginine, pI} = (9.04 + 12.48)/2 = 10.76$$

Because the pK_a values of the α-carboxylic acid groups of α-AAs are approximately 2.0–2.4 (Table 1.2), these groups are almost entirely in their carboxylate forms at pH > 3.5. Similarly, because the pK_a values of the α-amino groups of α-AA are approximately 9.0–10.0, these groups are almost entirely in their ammonium ion forms at pH < 8.0. Thus, at physiological pH (e.g., pH 7.4 in the plasma and fetal fluid and pH 7.0 in cytoplasm), the α-carboxylic acid and α-amino groups of α-AAs are completely ionized to take the zwitterion form. In their ionized state, glutamic acid and aspartic acid are often referred to as glutamate and aspartate, respectively.

AAs can be classified as neutral, basic, and acidic AAs, based on their net charges at neutral pH. Note that at neutral physiological pH, the side-chain $-NH_2$ group in asparagine, glutamine, and citrulline is not ionized and, therefore, has no electrical charge. The net charges of AAs at pH 1.5–3.5 (i.e., physiological pH in the luminal fluid of the stomach of monogastric animals, such as humans, pigs, rats, dogs, and chickens) are different from those at neutral pH. The net charges of AAs at pH 5–6.5 have important implications for their transport and metabolism by ruminal microbes in ruminants (e.g., cattle, sheep, and goats). The charges of AAs at pH > 8, which is substantially greater than the pH of fluids in the digestive tract, blood, cells, and tissues, have little physiological relevance in humans and other animals. Table 1.14 shows the charges and net charges of AAs at pH 7.0 and 2.0.

TABLE 1.14

Net Charges of Amino Acids in an Aqueous Solution at pH 7.0 and 2.0[a]

Amino Acids	Charges at pH 7.0				Charges at pH 2.0[b]			
	α-Acidic Group	α-Amino Group	Side Chain	Net Charge	α-Acidic Group	α-Amino Group	Side Chain	Net Charge
L-Alanine	−1	+1	0	0	−0.31	+1	0	+0.69
β-Alanine	−1	+1	0	0	0	+1	0	+1
γ-Aminobutyrate	−1	+1	0	0	0	+1	0	+1
β-Aminoisobutyrate	−1	+1	0	0	0	+1	0	+1
L-Asparagine	−1	+1	0	0	−0.49	+1	0	+0.51
L-Citrulline	−1	+1	0	0	−0.27	+1	0	+0.73
L-Cysteine	−1	+1	0	0	−0.48	+1	0	+0.52
L-Cystine	−1	+1	0	0	−1	+1	0	0
L-DOPA	−1	+1	0	0	−0.32	+1	0	+0.68
L-Glu-Na (MSG)	−	+1	−1	0	−	+1	0	+1
L-Glutamine	−1	+1	0	0	−0.40	+1	0	+0.60
Glycine	−1	+1	0	0	−0.31	+1	0	+0.69
L-Hydroxyproline	−1	+1	0	0	−0.55	+1	0	+0.45
L-Isoleucine	−1	+1	0	0	−0.30	+1	0	+0.70
L-Leucine	−1	+1	0	0	−0.32	+1	0	+0.68
L-Methionine	−1	+1	0	0	−0.34	+1	0	+0.66
L-Phenylalanine	−1	+1	0	0	−0.39	+1	0	+0.61
L-Proline	−1	+1	0	0	−0.50	+1	0	+0.50
L-Serine	−1	+1	0	0	−0.32	+1	0	+0.68
L-Taurine	−1	+1	0	0	−0.76	+1	0	+0.24
L-Threonine	−1	+1	0	0	−0.41	+1	0	+0.59
L-Tryptophan	−1	+1	0	0	−0.29	+1	0	+0.71
L-Tyrosine	−1	+1	0	0	−0.39	+1	0	+0.61
L-Valine	−1	+1	0	0	−0.34	+1	0	+0.66
L-Arginine	−1	+1	+1	+1	−0.40	+1	+1	+1.60
L-Histidine	−1	+1	+0.1	+0.1	−0.61	+1	0	+0.39
L-Homoarginine	−1	+1	+1	+1	−0.24	+1	+1	+1.76
L-Lysine	−1	+1	+1	+1	−0.40	+1	+1	+1.60
L-Ornithine	−1	+1	+1	+1	−0.53	+1	+1	+1.47
L-Aspartic acid	−1	+1	−1	−1	−0.57	+1	0	+0.43
L-Glutamic acid	−1	+1	−1	−1	−0.39	+1	0	+0.61
L-Phosphoarginine	−1	+1	−1	−1	−0.50	+1	−0.5	0
L-Selenocysteine	−1	+1	−1	−1	−0.24	+1	0[b]	+0.76

[a] When the acidic (e.g., the carboxyl or sulfuric acid) group is almost fully protonated (i.e., pH<pK_a by 2 or more units), it virtually has no charge. When the –NH$_2$, –NH or active N group is almost fully protonated (i.e., pH<pK_a by 2 or more units), it has a positive charge.

[b] See Table 1.13 for the calculation of the charges in amino acids based on the Henderson–Hasselbalch equation.

Data on the pI values of AAs help one understand the mechanisms responsible for the following: (1) buffering functions of AAs; (2) acid–base balance in physiological fluids; (3) transport of AAs by cells; (4) interorgan metabolism of AAs; (5) AA antagonism and imbalance; (6) protein structure and function; and (7) intracellular trafficking and location. With a pI of 6.07, as well as a pK_1 of 2.35 and a pK_2 of 9.78, glycine is a good buffer in the luminal fluid of the stomach, but makes a poor buffer in intracellular fluid with a pH of 7.0 or in blood with a pH of 7.4. By contrast, with a pH of 7.69, as well as a pK_3 of 6.04, histidine provides a good buffer in cells and blood under physiological conditions, under highly acidic or alkaline conditions. This explains, in part, why histidine is an abundant AA in hemoglobins and intramuscular dipeptides. Additionally, knowledge of pI values is useful for designing effective methods to analyze AAs and their products. For example, the different charges of free AAs at a given pH are the chemical basis for their separation by ion-exchange chromatography. Likewise, different charges of peptide-bound AAs allow for the separation of proteins and polypeptides by electrophoresis.

On the basis of their net charges at neutral pH, AAs are classified as neutral (net charge = 0), basic (net change ≥ +1), or acidic (net change ≤ −1). Thus, addition of an acidic or basic AA to a solution with a weak buffering capacity will substantially decrease or increase the pH of the solution, respectively. Similarly, intravenous infusion of large amounts of an acidic or basic AA into animals and humans will adversely disturb the acid–base balance of the body. Interestingly, supplementing an appropriate amount of an acidic (e.g., 1% glutamic acid) or basic (e.g., 1% arginine) AA to a corn- and soybean meal-based diet does not affect the pH in the lumen of the swine gastrointestinal tract. This is likely due to the highly acidic environment of the stomach (pH 2–2.5) and bicarbonate-containing secretions in the lumen of the small intestine.

1.3.5 Chemical Stability of AAs

1.3.5.1 Stability of Crystalline AAs

The crystalline forms of all AAs are stable at room temperature (i.e., 25°C) for at least 25 years without any detectable loss. This applies to L- and D-AAs, as well as proteinogenic and non-proteinogenic AAs. However, like all substances, AAs should be protected from light and should not be exposed to a high-humidity environment during storage (Ajinomoto® 2003). Anhydrous crystalline AAs (including asparagine, aspartate, glutamate, and glutamine) are stable at 105°C for 24 h without any detectable loss.

1.3.5.2 Stability of Free AAs in Water and Buffered Solutions at <0°C and ≤40°C

Except for cysteine and aminomalonic acid, AAs in water, buffered solutions (e.g., Krebs bicarbonate buffer), or deproteinized and neutralized biological samples are stable at −20°C for 3 months and stable at −80°C for 6 months without any detectable loss. Likewise, except for aminomalonic acid, AAs (including arginine, asparagine, aspartate, citrulline, cystine, glycine, lysine, methionine, phospho-arginine, proline, and tryptophan) are generally stable in aqueous solution at physiological pH and body temperature (e.g., 37°C in mammals and 40°C in birds), except for (1) cysteine, which undergoes rapid oxidation to cystine particularly in the presence of metal ions and the absence of reducing agents; (2) glutamine, whose amide and carboxyl groups spontaneously and slowly interact to form a cyclic product, the ammonium salt of pyrrolidone carboxylate (pyroglutamate; 5-oxo-proline; Furst et al. 1990), with the rate of this reaction occurring at a rate of <1%/day for 1 mM glutamine at pH 7.0 and 37°C; (3) glutamic acid, which undergoes spontaneous and slow intramolecular cyclization to form pyroglutamate (<0.2%/day for 1 mM glutamate at pH 7.0 and 37°C); and (4) aminomalonic acid, which is decarboxylated to glycine. At high concentrations, pyroglutamate is a neurotoxin. Note that glutamine is unstable on storage at 4°C or higher temperatures (e.g., 25°C or 37°C) in solution and, therefore, is not added as a free AA to total parenteral nutrition solution in clinical medicine.

The ratio of cystine to cysteine is approximately 10:1 in the plasma or serum of healthy individuals. Cystine is readily converted to cysteine inside the cell under physiological reducing conditions. N-Acetylcysteine (a water-soluble synthetic substance) is a stable precursor of cysteine for cultured cells and for intravenous or oral administration into humans and other animals. In chemical analysis, the thiol (–SH) group of cysteine can be protected by iodoacetic acid, whereas cystine can be readily reduced to cysteine by 2-mercaptoethanol. In contrast to cysteine, few means are available to protect glutamine from spontaneous cyclization in an aqueous solution. The chemical stability of AAs has important implications for the clinical nutrition of humans and other animals (Imseis et al. 2019).

1.3.5.3 Stability of Free AAs in Water at High Temperatures

All AAs, except for asparagine, cysteine, glutamate, glutamine, aminomalonic acid, and methionine, are stable in a neutral aqueous solution at 105°C for 24 h. Under these conditions, glutamine is completely decomposed; 40% asparagine, 15% glutamate, and 12% methionine are lost; and all cysteine is converted into cystine. The common product of the spontaneous degradation of glutamine and glutamate via intramolecular cyclization is pyroglutamate, whereas ammonia is also released from glutamine during this reaction. Similarly, asparagine undergoes intramolecular cyclization to form succinimide, which is subsequently deamidated to aspartate and ammonia (Catak et al. 2009). Thus, after a wet tissue (e.g., skeletal muscle, liver, fish, and shrimp) is placed in a 105°C oven for 24 h, glutamine is not detectable, and most of asparagine disappears. Therefore, free AAs in animal tissues should not be determined after they are dried in an oven.

1.3.5.4 Stability of Free AAs in Water under High Pressure and High Temperatures

Under high-pressure and high-temperature conditions in an autoclave, glutamine and asparagine are almost completely destroyed and cysteine is oxidized to cystine, but other AAs (including cystine) except for aminomalonic acid are stable. However, in a dipeptide form (e.g., L-alanyl-glutamine and glycyl-glutamine, as well as L-leucyl-asparagine and glycyl-asparagine), glutamine and asparagine are stable under these conditions. To prevent the loss of glutamine and asparagine under autoclaving conditions, a solution containing free glutamine and asparagine can be sterilized by passing the solution through a 0.2-μm filter before use for cell or tissue culture. Note that under autoclaving conditions, cysteine (2%, w/v) in deoxygenated water is stable at pH 4.9 but undergoes 8% and 17% losses at pH 7 and 8, respectively.

1.3.5.5 Stability of Free AAs in Strong Acid and Alkaline Solutions at ≤25°C

All proteinogenic AAs except glutamine, asparagine, and tryptophan are stable in 0.1 M HCl solution at ≤4°C for at least 3 months. Under these conditions, all non-proteinogenic AAs except aminomalonic acid are stable for at least 3 months. All AAs except for aminomalonic acid are stable in 1.5 M perchloric acid ($HClO_4$) at ≤25°C for at least 15 min and stable in 10% trichloroacetic acid at ≤25°C for at least 30 min. Under alkaline conditions (e.g., 4 M NaOH or KOH) at ≤25°C, tryptophan is stable for at least 24 h, aminomalonic acid is relatively stable, and other AAs are not stable.

1.3.5.6 Stability of Free AAs in Strong Acid and Alkaline Solutions at High Temperatures

Under standard conditions of acid hydrolysis (i.e., 6 M HCl, 110°C, and 24 h under nitrogen gas), changes in the following AAs occur: (1) all glutamine and asparagine are converted to glutamate and aspartate, respectively, with ammonia being a coproduct; (2) tryptophan is completely destroyed; (3) 20% of methionine undergoes oxidation to generate methionine sulfoxide; and (4) all aminomalonic acid is decarboxylated to glycine. Notably, under these conditions, other AAs are either highly stable (i.e., no detectable loss for alanine, arginine, cystine, glutamate, glycine, histidine, leucine, lysine, phenylalanine, and valine) or relatively stable (3% loss for aspartate and threonine; 5% loss for tyrosine and proline; and 10% loss for serine).

Under the conditions of alkaline hydrolysis at high temperatures (e.g., 105°C), most AAs (including arginine, asparagine, glutamine, glycine, histidine, serine, and threonine) are almost completely destroyed, and many AAs (e.g., cysteine, cystine, and methionine) are decomposed to a great extent. For example, heat treatment at alkaline pH converts (1) arginine to ornithine, urea, citrulline, and ammonia; (2) cysteine into dehydroalanine; (3) glutamine into glutamate and ammonia; and (4) asparagine into aspartate and ammonia. These conditions may occur during alkali refining of oils from soybeans, peanuts, and other foods. By contrast, tryptophan is stable and aminomalonic acid is relatively stable in alkaline solutions even at boiling temperatures. Thus, the analysis of tryptophan and aminomalonic acid in proteins can be successfully accomplished by alkaline hydrolysis in the presence of 4.2 M NaOH and 1% thiodiglycol (an antioxidant) at 105°C for 20 h.

1.3.6 Chemical Reactions of AAs

Knowledge about the chemical reactions of AAs is useful for their analysis and, therefore, in conducting AA research. Some of these reactions may occur in animals and may be of biochemical importance for understanding the safety of AAs in animals. Overall, chemical reactions of AAs are dependent upon the amino group, the carboxyl group, the side-chain, and the intact molecule (Hughes 2012).

1.3.6.1 Chemical Reactions of the Amino Group in α-AAs

The amino group of an α-AA is chemically active and participates in reactions with a variety of substances. These chemical reactions include acetylation, benzoylation, carbobenzoxylation, condensation, conjugation, deamination, dinitrophenylation, group protection, methylation, oxymethylation, and transamination (Table 1.15). Four of these reactions, conjugation, deamination, transamination, and oxymethylation, are briefly discussed herein because of their biological relevance and use in the analysis of AAs.

TABLE 1.15
Chemical Reactions Involving the Amino and Carboxyl Groups in α-Amino Acids (AAs)

Type of Reaction	Reagent	Product
(1) Involving the α-Amino Group		
Acetylation	Acetic anhydride [$(CH_3CO)_2O$] or Acetyl chloride (CH_3COCl)	N-Acetyl AA
Benzoylation	Benzoyl chloride (C_6H_5COCl)	N-Benzoyl AA
Carbobenzoxylation	Carbobenzoxy chloride ($C_6H_5CH_2OCOCl$)	N-Carbobenzoxy AA
Condensation	6-Aminoquinolyl-N-hydroxy-succinimidyl carbamate (AQC, $C_{14}H_{11}N_3O_4$)	AQC-AA derivatives (highly stable)
	4-Chloro-7-nitrobenzofurazan (NBD-Cl; $C_6H_2ClN_3O_3$)	NBD-AA
	Dansyl chloride ($C_{12}H_{12}ClNO_2S$)	AA derivatives (stable)
	9-Fluorenylmethyl chloroformate (FMOC; $C_{15}H_{11}ClO_2$)	FMOC-AA derivative (highly stable)
	o-Phthaldialdehyde [OPA; $C_6H_4(CHO)_2$] + ME	OPA-AA adduct (highly fluorescent)
	Phenylisothiocyanate (PITC, C_7H_5NS)	Phenylthiocarbamyl AA
Deamination	Nitrous acid (HNO_2)	Ammonia + hydroxyl acid
Dinitrophenylation	1-Fluoro-2,4-dinitrobenzene (FDNB; $C_6H_3FN_2O_4$)	2,4-Dinitrophenyl AA (yellow product)
Group Protection	t-Butyloxy carbamate [t-BOC; $(t-C_4H_9OCO)_2O$]	BOC-AA
	Aldehyde (RCHO)	Schiff base (C=N-)
Methylation	Dimethyl sulfate [$(CH_3)_2SO_4$] or methyl iodide (CH_3I)	N-methyl AA + betaine
Oxymethylation	Formaldehyde (HCHO)	N-Hydroxymethyl AA
Transamination	α-Ketoacid	α-AA (new) + α-ketoacid (new)
(2) Involving the Carboxyl Group		
Amidation	Ammonia	α-AA amide ($H_2NCHRCONH_2$)
Decarboxylation	Base [e.g., $Ba(OH)_2$] and heating	Amine

(Continued)

TABLE 1.15 (*Continued*)

Chemical Reactions Involving the Amino and Carboxyl Groups in α-Amino Acids (AAs)

Type of Reaction	Reagent	Product
Esterification	Base (ROH) and other reagents[a]	AA ester ($H_2NCHRCOOR'$)
Reduction	Lithium borohydride ($LiBH_4$) or sodium borohydride ($NaBH_4$)	Amino alcohol ($H_2NCHRCH_2OH$)
(3) Involving Both the Amino Acid and Carboxyl Groups		
Chelation	Minerals (e.g., Cu^{2+})	AA complex [e.g., ($H_2NCHRCOO)_2Cu$]
Cyclization	Potassium cyanate (KCNO)	Hydantoin (HNCHRCOCO–NH)
	Various reagents[b]	Diketopiperazine
Esterification and N^α-dehydrogenation	Base (R-OH), ethanol, and fatty acyl chloride	Ethyl-N^α-fatty acyl-AA
NCA formation	Phosgene ($COCl_2$)	NCA
Oxidative deamination (decarboxylation)	Ninhydrin, H_2O_2/Fe^{3+}, or other reagents[c]	Ammonia + aldehyde + CO_2
Racemization	Acetic anhydride	Azlactone
Peptide bond formation	NCA plus various reagents[d]	Peptides

Source: Greenstein, J.P. and M. Winitz. 1961. *Chemistry of Amino Acids*. John Wiley, New York; Meister, A. 1965. *Biochemistry of Amino Acids*. Academic Press, New York; and Ajinomoto® 2003. *Ajinomoto's Amino Acid Handbook*. Tokyo, Japan.

[a] Other reagents include 2,2-dimethoxypropane, absolute ethanol, and p-toluenesulfonic acid plus benzyl alcohol.

[b] Various reagents are used (e.g., N-butyloxy carbamate-phenylalanal, dichloroglyoxime, and imidazolin-2,4-5-trione) depending on experimental methods (Dinsmore and Beshore 2002).

[c] Other reagents include lead dioxide plus dilute sulfuric acid, sodium hypochlorite, or chloramine-T.

[d] Various reagents are used depending on experimental methods (Fridkin and Patchornik 1974).

Note: ME, 2-mercaptoethanol; NCA, N-carboxy amino acid anhydride.

1.3.6.1.1 Conjugation of the α-Amino Group of the AA with a Reagent

o-Phthalaldehyde (OPA, a nonfluorescent substance) is a reagent that reacts with primary AAs, β-AAs, and γ-AAs, as well as small peptides (e.g., alanyl-glutamine and glutathione). OPA was first chemically synthesized from α,α,α′,α′-tetrachloro-ortho-xylene by A. Colson and H. Gautier in 1887. In the 1970s, M. Roth and other chemists found that OPA reacts rapidly with a molecule containing a primary amino group at room temperature (e.g., 20°C–25°C) in the presence of 2-mercaptoethanol or 3-mercaptopropionic acid to form a highly fluorescent adduct. Proline does not react with OPA, and the reaction of cysteine or cystine with OPA is very limited. However, OPA does react readily with (1) 4-amino-1-butanol, which is produced from the oxidation of proline in the presence of chloramine-T and sodium borohydride at 60°C; and (2) S-carboxymethyl-cysteine, which is formed from cysteine in the presence of iodoacetic acid.

The OPA method is most widely used for AA analysis by high-performance liquid chromatography because of the following advantages: simple procedures for the preparation of samples, reagents, and mobile phase solutions; rapid formation of OPA derivatives and their efficient separation at room temperature (e.g., 20°C–25°C); high sensitivity of detection at picomole levels; easy automation of the instrument; few interfering side reactions; a stable chromatography baseline and accurate integration of peak areas; and rapid regeneration of guard and analytical columns. This method is suitable for the analysis of AAs in both tissues and protein hydrolysates.

As indicated previously, adequate knowledge of the chemistry of AAs is essential for studies of their biochemistry and nutrition through the development of reliable analytical methods. Some reagents react with the amino or imino group of AAs to yield stable derivatives with UV/VIS, fluorescence properties, or both (Table 1.16). This allows for direct analysis of imino acids (e.g., proline

TABLE 1.16
Reagents for Derivatization with Amino Acids (AAs) for Chromatographic Analysis via UV/VIS or Fluorescence Detection

Derivatizing Reagent	Reacting Group
(1) UV/VIS Detection	
Butylisothiocyanate (BITC)	Amino, imino, and carboxyl
Benzylisothiocyanate (BZITC)	Amino, imino, and carboxyl
4-Chloro-3,5-dinitrobenzotrifluoride (CDNBTF)	Amino, imino
4-Dimethylaminoazobenzene-4-sulfonyl chloride (DABSYL-Cl)	Amino, imino
Diethyl ethoxymethylenemalonate (DEEMM)	Amino, imino
2,4-Dinitrofluorobenzene (Sanger's reagent; DNFB)	Amino, imino
1-Fluoro-2,4-dinitrobenzene (FDNB)	Amino and imino
N,N-Diethyl-2,4-dinitro-5-fluoroaniline (FDNDEA)	Amino, imino
1-Fluoro-2-4-dinitrophenyl-5-L-alanine amide (Marfey's reagent) (FDNPAA)	Amino, imino
2,2-Dihydroxyindane-1,3-dione (ninhydrin)	Amino, imino, and carboxyl
1,2-Naphthoquinone-4-sulfonate (NQS)	Amino and imino
Copper oxide	Amino, imino, and carboxyl
4-Nitrophenylisothiocyanate (NPITC)	Amino, imino, and carboxyl
Phenylisothiocyanate (PITC)	Amino, imino, and carboxyl
(2) Fluorescence Detection	
3-(4-Carboxybenzoyl)-2-quinolinecarboxaldehyde (CBQCA)	Amino
Fluorescein-5-isothiocyanate (FITC)	Amino
9-Fluorenylmethyl chloroformate (FMOC-Cl)	Amino and imino
Fluorescamine (FRA)	Amino and imino
4-Chloro-7-nitrobenzofurazan (CNBF)[a]	Amino and imino
4-Fluoro-7-nitro-2,1,3-benzoxadiazole (NBD-F)	Amino and imino
Naphthalene-2,3-dialdehyde (NDA)[b]	Amino
o-Phthaldialdehyde (OPA)	Amino
4,7-Phenanthroline-5,6-dione (PAD)[c]	Amino
Styrene-divinylbenzene (SBD-P)	Amino and imino
(3) UV/VIS or Fluorescence Detection	
6-Aminoquinolyl-N-hydroxysuccinimidyl carbamate (AQC)	Amino and imino
4-Chloro-7-nitrobenzofurazan (CNBF)[a]	Amino and imino
1-Dimethylaminonaphthalene-5-sulfonyl chloride (Dansyl-Cl)	Amino and imino

[a] Also known as 7-chloro-4-nitrobenzo-2-oxa-1,3-diazole (NBD-Cl).
[b] Also known as naphthalene-2,3-dicarboxaldehyde (NDB).
[c] Also known as phanquinone.

and hydroxyproline) without prior opening of the pyrrolidine ring to improve detection limits and assay accuracy. Because imino acids are highly abundant as well as nutritionally and physiologically important in the animal, an ability to quantify them and all the AAs with a primary amino group is essential for the study of AA biochemistry and nutrition and to move the field forward.

The nitrogen-containing groups of certain AAs [particularly the ε-amino groups ($-NH_2$) of free and protein-bound lysine, the guanidino group of free and protein-bound arginine, and the ε-amino group of glutamine] can react with carbonyl compounds ($-HC=O$) of reducing sugars (e.g., glucose, fructose, or ribose) at elevated temperatures (e.g., >80°C) to form Amadori compounds via the Amadori rearrangement of the Schiff base. Further heating of the compounds results in the production of melanoidin polymers that give a brown color. The presence of salts in foods can accelerate the Maillard browning reaction.

1.3.6.1.2 Deamination of AAs

Removal of the α-amino group from an AA after treatment with nitrous acid to yield the corresponding hydroxy acid and nitrogen gas was recognized in the early 1910s. This reaction, known as the Van Slyke assay, was first used in 1911 by D.D. Van Slyke to determine AA concentrations. The nitrogen gas is measured by volumetric or manometric methods, and its production is directly proportional to the amount of the AA. Note that secondary AAs (e.g., proline and hydroxyproline) do not react with nitrous acid.

$$H_2N-CHR-COOH\ (AA) + HNO_2\ (Nitrous\ Acid) \rightarrow HO-CHR-COOH + N_2 + H_2O$$

An AA can undergo deamination to yield ammonia and the corresponding α-ketoacid in the presence of reactive carbonyls (e.g., alloxan, isatin, and quinones) or α-dicarbonyls (e.g., methylglyoxal and phenylglyoxal). In biology, deamination is catalyzed by D-AA deaminase (oxidase) and L-AA deaminase (oxidase). In 1909, O. Neubauer reported the deamination of α-AAs in the mammalian body. Enzyme-catalyzed deamination of AAs in animal tissues was discovered by H.A. Krebs in 1935. This biochemical reaction has important functions in neurological and immunological systems.

1.3.6.1.3 Transamination of AAs

Nonenzymatic transamination of AAs with an α-ketoacid occurs in response to heating. For example, α-aminophenyl-acetic acid ($C_6H_5CH(NH_2)COOH$) reacts with pyruvic acid in an aqueous solution to yield alanine, benzaldehyde (C_6H_5CHO), and CO_2. This chemical reaction was discovered in 1934 by R.M. Herbst and L.L. Engel, and is used to synthesize dipeptides, such as alanyl-alanine. Enzyme-catalyzed transamination of AAs is widespread in animals, plants, and microorganisms and plays an essential role in the synthesis and catabolism of many AAs.

1.3.6.1.4 Oxymethylation of AAs

In oxymethylation, the α-amino group of an AA reacts with formaldehyde to form an N-hydroxymethyl AA. This reaction was proposed by H. Schiff in 1899 and utilized in 1907 by S.P.L. Sörensen for AA analysis. In this method, excess formaldehyde is added to an AA solution, followed by titration with standard alkali to a strong red color with phenolphthalein as the indicator. It should be noted that (1) the AA must be dissolved in a colorless solution to prevent any interference of the assay; (2) cysteine, but not cystine, reacts with formaldehyde or 1,2-naphthoquinone-4-sodium sulfonate; and (3) many nitrogenous substances, including ammonia, peptides, primary amines (substances in which one hydrogen atom in ammonia is replaced by an alkyl group), nitrite, and nitrate, also react with formaldehyde. Thus, this method greatly overestimates concentrations of free AAs in animal products or tissue enzymatic hydrolysates.

$$H_2N-CHR-COOH + HCHO \rightarrow HOCH_2-NH-CHR-COOH$$

1.3.6.1.5   Keto–Enol Tautomerization and Amino–Imino Tautomerization

Keto–enol tautomerization (e.g., guanine and uric acid) or amino–imino (e.g., adenine and creatinine) tautomerization of AA metabolites spontaneously occurs in aqueous solutions due to the intramolecular migration of a hydrogen atom between the adjacent C and C groups or the adjacent C and N groups, respectively. The keto and enol forms or the amino and imino forms of substances are in chemical equilibrium. Both keto–enol and amino–imino tautomerization may occur in the same molecule (e.g., guanine or cytosine) that has both amino and carbonyl groups to increase its structural and chemical diversity (Singh et al. 2015). Tautomers are distinct chemical species and are important in AA metabolism.

$$
\underset{\text{Keto}}{-\overset{\overset{\text{O}}{\|}}{\text{C}}-\text{CH}_2-} \quad\underset{\substack{\text{Keto-Enol}\\\text{Tautomerization}}}{\rightleftharpoons}\quad \underset{\text{Enol}}{-\overset{\overset{\text{OH}}{|}}{\text{C}}=\text{CH}-} \; ; \quad \underset{\text{Amino}}{-\overset{\overset{\text{NH}_2}{|}}{\text{C}}=\text{N}-} \quad\underset{\substack{\text{Amino-Imino}\\\text{Tautomerization}}}{\rightleftharpoons}\quad \underset{\text{Imino}}{-\overset{\overset{\text{NH}}{\|}}{\text{C}}-\text{NH}-}
$$

1.3.6.2   Chemical Reactions of the Carboxyl Group in α-AAs

The carboxyl group of α-AAs is involved in several chemical reactions. These reactions include the following: amidation, decarboxylation, esterification, and reduction (Table 1.15). An example of amidation of an AA is the formation of glutamine from glutamate, whereas an example of decarboxylation of an AA is the conversion of histidine to histamine. AAs can be esterified by a base (e.g., NaOH). In addition, methyl, ethyl, and benzyl esters of many AAs can be chemically prepared using 2,2-dimethoxypropane, absolute ethanol, and p-toluenesulfonic acid plus benzyl alcohol, respectively. Esterification of an AA serves to block its α-carboxyl group from binding to undesirable substrates. Finally, α-AAs can be chemically converted into 1,2-amino alcohols. In these methods, modification of unprotected or *N*-protected α-AAs as the corresponding amino alcohols involves activation of the acid group to become an anhydride, acid fluoride, or active ester, followed by reduction with sodium borohydride. Alternatively, an AA can be reduced by sodium borohydride and iodine in tetrahydrofuran to form the corresponding alcohol.

1.3.6.3   Chemical Reactions of the Side Chain in α-AAs

The amino or carboxyl group of the side chain of α-AAs takes part in some chemical reactions. For example, the phenolic ring of tyrosine is iodinated under alkaline conditions to form iodinated tyrosine, whereas the ε-amino group of lysine and the guanidino group of arginine can participate in hydrogen bonding, methylation, and reactions with carbohydrates. The guanidination of free or protein-bound lysine with methylisourea generates homoarginine. In addition, the guanidino group of arginine, not its amino group, can react specifically with diketones. This reaction is used to determine a role for arginine residues in the stabilization of the tertiary and quaternary structure of proteins and in the allosteric and active sites of enzymes. Furthermore, the γ-amino group of asparagine can react with reducing carbohydrates, thereby providing key sites for N-linked glycosylation of proteins. Asparagine can also react with reactive carbonyls at high temperatures to generate acrylamide (a potential carcinogen), which is present in baked foods. Finally, the γ-amino group of asparagine and the ε-amino group of glutamine can undergo deamidation in the presence of an acid (e.g., 6 M HCl) at an elevated temperature (e.g., 110°C), whereas glutamine residues in proteins can be deamidated by transglutaminase I (in the presence of a primary amine) or transglutaminase II (in the presence of protein-bound lysine) to release NH_3. The transaminase-generated chemical bonds in the glutamine residues are highly resistant to proteases.

$$\text{Asparagine} + H_2O \rightarrow \text{Aspartate} + NH_4^+ \qquad (\text{heated acid})$$

$$\text{Glutamine} + H_2O \rightarrow \text{Glutamate} + NH_4^+ \qquad (\text{heated acid})$$

1.3.6.4 Chemical Reactions Involving Both the Amino and Carboxyl Groups of α-AAs

Because α-AAs contain both amino and carboxyl groups that are chemically active, they participate in some unique reactions, including chelation, cyclization, racemization, formation of N-carboxy anhydride, oxidative deamination (decarboxylation), and condensation (Table 1.15). These reactions yield AA-chelates, azlactone, diketopiperazine, N-carboxy AA anhydride (NCA), peptide bonds, and aldehyde. The structures of some products (including the copper–AA complex) generated from these reactions are illustrated as follows:

| Copper-AA chelate | Hydantoin | Azlactone | NCA | Diketopiperazine |

1.3.6.4.1 Chelation of AAs with Metals

Chelates of AAs with metals are used to efficiently supply an inorganic nutrient (e.g., Zn, Cu, and Fe) to animals. AAs have both ionizable carboxyl and amino groups, and therefore have the capacity to form metal complexes. This physicochemical property of AAs was discovered in 1854 when A. Gössmann first prepared the copper–leucine chelate. Subsequently, the copper complex of glycine in the ratio of 1:2 [(NH$_2$CH$_2$COO)$_2$Cu] was made in 1904 by mixing glycine in hot aqueous solution with an excess of copper carbonate. AA–mineral chelates are widely used as supplements in animal feeds and human food supplements (Ashmead 2012).

In the copper–glycine complex, a hydrogen atom in each glycine molecule is displaced by a single copper atom, and the metal forms coordinate covalent bonds with the amino groups of two glycine molecules. In contrast to solutions of the salts of the alkaline metals with glycine (e.g., sodium glycinate), aqueous solutions of the copper–glycine complex have virtually no conductivity (Greenstein and Winitz 1961). It is now known that only α- and β-AAs, but not γ- or δ-AAs, may form stable copper complexes and that their stability depends on the dissociation constant of the complexing nitrogen atom rather than simply the nature of the side chain. In addition to copper, α- and β-AAs can also form chelates with Ni^{2+}, Zn^{2+}, Co^{2+}, Fe^{2+}, Mn^{2+}, Mg^{2+}, and Ca^{2+} (Yamauchi et al. 2002). Examples include Zn-Met, Cu-Lys, and Mn-Gly that are now commercially available as feed additives for farm animals. For serine, threonine, and tyrosine, Ca^{2+} can form covalent bonds with all their functional groups (i.e., carboxyl, amino, and hydroxyl groups).

1.3.6.4.2 Esterification and N^α-dehydrogenation of α-AAs

An example for esterification and N^α-dehydrogenation of an α-AA is the chemical synthesis of lauric arginate (ethyl-N^α-lauroyl-L-arginate hydrochloride) from L-arginine monohydrochloride, ethanol, and lauroyl chloride (Ma et al. 2020). This reaction is initiated by thionyl chloride (SOCl$_2$)-catalyzed esterification of the carboxyl group of L-arginine hydrochloride with ethanol in the presence of a base (NaOH) to form ethyl arginine dihydrochloride, followed by its condensation with lauroyl chloride to finally yield lauric arginate. This substance is a novel cationic surfactant that has a potent antimicrobial effect. Thus, lauric arginate (e.g., 200 ppm) is now used as a safe preservative by the food and beverage industries. It may also be a useful feed additive to diets for animals (e.g., weanling pigs) to improve intestinal health and the efficiency of nutrient utilization.

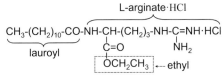

Ethyl-N^α-lauroyl-L-arginate hydrochloride

1.3.6.4.3   Oxidative Deamination (Decarboxylation) of AAs

Oxidative deamination (decarboxylation) of an AA to form ammonia, CO_2, and aldehyde in response to a mixture of lead dioxide and dilute sulfuric acid was first recognized by J. von Liebig in 1849. Such a reaction also occurs when AAs are treated with sodium hypochlorite or chloramine-T. The formation of the aldehyde is specific to the AAs under consideration, whereas ammonia and CO_2 is generated nonspecifically from all AAs. Another well-utilized oxidative deamination (decarboxylation) of an AA is its reaction with ninhydrin to yield colored products. This chemical reaction was discovered by S. Ruhemann in 1911, and its chemistry is very complex. First, an AA reacts with ninhydrin to form an intermediate amine, the corresponding aldehyde, carbon dioxide, and ammonia. Interestingly, the initial products vary with AAs. For example, the reaction of aspartate or cystine with ninhydrin yields 2 moles of CO_2, but the reaction of proline and hydroxyproline with ninhydrin does not generate ammonia. Second, the intermediate amine reacts with ninhydrin to yield indandione-2-N-2'-indanone enolate (Ruhemann's purple), hydrindantin (which can be detected by UV absorption), and ammonia. Third, hydrindantin reacts with ammonia to form Ruhemann's purple (blue-violet color with maximum absorption at 570 nm). Additionally, ammonia reacts with ninhydrin and the reduced ninhydrin to yield Ruhemann's purple. Overall, only the N atom of this pigment arises from α-AAs. Results of paper chromatography reveal that the reaction of proline or hydroxyproline with ninhydrin gives a yellow-colored product (maximum absorption at 440 nm), whereas a purple-blue color is formed with other AAs. In addition to AAs and ammonia, peptides can also react with ninhydrin to yield color products. To date, ninhydrin is used as a post-column derivatizing reagent to analyze AAs by ion-exchange chromatography.

$$\text{Ninhydrin} + \text{Amino acid} \rightarrow \text{RCHO}\left(\text{Aldehyde}\right) + CO_2 + H_2O + \text{Ruhemann's purple}$$

1.3.6.4.4   Condensation

At high temperatures, either two AAs or one AA and one AA metabolite can be condensed via a covalent single bond (not a peptide bond) to form a new AA through chemical reactions of their side chains. Such condensation does not involve the formation of a peptide bond. For example, heat and alkaline treatment of foods (e.g., temperature $\geq 60°C$; $pH \geq 10.5$) for 60 min results in the formation of (1) lanthionine and lysinoalanine from cystine plus cysteine and cysteine (or serine) plus lysine, respectively; and (2) 3-methyl-lanthionine and 3-methyl-lysinoalanine from threonine plus cysteine and threonine plus lysine, respectively (Figure 1.8). Other products include (1) ornithinoalanine formed from ornithine and alanine; (2) N-τ-histidinoalanine and N-π-histidinoalanine formed from histidine and alanine (e.g., the ratio of the N^τ- to the N^π-isomers in heated milk proteins being 8:1); and (3) phenylethylaminoalanine formed from β-phenylethylamine (a product of L-phenylalanine decarboxylation catalyzed by phenylalanine decarboxylase) and alanine (Figure 1.9). Such reactions, which also occur in peptide-bound lysine, threonine, serine, and cysteine, can reduce protein quality, because these AA derivatives are not hydrolyzed by any enzymes and have no nutritional value to animals. These chemical transformations are favored by high pH, high temperature, and prolonged exposure time, and the generation of lysinoalanine is reduced by the presence of SH-containing AAs, sodium sulfite, ascorbic acid, citric acid, and malic acid (Friedman 1999b).

  Lanthionine, lysinoalanine, and histidinoalanine occur naturally in some peptide antibiotics (produced by certain bacteria; widely used in food preservation; McAuliffe et al. 2001), as well as animal tissues (e.g., aorta, bone, dentin, and eyes with cataracts) and collagen proteins possibly due to the aging process (Friedman 1999b; Kanayama et al. 1987). Such peptide antibiotics (known as lantibiotics) include cinnamycin (a 19-AA tetracyclic polypeptide containing 3-methyl-lanthionine, lanthionine, and lysinoalanine that is produced by *Streptomyces cinnamoneus*); duramycin (a 19-AA tetracyclic polypeptide containing lanthionine and methyllanthionine that is produced by *Streptoverticillium cinnamoneus*); epidermin (a 21-AA heterodetic tetracyclic polypeptide containing lanthionine and methyllanthionine that is produced, as a sequence in a precursor protein, by *Staphylococcus epidermidis*); nisin (a 34-AA cationic polycyclic polypeptide

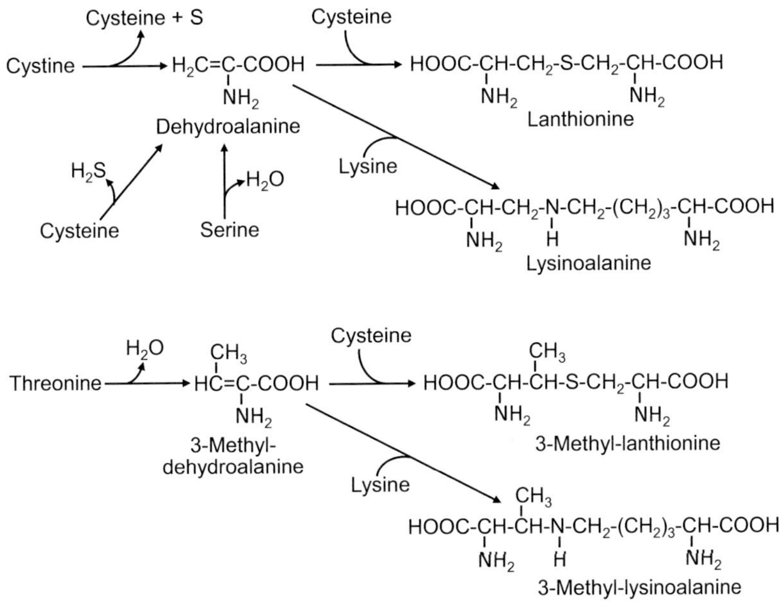

FIGURE 1.8 Formation of lanthionine, lysinoalanine, 3-methyl-lanthionine, and 3-methyl-lysinoalanine from free and peptide-bound amino acids after heat and alkaline treatment. Various amounts of these products commonly occur in proteins of foods processed under these conditions. Note that lanthionine and lysinoalanine occur naturally in certain peptide and antibiotics, as well as animal tissues (e.g., aorta, bone, dentin, and eyes with cataracts) and collagen proteins possibly due to the aging process.

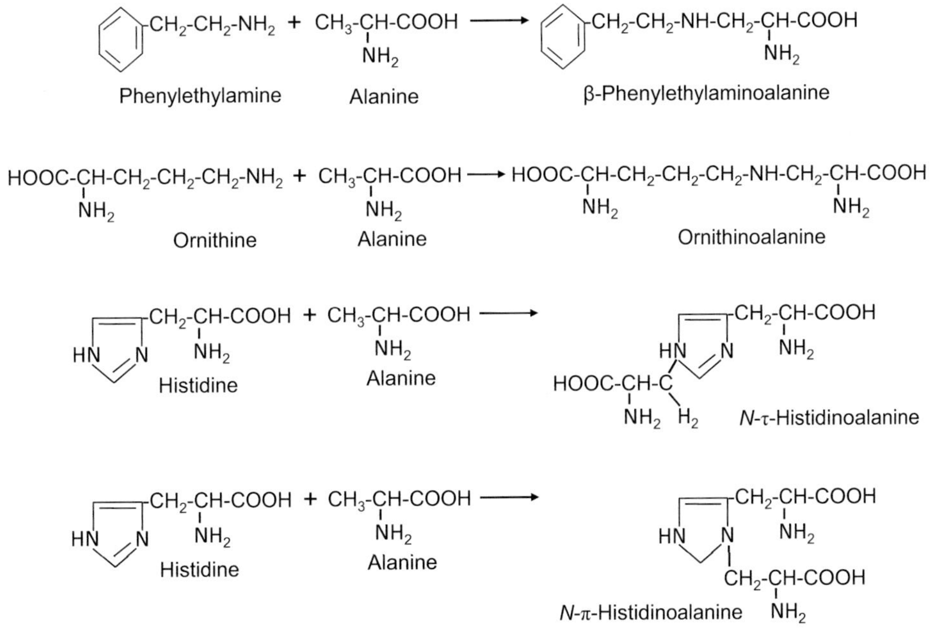

FIGURE 1.9 Formation of ornithinoalanine, histidinoalanine, and phenylethylaminoalanine from free and peptide-bound amino acids after heat and alkaline treatment. Various amounts of these products commonly occur in proteins of foods processed under these conditions. β-Phenylethylamine is a product of L-phenylalanine decarboxylation by phenylalanine decarboxylase. Note that histidinoalanine is present in animal tissues (e.g., aorta, bone, dentin, and eyes with cataracts) and collagen proteins possibly due to the aging process.

containing lanthionine, methyllanthionine, and didehydroalanine that is produced by *Streptococcus lactis*); and subtilin (a 32-AA cationic polypeptide containing lanthionine, 3-methyl-lanthionine, and dehydroalanine that is produced, as a sequence in a 56-AA precursor polypeptide, by *Bacillus subtilis*). The ratio of the N^τ- to the N^π-histidinoalanine in the calcium-binding phosphoproteins of the extrapallial fluid of certain bivalve mollusks is 3:1. Of note, the content of histidinoalanine in diseased eye lens (3.35 nmol/mg) is 66 times greater than that in normal eye lens (0.05 nmol/mg). In microbes and animal cells, the condensation of either two AAs or one AA and an AA metabolite may occur spontaneously at a very slow rate or catalyzed enzymatically (e.g., enzyme-catalyzed posttranslational modifications of proteins).

1.3.6.4.5 Peptide Synthesis

A carboxyl group of one AA can react with the amino group of another AA to form a peptide bond (–CONH–) with the loss of one molecule of H_2O (Figure 1.10). In 1907, E. Fischer synthesized a polypeptide of 18 AAs. N-Carboxy AA anhydride is an important activated derivative of AAs for the chemical synthesis of small peptides and proteins (Marglin and Merrifield 1970). Liquid-phase peptide synthesis is a classical method for peptide formation and is useful for large-scale production of peptides for industrial purposes. Solid-phase peptide synthesis, which was pioneered by R.B. Merrifield in 1963, is now widely used to synthesize peptides and proteins in the laboratory (Agouridas et al. 2020). The chemical synthesis of peptides proceeds in a C-terminal-to-N-terminal manner, with the N-termini being protected by either t-butyloxy carbamate (t-BOC) or 9-fluorenylmethyl chloroformate (FMOC-Cl). In general, peptides (e.g., glycyl-glutamine and alanyl-glutamine) consisting of either stable or unstable AAs are chemically stable in an aqueous solution at or below physiological temperatures (e.g., 37°C in mammals and 40°C in birds). This property of peptides is useful for their use in total parenteral nutrition, clinical therapy, and laboratory research.

Humans and other animals synthesize peptides (e.g., carnosine) from some AAs (including non-proteinogenic AAs), such as L-histidine and β-alanine, via non-ribosomal and non-mitochondrial peptide synthetases (e.g., carnosine synthetase). Peptide synthesis also occurs in microbes and plants. Peptides can be classified according to the number of their AA residues. An oligopeptide (oligo-, "few") consists of 2–20 AA residues. An oligopeptide containing ≤10 AA residues is also called a small peptide or small oligopeptide. An oligopeptide containing 11–20 AA residues is called a large peptide or large oligopeptide. A peptide that consists of ≥21 AA residues and does not have a three-dimensional structure is designated as a polypeptide. An example of a polypeptide is the β-amyloid peptide (involved in Alzheimer's disease) that contains approximately 40 AA residues. Some natural substances with nontypical peptide bonds [e.g., glutathione and N-pteroyl-L-glutamate (folate)] are beneficial for nutrition and physiology, whereas others [e.g., ergovaline (present in endophyte-infected Tall fescue – a cool-season grass) and phalloidine] are toxic to humans and other animals.

Peptide bond

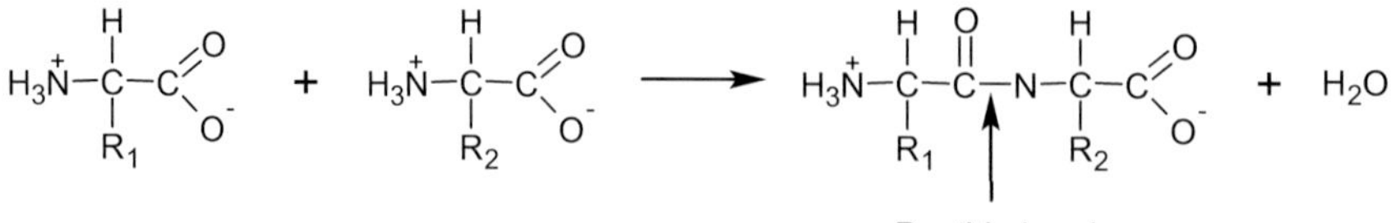

FIGURE 1.10 Synthesis of a dipeptide from two amino acids (AAs). R1 and R2 represent the side chains of the two AAs. With the loss of one H_2O molecule (one "H" atom from the α-amino group of an AA and the "–OH" from the carboxyl group of the other AA), a peptide bond (–CONH–) is formed. This reaction is used to produce peptides through chemical manufacturing and is catalyzed by enzymes in animal cells. Peptides are generally stable in an aqueous solution.

1.3.7 PROTEINS

In 1787, A.F. Fourcroy and colleagues recognized proteins [e.g., albumin (from egg whites and blood serum), fibrin, and wheat gluten] as a distinct class of biological molecules that can coagulate under heating or acid treatments. In 1838, the chemical composition (carbon, hydrogen, nitrogen, oxygen, phosphorus, and sulfur) of proteins (coined by J.J. Berzelius, a Swedish physician-chemist) was described by G.J. Mulder (a Dutch chemist) to be remarkably similar. The word protein originated from the Greek "proteios", meaning prime or primary. This is very appropriate, since proteins were then recognized by most scientists (e.g., Carl von Voit) to be the most fundamental component of tissues in animals, including humans. In 1840, J. von Liebig correctly proposed that proteins were made up of AAs. Over the past century, advanced physicochemical techniques aided in the determination of protein composition and structure (Hackenberger et al. 2020). A protein is a high-molecular-weight molecule consisting of α-AAs linked via peptide bonds and has a distinct three-dimensional structure (Jones 2012). A protein consists of one or more polypeptides. Nitrogen content in animal and food proteins ranges from 13% to 19%.

Proteins can be chemically synthesized like peptides. Humans and other animals have the machinery (including tRNA, mRNA, and enzymes) to synthesize proteins from AAs, including insulin, actin, myosin, hemoglobin, myoglobin, and collagen (see Chapter 8). Some proteins are hydrophilic, whereas some are hydrophobic. The largest and most abundant protein in animals is collagen. The healthy 70-kg adult human contains 15.1% protein (or 10.6 kg protein), including 3.72 kg collagen (Wu 2020b). The number of different proteins has been estimated to be approximately 100,000 in an animal and up to 50,000 in a plant (Sterck et al. 2007).

1.3.7.1 Determination of Protein Concentration

The acid and alkaline hydrolysis of protein yields free AAs, which are analyzed by an AA analyzer or using a chromatographic method (Lubec and Rosenthal 1990; Wu 1993). The molecular weights of AA residues (i.e., the molecular weights of an intact AA – 18) are used to calculate the amount of peptide-bound AAs. Alternatively, concentrations of proteins can be rapidly determined based on their interactions with specific reagents to generate colored substances, whose optical density is measured by a UV/VIS instrument (Markwell et al. 1978; Tal et al. 1985).

1.3.7.1.1 The Coomassie Brilliant Blue Dye

The Coomassie Brilliant Blue dye binds to proteins or large peptides (> 30 AA residues) under acidic conditions through (1) electrostatic interaction with protonated basic AAs (arginine, lysine, and histidine) and (2) hydrophobic associations with aromatic residues (e.g., phenylalanine and tyrosine). These reactions result in a spectral shift, such that the color of the Coomassie solution changes from brown (absorbance maximum 465 nm) to blue (absorbance maximum 610 nm). The change in color density is read at 595 nm and is proportional to the protein concentration in the solution. This method is very useful in protein identification and quantification (e.g., proteomics), but the Coomassie dye interacts differently with different proteins (Tal et al. 1985). Note that free AAs or peptides with <30 AAs do not react with the Coomassie dye reagents. A modified version of this method (Bradford 1976) does not suffer from interference with by Krebs–Henseleit bicarbonate buffer and, therefore, is suitable for determining protein concentrations in cell extracts and intact cells.

1.3.7.1.2 The Biuret Assay (the Piotrowski' Test)

Under alkaline conditions, the nitrogen atoms of two or more peptide bonds in proteins or polypeptides chelate with cupric (Cu^{2+}) ions in the reagent (9 g sodium potassium tartrate, 3 g copper sulfate·5 H_2O, and 5 g potassium iodide, all dissolved in order in 400 ml of 0.2 M NaOH, followed by the addition of water to a final volume of 1 L). This results in the reduction of Cu^{2+} to Cu^+ and the formation of a purple complex. The intensity of the color produced is stable and proportional to protein and peptide concentration in the solution. Free AAs do not interfere with the Biuret assay, and therefore, it is particularly useful for diluted whole tissue samples. However,

Tris and ammonia do interfere with this assay and, therefore, it should not be used for the analysis of protein in samples containing Tris buffer or a significant amount of ammonia (e.g., protein samples purified from ammonium sulfate precipitation). Note that the bicinchoninic acid (BCA) method, a modification of the Biuret assay, was developed to overcome the latter's shortcomings (Smith et al. 1985).

1.3.7.1.3 The Lowry Assay

The Lowry assay combines the reactions of copper ions with the nitrogen atoms of peptide bonds under alkaline conditions (the Biuret test), as well as the chemical oxidation of aromatic AA (phenylalanine, tryptophan, and tyrosine) and cysteine residues in proteins. This leads to the reduction of cupric ions (Cu^{2+}) to cuprous ions (Cu^+). The Cu^+ ions then react with the Folin–Ciocalteu reagent (phosphomolybdic/phosphotungstic acid) to produce a blue color that can be read at 650–750 nm. The blue color of the solution is intensified by the oxidation of aromatic AA residues in proteins and peptides. The color produced is stable and its intensity is proportional to the number of peptide bonds (Lowry et al. 1953). A modified version of this method does not suffer from interference with sucrose or EDTA (Markwell et al. 1978). Because the content of aromatic AAs and cysteine in proteins can affect the color intensity of the assay solution, the Lowry method may yield different results for the same quantity of animal and plant protein with different amounts of these four AAs.

1.3.7.2 Proteins versus Peptides

1.3.7.2.1 Distinctions between Peptides and Proteins

As noted previously, a peptide consists of two or more AA residues linked by peptide bonds, whereas a protein consists of one or more polypeptides. The dividing line between proteins and polypeptides is usually their molecular weight. Generally speaking, polypeptides with molecular weight greater than 8,000 (i.e., approximately 72 AA residues) are considered to be proteins. For example, growth hormone has 191 AAs with a molecular weight of ~22 kDa. Polypeptides with a molecular weight less than 8 kDa are considered to be peptides. Glucagon has 29 AA residues with a molecular weight of ~3,500 Da and is a polypeptide. However, this division between proteins and peptides on the basis of molecular weight is not absolute. For example, ubiquitin has 72 AA residues and a well-defined three-dimensional structure and, therefore, is a small protein. In addition, insulin (MW = ~5,700 Da) has 51 AA residues (20 in chain A and 31 in chain B) and a defined three-dimensional structure and, thus, is well recognized as a protein. The forces that contribute to the folded state of a protein include the hydrophobic effect, disulfide bond (-S-S-) formation, ionic interactions, hydrogen bonds, and van der Waals interactions. The formation and breakage of disulfide bonds between cysteine residues within proteins are catalyzed by protein disulfide isomerase, which localizes in the endoplasmic reticulum of eukaryotes and in the periplasm of bacteria. Not all proteinogenic AAs appear in proteins. For example, tryptophan is absent from insulin and all known collagen proteins, whereas cysteine/cystine is absent from type I collagen.

1.3.7.2.2 Separation of Peptides from Proteins

Peptides, like free AAs, are soluble in trichloroacetic acid (TCA; at a final concentration of 5%), perchloric acid ($HClO_4$, PCA; at a final concentration of 0.2 M), and 80% methanol, but these solutions precipitate proteins in animal cells and fluids (Li and Wu 2020; Moughan et al. 1990). Tungstic acid (1%) can precipitate small peptides consisting of ≥4 AA residues. Thus, PCA or TCA can be used along with tungstic acid to distinguish small and large peptides. Certain plant proteins with high proline content (e.g., zein, glidin, and hordein), which are called prolamines, are soluble in 70%–80% ethanol but insoluble in water or 100% ethanol. Furthermore, ammonium sulfate (e.g., at a final concentration of 35%) can precipitate proteins from a solution without altering their biological structure.

1.3.7.2.3 Extracellular Matrix Proteins and Glycosaminoglycans

The most abundant and largest proteins in swine, sheep, and chickens are collagens in the extracellular matrix, which account for approximately 29% and 35% of the total body protein at birth and in adult life, respectively (Li and Wu 2018). There are approximately 20 different types of collagen in the animal kingdom. Each mature collagen contains three polypeptide chains (called α chains) (Table 1.17), which may be the same or different and are organized in a triple-helical structure. In type I, II, and III collagens, each polypeptide is 300 nm long (corresponding to about 1000 AA residues). For example, in type I collagen, each of the two identical α1(I) chains consists of 1056 AA residues. The collagen molecules pack together side by side through an interchain cross-link between allysine residues formed by the extracellular lysyl oxidase to confer the strength, rigidity, and flexibility of connective tissue.

Interestingly, there is a Glycine–X–Y repeat in collagens, with proline being in the X or Y position but hydroxyproline only in the Y position. Thus, the collagen contains two dominant motifs: Glycine-Proline-X and Glycine-X-hydroxyproline, where X is any AA other than glycine, proline, or 4-hydroxyproline. On the molar basis, mammalian collagens contain approximately 1/3 glycine, 0.7/3 proline plus 4-hydroxyproline, and 1.3/3 other AAs (Table 1.18). In humans, collagen consists of 13.0 proline, 9.01 4-hydroxyproline, 0.09 3-hydroxyproline, and 33 glycine residues per 100 AA residues (or 13.3 g proline, 10.73 g 4-hydroxyproline, 0.11 g 3-hydroxyproline, and 25.8 g glycine residues per 100 g collagen) (Devlin 2006). On the gram basis, glycine, proline plus 4-hydroxyproline residues account for 20.7% and 24.5% of mammalian collagens, respectively (Table 1.19). Bone and skin collagens in bony fish (Actinopterygii) and cartilaginous fish (Elasmobranchii) contain slightly more glycine but substantially less proline and 4-hydroxyproline than those in mammals (Szpak, 2011). Thus, the content of 4-hydroxyproline in a collage product can be used to identify whether the product is derived from mammals or fish.

Based on the content of 4-hydroxyproline residue in bone or skin collagen (Table 1.20), an amount of this AA or the percentage of collagens in the total proteins in animals, tissues, and foods can be calculated as the content of protein-bound 4-hydroxyproline in an analyzed sample tissue (i.e., g/100 g tissue × 0.863 × the content of 4-hydroxyproline residue in collagens) (Table 1.21).

TABLE 1.17
The Major Types of Collagen in Animals[a]

Type	Composition	Arrangement	Representative Tissues
I	2 α1(I) chains + 1 α2(I) chain	Fibrils	Bone, dentin, interstitial tissues, ligaments, skin, and tendon
II	3 α1(II) chains	Fibrils	Cartilage and vitreous humor (eyeball)
III	3 α1(III) chains	Fibrils	Blood vessels, skeletal muscle, heart, and skin
IV	2 α1(IV) chains + 1 α2(IV) chain	Two-dimensional network	All basal laminae in tissues
V	3 α1(V) chains	Fibrils with GD	Bone, dentin, interstitial tissues, ligaments, skin, and tendon
VI	α1(VI) + α2(VI) + α3(VI) chains	Associated with type I collagen	Mainly extracellular matrix of skeletal muscle
IX	α1(IX) + α2(IX) + α3(IX) chains	Associated with type II collagen	Cartilage and vitreous humor (eyeball)

Source: Li, P. and G. Wu. 2018. *Amino Acids* 50:29-38.

[a] Individual α chains are identified by the following nomenclature: $\alpha n(N)_p$, where n is the identification number of the α chain, N is the collagen type, and *p* is the number of the polypeptide. For example, $\alpha 1(I)_2 \alpha 2(I)$ denotes a heterotrimer of type I collagen consisting of two identical α1 chains and one distinct α2 chain, whereas $[\alpha 1(II)]_3$ indicates three identical α1 chains of type II collagen.

Note: GD, globular N-terminal domain.

TABLE 1.18

Composition of Amino Acids (AAs) and Sugars in Collagens (AA or Sugar Residues/1,000 AA Residues)

Amino Acid	Type I		Type II	Type III	Type IV		Type V			Type VI			Type VII
	α1	α2	α1	α1	α1	α2	α1	α2	α3	α1	α2	α3	α1
Alanine	119	105	108	95	30	47	46	52	49	50	44	35	64
Arginine	49	51	52	48	22	42	45	50	42	59	68	83	48
Asp + Asn	46	45	36	42	45	50	50	51	42	87	81	85	51
Cysteine	0	0	0	2	2	3	0	0	1.3	10	6	14	6.7
Glu + Gln	77	70	95	71	88	64	91	84	98	119	108	110	105
Glycine	330	331	334	351	324	328	344	341	332	323	298	328	307
Histidine	4	10	2	6	6	7	8	11	14	7	9	11	3.1
5-OH-Lysine	10	12	18	6	49	39	35	24	43	57	67	47	41
3-OH-Proline	1.1	1.2	1.1	0	1	1	2.9	2.5	2.2	NR	NR	NR	0.1
4-OH-Proline	114	105	96	126	118	107	109	109	92	78	71	52	84
Isoleucine	8	16	11	13	32	39	19	16	20	15	20	27	10.5
Leucine	20	33	27	23	50	56	39	35	56	21	30	23	49
Lysine	27	20	20	29	7	5	20	18	15	8	17	19	18
Methionine	7	8	11	8	14	14	8	11	8.1	10	5	4	7.6
Phenylalanine	13	11	13	8	28	36	12	14	9.2	16	14	14	9.8
Proline	118	114	106	107	88	73	118	97	99	89	101	89	81
Serine	35	30	27	38	36	30	36	31	34	24	27	27	49
Threonine	18	18	22	13	20	28	19	26	19	14	16	19	26
Tryptophan	0	0	0	0	0	0	0	0	0	0	0	0	0
Tyrosine	2	3	1	3	8	6	2	2	2.4	15	10	11	28
Valine	19	35	19	15	32	25	25	24	29	18	19	20	35
Glucose	1	1	5	1	43	NR	18	10	17	NR	NR	NR	NR
Galactose	1	2	10	2	45	NR	30	14	24	NR	NR	NR	NR

Source: Burgeson, R.E. and N.P. Morris. 1987. In: *Connective Tissue Disease: Molecular Pathology of the Extracellular Matrix* (Uitto, J. and A.J. Perejda, eds.). Marcel Dekker Inc., New York, pp. 3–28, for all types of collagen except type VI; Chu, M.L., K. Mann, R. Deutzmann, D. Pribula-Conway, C.C. Hsu-Chen, M.P. Bernard, and R. Timpl. 1987. *Eur. J. Biochem.* 168:309–317, for the composition of all amino acids in type VI collagen, except cysteine and methionine; and Jander, R., J. Rauterberg, and R.W. Glanville. 1983. *Eur. J. Biochem.* 133:39–46, for the composition of cysteine and methionine in type VI collagen.

Note: 5-OH-Lysine, 5-hydroxylysine; 3-OH-Proline, 3-hydroxyproline; 4-OH-Proline, 4-hydroxyproline; NR, not reported.

Likewise, when foods are hydrolyzed by enzymes or some other means, the collagen proteins are degraded to yield peptides containing 4-hydroxyproline, and the content of this 4-hydroxyproline can be used to calculate the amount of the hydrolyzed collagens (Table 1.21). Let use the 30-day-old piglet as an example for the calculations.

1. Content of 4-hydroxyproline (based on intact MW) in the protein sample of the whole-body homogenate of a 30-day-old pig (A) = 0.433 g/100 g sample;
2. Content of 4-hydroxyproline residue in collagen (B) = 11.7 g/100 g collagen;
   Content of true protein in the sample of the whole-body homogenate of a 30-day-old pig (C) = 12.0 g/ 100 g sample;
3. Content of collagen in the piglet body (g/100 g; D) = A × 0.863 × 100/B = 0.433 × 100/11.7 = 3.70;
4. % of collagen in the total protein of the piglet body (g/g) = D × 100/C = 3.70 × 100/12.0 = 30.8.

TABLE 1.19

Composition of Amino Acids (AAs) in Mammalian and Fish Collagens (AA Residues/1,000 AA Residues)

	Bone			Skin		
Amino Acid	Mammalia (*n* = 23)	Bony Fish (*Actinopterygii*) (*n* = 12)	Cartilaginous Fish (*Elasmobranchii*) (*n* = 2)	Mammalia (*n* = 34)	Bony Fish (*Actinopterygii*) (*n* = 92)	Cartilaginous Fish (*Elasmobranchii*) (*n* = 17)
Alanine	115	119	117	109	114	114
Arginine	49	50	50	49	52	50
Asp + Asn	48	46	42	47	47	45
Cysteine	Trace	Trace	Trace	Trace	Trace	Trace
Glu + Gln	75	73	79	74	76	77
Glycine	330	343	339	329	339	332
Histidine	5	7	7	5	7	8
5-OH-Lysine	6	9	7	6	8	6
4-OH-Proline	95	72	77	95	67	74
Isoleucine	11	10	15	11	11	17
Leucine	26	22	21	24	23	23
Lysine	26	27	27	29	26	25
Methionine	4	13	11	6	13	13
Phenylalanine	14	14	14	13	14	12
Proline	119	105	97	126	108	109
Serine	35	42	44	36	46	46
Threonine	19	26	30	19	26	24
Tryptophan	0	0	0	0	0	0
Tyrosine	3	3	3	3	3	3
Valine	23	18	23	22	21	24
% of Nitrogen	15.3	15.5	15.4	15.3	15.5	15.4

Source: Szpak, P. 2011. *J. Archaeolog. Sci.* 38:3358–3372.
Note: 5-OH-Lysine, 5-hydroxylysine; 4-OH-Proline, 4-hydroxyproline.

In addition to mature collagens, mature elastin, glycosaminoglycans, and proteoglycans are also present in the extracellular matrix of connective tissue. Collagens and elastins are insoluble in water or strong alkaline solutions (e.g., 0.3 M NaOH), whereas glycosaminoglycans and proteoglycans are highly soluble in water or strong alkaline solutions. Elastin is about 1,000 times more flexible than collagens, and therefore, the main function of elastin is to maintain the elasticity of tissues. The composition of AAs in collagens (Table 1.18) and elastins (Table 1.22) is very different than that in non-collagen proteins. Note that the content of most AAs (including BCAAs, glutamate, glutamine, and lysine) in the various types of collagens (Table 1.18) and elastins (Table 1.22) is much lower than that in non-collagen proteins. For example, assuming leucine residue (the intact molecule – 18) accounts for 3.1% of the collagens in the whole-body of 30-day-old pigs and the body protein contains 6.93% leucine residue, the content of leucine residue in the non-collagen proteins of the body can be calculated to be 8.7%.

$3.1\% \times 0.308 + \chi \times 0.692 = 6.93\%$, where χ is the content (%) of leucine in non-collagen proteins.

$$\chi = (6.93\% - 3.1\% \times 0.308)/0.692 = 8.6\%.$$

TABLE 1.20

Amounts of Amino Acids (AAs) in Mammalian and Fish Collagens (g of AA Residue/100 g Collagen)[a]

Amino Acid	Bone			Skin		
	Mammalia ($n = 23$)	Bony Fish (*Actinopterygii*) ($n = 12$)	Cartilaginous Fish (*Elasmobranchii*) ($n = 2$)	Mammalia ($n = 34$)	Bony Fish (*Actinopterygii*) ($n = 92$)	Cartilaginous Fish (*Elasmobranchii*) ($n = 17$)
Alanine	8.93	9.34	9.11	8.44	8.89	8.86
Arginine	8.36	8.62	8.55	8.34	8.91	8.54
Asp + Asn	6.01	5.82	5.27	5.87	5.91	5.64
Cysteine	Trace	Trace	Trace	Trace	Trace	Trace
Glu + Gln	10.61	10.44	11.21	10.45	10.81	10.92
Glycine	20.56	21.61	21.19	20.45	21.23	20.72
Histidine	0.75	1.06	1.05	0.75	1.05	1.20
5-OH-Lysine	0.94	1.43	1.11	0.94	1.27	0.95
4-OH-Proline	11.73	8.99	9.54	11.71	8.32	9.16
Isoleucine	1.36	1.25	1.86	1.36	1.37	2.10
Leucine	3.21	2.75	2.60	2.96	2.86	2.85
Lysine	3.64	3.82	3.79	4.05	3.66	3.51
Methionine	0.57	1.88	1.58	0.86	1.87	1.87
Phenylalanine	2.25	2.27	2.26	2.08	2.26	1.93
Proline	12.62	11.26	10.32	13.33	11.51	11.58
Serine	3.33	4.04	4.20	3.42	4.40	4.38
Threonine	2.10	2.90	3.32	2.09	2.88	2.65
Tryptophan	0.00	0.00	0.00	0.00	0.00	0.00
Tyrosine	0.53	0.54	0.54	0.53	0.54	0.54
Valine	2.49	1.97	2.50	2.38	2.28	2.60

[a] Calculated on the basis of data in Table 1.19 and the molecular weights of amino acid residues.

Note: 5-OH-Lysine, 5-hydroxylysine; 4-OH-Proline, 4-hydroxyproline.

1.3.7.2.4   Myofibrillar Proteins

Actin and myosin are major intracellular proteins to form myofibrils along and regulatory proteins (e.g., tropomyosin, troponin, and actinin) in most animal cells (e.g., skeletal, cardiac, and smooth muscles). For example, actin and myosin comprise 65% and 2%–10% of the total cellular proteins in skeletal muscle and non-muscle cells, respectively (Rennie and Tipton 2000). Myofibrillar proteins are soluble in concentrated saline and extremely low-ionic-strength solutions, as well as strong alkaline solutions (e.g., 0.3 M NaOH), but are insoluble in typical physiological fluids. Actin has three α-isoforms (e.g., in the muscles), as well as β- and γ-isoforms (e.g., in both muscle and non-muscle cells). The actin isoforms differ by only a few AA residues and undergo posttranslational modifications (e.g., the methylation of His-73 of skeletal muscle α-actin to form 3-methyl-histidine). Of interest, actin can exist in monomeric globular (G-actin) and filamentous (F-actin) states. Myosin consists of six polypeptides: two heavy chains and two pairs of different light chains (essential light chains and regulatory light chains). Interestingly, both myosin and F-actin possess ATPase activity. In the resting state, actin and myosin filaments partially overlap each other in an interdigitating manner. When muscle contracts, the actin and the myosin slide past each other, with the required energy being provided through ATP hydrolysis. Besides contraction, actin and myosin also have other biological activities, such as cell motility, division, signaling, and organelle movement, as well as the maintenance of cell cytoskeleton and shape. Actin and myosin can be obtained from

TABLE 1.21

Content of Free, Peptide-Bound, and Protein-Bound Amino Acids, and Collagens in Animal- and Plant-Derived Feedstuffs (As-Fed Basis)[a]

| Sample | Total Amino Acids | Total Free Amino Acids | Amino Acids in Peptides and Proteins | | | Collagens | | |
			Total	Peptides	Proteins	Total	Partial Hydrolysates in Peptides	Proteins
Animal-Sourced Feedstuffs								
BSFM[b]	503.8	15.8	487.9	39.6	448.3	103.7	5.56	98.1
CBPM[b]	685.6	7.28	678.3	96.2	582.1	157.4	11.2	146.2
CVD[b]	798.3	60.9	737.4	459.0	278.4	132.8	117.0	15.8
Feather meal[b]	924.6	4.37	920.3	39.1	881.2	424.2	14.4	409.8
FM-M[c]	601.8	13.2	588.6	77.4	511.1	178.6	32.2	146.4
FM-P[c]	665.2	32.5	632.7	71.4	561.3	204.0	17.7	186.3
FM-SE[c]	703.6	48.1	655.5	131.6	523.8	213.1	64.8	148.3
SDPM[b]	590.0	232.2	357.8	180.1	177.7	45.7	28.7	17.0
PBM (PFG)[b]	642.0	14.7	627.3	78.7	548.6	191.3	11.7	179.6
SDPP[b]	864.0	10.3	853.7	49.7	804.0	1.47	0.02	1.45
SDEP[b]	630.1	2.35	627.7	52.5	575.2	1.89	0.01	1.88
Plant-Sourced Feedstuffs								
Algae SM	775.1	8.01	767.1	54.1	712.9	0.0	0.0	0.0
SBM	443.9	4.25	439.7	32.3	407.4	0.0	0.0	0.0
SPC	800.6	2.81	797.8	21.9	775.9	0.0	0.0	0.0

Source: Li, P. and G. Wu. 2020. *Amino Acids* 52:523–542.

[a] All values are expressed as g/kg feed. The content of collagen in the feedstuffs was calculated on the basis of their content of 4-hydroxyproline.

[b] The amount of collagens in the feedstuff from terrestrial animals was calculated as the content of 4-hydroxyproline in proteins or peptides (g/kg feed) × 100/11.7.

[c] The amount of collagens in the feedstuff from fish was calculated as the content of 4-hydroxyproline in proteins or peptides (g/kg feed) × 100/8.7.

Note: BSFM, black soldier fly larvae meal; CBPM, chicken by-product meal; CVD, chicken visceral digest; FM-M, fishmeal (United States Menhaden); FM-P, *fishmeal* (Peruvian anchovy); FM-SE, fishmeal (Southeast Asian miscellaneous marine fishes); Hyp, 4-hydroxyproline; PBM (PFG), poultry by-product meal (pet-food grade); PCA, perchloric acid; SBM, soybean meal; SDEP, spray-dried egg product; SDPM, spray-dried peptone from enzyme-treated porcine mucosal tissues; SDPP, spray-dried poultry plasma; SM, spirulina meal; SPC, soy protein concentrate.

the muscles by a technique involving homogenization in saline or buffer, the centrifugation of the homogenate to collect the myofibrillar pellets, their solubilization in 0.3 M NaOH and centrifugation to remove insoluble collagens, and the precipitation of myofibrillar proteins with 1.5 M PCA (Wilkinson et al. 2015). This basic method is very useful for studying the turnover of different proteins and, therefore, AA metabolism in skeletal, cardiac, and smooth muscles.

1.4 SUMMARY

AAs are unique organic substances widely present in nature. The history of their discoveries dates back to over 200 years ago when chemists identified AAs as components of protein and non-protein extracts. All proteinogenic AAs except glycine can have both L- and D-isomers. L-AAs are generally the most abundant physiological isomers and account for >99.9% of total AAs in the organisms,

TABLE 1.22

Composition of Amino Acids in Elastin (Residues/1,000 Amino Acid Residues)

Amino Acid	Porcine Elastin		Chicken Mature Elastin	Bovine Mature Elastin	Salmon Mature Elastin
	Soluble	Insoluble			
Alanine	187	181	177	228	126
Arginine	4	5	5	9	32
Asp + Asn	3	5	4	10	35
Cysteine	<1	<1	–	–	3
Glu + Gln	12	16	13	18	49
Glycine	245	256	361	320	387
Histidine	0	0	1	1	8
4-OH-Proline	7	8	19	9	10
Isoleucine	14	14	19	25	14
Leucine	41	41	50	62	47
Lysine	37	5	3	9	18
Methionine	0	0	0	trace	4
Phenylalanine	14	12	20	32	16
Proline	92	90	127	116	82
Serine	8	11	5	11	36
Threonine	10	11	7	11	37
Tryptophan	0	0	0	0	0
Tyrosine	14	12	11	9	46
Valine	103	92	166	127	48

Source: Li, P. and G. Wu. 2018. *Amino Acids* 50:29–38.

Note: 4-OH-Proline, 4-hydroxyproline; –, data are not available.

but some D-AAs (e.g., D-aspartate and D-serine) may have important functions, particularly in the neurological and immune systems of animals. Peptide bond-linked AAs and free AAs account for approximately 97% and 3% of the total AAs in animals, respectively. However, certain free AAs are abundant in the plasma (e.g., glutamine and glycine), skeletal muscle (e.g., glutamine, glutamate, and taurine), fetal fluids (e.g., arginine, ornithine, glutamine, and serine), and animal products (e.g., glutamine, glutamate, proline, and BCAAs in milk protein; and free glutamine, glutamate, and taurine in milk). In some plants, select AAs (e.g., glutamine and asparagine) are highly abundant in the free form, with free AAs representing 34.4% and 28.5% of the total AAs in potatoes and sweet potatoes, respectively. Dynamic changes in the concentrations of free AAs (particularly the arginine family of AAs) in the physiological fluids of animals during growth and development and under pathological conditions reveal an exciting aspect of multidisciplinary research on AAs. The diversity of AAs also lies in their different side chains, which confer their different chemical and biochemical properties (e.g., solubility, stability, reactions, and taste). The reactivity of the amino and carboxyl groups of AAs with select organic or inorganic reagents provides a basis for the analysis of AAs (including D-AAs) and peptides, which is necessary for comprehensive studies of AA biochemistry and nutrition. Free AAs and peptides can be separated from proteins (including myofibrillar and water-soluble proteins) through the precipitation of the proteins with TCA, PCA, 80% methanol, or ammonium sulfate. Collagen and non-collagen proteins represent about 30%–35% and 65%–70% of total proteins in postnatal animals (including humans), respectively, and differ substantially in their AA composition. Particularly, glycine, proline, and 4-hydroxyproline are abundant in collagens (e.g., those in meats, connective tissues, and bird feathers), but are relatively low in plant proteins. In this book, unless indicated otherwise, "AAs" refer to L-AAs and the letter "L-" is not used as the prefix before the name of individual L-AAs.

REFERENCES

Abe, H., N. Yoshikawa, M.G. Sarower, and S. Okada. 2005. Physiological function and metabolism of free D-alanine in aquatic animals. *Biol. Pharm. Bull.* 28: 1571–1577.

Agostinelli, E. 2020. Biochemical and pathophysiological properties of polyamines. *Amino Acids* 52:111–117.

Agostoni, C., B. Carratu, C. Boniglia, A.M. Lammardo, E. Riva, and E. Sanzini. 2000. Free glutamine and glutamic acid increase in human milk through a three-month lactation period. *J. Pediatr. Gastrointest. Nutr.* 31:508–512.

Agouridas, V., V. Diemer, and O. Melnyk. 2020. Strategies and open questions in solid-phase protein chemical synthesis. *Curr. Opin. Chem. Biol.* 31:1–9.

Ajinomoto®. 2003. *Ajinomoto's Amino Acid Handbook*. Ajinomoto Inc., Tokyo.

Alteheld, B., P. Stehle, and P. Fürst. 2004. Measurement of amino acid concentrations in biological fluids and tissues using reversed-phase HPLC-based methods. In: *Metabolic and Therapeutic Aspects of Amino Acids in Clinical Nutrition* (Cynober, L.A., ed). CRC Press, Boca Raton, FL. pp. 29–44.

Ashmead, H.D. 2012. *Amino Acid Chelation in Human and Animal Nutrition*. CRC Press, Boca Raton, FL.

Baldeón, M.E., J.A. Mennella, N. Flores, M. Fornasini, and A. San Gabriel. 2014. Free amino acid content in breast milk of adolescent and adult mothers in Ecuador. *SpringerPlus* 3:1–4.

Baslow, M.H. 1997. A review of phylogenetic and metabolic relationships between the acylamino acids, N-acetyl-L-aspartic acid and N-acetyl-L-histidine, in the vertebrate nervous system. *J. Neurochem.* 68:1335–1344.

Baslow, M.H. and D.N. Guilfoyle. 2015. N-acetyl-L-histidine, a prominent biomolecule in brain and eye of poikilothermic vertebrates. *Biomolecules* 5:635–646.

Beaumont, M. and F. Blachier. 2020. Amino acids in intestinal physiology and health. *Adv. Exp. Med. Biol.* 1265:1–20.

Bell, E.A. 1962. α, γ-Diaminobutyric acid in seeds of twelve species of Lathyrus and identification of a new natural amino-Acid, L-homoarginine, in seeds of other species toxic to man and domestic animals. *Nature* 193:1078–1079.

Berg, C.P. 1953. Physiology of D-amino acids. *Physiol. Rev.* 33:145–189.

Besant, P.G., P.V. Attwood, and M.J. Piggot. 2009. Focus on phosphoarginine and phospholysine. *Curr. Protein Peptide Sci.* 10:536–550.

Bischoff, R. and H. Schlüter. 2012. Amino acids – chemistry, functionality and selected non-enzymatic post-translational modifications. *J. Proteomics.* 75:2275–2296.

Braconnot, H. 1820. Sur la conversion des matières animales en nouvelles substances par le moyen de l'acide sulfurique. *Annales de Chimie et de Physique.* 13:113–125.

Bradford, M.M. 1976. A rapid and sensitive method for the quantitation of microgram quantities of protein utilizing the principle of protein-dye binding. *Anal. Biochem.* 72:248–254.

Brosnan, J.T. 2001. Amino acids, then and now – a reflection on Sir Hans Krebs' contribution to nitrogen metabolism. *IUBMB Life* 52:265–270.

Chamond, N., M. Goytia, N. Coatnoan, J.C. Barale, A. Cosson, W.M. Degrave, and P. Minoprio. 2005. Trypanosoma cruzi proline racemases are involved in parasite differentiation and infectivity. *Mol. Microbiol.* 58:46–60.

Cannon, P.R. 1945. Nutritional aspects of globulin metabolism. *J. Allergy Clin. Immunol.* 16:78–82.

Catak, S., G. Monard, V. Aviyente, and M.F. Ruiz-López. 2009. Deamidation of asparagine residues – direct hydrolysis versus succinimide-mediated deamidation mechanisms. *J. Phys. Chem. A* 113:1111–1120.

Closs, E.I., J.P. Boissel, A. Habermeier, and A. Rotmann. 2006. Structure and function of cationic amino acid transporters (CATs). *J. Membr. Biol.* 213:67–77.

Combet, C., C. Blanchet, C. Geourjon, and G. Deleage. 2000. NPS@: network protein sequence analysis. *Trends Biochem. Sci.* 25:147–150.

Copley, S.D., E. Frank, W.M. Kirsch, and T.H. Koch. 1992. Detection and possible origins of aminomalonic acid in protein hydrolysates. *Anal. Biochem.* 201:152–157.

Covenas, R., A. Mangas, M.L. Sanchez, D. Cadena, M. Husson, and M. Geffard. 2017. Generation of specific antisera directed against D-amino acids – focus on the neuroanatomical distribution of D-glutamate and other D-amino acids. *Folia Histochem. Cytobiol.* 55:177–189.

Crumpler, H.R., C.E. Dent, H. Harris, and R.G. Westall. 1951. β-Aminoisobutyric acid (α-methyl-β-alanine) – a new amino-acid obtained from human urine. *Nature* 167:307–308.

Davis, T.A., H.V. Nguyen, R. Garcia-Bravo, M.L. Fiorotto, E.M. Jackson, D.S. Lewis et al. 1994. Amino acid composition of human milk is not unique. *J. Nutr.* 124:1126–1132.

de Ruijter, A.J., A.H. van Gennip, H.N. Caron, S. Kemp, and A.B. van Kuilenburg. 2003. Histone deacetylases (HDACs) – characterization of the classical HDAC family. *Biochem. J.* 370:737–749.

Devlin, T.M. 2006. *Textbook of Biochemistry with Clinical Correlations.* Wiley-Liss Press, Hoboken, NJ.

Dinsmore, C.J. and D.C. Beshore. 2002. Recent advances in the synthesis of diketopiperazines. *Tetrahedron* 58:3297–3312.

Donn, G. and H. Köcher. 2012. Inhibitors of glutamine synthetase. In: *Herbicide Classes in Development – Mode of Action, Targets, Genetic Engineering, Chemistry* (Böger, P., K. Wakabayashi, and K. Hirai, eds). Springer, New York. 364 pp.

Ennor, A.H., J.F. Morrison, and H. Rosenberg. 1956. The isolation of phosphoarginine. *Biochem. J.* 62:358–361.

Errico, F., F. Napolitano, R. Nisticò, and A. Usiello. 2012. New insights on the role of free D-aspartate in the mammalian brain. *Amino Acids* 43:1861–1871.

Fernstrom, J.D., S.D. Munger, A. Sclafani, I.E. de Araujo, A. Roberts, and S. Molinary. 2012. Mechanisms for sweetness. *J. Nutr.* 142:1134S–1141S.

Fridkin, M. and A. Patchornik. 1974. Peptide synthesis. *Annu. Rev. Biochem.* 43:419–443.

Friedman, M. 1999a. Chemistry, nutrition, and microbiology of D-amino acids. *J. Agric. Food Chem.* 47:3457–3479.

Friedman, M. 1999b. Chemistry, biochemistry, nutrition, and microbiology of lysinoalanine, lanthionine, and histidinoalanine in food and other proteins. *J. Agric. Food Chem.* 47:1295–1319.

Fu, L., X. Wang, Y. Eyal, Y. She, L.J. Donald, K.G. Standing, and G. Ben-Hayyim. 2002. A selenoprotein in the plant kingdom. *J. Biol. Chem.* 277:25983–25991.

Furst, P., S. Albers, and P. Stehle. 1990. Glutamine-containing dipeptides in parenteral nutrition. *J. Parenteral. Enteral. Nutr.* 14:118S–124S.

Ghadimi, H. and P. Pecora. 1963. Free amino acids of different kinds of milk. *Am. J. Clin. Nutr.* 13:75–81.

Gilbreath, K.R., G.I. Nawaratna, T.A. Wickersham, M.C. Satterfield, F.W. Bazer, and G. Wu. 2019. Ruminal microbes of adult steers do not degrade extracellular L-citrulline and have a limited ability to metabolize extra-cellular L-glutamate. *J. Anim. Sci.* 97:3611–3616.

Gilbreath, K.R., F.W. Bazer, M.C. Satterfield, and G. Wu. 2021. Amino acid nutrition and reproductive performance in ruminants. *Adv. Exp. Med. Biol.* 1285:43–61.

Greenstein, J.P. and M. Winitz. 1961. *Chemistry of Amino Acids.* John Wiley, New York.

Grishin, D.V., D.D. Zhdanov, M.V. Pokrovskaya, and N.N. Sokolova. 2020. D-amino acids in nature, agriculture and biomedicine. *All Life* 13:11–22.

Hackenberger, C.P.R., P.E. Dawson, Y.-X. Chen, and H. Hojo. 2020. Modern peptide and protein chemistry – reaching new heights. *J. Org. Chem.* 85:1328–1330.

Hao, B., W. Gong, T.K. Ferguson, C.M. James, J.A. Krzycki, and M.K. Chan. 2002. A new UAG-encoded residue in the structure of a methanogen methyltransferase. *Science* 296:1462–1466.

Hara, R. and K. Kino. 2009. Characterization of novel 2-oxoglutarate dependent dioxygenases converting L-proline to *cis*-4-hydroxy-L-proline. *Biochem. Biophys. Res. Commun.* 379:882–886.

Hashimoto, A., S. Kumashiro, T. Nishikawa, T. Oka, K. Takahashi, T. Mito et al. 1993. Embryonic development and postnatal changes in free D-aspartate and D-serine in the human prefrontal cortex. *J. Neurochem.* 61:348–351.

Hayashi, K., Y. Fujii, R. Saito, H. Kanao, and T. Hino. 1966. The influence of measurement parameters on the specific rotation of amino acids. *Agric. Biol. Chem.* 30:1221–1237.

He, W.L. and G. Wu. 2020. Metabolism of amino acids in the brain and their roles in regulating food intake. *Adv. Exp. Med. Biol.* 1265:167–185.

He, W.L., P. Li, and G. Wu. 2021. Amino acid nutrition and metabolism in chickens. *Adv. Exp. Med. Biol.* 1285:81–107.

Heine, W.E. 1994. Qualitative aspects of protein in human milk and formula – amino acid patter. In: *Protein Metabolism during Pregnancy* (Räihä, N.C.R., ed). Raven Press, New York. pp. 121–132.

Hooi, M.Y.S. and R.J.W. Truscott. 2011. Racemisation and human cataract. D-Ser, D-Asp/Asn and D-Thr are higher in the lifelong proteins of cataract lenses than in age-matched normal lenses. *Age* 33:131–141.

Hou, Y.Q. and G. Wu. 2018. L-Glutamate nutrition and metabolism in swine. *Amino Acids* 50:1497–1510.

Hou, Y.Q., S.C. Jia, G. Nawaratna, S.D. Hu, S. Dahanayaka, F.W. Bazer, and G. Wu. 2015. Analysis of L-homoarginine in biological samples by HPLC involving pre-column derivatization with *o*-phthalaldehyde and *N*-acetyl-L-cysteine. *Amino Acids* 47:2005–2014.

Hou, Y.Q., W.L. He, S.D. Hu, and G. Wu. 2019. Composition of polyamines and amino acids in plant-source foods for human consumption. *Amino Acids* 51:1153–1165.

Hughes, A.B. 2012. *Amino Acids, Peptides and Proteins in Organic Chemistry.* Wiley-VCH Verlag Gmbh, Weinheim.

Huxtable, R.J. 1992. Physiological actions of taurine. *Physiol. Rev.* 72:101–163.

Imseis, E., Y. Liu, and J.M. Rhoads. 2019. Glutamine – general facilitator of gut absorption and repair. In: *Glutamine – Biochemistry, Physiology, and Clinical Applications* (Meynial-Denis, D., ed). CRC Press, Boca Raton, FL. pp. 149–165.

Jones, S. 2012. Computational and structural characterisation of protein associations. *Adv. Exp. Med. Biol.* 747:42–54.

Kanayama, T., Y. Miyanaga, K. Horiuchi, and D. Fujimoto. 1987. Detection of the cross-linking amino acid, histidinoalanine, in human brown cataractous lens protein. *Exp. Eye Res.* 44:165–169.

Kawai, M., Y. Sekine-Hayakawa, A. Okiyama, and Y. Ninomiya. 2012. Gustatory sensation of L- and D-amino acids in humans. *Amino Acids* 43:2349–2358.

Kim, P.M., X. Duan, A.S. Huang, C.Y. Liu, G.L. Ming, H. Song, and S.H. Snyder. 2010. Aspartate race-mase, generating neuronal D-aspartate, regulates adult neurogenesis. *Proc. Natl. Acad. Sci. USA.* 107:3175–3179.

Kimura, T., A. Hesaka, and Y. Isaka. 2020. D-Amino acids and kidney diseases. *Clin. Exp. Nephrol.* 24:404–410.

Klupczynska, A., P. Magdalena, Z.J. Kokot, and J. Matysiak. 2018. Application of metabolomic tools for studying low molecular-weight fraction of animal venoms and poisons. *Toxins (Basel)* 10:306.

Kreil, G. 1997. D-amino acids in animal peptides. *Annu. Rev. Biochem.* 66:337–345.

Kwon, H., T.E. Spencer, F.W. Bazer, and G. Wu. 2003. Developmental changes of amino acids in ovine fetal fluids. *Biol. Reprod.* 68:1813–1820.

Li, P. and G. Wu. 2018. Roles of dietary glycine, proline and hydroxyproline in collagen synthesis and animal growth. *Amino Acids* 50:29–38.

Li, P. and G. Wu. 2020. Composition of amino acids and related nitrogenous nutrients in feedstuffs for animal diets. *Amino Acids* 52:523–542.

Li, X.Y., S.X. Zheng, and G. Wu. 2021a. Nutrition and functions of amino acids in fish. *Adv. Exp. Med. Biol.* 1285:133–168.

Li, X.Y., T. Han, S.X. Zheng, and G. Wu. 2021b. Nutrition and functions of amino acids in aquatic crustaceans. *Adv. Exp. Med. Biol.* 1285:169–197.

Liu, Y.Y., X.J. Tian, B.K. He, T.K. Hoang, C.M. Taylor, E. Blanchard et al. 2019. *Lactobacillus reuteri* DSM 17938 feeding of healthy newborn mice regulates immune responses while modulating gut microbiota and boosting beneficial metabolites. *Am. J. Physiol.* 317:G824–G838.

Lowry, O.H., N.J. Rosebrough, A.L. Farr, and R.J. Randall. 1953. Protein measurement with the Folin phenol reagent. *J. Biol. Chem.* 193:265–275.

Lu, J. and A. Holmgren. 2008. Selenoproteins. *J. Biol. Chem.* 284:723–727.

Lubec, G. and G.A. Rosenthal (ed.) 1990. *Amino Acids – Chemistry, Biology and Medicine.* ESCOM Science Publisher B.V., Leiden.

Ma, Q., P.M. Davidson, and Q. Zhong. 2020. Properties and potential food applications of lauric arginate as a cationic antimicrobial. *Int. J. Food Microbiol.* 315:108417.

Mangas, A., R. Covenas, D. Bodet, M. Geffard, L.A. Aguilar, and J. Yajeya. 2007. Immunocyto-chemical visualization of D-glutamate in the rat brain. *Neurosci.* 144:654–664.

Marcus, F. and J.F. Morrison. 1964. The preparation of phosphoarginine – a comparative study. *Biochem. J.* 92:429–435.

Marglin, A. and R.B. Merrifield. 1970. Chemical synthesis of peptides and proteins. *Annu. Rev. Biochem.* 39:841–866.

Markwell, M.N.K., S.M. Haas, L.L. Bieber, and N.E. Tolbert. 1978. A modification of the Lowry pro-cedure to simplify protein determination in membrane and lipoprotein samples. *Anal. Biochem.* 87:206–210.

Masters, P.M., and M. Friedman. 1979. Racemization of amino acids in alkali-treated food proteins. *J. Agric. Food Chem.* 27:507–511.

Masumura, T., M. Sugahara, T. Noguchi, K. Mori, and Naito H. 1985. The effect of gizzerosine, a recently discovered compound in overheated fish meal, on the gastric acid secretion in chicken. *Poult. Sci.* 64:356-361.

McAuliffe, O., R.P. Ross, and C. Hill. 2001. Lantibiotics – structure, biosynthesis and mode of action. *FEMS Microbiol. Rev.* 25:285–308.

McNeal, C.J., C.J. Meininger, C.D. Wilborn, C.D. Tekwe, and G. Wu. 2018. Safety of dietary supplementation with arginine in adult humans. *Amino Acids* 50:1215–1229.

Meister, A. 1965. *Biochemistry of Amino Acids.* Academic Press, New York.

Morrison, J.F., D.E. Griffiths, and A.H. Ennor. 1957. The purification and properties of arginine phosphoki-nase. *Biochem. J.* 65:143–153.

Moughan, P.J., A.J. Darragh, W.C. Smith, and C.A. Butts. 1990. Perchloric and trichloroacetic acids as precipitants of protein in endogenous ileal digesta from the rat. *J. Sci. Food Agric.* 52:13–21.

Miyoshi, Y., R. Koga, T. Oyama, H. Han, K. Ueno, K. Masuyama et al. 2012. HPLC analysis of naturally occurring free D-amino acids in mammals. *J. Pharmaceut. Biomed. Analy.* 69:42–49.

Meyerhof, O. and K. Lohmann. 1928. Uber die naturlichen Guanidinophosphosauren (phosphagene) in der quergestreiften Muskulatur. II. Die physikalisch-chemischen Eigenschaften der Guanidinophosphosauren. *Biochem. Z.* 196:49–72.

Nagata, Y. 1999. D-Amino acids in nature. In: *Advances in BioChirality* (Pályi, G., C. Zucchi, and L. Caglioti, eds). Elsevier, New York. pp. 271–283.

Neinast, M., D. Murashige, and Z. Arany. 2019. Branched chain amino acids. *Annu. Rev. Physiol.* 81:139–164.

Neveux, N., P. David, and L. Cynober. 2004. Measurement of amino acid concentrations in biological fluids and tissues using ion exchange chromatography. In: *Metabolic and Therapeutic Aspects of Amino Acids in Clinical Nutrition* (Cynober, L.A., ed). CRC Press, Boca Raton, FL. pp. 17–28.

Nimura, Y. and H. Sato. 1982. Phosphoarginine content of the shrimp *Penaeus japonicus* with reference to the way of freezing. *Bull. Japn. Soc. Sci. Fish.* 48:725.

Nimura, Y. and H. Sato. 1983. Estimation of phosphoarginine in the muscle after enzymatic hydrolysis of free arginine. *Bull. Japn. Soc. Sci. Fish.* 49:1077–1081.

Nishikawa. T. 2011. Analysis of free D-serine in mammals and its biological relevance. *J. Chromatogr. B* 879:3169–3183.

Nishikawa, I., H. Yoshida, K. Ahiko, and A. Ueda. 1984. Free amino acid concentrations of human and cow's milk and effect of taurine supplementation to infant milk formulas on serum taurine levels of infants. *J. Jpn. Soc. Nutr. Food Sci.* 37:301–309.

Nunn, P.B., E.A. Bell, A.A. Watson, and R.J. Nash. 2010. Toxicity of non-protein amino acids to humans and domestic animals. *Nat. Prod. Commun.* 5:485–504.

O'Dowd, J.J., D.J. Robins, and D.J. Miller. 1988. Detection, characterisation, and quantification of carnosine and other histidyl derivatives in cardiac and skeletal muscle. *Biochim. Biophys. Acta* 967:241–249.

O'Dowd, J.J., M.T. Cairns, M. Trainor, D.J. Robins, and D.J. Miller. 1990. Analysis of carnosine, homocarnosine, and other histidyl derivatives in rat brain. *J. Neurochem.* 55:446–452.

O'Dowd, A., J.J. O'Dowd, J.J.M. O'Dowd, N. MacFarlane, H. Abe, and D.J. Miller. 1992. Analysis of novel imidazoles from isolated perfused rabbit heart by two high-performance liquid chromatographic methods. *J. Chromatogr.* 577:347–353.

Okazaki, T., T. Noguchi, K. Igarashi, Y. Sakagami, H. Seto, K. Mori et al. 1983. Gizzerosine, a new toxic substance in fish meal, causes severe gizzard erosion in chicks. *Agric. Biol. Chem.* 47:2852–2949.

Ota, N., S.S. Rubakhin, and J.V. Sweedler. 2014. D-Alanine in the islets of Langerhans of rat pancreas. *Biochem. Biophys. Res. Commun.* 447:328–333.

Patel, A.V., T. Kawai, L. Wang, S.S. Rubakhin, and J.V. Sweedler. 2017. Chiral measurement of aspartate and glutamate in single neurons by large-volume sample stacking capillary electrophoresis. *Anal. Chem.* 89:12375–12382.

Pruser, K.N. and N.E. Flynn. 2011. Acrylamide in health and disease. *Front. Biosci.* 3:S41–S51.

Radkov, A.D. and L.A. Moe. 2014. Bacterial synthesis of D-amino acids. *Appl. Microbiol. Biotechnol.* 98:5363–5374.

Rassin, D.K., J.A. Sturman, and G.E. Gaull. 1978. Taurine and other free amino acids in milk of man and other mammals. *Early Hum. Dev.* 2:1–13.

Remuzon, P. 1996. *trans*-4-Hydroxy-L-proline, a novel and versatile chiral starting block. *Tetrahedron* 52:13803–13835.

Rennie, M.J. and K.D. Tipton. 2000. Protein and amino acid metabolism during and after exercise and the effects of nutrition. *Annu. Rev. Nutr.* 20:457–483.

Roberts, L.D., P. Boström, J.F. O'Sullivan, R.T. Schinzel, G.D. Lewis, A. Dejam et al. 2014. Beta-aminoisobutyric acid induces browning of white fat and hepatic β-oxidation and is inversely correlated with cardiometabolic risk factors. *Cell Metab.* 19:96–108.

Rockstein, M. 1971. The distribution of phosphoarginine and phosphocreatine in marine invertebrates. *Biol. Bull.* 141:167–175.

Ryan, W.L. and I.C. Wells. 1964. Homocitrulline and homoarginine synthesis from lysine. *Science* 144:1122–1123

San Gabriel, A., E. Nakamura, H. Uneyama, and K. Torii. 2009. Taste, visceral information and exocrine reflexes with glutamate through umami receptors. *J. Med. Invest.* 56 Suppl:209–217.

Schell, M.J., O.B. Cooper, and S.H. Snyder. 1997. D-aspartate localizations imply neuronal and neuroendo-crine roles. *Proc. Natl. Acad. Sci. USA.* 94:2013–2018.

Singh, V., B.I. Fedeles, and J.M. Essigmann. 2015. Role of tautomerism in RNA biochemistry. *RNA* 21:1–13.

Smith, P.K., R.I. Krohn, G.T. Hermanson, A.K. Mallia, F.H. Gartner, M.D. Provenzano et al. (1985) Measurement of protein using bicinchoninic acid. *Anal. Biochem.* 150:76–85.

Solano, F. 2020. Metabolism and functions of amino acids in the skin. *Adv. Exp. Med. Biol.* 1265:187–199.

Srinivasan, G., C.M. James, and J.A. Krzycki. 2002. Pyrrolysine encoded by UAG in archaea – charging of a UAG-decoding specialized tRNA. *Science* 296:1459–1462.

Stadtman, T.C. 1996. Selenocysteine. *Annu. Rev. Biochem.* 65:83–100.

Sterck, L., S. Rombauts, K. Vandepoele, P. Rouzé, and Y. Van de Peer. 2007. How many genes are there in plants (… and why are they there)? *Curr. Opin. Plant Biol.* 10:199–203.

Sturman, J.A. 1993. Taurine in development. *Physiol. Rev.* 73:119–147.

Suryawan, A., M. Rudar, M.L. Fiorotto, and T.A. Davis. 2020. Differential regulation of mTORC1 activa-tion by leucine and β-hydroxy-β-methylbutyrate in skeletal muscle of neonatal pigs. *Am. J. Physiol.* 128:286–295.

Szpak, P. 2011. Fish bone chemistry and ultrastructure – implications for taphonomy and stable isotope analysis. *J. Archaeolog. Sci.* 38:3358–3372.

Tal, M., A. Silberstein, and E. Nusser. 1985. Why does Coomassie Brilliant Blue R interact differently with different proteins? *J. Biol. Chem.* 260:9976–9980.

Tallan, T.T., S. Moore, and W.H. Stein. 1956. *N*-acetyl-L-aspartic acid in brain. *J. Biol. Chem.* 219:257–264.

Togashi, M., E. Okuma, and H. Abe. 1998. HPLC determination of N-acetyl-L-histidine and its related compounds in fish tissues. *Fish. Sci.* 64:174–175.

Van Buskirk, J.J., W.M. Kirsch, D.L. Kleyer, R.M. Barkley, and T.H. Koch. 1984. Aminomalonic acid – identification in Escherichia coli and atherosclerotic plaque. *Proc. Natl. Acad. Sci. USA.* 81:722–725.

Van Sadelhoff, J.H.J., S.P. Wiertsema, J. Garssen, and A. Hogenkamp. 2020. Free amino acids in human milk – a potential role for glutamine and glutamate in the protection against neonatal allergies and infections. *Front. Immunol.* 11:1007.

Varanoske, A.N., J.R. Hoffman, D.D. Church, N.A. Coker, K.M. Baker, S.J. Dodd et al. 2017. β-Alanine supplementation elevates intramuscular carnosine content and attenuates fatigue in men and women similarly but does not change muscle L-histidine content. *Nutr. Res.* 48:16–25.

Vauquelin, L.N. and P.J. Robiquet. 1806. La découverte d'un nouveau principe végétal dans le suc des asperges. *Annales de Chimie.* 57:88–93.

Vickery, H.B. and C.A. Schmidt. 1931. The history of the discovery of the amino acids. *Chem. Rev.* 9:169–318.

Wagner, I. and H. Musso. 1983. New naturally occurring amino acids. *Angewandte Chemie Int. Ed. English* 22:816–828.

Watanabe, S., F. Fukumori, M. Miyazaki, S. Tagami, and Y. Watanabe. 2017. Characterization of a novel cis-3-hydroxy-L-proline dehydratase and a trans-3-hydroxy-L-proline dehydratase from bacteria. *J. Bacteriol.* 199:e00255-17.

Watford, M. 2000. Glutamine and glutamate metabolism across the liver sinusoid. *J. Nutr.* 130:983S–987S.

Watford, M. 2003. The ornithine cycle. *Biochem. Mol. Biol. Edu.* 31:289–297.

Weatherly, C.A., S. Du, C. Parpia, P.T. Santos, A.L. Hartman, and D.W. Armstrong. 2017. D-Amino acid levels in perfused mouse brain tissue and blood – a comparative study. *ACS Chem. Neurosci.* 8:1251–1261.

Wilkinson, D.J., J. Cegielski, B.E. Phillips, C. Boereboom, J.N. Lund, P.J. Atherton, and K. Smith. 2015. Internal comparison between deuterium oxide (D$_2$O) and L-[*ring*-^{13}C$_6$] phenylalanine for acute measure-ment of muscle protein synthesis in humans. *Physiol. Rep.* 3:e12433.

Wolosker, H., S. Blackshaw, and S.H. Snyder. 1999. Serine racemase – a glial enzyme synthesizing D-serine to regulate glutamate-N-methyl-D-aspartate neurotransmission. *Proc. Natl. Acad. Sci. USA.* 96:13409–13414.

Wong, M.L., I.A. Guzei, and L.L. Kiessling. 2012. An asymmetric synthesis of L-pyrrolysine. *Org. Lett.* 14:1378–1381.

Wright, C.E., H.H. Tallan, and Y.Y. Lin. 1986. Taurine – biological update. *Annu. Rev. Biochem.* 55:427–453.

Wright, J.L.C., R.K. Boyd, A.S.W. de Freitas, M. Falk, R.A. Foxall, W.D. Jamieson et al. 1989. Identification of domoic acid, a neuroexcitatory amino acid, in toxic mussels from eastern Prince Edward Island. *Can. J. Chem.* 67:481–490.

Wu, G. 1993. Determination of proline by reversed-phase high performance liquid chromatography with auto-mated pre-column *o*-phthaldialdehyde derivatization. *J. Chromatogr.* 641:168–175.

Wu, G. 2018. *Principles of Animal Nutrition.* CRC Press, Boca Raton, Florida.

Wu, G. 2020a. Metabolism and functions of amino acids in sense organs. *Adv. Exp. Med. Biol.* 1265: 201–216.

Wu, G. 2020b. Important roles of dietary taurine, creatine, carnosine, anserine and hydroxyproline in human nutrition and health. *Amino Acids* 52:329–360.

Wu, G., and D.A. Knabe. 1994. Free and protein-bound amino acids in sow's colostrum and milk. *J. Nutr.* 124:415–424.

Wu, G. and C.J. Meininger. 2008. Analysis of citrulline, arginine, and methylarginines using high-performance liquid chromatography. *Methods Enzymol.* 440:177–189.

Wu, G., T.L. Ott, D.A. Knabe, and F.W. Bazer. 1999. Amino acid composition of the fetal pig. *J. Nutr.* 129:1031–1038.

Wu, G., F.W. Bazer, G.A. Johnson, D.A. Knabe, R.C. Burghardt, T.E. Spencer et al. 2011. Important roles for L-glutamine in swine nutrition and production. *J. Anim. Sci.* 89:2017–2030.

Wu, G., H.R. Cross, K.B. Gehring, J.W. Savell, A.N. Arnold, and S. H. McNeill. 2016. Composition of free and peptide-bound amino acids in beef chuck, loin, and round cuts. *J. Anim. Sci.* 94:2603–2613.

Yamada, S. and M. Furuichi. 1990. N^α-Acetylhistidine metabolism in fish-I. Identification of N^α-acetylhistidine in the heart of rainbow trout *Salmo gairdneri*. *Comp. Biochem. Physiol. B* 97:539–541.

Yamauchi, O., A. Odani, and M. Takani. 2002. Metal-amino acid chemistry. Weak interactions and related functions of side chain groups. *J. Chem. Soc. Dalton Trans.* 2002:3411–3421.

Yang, H., X. Xiao, X. Zhao, and Y. Wu. 2015. Intrinsic fluorescence spectra of tryptophan, tyrosine and phenylalanine. *Proceedings of SPIE.* 10255:224–233.

Yang, Z., J.K. Htoo, and S.F. Liao. 2020. Methionine nutrition in swine and related monogastric animals – beyond protein biosynthesis. *Anim. Feed Sci. Technol.* 268:114608.

Yoshimura, T. and N. Esak. 2003. Amino acid racemases – functions and mechanisms. *J. Biosci. Bioengin.* 96:103–109.

Yoshimura, T. and M. Goto. 2008. D-Amino acids in the brain – structure and function of pyridoxal phosphate-dependent amino acid racemases. *FEBS J.* 275:3527–3537.

Zhang, Z., A.S. Adelman, D. Rai, J. Boettcher, and B. Lönnerdal. 2013. Amino acid profiles in term and pre-term human milk through lactation – a systematic review. *Nutrients* 5:4800–4821.

Zhang, Q., Y.Q. Hou, F.W. Bazer, W.L. He, E.H. Posey, and G. Wu. 2021. Amino acids in swine nutrition and production. *Adv. Exp. Med. Biol.* 1285:81–107.

Zhao, X., Z. Zhang, B. Hu, W. Huang, C. Yuan, and L. Zou. 2018. Response of gut microbiota to metabolite changes induced by endurance exercise. *Front. Microbiol.* 9:765.

2 Protein Digestion and Absorption of Peptides and Amino Acids

The digestion of dietary proteins and the absorption of their hydrolysis products [small peptides and free amino acids (AAs)] are the first two steps in their utilization by humans and other animals (Moughan 2003). Except for the absorption of intact immunoglobulins by the small intestine of mammalian neonates within the first days or weeks after birth (depending on species), dietary proteins have no nutritional value until they are hydrolyzed to small peptides and free AAs in the digestive tract (Blachier et al. 2013; Gardner 1975; Wu 1998). Thus, to nourish organisms, non-immunoglobulin proteins in food must undergo extracellular degradation by proteases and peptidases in the lumen of the stomach and small intestine.

Ruminants (e.g., cattle, sheep, and goats) and nonruminants (e.g., humans, dogs, pigs, and birds) differ greatly in the digestion of dietary protein. In ruminants, a well-developed rumen contains large amounts of anaerobic bacteria (10^{10}–10^{11}/mL), protozoa (10^5–10^6/mL), and fungi (10^3–10^4/mL), and together these cells convert food protein primarily into bacterial and protozoal proteins, as well as relatively small net amounts of ammonia, sulfate, free AAs, and small peptides (Wu 2018). In ruminant and nonruminant animals, the dietary and endogenous proteins that are not digested in the small intestine enter the large intestine (the last part of the digestive system) for fermentation via metabolic pathways similar to those in the rumen (Smith and Bryant 1979). In the large intestine of humans and other animals, anaerobic bacteria have high rates of AA utilization, but there is little or no absorption of microbial proteins (Tanksley and Knabe 1984; Bergen 2021).

The digestive system of the animal kingdom generally includes the mouth, teeth, tongue, pharynx, esophagus, stomach, small intestine, and large intestine, as well as accessory digestive organs (salivary glands, pancreas, liver, and gallbladder), and can vary greatly among different species (Wu 2018). For example, humans, dogs, cats, tigers, pigs, rats, and chickens (nonruminants) have a single stomach, whereas the stomachs of ruminants consist of four parts: rumen (containing a large number of different species of microbes), reticulum, omasum, and abomasum (true stomach). The digestive tract of humans is illustrated in Figure 2.1. Of note, most fish (e.g., Atlantic salmon, largemouth bass, and zebrafish) have a stomach, but some (e.g., carp, goldfish, and lungfish) do not (Li et al. 2021b). In crustaceans, the hepatopancreas secretes digestive enzymes and is the major site for the digestion of foods and the absorption of digestion products into the hemolymph (Li et al. 2021a).

In mammals, birds, fish, and crustaceans, the products of protein digestion (primarily small peptides and, to a lesser extent, free AAs) are either utilized by microorganisms in the gastrointestinal tract or absorbed into enterocytes (the columnar absorptive epithelial cells of the small intestine; Figure 2.2) via specific transporters (Bröer and Bröer 2017; Grimble 2000). Inside these cells, the oxidation of AAs is the major source of energy to support their high metabolic rates in mammals, birds, fish, and aquatic crustaceans (Li et al. 2021a, b; Wu 2018). The extensive catabolism of dietary AAs in the small intestine not only reduces the efficiency of the utilization of dietary proteins and AAs but also alters the pattern of AAs that enter the portal circulation (Yang and Liao 2019; Wu 1998). AAs that escape the small intestine to enter the large intestine have a lower nutritional value than those absorbed by the small intestine. This chapter highlights the key processes for protein digestion, absorption of the resulting small peptides and free AAs in mammals (ruminants

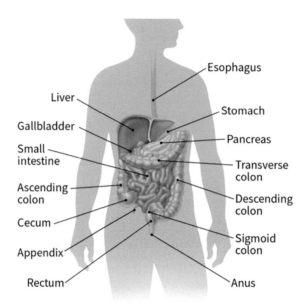

FIGURE 2.1 The digestive system of humans. Food enters the mouth, esophagus, stomach, small intestine, and large intestine. The digestion of dietary protein is initiated in the stomach, facilitated by secretions from the pancreas into the duodenum, and completed in the intestines. The jejunum is the major site for the absorption of the products of protein digestion. Non-human monogastric mammals have a digestive tract similar to that in humans. (Reproduced from a photo freely available in the public domain from American Cancer Society. 2020. https://www.cancer.org/cancer/gastrointestinal-carcinoid-tumor/detection-diagnosis-staging/signs-symptoms.html.)

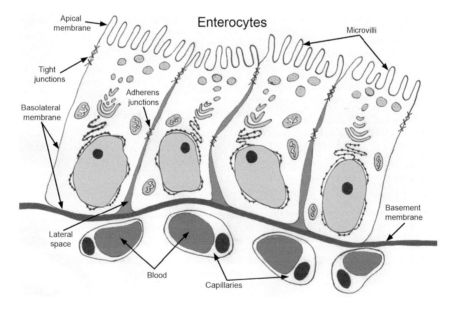

FIGURE 2.2 Anatomical relationships of the enterocytes (absorptive epithelial cells) with tight junctions in the small intestine. Each enterocyte has an apical membrane and a basolateral membrane. Before the gut closure, macromolecules (e.g., immunoglobulins) may pass the enterocyte through the tight junction. Amino acids are absorbed into the enterocyte by their transporters.

and nonruminants), birds, fish, and crustaceans, and the extensive recycling of nitrogen in the small and large intestines.

2.1 CLASSIFICATION AND CONTENT OF PROTEIN IN DIETS

2.1.1 CLASSIFICATION OF PROTEIN

Proteins can be classified on the basis of their structures (Table 2.1). There are four orders of protein structure: primary structure (the sequence of AAs along the polypeptide chain); secondary structure (the conformation of the polypeptide backbone); tertiary structure (the three-dimensional arrangement of protein); and quaternary structure (the spatial arrangement of polypeptide subunits). The forces stabilizing polypeptide aggregates are hydrogen and electrostatic bonds between AA residues, as well as disulfide linkages. Proteins in diets (based on plant and animal products), as well as proteins in the body, can be classified according to their overall shape (globular or fibrous), solubility in water (hydrophobic or hydrophilic), electric charge (acidic, basic, or neutral), three-dimensional structure (e.g., folded or unfolded), function (e.g., defense or conjugation), or attachments (simple or complex). For example, albumin, hemoglobin, G-actin, and protamines are globular proteins. Fibrous proteins include F-actin, myosin, collagens, elastin, α-keratins (wool and hair), and β-keratins (the feathers, skin, beaks, and scales of most birds and reptiles). Myosin is a unique protein as it is both fibrous and globular.

Proteins can also be classified on the basis of their physiological roles in animals (Table 2.2). For example, collagens are constituent structural proteins in animals and are highly rich in proline plus hydroxyproline and glycine, and are particularly abundant in the connective tissue (Li and Wu 2018). Mature collagens are insoluble in water. Collagen represents about one-third of the total proteins in the whole bodies of humans and other animals and is abundant in meat (Wu et al. 2016b). Therefore, knowledge of collagens is particularly important for the nutrition of carnivores and omnivores. In addition, foodstuffs with high percentages of water-insoluble protein are fish-meal, meat and bone meal, beet pulp, dried brewers grains, dried distillers grains, forages, sorghum, and soy hulls. Keratins are rich in cysteine, and wool protein contains approximately 4% sulfur. Most animal-sourced proteins, except for gelatin, provide adequate amounts and proper ratios of proteinogenic AAs, whereas most plant-sourced proteins contain inadequate amounts of one or more AAs and suboptimal ratios of AAs (Hou et al. 2019; Li and Wu 2020). A combination of gelatin with meat-, gut mucosa-, or blood-derived foodstuffs can result in complementary effects in the nutrition of humans and other animals. Note that there are no such terms as "fat protein" and "lean protein" in biochemistry, chemistry, or nutrition.

TABLE 2.1
Classification of Proteins as Simple or Complex Proteins in Animals and Foods

Protein	Chemical property	Source	Example
	(1) Simple Proteins		
Albumin	Soluble in water and saline, as well as acid alkaline solutions; precipitates in saturated ammonium sulfate; coagulates by heating	Animals and plants	Serum albumin (serum of animals), α-lactalbumin (milk), ovalbumin (egg white), and leucosin (wheat)
Fibrous protein	Insoluble in water, saline, acid, and alkaline solutions	Animals	Keratin (hair, horns, and nails), collagen (connective tissue), silk fibroin (silk), spongin (sponge), F-actin (muscles), myosin[a] (muscles), and gelatin[b]

(Continued)

TABLE 2.1 (*Continued*)

Classification of Proteins as Simple or Complex Proteins in Animals and Foods

Protein	Chemical property	Source	Example
Globulin	Insoluble in water; soluble in saline, as well as acid and alkaline solutions; precipitates in semi-saturated ammonium sulfate; coagulates by heating	Animals and plants	Serum globulin (serum of animals), β-lactoglobulin (milk), fibrinogen (serum of animals), G-actin (muscles), myosin[a] (muscles), and immunoglobulins (animals)
Glutelin	Insoluble in water; soluble in saline, as well as acid and alkaline solutions; insoluble in 80% ethanol; coagulable by heating	Cereal seeds (e.g., wheat, rye, barley, and rice)	Glutenin (wheat) and oryzenin (rice); one of the main proteins in the endosperm of cereal grains
Histone	Soluble in water, saline, and acid solution; highly basic protein (abundant in arginine and lysine); non-coagulable by heating	Animals	Thymus histone, erythrocyte histone, liver histone, placental histone, sperm histone, and scombrone (seminal vesicle)
Prolamin	Insoluble in water; soluble in saline and 80% ethanol, as well as acid and alkaline solutions	Cereal seeds	Gliadin (wheat), hordein (barley), and zein (corn)
Protamine	Soluble in water and saline; insoluble in ammonium solution; highly basic protein (highly abundant in arginine, lysine, and histidine); non-coagulable by heating	Sperm	Salmine (salmon), clupeine (herring), sturine (sturgeon), and scombrine (seminal vesicle)

(2) Complex Proteins

Protein	Chemical property	Source	Example
Chromoprotein	Bound to metals in organic pigments, such as iron in heme, copper in hemocyanin, and magnesium in chlorophyll	Animals, plants, and microbes	Hemoglobin (blood of animals), myoglobin (skeletal muscle), hemocyanin (the blood of invertebrates), catalase, and cytochrome C in mitochondria
Flavoprotein	Bound to FAD or FMN	Animals, plants, and microbes	Nitric oxide synthase, acyl-CoA dehydrogenase, and D-amino acid oxidase
Glycoprotein	Bound to saccharides	Animals, plants, and microbes	Ovomucin (egg white), seromucoid (the blood), membrane receptor proteins
Lipoprotein	Bound to lipids	Animals, plants, and microbes	Very low-density lipoprotein, low-density lipoprotein, and lipovitellin
Metalloprotein	Bound to one or more metals	Animals, plants, and microbes	Collagenase, calpain, carboxypeptidases A and B, and ceruloplasmin
Nucleic proteins	Bound to DNA and RNA	Animals, plants, and microbes	Nucleohistone (thymus), nucleoprotamine (sperm), and tobacco mosaic virus
Phosphoprotein	Proteins that contain phosphate groups	Animals, plants, and microbes	Casein (milk), vitellin (egg yolk), phosvitin (egg yolk), and phosphorylated proteins

Source: Ajinomoto® 2003. *Ajinomoto's Amino Acid Handbook*. Tokyo, Japan; Wu, G. 2018. *Principles of Animal Nutrition*, CRC Press, Boca Raton, FL.

[a] Myosin in muscles (skeletal, smooth, and cardiac muscles) is both a fibrous protein and a globular protein.

[b] A food protein obtained through the boiling of collagen.

TABLE 2.2

Classification of Proteins Based on Physiological Roles in Animals

Physiological Roles	Examples of Proteins
Acid–base balance (buffering)	Hemoglobin, myoglobin, and protamines (sperm)
Cell migration and signaling	Cell-surface receptors (e.g., integrins), actin (cytosol), FAK (cytosol), PI3K, calmodulin, adenylate cyclase, guanylate cyclase, GPCRs, and MTOR
Cell and tissue structures	Collagen, elastin, keratin, mucins, proteoglycans, and membrane proteins
Colloidal properties	Proteins in plasma (albumin and globulins), and caseins and whey proteins (milk)
Enzyme-catalyzed reactions	Arginase, nitric oxide synthase, creatine kinase, and glutamate dehydrogenase
Gene expression	DNA methylase, DNA-binding proteins, histones, repressor proteins, and STAT3
Hormone-mediated effects	Insulin, insulin receptor, IGF-1, membrane-bound G-protein, and HSL
Muscle contraction	F-Actin, G-actin, myosin, tropomyosin, troponins C, I, and T, and tubulin
Protective function	Blood clotting factors, immunoglobulins, interferons (τ and γ), and SOD
Storage of nutrients and O_2	Ceruloplasmin, FABs, ferritin, metallothionein, myoglobin, and perilipins
Transport of nutrients and O_2	Albumin, hemoglobin, plasma lipoproteins, CAT, GLUT, CrT, and PepT1

Note: CAT, cationic amino acid transporters; CrT, creatine transporter; FAK, focal adhesion kinase; GLUT, glucose transporters; GPCRs, G-protein-coupled receptors; HSL, hormone-sensitive lipase; IGF-1, insulin-like growth factor-I, MTOR, mechanistic target of rapamycin; PI3K, phosphoinositide 3-kinase; PepT1, peptide transporter 1; SOD, superoxide dismutase; STAT3, signal transducer and activator of transcription 3 (STAT3, a transcription factor).

Proteins have colloidal properties and differ in their solubilities in water. Water-soluble proteins are generally more rapidly digested than water-insoluble proteins. Like AAs, proteins exhibit characteristic isoelectric points and have buffering capacities mainly due to the presence of histidine residues (Chapter 1). All proteins can be denatured or structurally changed from their natural state by heat, acids, alkalis, alcohols, urea, and salts of heavy metals. The susceptibility of foodstuff proteins to heat damage during processing is increased in the presence of carbohydrates, owing to the Maillard reaction, which involves a condensation between the carbonyl group of a reducing sugar with the free amino group of an AA residue (e.g., lysine, arginine, and glutamine).

2.1.2 PROTEIN CONTENT OF FOODS OF ANIMAL AND PLANT ORIGIN

Either inadequate protein nutrition or an excess of dietary protein impairs the growth, development, health, and productivity of humans and other animals. In addition, over-consumption of protein is also uneconomical, because it is the most costly of the food nutrients. Thus, there has been a rich history of research on the protein content of foods of animal and plant origin. In 1742, the Italian chemist G.B. Beccari isolated gluten "of animal nature" from wheat flour. Sixty-four years later, the French chemist L.N. Vauquelin identified a high content of a gluten-like substance in soybeans. In 1841, the German chemist J. von Liebig analyzed protein content in foodstuffs. In the late 1880s, the French chemist P.E.M. Bertholet found that protein is the major constituent of dry matter (DM) in animal tissues. Protein constitutes 10%–23%, 16%–25%, and 30%–65% of diets (DM basis) for mammals, birds, and fish, respectively.

Historically, crude protein content in animal tissues and foodstuffs for humans and animals was calculated by multiplying the determined nitrogen content by a factor of 6.25 based on the average content of nitrogen (16%) in protein (Jones 1931). The Food and Drug Administration of the United States (2020) has long recognized that "Protein content may be calculated on the basis of the factor 6.25 times the nitrogen content of the food as determined by the appropriate method of analysis as given in the 'Official Methods of Analysis of the AOAC International', except when official AOAC procedures described in this paragraph (c)(7) require a specific factor other than 6.25". Total nitrogen is usually determined using the Kjeldahl method that was developed in 1883. Such an approach for quantifying protein in a diet or its ingredients may yield misleading results for the following reasons. First, different AAs have different nitrogen content, and the content of 16% nitrogen in protein is only an average but far from accurate for some proteins that contain less or more nitrogen (Chapter 1). Second, some nitrogenous compounds (e.g., ammonia, urea, amides, choline, betaine, purines, pyrimidines, nitrite, and nitrate) are neither proteins nor AAs. Crude protein content (nitrogen content×6.25) can be greatly overestimated by the presence of the non-AA substances and falsely elevated by nitrogen-rich and toxic compounds (e.g., melamine containing 66% nitrogen) in food. Thus, the composition of AAs in diets or ingredients must be determined to ensure foodstuff safety and quality. This goal can be easily and reliably achieved by using established analytical methods (e.g., high-performance liquid chromatography, gas chromatography, and mass spectrometry).

Melamine
($C_3H_6N_6$,
MW = 126.12 Da,
N = 66.7%)

Aminoguanidine
(CH_6N_4,
MW = 74.09 Da,
N = 75.6%)

Urea
(CH_4N_2O,
MW = 60.06 Da,
N = 46.6%)

Hydrazine
(N_2H_4,
MW = 32.05 Da,
N = 87.4%)

Ammonia
(NH_3,
MW = 17.03 Da,
N = 82.2%)

The content of protein in different foodstuffs varies between 4.5% and 96%, depending on source (Table 2.3). The content of true protein in most foodstuffs is about 15% lower than that of crude protein (Hou et al. 2019; Li et al. 2011; Li and Wu 2020). Interestingly, the content of true protein in some foodstuffs (soybean, soy protein concentrate, wheat flour, black soldier fly larvae meal, and meat and bone meal) is very similar to the content of crude protein. Differences between crude and true proteins are affected by the composition of individual AAs in foodstuffs. Based on the quantity and quality of protein, animal-sourced foods are generally superior to plant-sourced ones for the growth and health of humans, livestock (e.g., swine, cattle, sheep, and goats), poultry (e.g., chickens, turkey, and geese), fish, crustaceans (including shrimp, crayfish, and crabs), fur-bearing animals (foxes, racoon dogs, and mink), zoo animals, and companion animals (e.g., cats, dogs, and ferrets).

2.2 DEFINITIONS OF DIGESTION AND ABSORPTION

2.2.1 DIGESTION

Digestion is defined as the chemical disintegration of foodstuffs in the digestive tract into smaller molecules that are suitable for assimilation by the animal. The digestion of dietary protein is initiated in the stomach, facilitated by secretions from the pancreas into the lumen of the duodenum, and completed in the intestines. The term "AA digestibility" has traditionally referred to the hydrolysis of dietary protein to small peptides and free AAs in the lumen of the small intestine and to the disappearance of the AAs from the digestive tract. This process requires the action of proteases and peptidases in the lumen of the gastrointestinal tract (Table 2.4). The proteases and peptidases may originate from the animal itself or one of microbial origin. At present, the quantitative contribution of microbial enzymes (e.g., aspartic proteases, prolyl endopeptidease, and glutamine endoprotease) to the digestion of dietary protein in the gastrointestinal tract of humans and other animals is unknown. A dietary AA itself is not degraded by these digestive enzymes. Thus, protein digestibility refers to the percentage of protein in foodstuffs that is digested and absorbed by the animal. It is noteworthy that the concept of protein digestibility differs from that of dietary protein bioavailability. The latter represents the combined result of the digestion of dietary protein as well as the absorption and potential metabolism of the resultant AAs. AA bioavailability refers to the percentage of free or peptide-bound AAs that are digested, absorbed, and metabolically utilized

TABLE 2.3
Content of Protein and Other Nutrients in Foods for Humans and Other Animals

Food	Dry Matter (% of Wet Weight)	Nutrients in Dry Matter (% of Dry Matter)					
		Nitrogen	Crude Protein	Crude Lipids	Minerals	Carbohydrates	True Protein
(1) Foods for Humans							
Beef loin cut	30.8	11.7	73.4	20.0	3.46	3.14	67.9
Casein	91.7	15.4	96.0	---	2.92	1.08	94.0
Corn grain	18.3	1.62	10.1	5.18	1.35	83.4	8.85
Peanut	96.9	4.44	27.7	52.4	2.43	17.4	24.8
Pistachio nut	96.2	3.44	21.5	47.8	2.76	28.0	19.5
Potato	21.0	1.57	9.84	2.17	4.04	84.0	5.13[a]
Sorghum grain	89.1	1.81	11.3	3.87	2.68	82.2	9.88
Soybean	96.2	7.14	44.6	18.8	5.02	31.6	44.4
Soy protein concentrate	95.4	11.3	70.8	0.49	5.80	23.0	72.0
Sweet potato	22.9	1.11	6.91	0.90	4.13	88.1	4.53[a]
Wheat flour	95.1	2.35	13.4	1.48	0.75	84.4	13.4
White rice	90.7	1.32	8.25	0.36	0.40	91.0	7.25
(2) Foods for Farm and Companion Animals							
Algae spirulina meal	96.5	11.4	71.3	0.26	7.44	21.0	68.2
Black soldier fly larvae meal	95.3	7.05	44.1	35.2	6.53	14.2	44.0
Blood meal	91.8	14.3	97.6	1.10	1.15	0.15	96.2
Chicken by-product meal	98.0	11.1	69.4	13.6	12.6	4.29	59.2
Chicken visceral digest	93.2	11.7	73.0	9.19	12.9	5.84	67.3
Feather meal	95.8	15.2	95.3	3.67	0.91	0.16	81.6
Fishmeal (Menhaden)	92.8	10.8	67.3	12.0	20.3	0.41	54.3
Meat and bone meal	96.1	8.66	54.1	11.2	31.6	3.02	52.8
Peanut meal	91.8	7.65	47.8	4.04	5.58	42.6	38.2
SDPM	88.7	9.95	62.2	5.22	22.3	10.3	34.4[b]
Poultry by-product meal (PFG)	96.8	11.6	72.5	11.9	11.6	4.04	55.2
Soybean meal	89.2	8.32	52.0	1.05	6.37	40.6	42.4

Source: Li, P. and G. Wu. 2020. *Amino Acids* 52:523–542; Hou, Y.Q. et al. 2019. *Amino Acids* 51:1153–1165; Wu, G. et al. 2016b. *J. Anim. Sci.* 94:2603–2613.

Values are mean ± SEM, *n* = 6. The content of crude protein (%) was calculated as nitrogen content (%) multiplied by 5.70 for wheat flour or by 6.25 for other foods. The content of carbohydrates in dry matter was calculated by differences [i.e., 100 − (crude protein % + lipids % + minerals %)].

Note: PFG, pet-food grade; SDPM, spray-dried peptone from enzymes-treated porcine mucosal tissues.

[a] The product contains a large amount of free amino acids.

[b] Total peptides. As a result of enzymatic hydrolysis, this product contains a large amount of free amino acids.

for maintenance, growth, health, reproduction, or production. Therefore, the term "bioavailability" includes both "digestibility" and "metabolism". The digestion coefficient of free AAs in a foodstuff is 100%, but their bioavailability may be less than 100% depending on AA, dietary nutrient intake, and the physiological status of animals. Moreover, the processes of protein digestion and its products differ markedly between nonruminant species (including humans, dogs, cats, rats, pigs, horses, and chickens), which have one stomach (glandular structure), and ruminant species (e.g., cattle, deer, goats, and sheep), which have a more complex digestive system (Wu 2018). In ruminants, the glandular stomach (i.e., abomasum) is preceded by three organs (rumen, reticulum, and omasum) that support extensive digestion and fermentation of foodstuff proteins and AAs by

TABLE 2.4

Digestive Proteases and Peptidases in the Stomach and the Small Intestine

Enzyme	Site of Production	Recognized Amino Acid Residues in Peptide Bonds	pH of Optimal Activity
(1) Proteases in the Lumen of the Stomach			
Pepsins A, B, C, and D[a] (absent from stomach-less fish)	Mucosa of stomach	Aromatic and hydrophobic amino acids (most efficient)	1.8–2
Rennins (chymosins) A, B, and C[a] (some mammals; absent from birds, reptiles, humans, chimps, and fish)	Mucosa of stomach	Weak proteolytic activity; clot milk protein	1.8–2
(2) Proteases in the Lumen of the Small Intestine			
Trypsin[a]	Pancreas	Arginine and lysine	8–9
Chymotrypsins A, B, and C[a]	Pancreas	Aromatic amino acids and methionine	8–9
Elastase[a]	Pancreas	Aliphatic amino acids	8–9
Collagenase[a]	Pancreas	Imino acids	6.3–8.5
Carboxypeptidase A[b]	Pancreas	Aliphatic and aromatic amino acids	7.2
Carboxypeptidase B[b]	Pancreas	Basic amino acids (e.g., arginine and lysine)	8.0
Carboxypeptidase O (MB)[b]	Enterocytes	Acidic amino acids (e.g., glutamate and aspartate)	7.0
Aminopeptidases[b]	Enterocytes	Amino acids with free NH_2 groups	7.0–7.4
(3) Oligopeptidases, Tripeptidases, and Dipeptidases in the Lumen of the Small Intestine			
Oligopeptidase A	Enterocytes	A broad spectrum of oligopeptides	6.5–7.0
Oligopeptidase B	Enterocytes	Basic AAs in oligopeptides	6.5–7.0
Oligopeptidase P	Enterocytes	Pro or OH-Pro in oligopeptides	6.5–7.0
Dipeptidases	Enterocytes	Dipeptides (not containing imino acids)	6.5–7.5
Tripeptidases	Enterocytes	Dipeptides (not containing imino acids)	6.5–7.5
Prolidase I (dipeptidase)[c]	Enterocytes	Proline or hydroxyproline	7.2
Prolidase II (dipeptidase)[d]	Enterocytes	X-Hydroxyproline	8.0

Source: Lyons, P.J. and L.D. Fricker. 2011. *J. Biol. Chem.* 286:39023–39032; Wu, G. 2018. *Principles of Animal Nutrition.* CRC Press, Boca Raton, FL.

Note: MB, bound to the outside apical membrane of enterocytes through anchoring by glycosylphosphatidylinositol. Unlike carboxypeptidases A and B, which contain an N-terminal β-sheet-rich prodomain and are activated through the removal of the N-terminal prodomain, carboxypeptidase O does not appear to be regulated by proteolytic cleavage of an N-terminal peptide sequence.

[a] Endopeptidase (also called proteinase in the literature).

[b] Exopeptidase (a metalloprotease). Examples are (1) carboxypeptidases A, B, and O and (2) aminopeptidases A, B, N, L, and P. Aminopeptidases A, B, N, L, and P cleave an acidic AA (e.g., Asp or Glu), basic AA (e.g., Arg or Lys), neutral AA (e.g., Ala or Met), Leu, and Pro, respectively, from the N-terminus of a polypeptide. Aminopeptidase M removes any unsubstituted AA (including Ala and Pro) from the N-terminal position of a polypeptide; it is both an amino- and an imino-peptidase.

[c] Reacts with all imino dipeptides at high activity.

[d] Exhibits very low activity toward Gly-Pro and reacts with X (a non-glycine AA; e.g., methionine or phenylalanine)-hydroxyproline at high activity.

anaerobic microorganisms, as well as microbial metabolism and propagation. The major differences in the digestion of dietary protein between ruminants and nonruminants have important implications for their practical feeding. For example, diets for ruminants are formulated to feed the ruminal microbes and maximize microbial growth and microbial protein synthesis, whereas diets for nonruminants are designed to directly meet their nutritional needs.

2.2.2 ABSORPTION

Absorption refers to the movement of the products of digestion from the intestinal lumen into the enterocytes. There is limited or no absorption of dietary AAs in the stomach under normal feeding conditions. The absorption of the products of protein digestion (i.e., small peptides and free AAs) takes place along the length of the small intestine but primarily in the jejunum. AAs that are not utilized by the enterocytes enter the intestinal lamina propria, from which most AAs enter the portal vein (Figure 2.3) and a small proportion exits into lacteals (lymphatic capillaries in the intestine; Wu 2018). Some products of protein digestion are extensively metabolized by the intestinal mucosa, whereas others are readily transferred into the vascular system for utilization by the body. The cells responsible for absorption of protein digestion products (free AAs and small peptides) are the enterocytes. The concept that dietary protein was utilized by animals through the absorption of its constituent AAs in the forms of both small peptides and free AAs by the small intestine was initially proposed in 1959 by H. Newey and D.H. Smyth, and is now widely accepted after the cloning of intestinal peptide and AA transporters in the 1990s (Fei et al. 1994; Liang et al. 1995).

The enterocyte contains an apical (lumen-facing) membrane and a basolateral (blood-facing) membrane (Figure 2.2). The latter is mechanically supported by an underlying basement membrane. There is a lateral space between enterocytes resting on the basement membrane. Apical membranes of the enterocytes form the folded microvilli. An advantage of these microvilli is to increase the area for nutrient absorption. Absorption of small peptides and free AAs can occur through three routes. First, nutrients may pass completely through the enterocyte via transporters, entering at its apical membrane and leaving the cell through its basolateral membrane into the lateral intercellular space (transcellular absorption). Second, nutrients may move through the tight junctions directly into the lateral spaces (paracellular absorption). Third, small amounts of intact macromolecules (e.g., immunoglobulins and some other proteins that resist hydrolysis by gastrointestinal proteases)

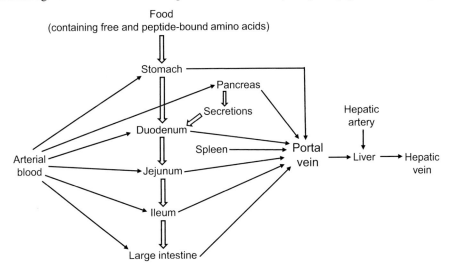

FIGURE 2.3 The portal vein-drained system in animals and the absorption of the products of protein digestion by the small intestine into the portal vein. The portal vein drains blood from the stomach, spleen, pancreas, small intestine, and large intestine [collectively called the portal-drained viscera (PDV)] into the liver. The PDV plus the liver is referred to as the splanchnic bed, which receives its blood supply from various branched arteries. The liver obtains approximately 70% and 30% of its blood supply from the portal vein and the hepatic artery, respectively. The blood leaves the liver via the hepatic vein. After dietary protein is digested in the lumen of the small intestine, its products (i.e., small peptides and free amino acids) are absorbed along the length of the gut (i.e., the duodenum, jejunum, and ileum) into the portal vein. Depending on the speed of gastric food passage, a limited amount of dietary free amino acids in the stomach may be directly absorbed through the gastric mucosa into the blood. The arrow "→" indicates the direction of blood flow.

can be absorbed by epithelial cells of the small intestine via clathrin- or receptor-mediated transcytosis (vesicular transport from one side of a cell to the other within a membrane-bound carrier) and are then exported through the basolateral membranes of enterocytes (Gardner 1975). Examples of transcytosis are the absorption, by the enterocytes, of proteins that resist degradation by proteases in the digestive tract, including (1) intact proteins (e.g., immunoglobulin G) via the neonatal Fc receptor-mediated ligand transport in mammalian neonates before the "*gut closure*" (e.g., within 48 h after birth in pigs); (2) intact bovine lactoferrins; and (3) the unusual transmissible prion protein (a misfolded and infectious protein consisting of approximately 250 AA residues) that causes bovine spongiform encephalopathy (mad-cow disease; Harris 1999). Intestinal absorption of intact proteins does not directly play a significant role in the protein nutrition of humans and other animals, but has important implications for health and disease.

2.3 PROTEIN DIGESTION AND ABSORPTION OF PEPTIDES AND AAs IN MONOGASTRIC ANIMALS

2.3.1 HISTORICAL PERSPECTIVE OF PROTEIN DIGESTION AND ABSORPTION

A series of studies with guinea pigs by Antoine Lavoisier (a French scientist) in the 1770s revealed that nutrients (including nitrogenous substances) in ingested food are utilized by the body. A British physician-chemist, William Prout, reported in 1824 that this digestive process was greatly facilitated by hydrochloric acid as the major acid in gastric juice. In 1836, T. Schwann discovered pepsin in the stomach as the first digestive enzyme of animal origin to hydrolyze protein and coined the name of this enzyme from the Greek word *pepsis*, meaning digestion. Approximately a half-century later, F. Hofmeister found in 1882 that the small intestine could cause the disappearance of a dietary protein (called "peptone" at that time). An important discovery was made in 1901 when O. Cohnheim reported that an enzyme, called "erepsin", isolated from the intestinal mucosa could break down the peptone to AAs. In 1903, Emil Fischer and his student Emil Abderhalden reported the hydrolysis of purified proteins (casein, edestin, hemoglobin, egg albumin, serum globulin, and fibrin) by pancreatic trypsin. They were puzzled by the same pattern of liberation of AAs: tyrosine first, followed by leucine, alanine, aspartic, and glutamate, and then the three basic AAs (arginine, histidine, and lysine), but no release of phenylalanine and proline. Meanwhile, E. Fischer and E. Abderhalden proposed that the hydrolysis of peptide bonds formed from phenylalanine or proline in a protein was resistant to trypsin. These results suggested the presence of enzymes to digest dietary protein, which was confirmed by O. Abderhalden and P. Rona who demonstrated in 1904 that mice fed either trypsin-digested casein hydrolysates or intact casein had the same rate of growth and survival. Similar findings were obtained for dogs in 1905. In the same year, Abderhalden proposed that dietary proteins (e.g., milk proteins such as casein, lactalbumin, and lactoglobulin) must be degraded in the digestive tract to a series of nonspecific building blocks (e.g., AAs) which are subsequently absorbed into the systemic circulation for the synthesis of specific proteins in the body. By 1912, it had already been shown that the main products of luminal protein digestion in animals were small peptides (London and Rabinowitsch 1912). D.D. van Slyke and G.M. Meyer (1913) reported that the products of protein digestion in the lumen of the canine small intestine are rapidly absorbed into the blood.

2.3.2 DIGESTION OF DIETARY PROTEIN IN THE GASTROINTESTINAL TRACT

It is clear from the above historic account that by the end of the 19th century, the physiological processes for the digestion of protein in ingested foods by higher animals had largely been discovered. Specifically, it was known that (1) dietary protein is degraded in the lumen of the stomach of higher animals to form smaller and more soluble aggregates without the formation of free AAs; (2) products of protein hydrolysis in the stomach and proteins that escape gastric breakdown are broken down to produce smaller and more soluble aggregates in the lumen of the upper small intestine through the action of pancreatic secretions; and (3) the smaller aggregates are hydrolyzed to generate free AAs because of secretions from both the pancreas and the small-intestinal mucosa. What was unknown at that time was the generation of large amounts of di- and tripeptides from dietary protein in the lumen of the digestive tract. The speed of the digestion of dietary protein is affected by its structure. For example, whey protein is digested faster than casein in adult humans (Boirie et al. 1997).

The digestion of dietary protein in monogastric animals is illustrated in Figure 2.4. In these animals, the digestion of dietary protein starts in the stomach (pH = approximately 2–3), where protein is denatured by hydrochloric acid, followed by digestion with proteases [pepsins A, B, and C, and rennins A, B, and C (in some mammals)]. Both pepsins and rennins are endopeptidases and have an ability to clot milk. Pepsins have been identified in the stomachs of mammals (including humans, pigs, and rats), birds, reptiles, adult amphibians, some species of fish (such as many tele-osts, including albacore, bluefin, cod, hake, perch, pink, salmon, and tuna), the sleeper shark, and the dogfish, but are absent from the larvae of frogs and toads as well as cyclostomes and the species of fish without a stomach (Steven and Hume 1995). Pepsin is not essential for the digestion of dietary protein, as indicated by the following evidence. First, pepsin is absent from larval amphibians and stomach-less fish, but these animals grow well when fed a diet consisting of intact protein as the sole source of AAs (Steven and Hume 1995). Second, humans with either achlorhydria (an inability to secrete pepsinogen and HCl by the gastric mucosa) or gastrectomy (the surgical removal of stomach) can maintain nitrogen balance when fed a diet consisting of protein as the primary source of AAs (Davenport 1982).

Rennin (also known as chymosin), which was first identified in the abomasum of calves, is secreted as prorennin (also known as prochymosin, an inactive enzyme) by the gastric chief cells into the lumen of the stomach of young mammals of some species, including the cat, cattle, dog, goat, horse, kangaroo, pig, porcupine, rat, sheep, and zebra, but is absent from birds, reptiles,

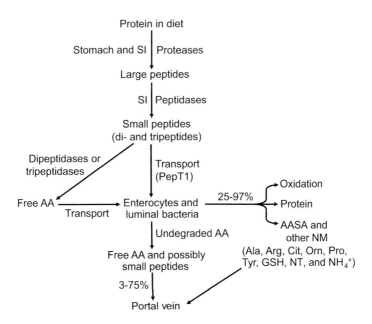

FIGURE 2.4 Digestion of dietary protein in the gastrointestinal tract of the small intestine in monogastric animals, including humans. All diet-derived AAs undergo various degrees of catabolism by luminal bacteria and some of them are oxidized by enterocytes. AA, amino acids; GSH, glutathione; AASA, amino acids that are synthesizable *de novo* in animal cells; NM, nitrogenous metabolites; NT, nucleotides; PepT1, H$^+$ gradient-driven peptide transporter 1; SI, the small intestine.

humans, chimps, and fish (Steven and Hume 1995). Gastric prorennin is activated by HCl through limited autocatalysis to rennin to facilitate the digestion of *k*-casein in milk. Specifically, rennin has a weak proteolytic activity but can cause the clotting of milk protein. Rennin liberates a glycopeptide from *k*-casein, and the remaining molecule (paracasein), along with calcium, forms a clot or curd which slows the passage of proteins in the intestinal tract. This allows additional time for the action of digestive proteolytic enzymes, thereby improving the utilization of milk proteins. Like pepsin, rennin is not essential for the digestion of dietary protein, as indicated by the fact that rennin is absent from birds, reptiles, humans, and fish, but these animals grow well when fed a diet consisting of intact protein as the sole source of AAs (Steven and Hume 1995).

The products of protein hydrolysis by pepsins, which are primarily large polypeptides and oligopeptides, as well as the rennin-processed milk protein (in some mammals), enter the lumen of the small intestine to be further hydrolyzed by specific proteases (including trypsin, chymotrypsin, elastase, carboxyl peptidases, and aminopeptidases) in an alkaline medium (owing to bile salts, pancreatic juice, and duodenal secretions). Enterokinase (an enzyme secreted by enterocytes) converts trypsinogen (a zymogen or proenzyme secreted by the pancreas) into trypsin (an active endopeptidase) through limited proteolysis (Figure 2.5). Trypsin activates other pancreatic proteases and peptidases, including chymotrypsin, elastase, and collagenase (endopeptidases) and carboxypeptidases A and B (exopeptidases) through limited proteolysis. Such a cascade of biochemical reactions is a characteristic of digestion in all postnatal animals. These enzymes occur in mammals (including humans, pigs, and rats), birds, reptiles, and amphibians and are essential for the digestion of dietary proteins in these species. In addition, Lyon and Fricker (2011) reported that the enterocytes of

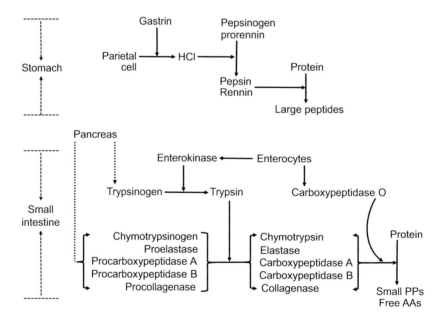

FIGURE 2.5 Generation of active proteases and peptidases in the gastrointestinal tract. Gastric inactive proteases [pepsinogen and prorennin (mammals)] are converted into active proteases by HCl through limited autocatalysis in the lumen of the stomach. Pepsinogen is also converted to pepsin by active pepsin. Inactive proteases and peptidases (zymogens) in the lumen of the small intestine are activated via the enterokinase-initiated, trypsin-mediated cascade of limited proteolysis. These enzymes play an important role in the gastrointestinal digestion of proteins and peptides. Note that (1) the pancreas secretes zymogens (trypsinogen, chymotrypsinogen, procarboxylases A and B, and procollagenase) into the lumen of the duodenum; (2) enterocytes of the small intestine secretes active enterokinase and active carboxypeptidase O; and (3) carboxypeptidases A, B, and O (metallopeptidases and exopeptidases) hydrolyze peptide bonds formed by aliphatic/aromatic, basic, and acidic AAs, respectively. FAA, free amino acids; PP, peptides.

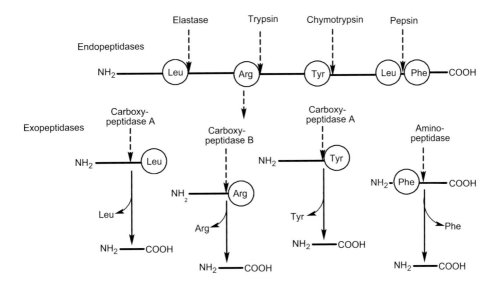

FIGURE 2.6 Hydrolysis of specific peptide bonds by digestive proteases in the stomach and small intestine of animals, including humans. Different proteases in the lumen of the gastrointestinal tract specifically cleave peptide bonds formed by basic, aromatic, aliphatic, or large neutral amino acids.

the mammalian and zebrafish small intestines secreted an active form of carboxypeptidase O that hydrolyzes peptide bonds formed by acidic AAs.

In the small intestine, the extracellular degradation of protein by trypsin, chymotrypsin, elastase, carboxypeptidases, and collagenase generates small peptides and considerable amounts of free AAs (Figure 2.6). Oligopeptides composed of more than three AA residues are further hydrolyzed extracellularly by peptidases (e.g., brush-border peptidases including aminopeptidases, dipeptidylcarboxypeptidase, and dipeptidylaminopeptidase IV; located mainly on the brush border of enterocytes and, to a lesser extent, in the intestinal lumen) to form tripeptides, dipeptides, and free AAs (Figure 2.4). Note that gut mucosa-derived proline peptidase specifically hydrolyzes proline-containing dipeptides (Sjostrom et al. 1973). Prolyl-4-hydroxyproline (Pro-Hyp, a product of Gly-Pro-Hyp degradation) can also be hydrolyzed to proline and 4-hydroxyproline by intestinal prolidase, which possesses a unique ability to degrade imidodipeptides (X-Pro or X-Hyp) in which a proline or 4-hydroxyproline residue is located at the C-terminal end (Lupi et al. 2008). Products of protein digestion in the lumen of the small intestine consist of approximately 20% free AAs and 80% of dipeptides plus tripeptides (Ganapathy et al. 2006).

Amounts and activities of proteases and peptidases in the gastrointestinal tract are affected by dietary factors. For example, increasing dietary protein levels stimulates the synthesis and secretion of proteolytic enzymes by the pancreas and small-intestinal mucosa. By contrast, the use of raw soybeans as ingredients for young animals (e.g., pigs, rats, and chicks) and juvenile fish results in growth impairment (Wu 2018). This is because soybeans and other leguminous seeds contain protease inhibitors, which inhibit the activities of digestive proteolytic enzymes, such as trypsin and chymotrypsin. Because protease inhibitors are heat-sensitive, soybeans must be heated at an appropriate temperature before they are used to feed animals. Furthermore, dietary phospholipids have beneficial effects on stimulating the secretion of peptidases by the enterocytes of the small intestine to enhance the digestion of dietary protein in animals (Wu 2018), including fish (Li et al. 2021b).

2.3.3 DEVELOPMENTAL CHANGES IN INTESTINAL DIGESTION AND ABSORPTION

There are developmental changes in the proteolytic digestive capacity in all animals. Let's use the pig as an example (Cranwell 1995). In the pig, gastric pepsinogens A and C are not expressed before birth and they appear after birth, and the amounts of the enzymes continue to increase gradually until at least day 160 of postnatal life. Gastric pepsinogen C is not expressed before birth and it appears soon after birth, and the amount of the enzyme increases gradually to the peak value at day 30 of postnatal life, declines thereafter until day 60 of postnatal life, and is leveled off until at least day 160 of postnatal life. By contrast, gastric prorennin is not expressed before day 65 of gestation, and the amount of prorennin increases rapidly between days 65 and 114 (term) of gestation to the peak value at birth and declines gradually to a nondetectable level at day 60 of postnatal life. In the small intestine, trypsin activity is low at birth, increases by 100% between days 0 and 28 of postnatal life, and thereafter increases rapidly by six-fold at day 56 of postnatal life. Chymotrypsin activity is also low at birth, increases by 200% between days 0 and 28 of postnatal life, and remains at the elevated level until at least day 42 of postnatal life. Thus, the pig is born with relatively low activities of gastric and pancreatic proteolytic enzymes, as well as relatively low concentrations of H^+ ions in the lumen of the stomach (e.g., pH = 3–5 in neonatal pigs as compared with pH = 2–3 in young adults), but a well-developed peptidase capacity (Cranwell 1995). Nonetheless, the neonatal piglet digests sow's milk protein well, with average AA digestibilities of 92%–100%, and has a high capacity to absorb free AAs and small peptides (Lin et al. 2009). By contrast, proteins of plant origin (e.g., corn and soy proteins) are digested to a lesser extent in the neonatal piglet than milk protein due to the presence of anti-nutritional factors, including cell walls and trypsin inhibitors. In early-weaned pigs (e.g., piglets weaned at 3 weeks of age) which often exhibit intestinal atrophy and inflammatory mucosa, the gastrointestinal tract has an impaired ability to digest dietary protein due to (1) reduced secretion of gastric juice and pancreatic juice; (2) reduced mass of the small intestine; and (3) stress- and starvation-induced abnormality in intestinal motility. By 6–8 weeks of age, the pig's digestive capacity is well developed to utilize plant protein-based diets. Similarly, in humans, the pancreatic secretion of protrypsinogen, prochymotrypsinogen, proelastase, and procollagenase into the small intestine is limited at birth but increases rapidly soon after birth (Sanderson and Walker 2000).

Total activities of proteases in the small intestine of chickens increase markedly between birth and 21 days of age (Noy and Sklan 1995). For example, total trypsin activity is five- to six-fold greater at day 10 than at day 1 post-hatching, and total chymotrypsin activity rises gradually from hatching to day 14 post-hatching and then remains constant until day 23 post-hatching. In chickens, total carboxypeptidase A activity peaks on the first day after hatching, declines during the first week post-hatching, and then remains at a constant level until 56 days post-hatching. As in mammals, intestinal peptidase activity is high in poultry at birth. When coupled with a functional gizzard to grind the ingested cereal grains, this developmental pattern of intestinal proteases and peptidases allows newly hatched birds to utilize a solid corn- and soybean meal-based diet, albeit at a lower rate (e.g., compared with older animals).

In all animals (including humans, birds, and fish with a stomach), gastric HCl activates pepsinogen to pepsin through limited autocatalysis, whereas zymogens (inactive proteases and peptidases) in the lumen of the small intestine (primarily the duodenum and jejunum) are activated via the enterokinase-initiated cascade of limited proteolysis, as noted previously. Pepsinogen is also converted to pepsin by active pepsin. Developmental changes in enterokinase activity vary with species (Sanderson and Walker 2000). For example, in humans, enterokinase is not expressed in the first 26 weeks of gestation, but intestinal enterokinase activity (mainly in the duodenum) increases between 26 and 40 weeks of gestation. In rats, intestinal enterokinase activity appears on day 20 of gestation (term = 21 days) and increases to the adult level by day 2 of postnatal life. In mice, enterokinase is not expressed before birth, but intestinal enterokinase activity appears soon after birth and reaches the adult level by 21 days of postnatal like.

As nonruminant mammals, birds, fish, and crustaceans grow after birth or hatching, luminal bacteria in their small intestines can be a significant source of proteases and peptidases for the hydrolysis of dietary proteins and peptides (Wu 2018). This can affect the digestion of dietary protein and the efficacy of dietary supplementation with food-grade proteases. The presence of the microbes may reduce the bioavailability of some dietary AAs in animals, while generating bioactive substances (e.g., polyamines) that are essential for intestinal cell growth and development. In addition, the foodstuff matrix can greatly influence the digestibility of dietary protein in developing animals and human infants (Gottlob et al. 2006; Moughan et al. 2014). In animals, including pigs (Yen et al. (2004) and fish (Li et al. 2021b), dietary free AAs appear in the portal circulation faster than the AAs derived from dietary protein.

2.3.4 DETERMINATION OF PROTEIN DIGESTIBILITY

The fecal digestibilities of dietary proteins were commonly measured in nutritional studies of monogastric animals in the 1930s–1960s. This method, which involves the collection of feces of the test animals within a period of time (e.g., 4 days), underestimates the true digestibilities of some AAs in dietary proteins (measured in the terminal ileum) but overestimates the true digestibilities of other AAs due to AA metabolism in the large intestine and an inadequate measure of endogenous AA flows (Knabe et al. 1989; Sauer and Ozimek 1986). For example, Rowan et al. (1994) reported that the true digestibilities of dietary AAs were greater than their apparent ileal or apparent fecal digestibility values in adult humans consuming a constant diet that consisted of cooked chicken meat, vegetables, fruits, bread, and dairy products (Table 2.5). In humans, the apparent fecal digestibility values for Arg, Asp, Gly, Phe, Pro, Ser, Thr, and Trp were higher than their apparent ileal values, but the apparent fecal digestibility of Met was lower than its apparent ileal value. Much evidence shows that the apparent ileal digestibilities of individual AAs in ingredient foodstuffs are erroneous and are not additive in animals fed a mixture of the foodstuffs (Stein et al. 2005).

Because the ileum is the last segment of the small intestine, the content of AAs in the diet and in the lumen of the distal ileum [often expressed on the basis of DM content] can be used to estimate the digestibility of dietary protein and its constituent AAs (Sauer et al. 2000). However, such values should be considered only as "apparent digestibility". This is due to the large flow of endogenous AAs into the lumen of the small intestine (g/kg of DM intake) as well as the microbial metabolism (synthesis and catabolism) of AAs in the lumen of the small intestine to possibly result in a net loss or gain of AAs to the animal. Values on the ileal endogenous flows (ileal losses) of AAs for humans, swine, and chickens are summarized in Table 2.6 and are affected by the physiological sate of animals and the dietary intakes of nutrients (including the type and amount of protein, digestible carbohydrate, and fiber; Moughan 2003; Yin et al. 2004). For example, a study with adult humans reported that compared to 30 g of milk protein, ingestion of 30 g soy protein increased the absolute amounts of the ileal endogenous flows of all AAs except for proline and decreased the absolute amount of the ileal endogenous flow of proline, while altering the patterns of AAs in the ileal endogenous flow (Gaudichon et al. 2002). In addition, increasing the dietary content of enzyme-hydrolyzed casein from 5% to 20% increased the ileal endogenous flows of all AAs, e.g., Arg (97%), Glu + Gln (266%), Gly (46%), His (169%), Ile, (128%), Leu (113%), Pro (171%), and Tyr (115%) (Hodgkinson et al. 2000). Similar results were reported for chickens (Adedokun et al. 2007; Ravindran et al. 2004). Furthermore, in the birds, the ileal endogenous flows of all AAs decreased markedly as the age increased from 5 to 21 days (Adedokun et al. 2007). By contrast, feeding enzyme-hydrolyzed casein to 15-kg pigs increasing the intake of a nitrogen-free diet by the 75-kg pig from 0.74 to 2.18 kg of dry matter/day reduces the ileal endogenous flows of many AAs [including Arg, Glu + Gln, His, Ile, Leu, and Tyr by 50%; Gly by 54%; and Pro by 35% (Moter and Stein 2004)].

The flow of endogenous AAs into the lumen of the ileum, if not corrected, leads to a substantial underestimation (25%–30%) of the true digestibility of dietary protein in the small intestine (Libao-Mercado et al. 2006; Moughan and Rutherfurd 2012a). Typical values for the true digestibilities of dietary protein and AAs in healthy adult humans are summarized in Table 2.7. Note that the true digestibility of milk protein in young mammals (e.g., piglets) is nearly 100% (Mavromichalis et al. 2001). When ileal endogenous AA flows are corrected for, the digestibility values are called "true" or sometimes "true ileal" digestibility coefficients (see below). In general, animal proteins are better

TABLE 2.5

True Ileal and Fecal Digestibilities (%) of Dietary Amino Acids and Nitrogen in Healthy Adult Humans and Growing Pigs

| Amino Acid | Meat- and Vegetable-Based Diet | | | | | Casein-Based Diet | | | |
| | Adult Humans[a] | | | Growing Pigs[a] | | Adult Humans[c] | | Growing Pigs[c] | |
	TID	AID[b]	AFD	TID	AID[b]	TID	AID	TID	AID
Alanine	98.9	88.1	87.9	98.0	88.9	95.1	84.2	96.2	88.0
Arginine	98.3	90.2	92.6	97.7	92.1	---	---	---	---
Asp + Asn	99.2	87.3	89.7	97.8	90.4	91.6	75.9	97.3	88.3
Cysteine	100	85.5	90.7	92.2	82.9	---	---	---	---
Glu + Gln	98.5	93.6	94.6	98.2	94.6	94.0	89.7	97.5	94.2
Glycine	92.4	71.5	86.5	90.5	77.9	---	---	---	---
Histidine	99.2	90.2	92.2	97.2	91.9	94.7	80.8	99.0	90.8
Isoleucine	99.5	90.9	90.6	97.6	92.8	94.1	83.8	97.2	92.2
Leucine	100	91.9	92.8	101[d]	94.7	97.2	90.0	98.9	94.3
Lysine	98.7	93.6	93.2	97.5	92.6	97.4	91.8	99.3	95.9
Methionine	98.4	93.1	83.3	96.0	90.5	---	---	---	---
Phenylalanine	99.9	89.6	91.3	97.5	91.0	96.3	88.9	99.2	95.7
Proline	101[d]	89.9	94.6	98.1	86.8	96.2	91.0	97.9	94.4
Serine	99.4	86.5	91.9	97.8	89.9	87.0	72.9	93.1	84.7
Threonine	105[d]	84.7	88.8	99.7	87.0	93.3	75.7	94.5	78.8
Tryptophan	99.1	76.7	82.6	96.8	80.0	---	---	---	---
Tyrosine	99.2	88.7	90.1	98.0	91.1	97.2	88.7	99.4	96.0
Valine	99.5	89.7	90.0	98.6	91.5	93.7	84.6	96.6	90.9
Total nitrogen	99.1	86.9	88.9	96.8	86.9	94.1	76.0	97.6	89.8

Note: AFD, apparent fecal digestibility; AID, apparent ileal digestibility; TID, true ileal digestibility.

[a] Humans (65-kg body weight) or pigs (25-kg body weight) consumed a constant diet consisting of cooked chicken meat, vegetables, fruits, bread, and dairy products for 7 days (Rowan et al. 1994).

[b] Endogenous flows of amino acids and nitrogen were not corrected for in the calculations.

[c] Humans (67 kg body weight) or pigs (40 kg body weight) consumed a constant diet consisting of 47% maltodextrin, 22% casein, 16% sucrose, and 15% soybean oil (Deglaire et al. 2009).

[d] TID should not exceed 100% but reported values from studies may be greater than 100% due to the experimental errors of measurement.

digested than plant proteins. Values for corn grains, soybean meal, sorghum, and meat and bone meal in pigs and chickens have previously been reported (Wu 2018). In diets consisting of different sources of protein feedstuffs, the proportional quantities of truly digestible AAs from each feed ingredient are generally additive, with the sum representing the quantities of truly digestible AAs from the constitutive feedstuffs (Moughan 2003; Stein et al. 2007).

$$\text{Apparent ileal digestibility of AA } (\%) = \big[(\text{AA intake} - \text{AA in ileal digesta})/\text{AA intake}\big] \times 100$$

$$\text{True ileal digestibility of AA } (\%)$$

$$= \big[(\text{AA intake} - (\text{AA in ileal digesta} - \text{total EIAA}))/\text{AA intake} \times 100,$$

where EIAA is the flow of endogenous AAs into the lumen of the small intestine.

The flow of endogenous AAs into the lumen of the ileum of humans and other animals occurs under both basal and diet-specific conditions (Miner-Williams et al. 2012; Moughan and Wolfe 2019).

TABLE 2.6
Endogenous Ileal Flows (Ileal Losses) of Amino Acids in Humans, Pigs, and Chickens

| Amino acid | Humans (Gaudichon et al. 2002)[a] | | Pigs | | | | | Poultry | | | |
	MP	SP	Kong et al. (2014)[b]	Moughan et al. (1992)[c]	Moter and Stein (2004)[d]	Zhai and Adeola (2011)[e]	Wu (2014)[f]	Golian et al. (2008)[g]	Ravindran et al. (2004)[h]	Kong & Adeola (2013)[i]	Wu (2014)[j]
					Ratio of Individual Amino Acid to Lysine (g/g)						
Alanine	1.37	0.95	1.11	1.40	1.45	1.08	1.25	1.25	1.40	0.91	1.31
Arginine	---	---	1.13	1.54	1.08	1.04	1.30	1.17	1.00	0.91	1.42
Asp + Asn	3.22	2.45	1.71	2.42	1.90	1.52	2.07	2.49	2.90	1.61	2.56
Cysteine	---	---	0.37	---	0.34	0.32	0.38	0.83	1.08	1.72	0.89
Glu + Gln	2.26	2.09	1.94	2.52	2.35	1.73	2.24	2.84	3.45	2.12	2.97
Glycine	2.78	1.67	2.83	5.32	2.77	2.60	2.96	1.42	2.43	1.04	2.38
Histidine	0.70	0.38	0.43	0.74	0.37	0.39	0.41	0.53	0.76	0.39	0.51
Isoleucine	1.11	0.67	0.69	0.74	0.85	0.63	0.72	1.16	1.37	0.86	1.20
Leucine	1.56	1.05	1.15	1.28	1.20	1.08	1.26	1.72	2.10	1.39	2.04
Lysine	1.00	1.00	1.00	1.00	1.00	1.00	1.00	1.00	1.00	1.00	1.00
Methionine	---	---	0.17	---	0.30	0.15	0.33	0.38	0.48	0.27	0.46
Phenylalanine	1.78[k]	1.29	0.67	0.76	0.72	0.63	0.71	2.43	1.37	0.79	0.88
Proline	2.52	1.09	8.14	11.4	9.69	7.45	9.48	1.67	---	1.07	1.85
Serine	2.00	0.64	1.15	1.76	1.28	0.82	1.26	1.98	2.03	1.13	2.02
Threonine	2.07	1.24	1.19	1.83	0.96	1.00	1.29	2.51	2.45	1.28	2.48
Tryptophan	---	---	0.38	---	0.23	0.24	0.24	0.41	0.45	0.11	0.43

(Continued)

TABLE 2.6 (*Continued*)
Endogenous Ileal Flows (Ileal Losses) of Amino Acids in Humans, Pigs, and Chickens

Amino acid	Humans (Gaudichon et al. 2002)[a]		Pigs					Poultry			
	MP	SP	Kong et al. (2014)[b]	Moughan et al. (1992)[c]	Moter and Stein (2004)[d]	Zhai and Adeola (2011)[e]	Wu (2014)[f]	Golian et al. (2008)[g]	Ravindran et al. (2004)[h]	Kong & Adeola (2013)[i]	Wu (2014)[j]
						Ratio of Individual Amino Acid to Lysine (g/g)					
Tyrosine	---	---	0.57	0.58	0.65	0.51	0.56	---	1.21	0.62	0.74
Valine	1.78	1.09	1.08	1.03	0.99	0.91	1.05	1.56	2.00	1.05	1.69

Note: MP, milk protein; SP, soy protein.

[a] Adult humans ingested a single meal of 30 g ^{15}N-labeled milk or soy protein, and the appearance of ^{15}N-labeled amino acids in the ileal digesta (using an ileal tube) was determined. The ileal endogenous flows of lysine were 2.7 and 5.5 mg/kg of body weight/day, respectively.

[b] Growing pigs (~70 kg) were fed a cornstarch-based nitrogen-free diet for 7 days (including 2 days of ileal digesta collection). The ileal endogenous flow of lysine was 365 mg/kg of dry matter intake.

[c] Growing pigs (~15 kg) were fed a wheaten cornflour-based nitrogen-free diet for 7 days (including 2 days of ileal digesta collection). Ideal digesta samples were hydrolyzed in 6 M HCl and 110° for 24 h. The ileal endogenous flow of lysine was 312 mg/kg of dry matter intake.

[d] Growing pigs (~75 kg) fitted with a cannula at the distal ileum were fed a cornstarch-based nitrogen-free diet for 7 days (including 2 days of ileal digesta collection) at ~30 g/kg of body weight/day. The ileal endogenous flow of lysine was 710 mg/kg of dry matter intake.

[e] Growing pigs (~75 kg) fitted with a cannula at the distal ileum were fed a cornstarch-based nitrogen-free diet for 7 days (including 2 days of ileal digesta collection). Ileal endogenous lysine flow was 427 mg/kg of dry matter intake.

[f] Growing pigs (18–23 kg) fitted with a cannula at the distal ileum were fed a cornstarch-based nitrogen-free diet at 12 g/kg of body weight for a 16-h period of food deprivation, and ileal digesta was obtained at 6 h after feeding. The ileal endogenous flow of lysine was 403 mg/kg of dry matter intake, respectively. The ratios of aspartate to asparagine and of glutamate to glutamine were 1:0.67 and 1:0.59, respectively.

[g] Broiler chicks (15 days of age) were fed a cornstarch-based nitrogen-free diet for 6 days before the ileal digesta was collected. The ileal endogenous flow of lysine was 173 mg/kg of dry matter intake.

[h] Broiler chicks (34 days of age) were fed a dextrose-based nitrogen-free diet for 4 days before the ileal digesta was collected. The ileal endogenous flow of lysine was 209 mg/kg of dry matter intake.

[i] Broiler chicks (21 days of age) were fed a cornstarch-based nitrogen-free diet for 4 days before the ileal digesta was collected. The ileal endogenous flow of lysine was 630 mg/kg of dry matter intake.

[j] Broiler chicks (21 days of age) were fed a cornstarch-based nitrogen-free diet at 25 g/kg of body weight for a 16-h period of food deprivation, and ileal digestae were obtained at 6 h after feeding. The ileal endogenous flow of lysine was 476 mg/kg of dry matter intake. The ratios of aspartate to asparagine and of glutamate to glutamine were 1:0.68 and 1:0.62, respectively.

[k] The value is the sum of phenylalanine and tyrosine.

TABLE 2.7
True Ileal Digestibilities (%) of Dietary Amino Acids and Nitrogen in Healthy Adult Humans

Amino Acid	Barley	Bread	Casein	CW	Corn Grain	Oats	Peas[a]	PP	Rice	Rice Bran	Sorghum	Soybean[a]	SPC	SWP	WF	WPC
Alanine	72	92	94	88	83	70	86	85	82	71	81	73	97	50	84	97
Arginine	83	93	97	87	86	88	96	91	90	82	85	90	100	53	95	99
Asp + Asn	76	90	95	89	81	73	86	81	85	69	81	84	97	51	87	98
Cysteine	81	87	90	91	82	72	---	74	97	65	78	---	91	47	93	99
Glu + Gln	87	93	96	88	86	83	96	85	91	79	88	87	98	51	96	98
Glycine	78	90	95	88	77	71	93	80	86	64	71	81	96	50	92	98
Histidine	82	92	97	87	84	85	74	85	99	77	81	76	97	47	95	89
Isoleucine	81	92	96	88	84	80	74	88	75	67	87	73	97	55	92	99
Leucine	82	93	97	88	88	82	82	90	81	67	88	80	97	51	94	99
Lysine	76	92	97	91	75	76	90	88	92	69	79	80	98	53	89	97
Methionine	83	93	97	89	86	82	95	90	86	73	87	72	96	64	93	99
Phenylalanine	83	88	98	88	86	84	72	89	86	68	89	80	97	53	95	99
Proline	91	91	97	88	87	77	100	93	99	61	69	71	96	47	96	95
Serine	81	93	91	88	86	75	87	85	93	70	84	86	97	47	94	93
Threonine	77	91	92	88	78	70	91	84	82	64	84	81	97	51	89	93
Tryptophan	80	90	97	85	76	77	---	78	89	72	87	---	---	47	91	---
Tyrosine	83	93	98	88	85	81	---	89	79	79	85	---	99	51	94	99
Valine	80	91	95	89	84	79	89	86	88	66	86	78	97	47	90	98
Protein	78	91	95	88	81	74	74	89	90	65	83	80	97	52	92	97

Source: Moughan, P.J. and S.M. Rutherfurd. 2012b. In: *Report of a Sub-Committee of the 2011 FAO Consultation on "Protein Quality Evaluation in Human Nutrition"*. FAO, Rome.

Note: CW, cheese whey (>27.5% crude protein); SPC, soy protein concentrate; PP, potato protein; SWP, sweet potato; WF, wheat flour; WPC, whey protein concentrate.

[a] Cooked. The true digestibility of protein was calculated as the average value for its constituent amino acids.

In the ileal digesta, the content of an AA consists primarily of three fractions: the undigested dietary AA, the basal EIAA ($EIAA_b$), and the diet-specific EIAA ($EIAA_s$). The basal ileal losses of AAs are influenced by the physiological state of animals but not by feed ingredient composition. By contrast, diet-specific ileal losses of AAs are induced by feed ingredient composition (e.g., the type and amount of protein, lipids, fiber, and anti-nutritional factors) and by interactions between the diet and the small intestine (intestinal secretion, integrity, local immune responses, and health). $EIAA_b$ can be measured by using (1) a cornstarch-based nitrogen-free diet; (2) the regression method ($EIAA_b$ is obtained when the intake of dietary protein in animals fed graded levels of protein is extrapolated to 0.0); or (3) the peptide alimentation technique (animals are fed a diet containing enzyme-hydrolyzed casein). If a nitrogen-free diet is used, $EIAA_b$ is usually estimated by determining the AA in ileal digesta and using an indigestible marker (e.g., 0.3% chromium oxide, Cr_2O_3) in the diet.

$$EIAA_b \, (g/kg \text{ of DM intake}) = AA \text{ in ileal digesta } (g/kg \text{ DM}) \times (\text{Marker in diet/Marker in digesta})$$

There are currently no reliable routine methods for directly determining $EIAA_s$ in animals. However, $EIAA_s$ may be estimated by subtracting $EIAA_b$ from total EIAA ($EIAA_t$). In this case, $EIAA_t$ can be estimated by using the homoarginine (hArg; Yin et al. 2015) or isotope tracer dilution technique (animals receive either a diet containing [^{15}N]AA-labeled protein or intravenous infusion of an [^{15}N]AA (e.g., [^{15}N]leucine; de Lange et al. 1990). The hArg method involves (1) the generation of hArg from lysine (nearly all peptide-bound lysine) in diets through the guanidination reaction of its ε-amino group with o-methylisourea (e.g., 0.3–0.6 mM) at 95°C under alkaline conditions; (2) consumption of the modified diet (containing hArg residues) by test animals (e.g., pigs); and (3) the analysis of hArg in the ileal digesta of the test animals.

$H_2N-CH_2-CH_2-CH_2-CH_2-CH-COOH$ — Guanidination → $HN-CH_2-CH_2-CH_2-CH_2-CH-COOH$

L-Lysine　　　O-Methylisourea　　　L-Homoarginine

The hArg method for the determination of endogenous AA flows in animals is based on the following principles: (1) a small but representative proportion of lysine in the diet can be converted into hArg in a guanidination reaction with methylisourea; (2) hArg is neither formed nor degraded in mammalian cells or microorganisms; (3) hArg is not a substrate for protein synthesis; (4) after digestion and absorption, hArg does not return to the small intestine; and (5) diet-derived hArg can be differentiated from endogenous AAs. The validity of these assumptions should be re-evaluated in view of the recent finding that hArg is synthesized from arginine and lysine in the whole bodies of animals (e.g., pigs and rats; Hou et al. 2016a), including their liver, kidneys, brain, and small intestine (Hou et al. 2015; Wu et al. 2016a). In addition, because leucine is catabolized by the small intestine (Chen et al. 2009), the appearance of intravenously administered ^{15}N-leucine in the lumen of the small intestine (e.g., distal ileum) may not accurately reflect the endogenous flow of leucine in the small intestine. This view is supported by the finding that the current ^{15}N-leucine infusion technique is not suitable for quantitative measurements of ileal endogenous AA flows in growing pigs (Leterme et al. 1998).

$$\text{True ileal digestibility of lysine } (\%) = \left[(\text{hArg in diet} - \text{hArg in ileal digesta})/\text{hArg in diet} \right] \times 100.$$

Total EIAA for lysine ($EIAA_{TLys}$) is estimated as the total flow of lysine in distal ileal digesta minus the flow of undigested dietary lysine.

$$\text{EIAA}_{\text{TLys}} = \text{Total Lys in ileal digesta} - \left[\text{Lys in diet} \times (1 - \text{True ileal digestibility of Lys (\%)})\right]$$

EIAA_t for the other AAs is calculated on the basis of $\text{EIAA}_{\text{TLys}}$ and the reported ratios of other AAs to Lys in endogenous secretions (mainly proteins), which are relatively constant in swine.

$$\text{EIAA}_t \text{for the other AAs} = \text{EIAA}_{\text{TLys}} \times \text{AA}_{\text{Literature}} / \text{Lys}_{\text{Literature}} \text{in endogenous proteins}$$

For growing pigs, EIAA_b values obtained with feeding a nitrogen-free diet or the regression method are similar (approximately 11 g crude protein/kg of DM intake) but 35% lower than those (17 g crude protein/kg of DM intake) obtained with the peptide alimentation technique. It appears that feeding either certain peptides or protein to humans and other animals can stimulate the flow of endogenous AAs into the lumen of the ileum (Moughan et al. 1992, 2007; Starck et al 2018), likely due to increases in (1) the secretion of pancreatic juice into the lumen of the small intestine; (2) the release of proteins, peptides, AAs, urea, and ammonia from enterocytes into the lumen of the small intestine; and (3) the synthesis of proteins, peptides, or AAs by microorganisms in the lumen of the small intestine. For consistency, feeding a nitrogen-free diet may be preferred over the other two methods to estimate EIAA_b. Normally, EIAA_b is relatively constant but EIAA_s is markedly affected by the composition of dietary ingredients. For example, EIAA_s is minimal in growing pigs fed a diet containing highly digestible protein (e.g., casein or egg protein) but can account for >50% of EIAA_t in response to a diet containing a high proportion of fiber or anti-nutritional factors (Stein et al. 2007).

As noted previously, the amount of nitrogen recovered at the distal ileum is influenced by many dynamic factors, including food matrix, protein digestibility, the absorption of peptides and AAs, secretions, and cell turnover. The ileal endogenous nitrogen consists of primarily protein and large polypeptide nitrogen, such as 60%–80% in pigs fed nitrogen-free diets (Moughan and Schuttert 1991) and rats fed nitrogen-free or low-protein diets (Butts et al. 1992; Moughan and Schuttert 1991), as well as 79% in humans fed a rapeseed protein isolate (Bos et al., 2007). Most (80%–90%) of the endogenous nitrogen that flows into the small intestine has been absorbed in the form of di- and tripeptides, as well as free AAs, urea, ammonia, and related metabolites by the time the digesta reaches the terminal ileum in pigs, rats, and humans (Moughan 2012). Besides the small intestine, there is also a substantial amount of endogenous nitrogen in the large intestine of humans and other animals (Starck et al. 2018), and typical values are presented in Table 2.6.

Recently, a concept of standardized ileal AA digestibility has been proposed to provide for some consistency in digestibility values. Previously determined values of the basal ileal endogenous flows of AAs are used to calculate the standardized ileal digestibilities of dietary AAs in animals. Accurate measurements of the basal ileal endogenous losses of AAs (including proper animal and AA analysis procedures) are crucial for the establishment of a reliable database of standardized ileal AA digestibilities for food ingredients. Values of standardized ileal AA digestibility are usually intermediate between apparent and true ileal AA digestibilities. As for true ileal AA digestibility, the proportional quantities of standardized ileal AA digestibility from each feed ingredient in a diet are generally additive (Fan et al. 1994; Moughan 2003). It has been recommended that standardized ileal AA digestibility values be used for feed formulation until more data on the true ileal AA digestibilities of feedstuffs are available in the literature (Stein et al. 2007). Note that the standardized ileal AA digestibility differs from the true ileal AA digestibility in that the former refers to the apparent ileal digestibility corrected for the basal ileal endogenous AA losses that have been reported for a given species.

Standardized ileal AA digestibility (%)

$$= \left[\text{AA intake} - \left(\text{AA in ileal digesta} - \text{EIAA}_b\right)\right] / \text{AA intake} \times 100$$

Measurements of fecal or ileal nitrogen and AA digestibility, as well as apparent and true nitrogen and AA digestibility, have very different nutritional significance, and therefore, caution should be exercised in data interpretation and use (Fuller and Tomé 2005). Measurements at the distal ileal can reflect losses of AAs from both dietary and endogenous origin, whereas measurements of AAs in feces can be useful for assessing whole-body nitrogen losses. In humans and other animals, there is active recycling of nitrogen (including AAs) between the gut (both the small and large intestines) and the systemic blood circulation. Because the measurements of endogenous AA flows and true digestibility require invasive surgical techniques, it is a challenge to directly assess either true ileal AA digestibility or AA bioavailability in humans. This difficulty can be overcome by using animal models, such as rats (FAO 1991, 2007, 2013) and swine (FAO 2013; Starck et al. 2018).

2.3.5 Absorption of Free AAs and Small Peptides by the Small Intestine

2.3.5.1 Transport of Free AAs via Transmembrane Transporters

The jejunum is the major site for the absorption of small peptides and free AAs, followed by the ileum and duodenum (Wu 2018). Major AA transporter systems and their proteins (many of which are not expressed by intestinal epithelia) are summarized in Table 2.8. In essence, free AAs in the lumen of the small intestine are taken up by enterocytes via several mechanisms: (1) simple diffusion (passive, non-saturable); (2) Na^+-independent systems (facilitated diffusion); and (3) Na^+-dependent systems (active transport) (Malandro and Kilberg 1996). Some transport proteins can use lithium to replace sodium, and a few of the transport proteins are H^+-driven. The Na^+-dependent AA transport requires energy (1 mol ATP/mol AA), as Na^+ that enters the cell is pumped out of the cell by Na-K ATPase in exchange for the entry of K^+ to maintain intracellular ion homeostasis. In animal cells, ATP binds Mg^{2+} to form the biologically active Mg-ATP complex for enzyme-catalyzed ATP-dependent reactions. AA transporters are highly expressed in the apical membranes of the enterocytes of humans and other animals, including sheep and cattle (Blachier et al. 2009; Howell et al. 2001). Based on sequence similarity, AA transporters are grouped into solute carrier (SLC) families. Eleven of them have been identified to date for animal cells (Closs et al. 2006; Kandasamy et al. 2018; Kantipudi et al. 2020). Interestingly, a lysosomal cystine transporter (cystinosin) has now been identified (SLC 66A4; NCBI 2020). Traditionally, AA transport systems have been classified according to substrate preference and Na^+ dependence. Uptake of ~60% of free AAs from the lumen of the small intestine into enterocytes is performed by Na^+-dependent AA transport systems (Ganapathy et al. 2006).

3 Na^+ (from inside the cell to outside the cell) + ATP^{4-} + H_2O ↔ 2 K^+ (from outside the cell to inside the cell) + ADP^{3-} + HPO_4^{2-} + H^+ (Na-K ATPase)

As a result of molecular cloning, contemporary classifications are usually based on gene family and Na^+ or H^+ dependence. Note that (1) more than one transporter can transport an AA; (2) Systems A and IMINO can transport aminoisobutyrate (AIB) and N-methylaminoisobutyrate (MeAIB), but Systems N, ASC, and NBB do not transport N-methylated substrates; (3) System N can use lithium (Li^+) to substitute Na^+; (4) Systems A and N are sensitive to inhibition by a low extracellular pH; and (5) System ASC is relatively insensitive to low pH. In recent years, some AA transporters, including System L transporters (LAT1 and LAT2), System N transporter (SNAT3), and a bidirectional Gln transporter (SLC1A5; in epithelial cells), may serve as transceptors, which are capable of sensing and signaling AA availability to a regulatory machinery [e.g., the mechanistic target of rapamycin (MTOR) pathway)] in cells.

2.3.5.2 Transport of AAs via the γ-Glutamyl Cycle

In 1973, A. Meister proposed that the γ-glutamyl cycle could function as a mechanism for transport of AAs across biological membranes (Figure 2.7). Note that the γ-carboxyl group of glutamate forms a peptide bond with the amino group of cysteine. This cycle has the following biochemical features: (1) the requirement of 3 mol ATP for the transport of 1 mol AA; (2) a 1:1 stoichiometry between GSH turnover and AA transport; (3) dependence of a membrane-bound enzyme, instead of a trans-membrane protein channel, for AA transport; (4) no requirement of Na^+ for cotransport of AAs;

TABLE 2.8

Transporters of Amino Acids and Related Substances in Animal Cells

Gene	Protein	Substrate(s)	System (Comment)
		(1) Na$^+$-Independent Systems for AA Transport	
SLC7A1	CAT-1	Basic L-AAs (Arg, His, Lys, Orn, HA, ADMA)	y$^+$ (uniporter; both AM and BM; UB)
SLC7A2	CAT-2 (2A and 2B)	Basic L-AAs (Arg, His, Lys, Orn, HA, ADMA, SDMA)	y$^+$ (uniporter; liver, pancreatic islets)
SLC7A3	CAT-3	Basic L-AAs (Arg, His, Lys, Orn)	y$^+$ (uniporter; brain, thymus, ovary, testes)
SLC7A5/ SLC3A2	LAT1/4F2hc[a]	Large neutral L-AAs (BCAAs, Gln, Met, Phe, Tyr, Trp); large neutral D-AAs	L1 (transport large neutral L- and D-AAs; localized to the BM of intestine and kidneys; participates in the efflux of large neutral L- and D-AAs); occurs in tissues
SLC7A6/ SLC3A2	y$^+$LAT2/4F2hc[b]	Basic L-AAs (Arg, Lys, His, Orn); BCAAs, Gln, Met	y$^+$L (Na$^+$-dependent for some neutral AAs); an arginine/glutamine exchanger
SLC7A7/ SLC3A2	y$^+$LAT1/4F2hc[b]	Basic L-AAs (Arg, Lys, His, Orn); *some neutral L-AAs (Ala, Cys, Gln, Leu, Met); Na$^+$-dependent for some neutral AAs; mediates ADMA efflux from cells*	y$^+$L (lysinuria, if defected; see above); occurs *mainly in the BM of epithelial cells in the* small intestine and kidney tubules
SLC7A8/ SLC3A2	LAT2/4F2hc[c]	All neutral L-AA (except proline); Gly	L2 (transport large neutral L; mainly localized to the BM of intestine and kidneys); does not transport D-Ser; also occurs in many tissues
SLC7A9/ SLC3A1	b$^{0,+}$AT/rBAT	L-Arg, L-Lys, L-Orn, L-Cystine; exchanges extracellular basic AAs and cystine with intracellular neutral AAs	b$^{0,+}$ (brain, kidney, small intestine; NIENB); on the AM of intestine and kidneys; does not transport D-Ser
SLC7A10/ SLC3A2	asc-AT1/4F2hc	Gly, small L-AAs (Ala, Ser, Cys, Thr); small D-AAs (e.g., Ala, Ser, Cys, Thr)	asc1 (localized to the BM of intestine and kidneys; participates in the efflux of Gly, as well as small L- and D-AAs)
SLC7A11/ SLC3A2	xCT/4F2hc[c]	L-Asp, L-Glu, and L-cystine exchanger	x^-_c, extracellular cystine/intracellular Glu; extracellular cystine/intracellular Asp
SLC7A12	asc-AT2	Gly, L-Ala, L-Ser, L-Cys, L-Thr	Asc
SLC16A10	TAT1	Aromatic L-AAs (Trp, Tyr, Phe); L-DOPA	T; the BA of intestine, kidney, and placenta
SLC36A1	PAT1/LYAAT1	Pro, Gly, Ala, GABA, MeAIB, β-Ala, Tau, Hyp	Imino (proton AAT); the AM of intestine, kidney, lung, and liver; other tissues
SLC36A2	PAT2/LYAAT2	Pro, Gly, Ala, GABA, MeAIB, β-Ala	Proton AAT; the AM of kidney and lung
SLC43A1	LAT3	Large neutral L-AAs (BCAAs, Met, Phe)	L
SLC43A2	LAT4	Large neutral L-AAs (BCAAs, Met, Phe)	L
		(2) Na$^+$-Dependent Systems for AA Transport	
SLC1A1	EAAT3	D-Asp, L-Asp, L-Glu, L-Cys, L-cystine	X$^-_{AG}$ (the AM of intestine, kidney, liver)
SLC1A2	EAAT2	D-Asp, L-Asp, L-Glu, L-Cys, L-cystine	X$^-_{AG}$ (the AM of liver)

(Continued)

TABLE 2.8 (*Continued*)
Transporters of Amino Acids and Related Substances in Animal Cells

Gene	Protein	Substrate(s)	System (Comment)
SLC1A3	EAAT1	D-Asp, L-Asp, L-Glu	X^-_{AG} (glia, neurons, retina, fibroblasts, myocytes; inner mitochondrial membrane in tissues as part of the malate shuttle)
SLC1A4	ASCT1	L-Ala, L-Ser, L-Cys, L-Thr; D-Ser	ASC (the AM of stomach, intestine, kidney, lung, and cornea); brain
SLC1A5	ASCT2 (ATB⁰)	L-AAs (Ala, Ser, Cys, Thr, Gln); D-Ser	ASC (the AM of intestine, kidney, lung, and other epithelial tissues); Na^+- and Cl^--coupled transporter
SLC1A6	EAAT4	D-Asp, L-Asp, L-Glu	X^-_{AG}
SLC1A7	EAAT5	D-Asp, L-Asp, L-Glu	X^-_{AG} (the AM of retina)
SLC3A1	rBAT	Trafficking subunit for HATs	HC-HAAT (cystinuria, if defected)
SLC3A2	4F2hc	Trafficking subunit for HATs	HC-HAAT
SLC6A1	GAT1	GABA	BETA (β); also requires Cl^-
SLC6A5	GLYT2	Gly, sarcosine	Gly
SLC6A6	TAUT	Taurine, GABA, β-Ala	BETA (β), TauT; also requires Cl^-
SLC6A7	PROT	Pro (in central nervous system)	Proline transporter
SLC6A9	GLYT1	Gly, sarcosine	Gly
SLC6A11	GAT3	GABA, betaine, taurine	BETA (β), TauT; also requires Cl^-
SLC6A12	BGT1	GABA, betaine	BETA (β); also requires Cl^-
SLC6A13	GAT2	GABA, betaine, Pro, β-Ala, Tau	BETA (β); also requires Cl^-
SLC6A14	ATB⁰,⁺	All neutral and cationic L-AAs, β-Ala; small and neutral D-AAs (e.g., D-Ala, D-Ser, D-Met, D-Leu, D-Trp)ᵈ	$B^{0,+}$ (Na^+- and Cl^--coupled transporter); localized to the AM of intestine and possibly kidneys; participates in the absorption of some L- and D-AAs
SLC6A15	B⁰AT2	L-Pro, L-BCAAs, L-Met	B^0
SLC6A17	NTT4/B⁰AT3	L-AAs (Leu, Met, Pro, Cys, Ala, Gln, Ser, His), Gly; possibly other neutral AAs	B^0 (brain, heart, skeletal muscle)
SLC6A18	XT2/B⁰AT3	Gly and L-Ala	Gly (the AM of kidney); also requires Cl^-
SLC6A19	B⁰AT1	All neutral L-AAs (including Gln, Trp, The, Phe, Tyr Met, BCAAs; brush border of small intestine)	NBB (B^0); small intestine, kidney, and placenta; Hartnup disease, if defected
SLC6A20	IMINO	Pro, OH-Pro; L-Cys, L-Ala, L-Leu, L-Met, L-Phe, Gly; sarcosine, pipecolate	IMINO; the AM of intestine, kidney, stomach, and choroid plexus; other tissues
SLC7A13	AGT1	L-Asp, L-Glu	Asp, Glu transporter
SLC17A6	VGLUT2	L-Glu	VGT
SLC17A7	VGLUT1	L-Glu	VGT
SLC17A8	VGLUT3	L-Glu	VGT
SLC25A2	ORC2 (ORNT2)	Basic L-AAs (Arg, Lys, His, Orn), and Cit; an exchanger of Orn/Cit	Orn/Cit carrier; Basic AA carrier in the mitochondria; also transport carnitine
SLC25A12	AGC1	L-Asp, L-Glu	Asp/Glu carrier; expressed in the skeletal muscle, heart, kidneys, and brain, but not in the liver

(Continued)

TABLE 2.8 (*Continued*)

Transporters of Amino Acids and Related Substances in Animal Cells

Gene	Protein	Substrate(s)	System (Comment)
SLC25A13	AGC2 (Citrin)	L-Asp and L-Glu (mitochondria)	Asp/Glu carrier; an exchanger of the mitochondrial Asp for the cytosolic Glu; broadly distributed in tissues, but mainly in the liver, kidney, heart, and intestine
SLC25A15	ORC1 (ORNT1)	Basic L-AAs (Arg, Lys, His, Orn), and Cit (mitochondria); an exchanger of Orn/Cit	Orn/Cit carrier; an exchanger of the cytosolic Orn for the mitochondrial Cit
SLC25A18	GC2	L-Glu	Glu carrier
SLC25A22	GC1	L-Glu	Glu carrier
SLC25A29	ORNT3	Basic AAs (Arg, Lys, Orn, His, HA)	Basic AA carrier in the mitochondria
SLC32A1	VIAAT	Gly, GABA	VGGT
SLC36A4	PAT4	L-Pro, L-Trp	Amino acid sensor
SLC38A1	SNAT1 (SAT1; ATA1; GlnT)	L-AAs (Gln, Ala, Asn, Cys, His, Met, Ser), Gly MeAIB, D-Ser	A (both AM and BM)
SLC38A2	SNAT2 (SAT2; ATA2)	Gly, L-AAs (Pro, Ala, Ser, Cys, Gln, Asn, His, Met), MeAIB, D-Ser	A (both AM and BM)
SLC38A3	SNAT3 (SN1)	L-Gln, L-Asn, L-Cit, L-His, L-Ala	N (Na^+- and H^+-coupled transporter)
SLC38A4	SNAT4 (SAT3; ATA3)	L-AAs (Ala, Ser, Cys, Gln, Asn, Met), Gly, MeAIB; no D-Ser	A; both AM and BM of the intestine; other tissues (liver and skeletal muscle)
SLC38A5	SNAT5 (SN2)	L-Gln, L-Asn, L-Cit, L-His, L-Ser, L-Ala, Gly	N (Na^+- and H^+-coupled transporter)
SLC66A4	Cystinosin	L-Cystine	LCT
NA	Unknown	L-Phe and L-Met	Phe; the AM of small intestine

		(3) Na^+-Dependent Transport of Substances Related to AAs		
SLC6A4	SERT	Serotonin, carnitine, and organic cations	5-HTT; also requires Cl⁻
SLC6A8	CRT	Creatine	Creatine; widespread in tissues; also requires Cl⁻
SLC22A5	OCTN2	L-Carnitine, acetyl-L-carnitine, organic cations (e.g., intestinal absorption of dietary substances)	High-affinity; AM; widespread in tissues; Na^+-independent for the transport of OC

		(4) Na^+-Independent Transport of Substances Related to AAs		
SLC15A1	PEPT1	Dipeptides and tripeptides (H^+-dependent)	the AM of intestine and renal tubules
SLC15A2	PEPT2	Dipeptides and tripeptides (H^+-dependent)	the AM of renal tubules; extraintestinal tissues
SLC22A1	OCT1	Organic cations (e.g., agmatine, serotonin, histamine, dopamine, norepinephrine, PA)	Mainly in the BM of liver; also in other tissues
SLC22A2	OCT2	Organic cations (e.g., agmatine, serotonin, histamine, dopamine, norepinephrine, PA)	Mainly in the BM of renal tubules; also in placenta, lung, brain, and intestine
SLC22A3	OCT3	Organic cations (e.g., agmatine, serotonin, histamine, dopamine, norepinephrine, PA)	Mainly in the BM of renal tubules; also broadly in tissues

(Continued)

TABLE 2.8 (*Continued*)

Transporters of Amino Acids and Related Substances in Animal Cells

Gene	Protein	Substrate(s)	System (Comment)
SLC22A4	OCTN1	Ergothioneine (an antioxidant from fungi and mycobacteria; not synthesized by animal cells)	the AM of intestine; neurons; requires H^+; does not transport carnitine

Source: Banjarnahor, S. et al. 2020. *J. Clin. Med.* 9:3975; Bröer, S. and M. Palacín. 2011. *Biochem. J.* 436:193–211; Hatanaka, T. et al. 2002. *Biochem. Biophys. Res. Commun.* 291:291–295; Hyde, R. et al. 2003. *Biochem. J.* 373:1–18; Kandasamy, P. et al. 2018. *Trends Biochem. Sci.* 43:752–789; Kantipudi, S. et al. 2020. *Int. J. Mol. Sci.* 21:7573; and Pochini, L. et al. 2014. *Front. Chem. Cell. Bioche*m. 2:61.

Note: AAs, amino acids; ADMA, asymmetric dimethylarginine; AM, apical membrane of the small intestine; BCAAs, branched-chain amino acids (leucine, isoleucine, and valine); BM, basolateral membrane of the small intestine; Cit, citrulline; EAAT1, excitatory amino acid transporter 1; 4F2hc, the heavy chain of the 4F2 cell surface antigen; GABA, γ-aminobutyric acid; HA, homoarginine; HAT, heteromeric AA transporters [e.g., the $b^{0,+}$AT1/rBAT consists of $b^{0,+}$AT1 (the light-chain with transport activity) and rBAT (heavy-chain mediating trafficking to the plasma membrane) linked by the disulfide bond]; HC-HAAT, the heavy chain of heteromeric AAT; 5-HTT, 5-hydroxytryptamine transporter; LAT1, L-type/large neutral amino acid transporter 1; LAT2, L-type/large neutral amino acid transporter 2; LCT, lysosomal cystine transporter; MeAIB, 2-methylaminoisobutyric acid; NA, not assigned; NBB, neutral brush border; NIENB, Na^+-independent exchanger of neutral/basic amino acids; OC, organic cations; OCT, organic cation transporter (polyspecific); Orn, ornithine; PAT, proton-coupled amino acid transporter; PA, polyamines (putrescne, spermidine, and spermine); rBAT, related to $b^{0,+}$ amino acid transporters; SDMA, symmetric dimethylarginine; TauT, taurine transporter; UB, ubiquitous; VGGT, vesicular Gly/GABA transporter; VGT, vesicular Glu transporter.

[a] LAT1 locates in the cytosol in the absence of 4F2hc and, upon combination with 4F2hc, translocates together to the plasma membrane. This transporter occurs in many tissues, e.g., the small intestine, kidneys, brain, mammary gland, ovary, testis, placenta, spleen, colon, blood–brain barrier, fetal liver, lymphocytes, and tumors. This transporter does not transport basic or acidic amino acids.

[b] This transporter transports basic and neutral amino acids in an Na^+-independent and Na^+-dependent manner, respectively.

[c] LAT2 locates in the cytosol in the absence of 4F2hc and, upon combination with 4F2hc, translocate together to the plasma membrane. This transporter localizes mainly in the basolateral membrane of the small intestine and kidney tubules, but also occurs in many other tissues, including the lung, heart, spleen, liver, brain, placenta, prostate, ovary, fetal liver, testis, and skeletal muscle.

[d] This transporter does not transport some D-AAs (e.g., Arg, Asn, Ile, Lys, and Val).

and (5) decrease in AA transport due to an inhibition of one of the enzymes in the γ-glutamyl cycle. On a theoretical basis, this γ-glutamyl cycle does not seem to be efficient for AA transport for the following reasons. First, the turnover of GSH has a high requirement for ATP. Note that only 1 mol ATP is required for the uptake of 1 mol of AA by a Na^+-dependent transporter. Second, γ-glutamyl transpeptidase has a poor affinity toward proline, and thus, the γ-glutamyl cycle plays only a minor role in proline transport by animal cells. It has been shown that the γ-glutamyl cycle is not a major mechanism for AA transport in mammalian cells, such as mammary epithelial, placental, and intestinal cells (Vina et al. 1989), but may contribute to the transport of some AAs by the endothelial cells of the blood–brain barrier (Hawkins and Vina 2016). These authors also suggest that the oxoproline formed is a potent activator of a number of AA transporters, including ASC and the EAATs.

2.3.5.3 Transport of Small Peptides by the Small Intestine

As noted previously, Newey and Smyth (1959) suggested that di- and tripeptides were transported by the small intestine across the apical membrane of the enterocyte into the cell. This concept had been largely established by 1975 based on both *in vitro* and vivo studies involving humans and other animals (Navab and Asatoor 1970; Silk et al. 1975a, b). About two decades later, the peptide transporter 1 (PepT1) gene (SLC15A1) was first cloned from rabbit tissues in 1994, providing definitive proof for the presence of peptide transport capacity by the small intestine

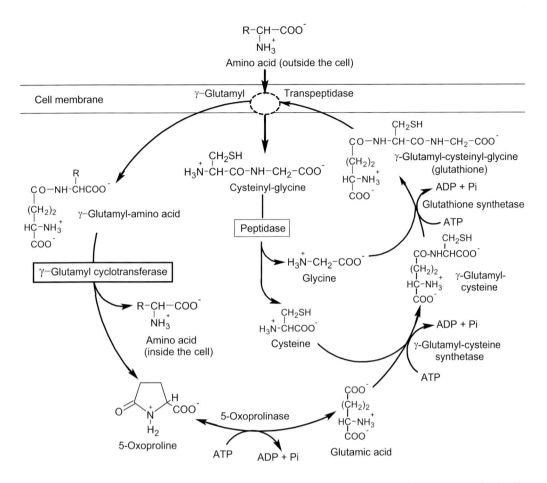

FIGURE 2.7 A proposed role for the γ-glutamyl cycle in the transport of amino acids (AAs) by animal cells. γ-Glutamyl transpeptidase is required for AA transport across the cell membrane. In general, 3 molecules of ATP would be required for the uptake of 1 molecule of AA. Experimental evidence shows that the γ-glutamyl cycle plays a minor role in AA transport by animal cells. (Adapted from Meister, A. 1973. *Science* 180:33–39.)

(Fei et al. 1994), followed immediately by the cloning of the human intestinal PepT1 (Liang et al. 1995). Subsequently, J.C. Matthews et al. (1996) demonstrated the expression of PepT1 in ruminant forestomach tissues by overexpressing size-fractionated mRNA isolated from the forestomach tissues of sheep that had classic PepT1 activity in *Xenopus laevis* oocytes. Five years later, PepT1 mRNA was isolated from sheep small intestine and cloned by Pan et al. (2001). To date, PepT1 has been cloned in many other animal species, including the Atlantic cod, cattle, chicken, dog, human, monkey, mouse, pig, rat, sheep, turkey, and zebrafish (Gilbert et al. 2008; Spanier 2014; Wang et al. 2017). In the small intestine, this peptide transporter is expressed primarily in the villus tip. PepT1 is a high-capacity, low-affinity peptide transporter with 12 transmembrane domains (Adibi 1997). It is encoded by the SLC15A1 gene and has broad specificity for dipeptides and tripeptides.

Dipeptides or tripeptides in the lumen of the small intestine can be directly transported into the enterocytes (i.e., the absorptive epithelial cells) through their apical membrane by H^+ gradient-driven (Na^+-independent) PepT1 (Daniel 2004). Neither free AAs nor peptides containing four or more AA residues are accepted as substrates for PepT1. The discovery of PepT1 in the small intestine helps to explain the findings that (1) the perfused human jejunum exhibited a kinetic absorptive advantage of di- and tripeptides over a mixture of the equivalent free AAs (Silk et al. 1975a); and (2) human patients with cystinuria (Silk et al. 1975b) and Hartnup disease (Navab and Asatoor 1970), which are characterized by genetic defects in the intestinal transport of certain free AAs, could obtain adequate AAs that were enterally provided as dipeptides. Clearly, hydrolysis of peptides on the mucosal brush border is not required for their uptake by the small intestine.

Compelling evidence indicates that the small intestine of humans (Adibi 1997) and other animals [including fish (Dabrowski et al. 2008)] transports small peptides (2–3 AA residues) at a faster rate than free AAs. When jejunal enterocytes (~5 mg cell protein) from 7-day-old pigs were incubated at 37°C in oxygenated (95% O_2/5% CO_2) Krebs bicarbonate buffer (pH 7.4) containing 5 mM alanyl-glutamine, about 60% of the dipeptide disappeared from the medium in 5 min (Haynes et al. 2009). The transport of di- and tripeptides or free AAs from the lumen into the enterocytes is associated with an influx of both Na^+ and water. Once inside enterocytes, the small peptides are hydrolyzed rapidly by intracellular peptidases to form free AAs, which are utilized in multiple pathways (Wu 1998). A small proportion of these peptides (e.g., di- and tripeptides containing proline or hydroxyproline) may exit the enterocytes via their basolateral membrane into the bloodstream (Osawa et al. 2018). Available evidence supports the view that a peptide transporter other than PepT1 is expressed in the basolateral membrane of the enterocytes for the movement of small peptides from inside the cell into the portal circulation. However, the identity of basolateral peptide transporters remains elusive.

Besides the small intestine, other tissues also contain transporters for small peptides so that di- and tripeptides in the plasma can be rapidly utilized in the body. Specifically, PepT1 is also present in the proximal kidney tubule, and PepT2 (encoded by the SLC15A2 gene) is widely expressed in extraintestinal tissues (including kidney tubules). In the kidneys, PepT2 has much higher affinity for small peptides than PePT1 and is also the predominant peptide transporter. The wide distribution of PepT2 in tissues explains why most of the intravenously administered di- and tripeptides disappear within a few minutes from the blood in humans and other animals (Furst et al. 1990).

The transport of small peptides offers distinct advantages over transport of free AAs. First, some free AAs are not highly stable (e.g., glutamine and cysteine) or have low solubility (e.g., tyrosine, tryptophan, and cysteine) in aqueous solutions. These shortcomings can be overcome by the delivery of small peptides (e.g., Ala-Gln, Gly-Gln, and Glu-Cys-Gly) so as to increase the availability of the constituent AAs to the body. Second, for equal molar concentrations of AAs, the use of dipeptides and tripeptides can reduce the osmolarity of free AAs by 50% and 67%, respectively. Third, dipeptides and tripeptides are absorbed faster and more efficiently by the intestine than free AAs. This can reduce catabolism of peptides by microorganisms in the lumen of the gastrointestinal tract and improve the balance of AA supply to the portal circulation. Thus, compared with intact proteins or a mixture of free AAs, addition of small peptides or hydrolyzed proteins to diets can offer a greater nutritional value to enhance protein retention, growth and development, and recovery from malnutrition and illness in humans and other terrestrial animals (Adibi 1997; Boza et al. 2000; Daenzer et al.; 2001; Dangin et al. 2001; Trocki et al. 1986). Likewise, free AA-based diets are generally inferior to protein- or peptide-based diets for the growth of fish (Dabrowski et al. 2010). However, because of their high costs, the use of small peptides as the sole source of dietary AAs is not sustainable practically in human or animal nutrition. Under some conditions, such as those encountered during the immediate post-enterectomy period, feeding a mixture of free AAs may be advantageous to intact protein for the nutritional support of individuals (Iglesias et al. 1994). In pigs, poultry, and fish, dietary supplementation with certain free AAs to achieve a balanced provision of AAs can improve their growth performance, feed efficiency, and health (Wu 2018).

2.3.6 NET BALANCE OF AAs ACROSS THE SMALL INTESTINE IN MONOGASTRIC ANIMALS

In humans and other animals, absorbed AAs have different metabolic fates in enterocytes (Wang et al. 2009; Wu 1998). Note that some AAs, such as chemically modified arginine and lysine that may be produced during the processing or cooking of food, may be absorbed as chemical complexes that are not utilized or metabolized by animals (Moughan 2003). It had been a long-standing belief that all dietary AAs entered the portal vein intact. However, this concept has recently been

TABLE 2.9

Percentages of Dietary Amino Acids (AAs) Entering the Portal Venous Blood in Young Swine (6–10 kg), Gestating Swine, and Adult Humans

AANA	Young Swine[a]	Gestating Swine[b]	Lactating Swine[c]	Adult Humans[d]	AASA	Young Swine[a]	Gestating Swine[b]	Lactating Swine[c]	Adult Humans[d]
Cysteine	69	71	72	---	Alanine	86	75	72	---
Histidine	71	69	71	---	Arginine	60	52	54	62
Isoleucine	66	56	58	70–80	Asparagine	74	75	75	---
Leucine	64	57	59	76–80	Aspartate	5	4	4	---
Lysine	55	65	66	70–82	Glutamate	3	3	3	4
Methionine	69	68	71	---	Glutamine	33	28	28	33
Phenylalanine	63	67	69	73–81	Glycine	69	71	71	---
Threonine	50	62	62	82	Proline	59	52	53	---
Tryptophan	75	70	71	---	Serine	66	71	74	---
Tyrosine	71	69	72	---	Taurine	100	100	100	100
Valine	65	56	57	70–80	β-Alanine	100	100	100	100

Source: Chapman, K.P. et al. 2013 *J. Nutr.* 143:290–294; Stoll, B. and D.G. Burrin. 2006. *J. Anim. Sci.* 84 (Suppl.):E60–E72; Wu, G. 1998. *J. Nutr.* 128:1249–1252; Wu, G. 2020. *Amino Acids* 52:329–360; Wu et al. 2010. In: *Dynamics in Animal Nutrition* (Doppenberg, J. and P. van der Aar, eds). Wageningen Academic Publishers, The Netherlands, pp. 69–98.

Note: AANA, amino acids that are not synthesized *de novo* in animal cells; AASA, amino acids that are synthesizable *de novo* in animal cells; ---, Data are not available.

[a] Young swine were fed a milk protein-based diet. The values include both the digestibility of dietary protein and the catabolism of AAs in the portal drained viscera.

[b] Gestating gilts were fed a corn- and soybean meal-based diet containing 12.2% crude protein. The values include both the digestibility of dietary protein and the bioavailability of orally administered free AAs.

[c] Lactating sows were fed a corn- and soybean meal-based diet containing 18% crude protein. The values include both the digestibility of dietary protein and the bioavailability of orally administered free AAs.

[d] The values refer to the percentages of orally administered free AAs entering the portal blood circulation.

challenged by findings from studies with young pigs that AAs in the enteral diet are degraded extensively by the small intestine in first pass (Table 2.9), with <20% of the extracted AAs being utilized for intestinal mucosal protein synthesis. Thus, an exciting new aspect of AA metabolism and nutrition is the finding that 20%–97% of dietary AAs may be catabolized by the small intestine of young, gestating, and lactating swine during the first pass (Hou et al. 2016b; van Goudoever et al. 2000; Stoll and Burrin 2006; Wu et al. 2010). For example, nearly all of glutamate and aspartate, 67%–70% of glutamine, 30%–40% of proline, and 35% of BCAAs in the enteral diet are catabolized by the small intestine of neonatal, weaned, and gestating swine. There is also evidence for extensive extraction (%) of dietary AAs by the portal-drained viscera (small intestine, large intestine, spleen, stomach, and pancreas) in healthy adult humans and infants: glutamine, 67%; glutamate, 96%; arginine (38%); leucine, 20%–30%; lysine, 30%; and phenylalanine, 27% (Matthews et al. 1993; van der Schoor et al. 2010; Wu 1998). The nitrogenous products of glutamate and glutamine metabolism in the small intestine of rats, pigs, sheep, cattle, and humans include ornithine, citrulline, arginine, proline, aspartate, and alanine (Chapter 3). Among AAs in regular diets, glutamate exhibits the highest rate of degradation in the small intestine of mammals, followed by glutamine, aspartate, and proline (Blachier et al. 2009; Wu 1998). The gut of postweaning mammals also degrades a substantial amount of dietary arginine and ornithine (Wu 1998). Likewise, the enterocytes of chickens extensively oxidize glutamate and aspartate for ATP production (He et al. 2018), as do the enterocytes of fish and crustaceans (Li et al. 2021a, b). The latter also actively degrade glutamine as a major metabolic fuel, such that the concentrations of this AA in their blood of hybrid striped bass or the hemolymph of shrimp are low relative to its dietary intake. Results of recent studies indicate that enterocytes of mammals, birds, fish, and shrimp can degrade BCAAs, but oxidation of lysine, methionine, phenylalanine, tryptophan, threonine, and histidine to CO_2 is absent or negligible in the enterocytes of mammals, birds, and fish (Chen et al. 2009; Li et al. 2020a,b).

The entire digestive tract of humans and other animals is colonized by a dense and highly complex community of microorganisms composed mainly of bacteria, the total number of which can exceed 10^{14} cells (Dai et al. 2011). Bacteria in the intestinal lumen and bacteria that are intimately associated with the gut mucosa can also take up and degrade free AAs and small peptides to generate ammonia, CO_2, polyamines, nucleotides, proteins, and other nitrogenous substances (including nitrite, nitrate, and GSH). These metabolites, which are produced from intestinal (combined enterocyte and microbial) AA catabolism, may enter the portal vein, the lumen of the small intestine, or synthetic/degradative pathways in enterocytes. Studies over the last decades have mainly focused on AA fermentation by diverse bacteria in the intestine. Among the AA-fermenting bacteria are strains that belong to the *Clostridium* clusters (including *Clostridium* spp., *Fusobacterium* spp., *Peptostreptococcus* spp., *Veillonella* spp., *Megasphaera elsdenii*, *Acidaminococcus fermentans*, *Selenomonas ruminantium*). They are the predominant AA-fermenting microbiota along the digestive tract. Phylogenetic analysis of the bacterial 16S rRNA gene sequences have shown that bacteria belonging to the *Clostridium* clusters, the *Bacillus–Lactobacillus–Streptococcus* group (including *Streptococcus* spp.) and *Proteobacteria* (including *Escherichia coli* and *Klebsiella* spp.) are abundant in the small intestine of humans and swine. Intestinal bacteria can degrade BCAAs and are primarily responsible for the catabolism of lysine, methionine, phenylalanine, tryptophan, threonine, and histidine in the small intestine (Chen et al. 2009). Results of recent studies with pigs indicate that bacteria in the lumen of the small intestine and those attached to the intestinal wall differentially metabolize AAs (Yang et al. 2014).

Intestinal metabolism of AAs has profound impacts on nutrition and health (Wu 1998; Yang and Liao. 2019). First, the catabolism of glutamine, glutamate, and aspartate provides most of the ATP needed to maintain gut integrity and function. Second, because elevated levels of glutamine, glutamate, and aspartate in the plasma exert a neurotoxic effect, their extensive catabolism by the small intestine is essential to the well-being and survival of organisms. Third, transformations of AAs in the intestine play an important role in regulating endogenous synthesis of AAs (e.g., citrulline, arginine, proline, and alanine) and modulating the availability of dietary AAs to extraintestinal tissues. Thus, the ratios of most AAs to lysine in diets differ markedly from those entering the portal vein from the small-intestinal lumen or appearing in the plasma and body proteins. The discrepancies in the patterns of AAs between diets and body proteins are particularly large for arginine, cysteine, glutamate, glutamine, glycine, histidine, methionine, proline, and serine. Therefore, ratios of these AAs to lysine in body proteins are not accurate estimates of their optimal dietary requirements by rapidly growing animals or infants.

2.3.7 Extensive Recycling of Nitrogen in the Intestine of Monogastric Animals

In monogastric animals, the diet is the major source of nitrogen in the lumen of the small intestine. The nitrogen can be in the forms of AAs, proteins, peptides, ammonia, urea, and other nitrogenous substances [including GSH, polyamines, purines, pyrimidines, nitrite, nitrate, uric acid, and nitrosylated products]. Dietary protein that is neither digested nor absorbed in the small intestine will enter the large intestine. The endogenous sources of nitrogen in the lumen of the small intestine include saliva, gastric secretions, sloughed cells, and cell debris originating from the stomach and intestine epithelium, bile, small-intestinal secretions, pancreatic secretions, mucus, microorganisms, and mesenteric arterial blood (Wu 2018). Note that intestinal mucins are particularly abundant in threonine (e.g., 23.0%, mol of threonine/100 mol of AAs; 17.62%, g of threonine/100 g of protein; Starck et al. 2018). There are also secretions of nitrogen-containing compounds from the circulation (e.g., glutamine, urea, and ammonia) into the small and upper large intestine. In both humans and other monogastric animals, some of the urea and ammonia are used to synthesize AAs in the lumen of the small and large intestines (Metges et al. 1999), but whether the amounts are nutritionally significant for the hosts remains largely unknown. Flows of sloughed colonocytes and colonized microbiota into the lumen of the large intestine, although the amounts are less than those from the upper gastrointestinal parts, also represent endogenous nitrogen (Fuller and Reeds 1998). Most of the endogenous nitrogen can be reabsorbed before reaching the terminal ileum and, to a much lesser extent, in the large intestine; this process is referred to as nitrogen recycling (Figure 2.8). In the lumen of the large intestine, AAs and peptides undergo extensive fermentation to yield ammonia, new AAs, methane, H_2S, and short-chain fatty acids.

In growing pigs and human infants, endogenous nitrogen flow leaving the small intestine (determined by collecting digesta at the terminal ileum) represents 30%–33% of dietary nitrogen intake and can be substantially increased in response to dietary anti-nutritional factors, high levels of fiber, as well as protein intake (Fuller and Reeds 1998). Approximately 75% and 15% of the nitrogen endogenously secreted from the upper gastrointestinal tract are reabsorbed by the small intestine and large intestine, respectively, into mucosal epithelial cells (Table 2.10). In adult humans, the endogenous flux of nitrogen into the small intestine appears to be 107% of dietary nitrogen

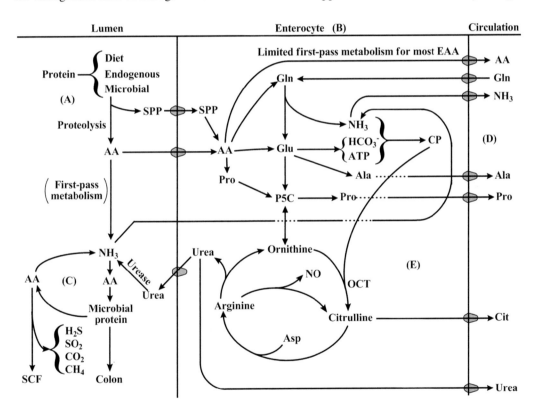

FIGURE 2.8 Nitrogen flows and recycling in the small intestine and colon. Most of the dietary nitrogen is absorbed into the enterocyte and then the systemic circulation. Both endogenous and undigested proteins, as well as intestine-derived amino acids (AAs), flow from the lumen of the small intestine into the large intestine where these nitrogenous substances undergo extensive fermentation to yield ammonia, AAs, methane, H_2S, and short-chain fatty acids. There is active recycling of N between the intestine and the extraintestinal tissues. EAA, nutritionally essential amino acids; CP, carbamoyl phosphate; SCFA, short-chain fatty acids; SPP, short peptides; and P5C, Δ^1-pyrroline-5-carboxylate. a, small intestine; b, enterocytes; c, liver; d, primarily large intestine. (Reproduced from Bergen, W.G. and G. Wu. 2009. *J. Nutr.* 139:821–825, with permission from the American Society of Nutrition.)

TABLE 2.10
Sources and Absorption of Nitrogen in the Lumen of the Pig Intestine

Source	Growing Pigs[a]	Adult Humans[b]
	(mg Nitrogen/kg body weight/day)	
Sources of Nitrogen in the Small Intestine		
Diet	1,530	200
Endogenous source	500	214
Saliva	14	3
Stomach	180	21
Bile	50	21
Pancreatic secretions	56	36
Small-intestinal secretions	100	133[c]
Microorganisms in the lumen	100	---
Absorption of Nitrogen in the Small Intestine	1,600	371
Flow from the Small Intestine to the Large Intestine	430	43
Secretions of Nitrogen into the Lumen of Large Intestine	65	243
Absorption of Nitrogen in the Large Intestine	320	257
Fecal Nitrogen Excretion	175	29

Source: Fuller, M.F. and P.J. Reeds. 1998. *Annu. Rev. Nutr.* 18:385–411; and Bergen, W.G. and G. Wu. 2009. *J. Nutr.* 139:821–825 for pigs; and from Jackson, A.A. 2000. In: *Proteins, Peptides and Amino Acids in Enteral Nutrition* (Furst, P, and V. Young, eds). Nestle Nutrition Workshop Series Clinical & Performance Program. Vol. 3. Karger AG, Basel. pp. 89–108; and Moughan, P.J. 2012. In: *Amino Acids in Human Nutrition and Health* (D'Mello, J.P.F, ed). CABI, Wallingford, UK. pp. 245–255 for adult humans.

[a] The 30–50 kg growing pig consuming an 18%-crude protein diet at the dry matter intake of 5.3% of body weight/day.

[b] Assuming the body weight of 70 kg. In the adult human, dietary intake of nitrogen is 14 g/day, the endogenous flux of nitrogen into the small intestine is 15 g/day, the amount of nitrogen absorbed by the small intestine is 26 g/day, the endogenous flux of nitrogen (e.g., from the intestinal secretions, epithelial enzymes, and sloughed cells), excluding the entry of nitrogen from the small intestine, into the large intestine is 17 g/day, the amount of nitrogen absorbed by the large intestine is 18 g/day, and the amount of fecal nitrogen is 2 g/day (Jackson 2000).

[c] Assuming the following fluxes into the lumen of the small intestine: 15% of the urea nitrogen produced by the liver (13 g N/day), namely 2 g urea N/day; mucus nitrogen, 2 g/day; the amount of nitrogen from epithelial enzymes and sloughed cells plus luminal microorganisms, 5.3 g/day.

intake (Jackson 2000), which is a much greater estimate than that in growing pigs (Table 2.10). Studies with pigs and humans indicate that 20%–25% of the urea synthesized in the liver enters, via the circulation, the lumen of the intestine (primarily the small intestine) where urea is hydrolyzed by microbial urease into ammonia and CO_2 (Jackson 2000). This is supported by the presence of urease in the small and large intestines of humans and other animals (Metges et al. 1999). Interestingly, the *in vivo* kinetics data indicate equal returns of urea carbon and nitrogen moieties to the urea pool, suggesting the presence of a metabolically significant rate of urea resynthesis in the epithelial cells of the intestine. In support of this view, G. Wu discovered in 1995 the synthesis of urea from both extracellularly and intracellularly generated ammonia in the enterocytes of postweaning pigs (see Chapter 6). Urea resynthesis in enterocytes helps to explain the apparent discrepancy in urea recycling between isotope dilution and mass balance studies (Wu 1995). In enterally fed humans, nitrogen cycling or salvage from the gut back into the body's AA pool is about 50% of dietary nitrogen intake. Extensive nitrogen recycling occurs at the expense of energy.

Among the endogenous AAs in the terminal ileum, the arginine-family of AAs (proline, glutamate plus glutamine, aspartate plus asparagine, and arginine) are most abundant, followed by (1) serine and glycine; (2) BCAAs; and (3) other AAs, including alanine and tyrosine (Table 2.6).

In response to the oral administration of $[^{15}N]NH_4Cl$, arginine is highly enriched with ^{15}N in humans (Patterson et al. 1995). This phenomenon can now be explained by arginine synthesis from ammonia, bicarbonate, ornithine (derived from glutamine, glutamate, and proline), and aspartate in enterocytes. Poor ^{15}N abundance of lysine and threonine may largely reflect the absence of catabolic pathways for their degradation initiated by a transaminase. Ammonia fixation initially involves glutamate dehydrogenase (GDH) to generate glutamate, which reacts with another ammonia molecule to form glutamine by glutamine synthetase (GS, Chapter 3). These two enzymes are abundant in bacteria but have low activities in intestinal mucosal cells (Li et al. 2009). Some of the ammonia is utilized by luminal microorganisms to grow (i.e., synthesize AAs and microbial protein). To varying degrees, such cells may be subsequently digested and the arising peptides and AAs may be absorbed, catabolized, or transported with the digesta flow to the large intestine. Evidence shows that the colonic epithelium is not a source of digestive enzymes and that protein/peptide hydrolysis in the colon is a principal function of microorganisms. Most likely, deamination and decarboxylation by colonic luminal microbes will out-compete any AA or peptide transporters in colonocytes for the substrates. Therefore, microorganisms in the intestinal lumen likely play a role in ammonia utilization through the synthesis of AAs, some of which can enter the lumen of the large intestine. Although AAs can arise from nitrogen cycling and microbial synthesis in the lumen of the large intestine, the actual net impact of this process on protein nutrition status appears to be limited in humans and other animals (Bergen and Wu 2009). Consistent with this view is the finding that when protein or free AAs were infused into the large intestine of growing pigs, most of the nitrogen disappearing from the gut was not retained in the body (Tanksley and Knabe 1984). This result indicates that the absorbed amount of free or peptide-bound AAs, if any, is nutritionally insignificant for protein synthesis in tissues. Because bacterial protein is the major product of nitrogen metabolism in the large intestine but is not absorbed by its epithelial cells, the protein and AAs that escape the small intestine into the hindgut likely have little nutritive value to the host, except for those species (e.g., rabbits, dogs, and gorillas) that have access to their own feces and practice coprophagy (eating feces; Wu 2018).

2.4   PROTEIN DIGESTION AND THE ABSORPTION OF PEPTIDES AND AAs IN RUMINANTS

2.4.1   Nutritional Significance of Protein Digestion in Ruminants

Before weaning, calves, lambs, and kids utilize dietary protein largely in the same manner as monogastric animals do. As soon as their forestomachs are functional, the preweaning ruminants also receive microbe-derived nutrients from their rumen. However, with the development of a fully functional rumen that contains different kinds of microorganisms, postweaning ruminants (e.g., cattle, sheep, and goat) are unique in their digestive physiology in that they can convert low quality feeds into organic molecules required for the synthesis of AAs, protein, glucose, and fatty acids (including short-chain fatty acids, conjugated linoleic acid, and odd-carbon number long-chain fatty acids; Schwab and Broderick 2017). Ruminants can also effectively utilize protein-derived AAs, ammonia, and carbon skeletons, as well as non-protein and non-AA nitrogen (e.g., urea and ammonia) for the synthesis of AAs and microbial protein in the rumen when the dietary supplies of fermentable carbohydrates and minerals (e.g., sulfur and cobalt) are not limited (Figure 2.9). Thus, ruminants can convert low-quality protein and non-protein materials into high-quality products (e.g., milk, meat, and wool) for human consumption and use without a need to compete with monogastric animals or humans for foods and natural resources (Bergen 2021). This underscores the nutritional and economic significance of the digestion of plant proteins by ruminants. An understanding of these processes will aid in increasing the supply of all AAs to the small intestine for absorption and utilization for tissue protein synthesis. Additionally, because the colon and cecum of humans also harbor large numbers of various strains of bacteria, knowledge about nitrogen metabolism in

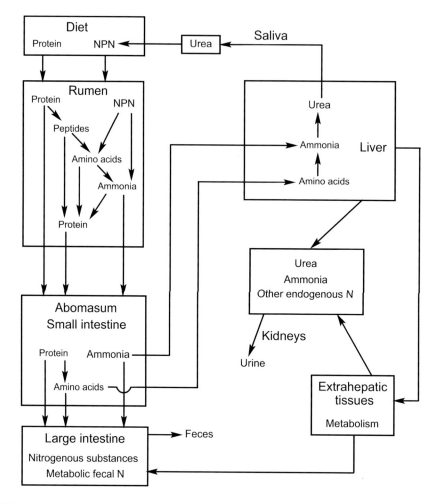

FIGURE 2.9 Utilization of dietary protein and non-protein nitrogen (NPN) by ruminants. Multiple organs participate in the conversion of dietary proteins into tissue proteins, ammonia, and urea. Some of the urea produced in the liver is recycled to the gastrointestinal tract where urea is hydrolyzed into ammonia by the luminal urease of bacterial origin. This ammonia enters the portal circulation and then the liver for ureagenesis.

the rumen has important implications for preventing human bowel diseases (e.g., colon cancer and inflammatory disorders).

2.4.2 DIGESTION OF DIETARY PROTEIN IN THE GASTROINTESTINAL TRACT

In ruminants fed a roughage diet, the rumen (normally pH 5.8–6.2) contains many different strains and species of bacteria, protozoa, and anaerobic fungi (Firkins et al. 2007). These microorganisms, primarily bacteria, release a variety of proteases, peptidases, and deaminases. The ruminal bacterial proteases, which are located on the outside cell surface and mainly cell-bound, are readily available to their extracellular substrates. Dietary protein is hydrolyzed by microbial proteases to form small peptides and free AAs (Figure 2.10). These products can be taken up by various species of microbes to produce (1) ammonia, microbial protein, and nitrogenous substances on the cell wall; (2) pyruvate and short-chain fatty acids (acetate, propionate, and butyrate); (3) branched-chain fatty acids (isobutyrate, isovaleric acid, and 2-methylbutyric acid from valine, isoleucine, and leucine, respectively); and (4) CO_2 and methane. Branched-chain fatty acids in the rumen serve as growth factors

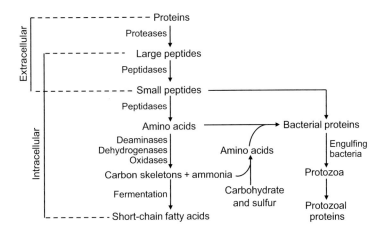

FIGURE 2.10 Synthesis of microbial proteins in the rumen of ruminants. Dietary proteins are hydrolyzed to form small peptides and amino acids (AAs). These AAs can be degraded to form ammonia and the corresponding α-ketoacids. Bacteria use small peptides, AAs, and ammonia to synthesize new proteins. CH_2O, fermentable carbohydrates; S, sulfur-containing precursors.

for microorganisms and as starting materials for the formation of long-chain branched fatty acids (Allison et al. 1962). By contrast, ruminal protozoa cannot utilize ammonia, but derive their nitrogen from bacteria by engulfing and digesting them with powerful intracellular proteases (optimal pH of 6.0–7.0; Foulkes and Leng 1988). Ruminal protein synthesis reaches a maximum level when ammonia (the sum of NH_4^+ and NH_3) concentrations in the ruminal fluid reach 5 mM (90 mg/L). This concentration can be achieved with diets containing 13% crude protein. In the rumen, 50%–80% of microbial N is derived from ammonia. Studies with ^{15}N have revealed that bacteria can derive up to 30% of their protein from sources (e.g., peptides and AAs) other than ammonia. The microbial protein content in the small intestine can be measured by assays of components associated with only microorganisms. Markers of microbial proteins include 2,6-diaminopimelic acid (characteristic of bacteria; Gilbreath et al. 2021) and 2-aminoethylphosphonic acid (characteristic of protozoa; Dufva et al. 1982). An alternative approach would be to measure the incorporation of [14]C-, [13]C-, [15]N-, or ^{35}S-labeled AAs into proteins in microbes. In ruminant nutrition, the microbial true protein and the dietary undegraded protein that passes intact through the rumen into the abomasum and small intestine for digestion are collectively referred to as metabolizable protein.

Many enzymes (including AA transaminases, AA hydroxylases, and AA decarboxylases) can initiate AA degradation in the rumen, ultimately leading to the production of ammonia and CO_2. However, AA deaminases, AA oxidases, and AA dehydrogenases can directly catalyze the production of ammonia and α-ketoacids from AAs in bacteria, protozoa, and the extracellular fluid of the rumen (Figure 2.11). AA deaminases are the principal enzymes whereby the amino groups of dietary AAs are lost irreversibly lost as ammonia in the rumen. The NADH and $FADH_2$, which are produced from AA dehydrogenases and AA oxidases, respectively, cannot be used for ATP production in the rumen via the electron transport system due to the anaerobic environment. Rates of the catabolism of AAs in the rumen are particularly high compared with animal tissues, which explain, in part, why their concentrations in ruminal fluid are very low, ranging from 1.3 μM for taurine to 44 μM for glutamate in steers (Gilbreath et al. 2020a). As noted above, the carbon skeletons of AAs are utilized, in part, for the synthesis of fatty acids. Some carbon skeletons of AAs are also utilized for the synthesis of new AAs (Broderick 1991).

The microbial population within the rumen has long been considered to have the capability to extensively degrade all dietary AAs (Owens and Basalan 2016; Tedeschi and Fox 2016). There is evidence that all the AAs studied to date (Ala, Arg, Asn, Asp, Cys, Gln, Gly, His, Ile, Leu, Lys, Met, Orn, Phe, Pro, Ser, Thr, Tyr, and Val) do not escape the rumen. For this reason, high-quality protein

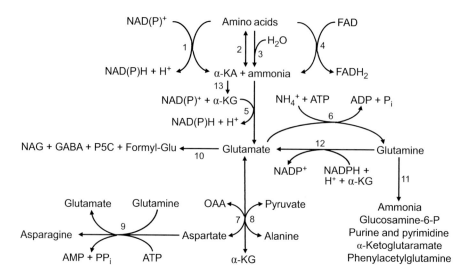

FIGURE 2.11 Production and utilization of ammonia by microorganisms in the rumen of ruminants. GABA, γ-aminobutyrate; Formyl-Glu, formylglutamate; α-KA, α-ketoacids; α-KG, α-ketoglutarate; NAG, *N*-acetylglutamate; P5C, Δ¹-pyrroline-5-carboxylate. The enzymes that catalyze the indicated reactions are (1) amino acid (AA) dehydrogenases; (2) AA transaminases; (3) AA deaminases; (4) AA oxidases; (5) glutamate dehydrogenase; (6) glutamine synthetase; (7) glutamate-oxaloacetate transaminase (aspartate transaminase); (8) glutamate-pyruvate transaminase (alanine transaminase); (9) asparagine synthetase; (10) enzymes for the syntheses of NAG, GABA, P5C, and Formyl-Glu from glutamate, which are catalyzed by NAG synthase, glutamate decarboxylase, γ-glutamyl kinase plus glutamyl semialdehyde dehydrogenase, and complex enzymes, respectively; (11) a series of enzymes required in multiple pathways; (12) glutamate synthase (also known as NADPH-dependent glutamine:α-ketoglutarate amidotransferase; glutamine + 2 α-ketoglutarate + NADPH + H⁺ → 2 glutamate + NADP⁺); and (13) enzymes for the conversion of α-ketoacids to α-ketoglutarate via various reactions. *Note*: NAG, *N*-acetyl-glutamate; OAA, oxaloacetate; P5C, Δ¹-pyrroline-5-carboxylate.

and crystalline AAs are generally encapsulated with lipids to protect them from attack by ruminal enzymes and microbes (Schwab and Broderick 2017). Of particular note, we recently discovered that although ruminal bacteria from adult cattle and adult sheep extensively degrade glutamine into glutamate and ammonia, and arginine into ornithine, proline, and ammonia, these cells have a limited ability to degrade extracellular glutamate and do not catabolize extracellular citrulline (Gilbreath et al. 2019, 2020b). There is a negligible uptake of glutamate and no detectable uptake of citrulline by the ruminal microbes. Similarly, when rumen-protected or unprotected citrulline is orally administered to the rumen of adult steers, none of the supplement is degraded in the rumen, and the oral administration of glutamine rapidly increases the concentration of glutamate in the ruminal fluid (Gilbreath et al. 2020a). Thus, in contrast to common belief, unprotected glutamate and citrulline can effectively escape the rumen of ruminants to enter the small intestine. This new knowledge advances the field of AA nutrition in ruminants and provides a novel biochemical basis for dietary supplementation with these two AAs to possibly enhance their growth and productivity (Brake et al. 2014; Gilbreath et al. 2021). These findings also have important implications for the nutrition of humans and other animals, such as dairy cows, horses, sheep, goats, deer, pigs, rabbits, rats, geese, turkey, chickens, fish, and crustaceans.

The proportion of the total dietary protein that is digested in the rumen varies from 70%–85% for most diets to 30%–40% for less soluble proteins (Firkins and Yu 2015). Rates of protein degradation in the rumen depend on residence time in the rumen, proteolytic activity of ruminal microorganisms, the type of protein, and the level of feeding. For example, certain proteins of animal origin (e.g., feather meal, meat and bone meal, and blood meal) are much more resistant to rumen degradation than plant proteins. About 90% of the total nitrogen in the ruminal content exists in an insoluble form (e.g., microbial proteins, smaller particles of undigested dietary protein, and sloughed ruminal epithelial cells). Nitrogen in the soluble pool (about 10% of the total ruminal nitrogen) consists of ammonia nitrogen (~70%) and a mixture of free AAs and peptides (Bergen 2021). Ammonia nitrogen is present in the rumen in concentrations ranging from 20 to 500 mg/L, depending on diet and time after feeding. Maximum concentrations of ammonia are usually reached about 2 h after the ingestion of a protein-containing diet. AA nitrogen and peptide nitrogen are present at either much lower (usually <20 mg/L; Schwab and Broderick 2017), similar, or even higher (Webb and Matthews 1994) concentrations in the rumen, depending on nutritional state. For example, the concentrations of AA nitrogen in the ruminal fluid range from 1.2 to 15 mg/L and 7.2 to 60 mg/L before and after feeding, respectively, whereas the concentrations of peptide nitrogen in the ruminal fluid range from 15 to 50 mg/L and 100 to 270 mg/L before and after feeding, respectively (Webb and Matthews 1994). Thus, feeding substantially increases the concentrations of AAs and peptides in the rumen.

In the presence of α-ketoacids (e.g., pyruvate, oxaloacetate, and α-ketoglutarate which are products of carbohydrate metabolism) and sulfur, ammonia is utilized by ruminal bacteria for the synthesis of new AAs and proteins (Chalupa 1972; Tyler 1978). The most important initial reaction for the microbial assimilation of ammonia is catalyzed by GDH to produce glutamate, which is then utilized to synthesize glutamine, alanine, aspartate, and asparagine by GS, glutamate-pyruvate transaminase, glutamate-oxaloacetate transaminase, and asparagine synthetase, respectively (Figure 2.11). Glutamate is also formed from glutamine and α-ketoglutarate (α-KG) by glutamate synthase. This glutamate family of AAs (glutamate, glutamine, alanine, aspartate, and asparagine) serves as substrates for the synthesis of all other AAs by microorganisms in the presence of fermentable carbohydrates and sulfur in the rumen (Chapter 3). Sulfur is needed for the synthesis of methionine and cysteine and can be supplied as sulfites (SO_3^{2-}), sulfates (SO_4^{2-}), or protein. Sulfate is converted to sulfide by ruminal microorganisms. The diets for ruminants should contain nitrogen and sulfur at a ratio of 10:1, 12:1, or 14:1, depending on their physiological states and expected productivity levels (Wu 2018). Under normal feeding conditions, the concentrations of free proteinogenic AAs in ruminal fluid are relatively low, ranging from 10 to 50 μM, partly due to active microbial protein synthesis in the rumen as well as the high turnover rates of AAs leaving the rumen. Also because of the extensive metabolism of most AAs in the rumen, diets and bacterial proteins have different AA profiles (Table 2.11).

2.4.3 DIGESTION OF NUCLEIC ACIDS IN THE RUMEN AND OTHER PARTS OF THE GASTROINTESTINAL TRACT

In the rumen, nucleic acids (5%–10% of dietary N) are degraded by nucleases (e.g., ribonucleases and deoxyribonucleases) into nucleotides, which are further hydrolyzed by nucleotidases and non-specific phosphatases into nucleosides and Pi (Nagaraja 2016). The nucleosides are degraded into (1) purine or pyrimidine bases plus ribose or deoxyribose by nucleosidases; or (2) purine or pyrimidine bases plus ribose-1-P by nucleoside phosphorylase. Purines are converted sequentially into uric acid, allantoin, allantoic acid, ureidoglycolic acid, and urea (a source for microbial AA synthesis) plus glyoxylate. Pyrimidine bases are metabolized to β-alanine, β-aminoisobutyrate, ammonia (a source for microbial AA synthesis), and CO_2. All of these products have been found in the rumen of ruminants (Vogels and Van der Driet 1976). Indeed, 42% of the ruminal coliform isolates are capable of growing on a medium that contains uric acid as the primary source of carbon and nitrogen. The predominant uricolytic organism is *Paracolobactrum aerogenoides*, but *S. ruminantium* can also use adenine and uric acid, but not allantoin, xanthine, or uracil, as nitrogen sources. The collective actions of ruminal bacteria benefit their ruminant hosts through the conversion of non-protein nitrogen (NPN) into ammonia, AAs, and protein.

TABLE 2.11

Composition of Amino Acids (AAs) in the Feeds, Ruminal Bacterial Protein, Plasma, and Skeletal Muscle Proteins of Adult Sheep and Cattle[a]

AAs	AAs in Feeds (g/100 g AAs)		AAs in Ruminal Bacterial Proteins (g/100 g AAs)[d]		Free AAs in Plasma (μmol/L)		AAs in Skeletal Muscle Proteins (g/100 AAs)[d]	
	Sheep[b]	Cattle[c]	Sheep[b]	Cattle[c]	Sheep[b]	Cattle[c]	Sheep[b]	Cattle[c]
Ala	6.53	8.02	6.74	6.72	182	181	5.52	5.55
Arg	5.91	5.18	5.03	5.01	190	121	6.58	6.57
Asn	5.13	4.71	5.34	5.36	33	31	4.16	4.18
Asp	5.83	6.58	6.74	6.75	11	5.4	5.15	5.16
Cys[e]	1.87	1.61	1.48	1.49	114	132	1.38	1.35
Gln	9.02	5.95	5.11	5.13	372	286	5.66	5.64
Glu	7.85	10.8	8.02	7.99	61	52	9.35	9.32
Gly	4.90	4.93	5.06	5.07	511	347	4.17	4.18
His	2.18	2.28	2.05	2.07	62	67	3.94	3.95
Ile	4.20	4.47	5.53	5.51	62	100	5.13	5.15
Leu	8.32	8.67	7.67	7.66	107	148	8.34	8.33
Lys	4.98	4.66	7.70	7.70	94	104	9.02	9.03
Met	1.63	1.79	2.42	2.40	24	27	3.18	3.17
Phe	4.90	5.30	5.13	5.16	36	51	4.19	4.18
Pro	7.93	4.90	3.67	3.66	156	184	4.06	4.08
Ser	5.05	4.56	4.65	4.62	75	67	4.38	4.41
Thr	3.81	4.78	5.52	5.57	60	62	4.61	4.59
Trp	1.24	1.53	1.39	1.38	39	49	1.26	1.25
Tyr	3.73	3.42	4.65	4.63	61	70	3.76	3.75
Val	4.98	5.91	6.08	6.11	128	224	5.96	5.94
Hyp	ND	ND	ND	ND	41	45	0.20	0.21

Source: Gilbreath et al. 2021. *Adv. Exp. Med. Biol.* 1285:43–61.

Note: Hyp, 4-hydroxyproline; ND, not detected.

[a] Adult Suffolk female sheep (60–65 kg) were fed a soybean hulls-, wheat middlings-, and corn-based diet (Gilbreath et al. 2020b), whereas adult Angus×Hereford steers (mean body weight of 538 kg) fitted with a ruminal cannula consumed daily 14.02 kg (dry matter) of Bermudagrass hay and 0.506 kg (dry matter) of dried distillers grains with solubles.

[b] Taken from Gilbreath et al. (2020b).

[c] Taken from Gilbreath et al. (2020a).

[d] Calculations were based on the molecular weights of intact amino acids.

[e] Total cysteine (cysteine plus ½ cystine).

The dietary nucleic acids that escape the rumen, as well as the bacterial and protozoal nucleic acids that leave the rumen, are hydrolyzed extracellularly to nucleotides in the small intestine by pancreatic nucleases (e.g., ribonuclease and deoxyribonuclease released from the pancreas) and by intestinal phosphodiesterases (released from the small intestine). Specific pancreatic nucleotidases and nonspecific phosphatases (released from the pancreas) further degrade nucleotides to nucleosides and phosphate. The digestibility of nucleic acids to nucleosides as well as purine and pyrimidine bases in the small intestine of ruminants is 80%–90% (Wu 2018).

The nucleosides and phosphate are transported, respectively, into the enterocytes by apical membrane Na$^+$-dependent nucleoside transporters (CNT1, selective for purine nucleoside; and CNT2, selective for pyrimidine nucleoside) and three Na$^+$-dependent phosphate transporters (NaPi2b, PiT1, and PiT2). The nucleosides that are not absorbed directly are degraded extracellularly by both pancreatic nucleosidases and small-intestinal mucosa-derived nucleoside phosphorylases to form purine or pyrimidine bases. The purine or pyrimidine bases are then transported by Na^+-dependent nucleobase transporters into the enterocytes. The small intestine of ruminants has a high capacity to absorb nucleosides and their bases (Stentoft et al. 2015).

Nucleic acid $+ H_2O \rightarrow$ Nucleotide (Nuclease; RNAse or DNAse)

Nucleotide $+ H_2O \rightarrow$ Nucleoside $+$ Pi (Nucleotidase)

Nucleoside $+ H_2O \rightarrow$ Purine or pyrimidine base $+$ Ribose or deoxyribose (Nucleosidase)

Nucleoside $+$ Pi $\rightarrow$ Purine or pyrimidine base $+$ Ribose-1-phosphate (Nucleoside phosphorylases)

2.4.4 ABSORPTION OF FREE AAS AND SMALL PEPTIDES BY THE SMALL INTESTINE

Microbial cells (bacteria and protozoa) containing proteins, peptides, and AAs, as well as undigested dietary protein, leave the reticulorumen and enter the omasum, abomasum (pH 2–3), and the small intestine. Digestion of proteins in the abomasum and small intestine of ruminants is qualitatively similar to that in the stomach and small intestine of monogastric animals (Huntington and Prior 1985; Wu 2018). However, there are some quantitative differences between ruminants and nonruminants. First, the amount of metabolic nitrogen (e.g., the nitrogen supplied from the pancreatic juice and bile into the duodenum, and the nitrogen from epithelial cells sloughed from the intestinal tract) in proportion to the amount of feed nitrogen is considerably greater in ruminants than in nonruminants. Second, due to high concentrations of short-chain fatty acids in the gastric fluid of the abomasum, the rate of neutralization of the digesta entering the duodenum is slower in ruminants than in monogastric animals. Third, in sharp contrast to simple-stomached animals, 50%–90% of the protein entering the small intestine is of microbial origin in ruminants, with the remainder being feed protein that has escaped degradation in the rumen. Fourth, activation and peak activity of pancreatic proteases occurs in the mid-jejunum in ruminants, rather than in the duodenum in simple-stomached animals. Fifth, the pancreatic juice of ruminants contains high activities of nucleases as a mechanism of adaptation to the high content of nucleic acids in microbial cells. Compared with monogastric animals, the concentrations of free AAs in the plasma of ruminants are much lower due to a lower intake of dietary protein (Table 2.11). Because of AA metabolism in extraintestinal tissues, the profiles of AAs in the plasma differ from those in tissues, such as skeletal muscle.

2.4.5 NITROGEN RECYCLING IN RUMINANTS AND ITS NUTRITIONAL IMPLICATIONS

The ammonia that is produced in the rumen but is not utilized for synthesis of AAs or polypeptides in microorganisms is absorbed into the blood circulation and converted into urea via the hepatic urea cycle (Figure 2.8). Ammonia in the ruminal fluid may also be utilized by ruminal epithelial cells for biosynthetic processes (including the production of urea, glutamate, and glutamine). The removal of ammonia is of physiological importance because it spontaneously takes up H^+ to form NH_4^+ to potentially increase the pH of the ruminal fluid. Ammonia in the plasma is taken up by the liver for the synthesis of urea (containing 46.7% nitrogen) via the urea cycle. Most of the urea is excreted into the urine. About 20% of the circulating urea is taken up by the intestine of ruminants where it is hydrolyzed by microbial urease to form ammonia plus CO_2 (Bergen 2021). Some urea in the blood also enters the rumen through the ruminal wall and by the secretion of salivary glands into the oral cavity (Archibeque et al. 2001). In the rumen, urea is hydrolyzed by microbial urease to form ammonia plus CO_2. Such a nitrogen recycling mechanism helps conserve ammonia for biosynthetic processes in the rumen. Because its hydrolysis to form ammonia by microbial urease, urea can be used as a source of nitrogen for the diets of ruminants (Reynolds and Kristensen 2008).

Urea is well utilized by ruminal microorganisms to synthesize AAs and protein when diets contain <13% crude protein. Results of extensive research indicate that urea may account for 15%–25% of crude protein in diets for beef cattle, cows, and sheep (Schwab and Broderick 2017).

Urea is a natural water-soluble substance in forages and is a major form of non-protein nitrogen in conventional ruminant diets. Corn silage and alfalfa may contain up to 50% and 20% of non-protein nitrogen, respectively (Wu 2018). Efficacy and safety of urea supplementation to diets for cattle and sheep depend on many factors, including (1) the dosage and frequency, (2) percentages of dietary carbohydrates and crude protein as well as their digestibilities in the rumen, and (3) adequate supply of phosphorus, sulfur, and trace minerals. It should be borne in mind that toxicity of ammonia and urea can occur when their concentrations in the rumen are very high. The underlying mechanisms involve (1) a substantial increase in the ruminal pH, leading to reductions in bacterial growth and synthetic activity in the rumen; (2) removal of α-KG from the Krebs cycle, thereby interfering with ATP production by cells and tissue, particularly those in the central nervous system; (3) disturbance of acid–base balance in the circulation; and (4) enhanced synthesis of glutamine, which inhibits the synthesis of nitric oxide (NO) from arginine in endothelial cells and, therefore, blood flow and oxygen supply to vital organs, particularly the brain. It is advantageous to supply urea as a liquid food supplement with higher concentrations of molasses and phosphoric acid. This is because (1) molasses serves as an energy source for microbial utilization of ammonia and protein synthesis and (2) phosphoric acid lowers the pH in the ruminal fluid.

2.4.6 Protecting High-Quality Protein and Crystalline AAs from Rumen Degradation

High-quality protein is required to support maximal growth, reproduction, and lactation performance of beef cattle, dairy cows, sheep, and goats (Wu 2018). However, not all dietary protein is utilized for microbial protein synthesis. Additionally, microbial protein synthesis requires large amounts of energy and the efficiency of energetic transformations for protein synthesis from AAs is usually less than 75%. Thus, it may be beneficial to protect high-quality protein or supplemental crystalline AAs (e.g., arginine, lysine, and methionine) in the diet from degradation in the rumen (Schwab and Broderick 2017). Several approaches have been developed to reduce the degradation of protein in the rumen. These methods include the treatment of protein by mild heating, chemical treatment, addition of polyphenolic phytochemicals, and physical encapsulation. In the small intestine, the coating lipids are readily broken down by lipase to release proteins or AAs. Similarly, supplemental AAs for ruminants should be protected from rumen degradation, and should be generally recognized as safe (GRAS) to ensure both high efficacy and safety. Rumen-protected AAs should be palatable and stable particularly when they are incorporated into silage- or forage-based total mixed rations.

2.4.6.1 Heating

Heating was one of the earliest methods that were used to protect high-quality protein (e.g., casein) from degradation in the rumen. This classic work was first reported in 1954. The underlying principle is based on the Maillard reaction (Figure 2.12). This involves the reaction between the free amino groups of certain AAs [particularly the ε-amino groups (–NH$_2$) of lysine residues in protein and the amino groups of free arginine and lysine] and carbonyl compounds (–HC=O), usually reducing sugars (e.g., glucose, fructose, or ribose). The initial reaction is the formation of a Schiff base, followed by Amadori rearrangement of the Schiff base to generate an Amadori compound. The formation of the Schiff base is reversible. However, further heating results in the production of melanoidin polymers that produce a brown color. The dark coloration of overheated hays and silages is symptomatic of the Maillard reaction. The modified lysine in the form of melanoidin polymers is nutritionally unavailable to animals. Therefore, excess heating of feed proteins poses a problem. If the heated proteins escape breakdown by proteases in the rumen, these proteins may also escape breakdown by proteases in the abomasum and the small intestine. The Maillard reaction, which can

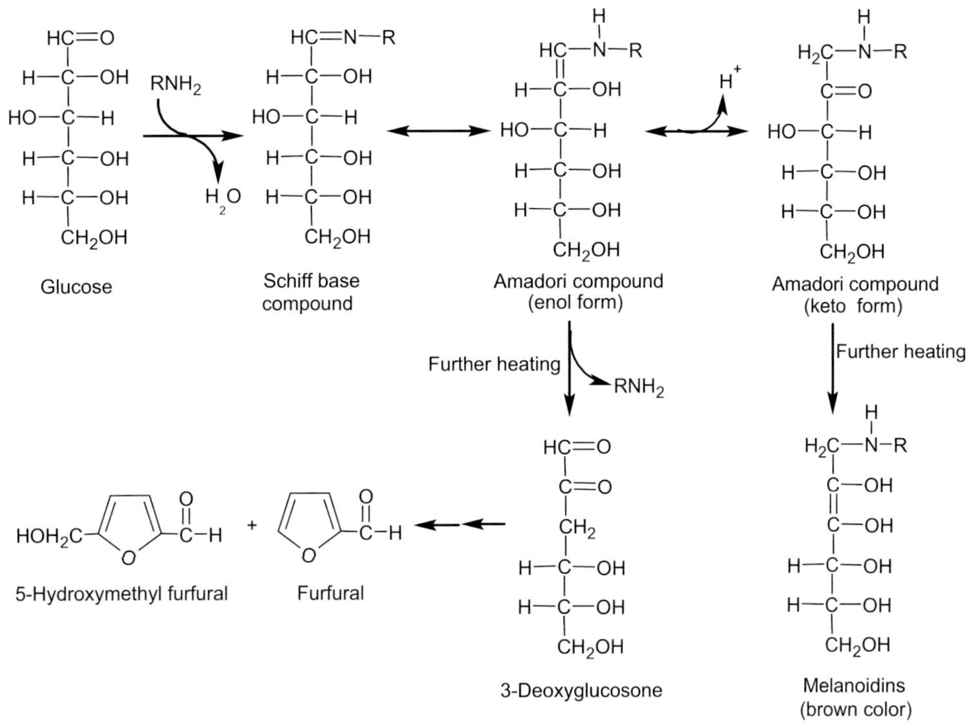

FIGURE 2.12 The Maillard reaction between amino acids and carbohydrates. RNH_2, a free amino acid (AA) or a peptide-bound amino acid (e.g., lysine or arginine). The formation of the Schiff base is reversible. However, in response to overheating, the modified AA in the form of melanoidin polymers is nutritionally unavailable to animals.

occur in the tissues (e.g., the blood) of animals at a low rate under hyperglycemic conditions, also has important implications for human nutrition and health.

2.4.6.2 Chemical Treatment

The main objective of chemical treatments of dietary proteins is to decrease protein solubility and decrease susceptibility of proteins to proteolysis in the rumen. An example of chemical treatment is the use of formaldehyde (HCHO), which has a carbonyl group (Waltz and Stern 1989). Therefore, a Maillard reaction occurs between AAs and formaldehyde. AAs whose α-amino groups (and side-chain NH_2 groups if any) have a high reactivity with formaldehyde include arginine, histidine, lysine, methionine, tryptophan, and tyrosine. Peptide bonds, as well as the amide groups of glutamine and asparagine, also react with formaldehyde. All of these reactions lead to reduced solubility of protein, and therefore decreased protein degradation in the rumen. An advantage of formaldehyde treatment is that most of the formaldehyde-protein reactions are unstable at low pH, such as the pH in the abomasum and the upper part of the small intestine. Therefore, formaldehyde-treated proteins are susceptible to degradation by proteases in the abomasum and the small intestine. A disadvantage of this method is that formaldehyde is a potential carcinogen, which poses hazards to the personnel who use formaldehyde and risks to the safety of animal products for human consumption.

2.4.6.3 Polyphenolic Phytochemicals

Natural phytochemicals that have been used to protect protein degradation in the rumen include tannins (polyphenolic compounds). Examples of these compounds include phloroglucinol, gallic acid, and catechin. They are water-soluble organic molecules.

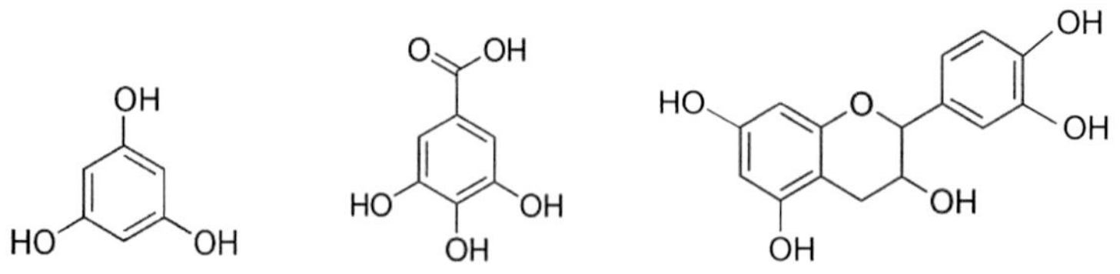

Phloroglucinol
(brown algae)

Gallic acid
(plants)

Catechin
(plants)

A chemical property of tannins is that they spontaneously react with proteins, primarily by hydrogen bonding, to form a water-insoluble complex (Naumann et al. 2017). Such a tannin–protein complex in diet is not susceptible to degradation by proteases at pH 5.5–6.5 (e.g., proteases in the rumen). However, at pH 2–3 (e.g., pH in the luminal fluid of the abomasum in ruminants), proteins are dissociated from the tannins and become available for degradation by proteases. Thus, the value of the supplemental tannins lies in the difference in the pH among the rumen, abomasum, and small intestine. Over the normal pH range in the rumen, the protein remains bound to the tannin. However, at a lower pH in the abomasum and the upper part of the small intestine, the protein is released from its tannin complex. Thus, high-quality proteins can be effectively protected from degradation in the rumen and become available for digestion in the abomasum and small intestine. In practice, tannins may be added directly to feedstuffs for ruminants. Note that tannins can also conjugate with free AAs or alkaloids to form a tannin–AA or tannin–alkaloid complex.

$$\text{Protein} + \text{Tannin} \rightarrow \text{Protein} - \text{Tannin complex}$$

(stable at pH 5.5 – 6.5; not attacked by proteases in the rumen of ruminants)

$$\text{Protein–Tannin complex} \rightarrow \text{Protein} + \text{Tannin}$$

(at pH 2 – 3; e.g., pH in the luminal fluid of the abomasum of ruminants)

2.4.6.4 Physical Encapsulation of Proteins or AAs

The idea of coating proteins originated from the observations in the 1970s that certain protein ingredients of animal origin are resistant to ruminal degradation (Tamminga 1979). The methods for physical encapsulation of proteins or AAs include spraying with the blood and the use of a hydrogenated lipid layer. In the first technique, protein supplements are sprayed with the blood, followed by heating the mixture to dryness. This procedure has been used to effectively coat the surface of proteins, which resists attack by ruminal microorganisms due, in part, to the poor colonization of the protein particles by ruminal bacteria. In the second approach, proteins or AAs are coated with hydrogenated lipids (e.g., lecithin or soy oils) to form microcapsules. Feeding an oil-coated linseed meal to young sheep has been reported to improve their N retention. Additionally, the entry of dietary protein to the abomasum is substantially increased in cattle fed rumen-protected soybeans that are prepared using the roasting and extrusion methods.

2.4.6.5 Inhibition of AA Degradation

The conversion of AAs to their carbon skeletons and ammonia is catalyzed by AA deaminases. Thus, an inhibition of AA breakdown in the rumen is expected to increase the availability of dietary AAs for absorption in the small intestine. In support of this view, dietary supplementation with an inhibitor of AA deaminases (e.g., diphenyliodonium chloride) can enhance the flow of high-quality protein from the rumen into the abomasum and the small intestine, thereby improving growth performance in beef cattle (Pineres et al. 1997). It should be noted that inhibition of AA deaminases would result in a decreased availability of ammonia for the synthesis of AAs by ruminal microorganisms and, therefore, is not beneficial for ruminants fed a diet containing low-quality and low-content protein.

2.4.7 DEGRADATION OF TOXIC AAs BY RUMINAL MICROBES

Microbes in the rumen can degrade some toxic AAs and their derivative in their diets, such as grass, legumes, and other plant species. For example, the ruminal microbes of sheep can decarboxylate diaminobutyrate (present in *Acacia angustissima*, a shrub legume) into diaminopropane via the vitamin B_6-dependent diaminobutyrate decarboxylase as a source of ammonia (Peng 2003). Thus, the adaptation of sheep to *Acacia angustissima* through a gradual increase in its intake levels can allow the animals to successfully utilize this high-protein plant without toxicity (Odenyo et al. 1997). Furthermore, mimosine (a toxic AA) is present in *Leucaena leucocephala* (a tropical leguminous shrub). The ruminal bacteria can metabolize mimosine into 3-hydroxy-4-(1H)-pyridone (a goitrogen) and 2,3-dihydroxy pyridine. Interestingly, there are geographic differences in the distribution of dihydroxypyridine-degrading ruminal bacteria among ruminants. Specifically, most ruminal microbes from cattle, sheep, and goats in the Virgin Islands and Haiti can degrade the dihydroxypyridines, but ruminal microbes from these ruminants in Iowa, as well as from cattle in Texas cannot catabolize dihydroxypyridines (Allison et al. 1990). Thus, an ability to utilize leucaena as a ruminant forage critically depends on the colonization of the rumen by bacteria that degrade dihydroxypyridines in certain plants. This knowledge has important implications for ruminant nutrition and production.

2.5 SUMMARY

Except for the absorption of milk-born intact immunoglobulins by the small intestine of neonates, dietary proteins have no nutritional value until they are digested to form short-chain peptides and free AAs in the digestive tract. In nonruminants, the digestion starts in the stomach (pH = ~2–3) where protein is first denatured by HCl and then hydrolyzed by proteases (e.g., pepsins A, B, and C, and rennins A, B, and C). The resulting large peptides enter the small intestine to undergo further degradation by proteases (e.g., trypsin, chymotrypsin, elastase, carboxyl peptidases, and aminopeptidases) in an alkaline medium (owing to the presence of bicarbonate in pancreatic juice and duodenal secretions). These enzymes release small peptides and considerable amounts of free AAs. Oligopeptides composed of more than three AA residues are broken down by peptidases to form tripeptides, dipeptides, and free AAs. Bacterial enzymes may also play a role in protein digestion. Major mechanisms for the intestinal absorption of AAs include both Na^+-dependent and Na^+-independent systems. Dipeptides and tripeptides are absorbed intact into the enterocytes of the small intestine through H^+ gradient-driven peptide transporters (mainly PepT1). Once inside the enterocytes, peptides are hydrolyzed by peptidases to form free AAs. Because substantial amounts of dietary AAs are catabolized by the small intestine in the first pass, only a portion of them (ranging from 3% to 74% depending on individual AAs) enters the portal circulation for utilization by extraintestinal tissues. In ruminants, dietary protein is hydrolyzed by ruminal microbial proteases to form small peptides and free AAs, which are further degraded to form ammonia, short-chain fatty acids, and CO_2. Small peptides, AAs, and ammonia are utilized by microorganisms in the presence of adequate energy supply (carbohydrates) to synthesize new AAs, protein, nucleic acids, and other nitrogenous substances. The most important initial reaction for microbial ammonia assimilation is catalyzed by GDH to produce glutamate, which is then utilized to synthesize glutamine, alanine, aspartate, and asparagine. These AAs serve as substrates for the synthesis of all other AAs by microorganisms in the presence of sulfur and ATP. Ruminal protozoa cannot utilize ammonia but derive their nitrogen by engulfing bacteria and digesting them with powerful intracellular proteases. Ammonia that cannot be fixed by ruminal microorganisms is absorbed into the blood for conversion into urea via the hepatic urea cycle. Ruminal microbial cells (bacteria and protozoa) containing proteins and AAs, as well as undigested dietary proteins, enter the abomasum and small intestine where the digestion of protein is similar to that in nonruminants. In both ruminants and nonruminants, the extensive recycling of nitrogen occurs in the intestine at the expense of energy to improve the efficiency of the utilization of the dietary AAs.

REFERENCES

Adedokun, S.A., C.M. Parsons, M.S. Lilburn, O. Adeola, and T.J. Applegate. 2007. Endogenous amino acid flow in broiler chicks is affected by the age of birds and method of estimation. *Poult. Sci.* 86:2590–2597.

Adibi, S.A. 1997. The oligopeptide transporter (PEPT1) in human intestine: biology and function. *Gastroenterology* 113:332–340.

Ajinomoto®. 2003. *Ajinomoto's Amino Acid Handbook*. Ajinomoto Inc., Tokyo, Japan.

Allison, M.J., M.P. Bryant, I. Katz, and M. Keeney. 1962. Metabolic function of branched-chain volatile fatty acids, growth factors for Ruminococci II. *J. Bacteriol.* 83:1084–1093.

Allison, M.J., A.C. Hammond, and R.J. Jones. 1990. Detection of ruminal bacteria that degrade toxic dihydroxypyridine compounds produced from mimosine. *Appl. Environ. Microbiol.* 56:590–594.

Archibeque, S.L., J.C. Burns, and G.B. Huntington. 2001. Urea flux in beef steers: effects of forage species and nitrogen fertilization. *J. Anim. Sci.* 79:1937–1943.

Banjarnahor, S., R.N. Rodionov, J. König, and R. Maas. 2020. Transport of L-arginine related cardiovascular risk markers. *J. Clin. Med.* 9:3975.

Bergen, W.G. 2021. Amino acids in beef cattle nutrition and production. *Adv. Exp. Med. Biol.* 1285:29–42.

Bergen, W.G. and G. Wu. 2009. Intestinal nitrogen recycling and utilization in health and disease. *J. Nutr.* 139:821–825.

Blachier, F., C. Boutry, C. Bos, and D. Tomé. 2009. Metabolism and functions of L-glutamate in the epithelial cells of the small and large intestines. *Am. J. Clin. Nutr.* 90:814S–821S.

Blachier, F., G. Wu, and Y.L. Yin. 2013. *Nutritional and Physiological Functions of Amino Acids in Pigs*. Springer, New York.

Boirie, Y., M. Dangin, P. Gachon, M.P. Vasson, J.L. Maubois, and B. Beaufrère. 1997. Slow and fast dietary proteins differently modulate postprandial protein accretion. *Proc. Natl. Acad. Sci. USA.* 94:14930–14935.

Bos, C., G. Airinei, F. Mariotti, R. Benamouzig, S. Bérot, J. Evrard et al. 2007. The poor digestibility of rapeseed protein is balanced by its very high metabolic utilization in humans. *J. Nutr.* 137:594–600.

Boza, J.J., D. Moënnoz, J. Vuichoud, A.R. Jarret, D. Gaudard-de-Weck, and O. Ballèvre. 2000. Protein hydrolysate vs free amino acid-based diets on the nutritional recovery of the starved rat. *Eur. J. Nutr.* 39:237–243.

Brake, D.W., E.C. Titgemeyer, and D.E. Anderson. 2014. Duodenal supply of glutamate and casein both improve intestinal starch digestion in cattle but by apparently different mechanisms. *J. Anim. Sci.* 92:4057–4067.

Broderick, G.A., R.J. Wallace, and E.R. Orskov. 1991. Control of rate and extent of protein degradation. In: *Physiological Aspects of Digestion and Metabolism in Ruminants* (Tsuda, T., Y. Sasaki, and R. Kawashima, eds). Academic Press, New York. pp. 541–592.

Bröer, S. and A. Bröer. 2017. Amino acid homeostasis and signalling in mammalian cells and organisms. *Biochem. J.* 474:1935–1963.

Bröer, S. and M. Palacín. 2011. The role of amino acid transporters in inherited and acquired diseases. *Biochem. J.* 436:193–211.

Butts, C.A., P.J. Moughan, and W.C. Smith. 1992. Protein nitrogen, peptide nitrogen and free amino-acid nitrogen in endogenous digesta nitrogen at the terminal ileum of the rat. *J. Sci. Food Agric.* 59:291–298.

Chalupa, W. 1972. Metabolic aspects of nonprotein nitrogen utilization in ruminant animal. *Fed. Proc.* 31:1152–1164.

Chapman, K.P., R. Elango, R.O. Ball, and P.B. Pencharz. 2013. Splanchnic first pass disappearance of threonine and lysine do not differ in healthy men in the fed state. *J. Nutr.* 143:290–294.

Chen, L.X., P. Li, J.J. Wang, X.L. Li, H.J. Gao, Y.L. Yin et al. 2009. Catabolism of nutritionally essential amino acids in developing porcine enterocytes. *Amino Acids* 37:143–152.

Closs, E.I., J.-P. Boissel, A. Habermeier, and A. Rotmann. 2006. Structure and function of cationic amino acid transporters (CATs). *J. Membr. Biol.* 213:67–77.

Cranwell, P.D. 1995. Development of the neonatal gut and enzyme systems. In: *The Neonatal Pig: Development and Survival* (M.A. Varley, ed). CAB International, Wallingford, Oxon, UK. pp. 99–154.

Dabrowski, K., B.F. Terjesen, Y. Zhang, J.M. Phang, and K.J. Lee. 2008. A concept of dietary dipeptides: a step to resolve the problem of amino acid availability in the early life of vertebrates. *J. Exp. Biol.* 208:2885–2894.

Dabrowski, K., Y.F. Zhang, K. Kwasek, P. Hliwa, and T. Ostaszewska. 2010. Effects of protein-, peptide- and free amino acid-based diets in fish nutrition. *Aquac. Res.* 41:668–683.

Daenzer, M., K.J. Petzke, B.J. Bequette, and C.C. Metges. 2001. Whole-body nitrogen and splanchnic amino acid metabolism differ in rats fed mixed diets containing casein or its corresponding amino acid mixture. *J. Nutr.* 131:1965–1972.

Dai, Z.L., G. Wu, and W.Y. Zhu. 2011. Amino acid metabolism in intestinal bacteria: links between gut ecology and host health. Front. Biosci. 16:1768–1786.

Dangin, M., Y. Boirie, C. Garcia-Rodenas, P. Gachon, J. Fauquant, P. Callier, O. Ballèvre, and B. Beaufrère. 2001. The digestion rate of protein is an independent regulating factor of postprandial protein retention. *Am. J. Physiol.* 280:E340–348.

Daniel, H. 2004. Molecular and integrative physiology of intestinal peptide transport. *Annu. Rev. Physiol.* 66:361–384.

Davenport, H.W. 1982. *Physiology of the Digestive Tract*, 5th ed. Year Book Medical Publishers, Chicago, IL.

de Lange, C.F.M., W.B. Souffrant, and W.C. Sauer. 1990. Real ileal protein and AA digestibilities in feedstuffs for growing pigs as determined with the ^{15}N-isotope dilution technique. *J. Anim. Sci.* 68:409–418.

Deglaire, A., C. Bos, D. Tomé, and P.J. Moughan. 2009. Ileal digestibility of dietary protein in the growing pig and adult human. *Br. J. Nutr.* 102:1752–1759.

Dufva, G.S., E.E. Bartley, M.J. Arambel, S.J. Galitzer, and A.D. Dayton. 1982. Content of 2-aminoethylphosphonic acid in feeds, bacteria and protozoa and its role as a rumen protozoal marker. *J. Anim. Sci.* 54:837–840.

Fan, M.Z., W.C. Sauer, R.T. Hardin, and K.A. Lien. 1994. Determination of apparent ileal AA digestibility in pigs: effect of dietary AA level. *J. Anim. Sci.* 72:2851–2859.

FAO (Food and Agriculture Organization of the United Nations). 1991. *Protein quality evaluation Report of Joint FAO/WHO Expert Consultation.* Rome, Italy.

FAO (Food and Agriculture Organization of the United Nations). 2007. *Protein and amino acid requirements in human nutrition. Report of a Joint WHO/FAO/UNU Expert Consultation.* Rome, Italy.

FAO (Food and Agriculture Organization of the United Nations). 2013. *Dietary protein quality evaluation in human nutrition. Report of an FAO Expert Consultation.* Rome, Italy.

FDA (U.S. Food and Drug Administration). 2020. CFR - Code of Federal Regulations Title 21. The information is available online and is current as of July 1, 2020. https://www.accessdata.fda.gov/scripts/cdrh/cfdocs/cfcfr/cfrsearch.cfm. Accessed on July 6, 2020.

Fei, Y.J., Y. Kanai, S. Nussberger, V. Ganapathy, F.H. Leibach, M.F. Romero et al. 1994. Expression cloning of a mammalian proton-coupled oligopeptide transporter. *Nature* 368:563–566.

Foulkes, D. and R.A. Leng. 1988. Dynamics of protozoa in the rumen of cattle. *Br. J. Nutr.* 59:429–436.

Firkins, J.L. and Z. Yu. 2015. How to use data on the rumen microbiome to improve our understanding of ruminant nutrition. *J. Anim. Sci.* 93:1450–1470.

Firkins, J.L., Z. Yu, and M. Morrison. 2007. Ruminal nitrogen metabolism: perspectives for integration of microbiology and nutrition for dairy. *J. Dairy Sci.* 90(E. Suppl.):E1–E16.

Fuller, M.F. and P.J. Reeds. 1998. Nitrogen cycling in the gut. *Annu. Rev. Nutr.* 18:385–411.

Fuller, M.F. and D. Tomé. 2005. In Vivo determination of amino acid bioavailability in humans and model animals. *AOAC Int.* 88:923–934.

Furst, P., S. Albers, and P. Stehle. 1990. Dipeptides in clinical nutrition. *Proc. Nutr. Soc.* 49:343–359.

Ganapathy, V., N. Gupta, and R.G. Martindale. 2006. Protein digestion and absorption. In: *Physiology of the Gastrointestinal Tract*, 4th edition, vol. 2 (Johnson, L.R., ed.). Academic Press, San Diego, CA, pp. 1667–1692.

Gardner, M.L.G. 1975. Absorption of amino acids and peptides from a complex mixture in the isolated small intestine of the rat. *J. Physiol.* 253:233–256.

Gaudichon, C., C. Bos, C. Morens, K.J. Petzke, F. Mariotti, J. Everwand et al. 2002. Ileal losses of nitrogen and amino acids in humans and their importance to the assessment of amino acid requirements. *Gastroenterology* 123:50–59.

Gilbert, E.R., E.A. Wong, and K.E. Webb, Jr. 2008. Peptide absorption and utilization: implications for animal nutrition and health. *J. Anim Sci.* 86:2135–2155.

Gilbreath, K.R., G.I. Nawaratna, T.A. Wickersham, M.C. Satterfield, F.W. Bazer, and G. Wu. 2019. Ruminal microbes of adult steers do not degrade extracellular L-citrulline and have a limited ability to metabolize extra-cellular L-glutamate. *J. Anim. Sci.* 97:3611–3616.

Gilbreath, K.R., G.I. Nawaratna, T.A. Wickersham, M.C. Satterfield, F.W. Bazer, and G. Wu. 2020a. Metabolic studies reveal that ruminal microbes of adult steers do not degrade rumen-protected or unprotected L-citrulline. *J. Anim. Sci.* 98:skz370.

Gilbreath, K.R., F.W. Bazer, M.C. Satterfield, J.J. Cleere, and G. Wu. 2020b. Ruminal microbes of adult sheep do not degrade extracellular L-citrulline. *J. Anim. Sci.* 98:skaa164.

Gilbreath, K.R., F.W. Bazer, M.C. Satterfield, and G. Wu. 2021. Amino acid nutrition and reproductive performance in ruminants. *Adv Exp. Med. Biol.* 1285:43–61.

Golian, A., W. Guenter, D. Hoehler, H. Jahanian, and C.M. Nyachoti. 2008. Comparison of various methods for endogenous ileal amino acid flow determination in broiler chickens. *Poult. Sci.* 87:706–712.

Gottlob, R.O., J.M. DeRouchey, M.D. Tokach, R.D. Goodband, S.S. Dritz, J.L. Nelssen et al. 2006. Amino acid and energy digestibility of protein sources for growing pigs. *J. Anim. Sci.* 84:1396–1402.

Grimble, G.K. 2000. Mechanisms of peptide and amino acid transport and their regulation. In: *Proteins, Peptides and Amino Acids in Enteral Nutrition* (Furst, P. and V. Young, eds). Nestle Nutrition Workshop Series Clinical & Performance Program. Vol. 3. Karger AG, Basel. pp. 63–88.

Harris, D.A. 1999. Cellular biology of prion diseases. *Clin. Microbiol. Rev.* 12:429–444.

Hatanaka, T., W. Huang, T. Nakanishi, C.C. Bridges, S.B. Smith, P.D. Prasad et al. 2002. Transport of D-serine via the amino acid transporter ATB$^{0,+}$ expressed in the colon. *Biochem. Biophys. Res. Commun.* 291:291–295.

Hawkins, R.A. and J.R. Vina. 2016. How glutamate is managed by the blood-brain barrier. *Biology* 5:37.

Haynes, T.E., P. Li, XL Li, K. Shimotori, H. Sato, N.E. Flynn et al. 2009. L-Glutamine or L-alanyl-L-glutamine prevents oxidant- or endotoxin-induced death of neonatal enterocytes. *Amino Acids* 37:131–142.

He, W.L., K. Furukawa, H. Leyva-Jimenez, C.A. Bailey, and G. Wu. 2018. Oxidation of energy substrates by enterocytes of 0- to 42-day-old chickens. *Poult. Sci.* 97 (E-Suppl. 1):3.

Hodgkinson, S.M., P.J. Moughan, G.W. Reynolds, and K.A.C. James. 2000. The effect of dietary peptide concentration on endogenous ileal amino acid loss in the growing pig. *Br. J. Nutr.* 83:421–430.

Hou, Y.Q., S.C. Jia, G. Nawaratna, S.D. Hu, S. Dahanayaka, F.W. Bazer, and G. Wu. 2015. Analysis of L-homoarginine in biological samples by HPLC involving pre-column derivatization with *o*-phthalaldehyde and *N*-acetyl-L-cysteine. *Amino Acids* 47:2005–2014.

Hou, Y.Q., S.D. Hu, S.C. Jia, G. Nawaratna, D.S. Che, F.L. Wang et al. 2016a. Whole-body synthesis of L-homoarginine in pigs and rats supplemented with L-arginine. *Amino Acids* 48:993–1001.

Hou, Y.Q., K. Yao, Y.L. Yin, and G. Wu. 2016b. Endogenous synthesis of amino acids limits growth, lactation and reproduction of animals. *Adv. Nutr.* 7:331–342.

Hou, Y.Q., W.L. He, S.D. Hu, and G. Wu. 2019. Composition of polyamines and amino acids in plant-source foods for human consumption. *Amino Acids* 51:1153–1165.

Howell, J.A., A.D. Matthews, K.C. Swanson, D.L. Harmon, and J.C. Matthews. 2001. Molecular identification of high-affinity glutamate transporters in sheep and cattle forestomach, intestine, liver, kidney, and pancreas. *J. Anim. Sci.* 79:1329–1336.

Huntington, G.B. and R.L. Prior. 1985. Net absorption of amino acids by portal-drained viscera and hind half of beef cattle fed a high concentrate diet. *J. Anim. Sci.* 60:1491–1499.

Hyde, R., P.M. Taylor, and H.S. Hundal. 2003. Amino acid transporters: roles in amino acid sensing and signalling in animal cells. *Biochem. J.* 373:1–18.

Iglesias, A.C., P.E. Portari, S. Zucoloto, and H. Vannucchi. 1994. Experimental short-bowel syndrome: free amino acid versus intact protein in nutritional support. *Nutr. Res.* 14:1831–1839.

Jackson, A.A. 2000. Nitrogen trafficking and recycling through the human bowel. In: *Proteins, Peptides and Amino Acids in Enteral Nutrition* (Furst, P. and V. Young, eds). Nestle Nutrition Workshop Series Clinical & Performance Program. Vol. 3. Karger AG, Basel. pp. 89–108.

Jones, D.B. 1931. Factors for converting percentages of nitrogen in foods and feeds into percentages of proteins. *Circular No. 183. United States Department of Agriculture*, Washington, D.C.

Kandasamy, P., G. Gyimesi, Y. Kanai, and M.A. Hediger. 2018. Amino acid transporters revisited: new views in health and disease. *Trends Biochem. Sci.* 43:752–789.

Kantipudi, S., J. Jeckelmann, Z. Ucurum, P.D. Bosshart, and D. Fotiadis. 2020. The heavy chain 4F2hc modulates the substrate affinity and specificity of the light chains LAT1 and LAT2. *Int. J. Mol. Sci.* 21:7573.

Knabe, D.A., D.C. LaRue, E.J. Gregg, G.M. Martinez, and T.D. Tanksley, Jr. 1989. Apparent digestibility of nitrogen and amino acids in protein feedstuffs by growing pigs. *J. Anim. Sci.* 67:441–458.

Kong, C. and O. Adeola. 2013. Ileal endogenous amino acid flow response to nitrogen-free diets with differing ratios of corn starch to dextrose in broiler chickens. *Poult. Sci.* 92:1276–1282.

Kong, C., D. Ragland, and O. Adeola. 2014. Ileal endogenous amino acid flow response to nitrogen-free diets with differing ratios of corn starch to dextrose in pigs. *Asian-Australas. J. Anim. Sci.* 27:1124–1130.

Leterme, P., B. Sève, and A. Thewis. 1998. The current ^{15}N-leucine infusion technique is not suitable for quantitative measurements of ileal endogenous AA flows in pigs. *J. Nutr.* 128:1961–1968.

Li, P. and G. Wu. 2018. Roles of dietary glycine, proline and hydroxyproline in collagen synthesis and animal growth. *Amino Acids* 50:29–38.

Li, P. and G. Wu. 2020. Composition of amino acids and related nitrogenous nutrients in feedstuffs for animal diets. *Amino Acids* 52:523–542.

Li, P., D.A. Knabe, S.W. Kim, C.J. Lynch, S.M. Hutson, and G. Wu. 2009. Lactating porcine mammary tissue catabolizes branched-chain amino acids for glutamine and aspartate synthesis. *J. Nutr.* 139:1502–1509.

Li, X.L., R. Rezaei, P. Li, and G. Wu. 2011. Composition of amino acids in feed ingredients for animal diets. *Amino Acids* 40:1159–1168.

Li, X.L., S.X. Zheng, and G. Wu. 2020a. Nutrition and metabolism of glutamate and glutamine in fish. *Amino Acids* 52:671–691.

Li, X.Y., S.X. Zheng, T. Han, F. Song, and G. Wu. 2020b. Effects of dietary protein intake on the oxidation of glutamate, glutamine, glucose and palmitate in tissues of largemouth bass (*Micropterus salmoides*) *Amino Acids* 52:1491–1503.

Li, X.Y., T. Han, S.X. Zheng, and G. Wu. 2021a. Nutrition and functions of amino acids in aquatic crustaceans. *Adv. Exp. Med. Biol.* 1285:169–197.

Li, X.Y., S.X. Zheng, and G. Wu. 2021b. Nutrition and functions of amino acids in fish. *Adv. Exp. Med. Biol.* 1285:133–168.

Liang, R., Y.-J. Fei, P.D. Prasad, S. Ramamoorthy, H. Han, T.L. Yang-Feng et al. 1995. Human intestinal H$^+$/peptide cotransporter. Cloning, functional expression, and chromosomal localization. *J. Biol. Chem.* 270:6456–6463.

Libao-Mercado, A.J., Y. Yin, J. van Eys, and C.F.M. de Lange. 2006. True ileal amino acid digestibility and endogenous ileal amino acid losses in growing pigs fed wheat shorts- or casein-based diets. *J. Anim. Sci.* 84:1351–1361.

Lin, C., D.C. Mahan, G. Wu, and S.W. Kim. 2009. Protein digestibility of porcine colostrum by neonatal pigs. *Livest. Sci.* 121:182–186.

London, E.S. and A.G. Rabinowitsch. 1912. Zum Chemismus der Verdauung und Resorption im tierischen Korper: Der Grad des Abbaues von verschiedenen Eiweissarten im Lumen des Magen-˝darmkanals. *Z. Phyziol. Chem.* 74:305–308.

Lupi, A., R. Tenni, A. Rossi, G. Cetta, and A. Forlino. 2008. Human prolidase and prolidase deficiency: an overview on the characterization of the enzyme involved in proline recycling and on the effects of its mutations. *Amino Acids* 35:739–752.

Lyons, P.J. and L.D. Fricker. 2011. Carboxypeptidase O is a glycosylphosphatidylinositol-anchored intestinal peptidase with acidic amino acid specificity. *J. Biol. Chem.* 286:39023–39032.

Malandro, M.S. and M.S. Kilberg. 1996. Molecular biology of mammalian amino acid transporters. *Annu. Rev. Biochem.* 65:305–336.

Matthews, D.E., M.A. Marano, and R.G. Campbell. 1993. Splanchnic bed utilization of glutamine and glutamic acid in humans. *Am. J. Physiol.* 264:E848–E854.

Matthews, J.C., E.A. Wong, P.K. Bender, J.R. Bloomquist, and K.E. Webb, Jr. 1996. Demonstration and characterization of dipeptide transport system activity in sheep omasal epithelium by expression of mRNA in Xenopus laevis oocytes. *J. Anim. Sci.* 74:1720–1727.

Mavromichalis, I., T.M. Parr, V.M. Gabert, and D.H. Baker. 2001. True ileal digestibility of amino acids in sow's milk for 17-day-old pigs. *J. Anim. Sci.* 79:707–713.

Metges, C.C., K.J. Petzke, A.E. El-Khoury, L. Henneman, I. Grant, S. Bedri et al. 1999. Incorporation of urea and ammonia nitrogen into ileal and fecal microbial proteins and plasma free amino acids in normal men and ileostomates. *Am. J. Clin Nutr.* 70:1046–1058.

Meister, A. 1973. On the enzymology of amino acid transport. *Science* 180:33–39.

Miner-Williams, W., A. Deglaire, R. Benamouzig, M.F. Fuller, D. Tomé, and P.J. Moughan. 2012. Endogenous proteins in terminal ileal digesta of adult subjects fed a casein-based diet. *Am. J. Clin. Nutr.* 96:508–515.

Moter, V. and H. H. Stein. 2004. Effect of feed intake on endogenous losses and amino acid and energy digestibility by growing pigs. *J. Anim. Sci.* 82:3518–3525.

Moughan, P.J. 2003. Amino acid availability: aspects of chemical analysis and bioassay methodology. *Nutr. Res. Rev.* 16:127–141.

Moughan P.J. 2012. Endogenous amino acids at the terminal ileum of the adult human. In: *Amino Acids in Human Nutrition and Health* (D'Mello, J.P.F., ed). CABI, Wallingford, UK. pp. 245–255.

Moughan, P.J. and S.M. Rutherfurd. 2012a. Gut luminal endogenous protein: implications for the determination of ileal amino acid digestibility in humans. *Br. J. Nutr.* 108 (Suppl. 2):S258–263.

Moughan, P.J. and S.M. Rutherfurd. 2012b. True ileal amino acid and protein digestibility (%) for selected human foods. In: *Report of a Sub-Committee of the 2011 FAO Consultation on "Protein Quality Evaluation in Human Nutrition"*. FAO, Rome.

Moughan, P.J. and G. Schuttert. 1991. Composition of nitrogen-containing fractions in digesta from the distal ileum of pigs fed a protein-free diet. *J. Nutr.* 121:1570–1574.

Moughan, P.J. and R.R. Wolfe. 2019. Determination of dietary amino acid digestibility in humans. *J. Nutr.* 149:2101–2109.

Moughan, P.J., G. Schuttert, and M. Leenaars. 1992. Endogenous amino acid flow in the stomach and small intestine of the young growing pig. *J. Sci. Food Agric.* 60:437–442.

Moughan, P.J., M.F. Fuller, K.S. Han, A.K. Kies, and W. Miner-Willams. 2007. Food-derived bioactive peptides influence gut function. *Int. J. Sport Nutr. Exerc. Metab.* 17:S5–S22.

Moughan, P.J., V. Ravindran, and J.O.B. Sorbara. 2014. Dietary protein and amino acids –Consideration of the undigestible fraction. *Poult. Sci.* 93:2400–2410.

Nagaraja, T.G. 2016. Microbiology of the rumen. In: *Rumenology* (Millen, D.D., M.D.B., Arrigoni, and R.D.L. Pacheco, eds). Springer, New York. pp. 39–61.

Naumann, H.D., L.O. Tedeschi, W.E. Zeller, and N.F. Huntley. 2017. The role of condensed tannins in ruminant animal production: advances, limitations and future directions. *Revista Bras. Zootec.* 46:929–949.

Navab. F. and A.M. Asatoor. 1970. Studies on intestinal absorption of amino acids and a dipeptide in a case of Hartnup disease. *Gut* 11:373–379.

NCBI. 2020. CTNS cystinosin, lysosomal cystine transporter [*Homo sapiens* (human)]. https://www.ncbi.nlm.nih.gov/gene?Db=gene&Cmd=DetailsSearch&Term=1497.

Newey, H. and D.H. Smyth. 1959. The intestinal absorption of some dipeptides. *J. Physiol.* 145:48–56.

Noy, Y. and D. Sklan. 1995. Digestion and absorption in the young chick. *Poult. Sci.* 74:366–373.

Odenyo, A.A., P.O. Osuji, O. Karanfil, and K. Adinew. 1997. Microbiological evaluation of Acacia angustissima as a protein supplement for sheep. *Anim. Feed Sci. Technol.* 65:99–112.

Osawa, Y., T. Mizushige, S. Jinno, F. Sugihara, N. Inoue, H. Tanaka, and Y. Kabuyama. 2018. Absorption and metabolism of orally administered collagen hydrolysates evaluated by the vascularly perfused rat intestine and liver in situ. *Biomed Res (Tokyo)* 39:1–11.

Owens, F.N. and M. Basalan. 2016. Ruminal fermentation. In: *Rumenology* (Millen, D.D., M.D.B., Arrigoni, and R.D.L. Pacheco, eds). Springer, New York. pp. 63–102.

Pan, Y., K. Webb, J. Bloomquist, and E. Wong. 2001. Expression of a cloned ovine gastrointestinal peptide transporter (oPepT1) in Xenopus oocytes induces uptake of oligopeptides in vitro. *J. Nutr.* 131:1264–1270.

Patterson, B.W., F. Carraro, S. Klein, and R.R. Wolfe. 1995. Quantification of incorporation of [^{15}N]ammonia into plasma amino acids and urea. *Am. J. Physiol.* 269:E508–E515.

Peng, H.H. 2003. *Rumen Microbial Degradation of Diaminobutyric Acid, a Non-Protein Amino Acid.* Ph.D. Thesis. University of Adelaide, Australia.

Pineres, M.A.R, W.C. Ellis, G. Wu, and S.C. Ricke. 1997. Effects of diphenyliodonium chloride on proteolysis and leucine metabolism by rumen microorganisms. *Anim. Feed Sci. Tech.* 65:139–149.

Pochini, L., M. Scalise, M. Galluccio, and C. Indiveri. 2014. Membrane transporters for the special amino acid glutamine: structure/function relationships and relevance to human health. *Front. Chem. Cell. Biochem.* 2:61.

Ravindran, V., L.I. Hew, G. Ravindran, and W.L. Bryden. 2004. Endogenous amino acid flow in the avian ileum: quantification using three techniques. *Br. J. Nutr.* 92:217–223.

Reynolds, C.K. and N.B. Kristensen. 2008. Nitrogen recycling through the gut and the nitrogen economy of ruminants: an asynchronous symbiosis. *J. Anim. Sci.* 86(14 Suppl):E293–E305.

Rowan, A.M., P.J. Moughan, M.N. Wilson, K. Maher, and C. Tasman-Jones. 1994. Comparison of the ileal and faecal digestibility of dietary amino acids in adult humans and evaluation of the pig as a model animal for digestion studies in man. *Br. J. Nutr.* 71:29–42.

Sanderson, I.R. and W.A. Walker. 2000. *Development of the Gastrointestinal Tract.* B.C. Decker Inc., London, UK.

Sauer, W.C. and L. Ozimek. 1986. Digestibility of amino acids in swine - results and their practical applications - a review. *Livest. Sci. Prod.* 15:367–388.

Sauer, W.C., M.Z. Fan, R. Mosenthin, and W. Drochner. 2000. Methods for measuring ileal amino acid digestibility in pigs. In: *Farm Animal Metabolism and Nutrition* (D'Mello, J.P.F., ed). CAPI Publishing, Wallingford, Oxon, UK. pp. 279–307.

Schwab, C.G. and G.A. Broderick. 2017. A 100-year review: protein and amino acid nutrition in dairy cows. *J. Dairy Sci.* 100:10094–10112.

Silk, D.B.A., P.D. Fairclough, N. J. Park, A.E. Lane, J.P. Webb, M.L. Clark, and A.M. Dawson. 1975a. A study of relations between the absorption of amino acids, dipeptides, water and electrolytes in the normal human jejunum. *Clin. Sci. Mol. Med.* 49:401–408.

Silk, D.B.A., D. Perrett, and M.L. Clark 1975b. Jejunal and ileal absorption of dibasic amino acids and an arginine containing dipeptide in cystinuria. *Gastroenterology* 68:1426–1432.

Sjostrom, H., O. Noren, and L. Josefsson. 1973. Purification and specificity of pig intestinal prolidase. *Biochim. Biophys. Acta* 327:457–470.

Smith, C.J. and M.P. Bryant. 1979. Introduction to metabolic activities of intestinal bacteria. *Am. J. Clin. Nutr.* 32:149–157.

Spanier, B. 2014. Transcriptional and functional regulation of the intestinal peptide transporter PEPT1. *J. Physiol.* 592:871–879.

Starck, C.S., R.R. Wolfe, and P.J. Moughan. 2018. Endogenous amino acid losses from the gastrointestinal tract of the adult human—A quantitative model. *J. Nutr.* 148:1871–1881.

Stein, H. H., C. Pedersen, A. R. Wirt, and R. A. Bohlke. 2005. Additivity of values for apparent and standardized ileal digestibility of amino acids in mixed diets fed to growing pigs. *J. Anim. Sci.* 83:2387–2395.

Stein, H.H., B. Sève, M.F. Fuller, P.J. Moughan, and C.F. de Lange. 2007. Amino acid bioavailability and digestibility in pig feed ingredients: terminology and application. *J. Anim. Sci.* 85:172–180.

Stentoft, C., B.A. Røjen, S.K. Jensen, N.B. Kristensen, M. Vestergaard, and M. Larsen. 2015. Absorption and intermediary metabolism of purines and pyrimidines in lactating dairy cows. *Br. J. Nutr.* 113:560–573.

Stevens, C.E. and I.D. Hume. 1995. *Comparative Physiology of the Vertebrate Digestive System*. Cambridge University Press, Cambridge, UK.

Stoll, B. and D.G. Burrin. 2006. Measuring splanchnic amino acid metabolism in vivo using stable isotopic tracers. *J. Anim. Sci.* 84 (Suppl.):E60–72.

Tamminga, S., 1979. Protein degradation in the forestomachs of ruminants. *J. Anim. Sci.* 49:1615–1625.

Tanksley, T.D. and D.A. Knabe. 1984. Ileal digestibilities of amino acids in pig feeds and their use in formulating diets. In: *Recent Advances in Animal Nutrition* (Cole D., ed). Butterworths, Wellington, UK. pp. 75–95.

Tedeschi, L.O. and D.G. Fox. 2016. *The Ruminant Nutrition System*. XanEdu, Acton, MA.

Trocki, O., H. Mochizuki, L. Dominioni, and J.W. Alexander. 1986. Intact protein versus free amino acids in the nutritional support of thermally injured animals. *JPEN* 10:139–145.

Tyler, B.M. 1978. Regulation of the assimilation of nitrogen compounds. *Annu. Rev. Biochem.* 47:1127–1162.

van Goudoever, J.B., B. Stoll, J.F. Henry, D.G. Burrin, and P.J. Reeds. 2000. Adaptive regulation of intestinal lysine metabolism. *Proc. Natl. Acad. Sci. USA.* 97:11620–11625.

van der Schoor, S.R.D., H. Schierbeek, P.M. Bet, M.J. Vermeulen, H.N. Lafeber, J.B. van Goudoever, and R.M. van Elburg. 2010. Majority of dietary glutamine is utilized in first pass in preterm infants. *Pediatr. Res.* 67:194–199.

van Slyke, D.D. and G.M. Meyer. 1913. The fate of protein digestion products in the body. III. The absorption of amino acids from the blood by the tissues. *J. Biol. Chem.* 16:197–212.

Vina, J.R., M. Palacin, I.R. Puertes, R. Hernandez, and J. Vina. 1989. Role of the γ-glutamyl cycle in the regulation of amino acid translocation. *Am. J. Physiol.* 257:E916–E922.

Vogels, G.D. and C. Van der Driet. 1976. Degradation of purines and pyrimidines by microorganisms. *Bacteriol. Rev.* 40:403–468.

Waltz, D.M. and M.D. Stern. 1989. Evaluation of various methods for protecting soya-bean protein from degradation by rumen bacteria. *Anim. Feed Sci. Technol.* 25:111–122.

Wang, W.W., S.Y. Qiao, and D.F. Li. 2009. Amino acids and gut function. *Amino Acids* 37:105–110.

Wang, J., X. Yan, R. Lu, X. Meng, and G. Nie. 2017. Peptide transporter 1 (PepT1) in fish: review. *Aquac. Fish.* 2:193–206.

Webb, K.E. Jr. and J.C. Matthews. 1994. Absorption of amino acids and peptides. In: *Principles of Protein Nutrition of Ruminants* (Asplund, M.J., ed). CRC Press, Boca Raton, FL. pp. 127–146.

Wu, G. 1995. Urea synthesis in enterocytes of developing pigs. *Biochem. J.* 312:717–723.

Wu, G. 1998. Intestinal mucosal amino acid catabolism. *J. Nutr.* 128:1249–1252.

Wu, G. 2014. Dietary requirements of synthesizable amino acids by animals: a paradigm shift in protein nutrition. *J. Anim. Sci. Biotechnol.* 5:34.

Wu, G. 2018. *Principles of Animal Nutrition*. CRC Press, Boca Raton, FL.

Wu, G. 2020. Important roles of dietary taurine, creatine, carnosine, anserine and 4-hydroxyproline in human nutrition and health. *Amino Acids* 52:329-360.

Wu, G., F.W. Bazer, R.C. Burghardt, G.A. Johnson, S.W. Kim, D.A. Knabe et al. 2010. Functional amino acids in swine nutrition and production. In: *Dynamics in Animal Nutrition* (Doppenberg, J. and P. van der Aar, eds). Wageningen Academic Publishers, The Netherlands. pp. 69–98.

Wu, Z.L., Y.Q. Hou, S.D. Hu, F.W. Bazer, C.J. Meininger, C.J. McNeal, and G. Wu. 2016a. Catabolism and safety of supplemental L-arginine in animals. *Amino Acids* 48:1541–1552.

Wu, G., H.R. Cross, K.B. Gehring, J.W. Savell, A.N. Arnold, and S. H. McNeill. 2016b. Composition of free and peptide-bound amino acids in beef chuck, loin, and round cuts. *J. Anim. Sci.* 94:2603–2613.

Yang, Z. and S.F. Liao. 2019. Physiological effects of dietary amino acids on gut health and functions of swine. *Front. Vet. Sci.* 6:169.

Yang, Y.X., Z.L. Dai, and W.Y. Zhu. 2014. Variations in the metabolism of amino acids by bacteria derived from different compartment of the pig small intestine. *Amino Acids* 46:252–253.

Yen, J.T., B.J. Kerr, R.A. Easter, and A.M. Parkhurst. 2004. Difference in rates of net portal absorption between crystalline and protein-bound lysine and threonine in growing pigs fed once daily. *J. Anim. Sci.* 82:1079–1090.

Yin, Y.L., R.L. Huang, A.J. Libao-Mercado, E.A. Jeaurond, M. Rademacher, and C.F.M. de Lange. 2004. Effect of including purified jack bean lectin in casein or hydrolyzed casein based diets on apparent and true ileal AA digestibility in the growing pig. *Anim. Sci.* 79:283–291.

Yin, J., W.K. Ren, Y.Q. Hou, M.M. Wu, H. Xiao, J.L. Duan et al. 2015. Use of homoarginine for measuring true ileal digestibility of amino acids in food protein. *Amino Acids* 47:1795–1803.

Zhai, H. and O. Adeola. 2011. Apparent and standardized ileal digestibilities of amino acids for pigs fed corn- and soybean meal-based diets at varying crude protein levels. *J. Anim. Sci.* 89:3626–3633.

3 Synthesis of Amino Acids

Since O. Neubauer postulated in 1909 that phenylalanine is converted to tyrosine in animals, research on amino acid (AA) synthesis has spanned over a century. The earlier work in this field involved primarily the N balance and growth of laboratory animals such as dogs and rats to infer which AA is synthesized in the body. In 1912, E. Abderhalden suggested that proline is synthesized in dogs because they could maintain a positive nitrogen balance and grow when fed a proline-free diet containing other AAs found in casein hydrolysates. By contrast, the dogs lost weight and died when fed tryptophan-free casein hydrolysates. On this basis, E. Abderhalden classified AAs as either nutritionally essential (indispensable) or non-essential (dispensable). An AA that is synthesized in the body at a rate to support nitrogen balance or growth was defined as a nutritionally non-essential AA (NEAA), whereas an AA that is not synthesized in the body was called a nutritionally essential AA (EAA; Rose 1957).

Beginning in 1924, W.C. Rose and coworkers published a series of landmark papers on AA nutrition and metabolism in rats and humans. These studies along with those of others (including A.E. Braunstein, F. Gowland Hopkins, H.A. Krebs, and D. Shemin) concluded that most animals can synthesize alanine, arginine, aspartate, cysteine, glutamate, glutamine, glycine, proline, serine, and tyrosine, but not isoleucine, leucine, lysine, methionine, phenylalanine, threonine, tryptophan, and valine. In the animal kingdom, AA synthetic pathways are now known to be cell-, tissue-, and species-specific (Blachier et al. 1993; Brosnan and Brosnan 2013; Wu 2009). Because most of the EAAs can be formed from their corresponding α-ketoacids *in vivo*, A. Meister (1965) indicated that it is the carbon skeletons of EAAs, not EAAs themselves, that cannot be synthesized in animals. Recent analysis of whole-genome sequences in a wide variety of eukaryotes reveals that deleterious mutations occurred during evolution for almost all the genes that were lost in AA synthetic pathways (Guedes et al. 2011). This may have nutritional and physiological significance in: (1) sparing phosphoenolpyruvate, D-erythrose-4-phosphate, and acetyl-CoA for the synthesis of glucose, nucleotides, and fatty acids, respectively; (2) reducing energy expenditure; and (3) minimizing the numbers of proteins and intermediary metabolites as well as metabolic complexity. Conversely, selective conservation of pathways for NEAA syntheses indicates that they are indispensable for the metabolic needs and survival of animals.

As indicated in Chapter 2, the lumens of the small and large intestines contain many different kinds of microbes, which form a complex ecosystem with their host animals. The interactions between intestinal epithelial cells and bacteria can profoundly influence intestinal mucosal integrity and function (Dai et al. 2011; Tomé et al. 2013). Thus, the metabolic activities of these bacteria have potential effects on host nutrition and health. Microorganisms in the lumen of the gastrointestinal tract of animals (including humans) can synthesize all protein AAs from ammonia, sulfur, and fermentable carbohydrates (the sources of appropriate carbon skeletons). These synthetic pathways are quantitatively important in ruminants (Bergen 2021) but nutritionally insignificant as a source of AAs for non-ruminants fed protein-adequate diets (Wu 2018). The objective of this chapter is to highlight AA synthesis in animals and gastrointestinal microbes. The old term "NEAA" has now been recognized as a misnomer in nutritional science and should be replaced by AASA (an AA that is synthesizable *de novo* in animal cells; Hou and Wu 2017). Although there is no *de novo* synthesis of cysteine and tyrosine (traditionally classified as NEAAs) in eukaryotes, this chapter introduces the metabolic pathways for the conversion of phenylalanine into tyrosine and of methionine into cysteine in humans and other animals.

3.1 SYNTHESIS OF AMINO ACIDS IN TISSUES AND CELLS OF HUMANS AND OTHER ANIMALS

3.1.1 OVERALL VIEW OF AMINO ACID SYNTHESIS

Rapidly growing neonates (e.g., piglets, lambs, kids, calves, and young rats) are useful animal models to study AA synthesis in human infants because they are very sensitive to changes in the endogenous provision of AAs. For mammalian species, milk had traditionally been thought to supply adequate amounts of all AAs to neonates. However, results of recent studies with lactating sows indicate that milk provides at most only 40% of arginine and proline for protein accretion in 7- to 21-day-old suckling pigs (Wu et al. 2004). Therefore, piglets must synthesize daily at least 60% of arginine and proline required by the body. Additionally, based on the concentrations of glycine and alanine in sow's milk, it meets at most 23% and 66%, respectively, of the piglet's needs for protein synthesis, which indicates that the neonate must synthesize daily at least 77% of glycine and 34% of alanine needed by its body (Wu et al. 2019). Interestingly, although aspartate plus asparagine and glutamate plus glutamine represent 23% and 42%, respectively, of total AASAs in sow's milk, this food provides at most only 8% and 9% of aspartate and glutamate for whole-body protein deposition in suckling piglets, respectively (Table 3.1). Similarly, a typical corn- and soybean meal–based diet cannot provide sufficient amounts of arginine, proline, aspartate, glutamate, glutamine, or glycine required for protein synthesis in postweaning growing pigs (Table 3.2).

In contrast to AASAs, more EAAs are provided from milk or weanling diets than are needed for protein accretion in young animals (Table 3.2). Similar results have been reported for gestating (Table 3.3) and lactating (Table 3.4) swine. Specifically, in gestating swine, Ala, Asn, and Ser are the only synthesizable AAs whose supplies in the diet exceed uterine uptake; therefore, other AASAs (including Arg, Glu, Gln, and Gly) must be synthesized by the gestating dam to support fetal growth and development (Hou et al. 2016a). In lactating sows, dietary Ala, Arg, Asn, Gly, and Ser exceed their output in milk, and they are synthesized via interorgan coordination for utilization by the mammary gland, but dietary Asp, Glu, Gln, and Pro cannot meet their output in milk, and these AAs must be synthesized *de novo* for milk production (Hou et al. 2016a).

Excess amounts of dietary EAAs are used to synthesize AASAs in young and adult animals (Figure 3.1). These reactions require ATP and/or cofactors (e.g., NADPH, NADH, and α-ketoacids). Dependence on EAAs to generate AASAs in animals is energetically inefficient in metabolism, and also produces ammonia (a toxic substance at elevated concentrations). Knowledge of AA synthesis in the body is important for the nutrition and health of humans and other animals (Closs et al. 2000; Cynober 2004; Felig 1975; Kalhan and Hanson 2012; Reeds 2000; Watford 2015), as well as the productivity of livestock, poultry, fish, and crustaceans (Belloir et al. 2015; Li et al. 2020 a, b; 2021 a, b).

3.1.2 CELL-, TISSUE-, AND SPECIES-SPECIFIC SYNTHESIS OF AMINO ACIDS IN HUMANS AND OTHER ANIMALS

Most mammals, including cattle, dogs, humans, pigs, rats, and sheep, can synthesize the following 11 proteinogenic AAs (alanine, arginine, aspartate, asparagine, cysteine, glutamate, glutamine, glycine, proline, serine, and tyrosine), as well as non-proteinogenic AAs (e.g., citrulline, ornithine, and taurine). All tissues in mammals can synthesize proline from arginine. Some mammals (e.g., cats, ferrets, mink, and tigers) and fish cannot synthesize arginine due to the lack of Δ^1-pyrroline-5-carboxylate (P5C) synthase for citrulline production in the body, particularly the enterocytes of the small intestine. Preterm mammals (including humans and pigs) have a limited ability to synthesize citrulline and, therefore, arginine; the underlying mechanisms remain largely unknown but may involve low expression of P5C synthase and *N*-acetylglutamate (NAG) synthase in the

TABLE 3.1

Utilization of Amino Acids (AAs) in Sow's Milk for Protein Accretion by 14-Day-Old Pigs[a]

AA	AA in sow's milk[b]	AA intake by pigs[c]	Dietary AA entering the portal vein[d]	AA content in pigs	AA accretion in proteins (g/day)[e]		
	(g/L)	(g/day)	(g/day)	(mg/g wet weight)	Whole body	Intestines (small and large)	Extraintestinal tissues
Alanine	1.97	1.80	1.38	8.85	2.08	0.10	1.98
Arginine	1.43	1.31	1.06	9.13	2.15	0.10	2.05
Asparagine	2.53	2.31	2.00	4.76	1.12	0.05	1.07
Aspartate	2.59	2.36	0.11	5.74	1.35	0.06	1.29
Cysteine	0.72	0.66	0.50	1.77	0.42	0.02	0.40
Glutamate	4.57	4.17	0.21	10.5	2.47	0.11	2.36
Glutamine	4.87	4.45	1.42	6.78	1.59	0.07	1.52
Glycine	1.12	1.02	0.82	15.2	3.57	0.16	3.41
Histidine	0.92	0.84	0.76	2.79	0.66	0.03	0.63
Isoleucine	2.28	2.08	1.41	4.75	1.12	0.05	1.07
Leucine	4.46	4.07	2.78	9.20	2.16	0.10	2.06
Lysine	4.08	3.73	3.09	8.11	1.91	0.09	1.82
Methionine	1.04	0.95	0.85	2.54	0.60	0.03	0.57
Phenylalanine	2.03	1.85	1.50	4.67	1.10	0.05	1.05
Proline	5.59	5.10	3.12	11.3	2.66	0.12	2.54
OH-Pro	1.04	0.95	0.86	4.96	1.17	0.05	1.12
Serine	2.35	2.15	1.72	5.97	1.40	0.06	1.34
Threonine	2.29	2.09	1.32	4.72	1.11	0.08	1.03
Tryptophan	0.66	0.60	0.52	1.47	0.35	0.02	0.33
Tyrosine	1.94	1.77	1.43	3.71	0.87	0.04	0.83
Valine	2.54	2.32	1.51	5.71	1.34	0.06	1.28
Total AAs	51.0	46.6	28.4	133	31.2	1.45	29.8

Source: Hou, Y.Q. et al. 2016a. *Adv. Nutr.* 7:331–342; Wu, G. et al. 2010. In: *Dynamics in Animal Nutrition* (Doppenberg, J. and P. van der Aar, eds). Wageningen Academic Publishers, The Netherlands, pp. 69–98.

Note: AAs, amino acids; OH-Pro, 4-hydroxyproline (not a substrate for proline or protein synthesis).

[a] The molecular weights of intact amino acids were used for all the calculations.

[b] Protein-bound plus free AAs in sow's whole milk obtained on days 7–21 of lactation.

[c] Milk consumption of 913 mL/day by 14-day-old pigs (3.9 kg body weight).

[d] Products of intestinal AA metabolism that enter the portal vein are not included.

[e] Calculated on the basis of a body weight gain of 235 g/day.

small intestine (Wu et al. 2004). Avian species cannot synthesize arginine due to the absence of endogenous synthesis of citrulline from glutamine, glutamate, or proline and have a limited ability to produce proline due to near absence or low activity of arginase in tissues. Likewise, birds cannot make adequate amounts of glycine to meet the need for the hepatic synthesis of uric acid.

While most animal species can make taurine from methionine or cysteine, cats have a limited ability to synthesize this sulfur-containing β-AA because of a deficiency of cysteine dioxygenase. Because taurine is absent from plants (Hou et al. 2019), cats, tigers, and carnivorous fish must be fed diets containing animal products or supplemental taurine (Che et al. 2021; Herring et al. 2021). Human infants (both term and preterm) cannot synthesize adequate amounts of taurine or cysteine

TABLE 3.2

Utilization of Dietary Amino Acids (AAs) for Protein Accretion in 30-Day-Old Postweaning Pigs[a]

AA	AA in diet[b] (g/kg)	AA intake by the Pig[c] (g/day)	Dietary AA entering the portal vein[d] (g/day)	AA content in the pig (mg/g wet weight)	AA accretion in proteins (g/day)[e]		
					Whole body	Intestines (small and large)	Extraintestinal tissues
Alanine	13.0	4.57	3.50	9.24	2.68	0.12	2.56
Arginine	13.2	4.64	2.50	9.52	2.76	0.13	2.63
Asparagine	9.40	3.30	2.44	5.06	1.47	0.06	1.41
Aspartate	13.2	4.64	0.23	6.02	1.75	0.08	1.67
Cysteine	3.74	1.32	0.91	1.86	0.54	0.02	0.52
Glutamate	17.2	6.04	0.21	11.9	3.45	0.15	3.30
Glutamine	18.4	6.46	1.79	7.20	2.09	0.09	2.00
Glycine	8.81	3.10	2.21	16.5	4.79	0.21	4.58
Histidine	5.73	2.01	1.43	2.92	0.85	0.04	0.81
Isoleucine	8.91	3.13	1.79	4.97	1.44	0.06	1.38
Leucine	17.8	6.25	3.63	9.61	2.79	0.13	2.67
Lysine	14.2	4.98	3.14	8.48	2.46	0.11	2.35
Methionine	3.58	1.26	0.89	2.63	0.76	0.03	0.73
Phenylalanine	9.93	3.49	2.37	4.82	1.40	0.06	1.34
Proline	15.8	5.55	2.91	12.1	3.51	0.15	3.36
OH-Pro	0.00	0.00	0.00	5.33	1.55	0.07	1.48
Serine	7.86	2.76	2.04	6.23	1.81	0.08	1.73
Threonine	8.52	2.99	1.79	4.93	1.43	0.08	1.35
Tryptophan	2.49	0.87	0.60	1.56	0.45	0.02	0.43
Tyrosine	7.62	2.68	1.89	3.82	1.11	0.05	1.06
Valine	9.96	3.50	1.94	5.93	1.72	0.07	1.65
Total AA	209	73.6	38.2	141	40.8	1.80	39.0

Source: Hou, Y.Q. et al. 2016a. *Adv. Nutr.* 7:331–342; Wu, G. et al. 2010. In: *Dynamics in Animal Nutrition* (Doppenberg, J. and P. van der Aar, eds). Wageningen Academic Publishers, The Netherlands, pp. 69–98.

Note: AAs, amino acids; BW, body weight; OH-Pro, 4-hydroxyproline.

[a] The molecular weights of intact amino acids were used for all the calculations. Based on the molecular weights of AA residues (molecular weights of intact AA - 18), true protein content in the body is 120 mg/g wet weight (or 12.0%).

[b] Corn- and soybean meal–based diet (protein-bound plus free AAs) containing 21.5% crude protein. Dry matter content in the diet was 89.5%.

[c] Feed intake (as-fed basis) is 45.0 g/kg body weight/day by 30-day-old pigs weaned at 21 days of age. The body weight of pigs at 30 days of age is 7.8 kg.

[d] Products of intestinal AA metabolism that enter the portal vein are not included.

[e] Calculated on the basis of a body weight gain of 290 g/day.

due to the underdevelopment of key enzymes for the pathways. Thus, complete infant formulas must be fortified with both arginine and taurine.

It is important to recognize that the synthesis of AAs occurs in a tissue- and cell-specific manner, requires energy, and also involves interorgan and compartmentalized metabolism of AAs. Some AASAs can be synthesized in certain tissues of animals, but not in others, due to the lack of one or more of the required enzymes. Tissue- and species-specific syntheses of AAs are summarized in Table 3.5 and are outlined in the following paragraphs.

TABLE 3.3

Metabolism of Amino Acids (AAs) in Gestating Gilts[a]

AA	AA in the diet[b] (g/kg)	Dietary AA entering the portal vein[c] (g/day)	Uterine uptake of AA (g/day)	AA accretion in fetuses[d] (g/day)	Uterine uptake of AA/ AA accretion in fetuses (g/g)	Extraintestinal metabolism of AA via non-protein synthesis pathways in maternal tissues[e]		
						Total amount (g/day)	Total nitrogen (mmol/day)	Total carbon (mmol/day)
(1) Catabolism of AAs Whose Carbon Skeletons Are Not Synthesized by Animal Cells (AANAs)								
Cysteine	2.30	3.28	2.02	1.36	1.49	1.92	15.9	47.5
Histidine	3.32	4.54	2.81	2.40	1.17	2.14	41.4	82.8
Isoleucine	5.08	5.70	4.16	3.28	1.27	2.42	18.5	111
Leucine	11.7	13.3	10.3	7.56	1.36	5.74	43.8	263
Lysine	5.81	7.48	7.62	6.61	1.15	0.87	11.9	35.7
Methionine	1.79	2.45	2.45	2.02	1.21	0.43	2.88	14.4
Phenylalanine	6.22	8.32	4.52	3.81	1.19	4.51	27.3	246
Threonine	4.94	6.07	4.82	3.61	1.34	2.46	20.7	82.6
Tryptophan	1.30	1.81	2.04	1.37	1.49	0.44	4.31	23.7
Tyrosine	4.49	6.19	3.40	2.54	1.34	4.70	25.9	234
Valine	6.52	7.27	5.85	4.55	1.29	2.72	23.2	116
Subtotal	53.5	66.4	50.0	39.1	---	28.3	236	1,257
(2) Net Synthesis, for Fetal Growth, of AAs Whose Carbon Skeletons Can Be Formed *de novo* by Animal Cells (AASAs)								
Alanine	7.76	11.7	8.91	7.23	1.23	13.6	152	457
Arginine	7.01	7.22	7.49	7.32	1.02	7.66[f]	44.0[f]	0
Asparagine	5.80	8.68	2.64	3.82	0.69	4.86	73.6	147
Aspartate	7.58	0.65	0.76	4.61	0.16	−3.96	−29.8	−119
Glutamate	10.7	0.74	4.20	9.22	0.46	−8.48	−57.6	−288
Glutamine	12.2	6.92	25.7	5.95	4.32	0.97	13.3	33.2

(Continued)

TABLE 3.3 (Continued)
Metabolism of Amino Acids (AAs) in Gestating Gilts[a]

AA	AA in the diet[b] (g/kg)	Dietary AA entering the portal vein[c] (g/day)	Uterine uptake of AA (g/day)	AA accretion in fetuses[d] (g/day)	Uterine uptake of AA/ AA accretion in fetuses (g/g)	Extraintestinal metabolism of AA via non-protein synthesis pathways in maternal tissues[e]		
						Total amount (g/day)	Total nitrogen (mmol/day)	Total carbon (mmol/day)
Glycine	5.50	7.76	16.2	13.8	1.18	−5.99	−79.8	−160
Proline	10.3	10.8	11.8	13.2[g]	0.89	0.16	1.39	6.90
Serine	4.52	7.14	5.75	4.71	1.22	2.43	23.1	69.4
Subtotal	71.4	61.6	83.5	69.8	---	11.2	141	147

Source: Hou, Y.Q. et al. 2016a. *Adv. Nutr.* 7:331–342.

Note: AAs, amino acids.

[a] The molecular weights of intact amino acids were used for all the calculations.

[b] Corn- and soybean meal–based diet containing 12.2% crude protein. Dry matter content in the diet was 89.8%.

[c] Calculated on the basis of feed intake (2 kg/day); the true ileal digestibility of 86% for each amino acid in the diet and the bioavailability (%) of orally administered AA entering the portal vein (Arg, 60; His, 80; Ile, 65; Leu, 66; Lys, 75; Met, 79; Phe, 78; Pro, 61; Thr, 72; Val, 65; Ala, 87; Asn, 87; Asp, 5; Cys, 83; Glu, 4; Gln, 33; Gly, 82; Ser, 83; Tyr, 80). Products of intestinal AA metabolism that enter the portal vein are not included.

[d] Calculated on the basis of 10 fetuses per gilt. The weight of the gilt at 110–140 d of gestation is 170 kg (130 kg maternal body weight + 40 kg conceptus).

[e] Rates of extraintestinal net catabolism of AAs whose carbon skeletons are not synthesized by animal cells are calculated as dietary AAs entering the portal vein – (accretion of AAs in the body + AAs formed from intestinal catabolism of dietary AAs). Rates of extraintestinal net synthesis of AAs whose carbon skeletons can be synthesized by animal cells are calculated as the accretion of AAs in the body – (dietary AAs entering the portal vein + AAs formed from intestinal catabolism of dietary AAs). The rates of AA formation from intestinal catabolism of dietary AAs (g/day) are estimated to be 9.10, 2.57, and 7.66 for Ala, Pro, and Arg, respectively, and to be negligible for other AAs. The sign "–" denotes the contribution of dietary AAs for extraintestinal AA synthesis in a cell- and tissue-specific manner.

[f] In pigs, citrulline (the precursor of Arg) is synthesized exclusively from Glu, Gln, and Pro exclusively in the small intestine, and citrulline is converted into arginine mainly in the extraintestinal tissues. Aspartate provides an amino group for arginine synthesis from citrulline.

[g] Including proline and its posttranslational derivative hydroxyproline for the calculation of extraintestinal balance of carbon and nitrogen balance.

TABLE 3.4

Metabolism of Amino Acids (AAs) in Lactating Sows[a]

AA	AA in the diet[b] (g/kg)	Dietary AA entering the portal vein[c] (g/day)	AA output in milk[d] (g/day)	Dietary AA entering the portal vein/AA output in milk (g/g)	Extraintestinal metabolism of AA via non-protein synthesis pathways[e]		
					Total amount (g/day)	Total nitrogen (mmol/day)	Total carbon (mmol/day)
(1) Catabolism of AAs Whose Carbon Skeletons Are Not Synthesized by Animal Cells (AANAs)							
Cysteine	3.04	13.0	6.13	2.12	6.87	56.7	170
Histidine	4.37	18.5	7.84	2.36	10.7	206	412
Isoleucine	7.44	25.5	19.4	1.31	6.07	46.3	278
Leucine	15.8	54.8	38.0	1.44	16.8	128	769
Lysine	9.00	35.4	34.8	1.02	0.64	8.70	26.2
Methionine	2.83	11.9	8.86	1.34	3.04	20.4	102
Phenylalanine	8.61	35.6	17.3	2.06	18.3	111	997
Threonine	6.53	24.0	19.5	1.23	4.49	37.7	151
Tryptophan	2.08	8.70	5.62	1.55	3.08	30.1	166
Tyrosine	6.95	29.6	16.5	1.79	17.1	94.5	850
Valine	8.17	27.7	21.6	1.28	6.06	51.7	259
Subtotal	74.8	285	196	---	93.1	791	4,180
(2) Net Synthesis, for Milk Production, of AAs Whose Carbon Skeletons Can Be Formed *de novo* by Animal Cells (AASAs)							
Alanine	9.35	42.4	16.8	2.53	−58.3	−655	−1,964
Arginine	10.8	34.5	12.2	2.83	34.8[f]	200[f]	0
Asparagine	7.68	34.0	21.6	1.58	−12.4	−188	−377
Aspartate	11.0	2.80	22.1	0.13	19.3	145	579
Glutamate	14.9	3.10	38.9	0.08	35.8	244	1,218
Glutamine	16.1	26.7	41.5	0.64	14.8	202	506

(*Continued*)

TABLE 3.4 (Continued)
Metabolism of Amino Acids (AAs) in Lactating Sows[a]

AA	AA in the diet[b] (g/kg)	Dietary AA entering the portal vein[c] (g/day)	AA output in milk[d] (g/day)	Dietary AA entering the portal vein/AA output in milk (g/g)	Extraintestinal metabolism of AA via non-protein synthesis pathways[e] Total amount (g/day)	Total nitrogen (mmol/day)	Total carbon (mmol/day)
Glycine	8.51	36.1	9.54	3.78	−26.6	−354	−708
Proline	14.3	45.0	56.5[g]	0.80	−0.21	−1.84	−9.20
Serine	8.31	36.5	20.0	1.82	−16.5	−157	−470
Subtotal	101	261	239	---	−9.30	−565	−1,225

Source: Hou, Y.Q. et al. 2016a. *Adv. Nutr.* 7:331–342.

Note: AAs, amino acids.

a The molecular weights of intact amino acids were used for all the calculations.

b Corn- and soybean meal–based diet containing 18% crude protein. Dry matter content in the diet was 89.8%.

c Calculated on the basis of feed intake (as-fed basis; 5.94 kg/day); the true ileal digestibility (%) of amino acids in the diet (Arg, 90; His, 89; Ile, 89; Lys, 88; Met, 90; Phe, 89; Pro, 87; Thr, 86; Trp, 87; Val, 88; Ala, 88; Asn, 86; Asp, 86; Cys, 87; Glu, 86; Gln, 84.0; Gly, 87; Ser, 89; Tyr, 90); and the bioavailability (%) of orally administered AA entering the portal vein (Arg, 60; His, 80; Ile, 66; Lys, 75; Met, 79; Phe, 78; Pro, 61; Thr, 72; Trp, 81; Val, 65; Ala, 87; Asn, 87; Asp, 5; Cys, 83; Glu, 4; Gln, 33; Gly, 82; Ser, 83; Tyr, 80). Products of intestinal AA metabolism that enter the portal vein are not included.

d Calculated on the basis of 9 piglets nursed by the lactating sow (174 kg body weight) and the average consumption of milk by the piglet at day 14 of lactation (246 mL milk/kg body weight/day). This amounts to a total production of 8.52 L milk/day per sow.

e Rates of extraintestinal net catabolism of AAs whose carbon skeletons are not synthesized by animal cells are calculated as dietary AAs entering the portal vein − (accretion of AAs in the body + AAs formed from intestinal catabolism of dietary AAs). Rates of extraintestinal net synthesis of AAs whose carbon skeletons can be synthesized by animal cells are calculated as the accretion of AAs in the body − (dietary AAs entering the portal vein + AAs formed from intestinal catabolism of dietary AAs). The rates of AA formation from intestinal catabolism of dietary AA (g/day) are estimated to be 32.7, 11.7, and 34.8 for Ala, Pro, and Arg, respectively, and to be negligible for other AAs. The sign "−" denotes the contribution of dietary AAs for extraintestinal AA synthesis in a cell- and tissue-specific manner.

f In pigs, citrulline (the precursor of Arg) is synthesized exclusively from Glu, Gln, and Pro exclusively in the small intestine, and citrulline is converted into arginine mainly in the extraintestinal tissues. Aspartate provides an amino group for arginine synthesis from citrulline.

g Including proline and its posttranslational derivative hydroxyproline for the calculation of extraintestinal balance of carbon and nitrogen balance.

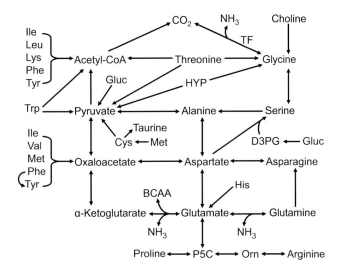

FIGURE 3.1 An overall view of metabolic transformations of nutritionally essential amino acids into nutritionally non-essential amino acids in animals. BCAA, branched-chain amino acids; D3GP, D-3-glyceraldehyde phosphate; HYP, hydroxyproline; P5C, Δ^1-pyrroline-5-carboxylate; Tau, taurine; and TF, tetrahydrofolate.

3.1.2.1 Synthesis of AAs in the Liver

This organ can synthesize many AASAs in a species-dependent manner (Hou et al. 2020). Under physiological conditions, there is no net synthesis of citrulline or arginine in the liver because (1) citrulline is immediately converted into arginine via argininosuccinate synthase (ASS) and argininosuccinate lyase (ASL) and (2) the arginine formed via the urea cycle is rapidly hydrolyzed to urea plus ornithine by hepatic arginase (Flynn et al. 2002). The liver cannot synthesize proline from glutamine or glutamate due to its lack of P5C synthase. However, in mammals, the liver can produce proline from arginine via arginase. The liver of all animals (including humans, pigs, chickens, cattle, sheep, rats, fish, and crustaceans) can synthesize aspartate, asparagine, glutamate, glutamine, cysteine, glycine, serine, and tyrosine from their respective precursor AAs. There is a species difference in the intracellular distribution of alanine transaminase in the liver, as this enzyme occurs primarily in the cytosol of the rat liver but is almost equally distributed between the mitochondria (54%) and cytosol (46%) in the pig liver (DeRosa and Swick 1975). In mammals and birds, branched-chain AAs (BCAAs) have a limited role in the direct synthesis of AAs in the liver because the hepatic activity of BCAA transaminase is negligible or absent under physiological conditions (Harper et al. 1984). In some fish, such as hybrid striped bass and largemouth bass, the liver plays a significant role in degrading BCAAs to form glutamate, alanine, glutamine, and aspartate (Li et al. 2020a). In most species (except for cats, tigers, and carnivorous fish), the liver can produce taurine from cysteine or cysteic acid.

3.1.2.2 Synthesis of Amino Acids in Skeletal Muscle, Heart, Brain, Lungs, and White Adipose Tissue

Alanine, aspartate, and glutamate can be synthesized from BCAAs (the donors of the amino group) and glucose-derived carbon skeletons in the skeletal muscle, heart, brain, lungs, and white adipose tissue of mammals, birds, and fish. These organs contain ATP-dependent glutamine synthetase [(GS), a cytosolic enzyme in mammals and the avian brain and skeletal muscle, but a mitochondrial enzyme in the avian liver] for converting glutamate and ammonia into glutamine, as well as alanine transaminase (localized in both the mitochondria and cytosol). Cytosolic alanine transaminase is the predominant form in the skeletal and cardiac muscles of pigs, rats, chickens, and guinea pigs for the formation of alanine from pyruvate (DeRosa and Swick 1975). In food-deprived or starved

TABLE 3.5

Syntheses of Amino Acids (AAs) in Sense and Non-sense Organs

AA	Sense organs					Non-sense organs											
	Eye	Ear	Nose	TG	Skin	Brain	SI	Liver	SM	Kidney	Heart	WA	Ovary	Testes	PL	MG	PAN
Alanine	+	+	+	+	+	+	+	+	+	+	+	+	+	+	+	+	+
Arginine[a]	+	+	+	+	+	+	+	−	+	+	+	+	+	+	+	+	+
Aspartate	+	+	+	+	+	+	+	+	+	+	+	+	+	+	+	+	+
Asparagine	+	?	?	?	+	+	+	+	?	+	?	?	?	+	+	+	+
Citrulline	−	−	−	−	−	−	+[d]	−	−	−	−	−	−	−	−	−	−
Cysteine[b]	−	−	−	−	−	−	−	+	−	−	−	−	−	−	−	−	−
GABA	+	−	−	−	−	+	−	−	−	−	−	−	−	−	−	−	−
Glutamate	+	+	+	+	+	+	+	+	+	+	+	+	+	+	+	+	+
Glutamine	+	?	+	?	+	+	+[e]	+	+	+	+	+	+	+	+	+	+
Glycine[c]	+	?	?	?	+	+	+[e]	+	+[e]	+	+	?	+	+	+	+	+
Proline	?	?	?	?	+	+	+	+	−	+	−	−	−	−	−	−	+
OH-Proline	+	+	+	+	+	+	+	+	+	+	+	+	+	+	+	+	+
Ornithine	+	+	+	+	+	+	+[d]	+	+	+	+	+	+	+	+[f]	+	+
Serine	?	?	?	?	+	+	+[e]	+	+[e]	+	+[e]	?	+	+	+	+	+
Tyrosine	?	?	?	?	+	−	+	+	−	+	−	−	−	−	−	+/−[g]	+

Source: Chen, J. et al. 2020. *Adv. Exp. Med. Biol.* 1265:57–70; He, W.L. and G. Wu et al. 2020. *Adv. Exp. Med. Biol.* 1265:167–185; Hou, Y.Q. et al. 2020. *Adv. Exp. Med. Biol.* 1265:21–37; Li, X.Y. et al. 2020b. *Adv. Exp. Med. Biol.* 1265:71–95; Wu, G. 2020. *Adv. Exp. Med. Biol.* 1265:201–216.

Note: "?", lack of data; "+", presence of the metabolic pathway; "−", lack of synthesis of an amino acid from precursors other than its α-ketoacid; GABA, γ-aminobutyrate; MG, mammary glands; OH-Pro, 4-hydroxyproline; PAN, pancreas; PL, placenta; SI, small intestine; SM, skeletal muscle; TG, tongue; WA, white adipose tissue.

[a] Synthesis of L-arginine from L-citrulline via argininosuccinate synthase and lyase in mammals and birds. This metabolic pathway may be absent from some carnivorous fish.

[b] Cys may be used for the synthesis of glutathione or conjugation with some biochemicals.

[c] Synthesis of glycine from 4-hydroxyproline and serine and catabolism of glycine via either conversion into serine by serine hydroxymethyltransferase or oxidative decarboxylation by the glycine cleavage system.

[d] Most mammals (including humans, pigs, cattle, sheep, dogs, rats, and mice). Some mammals (e.g., cats, tigers, and ferrets), birds, and carnivorous fish do not synthesize ornithine or citrulline from glutamine, glutamate, or proline.

[e] Low rate.

[f] Produced from arginine in the placentae of most species except for pigs. In the porcine placentae that have little arginase activity, ornithine is synthesized from proline via proline oxidase and ornithine aminotransferase.

[g] Species-specific expression. Enzyme activity is present in bovine and goat mammary tissues but is absent from porcine, rat, and guinea pig mammary tissues.

humans and other animals (e.g., rats, pigs, and chickens), alanine and glutamine, which constitute about 10% of total AAs in protein, account for approximately 50% of total AAs released by the skeletal muscle. Because of its large mass [40% and 45% of body weight (BW)] in neonates and adults, respectively), skeletal muscle is the major source of both alanine and glutamine in postabsorptive humans and other animals, including pigs, cattle, sheep, rats, and fish. The synthesis of glutamine from NH_3 and glutamate plays a major role in removing ammonia from the skeletal muscle, heart, lungs, and brain, with glucose being the primary source of the glutamate carbon skeleton (Chen et al. 2020; He and Wu 2020; Kowalski et al. 1997). The skeletal muscle, heart, brain, lungs, and white adipose tissue of humans and other animals lack enzymes for the *de novo* syntheses of citrulline and tyrosine, but can interconvert serine and glycine. Except for the brain, these tissues do not convert methionine into cysteine or taurine. By contrast, the brain has a limited ability to generate taurine from methionine and cysteine, but actively synthesizes γ-aminobutyrate (GABA) from glutamate (He and Wu 2020).

3.1.2.3 Synthesis of Amino Acids in the Small Intestine

The small intestine of most mammals can synthesize: (1) alanine, arginine, aspartate, asparagine, citrulline, ornithine, and proline from glutamate and glutamine; (2) glutamate from BCAAs plus glucose, glutamine, and proline; and (3) tyrosine from phenylalanine. In many mammalian species, the small intestine releases alanine, arginine, citrulline, ornithine, and proline in the postabsorptive state, indicating the net synthesis of these AAs by the gut. In the fed state, the small intestine of pigs also releases a substantial amount of tyrosine into the portal circulation. Because of the complex compartmentation of AA metabolism involving both the mitochondrion and cytoplasm, extracellular ornithine is poorly utilized for citrulline or arginine synthesis in enterocytes. Interconversion between serine and glycine occurs in the gut. The major cells responsible for these synthetic pathways are enterocytes. The mammalian small intestine has limited ability to synthesize glutamine due to a low activity of GS in enterocytes and other cell types. In contrast to mammals, the avian small intestine cannot synthesize ornithine, citrulline, arginine, or proline.

In some fish, such as hybrid striped bass and largemouth bass, the small intestine plays a significant role in converting: (1) BCAAs and glutamine into glutamate; (2) glutamate into alanine and aspartate; and (3) alanine into aspartate (Li et al. 2021a). This is also true for crustaceans, including shrimp and crabs (Li et al. 2021b). Such a metabolic pattern ensures that the small intestines of the aquatic animals have sufficient provision of metabolic fuels at all times for proper function.

3.1.2.4 Synthesis of Amino Acids in the Kidneys

The kidneys of mammals, birds, fish, and crustaceans can synthesize alanine, aspartate, glutamate, glycine, and serine and convert phenylalanine into tyrosine (Li et al. 2020b). There is a species difference in the renal expression of GS. Specifically, rat, rabbit, guinea pig, sheep, and cattle kidneys express GS, but cat, human, chicken, and pig kidneys lack this enzyme (Craan et al. 1982; Janicki and Goldstein 1969; Lemieux et al. 1976). Alanine transaminase activity is present in the kidneys of some species (e.g., humans, dogs, pigs, and guinea pigs) but has been reported to be relatively low in the rat kidneys (DeRosa and Swick 1975). There is also a species difference in the distribution of alanine transaminase activity between the mitochondria and cytosol in the kidneys, as are many aspects of AA metabolism. For example, this enzyme is exclusively a mitochondrial enzyme in the chicken kidneys but a cytosolic protein in the rat kidneys (albeit low activity), and occurs primarily in the mitochondria of the pig and guinea pig kidneys (DeRosa and Swick 1975). 4-Hydroxyproline is the major substrate for the renal synthesis of glycine. The kidneys contain ASS and ASL for converting citrulline into arginine. In mammals, these two enzymes are localized within the proximal convoluted tubules which express little arginase activity. In adults, approximately 60% of net arginine synthesis from citrulline occurs in the kidneys. However, this metabolic pathway may not occur in all fish (Li et al. 2020b). In birds and some species of fish, the kidneys play an important role in converting arginine into ornithine as a precursor for the production of polyamines.

3.1.2.5 Synthesis of Amino Acids in Endothelial Cells, Smooth Muscle Cells, Macrophages, and Lymphocytes

Cells of the immune and circulatory systems can synthesize alanine, aspartate, and glutamate from glutamine via the glutaminolysis pathway. These cells can also convert citrulline into arginine as a mechanism to conserve arginine at the expense of aspartate, thereby sustaining nitric oxide (NO) production by NO synthase. Furthermore, endothelial cells, smooth muscle cells, macrophages, and lymphocytes can transaminate BCAAs with α-ketoglutarate (α-KG) to form glutamate, which is utilized for the production of alanine and aspartate by glutamate–pyruvate transaminase and glutamate–oxaloacetate transaminase. However, all these cells do not synthesize: (1) citrulline from glutamine, glutamate, and proline; (2) tyrosine from phenylalanine; and (3) taurine from cysteine.

3.1.2.6   Synthesis of Amino Acids in Sense Organs

All sense organs (the eyes, ears, nose, tongue, and skin) can synthesize alanine, aspartate, glutamate, and hydroxyproline and convert citrulline into arginine (Solano 2020; Wu 2020a). The eyes and skin also produce asparagine, glutamine, and glycine, but little is known about these reactions in other sense organs. In addition, retinal cells in the eyes can decarboxylate glutamate to generate GABA (Chattopadhyaya et al. 2007). There is evidence that the skin can generate serine from glycine and glutamate plus glucose, as well as tyrosine from phenylalanine (Solano 2020; Wu 2020a). All the sense organs can form ornithine from arginine, but do not convert: (1) methionine into cysteine or (2) glutamine, glutamate, and proline into citrulline.

3.1.2.7   Synthesis of Amino Acids in Placentae, Mammary Glands, Ovaries, and Testes

The placentae, mammary glands, ovaries, and testes of all mammals, as well as ovaries and testes of all animals synthesize glutamate, glutamine, alanine, and aspartate, but not taurine or cysteine. In gestating mammals, the release of glutamine from the placenta contributes to a high ratio (>2) of fetal to maternal concentrations of glutamine in the plasma. In lactating mammals, the synthesis of glutamate, glutamine, and aspartate by mammary tissue contributes to their high abundance in milk. All these tissues can interconvert serine and glycine. The placentae, ovaries, and testes of all mammals (including humans, pigs, and sheep) lack phenylalanine hydroxylase activity (Fitzpatrick 1999; Lichter-Konecki et al. 1999). Interestingly, phenylalanine hydroxylase activity is present in bovine and goat mammary glands (Jorgensen and Larson 1968) but absent from rat, guinea pig, and porcine mammary glands.

3.1.3   Amino Acid Synthesis and Homeostasis in Humans and Other Animals

Interorgan synthesis of AAs affects: (1) the concentrations of AASAs and the ratios of AASAs to EAAs in the portal vein and systemic circulation; (2) endogenous provision of AASAs; and (3) the availability and patterns of AA substrates for intracellular synthesis of protein in animals. This notion is clearly illustrated from the results of studies involving both sow-reared pigs (Table 3.1) and postweaning (Table 3.2) pigs. For example, inhibition of intestinal ornithine, citrulline, and arginine synthesis for 12 h reduced the concentrations of ornithine, citrulline, and arginine in the plasma by 59%, 52%, and 76%, respectively, in 4-day-old sow-reared piglets (Flynn and Wu 1996). Likewise, inhibition of intestinal citrulline and arginine synthesis for 8 h reduced the concentrations of citrulline and arginine in the plasma by 26% and 22%, respectively, in 75-day-old pigs (Wu et al. 1997). Furthermore, local syntheses of some AASAs in certain tissues are essential for life because in healthy humans and many other animals the blood–brain barrier is impermeable to glutamate, aspartate, and GABA (neurotransmitters) in the blood and to the endogenous cerebral GABA; red blood cells do not take up extracellular glutamate (a constituent of glutathione); and the periportal hepatocytes of the liver do not extract glutamate from the blood (Hou and Wu 2018). Finally, due to the active metabolism of AAs in the whole body, the patterns of AAs in the plasma differ from those in diets and tissue proteins, as illustrated for both sow-reared and postweaning piglets (Table 3.6). Thus, protein nutrition should be based, in part, on an integrated biochemical and physiological approach to understanding whole-body AA synthesis and homeostasis relative to dietary AA intake.

NADH and NADPH participate in the reduction of some α-ketoacids to the corresponding α-AAs. The synthesis of some AAs plays an important role in removing H^+ within the cells to maintain acid–base balance, as shown in the following reactions:

$$\alpha\text{-Ketoglutarate}^{2-} + NH_3 + NADH + 2H^+ \rightarrow Glutamate^- + NAD^+$$

$$Glutamate^- + NH_3 + H^+ \rightarrow Glutamine$$

$$CO_2 + NH_3 + NADH + H^+ + Methylenetetrahydrofolate \rightarrow Glycine + NAD^+ + Tetrahydrofolate$$

$$Pyrroline\text{-}5\text{-}carboxylate^- + NADPH + 2H^+ \rightarrow Proline + NADP^+$$

TABLE 3.6

Patterns of Amino Acids (AAs) in Diets, Entry from Diets into the Portal Vein, Plasma, and Body Tissue Proteins of 14-Day-Old Sow-Reared Pigs and 30-Day-Old Postweaning Pigs[a]

AA	Patterns of AAs in the diet		Patterns of dietary AAs entering the portal vein		Patterns of free AAs in plasma		Patterns of AAs in the tissue proteins of the whole body	
	Sow's milk[b]	Weaning diet[c]	Milk-fed pigs[d]	Weaned pigs[e]	Milk-fed pigs[d,f]	Weaned diet[e,g]	Milk-fed pigs[f]	Weaned pigs[g]
Alanine	48	92	45	112	203	194	109	109
Arginine	35	93	34	80	73	120	113	112
Asparagine	62	66	65	78	39	42	59	60
Aspartate	63	93	4	7	7	7	71	71
Cysteine	18	26	16	29	59	69	22	22
Glutamate	112	121	7	7	67	86	130	140
Glutamine	119	130	46	57	228	290	84	85
Glycine	27	62	27	70	203	236	187	195
Histidine	23	40	25	46	44	60	34	34
Isoleucine	56	63	46	57	47	55	59	59
Leucine	109	125	90	116	71	97	113	113
Lysine	100	100	100	100	100	100	100	100
Methionine	25	25	28	28	36	33	31	31
Phenylalanine	50	70	49	76	46	50	58	57
Proline	137	111	101	93	198	212	201	205
OH-Pro	25	---	28	---	35	34	61	63
Serine	58	55	56	65	78	85	74	74
Threonine	56	60	43	57	91	104	58	58
Tryptophan	16	18	17	19	25	30	18	18
Tyrosine	48	54	46	60	90	98	44	45
Valine	62	70	49	62	104	121	70	70

Note: AAs, amino acids; OH-Pro, 4-hydroxyproline.

[a] Lysine is used as the reference value (100). The ratio of each AA to lysine is expressed as percentage (g/g × 100).

[b] Lysine content in sow's milk is 1.66% (g/g; dry matter basis).

[c] Corn- and soybean meal–based diet containing 21.5% crude protein. Lysine content in the diet is 1.59% (g/g; dry matter basis).

[d] Sow-reared 14-day-old pigs.

[e] Thirty-day-old pig weaned at 21 days of age to a corn- and soybean meal–based diet containing 21.5% crude protein.

[f] Suckling 14-day-old pigs. Lysine concentration in the plasma of blood samples obtained from the jugular vein at 1.5 h after feeding is 230 μM. See Table 3.1 for lysine content in the whole body.

[g] Thirty-day-old pig weaned at 21 days of age to a corn- and soybean meal–based diet containing 21.5% crude protein. Lysine concentration in the plasma of blood samples obtained from the jugular vein at 1.5 h after feeding is 186 μM. See Tables 3.1 and 3.2 for lysine content in the whole body.

There are species and age-dependent differences in AA synthesis (Table 3.7). However, clinical studies with both humans and animal models have convincingly shown that a lack or deficiency of the endogenous synthesis of AAs (e.g., arginine, glutamine, serine, and glycine) results in metabolic and neurological disorders, failure of embryonic implantation in the uterus, impairments of prenatal and postnatal growth and development, or even embryonic and neonatal deaths (Gantner et al. 2019; He et al. 2007; Le Douce et al. 2020; Spodenkiewicz et al. 2016). This indicates that: (1) the regular intake of AASAs in diets is insufficient for the growth, health, and survival of humans and

TABLE 3.7

Rates of the Syntheses of Amino Acids (AAs) in Humans and Other Animals

AA	Species	Nutritional state	Flux in arterial plasma[a]	Endogenous synthesis
			(μmol/kg of body weight/h)	
Arginine	Human infants	TPN	209	15
	Preterm infants	Fed (enterally)	461	42 (from proline)
	Adult humans	Fed (enterally)	73	5.2
	Neonatal pigs (3.9 kg BW)	Fed (enterally)	408	96
	Growing pigs (28 kg BW)	Fed (enterally)	319	65
	Adult rats	Fed (enterally)	479	65
	Adult dogs	Postabsorptive	225	9.4
Glutamine	Preterm human infants	Fasted	755	655
	Preterm human infants	Fed (enterally)	644	529
	AGA infants	Fasted	545	472
		Fed (enterally)	494	423
	SGA infants	Fasted	791	679
		Fed (enterally)	677	569
	Adult humans	Postabsorptive	348	245
	Young pigs	Fed (enterally)	934	328
Glutamate	Human infants	Fed (enterally)	607 (423–791)	482[b]
	Adult humans	Postabsorptive	83	67[c]
	Young pigs	Fed (enterally)	1,190	119
Glycine	Adult humans	Fed (enterally)	458	72
	Neonatal pigs	Fed (enterally)	≥1,770	≥668
	Adult rats	Fasted for 24 h	888	483[d]
		Diabetic (ALX)	732	327[d]
Proline	Adult humans	Fed (enterally)	128	39[c]
	Neonatal pigs	Fed (enterally)	448	215
Serine	Adult humans	Overnight fasted	150	110
	Adult rats	Fasted for 24 h	858	744[d]
		Diabetic (ALX)	630	516[d]

Source: Bertolo, R.F. and D.G. Burrin. 2008. *J. Nutr.* 138:2032S–2039S; Gersovitz, M. et al. 1980. *Metabolism* 29:1087–1094; Kalhan, S.C. and R.W. Hanson. 2012. *J. Biol. Chem.* 287:19786–19791; Parimi et al. 2002. *Am. J. Physiol.* 282:E618–E625; Parimi, P.S. et al. 2004. *Am. J. Clin. Nutr.* 79:402–409; Wu, G. and S.M. Morris Jr. 1998. *Biochem. J.* 336:1–17.

Note: AGA = appropriate for gestational age; ALX = alloxan-induced diabetes; SGA = small for gestational age; TPN = total parenteral nutrition.

[a] The flux of an amino acid in the arterial plasma is the sum of the entry of the amino acid into the plasma from the diet, the endogenous synthesis of the amino acid, and the release of the amino acid from protein degradation. Plasma flux = AA intake + AA synthesis + protein breakdown = AA oxidation + protein synthesis

[b] Estimated on the basis of the whole-body protein synthesis (20 g protein/kg BW/day, Stack et al. 1989) and the content of glutamate in the body (85 mg glutamate/g protein).

[c] Estimated on the basis of the rate of whole-body protein synthesis in adult humans (2.86 g protein/kg BW/day) and the content of glutamate in the body (85 mg glutamate/g protein).

[d] Estimated on the basis of the rate of whole-body protein breakdown in 24-h fasted adult rats (6.4 g protein/kg BW/day).

other animals; (2) the enormous importance of AA syntheses in maintaining the AA homeostasis of organisms; and (3) AASAs must be considered both nutritionally and physiologically essential for humans and other animals (Hou and Wu 2017).

3.1.4 ALTERATIONS IN THE RATES OF AMINO ACID SYNTHESIS IN DISEASE

The rates of AA synthesis in humans and other animals are altered under various pathological conditions. For example, infections decrease the rate of intestinal citrulline synthesis but increase the conversion of citrulline into arginine in the extraintestinal cells (e.g., activated macrophages and lymphocytes) and tissues (e.g., the kidneys and spleen) (Luiking et al. 2012; Morris 2009) while reducing the whole-body synthesis of glycine (Wang et al. 2013) and glutamine (Curthoys and Watford 1995) in mammals (including humans and pigs). By contrast, the *de novo* synthesis of arginine is reduced but the production of ornithine from arginine is increased in severely burned patients (Yu et al. 2001). Likewise, the rate of synthesis of proline is much lower than the rate of catabolism of proline in burned patients (Jaksic et al. 1991), and the results are summarized in Table 3.8. This necessitates dietary supplementation with proline to promote wound healing. In addition, the whole-body synthesis of alanine is enhanced in adult patients with insulin-dependent or non-insulin-dependent diabetes mellitus, resulting in increases in plasma alanine concentrations and glucose synthesis (Stumvoll et al. 1996; Hall et al. 1979). Furthermore, compared with control (normoglycemic) individuals with 5.9 mM glucose in the plasma, the rate of whole-body synthesis of glycine is decreased by 33% in hyperglycemic patients with insulin-dependent diabetes mellitus (15.2 mM glucose in the plasma) (Robert et al. 1985). Finally, acidosis impairs the synthesis of AAs by gastrointestinal bacteria (including those in the rumen and colon), whereas the cancer cells exhibit an increase in serine synthesis to drive oncogenesis (Amelio et al. 2014). Thus, AA synthesis is an expanding area of both nutritional and biomedical research.

TABLE 3.8
Rates of Whole-Body Metabolism of Proline in Adult Male Burned Patients and Healthy Control Individuals[a]

Variable	Male adult burned patients ($n = 5$)	Healthy individuals ($n = 6$)	P-value
Age, years	26.8 ± 2.7	19.8 ± 0.3	---
Body weight, kg	70.4 ± 3.6	80.3 ± 2.9	---
Energy intake, kcal/day	$3,521 \pm 243$	---	---
Protein intake, g/day	178 ± 6.8	---	---
Concentration of proline in the plasma, µmol/L	83.7 ± 7.9	130.8 ± 14.5	<0.05
Blood urea, mmol/L	2.35 ± 0.30	---	---
Serum creatinine, µmol/L	50 ± 0.6	---	---
Serum insulin, pmol/L	93 ± 8	43 ± 5	<0.05
Plasma leucine flux, µmol/kg BW/h	199.5 ± 27.6	86.1 ± 3.1	<0.01
Plasma proline flux, µmol/kg BW/h	136.8 ± 22.4	67.1 ± 3.1	<0.01
Whole-body oxidation of proline into CO_2, µmol/kg BW/h	29.4 ± 8.1	10.6 ± 0.5	<0.05
Whole-body synthesis of proline, µmol/kg BW/h	6.9 ± 11.7	16.2 ± 1.8	NS
Whole-body proline balance, µmol/kg BW/h	-22.4 ± 7.5	5.6 ± 4.1	<0.01

Source: Jaksic, T. et al. 1991. *Am. J. Clin. Nutr.* 54:408–413.

Note: BW = body weight; NS = statistically not significant ($P > 0.05$).

[a] The individuals were studied in the postabsorptive state. Values are means ± SEM.

3.2   GENERAL PATHWAYS FOR THE SYNTHESIS OF AMINO ACIDS IN ANIMAL CELLS

3.2.1   OVERALL PATHWAYS FOR THE SYNTHESIS OF AMINO ACIDS IN ANIMAL CELLS

The overall pathways for the syntheses of alanine, arginine, asparagine, aspartate, cysteine, glutamate, glutamine, glycine, proline, taurine, serine, and tyrosine in animal cells are illustrated in Figure 3.2. With the exception of arginine and taurine, pathways for the syntheses of these AAs were uniformly conserved in the animal kingdom (Wu 2009). Notably, except for arginine, cysteine, and taurine, only one or a few steps are required for the synthesis of most AAs.

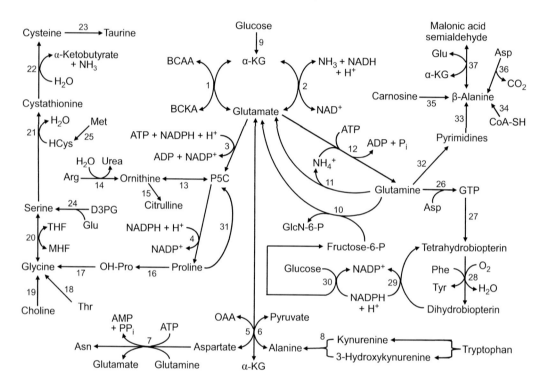

FIGURE 3.2   Synthesis of amino acids in animal tissues in a cell- and species-dependent manner. The enzymes catalyzing the indicated reactions are: (1) BCAA transaminase; (2) glutamate dehydrogenase; (3) P5C synthase; (4) P5C reductase; (5) aspartate transaminase; (6) alanine transaminase; (7) asparagine synthetase; (8) enzymes for tryptophan catabolism; (9) enzymes for converting glucose into α-KG; (10) glutamine:fructose-6-phosphate transaminase; (11) phosphate-activated glutaminase; (12) glutamine synthetase; (13) ornithine aminotransferase; (14) arginase; (15) ornithine carbamoyltransferase; (16) enzymes for protein synthesis, hydroxylation of peptide-bound proline, and protein degradation; (17) enzymes for converting hydroxyproline into glycine; (18) enzymes for converting threonine into glycine; (19) enzymes for converting choline into glycine; (20) serine hydroxymethyltransferase; (21) cystathionine β-synthase; (22) cystathionine γ-lyase; (23) enzymes for converting cysteine into taurine; (24) enzymes for converting D-3-phosphoglycerate and glutamate into serine; (25) enzymes for methionine catabolism; (26) enzymes for GTP synthesis; (27) enzymes for tetrahydrobiopterin synthesis; (28) phenylalanine hydroxylase; (29) dihydrobiopterin reductase; (30) enzymes of the pentose cycle; (31) proline oxidase; (32) enzymes for pyrimidine synthesis; (33) enzymes for pyrimidine catabolism; (34) enzymes for coenzyme A (CoA-SH) catabolism; (35) carnosinase; (36) aspartate decarboxylase; and (37) β-alanine-α-KG transaminase with malonic acid semialdehyde being produced from propionyl-CoA and malonyl-CoA semialdehyde. BCAA, branched-chain amino acid; BCKA, branched-chain α-ketoacid; D3PG, D-3-phosphoglycerate; GlcN-6-P, glucosamine-6-phosphate; HCys, homocysteine; MTH, N^5-N^{10}-methylene tetrahydrofolate; OH-Pro, hydroxyproline; OAA, oxaloacetate; P5C, Δ^1-Pyrroline-5-carboxylate; and THF, tetrahydrofolate.

Selective conservation of a metabolic pathway during evolution indicates its essentiality for the survival, growth, and reproduction of the organism. Pyruvate, oxaloacetate, and α-KG are the ultimate sources of the carbon skeletons of alanine, arginine, asparagine, aspartate, glutamate, glutamine, glycine, proline, and serine. In most cases, glutamate provides the amino group, and ATP supplies the energy for AA synthesis. Glutamine synthesis plays a central role in nitrogen metabolism (Curthoys and Watford 1995). Interestingly, there is evidence that liver GS is activated in a dose-dependent manner by high concentrations of α-KG (e.g., 5–30 mM; Tate and Meister 1971). However, the physiological significance of such a mechanism remains unclear because the concentration of this ketoacid in hepatocytes is well below 5 mM (Williamson and Brosnan 1974). Note that the accumulation of ammonia from the oxidative deamination of glutamate by glutamate dehydrogenase (GDH) is self-limiting in most cells because of the close-to-equilibrium nature of the reaction (Brosnan 2000).

Enzyme-catalyzed transamination of AAs in the biological system, discovered by A.E. Braunstein in 1937, is crucial for AA synthesis. While AA transaminases have broad substrate specificities for AAs and α-ketoacids, not all exogenous α-ketoacids can be used to form the corresponding AAs in organisms. For example, the oral administration of α-keto-ε-aminocaproic acid (the α-ketoacid of lysine; spontaneously cyclizes to Δ^1-piperidine-2-carboxylate) or α-keto-β-hydroxy-butyric acid (the α-ketoacid of threonine) is not effective in producing lysine or threonine in humans or other animals (Meister 1965). This is possibly because of: (1) extensive utilization of α-ketoacids by bacteria in the lumen of the small intestine and (2) the absence of a true transaminase for lysine and threonine in bacteria and animal cells.

3.2.2 HISTORICAL PERSPECTIVES OF AMINO ACID TRANSAMINATION

Because transamination plays a crucial role in AA synthesis, it is important to review the historical development of this field. Studies of AA transamination can be dated back to 1910 when F. Knoop reported that: (1) when α-keto-γ-phenylbutyric acid (or its α-hydroxy analog) was administered to dogs, some of the carbon skeleton was recovered in the urine as α-acetylamino-γ-phenylbutyric acid and (2) when DL-α-amino-γ-phenylbutyric acid was administered, some of its carbon was recovered as α-hydroxy-γ-phenylbutyric acid in urine. These results implied a reversible conversion of an α-AA to its corresponding α-ketoacid in animals. In 1930, D.M. Needham found that glutamate could be oxidized in muscle tissue extracts without the production of ammonia, suggesting a role for a biochemical reaction other than oxidative deamination in glutamate catabolism. In 1937, two Russian biochemists A.E. Braunstein and M.G. Kritzmann demonstrated that: (1) exogenous glutamate and endogenous lactate were utilized in equal amounts by extracts of pigeon muscle incubated aerobically and (2) in the absence of oxygen, glutamate disappeared from the incubation medium only when pyruvate was added. However, in both situations, the disappearance of glutamate was accompanied stoichiometrically by the formation of alanine. These authors proposed an enzyme-catalyzed, reversible reaction involving the transfer of an amino group between glutamate and alanine in tissues. In 1939, M.K. Karyagina confirmed the L-configuration of the AA produced in transamination. Subsequently, extensive studies established the biological importance of AA transamination in various tissues of animals (Cammarata and Cohen 1950).

3.3 SPECIFIC PATHWAYS FOR THE SYNTHESIS OF AMINO ACIDS IN HUMANS AND OTHER ANIMALS

3.3.1 SYNTHESIS OF ALANINE, GLUTAMINE, AND GLUTAMATE IN ANIMAL CELLS

H.A. Krebs described in 1935 the synthesis and degradation of glutamine in animal tissues. He also identified GS and glutaminase to catalyze these reactions, respectively. However, the sources of nitrogen in glutamate or glutamine were not fully understood until the seminal discovery of E.B.

Marliss and colleagues in 1971 reported that large amounts of glutamine are released by the skeletal muscle of obese humans. Using the rat model, A.L. Goldberg demonstrated in 1978 that BCAAs donate an amino group to α-KG to form glutamate, which is either amidated to produce glutamine or transaminated with pyruvate to yield alanine. The same reactions also occur in other species, including cattle, chickens, dogs, humans, pigs, and sheep. However, as noted previously, there is a species difference in the location of intracellular GS in that it is a cytosolic enzyme in mammalian cells and avian skeletal muscle, but is a mitochondrial protein in avian hepatocytes (Vorhaben and Campbell 1972). Mammalian GS consists of eight identical subunits, each containing an active site for the binding of glutamate, ammonia, and ATP (Krajewski et al. 2008; Tate et al. 1972). In all species, the ammonia utilized by GS is primarily derived from the blood, GDH (in some tissues), AA degradation, or the purine nucleotide cycle (particularly during exercise) (Figure 3.3), whereas glucose is the major source of α-KG for glutamate formation and of pyruvate for alanine synthesis when tissues (particularly skeletal muscle) respond well to insulin (Figure 3.2). As reported for the growing pigs (Ytrebø et al. 2006), some of the intramuscular glutamate can also come from glutamate uptake from the blood (e.g., 0.49–0.72 μmol glutamate/kg BW/min).

In skeletal muscle and white adipose tissue of fed or fasted animals, the catabolism of α-ketoacids of valine and isoleucine is relatively low due to a low activity of branched-chain α-ketoacid (BCKA) dehydrogenase. Thus, it is unlikely that these two BCAAs are a major source of α-KG or pyruvate for the formation of glutamate and alanine in the muscles and adipose tissues. In support of this view, there is little synthesis of glutamate, glutamine, or alanine in chicken skeletal muscle (Wu et al. 1989), porcine placenta (Self et al. 2004), and porcine mammary tissue (Li et al. 2009) incubated in glucose-free medium containing 0.25 mM leucine and 0.25 mM valine plus 0.25 mM isoleucine (physiological concentrations in the plasma). Likewise, GDH activity is low in skeletal muscle, and thus may not be a quantitatively significant source of ammonia. In the liver, the equilibrium of GDH favors the formation of ammonia and α-KG from glutamate.

$$\text{Glutamate} + NH_3 + ATP \rightarrow \text{Glutamine} + ADP + Pi \ (\text{GS; the MW of rat liver GS} = 44 \text{ kDa})$$

Glutamine and alanine are two major sources of nitrogen and carbon in the interorgan metabolism of AAs in mammals [including humans (Goldberg and Chang 1978; Nurjhan et al. 1995) and swine (Wu et al. 2011b)] and birds (Tinker et al. 1986). Skeletal muscle accounts for about 70% of total glutamine production in healthy adult humans, with 86% and 14% of the muscular contribution

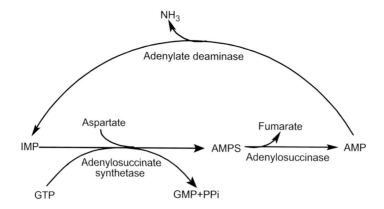

FIGURE 3.3 The purine nucleotide cycle in animals. This cycle is highly active in the skeletal muscle of humans and other animals during exercise. AMP, adenosine monophosphate; AMPS, adenosine monophosphate succinate; GTP, guanosine triphosphate; GMP, guanosine monophosphate; and IMP, inosine monophosphate.

being from *de novo* synthesis and proteolysis, respectively (Kuhn et al. 1999). Similar results were obtained for preterm infants (91% and 9% from *de novo* synthesis and proteolysis, respectively) and prepubertal boys (88% and 12% from *de novo* synthesis and proteolysis, respectively). In contrast to the muscle, there is little release of glutamine by the mammalian liver in the healthy state. However, under acidotic conditions, the liver becomes a net producer of glutamine, and its release by skeletal muscle is enhanced markedly to meet the increased demand of this AA by the kidneys for ammoniagenesis, which is necessary for the regulation of acid–base balance in the body (Welbourne 1987). Work involving mice with selective knockout of muscle GS confirms an important role for this enzyme and skeletal muscle in whole-body glutamine production and extrahepatic removal of ammonia, particularly in the fasting state (He et al. 2010).

Because the liver releases glucose which is taken up by skeletal muscle to form pyruvate (the carbon skeleton of alanine), L.E. Mallette, J.H. Exton, and C.R. Park proposed the glucose–alanine cycle between these two organs in 1969 (Figure 3.4). The amino group in alanine is derived primarily from glutamate, which is taken up from the blood (Marliss et al. 1971) or formed in the skeletal muscle from BCAAs (Goldberg and Chang 1978). Although there is no net contribution to glucose from the glucose–alanine cycle, this pathway fulfills the following functions: (1) carrying ammonia as alanine in a non-toxic form; (2) removing pyruvate from skeletal muscle, which allows for more ATP production from glucose because glycolysis-derived NADH can enter the mitochondria for oxidation via the electron transport system; (3) facilitating the conversion of muscle glycogen into glucose in the liver; and (4) maintaining a relatively high concentration of alanine in the liver to inhibit protein degradation. It is now known that an active glucose–alanine cycle also exists between the liver and cells of the immune system (e.g., lymphoid organs) and may play a role in defending the host against infectious disease.

The expression of mammalian GS is stimulated by glucocorticoids in a cAMP-dependent mechanism, indicating that the presence of a cAMP-responsive element in the GS gene. In cultured skeletal muscle cells, elevated extracellular concentrations of glutamine (>2 mM) stimulate the degradation of the GS protein (Wang and Watford 2007), but this feedback inhibition is unlikely to be a major factor for regulating glutamine homeostasis *in vivo* because glutamine (usually ~0.5–1 mM in the plasma) is constantly transported to all tissues via the blood circulation for active utilization.

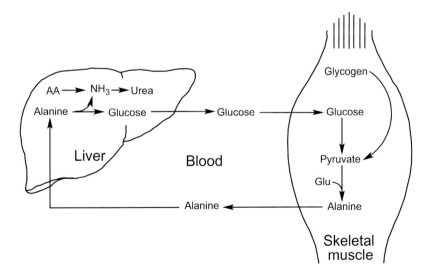

FIGURE 3.4 The glucose–alanine cycle. The liver releases glucose into the circulation. Skeletal muscle takes up arterial glucose for the generation of pyruvate, which is used for alanine synthesis via transamination. Skeletal muscle releases alanine which is converted into urea and glucose in the liver. There is no net synthesis of glucose by the glucose–alanine cycle when the source of pyruvate in the muscle is glucose.

Interestingly, such a phenomenon does not occur for GS in the brain and mature adipocytes. To date, no regulation of enzymatic activity through covalent modifications of protein has been reported for mammalian or avian GS.

3.3.2 Synthesis of Arginine, Citrulline, and Ornithine in Animal Cells

Nutritional studies (N balance and growth) in 1930 by W.C. Rose indicated that rats can synthesize arginine. Subsequently, H.J. Sallach, R.E. Koeppe, and W.C. Rose reported in 1951 the conversion of L-[U-^{14}C]glutamate into arginine and proline in rats. The 1970s–1990s witnessed groundbreaking research on arginine synthesis in mammals via the intestinal–renal axis. In their study of lipid metabolism, H.G. Windmueller and A.E. Spaeth serendipitously discovered in 1974 uptake of arterial glutamine and release of citrulline by rats' small intestine. After extensive investigation, these authors concluded in 1981 that the small intestine is the major source of circulating citrulline for endogenous synthesis of arginine in adult rats. This classical finding led to M.E. Jones's elucidation in 1983 of pathways for the intestinal synthesis of citrulline from glutamine via P5C synthase, but the responsible cell type in the small intestine was not identified. In humans, P5C synthase is encoded by the *ALDH18A1* gene in chromosome 10q24.1. Using both *in vivo* and *in vitro* techniques, J.T. Brosnan reported in 1990 that citrulline is quantitatively converted into arginine in the kidneys of adult rats and that this synthetic pathway is not affected by the dietary intake of arginine. There is also evidence that glutamine is a major AA for the synthesis of citrulline and arginine in young and adult humans (Ligthart-Melis et al. 2008).

Studies involving neonatal pigs have greatly expanded our knowledge of the crucial role for the intestinal synthesis of citrulline and arginine in animal growth. F. Blachier and colleagues identified in 1993 that carbamoyl phosphate, formed from bicarbonate (derived from ^{14}CO or ^{14}C-labeled glutamine oxidation) and ammonia, is incorporated into ^{14}C-arginine in the enterocytes of neonatal pigs. Using HPLC analysis of AAs, the conversion of glutamine and glutamate into ornithine, citrulline, and arginine in both pig and rat enterocytes was firmly established by G. Wu in 1994. In search for an explanation for the nutritional paradox that 7- to 21-day-old sow-reared piglets continue to grow despite a progressive and marked decline in intestinal production of citrulline from glutamine and glutamate, G. Wu discovered in 1997 the conversion of proline into both citrulline and arginine via proline oxidase in enterocytes of developing pigs. In contrast to the claim of some authors, the enterocytes of young and aging mice synthesize ornithine, citrulline, and arginine from glutamine and proline, as do the cells in rats and pigs (Posey et al. 2021). Quantitatively, proline is a major AA for the intestinal synthesis of citrulline and arginine in swine (Wu et al. 2018). The nutritional significance of this proline-dependent pathway was graphically illustrated by the subsequent work of R.O. Ball and P.B. Pencharz in 1999, who found that a deficiency of proline in the enteral diet resulted in arginine deficiency and death in neonatal pigs. Consistent with the findings from the swine studies (Wu 1997), Tomlinson et al. (2011) reported that proline is a major AA for the synthesis of citrulline and arginine in human infants. Studies with pigs indicate that the synthesis of citrulline and arginine from glutamine and proline in the enterocytes of pigs is not affected by supplementing 1% or 2% arginine to a corn- and soybean meal-based diet containing 1.35% arginine for 3 months (Wu et al. 2016).

It should be kept in mind that the entire molecule of P5C is incorporated into citrulline via ornithine aminotransferase (OAT) and ornithine carbamoyltransferase (OCT) in enterocytes. Thus, proline and glutamine provide their nitrogen and carbon skeletons for citrulline and arginine synthesis in the small intestine which expresses these two enzymes and P5C synthase (Flynn et al. 2002; Hu et al. 2008). A lack of knowledge or misunderstanding of these basic biochemical reactions can lead researchers to make erroneous conclusions regarding the contribution of proline or glutamine carbons to the endogenous synthesis of arginine. Results of both enzymatic and metabolic studies indicate that P5C synthase, NAG synthase, and proline oxidase are major regulatory enzymes in arginine synthesis in the small intestine (Figure 3.5).

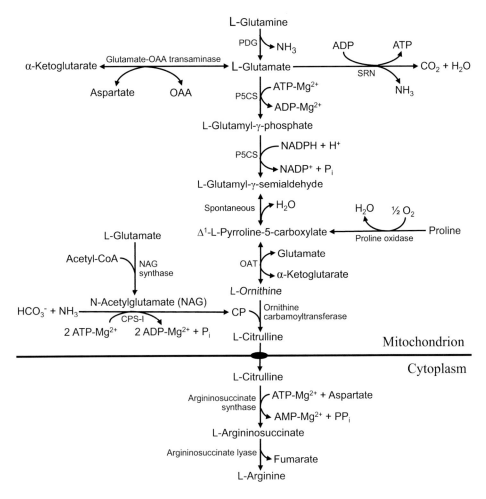

FIGURE 3.5 Arginine synthesis in most mammals including humans, pigs, rodents, and ruminants. There is no net synthesis of arginine by the liver under physiological conditions. The conversion of glutamine, glutamate, and proline into citrulline occurs exclusively in the mitochondria of enterocytes. Arginine is formed from citrulline in the cytoplasm of almost all cell types. In the neonatal small intestine, the near absence of arginase maximizes the output of arginine into the portal circulation. In adults, most of the intestine-derived citrulline is released into the portal circulation, bypasses the liver, and is extracted primarily by the kidneys for arginine synthesis. CP, carbamoyl phosphate; CPS-I, carbamoyl phosphate synthetase I; OAA, oxaloacetate; OAT, ornithine aminotransferase; PDG, phosphate-activated glutaminase; P5CS, Δ^1-pyrroline-5-carboxylate synthase (a bifunctional enzyme); and SRN, a series of enzyme-catalyzed reactions (Chapter 4).

There are species differences in the synthesis of citrulline and arginine among animals. For example, expressed per kg BW, neonatal pigs synthesize more arginine than human infants, and adult rats synthesize more arginine than adult humans (Table 3.7). Most mammals (e.g., humans, pigs, cattle, sheep, mice, and rats) synthesize both of the AAs from glutamate, glutamine, and proline via the intestinal–renal axis (Wu and Morris 1998). However, as noted previously, birds and some mammals (e.g., cats, mink, tigers, and ferrets) cannot synthesize arginine from glutamine or proline due to the near absence, lack of, or negligible activity of one or more enzymes (e.g., P5C synthase) in enterocytes (Herring et al. 2021; Rogers and Phang 1985; Wu and Morris 1998). This is also true for some carnivorous fish, such as hybrid striped bass and largemouth bass (Li et al. 2020a). Interestingly, Martinez et al. (2020, 2021) recently reported that enterocytes from newborn, young, and adult horses actively oxidized glutamine to CO_2 but did not synthesize citrulline and arginine from glutamine or proline. Thus, it is possible that unlike other mammalian livestock (e.g., swine, cattle, and sheep), horses may have little or no ability to synthesize de novo arginine and, therefore, arginine must be provided in equine diets for fetal and postnatal growth, development, and survival. This may explain why the milk of horses, like that of cats, must provide a large amount of arginine for their newborns, in contrast to humans, swine, cattle, sheep, and rats whose milk is all deficient in arginine (Davis et al. 1994; Wu and Knabe 1994) but whose offspring are capable of endogenous arginine synthesis to compensate for their inadequate intake of dietary arginine (Wu and Morris 1998; Wu et al. 2018).

3.3.3 Synthesis of Aspartate and Asparagine in Animal Cells

In all tissues of humans and other animals, aspartate is formed from glutamate or alanine (the donor of the amino group) and oxaloacetate (the source of the carbon skeleton) via transamination reactions. As noted previously, glutamate is generated from α-KG and ammonia by GDH, whereas alanine is produced from pyruvate via transamination with an AA (e.g., glutamate). Some of the extraintestinal tissues, mainly the liver and kidneys, express asparaginase to hydrolyze asparagine into aspartate and NH_4^+.

Most tissues possess asparagine synthetase [AS] (a cytosolic enzyme) to synthesize asparagine from aspartate and glutamine, but the basal expression level of the enzyme varies widely among different cell types (Lomelino et al. 2017). In contrast to prokaryotes, mammals express only one form of AS. The liver has the highest activity of AS among all organs. The mammalian AS (a class II glutamine amidotransferase) does not use aspartate and NH_4^+ as substrates, but rather requires glutamine as the source of nitrogen donor for the amidation of aspartate. This enzyme converts aspartate and ATP into the electrophilic β-aspartyl-AMP intermediate and also hydrolyzes glutamine into glutamate and ammonia, which attacks β-aspartyl-AMP to form asparagine. In contrast to normal mammalian cells, acute lymphoblastic leukemia cells and some other tumors do not express AS. Thus, leukemic cells must depend on extracellular asparagine for growth and survival.

$$\text{Aspartate} + \text{Glutamine} + \text{ATP} \rightarrow \text{Asparagine} + \text{Glutamate} + \text{AMP} + \text{PPi}$$

$$\left(\text{asparagine synthetase, Mg}^{2+}\right)$$

3.3.4 Synthesis of Cysteine and Taurine in Animal Cells

In studies to formulate an explanation for the large amounts of cystine in the urine from patients with cystinuria, E. Brand discovered in 1935 that cysteine is synthesized from methionine in mammals. Approximately 20 years later, taurine was identified in 1954 as a product of cysteine metabolism via the formation of cysteine sulfinic acid in rat liver.

The pathways for the synthesis of cysteine and taurine are illustrated in Figure 3.6. Note that serine contributes the carbon skeleton for the synthesis of cysteine from methionine (e.g., total flux of cysteine = ~40 μmol/kg BW/h; contribution of serine = ~5 μmol/kg BW/h in overnight-fasted adult humans; Kalhan and Hanson 2010). Over the past half-century, much research has been focused on species and developmental differences in cysteine and taurine syntheses. In cats, the conversion of cysteine into taurine is limited primarily due to a low activity of: (1) cysteine dioxygenase that oxidizes cysteine into cysteinesulfinate (cysteine sulfinic acid) and (2) cysteinesulfinate decarboxylase that catalyzes the formation of taurine from cysteinesulfinate (Morris and Rogers 1992). Like domestic cats, tigers, lions, and other felids (e.g., cheetah, puma, jaguar, and leopard) do not synthesize taurine (Herring et al. 2021). Interestingly, most dog species (carnivores) are able to synthesize taurine from cysteine in the liver (Hayes 1998). However, certain breeds of dogs [e.g., giant breed dogs (Newfoundland) and American Cocker Spaniels] and some individuals do not synthesize taurine due to genetic defects and must require a dietary source of taurine to maintain

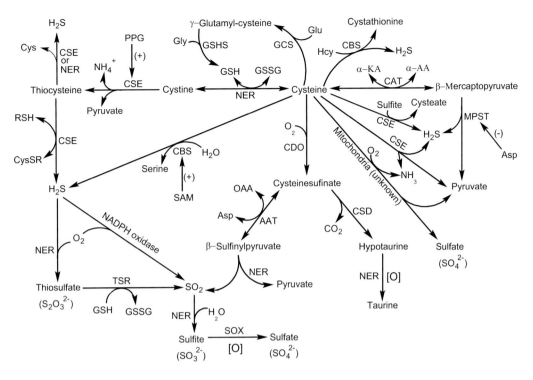

FIGURE 3.6 Cysteine and taurine syntheses in animal cells. The liver is the exclusive site for the conversion of methionine into cysteine, which is subsequently catabolized to form taurine. AAT, amino acid transaminase; CAT, cysteine aminotransferase; CBS, cystathionine-β-synthase; CDO, cysteine dioxygenase; CSD, cysteine sulfinate decarboxylase; CSE, cystathionine γ-lyase (also known as cystathionase); CysSR, cysteine–thiol complex; GCS, γ-glutamylcysteine synthase; GS, glutathione synthase; GSH, glutathione; GSSG, glutathione disulfide; α-KA, α-ketoacid; α-AA, α-amino acid; NER, non-enzyme–catalyzed reaction; OAA, oxaloacetate; PPG, propargylglycine (an irreversible inhibitor of cystathionine γ-lyase); RSH, a thiol-containing compound; SAM, S-adenosylmethionine; SOX, sulfite oxidase; and TSR, thiosulfate reductase.

health and prevent disorders, such as dilated cardiomyopathy and retinal lesions (Backus et al. 2003; Fascetti et al. 2003).

Compared with adult rats, adult humans or infants have a low rate of taurine synthesis due to exceedingly low activities of both cysteine dioxygenase and cysteinesulfinate decarboxylase (only about 0.1% of the value for rats; Sturman and Hayes 1980). Compared with livestock (e.g., cattle, pigs, and sheep) and poultry (e.g., chickens and ducks), humans also have a very low ability to synthesize taurine at any stage of life. Despite the relatively low rate of taurine synthesis, adult humans, but not infants, are resistant to a short-term deficiency of taurine in diets (Hayes and Sturman 1981; Huxtable 1992). This is likely because humans can conserve taurine through the reabsorption of hepatic bile acid–derived taurine from the lumen of the small intestine to the portal vein (Foley et al. 2019). Note that enterally derived cysteinesulfinate is extensively transaminated by the small intestinal mucosa to form β-sulfinylpyruvate. The latter spontaneously decomposes to pyruvate and SO_2 and, therefore, does not enter the liver for taurine synthesis (Stipanuk 2004). In contrast to enteral administration, parenterally or intraperitoneally administered cysteinesulfinate is an effective precursor of taurine in mammals (including cats and rats).

In addition to methionine, N-acetylcysteine (a chemically stable synthetic substance), cysteamine, and cystamine are effective precursors of cysteine in humans and other animals (Hou et al. 2015a). N-Acetylcysteine is readily taken up by cells where it is converted into cysteine by cytosolic deacetylase. Cystamine (2,2′-dithiobisethanamine; an analog of cystine) is an unstable linear aliphatic diamine with a disulfide linkage formed from the spontaneous oxidation of two cysteamine molecules and is a potentially toxic substance. Cysteamine is a product of the constitutive degradation of coenzyme A in all tissues, with the liver, brain, and heart being the major sites. Cystamine can be non-enzymatically reduced to cysteamine by glutathione. In animals, cysteamine is oxidized to hypotaurine by 2-aminoethanethiol dioxygenase. As noted previously, hypotaurine is oxidized to taurine. Under physiological conditions, cysteamine is quantitatively a minor substrate for taurine synthesis in animals without receiving dietary supplementation with the amine.

Cystamine (2,2′-dithiobisethanamine; $C_4H_{12}N_2S_2$; MW = 152.28)

Cysteamine + O_2 → Hypotaurine   (2-aminoethanethiol dioxygenase)

3.3.5   SYNTHESIS OF HOMOARGININE FROM ARGININE AND LYSINE IN ANIMAL CELLS

The liver and kidneys of humans and other animals (e.g., rats and pigs) synthesize L-homoarginine and ornithine from arginine and lysine via a putative mitochondrial enzyme called arginine:glycine amidinotransferase (AGAT; Hou et al. 2016b; Tsikas and Wu 2015). This enzyme catalyzes the transfer of the amidino group from L-arginine to L-lysine to form homoarginine. Homoarginine synthesis also occurs in some other tissues, such as the brain and small intestine to a lesser extent. The concentrations of homoarginine in the plasma, brain, kidney, and liver of adult rats are about 2, 1.5, 90, and 105 μM, respectively (Hou et al. 2015b). At present, little is known about homoarginine synthesis in birds, fish, or shrimp. The function of this arginine metabolite in tissues is unknown, but, as an analog of arginine, may play a role in regulating the synthesis of NO and creatine by neurons, hepatocytes, kidneys, and other cells.

3.3.6   SYNTHESIS OF GLYCINE AND SERINE IN ANIMAL CELLS

There is a rich history of studies on glycine and serine synthesis (Snell 1984). Using ^{15}N-labeled serine with ^{13}C in the carboxyl group, D. Shemin reported in 1945 interconversion between serine and glycine in rats and guinea pigs. Subsequent nutritional and isotopic studies in the 1950s led to the discovery that glycine is synthesized from both AAs and non-AA substrates in mammals, including pigs, rats, and humans. Specifically, these investigations showed that: (1) young animals could grow even though the diet did not contain glycine and (2) ^{15}N-glycine was greatly diluted due to the formation of new unlabeled glycine synthesized in the body. At the same time, biochemical studies with rats concluded that glycine is formed from: (1) serine, which is produced from glucose (the source of the carbon skeleton), and glutamate (the source of the amino group) via serine hydroxymethyltransferase (SHMT) through two divergent pathways involving phosphor- and non-phosphor-intermediates (Figure 3.7); (2) choline via the formation of sarcosine (Figure 3.8); and (3) threonine

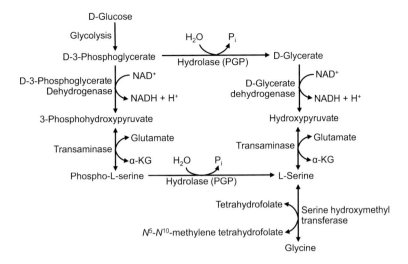

FIGURE 3.7 Serine and glycine synthesis from glucose and glutamate in animal cells. These synthetic pathways in mammals, birds, and fish are cell- and tissue-specific. The quantitative importance of endogenous serine and glycine syntheses relative to its needs varies with species. α-α-KG, α-ketoglutarate; and PGP, 3-phosphoglycerate phosphatase.

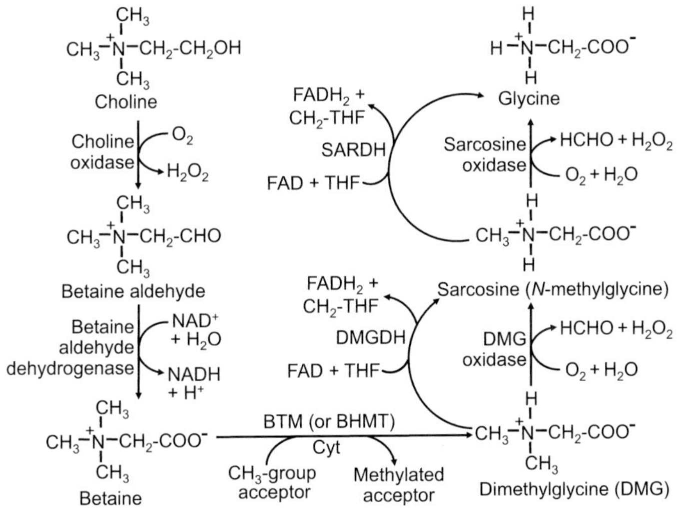

FIGURE 3.8 Glycine synthesis from choline in animals. Choline is present in animals, microbes, and plants primarily as phosphatidylcholine (lecithin) and, to a lesser extent, as free choline, sphingomyelin, choline plasmalogens, glycerophosphocholine, phosphocholine, and acetylcholine. In mammals, birds, and fish, this metabolic pathway occurs primarily in the liver and, to a much lesser extent, in the kidneys. Betaine is an intermediate in the conversion of choline into glycine. Except for betaine transmethylase [or betaine homocysteine methyltransferase (BHMT); a cytosolic enzyme in the liver and kidneys], all other enzymes are flavin adenine dinucleotide (FAD)-dependent flavoproteins and localize in the mitochondria of the liver and kidneys. Some of the glycine-generating enzymes are present in other tissues [e.g., BHMT in the testes, brain, and lungs]. Demethylation of dimethylglycine (a substance with fish-like odor) to sarcosine is catalyzed by dimethylglycine oxidase (EC 1.5.3.10) and dimethylglycine dehydrogenase (DMGDH; EC 1.5.99.2), whereas demethylation of sarcosine to glycine is catalyzed by sarcosine oxidase (EC 1.5.3.1) and sarcosine dehydrogenase (SARDH; EC 1.5.99.1). Of note, dimethylglycine dehydrogenase and sarcosine dehydrogenase (mitochondrial matrix enzymes) use tetrahydrobiopterin (THF) as the methylene (–CH$_2$) group acceptor to generate N^5,N^{10}-methylenetetrahydrofolate (CH$_2$–THF). Thus, choline catabolism to form glycine plays an important role in one-carbon metabolism. Cyt, cytosol; HCy, homocysteine; and Met, methionine.

TABLE 3.9

Relative Contributions of Milk versus Endogenous Synthesis to Meet the Glycine Requirement of 7-Day-Old Milk-Fed Piglets

	Amounts of glycine (mg/kg of body weight/day)
Glycine provision from sow's milk	311
Milk intake (0.78 L/day; 1.12 g/L of whole milk)	349
Undigestible glycine in sow's milk (11%)	38
Glycine requirements for growth and metabolic function	≥1,515
Body weight gain (200 g/day; 27.2 g protein)	1,216
Glycine oxidation to urea and carbon dioxide	96
Glycine utilization for creatine synthesis	46
Glycine utilization for purine synthesis	112
Glycine utilization for conjugation of bile acid	16
Glycine utilization for hepatic glutathione synthesis	13
Glycine utilization for hippuric acid production	11
Glycine utilization for heme synthesis	5
Glycine needed from endogenous synthesis	≥1,204
Dietary serine	81
Choline (via sarcosine)	36
Threonine (via threonine dehydrogenase)	33
4-Hydroxyproline from collagen degradation	272
4-Hydroxyproline from milk	336
Unknown substrate(s)	≥446

Source: Wang et al. 2013. *Amino Acids* 45:463–477; Wu, Z.L. et al. 2019. *Antioxid. Redox Signal.* 30:674–682.

via the threonine dehydrogenase pathway. Subsequent investigations in the 1990s identified the presence of these three pathways for glycine synthesis in pigs. Interestingly, these published results indicate that: (1) glycine synthesis from choline plus threonine contributes only ≤6% of the glycine needed by the young pig and (2) production of glycine from dietary serine represents only ≤7% of total glycine synthesis. Together, dietary serine, choline, and threonine contribute <12% of the glycine needed by young pigs (Table 3.9).

At present, substrates for ≥88% of the endogenous synthesis of glycine in milk-fed pigs have not been completely identified. Similarly, there was no detectable conversion of threonine into glycine in fasted or refed healthy newborn infants (Parimi et al. 2005). Of particular interest, J.T. Brosnan and colleagues reported in 1985 that the rat kidney converts 4-hydroxyproline (a product of collagen degradation) into glycine via 4-hydroxyproline oxidase (Figure 3.9). Alanine:glyoxylate aminotransferase catalyzes the nearly irreversible transfer of the amino group from alanine to glyoxylate, yielding glycine and pyruvate. This provides a novel mechanism for the conversion of 4-hydroxyproline and, therefore, proline, into glycine in animals. G. Wu and coworkers identified the presence of large amounts of free and peptide-bound 4-hydroxyproline in sow's milk and the piglet blood (Wu et al. 2019). Dietary and endogenous 4-hydroxyproline contributes to most (64%) of the total glycine synthesis in 3.9-day-old pigs (Wu et al. 2019). Likewise, the endogenous synthesis of glycine from 4-hydroxyproline plays an important role in maintaining the homeostasis of glycine in adult humans (Table 3.10). The net production of glycine by tissues depends on the activities of tetrahydrofolate-dependent SHMT and the methylenetetrahydrofolate-dependent glycine cleavage system. In the liver, high activities of both the glycine cleavage system and SHMT preclude this organ as a net releaser of glycine in the fed or postabsorptive state (Wu 2018). By contrast, in kidneys, the glycine cleavage system is not highly active in both young and adult animals (Lowry et al. 1985), thereby limiting the activity of SHMT and favoring the net production of glycine from hydroxyproline in the kidneys.

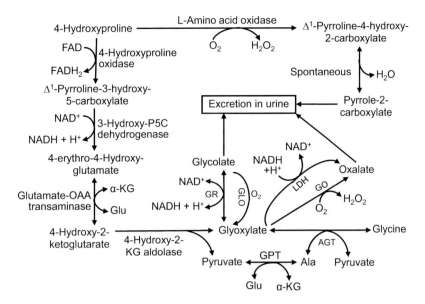

FIGURE 3.9 Glycine synthesis from 4-hydroxyproline in animal cells. This synthetic pathway occurs in mammals, birds, and fish in a cell- and tissue-specific manner. The kidneys, skeletal muscle, small intestine, and liver of animals can convert 4-hydroxyproline into glycine. AGT, alanine–glyoxylate aminotransferase; GLO, glycolate oxidase; GO, glycolate oxidase; GOT, glutamate–oxaloacetate transaminase; GPT, glutamate–pyruvate transaminase; GR, glyoxylate reductase; KG, ketoglutarate; P5C, Δ^1-pyrroline-5-carboxylate; LDH, lactate dehydrogenase; OAA, oxaloacetate; and Pyr, pyruvate.

TABLE 3.10
Relative Contributions of Diet versus Endogenous Synthesis to Meet the glycine Requirement of the 70-kg Healthy Adult Human[a]

Variable	Amount (g/day)
Dietary protein intake	52.5
Digestible glycine intake from the diet	1.42
Glycine intake from diet	1.58
Dietary glycine not digested (10%)	0.16
Metabolic needs for glycine	10.1
Heme synthesis	0.25
Creatine synthesis	1.00
Purine synthesis	0.25
Glutathione synthesis	0.57
Net serine synthesis	1.36
Bile salt synthesis	0.06
Hippurate synthesis	0.54
Irreversible loss through oxidation to CO_2	5.03
Urinary glycine loss	0.11
Sweat and dermal glycine loss	0.08
Ileal endogenous glycine loss	0.66
Colonic endogenous glycine loss	0.15
Glycine synthesis (calculated)	8.16
from serine	2.54
from dietary choline	0.107

(Continued)

TABLE 3.10 (*Continued*)

Relative Contributions of Diet versus Endogenous Synthesis to Meet the glycine Requirement of the 70-kg Healthy Adult Human[a]

Variable	Amount (g/day)
from threnoine	0.022
from endogenous sarcosine	0.142
from carnitine	0.006
from endogenous 4-hydroxyproline (Hyp)	5.34
Glycine synthesis (measured)	9.10
Dietary glycine intake meeting glycine needs	14%
Contribution of Hyp to whole-body glycine synthesis	59%

Source: Wu, G. 2020. *Amino Acids* 52:329–360.

[a] Adult humans consume 0.75 g protein/kg of body weight/day.

Because 4-hydroxyproline is used for glycine synthesis in humans and other animals, the excretion of 4-hydroxyproline in their urine is minimal (Li and Wu 2018). For example, in adult humans, the amounts of 4-hydroxyproline, oxalate, and glycolate excreted daily in the urine of adult humans are only 3–4, 1–3, and 10–20 mg, respectively (Knight et al. 2006). These authors have estimated that only about 5% of the collagen-derived 4-hydroxyproline is oxidized to oxalate and glycolate (Knight et al. 2006). Thus, it can be surmised that approximately 95% of the collagen-derived 4-hydroxyproline may be converted into glycine via the 4-hydroxyproline oxidase pathway in adult humans. The recent findings refute the traditional view that 4-hydroxyproline in its free or small peptide form is merely a metabolic waste in humans and other animals, including pigs (Bushinsky et al. 2002; Khan et al. 2006; Mandel et al. 2004).

The endogenous synthesis of glycine from 4-hydroxyproline, threonine, glucose plus glutamate, and choline in humans and other animals generates ATP (Table 3.11). When 1 mol 4-hydroxyproline, 1 mol threonine, 1 mol glucose plus 1 mol glutamate, or 1 mol choline is degraded to form 1 mol glycine (Wang et al. 2013), 4, 2.5, 2.5, or 2.5 mol ATP are produced, respectively. The yield of ATP is 60% greater with 4-hydroxyproline than any other substrates. However, the formation of 4-hydroxyproline from proline and of glutamate from other AAs requires energy (e.g., 6 mol ATP/mol 4-hydroxyproline, which includes 4 mol ATP for collagen synthesis and 2 mol ATP for collagen degradation). Oxidation of threonine (an AA that is not synthesized by animals but is barely adequate in their conventional diets) to glycine would reduce the use of threonine for protein synthesis and limit animal growth. For comparison, the removal of 1 mol ammonia as urea via the hepatic urea cycle requires 3.25 mol ATP, which is widely recognized as a pathway with a high energy cost (Wu 2018). Thus, direct provision of glycine, 4-hydroxyproline, and glutamate in diets can minimize the expenditure of energy for the endogenous synthesis of glycine.

The conventional diets provide barely sufficient serine and grossly inadequate glycine for protein synthesis in pigs (Tables 3.1–3.4), as well as humans and rats (Jackson 1991; Kalhan and Hanson 2012; Tabatabaie et al. 2010). The liver is the most active organ in the interconversion of glycine and serine through the vitamin B_6-dependent SHMT (Brosnan et al. 2015). This reaction plays an important role in intracellular one-carbon metabolism (Stover and Schirch 1990). There are two isoforms of SHMT: SHMT1 (cytosolic) and SHMT2 (mitochondrial). Due to the compartmentation of metabolic pathways, SHMT1 is involved in the syntheses of purines and thymidylate, as well as the net interconversion of glycine and serine depending on nutritional and physiological needs, whereas SHMT2 contributes to the production of formate from serine/glycine and one-carbon metabolism (Figure 3.10). Thus, SHMT is a useful indicator of DNA synthesis and cell growth (Bazer et al. 2021), as well as a potential target for thechemotherapy and intervention of cancers (Bouzidi et al. 2020).

The mitochondria and cytosol of hepatocytes readily convert serine and tetrahydrofolate into glycine and N^5,N^{10}-methylenetetrahydrofolate (Brosnan et al. 2020). Thus, the oral administration of

TABLE 3.11

Energy Expenditure for the Synthesis of Glycine, Proline, and 4-Hydroxyproline by Humans and Other Animals

Amino acid synthesis	Metabolic pathway	ATP production (mol/mol product)	ATP requirement (mol/mol product)
Glycine	4-Hydroxyproline to glycine	4	---
	Threonine to glycine	2.5	---
	Glucose plus glutamate to glycine	2.5	---
	Choline to glycine	2.5	---
Proline	Glutamine to proline (only in mammals)	---	8
	Glutamate to proline (only in mammals)	---	6
	Arginine to proline (in all animals)	---	2.5
4-Hydroxyproline	Proline to 4-hydroxyproline	---	6

Source: Li, P. and G. Wu. 2018. *Amino Acids* 50:29–38.

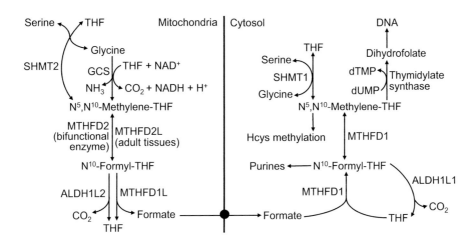

FIGURE 3.10 Interconversion of glycine and serine in the mitochondria and cytosol, as well as the related one-carbon unit metabolism and DNA synthesis, in animal cells. Tetrahydrofolate is required for the conversion of serine into glycine and also for the degradation of glycine via the glycine cleavage system. The net production of glycine by tissues depends on the activities of the tetrahydrofolate-dependent SHMT and the methylenetetrahydrofolate-dependent glycine cleavage system. Serine contributes one carbon for the mitochondrial formation of formate, which is used for the synthesis of purines and thymidylate. ALDH1L1, N^{10}-formyl-THF dehydrogenase (cytosolic); ALDH1L2, N^{10}-formyl-THF dehydrogenase (mitochondrial); dTMP, 2'-deoxythymidylate; dUMP, 2'-deoxyuridylate; GCS, glycine cleavage system; MTHFD1, methylene-THF dehydrogenase (cytosolic); MTHFD1L, mitochondrial monofunctional N^{10}-formyl-THF synthetase; MTHFD2, mitochondrial bifunctional methylene–THF dehydrogenase/methenyl–THF cyclohydrolase; MTHFD2L, mitochondrial isozyme of MTHFD2 in adult tissues; SHMT1, serine hydroxymethyltransferase-1 (cytosolic); SHMT2, serine hydroxymethyltransferase-2 (mitochondrial); and THF, tetrahydrofolate.

serine to humans and other animals markedly increases the concentration of glycine in the plasma. In overnight fasted adult humans, the flux of serine in the plasma is 150 μmol/kg BW/h, with its conversion into glycine and CO_2 being 26 and 12 μmol/kg BW/h, respectively (Kalhan and Hanson 2012). By contrast, animals have a limited ability to convert glycine into serine (Wang et al. 2013) possibly due to a low concentration of N^5,N^{10}-methylenetetrahydrofolate or other methyl group donors, such as *S*-adenosylmethionine, betaine, and choline in the cells. Note that in the mitochondria, the oxidation of glycine into ammonia plus CO_2 with the concomitant formation of

N^5,N^{10}-methylenetetrahydrofolate from tetrahydrofolate is coupled with the conversion of glycine into serine. Isotopic studies with adult humans have shown that virtually all of the methyl groups used for the remethylation of homocysteine into methionine in the whole body are derived from serine (Davis et al. 2004).

3.3.7 Synthesis of Methylarginines in Animal Cells

Because of their roles in the regulation of NO synthesis, there has been a growing interest in the metabolism of methylarginines in mammals. After arginine is incorporated into both cytoplasmic and nuclear proteins, arginine residues are methylated by a family of protein arginine N-methyltransferases (PRMTs). There are four major types of PRMTs that transfer the methyl group from S-adenosylmethionine to the guanidino group of arginine residues in protein substrates, resulting in the formation of both monomethylarginine residues in proteins and S-adenosylhomocysteine (Bedford and Clarke 2009). According to the attachment of methyl groups to specific guanidino nitrogen atoms of arginine residues in proteins, PRMTs are divided into four different types. Type I PRMTs (the most common type of PRMT) form ω-N^G-monomethyl-L-arginine (NMMA) from arginine residues in protein, as well as ω-N^G, N^G-dimethyl-L-arginine (asymmetrical dimethylarginine; ADMA) from NMMA residues in protein. Type II PRMTs generate ω-N^G, $N^{G'}$-dimethyl-L-arginine (symmetrical dimethylarginine; SDMA) from NMMA residues in protein and can also methylate NMMA from arginine residues in protein. Type III PRMTs form only ω-N^G-monomethylarginine from arginine residues in protein. Type IV PRMTs produce δ-N-methylarginine (δ-NMA) residues from arginine residues in protein, and this reaction was initially identified in yeast (Zobel-Thropp et al. 1998). These enzymes may play a role in receptor-mediated signaling and the transcriptional regulation of gene expression in cells. To date, nine mammalian genes for type I PRMTs have been identified and characterized, which include rat and human PRMT1; human PRMT2; rat and human PRMT3; and mouse coactivator-associated arginine methyltransferase 1. These enzymes differ in their substrate specificities, oligomerization properties, interaction with TIS21 (tissue plasminogen activator–induced sequence 21), and subcellular localization.

Thus, the posttranslational modification of protein-bound arginine residues results in the formation of NMMA, ADMA, SDMA, and δ-NMA residues (Figure 3.11). All PRMTs identified to date can monomethylate arginine residues in proteins. However, as indicated previously, further dimethylation of NMMA residues to form ADMA and SDMA residues is catalyzed by type I PRMT and type II PRMT, respectively. Most PRMT genes encode type I PRMT, but the Janus kinase–binding protein 1 and an estrogen receptor α-activator are members of type II PRMT. The arginine methylation reactions involve the modification of guanidino nitrogen or δ-nitrogen atoms and require S-adenosylmethionine. Thus, the synthesis of methylarginines is closely linked with one-carbon metabolism in humans and other animals.

When proteins are degraded by proteases and peptidases, free methylarginines (NMMA, ADMA, SDMA, and δ-NMA) are formed. A majority of free NMMA and ADMA produced in the body is metabolized by dimethylarginine dimethylaminohydrolase, of which two isoforms have recently been identified. Dimethylarginine dimethylaminohydrolase is widespread in mammalian tissues and cells, including the heart, brain, placenta, lung, liver, skeletal muscle, kidney, pancreas, and endothelial cells, and catalyzes the hydrolysis of the C–N bond in the methylated guanidino moiety of NMMA and ADMA to form citrulline and methylamines. Concentrations of free NMMA, ADMA, and SDMA in the plasma are low in healthy individuals (<1 μM), but can be elevated in patients with various cardiovascular and other disorders, such as obesity, diabetes, renal failure, hypercholesterolemia, atherosclerosis, schizophrenia, and multiple sclerosis, suggesting a role for dimethylarginines in these diseases. The concentrations of free δ-NMA in the plasma of healthy humans are about 30 nM (Martens-Lobenhoffer et al. 2016). At present, little is known about δ-NMA catabolism in humans and animals.

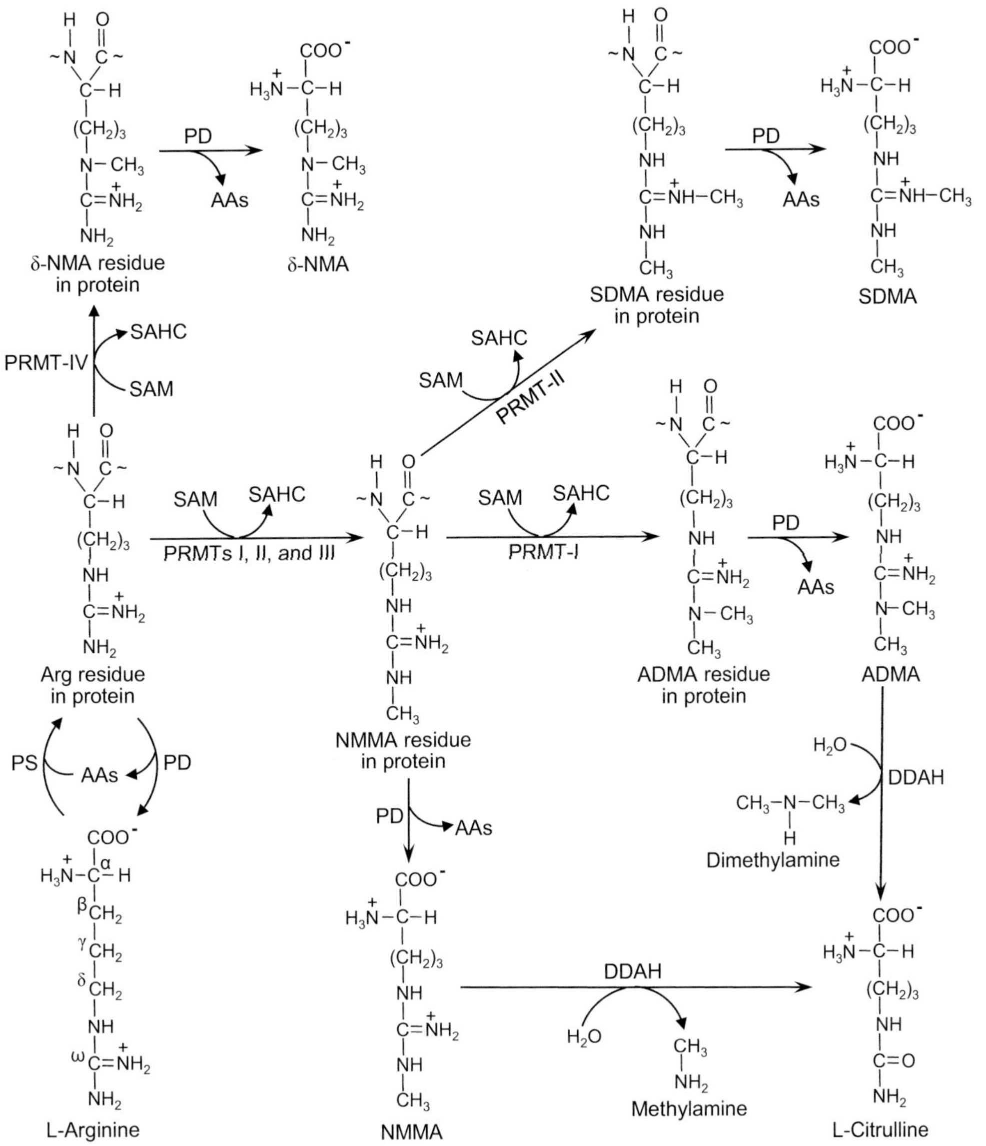

FIGURE 3.11 Synthesis of methylarginines from protein-bound arginine in animal cells. The liver and kidneys are two major organs for the production of methylarginines. In animals, alanine:glyoxylate aminotransferase 2 (the mitochondrial isoform of the enzyme) can transaminate ADMA and glyoxylate to form α-keto-δ-(N,N-dimethylguanidino)valeric acid and glycine (Rodionov et al. 2010). Arg, L-arginine; ADMA, asymmetrical ω-N^G,N^G-dimethyl-L-arginine (asymmetrical dimethylarginine); DDAH, dimethylarginine dimethylaminohydrolase; PRMTs, protein arginine N-methyltransferases; PRMT-I, type I protein arginine N-methyltransferase; PRMT-II, type II protein arginine N-methyltransferase; δ-NMA, δ-N-methylarginine; NMMA, N^G-monomethyl-L-arginine; PD, protein degradation; PS, protein synthesis; SAM, S-adenosylmethionine; SAHC, S-adenosylhomocysteine; and SDMA, symmetrical ω-N^G,$N^{G'}$-dimethyl-L-arginine (symmetrical dimethylarginine).

3.3.8   Synthesis of Proline and Hydroxyproline in Animal Cells

The unique structures of proline and its related metabolites are illustrated in Figure 3.12. Nutritional and biochemical studies in the 1930s by W.C. Rose and H.A. Krebs established that mammals can synthesize proline. It is now known that the synthesis of proline from glutamine, glutamate, arginine, and ornithine in animals is cell-, tissue- and species-specific and that substrate channeling plays an important role in proline synthesis in cells (Arentson et al. 2012; Phang et al. 2010). Specifically, all mammals can synthesize proline from arginine via arginase (both type I and type II), OAT, and P5C reductase, with the mammary tissue, small intestine (postweaning animals), liver, and kidneys being quantitatively the most active tissues. In mammary tissue, the activity of P5C reductase is at least 50-fold greater than that of P5C dehydrogenase, thereby favoring the conversion of arginine-derived P5C into proline rather than into glutamate and glutamine. The active synthesis of proline from arginine contributes to a high abundance of proline in milk proteins and also helps to prevent an irreversible loss of arginine carbons. In addition, the small intestine of postweaning pigs degrades approximately 40% of dietary arginine, 97% of dietary glutamate, and 70% of dietary glutamine to generate several AAs, including proline, as major nitrogenous products. Studies with jejunum-cannulated young pigs demonstrated a net release of proline from the small intestine of food-deprived piglets. *De novo* synthesis and hydrolysis of small peptides in enterocytes and in the intestinal lumen may be sources of this gut-derived proline. Compelling evidence shows that neonates cannot synthesize adequate amounts of proline to support their maximal growth (Ball et al. 1986; Wu et al. 2011a). Additionally, carnivores (e.g., cats and ferrets) lack P5C synthase in enterocytes and other cell types, and, therefore, cannot convert glutamine and glutamate into proline. Proline synthesis is particularly important for wound healing and remodeling of the extracellular matrix but requires a relatively large amount of energy. Note that the arginine pathway is the least expensive for proline synthesis in terms of energy cost, as compared with glutamate or glutamine (Table 3.11).

The occurrence of hydroxyproline residues in proteins (primarily collagens) results from the posttranslational hydroxylation of proline residues in the proteins. Namely, the hydroxylation of peptide-bound proline residues takes place after the collagens and other proteins are synthesized in ribosomes. In non-collagen proteins (including hypoxia-inducible transcription factor-α), only a limited number of proline residues are hydroxylated into 4-hydroxyproline residues. Specifically,

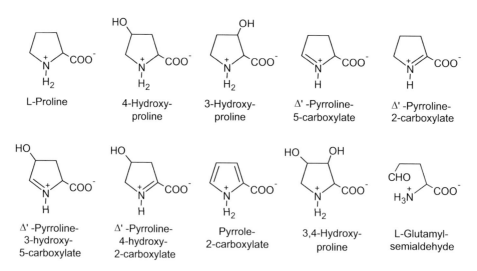

FIGURE 3.12 Chemical structures of proline and related substances in the non-ionized form. In animals, these substances exist in an L-form, and the physiological form of 4-hydroxyproline and 3-hydroxyproline is the *trans* configuration. Bacteria and plants contain D-proline. Both *trans-* and *cis*-4-hydroxy-L-proline are present in fungi.

proline residues in the collagen proteins are hydroxylated in the endoplasmic reticulum by collagen prolyl 4-hydroxylase or prolyl 3-hydroxylase in the presence of oxygen, ascorbic acid, α-KG, and Fe^{2+} (see Chapter 8). The ratio of 4-hydroxyproline to 3-hydroxyproline in collagen proteins is approximately 100:1. Both proline and 4-hydroxyproline are major AAs in the collagen proteins, which contain three chains of polypeptides (two α1 chains and one α2 chain) and are major extracellular components in connective tissues (e.g., skin, tendon, cartilage, vessels of the vascular system, and bone) (Wu et al. 2011a). The helical region of collagen comprises the repeat of Gly-X-Y, where proline can be in the X or Y position and hydroxyproline occurs only in the Y position. The unique ring structure of proline and hydroxyproline distinguishes them from other AAs in terms of rigidity, chemical stability, and biochemical reactions. Proline and hydroxyproline account for approximately 12.5% (g/g) of all proteins in animals at birth and in adult life, with the ratio of proline to hydroxyproline being 2.25:1. Thus, 31% of all proline residues in body proteins (primarily collagen) are hydroxylated after the polypeptides are synthesized. The percentage of hydroxyproline in the body increases markedly with fetal development and only slightly after birth. For example, the content of hydroxyproline (g/100 protein) is 0.84 and 3.64, respectively, in 40- and 114-day-old fetal pigs (term = 114 days), but is 3.76 and 3.86, respectively, in 14- and 180-day-old postnatal pigs (Wu et al. 2019). Note that hydroxyproline is not generated from free proline in humans or other animals.

Like other proteins in animals, collagens (present predominantly in the extracellular matrix) and proteins with 4-hydroxylprolyl and 3-hydroxylprolyl residues undergo continuous degradation. As a result, free 4-hydroxyproline and 3-hydroxyproline as well as small peptides containing hydroxyproline are generated from the degradation of these proteins (see Chapter 9). Matrix metalloproteinases (also called collagenases) are responsible for the hydrolysis of extracellular collagens in the connective tissue (Malemud 2006). Studies with pigs have shown that, in their plasma and sow's milk, 4-hydroxyproline exists mainly in the peptide-bound form (Table 3.12). A majority of

TABLE 3.12
Concentrations of 4-Hydroxyproline (Hyp) in Sow's Milk and in the Piglet Plasma, and 4-Hydroxyproline Intake by Sow-Reared Piglets

		Hyp in sow's milk			Hyp in piglet plasma	
	Milk intake	Free Hyp	Peptide-bound Hyp[‡]	Total intake of Hyp from milk by piglets	Free Hyp	Peptide-bound Hyp[‡]
Age of pigs (mean weight)	(mL/kg BW per day)	(μmol/L)	(mmol/L)	(mmol/kg BW per day)	(μmol/L)	(mmol/L)
1 day (1.4 kg)	193 ± 10[bd]	105 ± 5[a]	11.64 ± 0.70[a]	2.27 ± 0.12[b]	91 ± 6[b]	2.38 ± 0.11[b]
3 days (1.7 kg)	210 ± 12[bc]	98 ± 4[a]	9.74 ± 0.51[b]	2.07 ± 0.11[b]	86 ± 4[b]	2.51 ± 0.12[b]
7 days (2.5 kg)	307 ± 16[a]	82 ± 3[b]	9.02 ± 0.38[bc]	2.80 ± 0.13[a]	110 ± 7[a]	2.93 ± 0.14[a]
14 days (3.9 kg)	234 ± 14[b]	68 ± 2[c]	7.84 ± 0.36[c]	1.85 ± 0.08[c]	89 ± 4[b]	2.46 ± 0.10[b]
21 days (5.7 kg)	188 ± 12[cd]	55 ± 2[d]	6.29 ± 0.33[d]	1.19 ± 0.07[d]	80 ± 6[b]	2.32 ± 0.08[b]
28 days (7.7 kg)	170 ± 11[d]	56 ± 2[d]	6.26 ± 0.31[d]	1.06 ± 0.06[d]	86 ± 5[b]	2.25 ± 0.09[b]

Note: BW = body weight.

Values are means ± SEM, *n* = 10. Ten sows (offspring of Yorkshire × Landrace dams and Duroc × Hampshire sires) were fed a corn- and soybean meal–based gestation diet (containing 18% crude protein). On days 1, 3, 7, 14, 21, and 28 of lactation, milk samples were obtained from sows at 2 h after feeding, and blood samples were withdrawn from the jugular vein of piglets (three piglets/sow) into heparinized tubes at 1 h after suckling. Plasma samples of three piglets from the same sow were pooled. Milk and plasma samples were analyzed for free and peptide-bound hydroxyproline (Hyp) by using high-performance liquid chromatography (Wu et al. 1997).

[‡] Peptide-bound Hyp is in the form of glycine-proline-hydroxyproline. Data were analyzed by one-way analysis of variance and the Duncan multiple comparisons (Assaad et al. 2014).

[a-b] Within a column, means not sharing the same superscript letter differ ($P<0.05$).

4-hydroxyproline-containing peptides in enteral diets (including milk) are hydrolyzed by the small intestine into free 4-hydroxyproline (Chapter 2). Thus, most of the 4-hydroxyproline in the plasma is derived from collagen degradation in the body. The flux of 4-hydroxyproline in the plasma is greater in young than in older animals because of a higher rate of collagen turnover in the former (Wu et al. 2019).

3.3.9   Synthesis of Tyrosine in Animal Cells

As early as 1909, O. Neubauer postulated that phenylalanine is converted into tyrosine in animals. Based on their studies with perfused rat liver, Embden and Baldes reported in 1913 the synthesis of tyrosine from phenylalanine. Subsequently, the results from clinical experiments involving the oral administration of tyrosine or phenylalanine to patients with tyrosinosis led Grace Medes to conclude in 1932 that phenylalanine can be converted into tyrosine in humans. This conclusion was supported by W.C. Rose who demonstrated in 1934 that young rats could grow when fed a tyrosine-free diet containing phenylalanine. Interestingly, nutritional studies in the 1940s indicated that tyrosine can partially replace phenylalanine in the diets for young and adult animals, including rats and chicks. Biochemical studies in 1958 by S. Kaufman revealed that the hydroxylation of phenylalanine by phenylalanine hydroxylase requires BH4 and NADPH as essential cofactors (Kaufman 1987). This enzyme is allosterically activated by phenylalanine to enhance its hydroxylation (Fitzpatrick 1999; Hufton et al. 1995).

In humans and other animals, tyrosine synthesis takes place primarily in the liver and kidneys and, to a much lesser extent, in the pancreas, small intestine (at least in pigs), and skin (Table 3.5). Of particular note, there is evidence that the human kidneys synthesize an appreciable amount of tyrosine from phenylalanine (5.2 μmol/min) compared with that in the splanchnic bed (including the liver; 3.0 μmol/min) (Møller et al. 2000). Thus, in healthy adults, the kidneys may be the major site of tyrosine production. In addition, the mammary glands of ruminants (e.g., cows and goats; Jorgensen and Larson 1968), but not non-ruminants [e.g., pigs (Li et al. 2009; Zhang et al. 2019) as well as guinea pigs and rats (Jorgensen and Larson 1968)], contain phenylalanine hydroxylase activity for forming tyrosine from phenylalanine, indicating another species difference in AA metabolism among animals. Thus, the mammary tissue of lactating cows, but not rats, can synthesize milk protein when cultured in tyrosine-free medium containing all other canonical proteinogenic AAs (including phenylalanine; Jorgensen and Larson 1968). Many mammalian tissues do not possess phenylalanine hydroxylase activity, including the brain, heart, lung, salivary glands, skeletal muscle, spleen, and thymus (Tourian et al. 1969). A lack or near absence of the conversion of phenylalanine into tyrosine in the brain requires the presence of tyrosine in the blood circulation to meet the need for the production of tyrosine-derived neurotransmitters by this organ. At present, little is known about phenylalanine hydroxylase expression in the extrahepatic and extrarenal tissues of aquatic animals. Both phenylalanine and tyrosine are relatively abundant in animal and plant proteins (Li and Wu 2020).

3.3.10   Formation of β-Alanine in Animal Cells

β-Alanine is formed from six sources (Griffith 1986): (1) aspartate decarboxylation (primarily in bacteria); (2) hydrolysis of coenzyme A by a combination of several enzymes (phosphomonoesterase, phosphodiesterase, CoA pyrophosphatase, and a type of peptidase); (3) degradation of carnosine by carnosinase; (4) catabolism of pyrimidines through a series of reactions (Chapter 5); (5) transamination of malonic acid semialdehyde with glutamate (Figure 3.2); and (6) degradation of polyamines (Chapter 5). Concentrations of β-alanine in the plasma are generally much higher in ruminants than in non-ruminants (Kwon et al. 2003; Wu et al. 1995), suggesting an important contribution of bacteria to β-alanine synthesis in humans and other animals. β-Alanine is a limiting factor for the synthesis of anserine, balenine, and carnosine in the skeletal muscles of mammals, birds, and fish in a muscle fiber- and species-specific manner (Sale et al. 2010; Wu 2020b).

3.3.11 SYNTHESIS OF UNIQUE SULFUR-CONTAINING AMINO ACIDS IN FELIDAE SPECIES AND OTHER ANIMALS

Some Felidae species (e.g., the bobcat, ocelot, Chinese desert cat, kodkod, Siberian lynx, and domestic cat) synthesize three unique sulfur-containing AAs (Rutherfurd et al. 2002; Rutherfurd-Markwick et al. 2005). They are: felinine (2-amino-7-hydroxy-5,5-dimethyl-4-thiaheptanoic acid; (2*R*)-2-amino-3-[(3-hydroxy-1,1-dimethylpropyl)thio]propanoic acid]), isovalthine (2-amino-5-carboxy-6-methyl-4-thiaheptanoic acid), and isobuteine [2-amino-6-carboxy-4-thiaheptanoic acid; *S*-carboxyisopropylcysteine; and *S*-(2-methyl-2-carboxyethyl)cysteine]. Felinine, isovalthine, and isobuteine are unusual AAs in that they contain both a sulfur atom in the main chain and a branched side chain with a methyl group. In addition, certain felids (e.g., the domestic cat and lion), as well as humans with hypothyroidism and hypercholesterolemia and other select mammals (e.g., the rat, rabbit, guinea pig, and dog) produce isovalthine. Furthermore, the domestic cat, other select members of the Felidae family, and humans generate isobuteine.

HO–CH$_2$–CH$_2$–C(CH$_3$)(CH$_3$)–S–CH$_2$–CH(COOH)–NH$_2$ Felinine (C$_8$H$_{17}$O$_3$NS; MW = 207.29)

(H$_3$C)(H$_3$C)CH–CH(COOH)–S–CH$_2$–CH(COOH)–NH$_2$ Isovalthine (C$_8$H$_{15}$O$_4$NS; MW = 221.28)

H$_3$C–CH(COOH)–CH$_2$–S–CH$_2$–CH(COOH)–NH$_2$ Isobuteine (C$_7$H$_{13}$O$_4$NS; MW = 207.25)

The syntheses of felinine, isovalthine, and isobuteine require glutathione and either an isoprene unit or a branched-chain α-ketoacid (Figures 3.13 and 3.14). Specifically, in the livers of those species, glutathione conjugates with isopentenyl pyrophosphate (an intermediate of cholesterol biosynthesis), isovaleric acid (a metabolite of leucine), and possibly isobutyric acid (a metabolite of valine) to yield 3-methylbutanol-glutathione (3-mercaptobutanol-glutathionine; γ-glutamylfelinylglycine), *S*-(iso-propylcarboxymethyl)-glutathione, and *S*-(iso-ethylcarboxymethyl)-glutathione, respectively. These conjugation reactions are catalyzed by glutathione *S*-transferase in the cytosol of hepatocytes. The glutathione conjugates are released from the liver and transported in the blood to the kidneys, where they are metabolized via γ-glutamyl transferase (a membrane-bound enzyme in the proximal renal tubules) to form 3-methylbutanol-cysteinylglycine, *S*-(iso-propylcarboxymethyl)-cysteinylglycine, and *S*-(iso-ethylcarboxymethyl)-cysteinylglycine, respectively. These cysteinylglycine derivatives are hydrolyzed by dipeptidases (e.g., aminopeptidase M) in the cytosol of the proximal renal tubules to generate felinine, isovalthine, and isobuteine, respectively, with glycine as a coproduct. Some of the resultant sulfur-containing metabolites are locally *N*-acetylated by *N*-acetyltransferase to their corresponding acetyl derivatives (i.e., *N*-acetyl-felinine, *N*-acetyl-isovathine, and *N*-acetyl-isobuteine, respectively). Additionally, 3-methylbutanol-cysteinylglycine, *S*-(iso-propylcarboxymethyl)-cysteinylglycine, and *S*-(iso-ethylcarboxymethyl)-cysteinylglycine are hydrolyzed by the extracellular cauxin (a carboxylesterase secreted by the proximal straight renal tubules of the kidneys) in the lumen of the renal tubules and the bladder to yield felinine, isovalthine, and isobuteine, respectively, with glycine as a coproduct. In the cytosol of the proximal straight

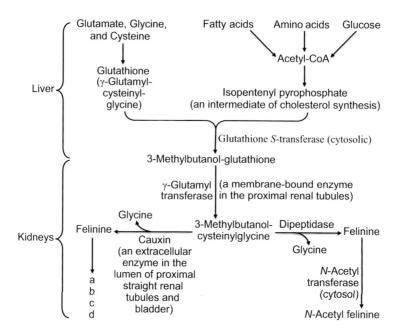

FIGURE 3.13 Synthesis and metabolism of felinine in some Felidae species through the cooperation of the liver and kidneys. In the liver of some Felidae species (e.g., the bobcat, ocelot, Chinese desert cat, kodkod, Siberian lynx, and domestic cat), glutathione S-transferase catalyzes the conjugation of glutathione with isopentenyl pyrophosphate to generate 3-methylbutanol-glutathione. The latter is released from the liver and transported in the blood to the kidneys, where it is metabolized via γ-glutamyl transferase (a membrane-bound enzyme in the proximal renal tubules) to form 3-methylbutanol-cysteinylglycine. This cysteinylglycine derivative is hydrolyzed by dipeptidases (e.g., aminopeptidase M) in the cytosol of the proximal renal tubules to generate felinine, with glycine as a coproduct. Felinine is locally N-acetylated by N-acetyltransferase to N-acetyl-felinine. Additionally, 3-methylbutanol-cysteinylglycine is hydrolyzed by the extracellular cauxin (a carboxylesterase secreted by the proximal straight renal tubules of the kidneys) in the lumen of the renal tubules and the bladder to yield felinine, with glycine as a coproduct. In the cytosol of the proximal straight renal tubules, feline is further metabolized into methylated products (a, b, c, and d). a = 3-mercapto-3-methyl-1-butanol; b = 3-mercapto-3-methylbutyl formate; c = 3-methyl-3-methylthio-1-butanol; and d = 3-methyl-3-(2-methyldisulfanyl)-1-butanol. Felinine and its derivatives are excreted in the urine.

renal tubules, felinine is further metabolized into 3-mercapto-3-methyl-1-butanol, 3-mercapto-3-methylbutyl formate, 3-methyl-3-methylthio-1-butanol, and 3-methyl-3-(2-methyldisulfanyl)-1-butanol. Similar modifications of isovalthine and isobuteine may also occur. Felinine, isovalthine, and isobuteine, as well as their derivatives are excreted in the urine (Herring et al. 2021).

Nutritional studies have shown that the syntheses of felinine, isovalthine, and isobuteine are influenced by dietary intakes of methionine and cysteine (Hendriks et al. 2008; Rutherfurd-Markwick et al. 2005), and possibly dietary lipids (in the case of felinine), leucine (in the case of isovalthine), and valine (in the case of isobutyrate) when the dietary provision of methionine, cysteine, glycine, and BCAAs is not limiting. Interestingly, the production of felinine by felids is gender-specific as its excretion in the urine is much higher in males than in females, but the urinary excretion of isovalthine by adult cats is not gender-specific (Hendriks et al. 2004). The biological significance of felinine, isovalthine, and isobuteine, as well as their derivatives remains largely elusive. It is possible that these sulfur-containing AAs and their metabolites serve as non-toxic, non-reactive, and relatively stable end products of methionine and cysteine to prevent excessive formation of toxic and highly acidic substances (e.g., H_2S, SO_2, and H_2SO_4) from methionine and cysteine. Of particular note, Miyazaki et al. (2008) have suggested that felinine is a territorial marker for intraspecies

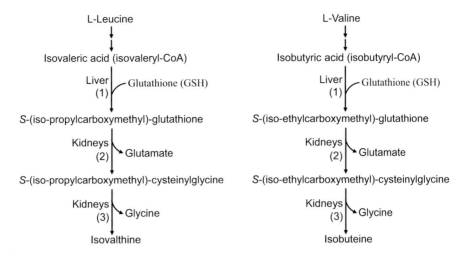

FIGURE 3.14   Synthesis of isovalthine and isobuteine in some Felidae species through the cooperation of the liver and kidneys. In the liver of some Felidae species (e.g., the bobcat, ocelot, Chinese desert cat, kodkod, Siberian lynx, and domestic cat), glutathione *S*-transferase catalyzes the conjugation of glutathione with isovaleric acid (a metabolite of L-leucine) or isobutyric acid (a metabolite of L-valine) to generate a glutathione derivative. The latter is released from the liver and transported in the blood to the kidneys, where it is metabolized via γ-glutamyl transferase (a membrane-bound enzyme in the proximal renal tubules) to form glutamate and a cysteinylglycine derivative. This cysteinylglycine derivative is hydrolyzed by dipeptidases (e.g., aminopeptidase M) in the cytosol of the proximal renal tubules to generate isovalthine or isobuteine, with glycine as a coproduct. Enzymes catalyzing the indicated reactions are: (1) glutathione *S*-transferase; (2) γ-glutamyl transferase (a membrane-bound enzyme); and (3) dipeptidases (e.g., aminopeptidase M).

communications and is also a putative precursor of a pheromone that serves as a chemical signal to attract females.

3.3.12   SYNTHESIS OF *N*-ACETYLATED AMINO ACIDS IN ANIMAL CELLS

As noted in Chapter 1, humans and other animals synthesize *N*-acetylated AAs, including *N*-acetylglutamate, *N*-acetyl-aspartate, *N*-acetyl-L-histidine, and *N*-acetyl-1-methylhistidine (*N*-acetylπ-methylhistidine) in a species- and tissue-specific manner. *N*-acetyl-glutamate is synthesized from acetyl-CoA and glutamate in the liver, enterocytes, and brain by *N*-acetyl-glutamate synthase. *N*-Acetyl-aspartate, *N*-acetyl-L-histidine (also known as N_α-acetyl-histidine), and *N*-acetyl-1-methylhistidine are synthesized from acetyl-CoA and the corresponding AA by aspartate, histidine, and 1-methylhistidine *N*-acetyltransferase, respectively (Baslow 1997); these enzymes are also known as *N*-acetyl-aspartate, *N*-acetyl-L-histidine, and *N*-acetyl-1-methylhistidine synthases, respectively. *N*-acetyl-glutamate, *N*-acetyl-aspartate, *N*-acetyl-L-histidine, and *N*-acetyl-1-methylhistidine synthases are all localized in the mitochondria of the specific tissues. Furthermore, the posttranslational acetylation of certain proteins can result in the release of *N*-acetylated AAs after their hydrolysis.

Acetyl-CoA + L-Glutamate → CoA + *N*-Acetyl-L-glutamate   (*N*-acetyl-glutamate synthase)

Acetyl-CoA + L-Aspartate → CoA + *N*-Acetyl-L-aspartate   (*N*-acetyl-aspartate synthase)

Acetyl-CoA + L-Histidine → CoA + *N*-Acetyl-L-histidine   (*N*-acetyl-histidine synthase)

Acetyl-CoA + 1-Methyl-L-histidine → CoA + *N*-Acetyl-1-methyl-L-histidine
   (*N*-acetyl-1-methyl-histidine synthase)

3.3.13 SYNTHESIS OF PHOSPHORYL AMINO ACIDS IN ANIMAL CELLS

Phosphoryl AAs occur in the blood and other tissues of mammals, birds, fish, and crustaceans. Some (e.g., phosphoserine, phosphothreonine, phosphotyrosine, N-phosphohistidine, and N-phosphoarginine, as well as phosphoethanolamine) of these substances are widespread in the animal kingdom (Attwood 2013), whereas others (e.g., phosphoarginine at millimolar concentrations in crustaceans) are distributed in a species-specific manner (Li et al. 2021b). There are reports that the concentrations of ethanolamine in the plasma of rats and humans range from 10 to 75 μM, depending on diets, as well as nutritional and physiological status (Baha et al. 1984; Kruse et al. 1985; Milakofsky et al. 1985). Protein serine/threonine, protein tyrosine kinases, protein histidine kinase, and protein arginine kinase can phosphorylate some serine/threonine, tyrosine, histidine, and arginine residues in proteins, respectively. The N-phosphorylation of a histidine residue in proteins involves the N1 or N3 atom of its imidazole group, whereas the N-phosphorylation of an arginine residue in proteins (e.g., histones) involves the two NH_2 groups of its guanidino group (Fuhrmann et al. 2015). Phosphoserine, phosphothreonine, phosphotyrosine, N-phosphohistidine, and N-phosphoarginine are released after the proteins that contain phosphorylated serine, threonine, tyrosine, histidine, and arginine residues are degraded by a combination of proteases and peptidases. In the crustaceans, arginine kinase acts on free L-arginine in the presence of ATP to directly generate a large amount of L-phosphoarginine and ADP (Chapter 1).

Serine → Protein → Phosphorylation of serine residues in protein → Phosphoserine

Threonine → Protein → Phosphorylation of threonine residues in protein → Phosphothreonine

Tyrosine → Protein → Phosphorylation of tyrosine residues in protein → Phosphotyrosine

Histidine → Protein → N-Phosphorylation of histidine residues in protein → N-Phosphohistidine

Arginine → Protein → N-Phosphorylation of arginine residues in protein → N-Phosphoarginine

L-Arginine (free) + ATP → L-Phosphoarginine + ADP   (arginine kinase; crustaceans)

Phosphoethanolamine (a precursor for the synthesis of phospholipids that are crucial for the structure and functions of cells) is synthesized from ethanolamine and ATP by ethanolamine kinase (an enzyme in the endoplasmic reticulum). Animal cells lack serine decarboxylase and, therefore, cannot directly produce ethanolamine from serine. However, humans and other animals are capable of synthesizing ethanolamine from serine and palmitoyl-CoA via the ceramide pathway in the endoplasmic reticulum (Figure 3.15). Phosphoethanolamine is converted into ethanolamine via the formation of phosphatidylethanolamine. In addition, the diets (free ethanolamine, phosphatidylethanolamine, and phosphatidylcholine) and intestinal microbes (via the serine decarboxylase and ceramide pathways) of an animal are also its sources of ethanolamine for metabolic utilization.

3.4 PATHWAYS FOR THE SYNTHESIS OF AMINO ACIDS IN MICROORGANISMS

The gastrointestinal tract of humans and other animals contains a large number of microbes, including diverse species of bacteria. The diversity of the bacteria and their metabolic redundancy make it easier for them to survive and interact with their neighboring species or eukaryotic hosts during transition along the length of the digestive tract. The outcomes of these interactions have important impacts on gut health, whole-body homeostasis, the development of diseases (e.g., obesity, diabetes, and stroke), and reproduction (Dai et al. 2015). When animals are food-deprived or consume protein-insufficient diets, AAs synthesized and absorbed in the large intestine may play a role in regulating whole-body nitrogen homeostasis (Mansilla et al. 2017). Microbes contain many

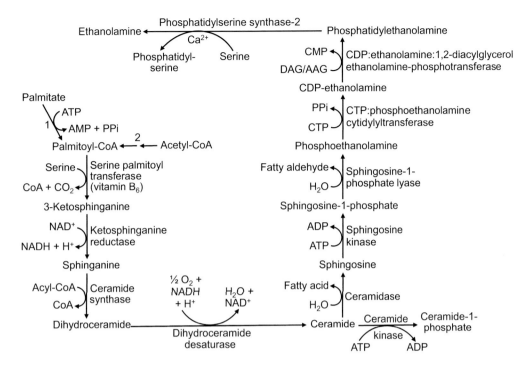

FIGURE 3.15 *De novo* synthesis of phosphoethanolamine and ethanolamine from serine and palmitoyl-CoA in animals. The conversion of serine and palmitoyl-CoA into ceramide, phosphoethanolamine, and ethanolamine occurs in the endoplasmic reticulum. The enzymes that catalyze the indicated reactions in the cytosol are: (1) palmitoyl-CoA synthase and (2) a series of enzymes for the synthesis of long-chain fatty acids from acetyl-CoA. AAG, 1-*O*-alkyl-2-acetyl-*sn*-glycerol; CTP, cytidine triphosphate; CDP, cytidine diphosphate; CMP, cytidine monophosphate; and DAG, diacylglycerol.

AA-synthesis enzymes that are absent from eukaryotic cells, including aspartokinase, aspartate semialdehyde dehydrogenase, chorismate synthase, chorismate mutase, homocitrate synthase, homoserine dehydrogenase, homoserine kinase, shikimate kinase, prephenate kinase, and threonine deaminase (Whitworth and Cock 2009). With recent advances in the science and technology of microbial AA synthesis, mutant or genetically engineered bacteria are now used for the large-scale production of AAs, such as arginine, citrulline, glutamate, glutamine, lysine, threonine, and tryptophan (D'Mello 2017).

3.4.1 Overall Pathways for the Synthesis of Amino Acids in Microorganisms

If dietary supplies of energy, carbon, nitrogen, and sulfur are sufficient, all AAs can be synthesized by microorganisms living in the rumen of ruminants and in the large intestine of monogastric species, including humans, rats, dogs, pigs, chickens, and horses (Bergen 2021; Metges 2000). Microbial synthesis of AAs also occurs in the lumen of the small intestine (Dai et al. 2015). Bacteria can adapt well to changes in extracellular provisions of nitrogenous substances to maintain their ecosystem and activities. As described in Chapter 2, ammonia, glutamate, and pyruvate are the ultimate substrates for syntheses of all non-sulfur AAs in bacteria. In the presence of serine, inorganic or organic sulfur can be used by these cells to produce cysteine and methionine (Campbell et al. 1997). The overall pathways for EAA syntheses by microorganisms are summarized in Figure 3.16. Note that many of these reactions depend on NADPH or NADH as a cofactor. Microbial synthesis of AAs appears to meet the maintenance needs of ruminants and their low levels of growth or productivity. However, results of recent studies clearly indicate that these synthetic pathways in

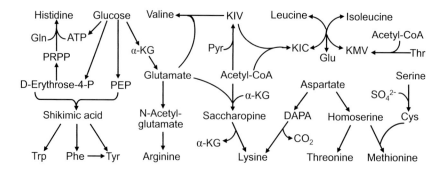

FIGURE 3.16 An overall view of pathways for the syntheses of nutritionally essential amino acids in microorganisms. DAPA, diaminopimelate; α-KG, α-ketoglutarate; KIC, α-ketoisocaproate; KIV, α-ketoisovalerate; KMV, α-keto-β-methylvalerate; PEP, phosphoenolpyruvate; PRPP, 5-phosphoribosyl-α-pyrophosphate; and Pyr, pyruvate.

the rumen are inadequate for the maximum growth of ruminants (e.g., beef cattle and sheep) or the maximum lactation of high-producing cows (Lapierre et al. 2006). Although microorganisms in the small and large intestines of monogastric animals are able to synthesize all AAs, it is unlikely that this is a quantitatively significant source of EAAs or AASAs due to the limited absorption of free AAs and no uptake of microbial protein (the major sink of nitrogen in bacteria) by colonocytes (Bergen and Wu 2009). Nonetheless, nitrogen and sulfur metabolism (e.g., the production of ammonia, hydrogen sulfide, and polyamines) in the large intestine plays an important role in gut integrity and health, as well as the pathogenesis of inflammatory bowel diseases and colon cancer in humans and other animals (Beaumont and Blachier 2020).

Note that some AA synthetic pathways that occur in animal cells are absent from microbes. For example, in contrast to the liver of humans and most of the other animals, microbes (including the gut microbiota) cannot synthesize taurine from cysteine (Dai et al. 2011). In addition, unlike animal tissues, microbes do not convert 4-hydroxyproline into glycine. Furthermore, bacteria lack arginine kinase for the direct synthesis of phosphoarginine from free arginine and ATP.

3.4.2 Pathways for the Synthesis of AASAs in Microorganisms

Microorganisms use either the same and/or different pathways as those found in animals to synthesize alanine, aspartate, glutamate, glutamine, glycine, proline, serine, and tyrosine. For example, like the mitochondrial dimethylglycine dehydrogenase in animals (Augustin et al. 2016), the cytosolic dimethylglycine dehydrogenase in bacteria oxidizes dimethylglycine to sarcosine in a flavin adenine dinucleotide (FAD)- and tetrahydrofolate-dependent manner (Leys et al. 2003). Additionally, AA synthetic pathways that are not found in mammals or birds may be present in microbes, such as bacteria and protozoa. Specific examples are provided in the following sections.

3.4.2.1 Synthesis of Glutamate and Glutamine

In contrast to animal cells, two molecules of glutamate can be formed from one molecule of glutamine plus one molecule of α-KG by NADPH-dependent glutamate synthase (also known as glutamine:α-KG amidotransferase; a complex iron-sulfur flavoprotein) in bacteria (e.g., *E. coli*) and plants. This enzyme requires four cofactors (FAD, flavin mononucleotide, iron, and sulfur) and possesses an iron-sulfur center in its catalytic site (Temple et al. 1998). This reaction is reversible. Thus, the NADP+-dependent glutamine synthesis plays an important role in the microbial assimilation of nitrogen and in generating NADPH for antioxidative reactions.

$$2\text{L-Glutamate} + \text{NADP}^+ \leftrightarrow \text{L-Glutamine} + \alpha\text{-KG} + \text{NADPH} + \text{H}^+$$

GDH and GS play essential roles in the utilization of ammonia for the microbial synthesis of gluta-mate and glutamine, respectively. Thus, much work has been done to understand the structures and catalytic mechanisms of these two enzymes. Most bacteria, including *Corynebacterium glutamicum, Escherichia coli, Salmonella typhimurium,* and *Synechocystis* PCC 6803, have the NADP+-dependent GDH isoform, which is a hexameric oligomer with 6 identical subunits (a subunit molecular weight of ~50 kDa). This type of GDH is encoded by the *gdhA* gene. Some bacteria (e.g., *Bacteroides fragilis* Bf1 and antarctic bacterium *Psychrobacter* sp.) possess two distinct isoforms of the GDH enzyme: NAD(P)+-dependent (encoded by *gdhA*) and NAD+-specific (encoded by *gdhB*). The NAD+-dependent GDH has either 6 identical subunits of ~48 KDa (e.g., *Clostridium symbiosum*) or 4 identical subunits of ~115 KDa (e.g., *Neurospora crassa*). In *Bacteroides fragilis*, the dual coenzyme-specific GDH is subjected to reversible inactivation and repression by ammonium. The hexameric enzymes are structurally similar and independent of their coenzyme specificity but differ to some extent in chemical, physical, and immunological properties (Hudson and Daniel 1993).

GS has a complex structure and unique regulatory mechanisms (Figure 3.17). GS in most bacteria (including *Escherichia coli*), which is encoded by *glnA,* consists of 12 identical 469-AA subunits (Eisenberg et al. 2000). Some bacteria, including *Rhizobium meliloti, Streptomyces viridochromogenes, Streptomyces coelicolor,* and *Frankia* sp., have a second form of GS encoded by *glnII*. A third isoform of GS, encoded by *glnT,* occurs in some bacteria, such as *Rhizobium meliloti* and *Rhizobium*

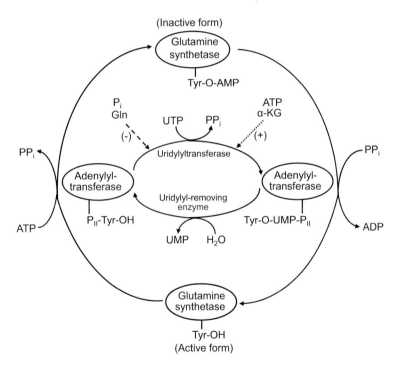

FIGURE 3.17 Regulation of bacterial glutamine synthetase (GS) activity by covalent adenylylation and deadenylylation under the control of a regulatory protein P_{II} through uridylylation and deuridylylation of adenylyltransferase. Adenylyltransferase forms a regulatory complex with P_{II}. Adenylylation of GS (tyrosine residue-397) by adenylyltransferase (when P_{II} is in the deuridylylated form) converts GS from an active to an inactive form. Deadenylylation of GS by adenylyltransferase (when P_{II} is in the deuridylylated form) converts GS from an inactive to an active form. Uridylyltransferase and uridylyl-removing enzyme, whose enzymatic activities are located on the same protein, respectively catalyze uridylylation and deuridylylation of P_{II} (tyrosine residue in the center part of the 110-amino acid residue protein). Glutamine and Pi inhibit uridylyltransferase and, therefore, GS. By contrast, α-ketoglutarate and ATP activate uridylyltransferase and, therefore, GS.

leguminosarum. Cyanobacterium has a different isoform of GS that is encoded by *glnN*. Microbial GS activity is regulated by covalent adenylylation of tyrosine-397 (inhibition) and deadenylylation (activation), with both enzymatic activities being catalyzed by the same protein known as adenylyl transferase. Adenylyl transferase acts in coordination with a tetrameric regulatory protein P_{II}. When a specific tyrosine residue in PII is uridylylated by the UTP-dependent uridylyltransferase, the adenylyl transferase-PII complex catalyzes the deadenylylation of GS to generate an active form of GS. The uridylyltransferase is activated by ATP and α-KG but inhibited by glutamine and Pi. When the attached uridine monophosphate group in PII is removed by the uridylyl-removing enzyme, the adenylyl transferase-PII complex catalyzes the adenylylation of GS to form an inactive form of GS. The adenylylation of GS is stimulated by glutamine and inhibited by α-KG. Of particular interest, the uridylyltransferase and uridylyl-removing enzyme activities are possessed by the same protein, which can be classified as a bifunctional protein. In addition to the covalent regulation of GS activity, this enzyme is inhibited, via allosteric mechanisms, by end products of microbial glutamine metabolism, including histidine, carbamoyl phosphate, ADP, AMP, and other nucleotides.

3.4.2.2 Synthesis of Arginine

Bacteria can synthesize arginine from glutamate via the metabolic pathways that are different from those in mammals. Specifically, P5C synthase is a bifunctional protein in mammals and catalyzes the formation of P5C from glutamate in the enterocytes of most mammals. By contrast, two separate enzymes are responsible for the conversion of glutamate into P5C in bacteria (Figure 3.18).

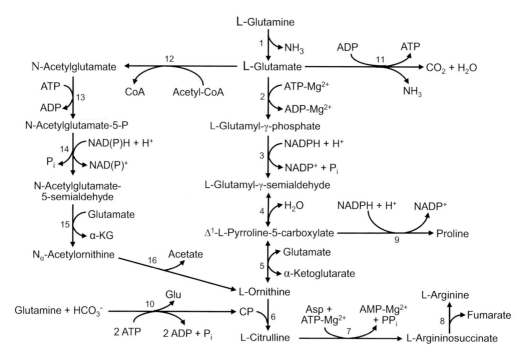

FIGURE 3.18 Ornithine and arginine synthesis from glutamate and glutamine in microorganisms. The enzymes catalyzing the indicated reactions are: (1) glutaminase (two isoforms: phosphate-independent and phosphate-activated); (2) γ-glutamyl kinase; (3) glutamyl-γ-phosphate dehydrogenase; (4) non-enzymatic reaction; (5) ornithine aminotransferase; (6) ornithine carbamoyltransferase; (7) argininosuccinate synthase; (8) argininosuccinate lyase; (9) pyrroline-5-carboxylate reductase; (10) carbamoyl phosphate synthetase II; (11) a series of enzyme-catalyzed reactions involving glutamate dehydrogenase, α-ketoglutarate dehydrogenase, and succinyl-CoA dehydrogenase; (12) *N*-acetylglutamate synthase; (13) acetylglutamate kinase; (14) *N*-acetyl-γ-glutamyl phosphate dehydrogenase; (15) *N*-acetylornithine-δ-aminotransferase; and (16) acetylornithine deacetylase.

Additionally, NAG is an allosteric activator of carbamoyl phosphate synthetase-I in the mammalian synthesis of ornithine, but is an intermediate in the production of *N*-acetylornithine and ornithine from glutamate in bacteria. Furthermore, the intestinal synthesis of citrulline and arginine involves two different compartments (the mitochondria and cytosol) of the same cell, whereas all reactions of the bacterial arginine synthesis occur in the same site (i.e., the cytoplasm).

3.4.2.3 Synthesis of Aspartate and Asparagine

In microbes, aspartate is produced from glutamate or alanine (the donor of the amino group) and oxaloacetate (the source of the carbon skeleton), with glutamate being formed from α-KG and ammonia by GDH and alanine being generated from pyruvate via transamination with AAs. Many prokaryotes express one or two forms of ATP-dependent AS, which requires either ammonia (AS-A) or glutamine (AS-B) as the source of the nitrogen donor for the amidation of aspartate (Lomelino et al. 2017). For example, *Escherichia coli* and *Klebsiella aerogenes* contain both AS-A and AS-B, whereas archaea (e.g., *Pyrococcus abyssi*) has a bacterial-type AS-A. Interestingly, some eukaryotes, such as *Leishmania* and *Trypanosoma* (parasites), also possess both AS-A and AS-B (Gowri et al. 2012). Either form of the enzyme converts aspartate and ATP into the β-aspartyl-AMP intermediate, which is then attacked by NH_3 to form asparagine. Like the mammalian AS, the N-terminal domain of the bacterial AS-B form has an ability to hydrolyze glutamine into glutamate and NH_4^+ and, therefore, the microbial enzyme is categorized as a class II glutamine amidotransferase. The AS-A in microbes and parasites uses the same substrates (i.e., ammonia and glutamate) for asparagine synthesis as does the AS in animal cells. In microbes, the formation of aspartate and asparagine plays an important role in the syntheses of other AAs for the cells to sustain their growth and survival. These microbial reactions are indicated as follows.

$$\text{Aspartate} + NH_4^+ + ATP \rightarrow \text{Asparagine} + AMP + PPi \left(\text{asparagine synthetase, AS-A}; Mg^{2+}\right)$$

$$\text{Aspartate} + \text{Glutamine} + ATP \rightarrow \text{Asparagine} + \text{Glutamate} + AMP + PPi$$

$$\left(\text{asparagine synthetase, AS-B}; Mg^{2+}\right)$$

3.4.2.4 Synthesis of Cysteine and Tyrosine

Microorganisms, but not animal cells, can form cysteine from serine and sulfate (Figure 3.19) or tyrosine from D-erythrose, phosphoenolpyruvate, and glutamate (see the section on EAA synthesis). All these precursors are produced from carbohydrates and ammonia as non-AA substrates. Note that sulfate is reduced to sulfite before the sulfur atom is incorporated into *O*-acetylserine to yield cysteine. The *de novo* synthesis of cysteine and tyrosine allows microbes to use ammonia and inorganic sulfur as their sole sources of nitrogen and sulfur, respectively, to grow and survive.

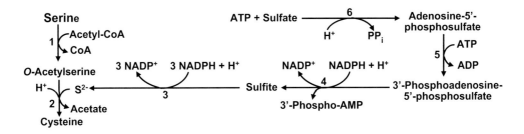

FIGURE 3.19 Cysteine synthesis from serine and inorganic sulfur in microorganisms. The enzymes catalyzing the indicated reactions are: (1) serine acetyltransferase; (2) *O*-acetylserine lyase; (3) sulfite reductase; (4) 3′-phosphoadenosine-5′-phosphosulfate reductase; (5) adenosine-5′-phosphosulfate kinase; and (6) ATP sulfurylase.

This is a unique advantage in the nutrition of ruminants, as well as the ecology and health of the intestinal microbiota in humans and other animals.

3.4.3 Pathways for the Synthesis of Essential Amino Acids in Microorganisms

Unlike animal cells, microorganisms are capable of producing all proteinogenic AAs (Umbarger 1978). The metabolic pathways have been established for microbial syntheses of: (1) BCAAs from pyruvate, α-ketobutyrate, and glutamate (Figure 3.20); (2) histidine from 5-phosphoribosyl-α-pyrophosphate and glutamine (Figure 3.21); (3) lysine, methionine, and threonine from aspartate, α-KG, and cysteine (Figure 3.22); and (4) phenylalanine, tyrosine, and tryptophan from phosphoenolpyruvate, erythrose-4-phosphate, and glutamate (or glutamine) (Figure 3.23). The common characteristics of these synthetic pathways are the requirements of multiple reactions, ATP, and glutamate. In addition, NADPH and NADH play an important role in the synthesis of EAAs. Interestingly, because animals can consume plants and other foods, one or more enzymes involved in EAA syntheses had been lost early in animal evolution (Payne and Loomis 2006). This adaptation mechanism may be of evolutionary advantages for animals because it helps: (1) eliminate the energy-dependent complex pathways for EAA syntheses, thereby conserving energy; (2) reduce the size of animal genomes and the metabolic costs of maintenance and growth; (3) minimize incidences of the inborn errors of AA metabolism; (4) spare energy and AA precursors (e.g., glutamate, glutamine, aspartate, asparagine, and alanine) for utilization by other pathways, such as protein synthesis and glucose synthesis in animals; (5) maximize the efficiency of nutrient utilization in animals by utilizing the preformed AAs in plants; and (6) establish interdependent relationships among species in the ecosystem involving animals, microorganisms, and plants.

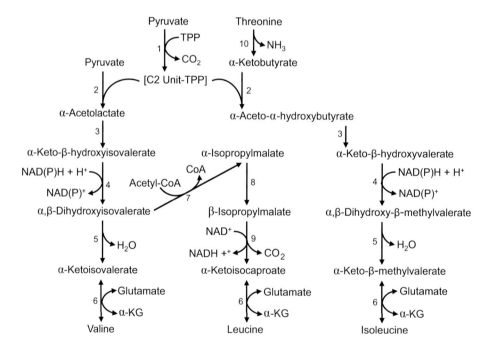

FIGURE 3.20 Synthesis of branched-chain amino acids in microorganisms. The enzymes catalyzing the indicated reactions are: (1) pyruvate dehydrogenase complex; (2) acetolactate synthase; (3) acetolactate mutase; (4) reductase; (5) dihydroxy acid dehydratase; (6) branched-chain amino acid transaminase; (7) α-isopropylmalate synthase; (8) isopropylmalate isomerase; (9) isopropylmalate dehydratase; and (10) threonine deaminase. α-KG, α-ketoglutarate and TPP, thiamine pyrophosphate.

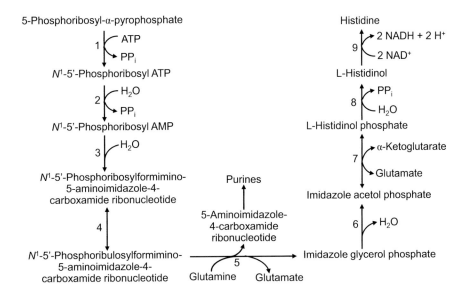

FIGURE 3.21 Histidine synthesis in microorganisms. The enzymes catalyzing the indicated reactions are: (1) ATP phosphoribosyl transferase; (2) pyrophosphohydrolase; (3) phosphoribosyl-AMP cyclohydrolase; (4) phosphoribosylformimino-5-aminoimidazole carboxamide ribonucleotide isomerase; (5) glutamine amidotransferase; (6) imidazole glycerol phosphate dehydratase; (7) L-histidine phosphate aminotransferase; (8) histidinol phosphate phosphatase; and (9) histidinol dehydrogenase.

The efficiency of EAA synthesis in microorganisms and plants is optimized by metabolic channeling, namely the intermediate of two reactions is directly transferred from the active site of one enzyme to another closely associated enzyme (Light and Anderson 2013). The channeling of intermediates can maintain a relatively high concentration of a substrate at the active site of its enzyme, prevent the loss or degradation of the intermediate by other enzymes, and, therefore, increase the rate of a metabolic pathway. A good example is tryptophan synthase, which has a tetrasubunit ($\alpha_2\beta_2$) structure and is a bifunctional enzyme (Dunn et al. 2008). The α units of tryptophan synthase catalyze the reversible conversion between indole-3-phosphate and indole plus glyceraldehyde-3-phosphate, whereas the β units of tryptophan synthase catalyze the irreversible step of the formation of tryptophan from indole and serine. Because indole is a hydrophobic substance, its immediate utilization by tryptophan synthase within the same protein can prevent a possible loss of indole from the bacterial cell by diffusing through the plasma and other membranes.

3.4.4 SYNTHESIS OF *N*-ACETYLATED AMINO ACIDS IN MICROORGANISMS

Microbes in the gastrointestinal tract synthesize *N*-acetylated AAs from free AAs through the action of *N*-acetylated AA synthetases (Liu et al. 2019). This enzyme uses an AA and acetyl-CoA as substrates and transfers the acetyl group of acetyl-CoA to the amino group of the AA. In addition, the α-amino group of some AA residues in proteins is *N*-acetylated by *N*-acetyltransferases (type I, II, III, and IV protein *N*-acetyltransferases). Furthermore, the ε-amino group of lysine in proteins is *N*-acetylated by N^ε-lysine *N*-acetyltransferases (formerly histone acetyltransferases) and also through a spontaneous non-enzymatic reaction with acetyl-CoA or acetyl phosphate (Wagner and Payne 2013). These enzymes transfer the acetyl group of acetyl-CoA (Ac-CoA) to the respective receptor in proteins. The *N*-acetylated proteins are degraded by proteases to release *N*-acetylated AAs. Note that similar reactions occur in eukaryotes (e.g., humans and other animals). In general, the N^α-amino acetylation of proteins is irreversible, whereas the N^ε-acetylation of lysyl residues in proteins can be deacetylated by deacetylases (e.g., type I, II, III, and IV protein deacetylases;

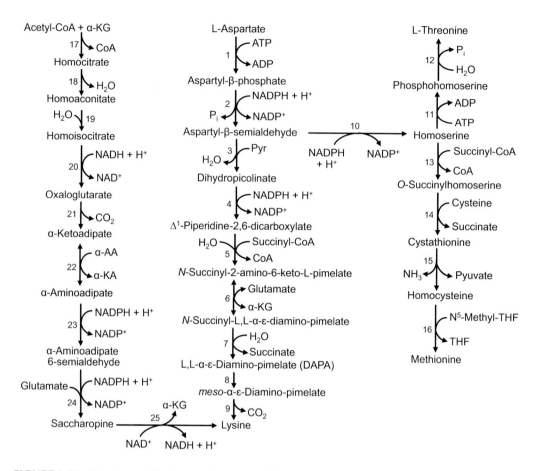

FIGURE 3.22 Syntheses of lysine, methionine, and threonine in microorganisms. The enzymes catalyzing the indicated reactions are: (1) aspartokinase; (2) aspartyl-β-phosphate dehydrogenase; (3) dihydropicolinate synthase; (4) dihydropicolinate synthase dehydrogenase; (5) N-succinyl-2-amino-6-keto-L-pimelate synthase; (6) succinyl-diaminopimelate aminotransferase; (7) succinyl-diaminopimelate desuccinylase; (8) diaminopimelate epimerase; (9) diaminopimelate decarboxylase; (10) aspartyl-β-semialdehyde dehydrogenase; (11) homoserine kinase; (12) threonine synthase; (13) homoserine acyltransferase; (14) cystathionine γ-synthase; (15) cystathionine β-lyase; (16) homocysteine methyltransferase; (17) homocitrate synthase; (18) homocitrate dehydratase; (19) homoaconitate hydratase (*lys2*); (20) homoisocitrate dehydrogenase; (21) oxaloglutarate decarboxylase; (22) aminoadipate aminotransferase; (23) aminoadipate reductase (*lys1 and lys7*); (24) saccharopine reductase; and (25) saccharopine dehydrogenase. In *E. coli*, reactions #1 and #10 are catalyzed by the same protein (a bifunctional protein).

VanDrisse and Escalante-Semerena 2019). Protein *N*-acetylation plays a role in regulating gene expression and protein synthesis in cells.

$$\text{AA(free)} + \text{Acetyl-CoA} \rightarrow N\text{-Acetylated AA} + \text{CoA} \qquad (N\text{-Acetylated AA synthetase})$$

$$\alpha\text{-Amino group in AA residues of protein} + \text{Acetyl-CoA} \rightarrow N\text{-Acetylated AA residues}$$

$$+ \text{CoA} \quad (\text{protein } N\text{-acetyltransferase})$$

$$\varepsilon\text{-Amino group in Lys residues of protein} + \text{Acetyl-CoA} \rightarrow N^{\varepsilon}\text{-Acetylated Lys residues of protein}$$

$$+ \text{CoA} \quad \left(N^{\varepsilon}\text{-lysine } N\text{-acetyltransferase}\right)$$

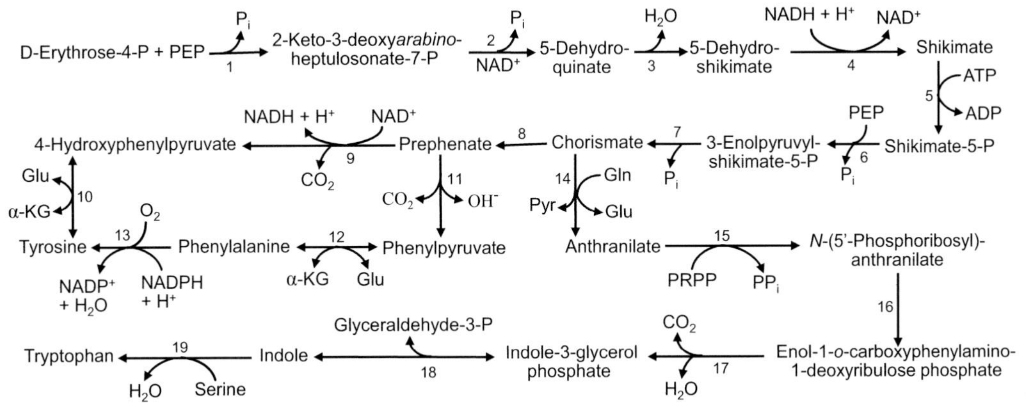

FIGURE 3.23 Syntheses of phenylalanine, tyrosine, and tryptophan in microorganisms. The enzymes catalyzing the indicated reactions are: (1) 2-keto-3-deoxy-D-arabinoheptulosonate-7-phosphate synthase; (2) dehydroquinate synthase (an NAD$^+$-activating reaction); (3) 5-dehydroquinate dehydratase; (4) 5-dehydroshikimate reductase; (5) shikimate kinase; (6) 3-enolpyruvylshikimate-5-phosphate synthase; (7) chorismate synthase; (8) chorismate mutase; (9) prephenate dehydrogenase; (10) aminotransferase; (11) prephenate dehydratase; (12) aminotransferase; (13) phenylalanine hydroxylase; (14) anthranilate synthase; (15) anthranilate phosphoribosyl transferase; (16) N-(5′-phosphoribosyl)-anthranilate isomerase; (17) indole-3-glycerol phosphate synthase; (18) tryptophan synthase (α-subunits); and (19) tryptophan synthase (β-subunits). α-KG, α-ketoglutarate; PEP, phosphoenolpyruvate; and PRPP, 5-phosphoribosyl-α-pyrophosphate.

ε-Amino group in Lys residues of protein + Acetyl-CoA → N^ε-Acetylated Lys residues of protein

$$+ \text{CoA} \quad (\text{non-enzymatic})$$

ε-Amino group in Lys residues of protein + Acetyl phosphate →

$$N^\varepsilon\text{-Acetylated Lys residues of protein} + \text{Pi} \quad (\text{non-enzymatic})$$

3.4.5 PATHWAYS FOR THE SYNTHESIS OF 2,6-DIAMINOPIMELIC ACID AND 2-AMINOETHYLPHOSPHONATE

Ruminal bacteria (like many species of bacteria in nature; Figure 3.22) and ruminal protozoa [like other species of protozoa (e.g., *Tetrahymena pyriformis*) Horiguchi and Kandatsu 1959] synthesize 2,6-diaminopimelic acid (also known as L, L-α-ε-diamino-pimelate, DAPA; Figure 3.22) and 2-aminoethylphosphonate, respectively, but these synthetic pathways are absent from mammalian and avian cells (Bergen 2021; Metcalf and van der Donk 2009). The precursors of DAPA are aspartate, pyruvate, succinyl-CoA, glutamate, and NADPH, whereas the precursors of 2-aminoethylphosphonate are phosphoenolpyruvate and alanine. All these substrates are produced from carbohydrates and ammonia in bacteria. It should be borne in mind that the presence of both the necessary enzymes and precursors is required for the bacterial synthesis of DAPA and the protozoal synthesis of 2-aminoethylphosphonate. Interestingly, the eggs of the freshwater snail *Helisoma* contain 95% of their phosphorus in the form of 2-aminoethylphosphonate-derived phosphonoglycans (Miceli et al. 1980). The content of 2-aminoethylphosphonate in protozoa and snails is influenced by its synthesis from phosphoenolpyruvate (a metabolite of glucose via glycolysis) and dephosphosrylarion into acetaldehyde plus phosphate (through the action of phosphonatase).

Phosphoenol-
pyruvate (PEP) → (PEP mutase) → Phosphono-
pyruvate (PnPyr) → (PnPyr decarboxylase, CO_2) → Phosphono-
acetaldehyde → (AEP transaminase, Ala, Pyr) → 2-Aminoethyl-
phosphonate (AEP)

3.4.6 Pathways for the Synthesis of Phosphoryl Amino Acids in Microorganisms

The synthesis of phosphoserine, phosphothreonine, phosphotyrosine, N-phosphohistidine, and N-phosphoarginine in microbes occurs via the metabolic pathways similar to those in animal cells as described previously. The protein AA phosphorylation is reversible (Fuhrmann et al. 2015). Of note, Elsholz et al. (2012) detected 121 arginine phosphorylation sites in 87 proteins in the Gram-positive model organism *Bacillus subtilis in vivo*. The phosphorylation of AAs in proteins plays a crucial role in the regulation of critical cellular processes in bacteria, such as protein degradation and stress responses, as well as cell growth and survival (Fuhrmann et al. 2015).

Bacteria (like plants), but not animal cells, express serine decarboxylase to generate ethanol-amine from serine, although both prokaryotes and eukaryotes express ethanolamine kinase (an enzyme in the endoplasmic reticulum) to convert ethanolamine and ATP and phosphoethanolamine and ADP (Figure 3.15). Serine decarboxylation is highly active in the gastrointestinal bacteria of animals, including those in the rumen of ruminants. Thus, the plasma concentrations of ethanol-amine in ruminants (e.g., 25 to 40 µM in adult cattle and sheep) are usually greater than those in non-ruminants (e.g., 10–20 µM in adult pigs).

L-Serine → (Serine decarboxylase (bacteria and plants), CO_2) → Ethanolamine (EA) → (EA kinase (both prokaryotes and eukaryotes), ATP, ADP) → Phosphoethanolamine

3.5 SYNTHESIS OF D-AAs FROM L-AAs IN ANIMAL CELLS AND MICROORGANISMS

3.5.1 Human and Other Animals

Free D-AAs occur in both vertebrates (including humans and rats; Graham et al. 2019) and inverte-brates (including silkworm and the acorn worm; Uda et al. 2016, 2019). AA racemases (also known as D-AA racemases) convert free L-AAs into D-AAs and are the major source of D-AAs in the organisms. Racemases catalyze the stereochemical inversion around the asymmetric carbon atom in a substrate (e.g., alanine, aspartate, glutamate, proline, and serine) with only one center of asym-metry. Most AA racemases (including D-alanine racemase, D-aspartate racemase, D-glutamate racemase, D-proline racemase, and D-serine racemase) depend on pyridoxal-5′-phosphate for cat-alytic activity (Table 3.13). These enzymes localize in the cytoplasm with their respective sub-strates. Most D-AA racemases depend on vitamin B_6 for reactions involving a deprotonation of the substrate at the α-position to form an anionic intermediate and a subsequent reprotonation in the opposite stereochemical sense. Vitamin B_6-independent D-AA racemases require thiol/thiolate to convert L-AAs into D-AAs. Thus, B_6-dependent and B_6-independent D-AA racemases use different reaction mechanisms for the spatial rearrangement of the α-hydrogen in the corresponding AAs. To date, D-aspartate racemase and D-serine racemase have been cloned in mammals and invertebrates (Uda et al. 2019). These two enzymes are widely distributed in the animal kingdom.

TABLE 3.13

Vitamin B_6-Dependent and Independent D-Amino Acid Racemases in Animal Cells and Microorganisms

Enzyme	Expression				Requirement for vitamin B_6			
	Mammalian cells	Aquatic animals & silkworms	Bacteria & archaea	Fungi	Mammalian cells	Aquatic animals & silkworms	Bacteria & archaea	Fungi
D-Alanine racemase	No	Yes	Yes	Yes	---	Yes	Yes	Yes
D-Arginine racemase	? (unknown)	?	Yes	?	?	?	Yes	?
D-Aspartate racemase	Yes (e.g., brain)	Yes	Yes	Yes	Yes	Yes	No	Yes
D-Glutamate racemase	?	?	Yes	?	?	?	No	?
D-Proline racemase	?	Yes	Yes	Yes	?	No	No	No
D-Serine racemase	Yes (e.g., brain)	Yes	Yes	Yes	Yes	Yes	Yes	Yes
Ls-Maly[a]	--- (not applicable)	---	Yes[a]	---	---	---	Yes	---
Yge A[b]	---	---	Yes[b]	---	---	---	No	---
Racx[c]	---	---	Yes[c]	---	---	---	No	---

Source: Kato, S. and T. Oikawa. 2018. *Front. Microbiol.* 9:403; Miyamoto, T. et al. 2017. *Amino Acids.* 49:1885–1894; Yoshimura, T. and N. Esak. 2003. *J. Biosci. Bioengin.* 96:103–109; Yoshimura, T. and M. Goto. 2008. *FEBS J.* 275:3527–3537.

[a] A bifunctional protein isolated from *Lactobacillus sakei* strain LK-145. This enzyme has both AA racemase and cystathionine β-lyase activities. It can convert some L-AAs (e.g., Ala, Arg, Asn, Glu, Gln, His, Leu, Lys, Met, Ser, Thr, Trp, and Val) at various rates.

[b] YgeA prefers to use L-homoserine as its substrate, but also converts other L-AAs (including Met, Leu, Val, His, Asn, Ile, Ser, Ala, Gln, and Phe) into D-AAs.

[c] Racx prefers to use basic L-AAs (Arg, Lys, and Orn) as its substrate, but also converts some other L-AAs (including His, Ala, Tyr, Phe, Ser, Gln, Met, Asn, and homoserine) into D-AAs.

D-Amino acid ↔ L-Amino acid   (amino acid racemase)

All animals express D-aspartate racemase, which converts free L-aspartate into D-aspartate in certain tissues (e.g., the brain). Recently, P.M. Kim and colleagues obtained and cloned the mammalian D-aspartate racemase in 2010. These authors also cloned the first mammalian D-aspartate racemase (Kim et al. 2010). The K_m of recombinant D-aspartate racemase for L-aspartate is 3.1 mM and the V_{max} is 0.46 μmol/mg/min at the optimum pH of 7.5 and the optimum temperature of 37°C. Both D-aspartate and D-aspartate racemase are concentrated in: (1) pinealocytes of the pineal gland; (2) pituicytes of the posterior pituitary gland; (3) epinephrine-producing chromaffin cells of the medulla of the adrenal glands; and (4) elongated spermatids of the testes. In the brain, endogenously synthesized D-aspartate is important for neurological function because the entry of D-AAs from the peripheral circulation into this organ appears to be limited by the blood–brain barrier. In addition to nervous tissues, D-aspartate racemase has been reported in the kidney and liver of mammals, which is in keeping with the presence of D-aspartate in these organs. D-Aspartate racemase can use L-glutamate as a substrate to generate D-glutamate (Uda et al. 2019) and D-serine racemase can use L-alanine as a substrate to produce D-alanine (Uo et al. 1998), but the rates of D-glutamate and D-alanine syntheses are much lower than those for D-aspartate and D-alanine syntheses, respectively.

D-Serine racemase converts free L-serine into D-serine. This enzyme does not use glycine as a substrate but is competitively inhibited by high levels of glycine. In 1999, H. Wolosker and coworkers isolated and cloned, for the first time, D-serine racemase in mammals. This enzyme is enriched in rat's brain where it occurs in glial cells that possess high levels of D-serine. D-serine racemase has a striking similarity to the serine/threonine dehydratase enzyme of *E. coli*, rather than a similarity to classical AA racemases. Mg-ATP appears to stabilize the folding of D-serine racemase. In the rat brain, the K_m of serine racemase for L-serine is approximately 10 mM with a V_{max} of 5 μmol/mg protein per h. The enzyme can also convert D-serine to L-serine but with lesser affinity, as the K_m in this direction is approximately 60 mM. In addition to mammals, D-serine racemase has been detected in fungi, plants, and invertebrates.

3.5.2 Microorganisms

3.5.2.1 Amino Acid Racemases

As noted in Chapter 1, bacteria possess a peptidoglycan layer in the cell wall that typically contains D-alanine and D-glutamic acid, as well as various non-canonical D-AAs. These D-AAs play an important role in peptidoglycan remodeling, the inhibition of biofilm formation, and the triggering of biofilm disassembly (Cava et al. 2011a, b). In addition, bacteria synthesize D-AAs as a common survival strategy for adapting to environmental changes.

The available evidence shows that microorganisms have a greater capacity to synthesize D-AAs than eukaryotes primarily through the action of D-AA racemases (Aliashkevich et al. 2018). For example, bacteria and archaea (a domain of single-celled organisms) express D-alanine racemase, D-arginine racemase, aspartate racemase, glutamate racemase, proline racemase, and serine racemase (Yoshimura and Esak 2003). In general, D-AA racemases are classified into two groups: vitamin B_6-dependent and independent enzymes (Table 3.13). As in animals, most of the microbial D-AA racemases depend on vitamin B_6 for enzymatic activity, but some do not have a requirement for this coenzyme. Those B_6-independent D-AA racemases contain two cysteine residues at the catalytic site. D-AAs play an important role in the structure, growth, and function of microbes.

L-Proline ↔ D-Proline   (proline racemase; also known as D-proline racemase)

Bacterial D-alanine racemase is arguably the most studied D-AA racemase because of its essential role in cell survival (Kawakami et al. 2018; Walsh 1989). D-Alanine racemase converts free

L-alanine into D-alanine, which is a key building block in the biosynthesis of the peptidoglycan layer in bacterial cell walls. This enzyme (K_m for D-alanine = 8.5 mM) was discovered in *Streptococcus faecalis* by W.A. Wood and I.C. Gunsalus in 1951, based on the report of J.T. Holden and E.E. Snell in 1949, that D-alanine and L-alanine were interconverted in these cells. D-Alanine racemases are ubiquitous among microorganisms and also present in certain invertebrates, but are typically absent from mammals, birds, and fish. Bacteria (e.g., *Streptococcus faecalis, Mycobacterium tuberculosis, E. coli, Listeria monocytogenes*, and *Bacillus anthracis*) and invertebrates (e.g., *Corbicula japonica*, a brackish water species, and crayfish) use D-alanine to grow. Thus, D-alanine racemase is an attractive target for the development of novel antimicrobials in both medicine and livestock production.

Some microbial D-AA racemases use a broad group of L-AAs as substrates. For example, the RacX from *Bacillus subtilis* and YgeA from *Escherichia coli* MG1655 have been shown to be novel D-AA racemases with broad-substrate specificity (Miyamoto et al. 2017). Specifically, YgeA has the highest racemization activity for L-homoserine, but also converts other L-AAs (including Met, Le, Val, His, Asn, Ile, Ser, Ala, Gln, and Phe) into D-AAs. Similarly, Racx prefers to use basic L-AAs (Arg, Lys, and Orn) as substrates, but also converts some other L-AAs (including His, Ala, Tyr, Phe, Ser, Gln, Met, Asn, and homoserine) into D-AAs. Of note, both YgeA and Racx do not appear to require vitamin B_6 as a cofactor. Furthermore, Kato and Oikawa (2018) recently reported that *Ls*-MalY from *Lactobacillus sakei* LT-13 is a vitamin B_6-dependent bifunctional enzyme that has both AA racemase and cystathionine β-lyase activities. This enzyme can convert some L-AAs (e.g., Ala, Arg, Asn, Glu, Gln, His, Leu, Lys, Met, Ser, Thr, Trp, and Val) into D-AAs at various rates.

3.5.2.2 Amino Acid Epimerases

Epimerases catalyze the stereochemical inversion of the configuration around an asymmetric carbon atom in a substrate (e.g., 4-hydrocyproline and 3-hydroxyproline) with more than one center of asymmetry. Collagen proteins in animals contain L-4-hydroxyproline and L-3-hydroxyproline, whereas these two AAs also occur in microbes (Chapter 1). In recent years, D-hydroxyproline has received growing attention from biomedical scientists because of its potential role in regulating collagen synthesis and inhibiting tumor growth. Recent studies have shown that microbes express 4-hydroxyproline epimerase (interconverting *trans*-4-hydroxy-L-proline into *cis*-4-hydroxy-D-proline) and 3-hydroxyproline epimerase (interconverting *trans*-3-hydroxy-L-proline into *cis*-3-hydroxy-D-proline) (Watanabe et al. 2015). Interestingly, archaea express a bifunctional proline racemase/hydroxyproline epimerase that can interconvert: (1) L-proline and D-proline; (2) *trans*-4-hydroxy-L-proline and *cis*-4-hydroxy-D-proline; and (3) t*rans*-3-hydroxy-L-proline and *cis*-3-hydroxy-D-proline (Watanabe et al. 2015). Like proline racemase, 4-hydroxyproline epimerase and 3-hydroxyproline epimerase do not require *pyridoxal phosphate* as a cofactor.

Trans-4-hydroxy-L-proline ↔ Cis-4-hydroxy-D-proline (4-hydroxyproline epimerase)

Trans-3-hydroxy-L-proline ↔ Cis-3-hydroxy-D-proline (3-hydroxyproline epimerase)

3.6 CONVERSION OF D-AAs INTO L-AAs IN ANIMAL CELLS AND MICROORGANISMS

3.6.1 Humans and Other Animals

Animal cells lack D-AA transaminase activity under physiological conditions (Greenstein and Winitz 1961; Meister 1965). Therefore, D-AAs do not undergo transamination reactions in mammalian, avian, or other vertebrate cells. Although Kakimoto et al. (1969) reported the presence of D-β-aminoisobutyrate:pyruvate aminotransferase in the liver of rats, guinea pigs, and pigs to metabolize D-β-aminoisobutyrate (a physiological metabolite of pyrimidines), the enzyme assay

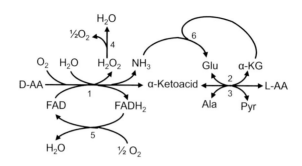

FIGURE 3.24 Conversion of D-AAs into L-AAs in the animal body. The bacteria of the intestine and animal tissues contribute to the conversion of D-AAs into L-AAs in the body. The enzymes that catalyze the indicated reactions are: (1) D-AA oxidase; (2) L-glutamate transaminase; (3) L-alanine transaminase; (4) catalase; (5) enzymes of the mitochondrial electron transport system; and (6) glutamate dehydrogenase (an NAD$^+$-dependent enzyme). Glu, glutamate; α-KG, α-ketoglutarate; and Pyr, pyruvate.

conditions involved an exceedingly high concentration of D-β-aminoisobutyrate (25 mM; ≥5,000 times its physiological concentration in the plasma) as a substrate. Thus, the physiological relevance of the result is questionable. However, many animal tissues (e.g., liver, kidney, brain, and heart) contain D-AA oxidases (oxidoreductases) to oxidize D-AAs to their corresponding α-ketoacids (Zhang et al. 2015). Subsequently, L-AA transaminases catalyze the conversion of these α-ketoacids and glutamate (or alanine) into the corresponding L-α-AA and α-KG (or pyruvate) (Figure 3.24). Let's take the conversion of D-methionine to L-methionine in animal cells as an example:

1. D-Methionine + O_2 + H_2O + FAD → α-Keto-γ-methylthiobutyrate + $FADH_2$ + H_2O_2

2. α-Keto-γ-methylthiobutyrate + L-Glutamate ↔ L-Methionine + α-Ketoglutarate

3.6.2 MICROORGANISMS

C.B. Thorne and coworkers discovered the presence of D-AA aminotransferases in the cell-free extract of *Bacillus subtilis* and *Bacillus anthracis* in 1955. They identified that these enzymes required vitamin B_6 as an essential cofactor. D-AA aminotransferases were subsequently demonstrated in extracts of bacteria, such as *Rhodospirillum rubrum*, *Bacillus sphaericus*, and *Bacillus licheniformis*.

Like animal cells, bacteria in the lumen of the small intestine express both D-AA oxidases and L-AA transaminases and, therefore, can convert D-AAs to L-AAs. The microbes in the large intestine likely play a minor role in supplying D-AA as usable L-AAs to the animal hosts. Notably, in contrast to animal cells, bacteria possess D-AA transaminases to produce α-ketoacids from D-AAs. These α-ketoacids are transaminated by L-AA transaminases to generate new L-α-AAs. Let's use D-tryptophan as an example to illustrate a role for the transamination of a D-AA in the production of an L-α-AA in bacteria:

1. D-Tryptophan + α-Ketoglutarate (or Pyruvate) ↔ Indole-3-pyruvate + L-Glutamate (or L-Alanine)

2. Indole-3-pyruvate + L-Glutamate (or L-Alanine) ↔ L-Tryptophan + α-Ketoglutarate (or Pyruvate)

The conversion of dietary D-AAs to L-AAs in the whole body can take place both in the luminal bacteria of the small intestine and, after the absorption of D-AAs into the portal vein, in animal tissues. Because the final steps for the syntheses of L-arginine, L-cysteine, L-lysine, and L-threonine do not involve AA transaminases, D-arginine, D-cysteine (D-cystine), D-lysine, or D-threonine are

TABLE 3.14

Efficiency of Utilization of D-Amino Acids (D-AAs) by Humans and Other Animals

D-AA	Chick	Rat	Mouse	Dog	Human	Pig
	Percentage of the value for the L-isomer					
Arginine	0	0	0	0	0	0
Cysteine (or cystine)	0	0	0	0	0	0
Histidine	10	22	10	---	---	---
Isoleucine (*2R, 3R*)	0	0	0	---	0	0
Alloisoleucine (*2R, 3S*)	60	---	---	---	---	---
Leucine	100	50	15	---	0	---
Lysine	0	0	0	0	0	0
Methionine	90	90	75	100	36	100
Phenylalanine	75	70	52	---	50	---
Threonine[a]	0	0	0	---	0	0
Tryptophan	20	100	30	36	0	80
Tyrosine	100	100	---	---	0	100
Valine	70	15	5	---	---	---

Source: Baker, D.H. 1994. In: *Amino Acids in Farm Animal Nutrition* (D'Mello, J.P.F., ed). CAB International, Wallingford, Oxon, UK. pp. 37–61; Lewis, A.J. and D.H. Baker. 1995. In: *Bioavailability of Nutrients for Animals: Amino Acids, Minerals, Vitamins* (C.B. Ammerman, D.H. Baker and A.J. Lewis, eds). Academic Press, San Diego. pp. 65–81.

Note: "---", data are not available.

[a] D-allothreonine (*2R, 3R*).

not precursors for L-AAs in all the animal species studied (Figure 3.4). Thus, except for D-arginine, D-cysteine (D-cystine), D-lysine, and D-threonine, all of the D-AAs can be converted to their corresponding L-AAs in animals, but the rates vary greatly with D-AAs, dietary content of L-AAs, developmental stage, and species. The efficiency of utilization of some D-AAs by animals is shown in Table 3.14. At present, little is known about the production of L- AASAs from their corresponding D-AAs in animals.

3.7   CONVERSION OF α-KETOACIDS INTO L-AAs IN ANIMAL CELLS AND MICROORGANISMS

As noted previously, L-AA transaminases are widely distributed in humans and animals, as well as microbes (e.g., bacteria). These enzymes have a broad specificity for L-α-AA and reversibly interconvert most of α-ketoacids and L-α-AA in all the organisms. Because the final steps for the syntheses of L-Arg, L-Cys, and Gly in animal cells or of L-Lys and L-Thr in microbes do not involve transamination, these AAs do not generate their α-ketoacids in the organisms. Thus, except for five AAs (L-Arg, L-Cys, L-Lys, L-Thr, and Gly), all canonical proteinogenic AAs can be formed from their α-ketoacids through L-AA transaminases. An α-ketoacid (KA_1) transaminates with an α-AA (AA_2, usually Glu) to generate a new α-AA (AA_1) and a new α-ketoacid (KA_2). Because Glu is synthesized from ammonia and α-KG, the conversion of an α-ketoacid into its corresponding L-AA drives the disposal of ammonia for the production of a new L-AA. Therefore, in response to the administration of an α-ketoacid (e.g., α-ketoisocaproate or *p*-hydroxyphenylpyruvate), tissues and the whole body can readily synthesize the corresponding L-α-AA (e.g., L-leucine or L-tyrosine). In addition, ammonia and α-KG can be converted into L-glutamate by GDH in tissues (primarily the liver), when the concentrations of the substrates are relatively high. Based on this biochemical principle, the oral or intravenous administration of α-ketoacids can beneficially

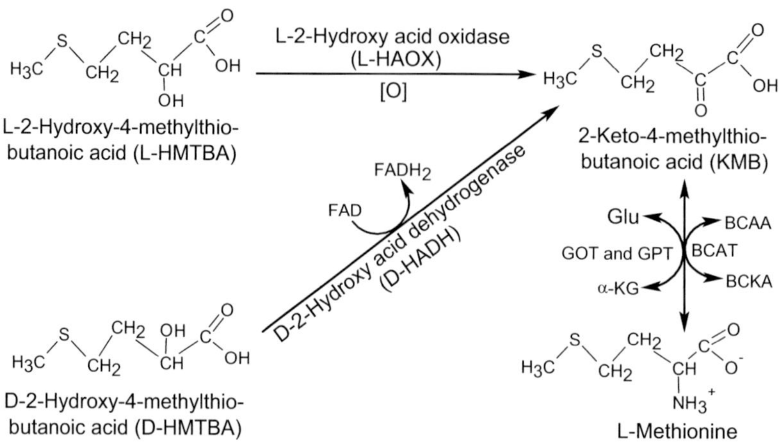

FIGURE 3.25 Synthesis of methionine from its hydroxy ketoacids in humans and other animals, as well as microorganisms. Enzymes for these reactions occur widely in the animal kingdom and microbes (including bacteria). The conversion of L-2-hydroxy-4-methylthiobutanoic acid and D-2-hydroxy-4-methylthiobutanoic acid into L-methionine requires the cooperation of multiple organs, which include primarily the liver, kidneys, and skeletal muscle. This pathway also occurs in intestinal microbes. The α-ketoacid analogs of methionine are effectively converted into L-methionine in mammals, birds, fish, and shrimp.

reduce the concentrations of ammonia in the plasma and provide L-AAs to humans or other animals with hyperammonenia (Mitch 1980; Walser 1984), endotoxin-induced inflammation (Wang et al. 2016), intestinal dysfunction (Hou et al. 2011), and insulin resistance (Tekwe et al. 2019), or fed a low-protein diet (Chen et al. 2018).

$$\alpha\text{-Ketoacid}\left(\text{KA}_1; \text{e.g., Pyr}\right) + \alpha\text{-AA}\left(\text{AA}_2, \text{e.g., Glu}\right) \leftrightarrow \alpha\text{-AA}\left(\text{AA}_1; \text{e.g., Ala}\right)$$

$$+ \alpha\text{-Ketoacid}\left(\text{KA}_2; \text{e.g., }\alpha\text{-KG}\right)$$

α-Ketoacid analogs of methionine are widely used as a source of AAs in farm animals because of technical challenges to manufacture methionine through microbial fermentation (Yang et al. 2020). In recent years, two α-hydroxy acids related to methionine (L-2-hydroxy-4-methylthiobutanoic acid and D-2-hydroxy-4-methylthiobutanoic acid) have been used as the precursors of L-methionine through the formation of α-keto-γ-methylthiobutyrate in farm animals (Figure 3.25). These α-hydroxy acids in diets are absorbed by the small intestine mainly through monocarboxylate transporter-1, which is coupled with the action of Na⁺/H⁺ exchanger (NHE3). L-2-Hydroxy acid oxidase (a H_2O_2-producing flavoenzyme in peroxisomes of tissues, mainly the liver and kidneys) oxidizes L-2-hydroxy-4-methylthiobutanoic acid into α-keto-γ-methylthiobutyrate, whereas D-2-hydroxy acid dehydrogenase (a H_2O_2-producing flavoenzyme in the mitochondria of tissues, mainly the liver and kidneys) converts D-2-hydroxy-4-methylthiobutanoic acid into α-keto-γ-methylthiobutyrate (Zhang et al. 2015). The latter is transaminated with an α-AA (e.g., glutamate and a BCAA) to form L-methionine. The choice of an L-methionine precursor as a feed additive for livestock, poultry, fish, and shrimp depends on its cost (compared with other sources of preformed L-methionine, such as meat & bone meal, intestinal mucosal protein, and blood meal) and diets.

3.8   SUMMARY

Microorganisms in the lumen of the gastrointestinal tract can synthesize all AAs from ammonia, carbohydrates, and sulfur. These synthetic pathways are quantitatively important in ruminants (e.g., cows, cattle, sheep, and goats) but nutritionally insignificant in non-ruminants (e.g., humans, dogs, pigs, and rats). The animal kingdom cannot synthesize *de novo* isoleucine, leucine, lysine, methionine, phenylalanine, threonine, tryptophan, and valine from nitrogenous precursors, carbohydrates, and sulfur. Thus, these AAs must be provided in the diets of animals, and are classified as EAAs. By contrast, all animals can form alanine, aspartate, cysteine, glutamate, glutamine, glycine, serine, and tyrosine, and these AAs have historically not received much attention from nutritionists and were traditionally classified as AASAs. As examples, the quantitative aspects of the whole-body syntheses of glutamate (Figure 3.26) and glutamine (Figure 3.27) are illustrated for milk-fed young pigs. The syntheses of arginine, citrulline, ornithine, proline, and taurine are species-specific and must be quantified to guide conceptual development and nutritional practice. Specifically, most mammals (including humans, pigs, and rats) can synthesize arginine, citrulline, and ornithine from glutamate, glutamine, and proline via the metabolism of enterocytes in the small intestine, but these synthetic pathways are absent from carnivores, birds, and possibly most aquatic animals. In avian species, proline synthesis is limited due to the absence of P5C and a low activity of arginase. Except for most carnivores (e.g., cats and tigers), all animals can synthesize taurine from methionine or cysteine. Interestingly, some Felidae species synthesize felinine, isovalthine, and isobuteine as unique sulfur-containing AAs. In all animals, AA syntheses require not only substrates but also cofactors (e.g., NADH, NADPH, FAD, pyruvate, oxaloacetate, and α-KG), which should be taken into consideration when metabolically engineering pathways and developing transgenic animals expressing AA-synthetic enzymes. As the resources of protein and L-AAs have become more and more scarce but the demands for L-AAs are increasing in human consumption, as

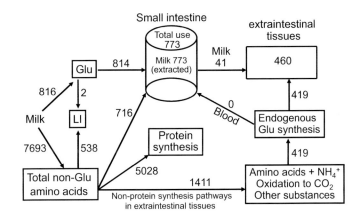

FIGURE 3.26 Whole-body synthesis of glutamate (Glu) in milk-fed young pigs. Values are expressed as mg/kg body weight (BW)/day. The pig (7.92 kg BW) consumes 816 mg Glu/kg BW/day from milk (true ileal digestibility of Glu = 99.7%) and gains 293 g BW/day. The total content of amino acids (AAs) in the milk is 50 g/L and milk intake by piglets is 170 mL/kg BW/day. True ileal digestibility of non-Glu AAs is 93%. There is no net flux of arterial plasma Glu into the small intestine. Utilization of dietary (milk) Glu by the small intestine in first pass is 773 mg/kg BW/day ($814 \times 95\% = 773$), with the total use of Glu by the small intestine being 773 mg/kg BW/day. The entry of dietary (milk) Glu into portal vein is 41 mg/kg BW/day ($814 \times 5\% = 41$). Utilization of non-Glu AAs in the body is calculated on the basis of the following: intake of non-Glu AAs from milk (7,693 mg/kg BW/day), non-Glu AAs entering large intestine (538 mg/kg BW/day = $7,693 \times 7\% = 538$), the amount of non-Glu AAs available to the small intestine (7,155 mg/kg BW/day = $7,693 - 538 = 7,155$), the rate of the degradation of non-Glu AAs by the small intestine (10% of non-Glu AAs in the lumen of the small intestine; 716 mg/kg BW/day = $7,155 \times 10\% = 716$), the needs for non-Glu AAs for whole-body protein synthesis (5,028 mg/kg BW/day), and the amount of non-Glu AAs available for oxidation and AA synthesis in the body = 1,411 mg/kg/day ($7,155 - 716 - 5,028 = 1,411$). To meet the needs for Glu for utilization by extraintestinal tissues (460 mg/kg BW/day), the endogenous synthesis of Glu is 419 mg/kg BW/day ($460 - 41 = 419$). LI, large intestine. (Adapted from Hou, Y.Q. and G. Wu. 2018. *Amino Acids* 50:1497–1510.)

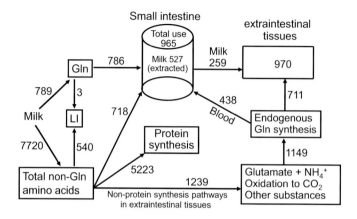

FIGURE 3.27 Whole-body synthesis of glutamine (Gln) in milk-fed young pigs. Values are expressed as mg/kg body weight (BW)/day. The pig (7.92 kg BW) consumes 789 mg Gln/kg BW/day from milk (true ileal digestibility of Gln = 99.7%) and gains 293 g BW/day. The total content of amino acids (AAs) in the milk is 50 g/L and milk intake by piglets is 170 mL/kg BW/day. True ileal digestibility of non-Gln AA is 93%. Net flux of arterial plasma Gln into the small intestine is 438 mg/kg BW/day. Utilization of dietary (milk) Gln by the small intestine in first pass is 527 mg/kg BW/day ($786 \times 67\% = 527$) and uptake of arterial plasma Gln by the small intestine is 438 mg/kg BW/day, with the total use of Gln by the small intestine being 965 mg/kg BW/day. Entry of dietary (milk) Gln into portal vein is 259 mg/kg BW/day ($786 \times 33\% = 259$). Utilization of non-Gln AAs is calculated on the basis of the following: intake of non-Gln AAs from milk (7,720 mg/kg BW/day), non-Gln AAs entering large intestine (540 mg/kg BW/day = $7,720 \times 7\% = 540$), the amount of non-Gln AAs available to the small intestine (7,180 mg/kg BW/day = $7,720 - 540 = 7,180$), the rate of the degradation of non-Gln AAs by the small intestine (10% of non-Gln AAs in the lumen of the small intestine; 718 mg/kg BW/day = $7,180 \times 10\% = 718$), the needs for non-Gln AAs for whole-body protein synthesis (5,223 mg/kg BW/day), and the amount of non-Gln AAs available for oxidation and Gln synthesis = 1,239 mg/kg/day ($7,180 - 718 - 5,223 = 1,239$). To meet the needs for Gln for utilization by extraintestinal tissues (970 mg/kg BW/day), the endogenous synthesis of Gln = 1,149 mg/kg BW/day ($438 + 711 = 1,149$). LI, large intestine. (Adapted from Wu et al. 2011b. *J. Anim. Sci.* 89:2017–2030.)

well as global livestock, poultry, and aquaculture production, there is growing interest in the use of D-AAs (e.g., D-methionine and D-tryptophan) or α-ketoacids as precursors of L-AAs. Likewise, the recent discovery that D-AAs (e.g., D-aspartate and D-serine) are synthesized from their L-isomers by racemases in animals has opened a new avenue to study the mechanisms for the regulation of these novel synthetic pathways and the physiological significance of D-AAs. While it had traditionally been assumed that animals could adequately synthesize all NEAAs to support maximal growth and development, results of recent studies involving pigs, rats, poultry, and fish indicate that this assumption is invalid. The century-old term "NEAA" has now been recognized as a misnomer in nutritional sciences and should be replaced by AASA in nutrition research and practices.

REFERENCES

Aliashkevich, A., L. Alvarez, and F. Cava. 2018. New insights into the mechanisms and biological roles of D-amino acids in complex eco-systems. *Front. Microbiol.* 9:683.

Amelio, I., F. Cutruzzolá, A. Antonov, M. Agostini, and G. Melino. 2014. Serine and glycine metabolism in cancer. *Trends Biochem. Sci.* 39:191–198.

Arentson, B.W., N. Sanyal, and D.F. Becker. 2012. Substrate channeling in proline metabolism. *Front. Biosci.* 17:375–388.

Assaad, H., L. Zhou, R.J. Carroll, and G. Wu. 2014. Rapid publication-ready MS-Word tables for one-way ANOVA. *SpringerPlus* 3:474.

Attwood, P.V. 2013. Histidine kinases from bacteria to humans. *Biochem. Soc. Trans.* 41:1023–1028.

Augustin, P., A. Hromic, T. Pavkov-Keller, K. Gruber, and P. Macheroux. 2016. Structure and biochemical properties of recombinant human dimethylglycine dehydrogenase and comparison to the disease-related H109R variant. *FEBS J.* 283:3587–3603.

Backus, R.C., G. Cohen, P.D. Pion, K.L. Good, Q.R. Rogers, and A.J. Fascetti. 2003. Taurine deficiency in Newfoundlands fed commercially available complete and balanced diets. *J. Am. Vet. Med. Assoc.* 223:1130–1136.

Baha, S., Y. Watanahe, F. Gejyo, and M. Arkawa. 1984. High-performance liquid chromatographic determination of serum aliphatic amines in chronic renal failure. *Clin. Chim. Acta.* 136:49–56.

Baker, D.H. 1994. Utilization of precursors for L-amino acids. In: *Amino Acids in Farm Animal Nutrition* (D'Mello, J.P.F., ed). CAB International, Wallingford, Oxon, UK. pp. 37–61.

Ball, R.O., J.L. Atkinson, and H.S. Bayley. 1986. Proline as an essential amino acid for the young pig. *Br. J. Nutr.* 55:659–668.

Baslow, M.H. 1997. A review of phylogenetic and metabolic relationships between the acylamino acids, *N*-acetyl-L-aspartic acid and *N*-acetyl-L-histidine, in the vertebrate nervous system. *J. Neurochem.* 68:1335–1344.

Bazer, FW, H. Seo, G.A. Johnson, and G. Wu. 2021. One-carbon metabolism and development of the conceptus during pregnancy: lessons from studies with sheep and pigs. *Adv. Exp. Med. Biol.* 1285:1–15.

Beaumont, M. and F. Blachier. 2020. Amino acids in intestinal physiology and health. *Adv. Exp. Med. Biol.* 1265:1–20.

Bedford, M.T. and S.G. Clarke. 2009. Protein arginine methylation in mammals: who, what, and why. *Mol. Cell.* 33:1–13.

Belloir, P., M. Lessire, C. Berri, W. Lambert, E. Corrent, and S. Tesseraud. 2015. Revisiting amino acid nutrition. In: *Proceedings of 20th European Symposium on Poultry Nutrition*. Prague, Czech Republic. pp. 1–8.

Bergen, W.G. 2021. Amino acids in beef cattle nutrition and production. *Adv. Exp. Med. Biol.* 1285:29–42.

Bergen, W.G. and G. Wu. 2009. Intestinal nitrogen recycling and utilization in health and disease. *J. Nutr.* 139:821–825.

Bertolo, R.F. and D.G. Burrin. 2008. Comparative aspects of tissue glutamine and proline metabolism. *J. Nutr.* 138:2032S–2039S.

Blachier, F., H. M'Rabet-Touil, L. Posho L, B. Darcy-Vrillon, and P.H. Duée. 1993. Intestinal arginine metabolism during development. Evidence for de novo synthesis of L-arginine in newborn pig enterocytes. *Eur. J. Biochem.* 216:109–117.

Bouzidi, A., M.C. Magnifico, A. Paiardini, A. Macone, G. Boumis, G. Giardina et al. 2020. Cytosolic serine hydroxymethyltransferase controls lung adenocarcinoma cells migratory ability by modulating AMP kinase activity. *Cell Death Dis.* 11:1012.

Brosnan, J.T. 2000. Glutamate, at the interface between amino acid and carbohydrate metabolism. *J. Nutr.* 130:988S–990S.

Brosnan, J.T. and Brosnan, M.E. 2013. Glutamate: a truly functional amino acid. *Amino Acids.* 45:413–418.

Brosnan, M.E., L. MacMillan, J.R. Stevens, and J.T. Brosnan. 2015. Division of labour: how does folate metabolism partition between one-carbon metabolism and amino acid oxidation? *Biochem. J.* 472:135–146.

Brosnan, M.E., G. Tingley, L. MacMillan, B. Harnett, T. Pongnopparat, J.D. Marshall, and J.T. Brosnan. 2020. Plasma formate is greater in fetal and neonatal rats compared with their mothers. *J. Nutr.* 150:1068–1075

Bushinsky, D.A., J.R. Asplin, M.D. Grynpas, A.P. Evan, W.R. Parker, K.M. Alexander, and F.L. Coe. 2002. Calcium oxalate stone formation in genetic hypercalciuric stone-forming rats. *Kidney Int.* 61:975–987.

Cammarata, P.S. and P.P. Cohen. 1950. The scope of the transamination reaction in animal tissues. *J. Biol. Chem.* 187:439–452.

Campbell, C.G., Titgemeyer. E.C., and St-Jean, G. 1997. Sulfur amino acid utilization by growing steers. *J. Anim. Sci.* 75:230–238.

Cava, F., H. Lam, M.A. de Pedro, and M.K. Waldor. 2011a. Emerging knowledge of regulatory roles of D-amino acids in bacteria. *Cell. Mol. Life Sci.* 68:817–831.

Cava, F., M.A. de Pedro, H. Lam, B.M. Davis, and M.K. Waldor. 2011b. Distinct pathways for modification of the bacterial cell wall by non-canonical D-amino acids. *EMBO J.* 30:3442–3453.

Chattopadhyaya, B., G. Di Cristo, C.Z. Wu, G. Knott, S. Kuhlman, Y. Fu et al. 2007. GAD67-mediated GABA synthesis and signaling regulate inhibitory synaptic innervation in the visual cortex. *Neuron* 54:889–903.

Che, D.S., P.S. Nyingwa, K.M. Ralinala, G.M.T. Maswanganye, and G. Wu. 2021. Amino acids in the nutrition, metabolism, and health of domestic cats. *Adv. Exp. Med. Biol.* 1285:217–231.

Chen, J., W. Su, B. Kang, Q. Jiang, Y. Zhao, C. Fu, and K. Yao. 2018. Supplementation with α-ketoglutarate to a low-protein diet enhances amino acid synthesis in tissues and improves protein metabolism in the skeletal muscle of growing pigs. *Amino Acids* 50:1525–1537.

Chen, J.Q., Y.H. Jin, Y. Yang, Z.L. Wu, and G. Wu. 2020. Epithelial dysfunction in lung diseases: effects of amino acids and potential mechanisms. *Adv. Exp. Med. Biol.* 1265:57–70.

Closs, E.I., J.S. Scheld, M. Sharafi, and U. Förstermann. 2000. Substrate supply for nitric-oxide synthase in macrophages and endothelial cells: role of cationic amino acid transporters. *Mol. Pharmacol.* 57:68–74.

Craan, A.G., G. Lemieux, P. Vinay and A. Gougoux. 1982. The kidney of chicken adapts to chronic metabolic acidosis: in vivo and in vitro studies. *Kidney Int.* 22:103–111.

Curthoys, N.P. and Watford, M. 1995. Regulation of glutaminase expression and glutamine metabolism. *Annu. Rev. Nutr.* 15:133–159.

Cynober, L.A. (ed.) 2004. *Metabolic and Therapeutic Aspects of Amino Acids in Clinical Nutrition.* CRC Press, Boca Raton, FL.

Dai, Z.L., G. Wu and, W.Y. Zhu. 2011. Amino acid metabolism in intestinal bacteria: links between gut ecology and host health. *Front. Biosci.* 16:1768–1786.

Dai, Z.L., Z.L. Wu, S.Q. Hang, W.Y. Zhu, and G. Wu. 2015. Amino acid metabolism in intestinal bacteria and its potential implications for mammalian reproduction. *Mol. Hum. Reprod.* 21:389–409.

Davis, T.A., H.V. Nguyen, R. Garcia-Bravo, M.L. Fiorotto, E.M. Jackson, D.S. Lewis et al. 1994. Amino acid composition of human milk is not unique. *J. Nutr.* 124:1126–1132.

Davis, S.R., Stacpoole, P.W., J. Williamson, L.S. Kick, E.P. Quinlivan, B.S. Coats et al. 2004. Tracer-derived total and folate-dependent homocysteine remethylation and synthesis rates in humans indicate that serine is the main one-carbon donor. *Am. J. Physiol.* 286:E272–279.

DeRosa, G. and R.W. Swick. 1975. Metabolic implications of the distribution of the alanine aminotransferase isoenzymes. *J. Biol. Chem.* 250:7961–7967.

D'Mello, J.P.F. 2017. *The Handbook of Microbial Metabolism of Amino Acids.* CABI, Wallingford, UK.

Dunn, M.F., Niks, D., Ngo, H., Barends, T.R., and Schlichting, I. 2008. Tryptophan synthase: the workings of a channeling nanomachine. *Trends Biochem. Sci.* 33:254–264.

Eisenberg, D., Gill, H.S., Pfluegl, G.M., and Rotstein, S.H. 2000. Structure-function relationships of glutamine synthetases. *Biochim. Biophys. Acta* 1477:122–145.

Elsholz, A.K.W., K. Turgay, S. Michalik, B. Hessling, K. Gronau, D. Oertel, U. Mäder et al. 2012. Global impact of protein arginine phosphorylation on the physiology of *Bacillus subtilis. Proc. Natl. Acad. Sci. USA.* 109:7451–7456.

Fascetti, A.J., J.R. Reed, Q.R. Rogers, and R.C. Backus. 2003. Taurine deficiency in dogs with dilated cardiomyopathy: 12 cases (1997–2001). *J. Am. Vet. Med. Assoc.* 223:1137–1141.

Felig, P. 1975. Amino acid metabolism in man. *Annu. Rev. Biochem.* 44:933–955.

Fitzpatrick, P.F. 1999. Tetrahydropterin-dependent amino acid hydroxylases. *Annu. Rev. Biochem.* 68:355–381.

Flynn, N.E., and G. Wu. 1996. An important role for endogenous synthesis of arginine in maintaining arginine homeostasis in neonatal pigs. *Am. J. Physiol.* 271:R1149–R1155.

Flynn, N.E., C.J. Meininger, T.E. Haynes, and G. Wu. 2002. The metabolic basis of arginine nutrition and pharmacotherapy. *Biomed. Pharmacother.* 56:427–438.

Foley, M.H., S. O'Flaherty, R. Barrangou, and C.M. Theriot. 2019. Bile salt hydrolases: gatekeepers of bile acid metabolism and host-microbiome crosstalk in the gastrointestinal tract. *PLoS Pathog.* 15:e1007581.

Fuhrmann, J., K.W. Clancy, and P.R. Thompson. 2015. Chemical biology of protein arginine modifications in epigenetic regulation. *Chem. Rev.* 115:5413–5461.

Gantner, M.L., K. Eade, M. Wallace, M.K. Handzlik, R. Fallon, J. Trombley et al. 2019. Serine and lipid metabolism in macular disease and peripheral neuropathy. *N. Engl. J. Med.* 381:1422–1433.

Gersovitz, M., D. Bier, D. Matthews, J. Udall, H.N. Munro, and V.R. Young. 1980. Dynamic aspects of whole body leucine metabolism: influence of protein intake in young adult and elderly males. *Metabolism* 29:1087–1094.

Goldberg, A.L. and T.W. Chang. 1978. Regulation and significance of amino acid metabolism in skeletal muscle. *Fed. Proc.* 37:2301–2307.

Gowri, V.S., I. Ghosh, A. Sharma, and R. Madhubala. 2012. Unusual domain architecture of aminoacyl tRNA synthetases and their paralogs from *Leishmania major. BMC Genomics* 13:621.

Graham, D.L., M.L. Beio, D.L. Nelson, and D.B. Berkowitz. 2019. Human serine racemase: key residues/active site motifs and their relation to enzyme function. *Front. Mol. Biosci.* 6:8.

Greenstein, J.P. and M. Winitz. 1961. *Chemistry of Amino Acids*. John Wiley, New York.

Griffith, O.W. 1986. Beta-amino acids: mammalian metabolism and utility as alpha-amino acid analogues. *Annu. Rev. Biochem.* 55:855–878.

Guedes, R.L.M., F. Prosdocimi, G.R. Fernandes, L.K. Moura, H.A.L. Ribeiro, and J.M. Ortega. 2011. Amino acids biosynthesis and nitrogen assimilation pathways: a great genomic deletion during eukaryote evolution. *BMC Genomics* 12(Suppl. 4):S2.

Hall, S.E.H., J.T. Braaten, J.B.R. McKendry, T. Bolton, D. Foster, and M. Berman. 1979. Normal alanine-glucose relationships and their changes in diabetic patients before and after insulin treatment. *Diabetes* 28:737–745.

Harper, A.E., R.H. Miller, and K.P. Block. 1984. Branched-chain amino acid metabolism. *Annu. Rev. Nutr.* 4:409–454.

Hayes, K.C. 1998. Taurine nutrition. *Nutr. Res. Rev.* 1:99–113.

Hayes, K.C. and J.A. Sturman. 1981. Taurine in metabolism. *Annu. Rev. Nutr.* 1:401–425.

He, W.L. and G. Wu. 2020. Metabolism of amino acids in the brain and their roles in regulating food intake. *Adv. Exp. Med. Biol.* 1265:167–185.

He, Y., T.H.M. Hakvoort, J.L.M. Vermeulen, W.H. Lamers, and M.A. van Roon. 2007. Glutamine synthetase is essential in early mouse embryogenesis. *Devel. Dynamics* 236:1865–1875.

He, Y., T.B. Hakvoort, S.E. Kohler, J.L. Vermeulen, D.R. de Waart, C. de Theije et al. 2010. Glutamine synthetase in muscle is required for glutamine production during fasting and extrahepatic ammonia detoxification. *J. Biol. Chem.* 285:9516–9524.

Hendriks, W.H., R. Vather, S.M. Rutherfurd, K. Weidgraaf, and K.J. Rutherfurd-Markwick. 2004. Urinary isovalthine excretion in adult cats is not gender dependent or increased by oral leucine supplementation. *J. Nutr.* 134:2114S–2116S.

Hendriks, W.H., K.J. Rutherfurd-Markwick, K. Weidgraaf, R.H. Morton, and Q.R. Rogers. 2008. Urinary felinine excretion in intact male cats is increased by dietary cystine. *Br. J. Nutr.* 100:801–809.

Herring, C.M., F.W. Bazer, and G. Wu. 2021. Amino acid nutrition for optimum growth, development, reproduction, and health of zoo animals. *Adv. Exp. Med. Biol.* 1285:233–253.

Horiguchi, M. and M. Kandatsu. 1959. Isolation of 2-aminoethane phosphonic acid from rumen protozoa. *Nature* 184:12:901–902.

Hou, Y.Q. and G. Wu. 2017. Nutritionally nonessential amino acids: a misnomer in nutritional sciences. *Adv. Nutr.* 8:137–139.

Hou, Y.Q. and G. Wu. 2018. L-Glutamate nutrition and metabolism in swine. *Amino Acids* 50:1497–1510.

Hou, Y.Q., L. Wang, B.Y. Ding, Y.L. Liu, H.L. Zhu, J. Liu et al. 2011. Alpha-ketoglutarate and intestinal function. *Front. Biosci.* 16:1186–1196.

Hou, Y.Q., L. Wang, D. Yi, and G. Wu. 2015a. N-acetylcysteine and intestinal health: a focus on mechanisms of its actions. *Front. Biosci.* 20:872–891.

Hou, Y.Q., S.C. Jia, G. Nawaratna, S.D. Hu, S. Dahanayaka, F.W. Bazer, and G. Wu. 2015b. Analysis of L-homoarginine in biological samples by HPLC involving pre-column derivatization with *o*-phthalaldehyde and *N*-acetyl-L-cysteine. *Amino Acids* 47:2005–2014.

Hou, Y.Q., K. Yao, Y.L. Yin, and G. Wu. 2016a. Endogenous synthesis of amino acids limits growth, lactation and reproduction of animals. *Adv. Nutr.* 7:331–342.

Hou, Y.Q., S.D. Hu, S.C. Jia, G. Nawaratna, D.S. Che, F.L. Wang et al. 2016b. Whole-body synthesis of L-homoarginine in pigs and rats supplemented with L-arginine. *Amino Acids* 48:993–1001.

Hou, Y.Q., W.L. He, S.D. Hu, and G. Wu. 2019. Composition of polyamines and amino acids in plant-source foods for human consumption. *Amino Acids* 51:1153–1165.

Hou, Y.Q., S.D. Hu, X.Y. Li, W.L. He, and G. Wu. 2020. Amino acid metabolism in the liver: nutritional and physiological significance. *Adv. Exp. Med. Biol.* 1265:21–37.

Hu, C.A., S. Khalil, S. Zhaorigetu, Z. Liu, M. Tyler, G. Wan, and D. Valle. 2008. Human delta¹-pyrroline-5-carboxylate synthase: function and regulation. *Amino Acids* 35:665–672.

Hufton, S.E., I.G. Jennings, and G.H. Cotton. 1995. Structure and function of the aromatic amino acid hydroxylase. *Biochem. J.* 311:353–366.

Hudson, R.C. and R.M. Daniel. 1993. L-glutamate dehydrogenases: distribution, properties and mechanism. *Comp. Biochem. Physiol. B.* 106:767–792.

Huxtable, R.J. 1992. Physiological actions of taurine. *Physiol. Rev.* 72:101–163.

Jackson, A. 1991. The glycine story. *Eur. J. Clin. Nutr.* 45:59–65.

Jaksic, T., D.A. Wagner, J.F. Burke, and V.R. Young. 1991. Proline metabolism in adult male burned patients and healthy control subjects. *Am. J. Clin. Nutr.* 54:408–413.

Janicki, R.H. and L. Goldstein. 1969. Glutamine synthetase and renal ammonia metabolism. *Am. J. Physiol.* 216:1107–1110.

Jorgensen, G.N. and B.L. Larson. 1968. Conversion of phenylalanine to tyrosine in the bovine mammary secretory cell. *Biochim. Biophys. Acta* 165:121–126.

Kalhan, S.C. and R.W. Hanson. 2012. Resurgence of serine: an often neglected but indispensable amino acid. *J. Biol. Chem.* 287:19786–19791.

Kakimoto, Y., K. Taniguchi, and I. Sano. 1969. D-β-aminoisobutyrate:pyruvate aminotransferase in mammalian liver and excretion of β-aminoisobutyrate by man. *J. Biol. Chem.* 244:335–340.

Kato, S. and T. Oikawa. 2018. A novel bifunctional amino acid racemase with multiple substrate specificity, MalY from *Lactobacillus sakei* LT-13: genome-based identification and enzymological characterization. *Front. Microbiol.* 9:403.

Kaufman, S. 1987. Enzymology of the phenylalanine-hydroxylating system. *Enzyme* 38:286–295.

Kawakami, R., T. Ohshida, H. Sakuraba, and T. Ohshima. 2018. A novel PLP-dependent alanine/serine racemase from the hyperthermophilic archaeon *Pyrococcus horikoshii* OT-3. *Front. Microbiol.* 9:1481.

Khan, S.R., P.A. Glenton, and K.J. Byer. 2006. Modeling of hyperoxaluric calcium oxalate nephrolithiasis: experimental induction of hyperoxaluria by hydroxy-L-proline. *Kidney Int.* 70:914–923.

Kim, P.M., X. Duan, A.S. Huang, C.Y. Liu, G.L. Ming, H. Song, and S.H. Snyder. 2010. Aspartate racemase, generating neuronal D-aspartate, regulates adult neurogenesis. *Proc. Natl. Acad. Sci. USA.* 107:3175–3179.

Knight, J., J. Jiang, D.G. Assimos, and R.P. Holmes. 2006. Hydroxyproline ingestion and urinary oxalate and glycolate excretion. *Kidney Int.* 70:1929–1934.

Kowalski, T.J., G. Wu, and M. Watford. 1997. Rat adipose tissue amino acid metabolism in vivo as assessed by microdialysis and arterio-venous techniques. *Am. J. Physiol.* 273:E613–E622.

Krajewski, W.W., R. Collins, L. Holmberg-Schiavone, T.A. Jones, T. Karlberg, and S.L. Mowbray. 2008. Crystal structures of mammalian glutamine synthetases illustrate substrate-induced conformational changes and provide opportunities for drug and herbicide design. *J. Mol. Biol.* 375:317–328.

Kruse, T., H. Reiber, and V. Neuhoff. 1985. Amino acid transport across the human blood-CSF barrier. *J. Neurol. Sci.* 70:129–138.

Kuhn, K.S., K. Schuhmann, P. Stehle, D. Darmaun, and P. Fürst. 1999. Determination of glutamine in muscle protein facilitates accurate assessment of proteolysis and de novo synthesis–derived endogenous glutamine production. *Am. J. Clin. Nutr.* 70:484–489.

Kwon, H., T.E. Spencer, F.W. Bazer, and G. Wu. 2003. Developmental changes of amino acids in ovine fetal fluids. *Biol. Reprod.* 68:1813–1820.

Lapierre, H., D. Pacheco, R. Berthiaume, D.R. Ouellet, C.G. Schwab, P. Dubreuil et al. 2006. What is the true supply of amino acids for a dairy cow? *J. Dairy Sci.* 89 (Suppl 1):E1–E14.

Le Douce, J., M. Maugard, J. Veran, S.H.R. Oliet, A. Panatier, G. Bonvento et al. 2020. Impairment of glycolysis-derived L-serine production in astrocytes contributes to cognitive deficits in Alzheimer's disease. *Cell Metab.* 31:503–517.

Lemieux, G., G. Baverel, P. Vinay, and P. Wadoux. 1976. Glutamine synthetase and glutamyltransferase in the kidney of man, dog and rat. *Am. J. Physiol.* 231:1068–1073.

Lewis, A.J. and D.H. Baker. 1995. Bioavailability of D-amino acids and DL-hydroxy-methionine. In: *Bioavailability of Nutrients for Animals: Amino Acids, Minerals, Vitamins* (Ammerman, C.B., D.P. Baker, and A.J. Lewis, eds). Academic Press, San Diego. pp. 65–81.

Leys, D., J. Basran, N.S. Scrutton. 2003. Channelling and formation of 'active' formaldehyde in dimethylglycine oxidase. *EMBO J.* 22:4038–4048.

Li, P. and G. Wu. 2018. Roles of dietary glycine, proline and hydroxyproline in collagen synthesis and animal growth. *Amino Acids* 50:29–38.

Li, P. and G. Wu. 2020. Composition of amino acids and related nitrogenous nutrients in feedstuffs for animal diets. *Amino Acids* 52:523–542.

Li, P., D.A. Knabe, S.W. Kim, C.J. Lynch, S.M. Hutson, and G. Wu. 2009. Lactating porcine mammary tissue catabolizes branched-chain amino acids for glutamine and aspartate synthesis. *J. Nutr.* 139:1502–1509.

Li, X.L., S.X. Zheng, and G. Wu. 2020a. Nutrition and metabolism of glutamate and glutamine in fish. *Amino Acids* 52:671–691.

Li, X.Y., S.X. Zheng, and G. Wu. 2020b. Amino acid metabolism in the kidneys: nutritional and physiological significance. *Adv. Exp. Med. Biol.* 1265:71–95.

Li, X.Y., S.X. Zheng, and G. Wu. 2021a. Nutrition and functions of amino acids in fish. *Adv. Exp. Med. Biol.* 1285:133–168.

Li, X.Y., T. Han, S.X. Zheng, and G. Wu. 2021b. Nutrition and functions of amino acids in aquatic crustaceans. *Adv. Exp. Med. Biol.* 1285:169–197.

Lichter-Konecki, U., C.M. Hipke, and D.S. Konecki. 1999. DS. Human phenylalanine hydroxylase gene expression in kidney and other nonhepatic tissues. *Mol. Genet. Metab.* 67:308–316.

Ligthart-Melis, G.C., M.C.G. van de Poll, P.G. Boelens, C.H.C. Dejong, N.E.P. Deutz, and P.A.M. van Leeuwen. 2008. Glutamine is an important precursor for de novo synthesis of arginine in humans. *Am. J. Clin. Nutr.* 87:1282–1289.

Light, S.H. and W.F. Anderson. 2013. The diversity of allosteric controls at the gateway to aromatic amino acid biosynthesis. *Protein Sci.* 22:395–404.

Liu, Y.Y., X.J. Tian, B.K. He, T.K. Hoang, C.M. Taylor, E. Blanchard et al. 2019. *Lactobacillus reuteri* DSM 17938 feeding of healthy newborn mice regulates immune responses while modulating gut microbiota and boosting beneficial metabolites. *Am. J. Physiol.* 317:G824–838.

Lomelino, C.L., J.T. Andring, R. McKenna, and M.S. Kilberg. 2017. Asparagine synthetase: function, structure, and role in disease. *J. Biol. Chem.* 292:19952–19958.

Lowry, M., D.E. Hall, and J.T. Brosnan. 1985, Increased activity of renal glycine-cleavage-enzyme complex in metabolic acidosis. *Biochem. J.* 231:477–480.

Luiking, Y.C., G.A. Ten Have, R.R. Wolfe, and N.E. Deutz. 2012. Arginine de novo and nitric oxide production in disease states. *Am. J. Physiol.* 303:E1177–E1189.

Malemud, C.J. 2006. Matrix metalloproteinases (MMPs) in health and disease: an overview. *Front. Biosci.* 11:1696–1701.

Mallette, L.E., J.H. Exton, and C.R. Park. 1969. Control of gluconeogenesis from amino acids in the perfused rat liver. *J. Biol. Chem.* 244:5713–5723.

Mandel, N.S., J.D. Henderson, L.Y. Hung, D.F. Wille, and J.H. Wiessner. 2004. A porcine model of calcium oxalate kidney stone disease. *J. Urol.* 171:1301–1303.

Mansilla, W.D., D.A. Columbus, J.K. Htoo, and C.F.M. de Lange. 2015. Nitrogen absorbed from the large intestine increases whole-body nitrogen retention in pigs fed a diet deficient in dispensable amino acid nitrogen. *J. Nutr.* 145:1163–1169.

Mansilla, W.D., J.K. Htoo, and C.F.M. de Lange. 2017. Replacing dietary nonessential amino acids with ammonia nitrogen does not alter amino acid profile of deposited protein in the carcass of growing pigs fed a diet deficient in nonessential amino acid nitrogen. *J. Anim. Sci.* 95:4481–4489.

Marliss, E.B., T.T. Aoki, T. Pozefsky, A.S. Most, and G.F. Cahill. 1971. Muscle and splanchnic glutamine and glutamate metabolism in postabsorptive and starved man. *J. Clin. Invest.* 50:814–817.

Martens-Lobenhoffer, J., S.M. Bode-Böger, and B. Clement. 2016. First detection and quantification of N^δ-monomethylarginine, a structural isomer of N^G-monomethylarginine, in humans using MS. *Anal. Biochem.* 493:14–20.

Martinez, R.E., J.L. Leatherwood, A.N. Bradbery, M.L. Much, B.L. Silvers, E.A. Posey et al. Equine enterocytes actively oxidize L-glutamine but do not synthesize L-citrulline and L-arginine from L-glutamine or L-proline in vitro. *J. Anim.* Sci. 98:90–91.

Martinez, R.E., J.L. Leatherwood, A.N. Bradbery, B.L. Silvers, E.A. Posey, W.L. He, and G. Wu. 2021. Enterocytes from mature horses do not produce arginine or citrulline from glutamine or proline *in vitro*. The Annual Meeting of the Equine Science Society. June 2021.

Meister, A. 1965. *Biochemistry of Amino Acids*. Academic Press, New York.

Metcalf, W.W. and W.A. van der Donk. 2009. Biosynthesis of phosphonic and phosphinic acid natural products. *Annu. Rev. Biochem.* 78:65–94.

Metges, C.C. 2000. Contribution of microbial amino acids to amino acid homeostasis of the host. *J. Nutr.* 130:1857S–1864S.

Miceli, M.V., T.O. Henderson, and T.C. Myers. 1980. 2-Aminoethylphosphonic acid metabolism during embryonic development of the planorbid snail *Helisoma*. *Science* 209:1245–47.

Milakofsky, L., T.A. Hare, J.M. Miller, and W.H. Vogel. 1985. Rat plasma levels of amino acids and related compounds during stress. *Life Sci.* 36:753–761.

Mitch, W.E. 1980. Metabolism and metabolic effects of ketoacids. *Am. J. Clin. Nutr.* 33:1642–1648.

Møller, N., S. Meek, M. Bigelow, J. Andrews, and K.S. Nair. 2000. The kidney is an important site for in vivo phenylalanine-to-tyrosine conversion in adult humans: a metabolic role of the kidney. *Proc. Natl. Acad. Sci. USA*. 97:1242–1246.

Morris, J.H. and Q.R. Rogers. 1992. The metabolic basis for the taurine requirement of cats. *Adv. Exp. Med. Biol.* 315:33–44.

Morris SM Jr. 2009. Recent advances in arginine metabolism: roles and regulation of the arginases. *Br. J. Pharmacol.* 157:922–930.

Miyazaki, M., T. Yamashita, H. Taira, and A. Suzuki. 2008. The biological function of cauxin, a major urinary protein of the domestic cat. In: *Chemical Signals in Vertebrates*, Vol. 11 (Hurst, J.L., R.J. Beynon, S.C. Roberts, and T.D. Wyatt, eds). Springer, New York. pp. 51–60.

Miyamoto, T., M. Katane, Y. Saitoh, M. Sekine, and H. Homma. 2017. Identification and characterization of novel broad-spectrum amino acid racemases from *Escherichia coli* and *Bacillus subtilis*. *Amino Acids* 49:1885–1894.

Nurjhan, N., A. Bucci, G. Perriello, M. Stumvoll, G. Dailey, Bier, D.M. et al. 1995. Glutamine: a major gluconeogenic precursor and vehicle for interorgan carbon transport in man. *J. Clin. Invest.* 95:272–277.

Parimi, P.S., S. Devapatla, L. Gruca, A.M. O'Brien, R.W. Hanson, and S.C. Kalhan. 2002. Glutamine and leucine nitrogen kinetics and their relation to urea nitrogen in newborn infants. *Am. J. Physiol.* 282:E618–E625.

Parimi, P.S., S. Devapatla, L.L. Gruca, S.B. Amini, R.W. Hanson, and S.C. Kalhan. 2004. Effect of enteral glutamine or glycine on whole-body nitrogen kinetics in very-low-birth-weight infants. *Am. J. Clin. Nutr.* 79:402–409.

Parimi, P.S., L.L. Gruca, and S.C. Kalhan. 2005. Metabolism of threonine in newborn infants. *Am. J. Physiol.* 289:E891–895.

Payne, S.H. and W.F. Loomis. 2006. Retention and loss of amino acid biosynthetic pathways based on analysis of whole-genome sequences. *Eukaryotic Cell* 5:272–276.

Phang, J.M., W. Liu, and O. Zabirnyk. 2010. Proline metabolism and microenvironmental stress. *Annu. Rev. Nutr.* 21;30:441–63.

Posey, E.A., F.W. Bazer, and G. Wu. 2021. Protein nutrition in humans and other animals. *Adv. Exp. Med. Biol.* (in press)

Reeds, P.J. 2000. Dispensable and indispensable amino acids for humans. *J. Nutr.* 130:1835S–1840S.

Robert, J.J., B. Beaufrere, J. Koziet, J.F. Desjeux, D.M. Bier, V.R. Young, and H. Lestradet. 1985. Whole body de novo amino acid synthesis in type I (insulin-dependent) diabetes studied with stable isotope labeled leucine, alanine, and glycine. *Diabetes* 34:67–73.

Rodionov, R.N., D.J. Murry, S.F. Vaulman, J.W. Stevens, and S.R. Lentz. 2010. Human alanine-glyoxylate aminotransferase 2 lowers asymmetric dimethylarginine and protects from inhibition of nitric oxide production. *J. Biol. Chem.* 285:5385–5391.

Rogers, Q.R. and J.M. Phang. 1985. Deficiency of pyrroline-5-carboxylate synthase in the intestinal mucosa of the cat. *J. Nutr.* 115:146–150.

Rose, W.C. 1957. The amino acid requirements of adult man. *Nutr. Abstr. Rev. Ser. Hum. Exp.* 27:631–647.

Rutherfurd, K.J., S.M. Rutherfurd, P.J. Moughan, and W.H. Hendriks. 2002. Isolation and characterization of a felinine-containing peptide from the blood of the domestic cat (*felis catus*). *J. Biol. Chem.* 277:114–119.

Rutherfurd-Markwick, K.J., Q.R. Rogers, and W.H. Hendriks. 2005. Mammalian isovalthine metabolism. *J. Anim. Physiol. Anim. Nutr. (Berl)* 89:1–10.

Sale, C., B. Saunders, and R.C. Harris. 2010. Effect of beta-alanine supplementation on muscle carnosine concentrations and exercise performance. *Amino Acids* 39:321–333

Self, J.T., T.E. Spencer, G.A. Johnson, J. Hu, F.W. Bazer, and G. Wu. 2004. Glutamine synthesis in the developing porcine placenta. *Biol. Reprod.* 70:1444–1451.

Snell, K. 1984. Enzymes of serine metabolism in normal, developing and neoplastic rat tissues. *Adv. Enzyme Regul.* 22:325–400.

Solano, F. 2020. Metabolism and functions of amino acids in sense organs. *Adv. Exp. Med. Biol.* 1265:187–199.

Spodenkiewicz, M., C. Diez-Fernadez, V. Rufenacht, C. Gemeperle-Britschgi, and J. Haberle. 2016. Minireview on glutamine synthetase deficiency, an ultra-rare error of amino acid biosynthesis. *Biology* 5:50.

Stack, T., P.J. Reeds, T. Preston, S. Hay, D.J. Lloyd, and P.J. Aggett. 1989. [15]N tracer studies of protein metabolism in low birth weight preterm infants: a comparison of ^{15}N glycine and ^{15}N yeast protein hydrolysate and of human milk- and formula-fed babies. *Pediatr. Res.* 25:167–172.

Stipanuk, M.H. 2004. Sulfur amino acid metabolism: pathways for production and removal of homocysteine and cysteine. *Annu. Rev. Nutr.* 24:539–577.

Stover, P. and V. Schirch. 1990. Serine hydroxymethyltransferase catalyzes the hydrolysis of 5,10-methenyltetrahydrofolate to 5-formyltetrahydrofolate. *J. Biol. Chem.* 265:14227–33.

Stumvoll, M., G. Perriello, N. Nurjhan, S. Welle, J. Gerich, A. Bucci et al. 1996. Glutamine and Alanine Metabolism in NIDDM. *Diabetes* 45:863–868.

Sturman, J.A. and K.C. Hayes. 1980. The biology of taurine in nutrition and development. *Adv. Nutr. Res.* 3:231–239.

Tate, S.S. and A. Meister. 1971. Regulation of rat liver glutamine synthetase: activation by alpha-ketoglutarate and inhibition by glycine, alanine, and carbamyl phosphate. *Proc. Natl. Acad. Sci. USA.* 68:781–785.

Tabatabaie, L., L.W. Klomp, R. Berger, and T.J. de Koning. 2010. L-Serine synthesis in the central nervous system: a review on serine deficiency disorders. *Mol. Genet. Metab.* 99:256–262.

Tate, S.S., F.Y. Leu, and A. Meister. 1972. Rat liver glutamine synthetase. *J. Biol. Chem.* 247:5312–5321.

Tekwe, C.D., K. Yao, J. Lei, X.L. Li, A. Gupta, Y.Y. Luan et al. 2019. Oral administration of α-ketoglutarate enhances nitric oxide synthesis by endothelial cells and whole-body insulin sensitivity in diet-induced obese rats. *Exp. Biol. Med.* 244:1081–1088.

Temple, S.J., C.P. Vance, and J.S. Gantt. 1998. Glutamate synthase and nitrogen assimilation. *Trends Plant Sci.* 3:51–56.

Tinker, D.A., J.T. Brosnan, and G.R. Herzberg. 1986. Interorgan metabolism of amino acids, glucose, lactate, glycerol and uric acid in the domestic fowl (*Gallus domesticus*). *Biochem. J.* 240:829–836.

Tsikas, D. and G. Wu. 2015. Homoarginine, arginine, and relatives: analysis, metabolism, transport, physiology, and pathology. *Amino Acids* 47:1697–1702.

Tomé, D., M. Gotteland, B. Pierre Henri, M. Andriamihaja, Y. Sanz, F. Blachier, and A.M. Davila. 2013. Intestinal luminal nitrogen metabolism: role of the gut microbiota and consequences for the host. *Pharmacol. Res.* 69:114–126.

Tomlinson, C., M. Rafii, M. Sgro, R.O. Ball, and P. Pencharz. 2011. Arginine is synthesized from proline, not glutamate, in enterally fed human preterm neonates. *Pediatr. Res.* 69:46–50.

Tourian, A., J. Goddard, and T.T. Puck. 1969. Phenylalanine hydroxylase activity in mammalian cells. *J. Cell. Physiol.* 73:159–170.

Uda, K., K. Abe, Y. Dehara, K. Mizobata, N. Sogawa, Y. Akagi et al. 2016. Distribution and evolution of the serine/aspartate racemase family in invertebrates. *Amino Acids* 48:387–402.

Uda, K., N. Ishizuka, Y. Edashige, A. Kikuchi, A.D. Radkov, and L.A. Moe. 2019. Cloning and characterization of a novel aspartate/glutamate racemase from the acorn worm Saccoglossus Kowalevskii. *Comp. Biochem. Physiol.* 232:87–92.

Umbarger, H.E. 1978. Amino acid biosynthesis and its regulation. *Annu. Rev. Biochem.* 47:533–606.

Uo, T., T. Yoshimura, S. Shimizu, and N. Esaki. 1998. Occurrence of pyridoxal 5'-phosphate-dependent serine racemase in silkworm, Bombyx Mori. *Biochem. Biophys. Res. Commun.* 246:31–34.

VanDrisse, C.M. and J.C. Escalante-Semerena. 2019. Protein acetylation in bacteria. *Annu. Rev. Microbiol.* 73:111–132.

Vorhaben, J.E. and J.W. Campbell. 1972. Glutamine synthetase a mitochondrial enzyme in uricotelic species. *J. Biol. Chem.* 247:2763–2767.

Wagner, G.R. and R.M. Payne. 2013. Widespread and enzyme-independent N^ϵ-acetylation and N^ϵ-succinylation of proteins in the chemical conditions of the mitochondrial matrix. *J. Biol. Chem.* 288:29036–29045.

Walser, M. 1984. Rationale and indications for the use of α-keto analogues. *J. Parent. Ent. Nutr.* 8:37–41.

Walsh, C.T. 1989. Enzymes in the D-alanine branch of bacterial cell wall peptidoglycan assembly. *J. Biol. Chem.* 264:2393–2396.

Wang, X. and M. Watford. 2007. Glutamine, insulin and glucocorticoids regulate glutamine synthetase expression in C2C12 myotubes, Hep G2 hepatoma cells and 3T3 L1 adipocytes. *Biochim. Biophys. Acta* 1770:594–600.

Wang, W.W., Z.L. Wu, Z.L. Dai, Y. Yang, J.J. Wang, and G. Wu. 2013. Glycine metabolism in animals and humans: implications for nutrition and health. *Amino Acids* 45:463–477.

Wang, L., D. Yi, Y.Q. Hou, B.Y. Ding, K. Li, B.C. Li et al. 2016. Dietary supplementation with α-ketoglutarate activates mTOR signaling and enhances energy status in skeletal muscle of lipopolysaccharide-challenged piglets. *J. Nutr.* 146:1514–1520.

Watanabe, S., Y. Tanimoto, H. Nishiwaki, and Y. Watanabe. 2015. Identification and characterization of bifunctional proline racemase/hydroxyproline epimerase from archaea: discrimination of substrates and molecular evolution. *PLoS One* 10:e0120349.

Watford, M. 2015. Glutamine and glutamate: nonessential or essential amino acids? *Anim. Nutr.* 1:119–122.

Welbourne, T.C. 1987. Interorgan glutamine flow in metabolic acidosis. *Am. J. Physiol.* 253:F1069–F1076.

Whitworth, D.E. and Cock, P.J. 2009. Evolution of prokaryotic two-component systems: insights from comparative genomics. *Amino Acids.* 37:459–466.

Williamson, D.H. and J.T. Brosnan, 1974. Concentrations of metabolites in animal tissues. In: *Methods of Enzymatic Analysis* (Bergmeyer, H.U., ed). Vol 4, Academic Press, New York. pp. 2266–2302.

Wolosker, H., S. Blackshaw, and S.H. Snyder. 1999. Serine racemase: a glial enzyme synthesizing D-serine to regulate glutamate-N-methyl-D-aspartate neurotransmission. *Proc. Natl. Acad. Sci. U.S.A.* 96:13409–13414.

Wu, G. 1997. Synthesis of citrulline and arginine from proline in enterocytes of postnatal pigs. *Am. J. Physiol.* 272:G1382–G1390.

Wu, G. 2009. Amino acids: metabolism, functions, and nutrition. *Amino Acids* 37:1–17.

Wu, G. 2018. *Principles of Animal Nutrition*. CRC Press, Boca Raton, FL.

Wu, G. 2020a. Metabolism and functions of amino acids in sense organs. *Adv. Exp. Med. Biol.* 1265:201–217.

Wu, G. 2020b. Important roles of dietary taurine, creatine, carnosine, anserine and hydroxyproline in human nutrition and health. *Amino Acids* 52:329–360.

Wu, G. and D. A. Knabe. 1994. Free and protein-bound amino acids in sow's colostrum and milk. *J. Nutr.* 124:415–424.

Wu, G. and S.M. Morris, Jr. 1998. Arginine metabolism: nitric oxide and beyond. *Biochem. J.* 336:1–17.

Wu, G., J.R. Thompson, G. Sedgwick, and M. Drury. 1989. Formation of alanine and glutamine in chick (*Gallus domesticus*) skeletal muscle. *Comp. Biochem. Physiol.* 93B:609–613.

Wu, G., F.W. Bazer, and W. Tuo. 1995. Developmental changes of free amino acid concentrations in fetal fluids of pigs. *J. Nutr.* 125:2859–2868.

Wu, G., P.K. Davis, N.E. Flynn, D.A. Knabe, and J.T. Davidson. 1997. Endogenous synthesis of arginine plays an important role in maintaining arginine homeostasis in postweaning growing pigs. *J. Nutr.* 127:2342–2349.

Wu, G., D.A. Knabe and S.W. Kim. 2004. Arginine nutrition in neonatal pigs. *J. Nutr.* 134:2783S–2390S.

Wu, G., F.W. Bazer, R.C. Burghardt, G.A. Johnson, S.W. Kim, D.A. Knabe et al. 2010. Functional amino acids in swine nutrition and production. In: *Dynamics in Animal Nutrition* (Doppenberg, J. and P. van der Aar, eds). Wageningen Academic Publishers, The Netherlands, pp. 69–98.

Wu, G., F.W. Bazer, R.C. Burghardt, G.A. Johnson, S.W. Kim, D.A. Knabe et al. 2011a. Proline and hydroxy-proline metabolism: implications for animal and human nutrition. *Amino Acids* 40:1053–1063.

Wu, G., F.W. Bazer, G.A. Johnson, D.A. Knabe, R.C. Burghardt, T.E. Spencer et al. 2011b. Important roles for L-glutamine in swine nutrition and production. *J. Anim. Sci.* 89:2017–2030.

Wu, Z.L., Y.Q. Hou, S.D. Hu, F.W. Bazer, C.J. Meininger, C.J. McNeal, and G. Wu. 2016. Catabolism and safety of supplemental L-arginine in animals. *Amino Acids* 48:1541–1552.

Wu, G., F.W. Bazer, G.A. Johnson, and Y.Q. Hou. 2018. Arginine nutrition and metabolism in growing, gestating and lactating swine. *J. Anim. Sci.* 96:5035–5051.

Wu, Z.L., Y.Q. Hou, Z.L. Dai, C.A. Hu, and G. Wu. 2019. Metabolism, nutrition and redox signaling of hydroxyproline. *Antioxid. Redox Signal.* 30:674–682.

Yang, Z., J.K. Htoo, and S.F. Liao. 2020. Methionine nutrition in swine and related monogastric animals: beyond protein biosynthesis. *Anim. Feed Sci. Technol.* 268:114608.

Yoshimura, T. and M. Goto. 2008. D-Amino acids in the brain: structure and function of pyridoxal phosphate-dependent amino acid racemases. *FEBS J.* 275:3527–3537.

Yoshimura, T. and N. Esak. 2003. Amino acid racemases: functions and mechanisms. *J. Biosci. Bioengin.* 96:103–109.

Ytrebø, L.M., S. Sen, C. Rose, G.A.M. Ten Have, N.A. Davies, S. Hodges et al. 2006. Interorgan ammonia, glutamate, and glutamine trafficking in pigs with acute liver failure. *Am. J. Physiol.* 291:G373–G381.

Yu, Y.-M., C.M. Ryan, L. Castillo, X.-M. Lu, L. Beaumier, R.G. Tompkins, and V.R. Young. 2001. Arginine and ornithine kinetics in severely burned patients: increased rate of arginine disposal. *Am. J. Physiol.* 280:E509–E517.

Zhang, S., E.A. Wong, and E.R. Gilbert. 2015. Bioavailability of different dietary supplemental methionine sources in animals. *Front. Biosci.* E7:478–490.

Zhang, J.M., W.L. He, D. Yi, D. Zhao, Z. Song, Y.Q. Hou, and G. Wu. 2019. Regulation of protein synthesis in porcine mammary epithelial cells by L-valine. *Amino Acids* 51:717–726.

Zobel-Thropp, P., J.D. Gary, and S. Clarke. 1998. δ-*N*-Methylarginine is a novel posttranslational modification of arginine residues in yeast proteins. *J. Biol. Chem.* 273:29283–29286.

4 Degradation of Amino Acids

Catabolism of amino acids (AAs) occurs in humans and other animals regardless of their nutritional states, with the rates being the highest immediately after feeding (Jungas et al. 1992). Because physiological concentrations of AAs are readily soluble in water (a major component of the body) and accumulation of large amounts of free AAs in the body can substantially increase the osmolarity of physiological fluids, most of the AAs in excess of the needs for the synthesis of protein and other biologically active substances are degraded in a cell- and tissue-specific manner (Krebs 1972). The major products of AA catabolism are CO_2, water, ammonia, urea, uric acid, pyruvate, and acetyl-CoA, with the metabolic fates of pyruvate (e.g., glucose or fatty acid synthesis) and acetyl-CoA (oxidation to CO_2 or fatty acid synthesis) depending on nutritional, physiological, and pathological states (Wu 2020b,c). Nonetheless, in cells or tissues constantly exposed to elevated concentrations of AAs (e.g., glutamine, taurine, and β-alanine), intracellular concentrations can be greatly increased. For example, increasing extracellular concentrations of glutamine from 0.5 to 15 mM dose-dependently augments its intracellular concentrations from 6 to 36 mM in chicken skeletal muscle (Wu and Thompson 1990). This is in contrast to the common belief that regardless of their source, the AAs not immediately incorporated into new proteins are rapidly degraded in animals.

The degradation of AAs to regulate their homeostasis in the body and generate bioactive metabolites [e.g., nitric oxide (NO), taurine, dopamine, serotonin, and H_2S] fulfills important physiological functions in organisms (Bröer and Bröer 2017; Closs et al. 2006; Wester et al. 2015). Interestingly, it has been known for more than a century that, in omnivorous animals (including humans) consuming a normal meal with protein, carbohydrate, and lipids, the catabolism of any excess AAs (i.e., AAs not needed for maintenance and growth) takes precedence over the degradation of carbohydrate and fatty acids (Hämäläinen and Helme 1907; Lusk 1921). In addition, the whole-body degradation of AAs is enhanced in some physiological (e.g., exercise and responses to cold stress) and pathological (e.g., cancer and infection) states and is reduced in response to low protein or low AA intake and food deprivation (Meredith et al. 1986; Wu 2009; Zhao et al. 1986). Even when there is no exogenous provision of AAs (e.g., fasting and consumption of a nitrogen-free diet), AAs undergo oxidation to produce ammonia because the constitutive enzymes are not entirely inhibited (Meijer et al. 1990).

It should be borne in mind that although some cell types (e.g., the enterocytes of mammals, birds, fish, and crustaceans) depend on the oxidation of certain AAs (glutamate, aspartate, and glutamine) as the major source of energy, the use of AAs as metabolic fuels is energetically inefficient in mammals and birds, as compared with the oxidation of glucose and fatty acids. However, the energetic efficiency of AA oxidation for ATP production in animal species (e.g., fish) that directly excrete ammonia into the surrounding environment is only moderately lower than that for glucose and fatty acids, because this route of ammonia disposal is largely energy-independent (Li et al. 2021a). Pathways for AA degradation in animals and gastrointestinal microbes will be highlighted in this chapter.

4.1 GENERAL CHARACTERISTICS OF AA DEGRADATION IN ANIMAL CELLS

4.1.1 Overall View of AA Catabolism

Dietary proteins are terminally hydrolyzed by proteases and peptidases into small peptides (di- and tri-peptides) and free AAs in the small intestine (Chapter 2). Most of these products are taken up by the mucosal cells (primarily enterocytes) of the small intestine, and some are taken up by microbes present in the gut. Small peptides and AAs are degraded by the small intestine (mucosal cells, microbes, and both) at various rates during the first pass into the portal circulation. In the blood, all canonical proteinogenic AAs and most of non-proteinogenic AAs are transported in the unbound form, and a few (e.g., homocysteine) occurs as a complex with protein. In humans and other animals (e.g., horses and rats), erythrocytes (red blood cells) may play a role in the transport of AAs to tissues (Felig et al. 1973; Thorn et al. 2020).

A major difference between AAs and other macronutrients (fat and carbohydrate) is that AAs contain nitrogen and sulfur. In nature, nitrogen in substances exists in various oxidation states: $+5$ (NO_3^-, nitrate), $+3$ (NO_2^-, nitrite), $+2$ (NO), 0 (N_2), -3 (NH_3, urea, and the $-NH_2$ group in AAs). Except for N_2, all of these forms of nitrogen are produced from AA oxidation by animals. Thus, nitrogen actively participates in metabolic transformations. Similarly, sulfur has multiple oxidation states: -2 [H_2S (hydrogen sulfide), sulfides, and cysteine thiols ($-SH$; cysteine, methionine, and glutathione)], -1 ($-S-S-$; cystine), 0 [sulfur and RSO^- (sulfenic acid)], $+1$, $+2$ [RSOH (sulfinic acid) and cysteine sulfinic acid], $+3$, $+4$ [SO_2 (sulfur dioxide), sulfites, $RS(O)_2OH$ (sulfonic acid), and taurine (sulfonate)], $+5$, and $+6$ [SO_4^{2-} (sulfate) and sulfuric acid]. The major sulfur-containing products of the catabolism of sulfur AAs are SO_4^{2-}, H_2S, SO_2, and, in most animal species, taurine.

The carbon skeletons of AAs have metabolic fates similar to those of glucose and fatty acids, but the oxidation of sulfur is unique to AAs. In humans and other animals regularly consuming normal meals without any excess, all of the nitrogen, sulfur, and carbon of dietary AAs are metabolized daily for replacement and/or growth of tissues. However, when an excess amount of dietary protein is ingested, most of its nitrogen and sulfur are excreted gradually within days but some of its carbon is retained as glycogen and fats (Krebs 1972). This is clearly illustrated by the early finding of Hämäläinen and Helme (1907) that, in adult humans ingesting a protein and energy-adequate diet plus an additional 320 g veal, 61% of the extra nitrogen was eliminated on the first day, 26% on the second day, and the remaining 13% on the third day, whereas 74% of the extra sulfur was excreted on the first day, and protein was partly oxidized for ATP production and partly converted into carbohydrates (glucose and glycogen) and lipids (fatty acids and triglycerides). This indicates a dynamic pattern of dietary AA metabolism in the body. Note that most of AA-degrading enzymes (e.g., tyrosine transaminase, ornithine transaminase, arginase, glutaminase, asparaginase, glutamate:pyruvate transaminase, phenylalanine hydroxylase, and tryptophan pyrrolase) are inducible by high protein or AA intake and by elevated concentrations of hormones in the blood (e.g., glucagon and cortisol; Krebs 1972).

4.1.2 Catabolic Pathways of AAs and Their Major Metabolites

Because of differences in side chains, individual AAs have their own transporters (Bröer and Bröer 2017; Closs et al. 2006) and unique catabolic pathways (Krebs 1964). However, the catabolism of many AAs shares a number of common steps to generate pyruvate, oxaloacetate, α-KG, fumarate, succinyl-CoA, and acetyl-CoA (Figure 4.1). In addition to transamination, other reactions also play an important role in initiating AA degradation (Table 4.1). Complete oxidation of many AAs requires inter-organ cooperation. Based on the rate of oxygen consumption by the human liver, Jungas et al. (1992) have suggested that little or none of AA carbons are completely oxidized into CO_2 in this organ. Metabolites of AAs include ammonia, CO_2, urea, uric acid, acetyl-CoA, long-chain and short-chain fatty acids, formate, glucose, H_2S, ketone bodies, NO, polyamines, and other nitrogenous substances, with each having enormous biological importance (see Chapter 11). In an aqueous solution, free ammonia (NH_3) is at equilibrium with ammonium ion (NH_4^+; $pK_a = 9.2$). At pH 7.4 and 37°C, approximately 1.6% and 98.4% of ammonia exists as free NH_3 and ammonium ion, respectively. In this book, free NH_3 and NH_4^+ are collectively referred to as ammonia.

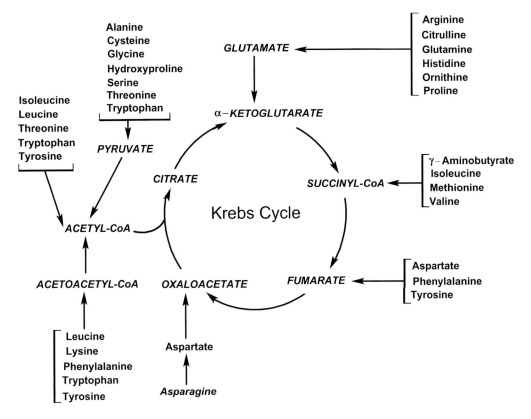

FIGURE 4.1 An overall view of amino acid catabolism in humans and other animals. Different metabolic pathways for the catabolism of amino acids converge to common intermediates (α-KG, oxaloacetate, and pyruvate) that feed into the Krebs cycle in tissues. Different amino acids have different metabolic fates in the body.

$$NH_3 + H^+ \rightleftharpoons NH_4^+$$

$$pH = pK_a + \log\left([NH_3]/[NH_4^+]\right)$$

pK_a of the ammonium ion = 9.2 at 37°C

$[NH_3]/[NH_4^+] = 0.016$ at pH 7.40

$[NH_3] = 1.6\%; [NH_4^+] = 98.4\%$

In the fed state, oxidation to CO_2 and water for ATP production is a metabolic fate of the carbon skeletons of the AAs not used for storage or peptide synthesis. In the Krebs cycle, oxaloacetate serves as a substrate of citrate synthase to introduce acetyl-CoA into the cycle and there is extensive randomization of both carbons and hydrogens due to the symmetrical nature of the succinate molecule (Figure 4.2). The major function of the Krebs cycle is to oxidize acetyl-CoA, generating CO_2, NADH + H^+, FADH$_2$, and GTP. Subsequently, NADH and FADH$_2$ are oxidized via the mitochondrial electron transport system to produce ATP and water. Note that none of the intermediates of the Krebs cycle (including oxaloacetate) undergo net oxidation to CO_2 and water via the cycle. Rather, all intermediates of the Krebs cycle are regenerated through the cyclic process. Thus, complete oxidation of AAs occurs only if their carbons are ultimately converted to acetyl-CoA.

$$C_3H_4O_3\left(\text{Pyruvate}\right) + 2.5O_2 \rightarrow 3CO_2 + 2H_2O \left(\text{heat of combustion, } \Delta H = 1,165 \text{ J/mol}\right)$$

TABLE 4.1

Reactions Initiating the Catabolism of Amino Acids in Animals

Reactions	Examples	
Amidotransferation	Glutamine + F6P → Glucosamine-6-phosphate + Glutamate	(1)
Cleavage	Glycine + NAD$^+$ + THF ↔ MTHF + CO$_2$ + NH$_3$ + NADH + H$^+$	(2)
Condensation	Methionine + Mg-ATP → S-Adenosylmethionine + Mg-PPi + Pi	(3)
Deaminated oxidation (FAD)	D-Amino acid + O$_2$ + H$_2$O → α-Ketoacid + H$_2$O$_2$ + NH$_3$	(4)
	L-Amino acid + O$_2$ + H$_2$O → α-Ketoacid + H$_2$O$_2$ + NH$_3$	(5)
Deamination	Leucine + ½ O$_2$ → α-Ketoacid + NH$_3$	(6)
Decarboxylation (PLP)	Ornithine → Putrescine + CO$_2$	(7)
Dehydration	Serine → Aminoacrylate + H$_2$O	(8)
Dehydrogenation	Threonine + NAD$^+$ → 2-Amino-3-ketobutyrate + NADH + H$^+$	(9)
Dioxygenation	Cysteine + O$_2$ → Cysteinesulfinate	(10)
Hydrolysis[a]	Arginine + H$_2$O → Ornithine + Urea	(11)[a]
Hydrolysis[b]	Glutamine + H$_2$O → Glutamate + NH$_3$	(12)[b]
Hydroxylation	Arginine + O$_2$ + BH4 + NADPH + H$^+$ → NO + BH4 + Citrulline + NADP$^+$	(13)
One-carbon unit transfer	Glycine + MTHF ↔ Serine + THF	(14)
Oxidation (FAD)	Proline + ½ O$_2$ → Pyrroline-5-carboxylate + H$_2$O	(15)
Oxidative deamination	Glutamate + NAD$^+$ ↔ α-Ketoglutarate + NH$_3$ + NADH + H$^+$	(16)
Reduction	Lysine + α-Ketoglutarate + NADPH + H$^+$ → Saccharopine + NADP$^+$	(17)
Transamination (PLP)	Leucine + α-Ketoglutarate ↔ α-Ketoisocaproate + Glutamate	(18)

Enzymes that catalyze the indicated reactions are as follows: (1) glutamine:fructose-6-phosphate transaminase; (2) glycine synthase (glycine cleavage system); (3) S-adenosylmethionine synthase; (4) D-amino acid oxidase; (5) D-amino acid oxidase; (6) deaminase; (7) ornithine decarboxylase; (8) serine dehydratase; (9) threonine dehydrogenase; (10) cysteine dioxygenase; (11) arginase; (12) glutaminase; (13) NO synthase; (14) hydroxymethyltransferase; (15) proline oxidase; (16) glutamate dehydrogenase; (17) lysine:α-ketoglutarate reductase; and (18) BCAA transaminase. F6P, fructose-6-phosphate; MTHF, N^5-N^{10}-methylene-THF; NO, nitric oxide; THF, tetrahydrofolate. BH4, tetrahydrobiopterin (required for the hydroxylation of arginine, phenylalanine, tyrosine, and tryptophan).

[a] Amidinohydrolysis.

[b] Deamidation.

$$\text{Pyruvate} + \text{NAD}^+ \rightarrow \text{Acetyl-CoA} + \text{NADH} + \text{H}^+ \quad \left(\text{pyruvate dehydrogenase; 2.5 ATP}\right)$$

$$\text{Acetyl-CoA} \rightarrow 2\,\text{CO}_2 + 2\,\text{H}_2\text{O} + \text{CoA} \quad \left(\text{Krebs cycle and the electron transport system; 10 ATP}\right)$$

The metabolic fates of nitrogen, sulfur, and carbon skeletons of AAs vary among cells, tissues, and species. In all animals, the conversion of oxaloacetate into pyruvate involves (1) phosphoenolpyruvate carboxykinase (PEPCK), which catalyzes the decarboxylation of oxalo-acetate to form phosphoenolpyruvate; (2) pyruvate kinase, which generates pyruvate from phos-phoenolpyruvate; and NAD$^+$- or NADP$^+$-linked malic enzyme (Figure 4.3). However, whether AAs may be substrates for glucose synthesis critically depends on the intracellular localization of PEPCK in the liver and kidneys of animal species (Watford 1985). PEPCK is present exclusively in the mitochondria (the liver of pigeons, chickens, and rabbits) or cytoplasm (rats, mice, and golden hamsters), or even both compartments (humans, cattle sheep, pigs, guinea pigs, and frogs, as well as the kidneys of chickens), depending on species and cell type. Because NADH is required for the conversion of phosphoenolpyruvate into glucose in the cytoplasm, the presence of cytosolic PEPCK allows for the generation of NADH and, therefore, the synthesis of glucose from AA catabolism.

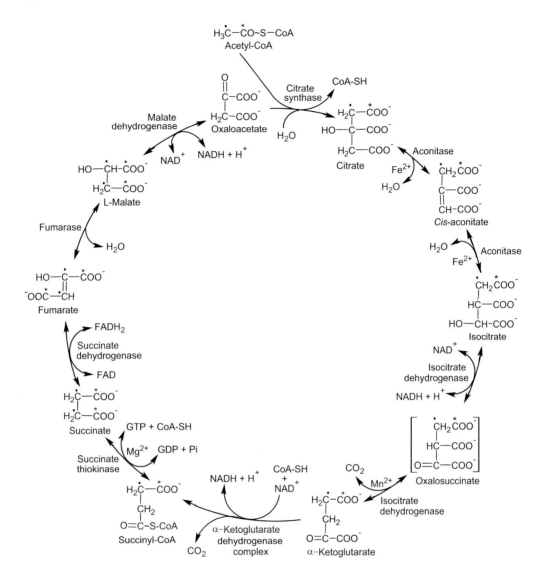

FIGURE 4.2 The Krebs cycle (citric acid cycle) in humans and other animals. The carboxyl and methyl carbons of acetyl-CoA are shown with labels designated by symbols "*" and "·", respectively. In the first turn of the cycle, two molecules of CO_2 are produced, which are derived from the oxaloacetate portion of citrate but not the acetyl-CoA that immediately enters the cycle. Because succinate is a symmetric compound and because succinate dehydrogenase does not differentiate between its two carboxyl groups, "randomization" of label occurs at this step such that all four carbons of succinate, fumarate, malate, and oxaloacetate are labeled after one turn of the cycle. The carboxyl and methyl carbons of acetyl-CoA are completely lost as CO_2 after two and fifteen turns of the cycle, respectively.

By contrast, the presence of PEPCK solely in the mitochondria does not allow for the generation of NADH; therefore, little glucose is formed from AA catabolism in this instance. In other words, mitochondrial PEPCK does not support glucose synthesis from AAs. This concept is supported by the finding of Watford et al. (1981) that alanine, aspartate, glutamate, glutamine, glycine, proline, or serine (5 mM each, which is approximately 5–20 times physiological concentrations in the plasma) is a poor substrate for gluconeogenesis in the chicken liver which expresses PEPCK only in the mitochondria. However, these AAs are effective precursors for glucose production in the chicken kidneys which express PEPCK in both the cytoplasm and mitochondria.

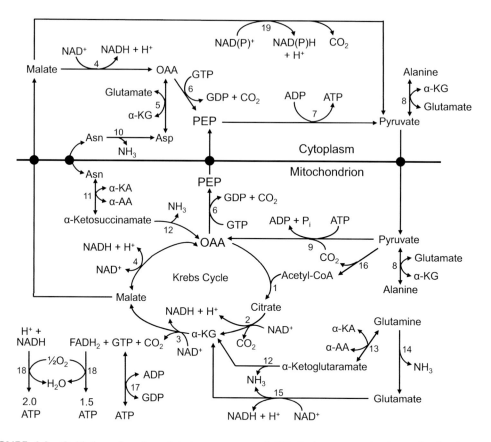

FIGURE 4.3 Oxidation of oxaloacetate to pyruvate and CO_2 in humans and other animals. Complete oxidation of amino acid-derived oxaloacetate to CO_2 occurs through its conversion to pyruvate that involves both mitochondria and the cytoplasm of cells. Pyruvate enters the mitochondria and is decarboxylated to form acetyl-CoA. α-KG, α-ketoglutarate; OAA, oxaloacetate; PEP, phosphoenolpyruvate. The enzymes that catalyze the indicated reactions are as follows: (1) citrate synthase; (2) aconitase and isocitrate dehydrogenase; (3) α-KG dehydrogenase, succinate dehydrogenase, and fumarase; (4) malate dehydrogenase; (5) aspartate transaminase; (6) phosphoenolpyruvate carboxykinase; (7) pyruvate kinase; (8) alanine transaminase; (9) pyruvate carboxylase; (10) asparaginase; (11) asparagine transaminase; (12) ω-amidase; (13) glutamine transaminase; (14) phosphate-activated glutaminase; (15) glutamate dehydrogenase; (16) pyruvate dehydrogenase; (17) nucleoside-diphosphate kinase; (18) enzymes of the mitochondrial electron transport system; and (19) NAD^+- or $NADP^+$-linked malic enzyme.

4.1.3 ENERGETIC EFFICIENCIES OF AA CATABOLISM

On a molar basis, the oxidation of AAs to CO_2 and water is less efficient for ATP production than the oxidation of fat and glucose to CO_2 and water (Table 4.2). Calculations for ATP production from the oxidation of selective AAs in mammals are provided for glutamine (Table 4.3), arginine (Table 4.4), and leucine (Table 4.5). On average, the biological oxidation of 100 g protein generates a net amount of 20 mol ATP in these animals. The efficiency of energy transfer from AAs to ATP ranges from 23.8% for methionine to 49.1% for threonine, in comparison with that for pyruvate (55.4%). However, glutamine is a preferred major fuel for rapidly dividing cells (e.g., enterocytes and tumors), cells with great division potential (e.g., lymphocytes), and certain metabolically active cells and tissues (e.g., monocytes, macrophages, and kidney). Provision of NH_3 from an abundant neutral AA to rapidly remove both diet-derived and endogenously generated H^+ for the regulation of acid-base balance may be an important reason for the extensive catabolism of glutamine by these cells and tissues in animals, including humans, swine, birds, ruminants, rats, and fish.

Some animals (e.g., ammoniotelic fish) secrete ammonia to the surrounding environments as the nitrogenous product of AA catabolism (Jürss and Bastrop 1995). Because no energy is required for ammonia disposal, the use of AAs as metabolic fuels is highly efficient in these organisms. Additionally, because carnivorous fish consume animal-source foods containing 65%–70% protein (on a dry matter basis) but a limited amount of glucose, AAs (primarily glutamate, glutamine and aspartate, and, to a much lesser extent, alanine and leucine) are extensively oxidized in their tissues (e.g., the proximal intestine, liver, kidneys, and skeletal muscles) for ATP production (Jia et al. 2019; Li et al. 2020a; Van Der Schoor et al. 2002). Because some ammoniotelic-secreting species (e.g., largemouth bass; Li et al. 2020b) cannot tolerate a high dietary content of highly digestible carbohydrates (e.g., starch) with the occurrence of hepatic glycogenosis (a metabolic disease; Li et al. 2021a), they have developed a strategy to preferentially use AAs as the major energy substrate. The energetic efficiencies of AA oxidation for ATP production in ammoniotelic species are greater than those in mammals and birds (Table 4.2). Thus, in fish, the efficiency of energy transfer from glutamate and glutamine to ATP production via biological oxidation is only 6.5% and 18% lower than that for glucose oxidation, respectively.

TABLE 4.2
Energetic Efficiency of the Oxidation of Amino Acids (AAs), Protein, and Other Substrates in Mammals, Birds, and Fish

| Nutrients | Combustion Energy kJ per | | Net ATP Production[a] | | | | | | Efficiency of Energy Transfer to ATP[b] % | | |
| | mol | g | Mammal | Bird | Fish | Mammal | Bird | Fish | Mammal | Bird | Fish |
			mol/mol			mol/g					
Alanine	1,577	17.7	13.0	10.25	15.0	0.146	0.115	0.168	42.5	33.5	49.1
Arginine	3,739	21.5	23.5	18.0	27.5	0.135	0.103	0.158	32.4	24.8	37.9
Asparagine	1,928	14.6	11.0	5.50	15.0	0.083	0.042	0.113	29.4	14.7	40.2
Aspartate	1,601	12.0	13.0	10.25	15.0	0.098	0.077	0.113	42.0	33.1	48.3
Citrulline	3,392	19.4	21.5	16.0	25.5	0.123	0.091	0.146	32.7	24.3	38.7
Cysteine	2,249	18.6	10.5	7.75	12.5	0.087	0.064	0.102	24.0	17.7	28.7
Glutamate	2,244	15.3	20.5	17.75	22.5	0.139	0.121	0.153	47.0	40.7	51.6
Glutamine	2,570	17.6	18.5	13.0	22.5	0.127	0.089	0.154	37.1	26.1	45.1
Glycine[c]	973	13.0	7.0	4.25	9.0	0.093	0.057	0.120	37.0	22.5	47.6
Histidine	3,213	20.7	16.5	8.25	22.5	0.106	0.053	0.145	26.5	13.3	36.1
Isoleucine	3,581	27.3	33.5	30.75	35.5	0.255	0.234	0.271	48.3	44.3	51.2
Leucine	3,582	27.3	32.5	29.75	34.5	0.248	0.227	0.263	46.8	42.9	49.7
Lysine[d]	3,683	25.2	30.0	24.5	34.0	0.205	0.168	0.232	42.0	34.3	47.6
Methionine	3,245	23.0	15.0	12.25	17.0	0.101	0.082	0.114	23.8	18.4	27.0
Ornithine	3,030	22.9	23.5	18.0	27.5	0.177	0.136	0.208	40.1	30.7	46.9
Phenylalanine	4,647	28.1	32.0	29.25	34.0	0.194	0.177	0.206	35.6	32.5	37.8
Proline	2,730	23.7	23.0	20.25	25.0	0.200	0.176	0.217	43.5	38.3	47.3
Serine	1,444	13.7	10.5	7.75	12.5	0.100	0.074	0.119	37.6	27.8	44.8
Threonine[e]	2,053	17.2	19.5	16.75	21.5	0.164	0.141	0.180	49.1	42.2	54.1
Tryptophan	5,628	27.6	35.5	30.0	39.5	0.174	0.147	0.194	32.5	27.5	36.2
Tyrosine	4,429	24.4	34.5	31.75	36.5	0.191	0.175	0.202	40.2	37.1	42.5
Valine	2,922	25.0	26.0	23.25	28.0	0.222	0.198	0.239	45.9	41.0	49.4
Protein[f]	2,260	22.6	20.0	16.7	22.4	0.200	0.167	0.224	45.7	38.1	51.1
Glucose	2,803	15.6	30.0	30.0	30.0	0.167	0.167	0.167	55.3	55.3	55.3

(Continued)

TABLE 4.2 (*Continued*)

Energetic Efficiency of the Oxidation of Amino Acids (AAs), Protein, and Other Substrates in Mammals, Birds, and Fish

Nutrients	Combustion Energy kJ per		Net ATP Production[a] mol/mol			Net ATP Production[a] mol/g			Efficiency of Energy Transfer to ATP[b] %		
	mol	g	Mammal	Bird	Fish	Mammal	Bird	Fish	Mammal	Bird	Fish
Starch[g]	2,779	17.2	30.0	30.0	30.0	0.185	0.185	0.185	55.7	55.7	55.7
Palmitate	9,791	38.2	106	106	106	0.414	0.414	0.414	55.9	55.9	55.9
Fat[h]	31,676	39.3	336.5	336.5	336.5	0.417	0.417	0.417	54.8	54.8	54.8
Pyruvate	1,165	13.2	12.5	12.5	12.5	0.142	0.142	0.142	55.4	55.4	55.4
Acetoacetate	1,775	17.4	19	19	19	0.186	0.186	0.186	55.2	55.2	55.2
β-hydroxybutyrate	2,039	19.6	21.5	21.5	21.5	0.207	0.207	0.207	54.4	54.4	54.4

[a] Based on (1) production of 2.5 mol ATP from oxidation of 1 mol NADH or NADPH to H_2O, and (2) production of 1.5 mol ATP from oxidation of 1 mol $FADH_2$ to H_2O. Thus, complete oxidation of 1 mol acetyl-CoA to CO_2 and H_2O via the Krebs cycle and the mitochondrial electron transport system results in the net production of 10 mol ATP. Net production of ATP from AA oxidation is calculated as total ATP production minus the amounts of ATP required for AA catabolism (including the urea cycle). Conversion of 1 mol NH_3 into 0.5 mol urea via the urea cycle consumes 2 mol ATP. Conversion of 1 mol NH_3 to 0.25 mol uric acid consumes 2.75 mol ATP.

[b] Calculated on the basis of 51.6 kJ/mol for one high-energy bond in ATP (mol of net ATP production/mol substrate × 51.6 kJ/mol ÷ combustion energy of kJ/mol substrate × 100%).

[c] When 1 mol glycine is catabolized by the glycine cleavage system, 1 mol ATP is produced. When 1 mol glycine is converted to serine and then oxidized, 13 mol ATP are produced. Because N^5-N^{10}-methylene-tetrahydrofolate, which donates one carbon unit for converting glycine to serine, is formed from tetrahydrofolate via reactions that consume 3.5 mol ATP, this amount is subtracted in the calculation of net ATP production from glycine oxidation via the serine pathway.

[d] Calculated on the basis of lysine catabolism via the lysine-α-ketoglutarate reductase pathway.

[e] Calculated on the basis of threonine catabolism via the threonine dehydrogenase pathway.

[f] Assuming that the average molecular weight of an AA residue in protein is 100.
   Protein oxidation: $C_{4.3}H_7O_{1.4}N_{1.2} \rightarrow 0.6\ CH_4N_2O + 3.7\ CO_2 + 2.3\ H_2O$

[g] The average molecular weight of glucose residue in starch is 162.

[h] Tripalmitoylglycerol is used as an example.

TABLE 4.3

ATP Production from the Oxidation of Glutamine in Mammals

Reactions	ATP production
A. Mitochondria (Glutamine to Malate)	
(1) Glutamine + $H_2O \rightarrow$ Glutamate + NH_4^+	0
(2) Glutamate + $NAD^+ \rightarrow NH_4^+$ + α-KG + NADH + H^+	2.5
(3) 2 NH_4^+ + HCO_3^- + 3 ATP → Urea + 2 ADP + 1 AMP + 2 Pi + PPi (equivalent to 4 high-energy bonds)	−4
(4) α-KG + CoA + $NAD^+ \rightarrow$ Succinyl-CoA + CO_2 + NADH + H^+	2.5
(5) Succinyl-CoA + GDP + Pi → Succinate + GTP	1
(6) Succinate + FAD → Fumarate + $FADH_2$	1.5
(7) Fumarate + $H_2O \rightarrow$ Malate	0

(Continued)

TABLE 4.3 (*Continued*)
ATP Production from the Oxidation of Glutamine in Mammals

Reactions	ATP production
B. Cytoplasm (Malate to Pyruvate)	
(8) Malate + NAD$^+$ → Oxaloacetate + NADH + H$^+$	2.5
(9) Oxaloacetate + GTP → Phosphoenolpyruvate + CO$_2$ + GDP	−1
(10) Phosphoenolpyruvate + ADP → Pyruvate + ATP	1
C. Mitochondria (Pyruvate to CO$_2$ and H$_2$O)	
(11) Pyruvate + NAD$^+$ → Acetyl-CoA + CO$_2$ + NADH + H$^+$	2.5
(12) Acetyl-CoA + 2 H$_2$O $_+$ 3 NAD$^+$ + FAD + GDP + Pi → 2 CO$_2$ + 3 NADH + 3 H$^+$ + FADH$_2$ + GTP + CoA	10
D. Net Reaction	
C$_5$H$_{10}$N$_2$O$_3$ + 4.5 O$_2$ → CH$_4$N$_2$O + 4 CO$_2$ + 3 H$_2$O + 1 Urea	18.5

α-KG, α-ketoglutarate.

TABLE 4.4
ATP Production from the Oxidation of Arginine via the Arginase Pathway in Mammals

Reactions	ATP Production
A. Mitochondria and Cytoplasm	
(1) Arginine + H$_2$O → Urea + Ornithine	0
B. Mitochondria (Ornithine to Malate)	
(2) Ornithine + α-KG → P5C + Glutamate	0
(3) Glutamate + NAD$^+$ → NH$_4^+$ + α-KG + NADH + H$^+$	2.5
(4) P5C + NADP$^+$ → Glutamate + NADPH + H$^+$	2.5
(5) Glutamate + NAD$^+$ → NH$_4^+$ + α-KG + NADH + H$^+$	2.5
(6) α-KG + NAD$^+$ + CoA → Succinyl-CoA + CO$_2$ + NADH + H$^+$	2.5
(7) Succinyl-CoA + GDP + Pi → Succinate + GTP + CoA	1
(8) Succinate + FAD → Fumarate + FADH$_2$	1.5
(9) Fumarate + H$_2$O → Malate	0
(10) 2 NH$_4^+$ + HCO$_3^-$ + 3 ATP → Urea + 2 ADP + 1 AMP + 2 Pi + PPi (equivalent to 4 high-energy bonds)	−4
C. Cytoplasm (Malate to Pyruvate)	
(11) Malate + NAD$^+$ → Oxaloacetate + NADH + H$^+$	2.5
(12) Oxaloacetate + GTP → Phosphoenolpyruvate + CO$_2$ + GDP	−1
(13) Phosphoenolpyruvate + ADP → Pyruvate + ATP	1
D. Mitochondria (Pyruvate to CO$_2$ and H$_2$O)	
(14) Pyruvate + NAD$^+$ + CoA → Acetyl-CoA + CO$_2$ + NADH + H$^+$	2.5
(15) Acetyl-CoA + 2 H$_2$O + 3 NAD$^+$ + FAD + GDP + Pi → 2 CO$_2$ + 3 NADH + 3 H$^+$ + FADH$_2$ + GTP + CoA	10
E. Net Reaction	
C$_6$H$_{14}$N$_4$O$_2$ + 5.5 O$_2$ → 2 CH$_4$N$_2$O + 4 CO$_2$ + 3 H$_2$O + 2 Urea	23.5

α-KG, α-ketoglutarate; P5C, Δ^1-pyrroline-5-carboxylate.

TABLE 4.5
ATP Production from the Oxidation of Leucine in Mammals

Reactions	ATP Production
A. Mitochondria and Cytoplasm (Leucine to KIC)	
(1) Leucine + α-KG $\rightarrow$ KIC + Glutamate	0
B. Mitochondria (KIC to CO_2 and H_2O)	
(2) Glutamate + NAD^+ $\rightarrow$ NH_4^+ + α-KG + NADH + H^+	2.5
(3) NH_4^+ + 1.5 ATP $\rightarrow$ 0.5 Urea + 1 ADP + 0.5 AMP + 1 Pi + 0.5 PPi	-2
(4) KIC + CoA + NAD^+ $\rightarrow$ Isovaleryl-CoA + CO_2 + NADH + H^+	2.5
(5) Isovaleryl-CoA + FAD $\rightarrow$ β-Methylcrotonyl-CoA + $FADH_2$	1.5
(6) β-Methylcrotonyl-CoA + ATP + CO_2 + H_2O $\rightarrow$ β-Methylglutaconyl-CoA + ADP + Pi	-1
(7) β-Methylglutaconyl-CoA + H_2O $\rightarrow$ HMG-CoA	0
(8) HMG-CoA $\rightarrow$ Acetyl-CoA + Acetoacetate	
(9) Acetyl-CoA + 2 O_2 + 3 NAD^+ + FAD + GDP + Pi $\rightarrow$ 2 CO_2 + 4 H_2O + 3 NADH + 3 H^+ + $FADH_2$ + GTP + CoA	10
(10) Acetoacetate + Succinyl-CoA $\rightarrow$ Acetoacetyl-CoA + Succinate	0
(11) Succinate + GTP + CoA $\rightarrow$ Succinyl-CoA + GDP	-1
(12) Acetoacetyl-CoA $\rightarrow$ 2 Acetyl-CoA	
(13) 2 Acetyl-CoA + 4 H_2O + 6 NAD^+ + 2 FAD + 2 GDP + 2 Pi $\rightarrow$ 4 CO_2 + 6 NADH + 6 H^+ + 2 $FADH_2$ + 2 GTP + 2 CoA	20
C. Net Reaction	
$C_6H_{13}NO_2$ + 7.5 O_2 $\rightarrow$ 0.5 CH_4N_2O + 5.5 CO_2 + 5.5 H_2O + 0.5 Urea	32.5

KIC, α-ketoisocaproate; α-KG, α-ketoglutarate.

$$\text{Glutamate: } C_5H_9NO_4 + 4.5O_2 \rightarrow NH_3 + 5CO_2 + 3H_2O \left(ATP/CO_2 = 4.5; \text{ mol/mol} \right)$$

$$\text{Glutamine: } C_5H_{10}N_2O_3 + 4.5O_2 \rightarrow 2NH_3 + 5CO_2 + 2H_2O \left(ATP/CO_2 = 4.5; \text{ mol/mol} \right)$$

$$\text{Alanine: } C_3H_7NO_2 + 3O_2 \rightarrow NH_3 + 3CO_2 + 2H_2O \left(ATP/CO_2 = 5; \text{ mol/mol} \right)$$

$$\text{Aspartate: } C_4H_7NO_4 + 3O_2 \rightarrow NH_3 + 4CO_2 + 2H_2O \left(ATP/CO_2 = 3.75; \text{ mol/mol} \right)$$

$$\text{Leucine: } C_6H_{13}NO_2 + 7.5O_2 \rightarrow NH_3 + 6CO_2 + 5H_2O \left(ATP/CO_2 = 5.75; \text{ mol/mol} \right)$$

$$\text{Palmitate: } C_{16}H_{32}O_2 + 23O_2 \rightarrow 16CO_2 + 16H_2O \left(ATP/CO_2 = 6.625; \text{ mol/mol} \right)$$

$$\text{Glucose: } C_6H_{12}O_6 + 6O_2 \rightarrow 6CO_2 + 6H_2O \left(ATP/CO_2 = 5; \text{ mol/mol} \right)$$

4.1.4 CELL-, TISSUE-, AND SPECIES-SPECIFIC DEGRADATION OF AAS

Degradation of AAs is catalyzed by specific enzymes, whose distribution and, therefore, the catabolic pathways of AAs vary greatly among different cells, tissues, and species (Table 4.6).

TABLE 4.6

Degradation of Amino Acids (AAs) in Sense and Non-Sense Organs

AA	Sense Organs					Non-Sense Organs											
	Eye[a]	Ear	Nose	TG	Skin[b]	Brain	SI	Liver	SM	Kidney	Heart	WA	Ovary	Testes	PL	MG	PAN
Alanine	+	+	+	+	+	+	+	+	+	+	+	+	+	+	+	+	+
Arginine[c]	+	+	+	+	+	+	+	+	+	+	+	+	+	+	+	+	+
Aspartate	+	+	+	+	+	+	+	+	+	+	+	+	+	+	+	+	+
Asparagine	+	?	?	?	?	+	–	+	–	+	–	–	+[f]	+	+	–	+
Citrulline[d]	+	+	+	+	+	+	+	+	+	+	+	+	+	+	+	+	+
Cysteine[e]	?	?	?	?	?	+	–	+	–	+	–	–	–	–	–	–	+
GABA	+	?	?	?	?	+	–	+	–	+	–	–	–	–	–	–	–
Glutamate	+	+	+	+	+	+	+	+	+	+	+	+	+	+	+	+	+
Glutamine	+	+	+	+	+	+	+	+	+	+	+	+	+	+	+	+	+
Glycine[c]	+	?	?	?	+	+	+	+	–	+	–	–	+	+	+	+	+
Histidine	?	?	?	?	+	+	–	+	–	–	–	–	–	–	–	–	+
Isoleucine	+	+	+	+	+	+	+	–[g]	+	+	+	+	+	+	+	+	+
Leucine	+	+	+	+	+	+	+	–[g]	+	+	+	+	+	+	+	+	+
Lysine	?	?	?	?	+	+[h]	–	+	–	+[h]	–	–	–	–	–	–	–
Methionine	?	?	?	?	+	+[h]	+[h]	+	–	+[h]	–	–	+[h]	+[h]	+[h]	+[h]	+[h]
Phenylalanine	+	?	?	?	+	–	+	+	–	+	–	–	–	–	–	+/–[i]	+
Proline	?	?	?	?	+	+	+	+	–	+	–	–	+	+	+	–	+
OH–proline	?	?	?	?	+	+	+	+	+	+	–	+	+	+	+	+	–
Ornithine	+	+	+	+	+	+	+	+	+	+	+	+	+	+	+	+	+
Serine	+	?	?	?	+	+	+	+	–	+	–	–	+	+	+	+	+
Threonine	?	?	?	?	?	–	–	+	–	+	–	–	–	–	–	–	+
Tryptophan	+	?	?	?	+	+	+	+	–	+	–	–	+	+	+	+[h]	+
Tyrosine	+	?	?	?	+	+	–	+	–	+	–	–	+	+	+	+	+
Valine	+	+	+	+	+	+	+	–[g]	+	+	+	+	+	+	+	+	+

Source: Chen, J. et al. 2020. *Adv. Exp. Med. Biol.* 1265:57–70; He, W.L. et al. 2020. *Adv. Exp. Med. Biol.* 1265:167-18; Hou, Y.Q. et al. 2020. *Adv. Exp. Med. Biol.* 1265:21–37; Li, X.Y. et al. 2020b. *Adv. Exp. Med. Biol.* 1265:71–95; Wu, G. 2020a. *Adv. Exp. Med. Biol.* 1265:201–216.

[a] Metabolites include melanin and dopamine (from phenylalanine and tyrosine), and serotonin and melatonin (from tryptophan).

[b] Metabolites include melanin and dopamine (from phenylalanine and tyrosine), serotonin and melatonin (from tryptophan), as well as urocanic acid and histamine (from histidine).

[c] Rates of degradation of L-arginine vary among animal species, tissues, and cell types.

[d] Citrulline is converted into arginine, which is subsequently degraded via arginase, nitric oxide synthase, and other tissue-specific enzymes.

[e] Cysteine may be used for the production of H_2S, the synthesis of glutathione, or conjugation with some biochemicals. Glutathione synthesis and conjugation occur virtually in all tissues, but are not considered as pathways for cysteine catabolism.

[f] Present in ovarian tumors.

[g] Degradation of branched-chain amino acids in the liver of mammals and birds is nearly absent under physiological conditions, but is relatively active in the liver of fish.

[h] Very low rates for either partial degradation or complete oxidation to CO_2.

[i] Species-specific expression. Enzyme activity is present in bovine and goat mammary tissues but is absent from porcine, rat, and guinea pig mammary tissues.

Note: "?", lack of data; "+", presence of the metabolic pathway; "–", lack of synthesis of an amino acid from precursors other than its α-ketoacid; GABA, γ-aminobutyrate; MG, mammary glands; PAN, pancreas; PL, placenta; SI, small intestine; SM, skeletal muscle; TG, tongue; WA, white adipose tissue.

Thus, like AA synthesis, catabolism of most AAs occurs in a tissue- and cell-specific manner. Due to the complex compartmentation of AA degradation in cells, extracellularly and intracellularly derived AAs may have very different metabolic fates. Additionally, rates of degradation of AAs are critically dependent on their extracellular concentrations. For reversible reactions, AA catabolism is also influenced by their equilibrium. For most AAs, the cooperation of multiple organs is required for their biological oxidation in the presence of oxygen to CO_2, NH_3, and water, with NH_3 being further oxidized primarily to urea in mammals and uric acid in uricotelic species (e.g., birds; Chapter 6). Ammonia (a gas) and urea have much higher solubilities in water (18.8 and 12.9 mol/L at 37°C and 1 atmosphere, respectively) than CO_2 (a gas; 22.7 mmol/L), O_2 (a gas; 1.0 mmol/L), and uric acid (0.36 mmol/L) under the same conditions (Engineering ToolBox 2008). If CO_2 and other metabolically generated gasses (e.g., NH_3 and NO) are expired efficiently from the body, their production does not affect the volume of tissues or animals.

In humans and other animals, alanine, aspartate, glutamate, arginine, and ornithine can be degraded by all types of cells and tissues, but the rates of their degradation vary considerably. Except for the placenta, mammary gland, and mature erythrocytes, all types of cells and tissues (including skeletal muscle and heart) can degrade glutamine via the phosphate-activated glutaminase pathway (Wu et al. 2011a). With exception of the liver, all other organs and cells can initiate BCAA transamination and can decarboxylate the α-ketoacids of BCAAs. All of the other AAs can be degraded in the liver but net degradation may not always occur depending on their extracellular concentrations. For example, there was no net degradation of physiological levels of glutamine (0.5 to 1 mM in the perfusion medium) in the perfused rat liver (Lund and Watford 1976). However, net degradation of glutamine occurs in the liver when its extracellular concentration exceeds 1 mM. Hepatic AA catabolism is regulated by dietary intakes of nutrients (e.g., protein, lipids, and carbohydrate) and hormones (e.g., insulin and glucagon) (Wester et al. 2015). Among extrahepatic tissues and cells, only the kidneys and small intestine can degrade phenylalanine to form tyrosine. Because the catabolism of some AAs in the liver produces acetoacetate, which does not undergo oxidation in hepatocytes, this metabolite is oxidized into CO_2 and water by extrahepatic tissues and cells. All AA transaminases and AA decarboxylases depend on vitamin B_6 for their catalytic activities. Vitamin B_6 is also required for the activities of threonine aldolase, some D-AA racemases, cystathionase, cystathionine synthase, the glycine cleavage system, kynureninase (kynurenine hydrolase), kynurenine transaminase, methionine synthetase, and serine hydroxymethyl transferase. Note that the presence of mRNA levels for enzymes for AA degradation in cells or tissues does not necessarily mean that the related metabolic pathways actually occur. To provide definitive evidence, the conversion of AAs to their degradation products must be measured under physiologically relevant conditions. The rates of whole-body catabolism of some AAs in humans and other animals are summarized in Table 4.7. It appears that in the fed state, glutamine has the highest rate of whole-body catabolism in healthy adults, followed by arginine and glycine.

4.1.5 Age-Dependent Changes in AA Catabolism

The rates of the degradation of most AAs generally decrease with age in both humans and other animals (Waterlow and Stephen 1967; Wu 2018), and the response to advanced age is affected by the physiological state and dietary AA intake (i.e., dietary ingredients and their AA content). This is illustrated by the catabolism of absorbed dietary AAs (those that are not synthesized de novo) in the whole bodies of neonatal, weanling, gestating, and lactating swine (Table 4.8). However, arginine metabolism in pre-weaning mammals is now known to be one exception, because expression of arginase in extrahepatic tissues is low or negligible before weaning but is induced by glucocorticoids during weaning (Wu et al. 2000b). The near absence of arginase in the small intestine of pre-weaning mammals (e.g., pigs and mice) minimizes arginine degradation and maximizes the output of diet- and enterocyte-derived arginine into the portal circulation (Wu et al. 1996). This is nutritionally and physiologically significant for neonatal survival and growth, because the milk of most mammals (except for cats and horses) is severely deficient in arginine (Chapter 3).

TABLE 4.7

Rates of the Catabolism of Amino Acids (AAs) in Humans and Other Animals

AA	Species	Nutritional State	Endogenous Flux[a] (μmol/kg BW/h)	Degradation (μmol/kg BW/h)
Arginine	Human infants	Total parenteral nutrition	173	34
	Preterm infants	Fed (enterally)	461	29[b]
	Adult humans	Fed (enterally)	58	20
	Neonatal pigs (3.9 kg BW)	Fed (enterally)	315	79
	Growing pigs (28 kg BW)	Fed (enterally)	254	63
	Adult rats	Fed (enterally)	424	122
Cysteine	Adult humans	Fasted for 12 h	36–47	5.3
Glutamine	Preterm human infants	Fasted	755	463[b]
	Preterm human infants	Fed (enterally)	619	327[b]
	AGA infants	Fasted	545	253[b]
		Fed (enterally)	488	196[b]
	SGA infants	Fasted	791	499[b]
		Fed (enterally)	671	379[b]
	Adult humans	Post-absorptive	348	306[c]
	Young pigs	Fed (enterally)	860	528
	Adult rats	Post-absorptive	1,959	1,089–1,338
		Septic, post-absorptive	2,331	1,232
Glutamate	Human infants	Fed (enterally)	605 (421–789)	155[b]
	Adult humans	Post-absorptive	83	15
	Young pigs	Fed (enterally)	1,179	316
Glycine	Adult humans	Fed (enterally)	445	81
	Neonatal pigs	Fed (enterally)	≥1,600	167
	Adult rats	Post-absorptive	660	262[d]
		Fasted (for 24 h)	888	553[e]
		Diabetic (ALX)	732	397[e]
Isoleucine	Adult rats	Post-absorptive	180	108[d]
Leucine	AGA infants	Fed (enterally)	98	51
	SGA infants	Fed (enterally)	151	67
	Adult humans	Fasted for 12 h	101	15
		Fed (enterally)	96	40
		Post-absorptive (14-h fast)	87	16
	Adult rats	Post-absorptive	521	320
		Septic, post-absorptive	628	413
Lysine	Adult humans	Fed (enterally)	71	28
		Fed (2 to 100 mg Lys/kg BW/day)	46	5–31
	Adult rats	Post-absorptive state (AP)	840	728[d]
Methionine	Adult humans	Fasted for 12 h	16	12
		Fasted for 10 h	19	10
		Fed	41	34
Phe	Adult humans	Fasted for 12 h	45	9.3
		Fed (enterally)	44–52	15
Proline	Preterm infants	Fed (enterally)	237	–
	Adult humans	Fed (enterally)	115	52[c]
	Neonatal pigs	Fed (enterally)	424	228
Serine	Adult humans	Fasted (overnight)	150	115
	Adult rats	Fasted for 24 h	858	764[e]
		Diabetic (ALX)	630	536[e]

(Continued)

TABLE 4.7 (*Continued*)
Rates of the Catabolism of Amino Acids (AAs) in Humans and Other Animals

AA	Species	Nutritional State	Endogenous Flux[a] (μmol/kg BW/h)	Degradation (μmol/kg BW/h)
Threonine	Preterm infants	Fed (enterally)	211	15
	Adult humans	Fed (enterally)	90	16
Tyrosine	Adult humans	Fasted for 12 h	42–48	7.5
		Fed (enterally)	31–40	10
Valine	Adult humans	Post-absorptive (14-h fast)	80	12
	Adult rats	Post-absorptive	430	336[d]

Source: Beaufrere, B. et al. 1989. *Am. J. Physiol.* 257:E712–721; Beaufrere, B. et al. 1992. *Am. J. Physiol.* 263:E214–E220; Bertolo, R.F. and D.G. Burrin. 2008. *J. Nutr.* 138:2032S–2039S; Borgonha, S. et al. 2002. *Am. J. Clin. Nutr.* 75:698–704; Chapman, K.P. et al. 2013. *J. Nutr.* 143:290–294; Cortiella, J. et al. 1992. *Am. J. Clin. Nutr.* 56:517–525; Dasarathy, J. et al. 2010. *Am. J. Clin. Nutr.* 91:357–365; Denne, S.C. et al. 1991. *Pediatr. Res.* 30:23–27; Fukagawa, N. et al. 1998. *Am. J. Clin. Nutr.* 68:380–388; Gersovitz, M. et al. 1980. *Metabolism* 29:1087–1094; Kalhan, S.C. and R.W. Hanson. 2012. *J. Biol. Chem.* 287:19786–19791; Kuhn, K.S et al. 1999. *Am. J. Clin. Nutr.* 70:484–489; Meredith, C.N. et al. 1986. *Am. J. Clin. Nutr.* 43:787–794; Parimi et al. 2002. *Am. J. Physiol.* 282:E618–E625; Parimi, P.S. et al. 2004. *Am. J. Clin. Nutr.* 79:402–409; Raguso, C.A. et al. 2000. *Am. J. Clin. Nutr.* 71:491–499; Rennie, M.J. et al. 1982. *Clin. Sci.* 63:519–523; Squires, E.J. and J.T. Brosnan. 1983. *Biochem. J.* 210:277–280; Staten, M.A. et al. 1984. *Am. J. Clin. Nutr.* 40:1224–1234; Tomlinson, C. et al. 2011. *Pediatr. Res.* 69:46–50; Van Der Schoor, S.R.D. et al. 2007. *Am. J. Clin. Nutr.* 86:1132–1138; Van Der Schoor, S.R.D. et al. 2010. *Pediatr. Res.* 67:194–199; Waterlow, J.C. and J.M.L. Stephen. 1967. *Clin. Sci.* 33:489–506; Wu, G. and S.M. Morris Jr. *Biochem. J.* 1998. 336:1–17; Wu, Z.L. et al. 2016. *Amino Acids* 48:1541–1552; Yoshida, S. et al. 1991. *Biochem. J.* 276:405–409.

[a]   The endogenous flux of an amino acid is the sum of the entry of the amino acid into the plasma from the endogenous synthesis of the amino acid and the release of the amino acid from protein degradation, and is estimated on the basis of the flux of the amino acid in the arterial plasma minus the intake of the amino acid from diet. In the fasting or post-absorptive state, the intake of the amino acid from diet is considered to be zero. Plasma flux = AA intake + AA Synthesis + Protein breakdown = AA oxidation + Protein synthesis.

[b]   Estimated on the basis of the rate of whole-body protein synthesis in preterm infants (20 g protein/kg BW/day; Stack et al. 1989). The infants gained 15 g of BW/kg BW/day.

[c]   Estimated on the basis of the rate of whole-body protein synthesis in adult humans (2.86 g protein/kg BW/day).

[d]   Estimated on the basis of the rate of whole-body protein synthesis in adult rats (6.3 g protein/kg BW/day; Waterlow and Stephen 1967).

[e]   Estimated on the basis of the rate of whole-body protein synthesis in adult rats (5.3 g protein/kg BW/day).

Note: BW = body weight.

4.1.6   HALF-LIVES OF AAS IN THE BLOOD PLASMA OF HUMANS AND OTHER ANIMALS

The half-life ($T_{1/2}$) of an AA in the blood plasma is defined as the time required for the concentration or amount of the AA in the plasma to be reduced by 50% (Böger and Bode-Böger (2001). To date, there is a limited database on the half-lives of AAs in the blood circulation of humans and other animals. Just like the whole-body catabolism of AAs, their half-lives in the plasma vary substantially among different species at different physiological and pathological states (Lassala et al. 2009; Parimi et al. 2005; Wu et al. 2007). This is clearly illustrated by findings from studies with laboratory and farm animals, as well as humans (Table 4.9). In general, the half-lives of AAs (ranging from 0.63 to 1.88 h) in the plasma increase with advanced age, but are shorter during pregnancy than in the non-pregnancy state. In addition, different AAs have different half-lives in the plasma. For example, the values for arginine, glutamine, and glycine are much lower than those for aspartate, citrulline, glutamate, leucine, lysine, and proline in pigs, and similar qualitative results are obtained for arginine, citrulline, glutamine, leucine, and proline in sheep and rats.

TABLE 4.8
Catabolism of Absorbed Dietary Amino Acids (that are not synthesized *De Novo*) in the Whole Bodies of Neonatal, Weanling, Gestating, and Lactating Swine

Amino Acid	Extra-Intestinal Catabolism (g/day)					Extra-Intestinal Catabolism (mg/kg BW/day)				
	Sow-Reared Pigs (14 days of age; 3.9 kg BW)[a]	Weaned Pigs (30 days of age; 7.8 kg BW)[b]	180-Day-Old Pigs (117 kg BW)[c]	Gestating Gilts (maternal BW = 130 kg)[d]	Lactating Sows (maternal BW = 174 kg)[e]	Sow-Reared Pigs (14 days of age; 3.9 kg BW)[a]	Weaned Pigs (30 days of age; 7.8 kg BW)[b]	180-Day-Old Pigs (117 kg BW)[c]	Gestating Gilts (maternal BW = 130 kg)[d]	Lactating Sows (maternal BW = 174 kg)[d]
Cys	0.13	0.56	5.84	2.08	9.58	34	71	34	15	56
His	0.18	0.94	8.23	2.92	15.3	46	120	48	21	90
Ile	0.75	1.31	13.7	4.65	19.9	193	169	80	34	117
Leu	1.55	2.71	29.8	11.1	45.5	396	347	175	81	268
Lys	1.52	1.72	14.7	1.41	12.3	389	221	87	10	72
Met	0.34	0.36	4.70	0.62	6.27	87	46	28	4.5	37
Phe	0.57	1.64	16.4	6.02	28.2	146	210	97	44	166
Thr	0.65	1.05	11.2	3.59	13.9	166	135	66	26	82
Trp	0.23	0.28	3.69	0.50	5.13	59	36	22	3.7	30
Tyr	0.72	1.25	13.6	4.57	20.6	186	160	80	33	121
Val	0.68	1.26	14.4	5.31	21.1	174	161	85	39	124

Source: Hou, Y.Q. et al. 2016. *Adv. Nutr.* 7:331–342.

[a] Pigs were nursed by sows fed a diet containing 18% crude protein. The 14-day-old piglet (3.9 kg of BW) consumed 913 mL of milk/day and gained 235 g of BW/day.

[b] Pigs were weaned at 21 days of age to a corn- and soybean meal-based diet containing 21.5% crude protein. The 30-day-old weaned pig (7.8 kg of BW) consumed 351 g of diet/day and gained 290 g of BW/day.

[c] Pigs were fed a corn- and soybean meal-based diet containing 14% crude protein. The 180-day-old pig (117 kg of BW) consumed 3.39 kg of diet/kg BW/day and gained 0.85 kg of BW/day. Data were calculated as described by Hou et al. (2016).

[d] Days 110–114 of gestation. The gilt gestated ten live fetuses, was fed a corn- and soybean meal-based diet containing 12.2% crude protein, and consumed 2 kg of diet/day. The weight of the gilt at days 110–114 of gestation was 170 kg (130 kg of maternal BW + 40 kg of conceptuses). AA accretion in the fetus during days 110–114 of gestation (g/day) is as follows: Cys, 1.36; His, 2.40; Ile, 3.28; Leu, 7.56; Lys, 6.61; Met, 2.02; Phe, 3.81; Thr, 3.61; Trp, 1.37; Tyr, 2.54; and Val, 4.55. AA accretion in maternal tissues during days 110 to 114 of gestation (g/day) is as follows: Cys, 0.49; His, 0.77; Ile, 1.31; Leu, 2.53; Lys, 2.23; Met, 0.69; Phe, 1.27 Thr, 1.30; Trp, 0.41; Tyr, 1.00; and Val, 1.56.

[e] Day 14 of lactation. The lactating sow (170 kg of BW) nursed nine piglets, was fed a corn- and soybean meal-based diet containing 18% crude protein, and consumed 5.94 kg diet/day.

TABLE 4.9
Half-Lives of Amino Acids in the Blood Plasma of Laboratory and Farm Animals[a]

Amino Acid	Pigs							Rats		Sheep			Humans (Adult)[h]
	8-Day-Old[b,c]	14-Day-old[b,c]	35-Day-Old[b,c]	6-mo Old[b]	11-Month[b]	Gestating Day 80[b]	Gestating Day 105[b,c]	Non-Diabetic (Adult)[b,d]	Diabetic (BB Rats, Adult)[b,d,e]	NP (Adult)[b]	Gestating[b,f,g] Day 105	Day 135	
L-Arginine	0.65	0.66	0.67	0.83	1.06	0.75	0.71	0.76	0.65	1.04	0.74	0.76	~1.0
L-Aspartate	1.03	1.06	1.12	1.44	1.69	1.20	1.08	–	–	1.61	1.10	1.08	–
L-Citrulline	1.25	1.27	1.31	1.60	1.82	1.45	1.38	1.46	1.48	1.88	1.47	1.49	1.0
L-Glutamate	1.02	1.08	1.19	1.42	1.70	1.28	1.14	–	–	1.64	1.22	1.19	0.5
L-Glutamine	0.63	0.64	0.66	0.79	0.95	0.70	0.67	0.70	0.69	0.93	0.71	0.72	~1.0
Glycine	0.67	0.68	0.70	0.81	0.98	0.73	0.70	0.74	0.62	0.94	0.73	0.72	1.05
L-Leucine	1.04	1.16	1.28	1.48	1.67	1.33	1.24	1.15	1.54	1.46	1.12	1.10	0.57–1.0[i]
L-Lysine	1.22	1.24	1.33	1.52	1.70	1.30	1.21	–	–	–	–	–	–
L-Proline	0.91	0.92	0.95	1.10	1.25	0.96	0.90	1.37	1.33	1.28	0.95	0.93	–

[a] Values (the means) are expressed as hours.

[b] Determined as described by Wu et al. (2007).

[c] Wu et al. (2007, 2010).

[d] 100–105 days of age.

[e] 30 days after onset of diabetes.

[f] singleton pregnancy.

[g] Wu et al. (2007).

[h] Bratusch-Marrain et al. (1980), FDA (2004), Hahn et al. (1989).

[i] 0.57h in healthy adults, and 1.0h in adults with insulin-dependent diabetes (Bratusch-Marrain et al. 1980).

Note: mo, month; NP, non-pregnant; –, Data are not available.

4.1.7 ALTERATIONS IN THE RATES AND PATTERNS OF AA CATABOLISM IN DISEASE

The rates and patterns of AA catabolism in humans and other animals are altered under various pathological conditions (Hou et al. 2020; Li et al. 2020b; Newsholme et al. 2011). For example, infections increase the rates of whole-body and tissue-specific catabolism of arginine, glutamine, glycine, proline, and tryptophan in mammals (including humans, pigs, and rats) to increase the generation of NO, ammonia, and urea, while reducing the production of creatine from arginine and glycine, of arginine from glutamine and proline, and of serotonin from tryptophan (Deutz et al. 1992; Field et al. 2000; Förstermann and Münzel 2006; Le Floc'h et al. 2011; Luiking et al. 2012; Morris 2009). In addition, the whole-body and intramuscular degradation of BCAAs is impaired in persons with obesity or diabetes, leading to increases in their plasma concentrations (Yang et al. 2015). Furthermore, compared with control (nondiabetic) individuals, the rates of whole-body turnover of alanine and its conversion into glucose are increased but the rates of whole-body turnover of glutamine are unaltered (with an increase in the conversion of glutamine into glucose and a decrease in its oxidation to CO_2) in patients with noninsulin-dependent diabetes mellitus (Stumvoll et al. 1996); these data are summarized in Table 4.10. Similar results have been reported for patients with insulin-dependent diabetes mellitus (Hall et al. 1979; Hankard et al. 2000). Finally, both acidosis and cancer stimulate the whole-body catabolism of glutamine and BCAAs in humans and animal models in an attempt to regulate pH and energy homeostasis as well as the production of ammonia and alanine (Curthoys and Watford 1995). Thus, AA catabolism is an active field of both nutritional and biomedical research.

TABLE 4.10
Rates of Whole-Body Catabolism of Glutamine and Alanine in Adult Humans with NonInsulin-Dependent Diabetes Mellitus (NIDDM)[a]

Variable	Control (Nondiabetic) individuals ($n = 18$)	NIDDM Patients ($n = 14$)	P-value
Age, Years	48.4 ± 1.7	54.8 ± 2.3	NS
Body weight, kg	81.5 ± 2.8	87.7 ± 3.1	NS
Body mass index, kg/m²	27.7 ± 1.0	28.1 ± 1.0	NS
Plasma glucose, mM	5.2 ± 0.1	11.0 ± 0.8	<0.001
Plasma glutamine (Gln), mM	0.61 ± 0.03	0.58 ± 0.03	0.59
Plasma glutamate, mM	0.066 ± 0.004	0.077 ± 0.006	0.52
Plasma alanine (Ala), mM	0.33 ± 0.02	0.37 ± 0.02	0.16
Plasma free fatty acids, mM	0.707 ± 0.046	0.751 ± 0.038	0.27
Plasma insulin, pmol/L	60 ± 8	72 ± 13	0.28
Plasma C-peptide, nmol/L	0.42 ± 0.04	0.52 ± 0.05	0.10
Plasma glucagon, ng/L	92 ± 6	126 ± 9	0.006
Whole-body phenylalanine appearance, μmol/kg BW/min	0.68 ± 0.05	0.64 ± 0.03	0.53
Whole-body turnover, μmol/kg BW/min			
Glutamine	4.81 ± 0.23	4.40 ± 0.31	0.41
Alanine	4.54 ± 0.24	5.64 ± 0.33	0.02
Conversion into glucose, μmol/kg BW/min			
Glutamine	0.57 ± 0.04	1.08 ± 0.10	0.001
Alanine	1.02 ± 0.09	1.56 ± 0.17	0.008
Conversion of glutamine into alanine, μmol Gln/kg BW/min	0.10 ± 0.01	0.34 ± 0.04	0.001
Formation of Ala from glutamine, μmol Ala/kg BW/min	0.17 ± 0.02	0.57 ± 0.07	0.001
Oxidation of glutamine to CO_2, μmol Gln/kg BW/min	2.84 ± 0.27	1.84 ± 0.15	0.03
Release from the forearm, μmol/kg BW/min			
Glutamine	−0.77 ± 0.05	−0.62 ± 0.09	0.008

(Continued)

TABLE 4.10 (*Continued*)

Rates of Whole-Body Catabolism of Glutamine and Alanine in Adult Humans with NonInsulin-Dependent Diabetes Mellitus (NIDDM)[a]

Variable	Control (Nondiabetic) individuals (*n* = 18)	NIDDM Patients (*n* = 14)	*P*-value
Alanine	−0.45 ± 0.04	−0.39 ± 0.04	0.35
Uptake from the blood into the forearm, μmol/kg BW/min			
Glutamine	0.44 ± 0.04	0.43 ± 0.08	0.92
Alanine	0.29 ± 0.03	0.26 ± 0.04	0.43
Net balance across the forearm, μmol/kg BW/min			
Glutamine (net release)	−0.33 ± 0.03	−0.19 ± 0.04	0.02
Alanine (net release)	−0.15 ± 0.02	−0.14 ± 0.02	0.78
Uptake of glucose from blood into the forearm, μmol/kg BW/min	0.76 ± 0.08	0.76 ± 0.13	0.99
Fractional extraction by the forearm, %			
Glutamine	23.7 ± 1.5	20.8 ± 2.3	0.017
Alanine	29.8 ± 2.7	27.0 ± 4.0	0.16

Source: Stumvoll, M. et al. 1996. *Diabetes* 45:863–868.

[a] Overnight-fasted individuals (nine males and nine females in the control group; nine males and five females in the NIDDM group) were used for the study. Values are means ± SEM.

Note: BW, body weight; NS, statistically not significant (*P* > 0.05).

4.2 PATHWAYS FOR THE DEGRADATION OF AAs IN ANIMAL CELLS

4.2.1 HISTORICAL PERSPECTIVES

A major product of AA catabolism is ammonia. It has been known as a metabolite of animals (including humans) since the Middle Ages. However, how ammonia was produced in the body was a mystery until the late 1700s and the 1800s when chemists and physicians had interest in studying the components of proteins in foodstuffs and their utilization by animals and humans. In 1794, the French chemist Antoine Lavoisier proposed that the oxidation of organic substances (including AAs) to CO_2 and water would be a source of ammonia produced by the body. Due to the lack of analytical techniques to quantify most nitrogenous products, metabolic pathways for AA degradation were largely unknown at the end of the 19th century. In the early 1900s, it was discovered that AAs are oxidized into α-ketoacids and ammonia by deaminases and that ammonia is subsequently converted into urea and uric acid in mammals but exclusively to uric acid in avian species. In the 1930s when stable isotopes (e.g., ^{15}N-,^{13}C- or ^2H-labeled AAs) became available for use in biochemical research, they provided scientists with a powerful tool to initiate studies aimed at elucidating detailed pathways for AA catabolism in organisms (Borsook and Dubnoff 1943). Meanwhile, classic biochemical techniques were used to identify new enzymes for the degradation of AAs, primarily glutamate and glutamine (Krebs 1935). Progress in this endeavor was greatly facilitated by the availability of radioactive tracers (e.g., ^{14}C- or ^3H-labeled AAs) in the 1940s. Thus, by the early 1960s, pathways for AA metabolism had largely become known and were elegantly summarized by Hans A. Krebs in his chapter published in the book entitled *Mammalian Protein Metabolism* edited by H. Munro and J.B. Allison in 1964. The discovery of the synthesis of NO from arginine via NO synthases in the 1980s renewed interest in AA catabolism.

4.2.2 CATABOLISM OF ALANINE, ASPARTATE, ASPARAGINE, GLUTAMATE, AND GLUTAMINE

The pioneering work of biochemists in the early 20th century on the intermediary metabolism of alanine, aspartate, asparagine, and glutamate laid a foundation for subsequent studies of AA catabolism in animals. Specifically, L. Knopf, A.I. Ringer, and G. Lusk discovered the conversion of asparagine, glutamate, and aspartate to glucose in animals, respectively, in 1903, 1908, and≈1910. Similar observations were confirmed by studies with diabetic dogs by H.D. Dakin in 1913. Meanwhile, Dakin found that alanine was also readily converted into glucose in the canine liver. A series of papers of H.A. Krebs in the 1930s greatly advanced the field of AA catabolism by discovering glutamine synthesis from glutamate and ammonia, as well as glutamine degradation via the kidney-type glutaminase (now known as GLS1) and the liver-type glutaminase (now known as GLS2) (Watford 2015). In addition, alanine, aspartate, and glutamate were found to participate in intracellular transamination in animal tissues. Subsequently, glutamate was recognized as an excitatory neurotransmitter in the brain in the 1960s. It was discovered in the 1970s–1990s that dietary glutamate is almost completely degraded by the small intestine of the mammals studied including rats, humans, pigs, cattle, and sheep) in first-pass metabolism and, therefore, does not enter the portal circulation in significant quantities. This seminal finding substantially expanded our knowledge about the utilization of dietary glutamate by mammals and helped scientists to understand the safety of consumption of monosodium glutamate by humans and other animals as a flavor enhancer and physiological regulator of intestinal function.

$$Glutamine + H_2O \rightarrow Glutamate + NH_4^+$$

$$\left[glutaminase \left(a\ mitochondrial\ enzyme \right);\ present\ in\ most\ tissues \right]$$

$$Asparagine + H_2O \rightarrow Aspartate + NH_4^+$$

$$\left[asparaginase \left(a\ cytosolic\ enzyme \right);\ expressed\ in\ most\ of\ extra-intestinal\ tissues \right]$$

4.2.2.1 Enzyme-Catalyzed Reactions for the Initiation of Glutamine, Glutamate, Aspartate, and Alanine Catabolism

Since H.G. Windmueller and A.E. Spaeth reported (1975, 1976) that the rat's small intestine utilizes large amounts of both luminal and arterial glutamine as well as luminal aspartate and glutamate as major metabolic fuels, there has been growing interest in the use of glutamine to improve the gut function of animals (including humans) in the last four decades. Subsequent work by these authors has revealed the extensive catabolism of luminal glutamate and aspartate by the small-intestinal mucosa of adult rats. The degradation of glutamine is initiated primarily by phosphate-activated glutaminase, a mitochondrial enzyme expressed in most tissues (Curthoys and Watford 1995). Interestingly, although asparagine differs from glutamine by one $-CH_2$ unit, the small intestine does not degrade asparagine (Windmueller and Spaeth 1976). The metabolic fates of glutamine, glutamate, and aspartate in the rat small intestine and porcine enterocytes are summarized in Table 4.11. Additionally, the findings in the 1980s that glutamine stimulates muscle protein synthesis and lymphocyte proliferation led to extensive laboratory and clinical research on glutamine turnover, physiology, and nutrition in the 1990s and 2000s. Glutamine is now known to be an abundant AA in physiological fluids (e.g., the plasma, milk, fetal fluid, and skeletal muscle), a major vehicle for interorgan metabolism of both carbon and nitrogen, a key regulator of gene expression, and an essential precursor for the synthesis of molecules [including nucleotides, amino sugars, and $NAD(P)^+$] (see Chapter 11).

Transamination plays an important role in initiating the degradation of alanine, aspartate, and glutamate to yield pyruvate, oxaloacetate, and α-KG, respectively (Figure 4.3). These α-ketoacids are oxidized to CO_2 and water via conversion into acetyl-CoA through cooperation between the cytosol and mitochondria. Alanine transaminase (also known as glutamate-pyruvate transaminase) and aspartate transaminase (also known as glutamate-oxaloacetate transaminase) are abundant in the mitochondria and/or the cytoplasm of most mitochondria-containing cells, particularly

TABLE 4.11

The Metabolic Fates of the Carbons of Luminal Amino Acids by the Small Intestine of Adult Rats and Young Pigs

Metabolite	The Small Intestine of Adult Rats				The Small Intestine of 29-Day-Old-Pigs Reared by Sows				The Small Intestine of 58-Day-Old Weaned Pigs			
	Gln[a]	Glu	Asp[b]	Arg[c]	Gln	Glu	Asp[d]	Pro	Gln	Glu	Arg	Pro
	% of Total Catabolized Amino Acid Carbon in Product											
CO_2	56	64	51	14	52	52	48	1.6	46.3	49.1	0.9	1.6
Lactate	16	16	20	–	3.6	3.9	4.0	0.0	4.8	5.2	0.0	0.0
Proline	5.8	4.1	1.7	13	5.2	5.2	0.0	–	2.4	2.0	57	–
Citrulline	4.4	3.2	1.1	17	4.1	4.1	0.0	56	13.3	8.1	4.0	57
Alanine	4.0	3.3	8.0	1.1	6.8	6.5	21	0.0	6.7	7.0	0.0	0.0
Ornithine	2.1	1.0	0.4	32	0.50	0.50	0.0	38	1.6	1.2	38	37
Arginine	–	–	–	–	0.80	0.80	0.0	4.4	3.3	2.4	–	4.4
Glutamine	–	0.3	–	–	–	0.0	0.0	0.0	–	–	0.0	0.0
Glutathione	–	–	–	–	4.6	11.7	0.0	0.0	6.0	7.7	0.0	0.0
Aspartate	–	–	–	–	7.0	7.1	–	0.0	6.5	7.5	0.0	0.0
Asparagine	–	–	–	–	0.5	0.4	0.2	0.0	0.3	0.2	0.0	0.0
Other OA	4	3	2.9	4.4	7.7	7.7	27	0.0	8.9	9.5	0.0	0.0

Source: Hou, Y.Q. and Wu. 2018. *Amino Acids* 50:1497–1510; Wu, G. 1998. *J. Nutr.* 128:1249–1252; Windmueller, H.G. and A.E. Spaeth. 1975. *Arch. Biochem. Biophys.* 171:662–672; Windmueller, H.G. and A.E. Spaeth. 1976. *Arch. Biochem. Biophys.* 175:670–676; Wu, G. 1997. *Am. J. Physiol.* 272:G1382–G1390; Wu, G. 1998. *J. Nutr.* 128:1249–1252; Wu, G. et al. 2011. *J. Anim. Sci.* 89:2017–2030; Wu, G. et al. 1996. *Am. J. Physiol.* 271:G913–G919; Wu G. (unpublished work).

[a] 2.5% of glutamine carbon appeared in glutamate.

[b] 1.2% of aspartate carbon appeared in glutamate.

[c] 1.2% of arginine carbon appeared in glutamate.

[d] Determined as described by Wu (1997).

Note: OA, organic acids (α-KG, malate, pyruvate, and succinate) other than amino acids and lactate.

hepatocytes and enterocytes. Thus, the activities of these two enzymes in serum are often determined to assess hepatic injury in clinical medicine. In addition, glutamine transaminases L and K, which convert glutamine to α-ketoglutaramate (Figure 4.3), are ubiquitous in both mitochondria and the cytoplasm of animal tissues (including skeletal muscle, liver, and kidneys; Cooper and Meister 1981). α-Ketoglutaramate undergoes hydrolysis by ω-amidase (expressed in both mitochondria and the cytoplasm of mitochondria-containing cells) to form α-KG and NH_3 (Cooper et al. 2016). As shown in Table 4.2, glutamine has a lower value of energetic efficiency than glutamate in animals (37% vs. 47%) because additional two ATP are required for converting the glutaminase-generated ammonia to urea.

In addition to transamination, the dehydrogenation of glutamate by GDH results in the production of α-KG plus ammonia. Although GDH catalyzes the interconversion of glutamate into α-KG and ammonia, the equilibrium of this reaction at physiological concentrations of substrates and products favors the production of ammonia in the liver to facilitate its detoxification as urea (in mammals) and uric acid (in birds). GDH is a major enzyme that directly produces ammonia from AA catabolism in many cell types (primarily hepatocytes and renal tubules), but its activity is low in the small intestine, skeletal muscle, and heart of mammals and birds. In fish and crustaceans, the proximal intestine, liver, skeletal muscle, and kidneys express high GDH activity to catabolize glutamate as a major metabolic fuel (Li et al. 2021a). Interestingly, this enzyme is allosterically activated by L-leucine and ADP but inhibited by GTP, which has important implications for the regulation of glutamate metabolism and hormone secretion.

Decarboxylation of glutamate by glutamate decarboxylase produces GABA in tissues (Figure 4.4). This enzyme is particularly abundant in the brain and the pancreas. In mammals, glutamate decarboxylase exists in two isoforms, which are encoded by two different genes: *GAD1* (the brain) and *GAD2* (the pancreas). GAD1 and GAD2 proteins have molecular weights of 67 and 65 kDa, respectively. GABA is further degraded to either succinate by succinate semialdehyde dehydrogenase or γ-hydroxybutyrate (Figure 4.4). In the brain, the production and catabolism of GABA from glutamate occur in neurons and glial cells, respectively (Figure 4.5), with the glutamate being synthesized from BCAAs and glutamine in a cell-specific manner. This is crucial for brain function, because the blood-brain barrier is not permeable to GABA and glutamate (He and Wu 2020). These highly cell-specific events play an important role in neurotransmission.

Besides glutamine transaminases, glutamine:fructose-6-phosphate transaminase (GFAT; a cytosolic enzyme) catalyzes the formation of glutamate from glutamine in all cell types, as noted in Chapter 3. GFAT is particularly abundant in red blood cells (Zhang et al. 2021) and endothelial cells (Wu et al. 2001). This reaction may be the major source of glutamate in red blood cells that do not take up extracellular glutamate. Glutamine donates the amide group (-NH$_2$) for the synthesis of UDP-*N*-acetylglucosamine (see Chapter 11), which is a precursor for the formation of

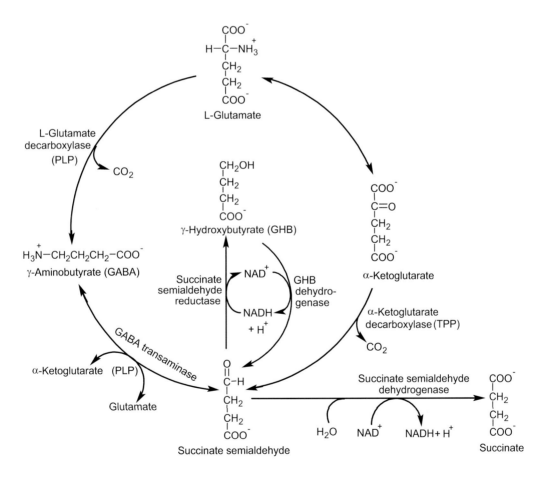

FIGURE 4.4 Catabolism of γ-aminobutyrate in humans and other animals. PLP, pyridoxal phosphate; TPP, thiamine pyrophosphate. PLP is a cofactor for glutamate decarboxylase and γ-aminobutyrate transaminase, whereas TPP is required by α-ketoglutarate decarboxylase for catalytic activity.

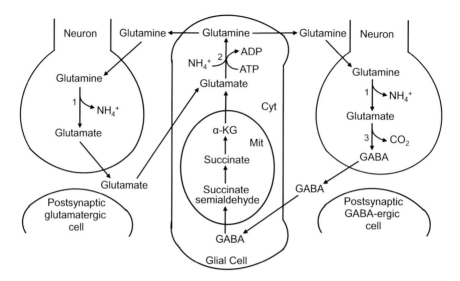

FIGURE 4.5 Cell-specific production and catabolism of GABA in the brain of humans and other animals. A synapse (a small gap between two cells) allows for the first cell (the presynaptic cell) to communicate with the second cell (the postsynaptic cell) through a chemical signal (e.g., glutamate or GABA). These neurotransmitters act on the postsynaptic cell through specialized protein molecules called neurotransmitters receptors. In the brain, neurons produce and release glutamate and GABA into synapses from which these two amino acids are taken up by glial cells to form glutamine or succinate, respectively. Within mitochondria, succinate can be metabolized to α-ketoglutarate which is subsequently converted into glutamate by glutamate dehydrogenase. The enzymes that catalyze the indicated reactions are as follows: (1) phosphate-activated glutaminase (mitochondrial enzyme); (2) glutamine synthetase (cytosolic enzyme); and (3) glutamate decarboxylase (a pyridoxal phosphate-dependent cytosolic enzyme). GABA, γ-aminobutyrate; α-KG = α-ketoglutarate; Mit, mitochondrion; Cyt, cytoplasm.

all macromolecules containing amino sugars (including membrane hormone receptors, hyaluronic acid, chondroitins, heparin, and mucins). Thus, the hexosamine-synthetic pathway is essential to cell growth, development, and function, as well as the structure of the extracellular matrix that contains large amounts of glycosaminoglycans.

4.2.2.2 Kidney- and Liver-Type Glutaminases

Phosphate-activated glutaminase (a mitochondrial enzyme) is quantitatively the major enzyme for initiating glutamine degradation in nearly all mitochondria-containing mammalian cells. The lack of this enzyme in the placenta and mammary glands maximizes the transfer of glutamine from the mother to the fetus and from the maternal blood to milk, respectively. Of particular note, the avian liver has little or no glutaminase activity (Coon and Balling 1984; Wu et al. 1998), which minimizes glutamine degradation to ammonia and CO_2 so as to maximize the availability of glutamine for uric acid synthesis. Glutaminase has two isoforms: the hepatic protein (~66.3 kDa) and the renal protein (~73.5 kDa) that are encoded by two different genes and differ in biochemical properties (Curthoys and Watford 1995). Glutaminase in extrahepatic tissues and cells is the kidney-type enzyme. Differences in catalytic kinetics and regulation between kidney- and liver-type glutaminases, as originally noted by H.A. Krebs in 1935, are summarized as follows:

Kidney-Type Glutaminase:

    a. does not require NH_3 for activation
    b. has low K_m for glutamine and low affinity for phosphate
    c. is subject to inhibition by low [glutamate]

Liver-Type Glutaminase:

    a. absolutely requires NH_3 for activation
    b. has high K_m for glutamine and high affinity for phosphate
    c. is not affected by low [glutamate]

The glutamine-derived glutamate is degraded as described previously. In many cells types, including cells of the immune system (e.g., lymphocytes, macrophages, and natural killer cells), oxidation of glutamate is incomplete, producing relatively large amounts of aspartate and alanine (Field et al. 2000; Newsholme et al. 1985). The importance of high rates of glutamine hydrolysis to glutamate, aspartate, alanine, and ammonia in cells, which is known as glutaminolysis (Figure 4.6), remains obscure, but may provide aspartate and ATP for syntheses of purine and pyrimidine nucleotides. Note that glutamine is only partially catabolized via glutaminolysis possibly to conserve its nitrogen and carbon. In the small intestine of most mammals, glutamate is used to produce ATP, alanine, ornithine, proline, citrulline, and arginine, as discussed in Chapter 3. Although glucose had long been considered to be the sole metabolic fuel for immunocytes, the work of E.A. Newsholme in the 1980s led to the recognition that glutamine is extensively degraded via glutaminolysis in lymphocytes and macrophages. Subsequent studies by G. Wu and colleagues concluded that glutamine contributes approximately 50% of ATP to these cells. It is now known that dietary glutamate, aspartate, and glutamine plus arterial glutamine provide approximately 80% of ATP to the small-intestinal mucosae in mammals, chickens, fish, and crustaceans (Li et al. 2020a,c; 2021a,b). Recently, Sakai et al. (2020) reported that a human intestinal epithelial cell monolayer (Caco-2 cells) completely metabolized luminal ^{13}C- and ^{15}N-labeled glutamate.

Although the mammalian liver contains high glutaminase activity, oxidation of physiological concentrations of glutamine by the rat liver is limited (Lund and Watford 1976). To explain this phenomenon, D. Haussinger proposed in 1990 an intercellular glutamine-glutamate cycle between periportal and perivenous hepatocytes in the liver (Figure 4.7). Periportal and perivenous hepatocytes are located near the portal vein and hepatic vein, respectively, representing approximately 90%–95% and 5%–10% of total hepatocytes in the liver. When extracellular glutamine is <1 mM, it is converted to glutamate and NH_3 in periportal hepatocytes and can be resynthesized from glutamate and NH_3 in perivenous hepatocytes. The intercellular glutamine-glutamate cycle consumes energy (one mole of ATP per mole of glutamine turnover), but has important physiological significance. First, this cycle can scavenge ammonia by the high-affinity glutamine synthetase and maintain low concentrations of ammonia in the plasma. Second, this cycle can help adjust ammonia flux into either urea or glutamine according to the needs for regulation of the acid-base balance. At normal pH, there is no release of glutamine by the liver. However, at pH < 7.4, the hydrolysis of glutamine into glutamate and ammonia is decreased and the formation of glutamine from glutamate and ammonia is increased, thereby resulting in the release of glutamine from the liver.

4.2.2.3 Asparaginase

Asparagine is hydrolyzed by asparaginase (a cytosolic enzyme) to form aspartate and ammonia (McGee et al. 1971). This enzyme is virtually absent from the small intestine (as noted previously) and skeletal muscle, but is expressed predominantly in the liver and, to a much lesser extent, kidneys, with a K_m value of 4.7 mM for asparagine. The activity of asparaginase is relatively low in the pancreas, brain, lung, spleen, heart, eyes, testis, ovaries, and placenta. Studies with rats have shown that hepatic asparaginase activity is barely detectable at birth, increases rapidly within 1 week, and continues to rise until 3 weeks of age (McGee et al. 1971). In adults, asparaginase activity in the kidneys is about 25% of that in the liver. The tissue distribution of asparaginase differs greatly from that of glutaminase (a mitochondrial enzyme), despite the similar chemical structures of asparagine and glutamine. This reflects different functions of these two enzymes in metabolism and physiology. For example, although both glutamine and asparagine promote cancer cell proliferation, the former is a major metabolic fuel and the latter is an AA exchange factor in tumors (Krall et al. 2016).

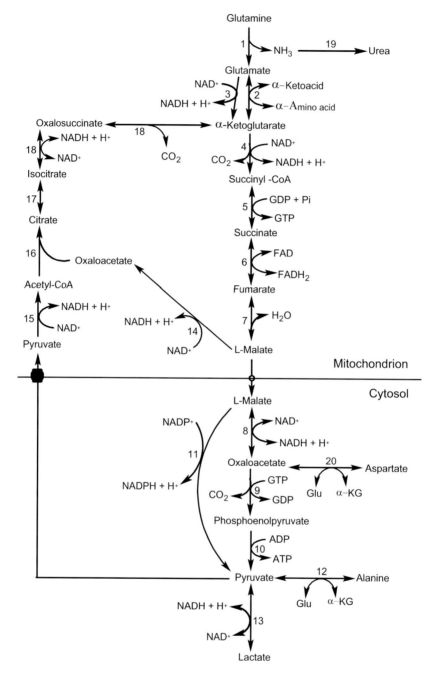

FIGURE 4.6 Catabolism of glutamine in animal cells with the mitochondria. This metabolic pathway occurs in humans and other animals. The enzymes that catalyze the indicated reactions are as follows: (1) phosphate-activated glutaminase; (2) glutamate transaminase; (3) glutamate dehydrogenase; (4) α-ketoglutarate dehydrogenase; (5) succinate thiokinase; (6) succinate dehydrogenase; (7) fumarase; (8) NAD⁺-linked malate dehydrogenase (cytoplasm); (9) phosphoenolpyruvate carboxykinase; (10) pyruvate kinase; (11) NADP⁺-linked malate dehydrogenase; (12) glutamate-pyruvate transaminase; (13) lactate dehydrogenase; (14) NAD⁺-linked malate dehydrogenase (mitochondria); (15) pyruvate dehydrogenase; (16) citrate synthase; (17) aconitase; (18) isocitrate dehydrogenase; (19) the conversion of ammonia into urea via the urea cycle (see Chapter 6); and (20) glutamate-oxaloacetate transaminase. Glutamine degradation to form glutamate, aspartate, and alanine is known as glutaminolysis.

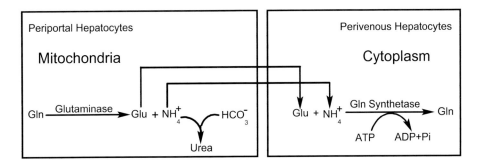

FIGURE 4.7 Intercellular glutamine-glutamate cycle involving periportal and perivenous hepatocytes in the mammalian liver. Ammonia that is not converted into urea in periportal hepatocytes is utilized to synthesize glutamine in perivenous hepatocytes.

In this role, intracellular asparagine exchanges with extracellular AAs and regulates the uptake of AAs, particularly arginine, histidine, and serine. Like glutaminase, mammalian asparaginase is inducible by glucocorticoids. Unlike glutaminase, asparaginase is not found in the mitochondria of cells in young or adult animals (McGee et al. 1971).

In contrast to normal mammalian cells, asparaginase is undetectable in leukemia cells and transplanted neoplasias with high glutaminase activity (Richards and Kilberg 2006). Because acute lymphoblastic leukemia cells and some other tumors do not synthesize asparagine, they must depend on extracellular asparagine for growth and survival. Thus, depriving these cells of extracellular asparagine through the administration of exogenous asparaginase can result in their death by inducing apoptosis and limiting protein synthesis. This is the principle underlying the use of *E. coli*-derived asparaginase (intravenous, intramuscular, or subcutaneous injection) to treat patients with acute lymphoblastic leukemia cells or other types of cancers (Broome 1981).

4.2.3 Catabolism of Arginine, Citrulline, and Ornithine

Work on arginine catabolism is dated back to 1904 when arginase was discovered by A. Kossel and H.D. Dakin to hydrolyze this AA to ornithine and urea. Physiological and nutritional studies between the late 1930s and the 1970s identified important roles for arginine in the synthesis of creatine, ammonia detoxification, and maintenance of nitrogen balance in young mammals and carnivores. During the 1950s, arginine was found to exist also as phosphoarginine (a hydrogen atom in the guanidino group was replaced by a phosphate group) in skeletal muscles from various invertebrate animals, where phosphoarginine functions to store biological energy like phosphocreatine in vertebrate species (Chapters 1 and 3). Since the discovery of NO synthesis from L-arginine by tetrahydrobiopterin (BH4)-dependent NO synthase (NOS) in mammalian cells in 1987 (Figure 4.9), there has been growing interest in arginine biochemistry, nutrition, and physiology.

4.2.3.1 Multiple Enzymes for the Initiation of Arginine Catabolism

Arginine catabolism occurs via multiple pathways, generating NO, ornithine, urea, polyamines, proline, glutamate, creatine, agmatine, CO_2, and water (Wu and Morris 1998). These pathways are initiated by arginases, three isoforms of the NOS, arginine decarboxylase (Figure 4.8), and arginine:glycine amidinotransferase (Chapter 5). Certain animals, such as carnivorous fish, may possess arginine deiminase to hydrolyze arginine into citrulline and ammonia, but this metabolic pathway remains to be established. In mammals, the arginase pathway is quantitatively most important for arginine degradation and responsible for the oxidation of arginine to CO_2 and H_2O, with an energetic efficiency of approximately 30% (Table 4.2). For example, the arginase pathway

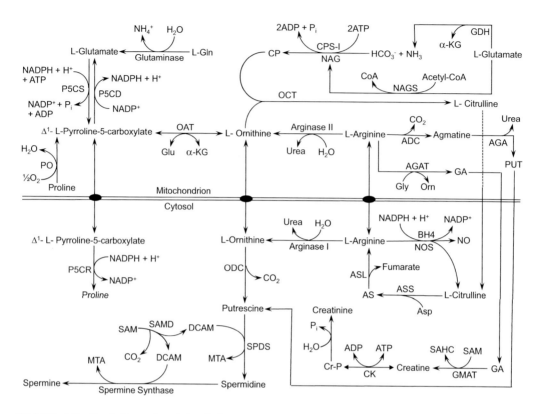

FIGURE 4.8 Catabolism of arginine in humans and other animals. Multiple enzymes initiate arginine catabolism in cells. Most enzymes that degrade arginine are cell- and tissue-specific. ADC, arginine decarboxylase; AGA, agmatinase; AGAT, arginine:glycine amidinotransferase; ASL, argininosuccinate lyase; ASS, argininosuccinate synthase; AS, argininosuccinate; Asp, aspartate; BH$_4$, (6R)-5,6,7,8-tetrahydro-L-biopterin; CP, carbamoyl phosphate; CPS-I, carbamoyl phosphate synthetase-I (ammonia); DCAM, decarboxylated S-adenosylmethionine; Glu, glutamate; Gln, glutamine; GDH, glutamate dehydrogenase; GA, guanidinoacetate; GMAT, guanidinoacetate N-methyltransferase; CK, creatine kinase; Cr-P, creatine-phosphate; α-KG, α-ketoglutarate; MTA, methylthioadenosine; NAG, N-acetylglutamate; NAGS, N-acetylglutamate synthase; NO, nitric oxide; NOS, nitric oxide synthase; OAT, ornithine aminotransferase; OCT, ornithine carbamoyltransferase; ODC, ornithine decarboxylase; PO, proline oxidase; PUT, putrescine; P5CD, pyrroline-5-carboxylate dehydrogenase; P5CR, pyrroline-5-carboxylate reductase; P5CS, pyrroline-5-carboxylate synthase; SAM, S-adenosylmethionine; SAMD, S-adenosylmethionine decarboxylase; SAHC, S-adenosylhomocysteine; SPDS, spermidine synthase.

is responsible for the catabolism of 99% of arginine in the small intestine, as well as 76%–85% and 81%–96% arginine in extra-intestinal tissues of postweaning pigs and adult rats, respectively (Wu et al. 1996, 2016). Quantitatively, <1% and 2% of metabolized arginine is utilized for polyamine synthesis and constitutive NO production, respectively, in mammalian cells. Some of the NO generated in the body is exhaled through the lungs (Kharitonov et al. 1995), whereas some is oxidized to nitrite and nitrate for urinary excretion (Wu and Morris 1998). Because guanidinoacetate (a product of arginine:glycine amidinotransferase) is neurotoxic, it must be converted to a nontoxic substance, namely creatine, which has both metabolic and regulatory roles. There is complex compartmentation of arginine degradation at cellular, tissue, and whole-body levels.

Arginine + H$_2$O → Citrulline + NH$_4^+$ (arginine deiminase, possible present in certain animals)

4.2.3.2 Arginases

Much of our current knowledge on the molecular regulation of arginase expression has been produced by the extensive studies of S.M. Morris Jr. (2009) and other researchers. Type-I arginase is expressed abundantly in hepatocytes and to a limited extent, in extrahepatic cells, including enterocytes of postweaning mammals, endothelial cells, mammary epithelial cells, macrophages, and primate red blood cells. By contrast, Type-II arginase is widely expressed at relatively low levels in virtually all mitochondria-containing extrahepatic cells (including neuronal, renal, vascular, and muscle cells) and plays an important role in regulating the synthesis of NO, proline, and polyamines. Arginases I and II are encoded by two different genes and differ in their biochemical and immunological properties. In animals, the arginine-derived ornithine undergoes either transamination by ornithine aminotransferase (a mitochondrial enzyme) to generate Δ^1-pyrroline-5-carboxylate (P5C; a precursor for the mitochondrial synthesis of glutamate and the cytosolic production of proline) or decarboxylation to form putrescine (Wu 1998; Hou and Wu 2018). Concentrations of polyamines depend on the rates of their synthesis and degradation. Pathways for the catabolism of polyamines will be described in Chapter 5.

Arginase expression varies with tissue and species. One example is that arginase activity is absent from rapidly growing porcine placentae and enterocytes of suckling piglets (Wu et al. 1996), but is very high in the small intestine of postweaning mammals (Windmueller and Spaeth 1976). These metabolic strategies help maximize the supply of arginine from mother to fetus and from maternal milk to the systemic circulation of neonates, while also providing polyamines for the small-intestinal mucosae of weaned mammals (Wu 1998). Thus, in the placenta and small intestine, both of which grow rapidly, proline is the major source of ornithine for polyamine synthesis (Wu et al. 2000a, 2005). By contrast, a relatively high arginase activity is expressed in ovine placentae to compensate for lower concentrations of proline in the ovine maternal plasma. This species difference in placental arginase expression contributes to an unusual abundance of arginine (e.g., 4–6 mM at Day 40 of gestation) in porcine allantoic fluid but much lower concentrations of arginine (e.g., 0.82 mM at Day 60 of gestation) in ovine allantoic fluid. Interestingly, citrulline is unusually abundant (e.g., 10 mM at Day 60 of gestation) in ovine allantoic fluid as an effective precursor for arginine generation in the conceptus. Available evidence shows that arginase is expressed in human and rat placentae. Notably, the lactating mammary gland in all species studied (including cattle, pig, rat, and sheep) expresses a high level of arginase, resulting in arginine deficiency but relatively high abundances of both proline and polyamines in the milk.

Because arginase II and OAT are localized in the mitochondria, arginine and ornithine enter this organelle from the cytoplasm via the mitochondrial basic AA carriers (BAC). Some of these transporters have been identified as follows: ORNT1 (SLC25A15), ORNT2 (SLC25A2), and ORNT3 (SLC25A29; Camacho and Rioseco-Camacho 2009). ORNT1 (primarily an antiporter), which exchanges the mitochondrial citrulline for the cytosolic ornithine, is expressed in most tissues, with the highest abundances being in the liver, pancreas, lung, and kidney. ORNT2 (primarily an antiporter) is more restricted to the liver, testes, spleen, lung, and pancreas (Gutiérrez-Aguilar and Baines 2013), but has a broader specificity than ORC1 and also uses L- and D-histidine, L-homoarginine, and D-isomers of ornithine, lysine, and ornithine as substrates (Fiermonte et al. 2003). ORNT3 (a uniporter) is expressed widely in tissues, including the small intestine, colon, heart, brain, liver, lung, and kidney (Monné et al. 2019). ORNT3 transports arginine and lysine and to a much lesser extent, ornithine and histidine from the cytosol into the mitochondria, with the K_m of 0.4 and 0.7 mM for arginine and lysine, respectively (Monné et al. 2019). Available evidence shows that ORNT3 is the primary transporter of arginine across the mammalian mitochondrial membrane (Porcelli et al. 2014).

4.2.3.3 NO Synthases

There are three isoforms of the NOS: NOS1, NOS2, and NOS3 that differ greatly in biochemical properties and tissue distribution (Table 4.12). The NOS1 isoform (also known as nNOS) was first discovered in 1990 in neuronal tissues, the NOS2 isoform (also known as iNOS) was originally found in 1991 to be inducible under certain conditions in macrophages, and the NOS3 isoform

TABLE 4.12

Compartmentation, Biochemical Properties, and Gene Structure of the NOS Isoforms in Animal Tissues

Tissue	nNOS (NOS1)	iNOS (NOS2)	eNOS (NOS3)
(1) Tissue Distribution			
Blood vessel	Weakly expressed	Weakly expressed	Cytoplasm, PMC
Brain	Cytoplasm, RER PM, mitochondria	Primarily cytoplasm	Cytoplasm, PMC
Brown adipose	Weakly expressed in cytoplasm	Cytoplasm, nucleus	Cytoplasm, nucleus, PMC, membrane caveolae
Heart	Mitochondria, SR	Primarily cytoplasm	PTC, sarcoplasm
Kidney	Mitochondria	Primarily cytoplasm	Cytoplasm, PMC
Liver	Mitochondria	Primarily cytoplasm in periportal hepatocytes	Cytoplasm, PMC in hepatocytes
Placenta	Weakly expressed	Absent	Cytoplasm, PMC
Skeletal muscle	Mitochondria, sarcoplasm, SM	Sarcoplasm, SM	Sarcoplasm, SR, SM caveolae
White adipose	Weakly expressed in cytoplasm	Cytoplasm, plasma membrane	Cytoplasm, PMC
(2) Chromosome, Gene Size, and Gene Structure			
Chromosome	12	17	7
Gene size	160 kb	37 kb	21 kb
Gene structure	29 Exons, 28 introns	26 Exons, 25 introns	26 exons, 25 introns
(3) Protein Structure, Molecular Weight, and Enzyme Kinetics			
Protein structure	Homodimer	Homodimer	Homodimer
Molecular weight	160 kDa/monomer	125–130 kDa/monomer	135 kDa/monomer
K_m (arginine)	3–16 μM	3–16 μM	2.9 μM
K_m (BH4)	0.2–0.3 μM	1.6 μM	0.2–0.3 μM
K_m (NADPH)	3–5 μM	0.2–1 μM	3.0 μM

Source: Wu, G. and S.M. Morris, Jr. 1998. *Biochem. J.* 336:1–17; Alderton, W.K. et al. 2001. *Biochem. J.* 357:593–615.

Note: BH4, tetrahydrobiopterin; eNOS, endothelial NO synthase; iNOS, inducible NO synthase; nNOS, neuronal NO synthase; PM, postsynaptic membrane; PMC, plasma membrane caveolae; PTC, plasmalemmal and T-tubular caveolae; RER, rough endoplasmic reticulum; SM, sarcolemmal membrane; SR, sarcoplasmic reticulum.

(also known as eNOS) was first identified in 1991 in endothelial cells. Both NOS1 and NOS3 are Ca^{2+}-dependent and constitutively expressed, whereas NOS2 is Ca^{2+}-independent and expressed abundantly in response to immunological challenges. The NOS isoforms can be present in the plasma membrane caveolae, cytoplasm, nucleus, rough endoplasmic reticulum, and mitochondria, depending on isoform and cell type.

The NOS isoforms are encoded by three different genes, have 51%–57% homology in nucleotide sequences, and require arginine, O_2, BH4, NADPH, calmodulin, FMN, and FAD for NO synthesis. Arginine, BH4, and heme promote and stabilize the active dimeric form of all isoforms of the NOS. Additionally, BH4 plays a redox role in NOS catalysis. Specifically, BH4 donates an electron to form a BH4 radical, which then returns to the reduced state by accepting an electron from a flavin in the reductase domain of NOS. BH4 is synthesized *de novo* from GTP in all cell types, with GTP cyclohydrolase I as the first and rate-controlling enzyme (Figure 4.9). Sepiapterin (a synthetic chemical) can be readily converted into BH4 via the "salvage pathway" in all cells, and this pathway has been exploited experimentally to treat endothelial dysfunction

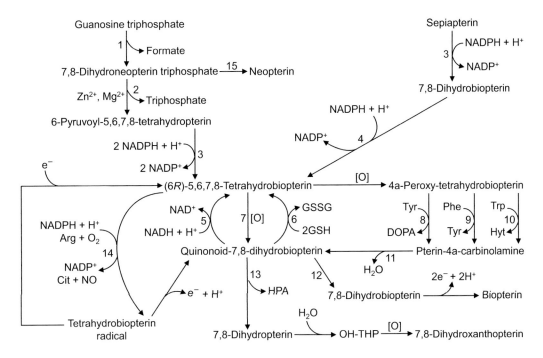

FIGURE 4.9 Synthesis of tetrahydrobiopterin via both *de novo* and salvage pathways in humans and other animals. Enzymes that catalyze the indicated reactions are as follows: (1) GTP cyclohydrolase I; (2) 6-pyruvoyl tetrahydropterin synthase; (3) sepiapterin reductase; (4) dihydrofolate reductase; (5) dihydropteridine reductase; (6) reduction by reduced glutathione; (7) oxidation by reactive oxygen and nitrogen species; (8) tyrosine hydroxylase; (9) phenylalanine hydroxylase; (10) tryptophan hydroxylase; (11) pterin-4a-carbinolamine dehydratase; (12) nonenzymatic rearrangement; (13) nonenzymatic loss of the alkyl side chain; (14) NO synthase; and (15) phosphatases. Arg, arginine; Cit, citrulline; DOPA, 3,4-dihydroxyphenylalanine; GSH, glutathione; GSSG, glutathione disulfide (oxidized glutathione); HPA, 2-hydroxy-propionaldehyde ($CH_3CHOHCHO$); Hyt, 5-hydroxytryptophan; OH-THP, 6-hydroxy-5,6,7,8-tetrahydropterin; Trp, tryptophan; Tyr, tyrosine.

associated with BH4 deficiency. Thus, since the initial description of a pteridine in butterflies by F.G. Hopkins in 1889, research on BH4 and its related substances (Figure 4.10) has greatly advanced AA biochemistry and nutrition.

NOS and arginase compete for arginine in cell metabolism (Blachier et al. 2011; Wu and Morris 1998). Therefore, relative changes in their enzymatic activities serve as major determinants of NO and polyamine production in many cell types, including endothelial cells, macrophages, smooth muscle cells, astrocytes, bacteria, and parasites. A marked elevation in arginase activity provides a mechanism responsible for the survival of immunologically challenged parasites and bacteria.

4.2.3.4 The Arginine Paradox for NO Synthesis

The K_m values of NOS for arginine have been reported to be 3–20 μM (≤10% of intracellular arginine concentrations) depending on isoforms (e.g., 2.9 μM for eNOS). For comparison, intracellular concentrations of arginine are usually 0.5–2 mM in extrahepatic cells exposed to 0.1–0.2 mM extracellular arginine, which are the usual physiological concentrations in the plasma of healthy post-absorptive humans and animals, depending on species. Thus, in extrahepatic cells, intracellular concentrations of arginine are usually 5–10 times those found in the plasma or culture medium. Even in mammalian hepatocytes with an exceedingly high arginase activity, intracellular concentrations of arginine are normally 50–100 μM, depending on species and extracellular concentrations of arginine. Therefore, in animal cells exposed to 0.05 mM extracellular arginine, NOS is already well saturated with its substrate arginine and the enzyme-catalyzed reaction would not be affected

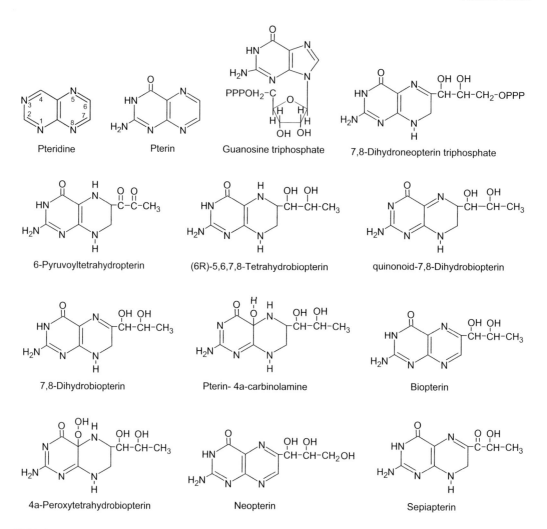

FIGURE 4.10 Chemical structures of tetrahydrobiopterin and related pterins. Except for sepiapterin (a synthetic substance), all other compounds are produced by animals. Tetrahydrobiopterin almost exclusively participates in the hydroxylation of arginine, aromatic amino acids (phenylalanine, tyrosine, and tryptophan), and related substances in humans and other animals. Sepiapterin is a substrate for tetrahydrobiopterin synthesis in animal cells. Biopterin is a useful indicator of immune activation in mammals and birds, whereas an elevated ratio of dihydrobiopterin to tetrahydrobiopterin suggests the presence of oxidative stress in animal cells. Some pterins (e.g., biopterin and neopterin) contribute to pigmentation in certain animals (e.g., insects and birds) and also serve as intra-species communication signals.

by an extracellular concentration of arginine greater than 0.05 mM. However, increasing extracellular concentrations of arginine from 0.05 to 10 mM dose-dependently increases NO production by endothelial cells, activated macrophages, and other cell types. This phenomenon has been termed "the arginine paradox" for NO synthesis. This paradox can now be explained satisfactorily by arginine-induced changes in the amounts of NOS or cofactors. For example, in cells (e.g., cytokine-stimulated astrocytes), arginine promotes the translation of NOS1 mRNA and increases the amount of iNOS, thereby enhancing NO synthesis. In endothelial cells, arginine has no effect on eNOS abundance but augments the expression of GTP cyclohydrolase I for BH4 synthesis, thereby stimulating NO generation (Wu et al. 2004).

4.2.3.5   Arginine Decarboxylase

Arginine decarboxylase (a mitochondrial enzyme) was discovered in the rat brain in 1994 and is the most recent addition to a family of mammalian arginine-metabolic enzymes. This enzyme catalyzes the synthesis of agmatine from arginine in the rat brain, liver, kidney, adrenal gland, macrophages, and other cell types. Agmatine was initially identified as an endogenous agonist at imidazoline receptors in the brain and was subsequently found to be an inhibitor of NOS. In cells expressing arginine decarboxylase, agmatine is decarboxylated by agmatinase (a mitochondrial enzyme) to produce putrescine (Figure 4.8), and this may be a novel path for polyamine synthesis in animal cells. There are species and perhaps developmental differences in the tissue distribution of arginine decarboxylase activity. For example, arginine decarboxylase or agmatinase activity is absent from porcine enterocytes (Wu et al. 1996, 2005). By contrast, low levels of both enzymes are expressed in the liver and ovine conceptuses (Wang et al. 2014). Additionally, agmatinase is present constitutively in some cell types (e.g., the RAW 264.7 murine macrophage line), and its expression can be induced by lipopolysaccharide (Sastre et al. 1998) and the hepatitis B virus (Mistry et al. 2002), suggesting a role for this enzyme in the pathogenesis of this liver disease. Because arginase activities are much higher than those of arginine decarboxylase or agmatinase in rat tissues, changes in arginase activities will likely have a much greater impact on mammalian synthesis of NO and polyamines, compared with arginine decarboxylase. At present, almost nothing is known about the properties of mammalian arginine decarboxylase or agmatinase nor agmatine metabolism *in vivo*.

4.2.3.6   Syntheses of Polyamines and Creatine from Arginine

Arginine-derived ornithine can be converted to putrescine, spermidine, and spermine via ornithine decarboxylase (ODC), spermidine synthase, and spermine synthase in almost all cell types (Chapter 5). As noted previously, ornithine can also be utilized for the synthesis of proline (Figure 4.8), which is used as a major substrate for the production of putrescine in the small intestine of neonatal mammals and in the placenta. In the tissues of some mammals (e.g., the conceptuses of sheep), an alternative source of putrescine is arginine decarboxylase, as described above. Specifically, arginine is decarboxylated by arginine decarboxylase to yield agmatine, which is hydrolyzed by agmatinase to putrescine (Chapter 5). This metabolic pathway, however, is absent from the small intestine and placenta of swine. In humans and other terrestrial animals, large amounts of creatine are formed from arginine, glycine, and methionine via inter-organ metabolism in animals, and these pathways will be described in Chapter 5.

4.2.4   Catabolism of BCAAs

Early in 1906, G. Embden recognized that leucine is converted into acetoacetate and β-hydroxybutyrate in mammals. By contrast, A.I. Ringer reported in 1913 that valine is converted into glucose via succinate as an intermediate, indicating a different metabolic pathway than leucine. Subsequently, N.L. Edson found in 1935 that isoleucine can be metabolized to either glucose or ketone bodies in animals, depending on experimental conditions. It was long assumed without much evidence that BCAAs were catabolized extensively in the liver. This assumption was questioned in 1965 by the observation that concentrations of BCAAs in the plasma did not change in dogs without a liver for up to 22h, suggesting that the liver is not a site for BCAA catabolism. This conclusion was subsequently supported by the finding that the liver has a very low activity of BCAA transaminase in the presence of physiological concentrations of BCAAs. Thus, in mammals and birds, the liver plays a minor role in BCAA degradation (Krebs 1972). In contrast to the liver, skeletal muscle had long been considered to be a relatively inert protein reservoir until 1961 when P. Johnson reported for the first time that[14]CO_2 is produced from L-[1-^{14}C]leucine by the rat diaphragm. Subsequent work established skeletal muscle as the major site for BCAA transamination in the body. Based on isotopic and enzymological studies, H.A. Krebs proposed in 1964 that BCAA catabolism shares the first three common steps (Figure 4.11): transamination, oxidative decarboxylation, and acyl-CoA dehydrogenation. The first two reactions are now known to be highly tissue-specific.

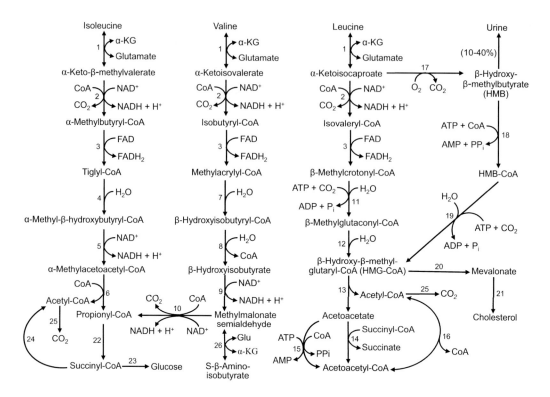

FIGURE 4.11 Catabolism of branched-chain amino acids (BCAAs) in humans and other animals. In mammals and birds, the transamination of BCAAs is initiated in their non-hepatic tissues (e.g., the skeletal muscle, intestine, heart, kidneys, brain, and mammary glands), with some of their α-ketoacids being decarboxylated to acyl-CoA in the same tissues. Because these tissues have a relatively low activity of branched-chain α-ketoacid dehydrogenase, most of the α-ketoacids are released to the blood for uptake and degradation by the liver. In some fish, their liver is a significant site for BCAA transamination. In all animals, inter-organ cooperation plays an important role in the complete oxidation of BCAAs to CO_2. Note that tiglyl-CoA, a metabolite of isoleucine, is also known as α-methylcrotonoyl-CoA or α-methylcrotonoyl-CoA, which differs from β-methylcrotonoyl-CoA, a metabolite of leucine. The enzymes that catalyze the indicated reactions are as follows: (1) BCAA transaminase; (2) branched-chain α-ketoacid dehydrogenase; (3) acyl-CoA dehydrogenase; (4) enoyl-CoA hydratase; (5) β-hydroxyacyl-CoA dehydrogenase; (6) acetyl-coA acetyltransferase; (7) enoyl-CoA hydratase; (8) β-hydroxyisobutyryl-CoA hydrolase; (9) β-hydroxyisobutyrate dehydrogenase; (10) methylmalonate semialdehyde dehydrogenase; (11) β-methylcrotonoyl-CoA carboxylase (a biotin-dependent enzyme); (12) β-methylglutaconyl-CoA hydratase; (13) HMG-CoA lyase; (14) 3-ketoacid CoA transferase; (15) succinyl-CoA:3-ketoacid CoA transferase; (16) acetoacetyl-CoA thiolase; (17) α-ketoisocaproate dioxygenase; (18) HMB-CoA synthase; (19) HMB-CoA carboxylase; (20) HMG-CoA reductase (an NADPH-dependent enzyme); (21) enzymes for cholesterol synthesis; (22) a series of enzymes for conversion of propionyl-CoA to succinyl-CoA [propionyl-CoA carboxylase (biotin), methylmalonyl-CoA racemase, and methylmalonyl-CoA isomerase (vitamin B_{12})]; (23) enzymes for gluconeogenesis; (24) enzymes for conversion of succinyl-CoA to acetyl-CoA; (25) enzymes of the Krebs cycle; and (26) β-aminoisobutyrate transaminase.

4.2.4.1 BCAA Transaminases

Two isoforms of BCAA transaminase (mitochondrial and cytosolic) have been identified in animal tissues (including skeletal muscle, small intestine, adipose tissue, mammary gland, placenta, kidneys, heart, and brain), which use α-KG as the major acceptor of the amino group (Table 4.13). This enzyme accepts all three BCAAs as substrates but has little activity with pyruvate and none with oxaloacetate. In the mammalian and avian livers, the mitochondria have little or low activity of BCAA transaminase (Harper et al. 1984). In mammals and birds, the level of the cytosolic enzyme protein in the liver

TABLE 4.13

Branched-Chain Amino Acid (BCAA) Transaminases and Branched-Chain α-Ketoacid (BCKA) Dehydrogenase in Mammalian Cells

Enzyme	Molecular Mass	Cofactor or Prosthetic Group
BCAA Transaminase		
Mitochondrial	41 kDa/monomer (homodimer)	Pyridoxal phosphate
Cytosolic	43 kDa/monomer (homodimer)	Pyridoxal phosphate
BCKA Dehydrogenase Complex		
BCKA decarboxylase (E1)	$\alpha_2\beta_2$ (1.7×10^2 kDa)	TPP
α-Subunit	46.5 kDa	Mg^{2+}
β-Subunit	37.2 kDa	
Dihydrolipoyl transacylase (E2)	α_{24} (1.12×10^6 kDa)	Lipoic acid
Subunit	46.518 kDa	
Dihydrolipoyl dehydrogenase (E3)	1.1×10^2 kDa	FAD
Subunit	55 kDa	
BCKD kinase	43 kDa/monomer (homodimer)	Mg^{2+}
BCKD phosphatase	4.6×10^2 kDa	Mn^{2+}
Subunit (catalytic)	33 kDa	

Source: Brosnan, J.T. and M.E. Brosnan. 2006. *J. Nutr.* 136: 207S–211S; Harper, A.E. et al. 1984. *Annu. Rev. Nutr.* 4: 409–454; Islam, M.M. et al. 2007. *J. Biol. Chem.* 282:11893–11903; and Reed et al. In: *Metabolic Interconversion of Enzymes* (Holzer, H., ed.). Springer, New York. pp 124–133.

Note: BCKA, branched-chain α-ketoacid; BCKD, branched-chain α-ketoacid dehydrogenase; TPP, thiamine pyrophosphate.

is also much lower than that in the skeletal muscle, kidney, heart, and small intestine. Thus, at physiological concentrations of BCAAs, their transamination in the liver of terrestrial mammals and birds is rather limited. This ensures that most of the dietary BCAAs are available to extrahepatic tissues for: (1) the synthesis of glutamate, glutamine, and alanine; and (2) the activation of the mechanistic target of the rapamycin signaling pathway to stimulate protein synthesis. Results of recent studies indicate that BCAAs are actively transaminated in the liver and other major tissues of some fish [e.g., largemouth bass and hybrid striped bass (carnivorous fish), as well as zebrafish], shrimp, and crustaceans, including the intestine, kidneys, and skeletal muscle (Li et al. 2021a,b). Due to the large size of skeletal muscle, this tissue is the major site for BCAA transamination in the body (Hutson et al. 2005).

Considerable oxidation of BCKAs occurs in extrahepatic tissues. For example, 28%, 29%, and 22% of the transaminated leucine are released as α-ketoisocaproate (KIC) from the skeletal muscle of 10-day-old fed, 12-h fasted, and 24-h fasted chicks, respectively, whereas 72%, 71%, and 78% of the transaminated leucine are oxidized into CO_2, respectively (Wu and Thompson 1987). In addition, about 40% of the transaminated BCAAs (leucine, isoleucine, and valine) is released as BCKAs from the lactating porcine mammary tissue, about 60% of the transaminated BCAAs is oxidized into CO_2, and 68% of the decarboxylated BCKAs is oxidized into CO_2 (Li et al. 2009). Furthermore, ~70% of the transaminated BCAAs (leucine, isoleucine, and valine) is released as BCKAs from the enterocytes of 50-day-old pigs, 30% the transaminated BCAAs is oxidized into CO_2, and 60% of the decarboxylated BCKAs is oxidized into CO_2. By contrast, 81–91% of the transaminated BCAAs (leucine, isoleucine, and valine) is released as BCKAs from porcine placentae, and 9–19% of the transaminated BCAAs is oxidized into CO_2 (Table 4.14), depending on gestational age. Clearly, the porcine placentae release most of the BCAA-derived BCKAs.

TABLE 4.14

Degradation of Branched-Chain Amino Acids in Porcine Placentae on Different Days of Gestation

	Days of Gestation								
	20	30	35	40	45	50	60	90	110
Leucine									
Decarboxylation[a]	0.05	0.09	0.20	0.27	0.16	0.09	0.08	0.08	0.08
Net KIC production[a]	0.43	0.63	1.10	1.64	1.07	0.84	0.63	0.61	0.61
Net transamination[a]	0.48	0.72	1.30	1.91	1.23	0.93	0.71	0.69	0.68
% of Transaminated leucine released as KIC	89.6	87.5	84.6	85.9	87.0	90.3	88.7	88.4	89.7
% of Transaminated leucine oxidized to CO_2	10.4	12.5	15.4	14.1	13.0	9.7	11.3	11.6	10.3
Isoleucine									
Decarboxylation[a]	0.04	0.12	0.17	0.23	0.13	0.07	0.07	0.06	0.06
Net KMV production[a]	0.35	0.52	0.84	1.29	0.86	0.65	0.49	0.53	0.52
Net transamination[a]	0.39	0.64	1.01	1.52	0.99	0.72	0.56	0.59	0.58
% of Transaminated isoleucine released as KMV	89.7	81.3	83.2	84.9	86.9	90.3	87.5	89.8	89.7
% of Transaminated isoleucine oxidized to CO_2	10.3	18.8	16.8	15.1	13.1	9.7	12.5	10.2	10.3
Valine									
Decarboxylation[a]	0.02	0.07	0.09	0.15	0.08	0.05	0.05	0.04	0.05
Net KIV production[a]	0.21	0.35	0.59	0.87	0.57	0.44	0.34	0.34	0.33
Net transamination[a]	0.23	0.42	0.68	1.02	0.65	0.49	0.39	0.38	0.38
% of Transaminated valine released as KIV	91.3	83.3	86.8	85.3	87.7	89.8	87.2	89.5	86.8
% of Transaminated valine oxidized to CO_2	8.7	16.7	13.2	14.7	12.3	10.2	12.8	10.5	13.2

Source: Self, J.T. et al. 2004. *Biol. Reprod.* 70:1444-1451.

[a] Mean values, expressed as nmol/mg tissue per 2 h.

Note: KIC, α-ketoisocaproic acid; KIV, α-ketoisovaleric acid; KMV, α-keto-β-methylvaleric acid.

4.2.4.2 BCKA Dehydrogenase

In contrast to BCAA transaminase, the activity of BCKA dehydrogenase (a mitochondrial enzyme), which decarboxylates BCKA (products of BCAA transamination) to form acyl-CoA, is particularly high in the liver but much lower in other tissues (including skeletal muscle, small intestine, adipose tissue, mammary gland, placenta, kidneys, heart, and brain; Harris et al. 2004). Thus, most of the BCKA produced by extrahepatic tissues is released to the circulation for uptake and catabolism by the liver. The BCKA dehydrogenase complex, which is similar to the pyruvate dehydrogenase complex and the α-KG dehydrogenase complex, consists of BCKA decarboxylase (E_1 which requires thiamine pyrophosphate as a cofactor), dihydrolipoamide acyltransferase (E_2 which requires lipoate and coenzyme A as cofactors), and dihydrolipoamide dehydrogenase (E_3 which requires FAD and NAD^+ as cofactors; Table 4.13). The BCKA dehydrogenase E1 is composed of two subunits: E1a and E1b. The oxidative decarboxylation of BCKA is regulated by both allosteric and covalent mechanisms. BCKA dehydrogenase is inhibited by phosphorylation and activated by dephosphorylation. Allosteric inhibition of BCKA dehydrogenase kinase by BCKA [particularly by α-ketoisocaproate (KIC, the α-ketoacid of leucine)] provides a mechanism for promoting the catabolism of excess BCAAs and conserving low concentrations of BCAAs.

4.2.4.3 KIC Dioxygenase

Besides BCKA dehydrogenase, approximately 5%–10% of KIC is degraded by KIC dioxygenase in the cytosol of the liver to generate β-hydroxy-β-methylbutyrate (HMB). KIC dioxygenase is an O_2-dependent, Fe^{2+}-containing non-heme oxygenase. This enzyme was initially discovered by P.J.

Sabourin and L.L. Bieber in 1981. In contrast to many other oxygenases, KIC dioxygenase does not use α-ketoglutarate as a substrate. As noted by K. Bloch in 1954, HMB is metabolized to β-hydroxy-β-methylglutaryl-CoA in hepatocytes, which is the precursor of acetyl-CoA, acetoacetate, and cholesterol. Dietary supplementation with HMB has been reported to enhance protein synthesis in skeletal muscle via yet unknown mechanisms (Kao et al. 2016).

4.2.4.4 Other Enzymes for the Degradation of BCKAs

After the step of acryl-CoA dehydrogenation, the carbon skeletons of leucine, isoleucine, and valine are degraded by different enzymes, which are all located in the mitochondria. Specifically, acetyl-CoA plus acetoacetate, succinyl-CoA, and acetyl-CoA plus succinyl-CoA are produced from leucine, valine, and isoleucine, respectively. Because the liver cannot utilize acetoacetate due to the lack of 3-ketoacid CoA transferase, this metabolite must be converted into β-hydroxybutyrate and the two ketone bodies are subsequently oxidized by extrahepatic tissues. The catabolism of valine also generates β-aminoisobutyrate, whose excretion in urine is increased in patients with neoplastic disease. Based on the metabolic fate of BCAAs, leucine is strictly ketogenic, valine is glucogenic, and isoleucine is both ketogenic and glucogenic. As illustrated with leucine as an example (Table 4.5), BCAAs are among the AAs with a relatively high value of energetic efficiency (47%) in animals. This may explain why the liver of some fish species (e.g., largemouth bass and hybrid striped bass) and crustaceans has a relatively high rate of BCAA degradation (Li et al. 2021a.b).

The isoleucine- and valine-derived propionyl-CoA is further metabolized in the mitochondria of hepatocytes to D-methylmalonyl-CoA by propionyl-CoA carboxylase, a biotin-dependent enzyme (Figure 4.12). The intramolecular rearrangement of D-methylmalonyl-CoA by methylmalonyl-CoA racemase (epimerase) and methylmalonyl-CoA isomerase (mutase) generates D-methylmalonyl-CoA and L-methylmalonyl-CoA, respectively (Figure 4.12). D-Methylmalonyl-CoA is hydrolyzed by the mitochondrial D-methylmalonyl-CoA hydrolase (Kovachy et al. 1983). This enzyme is specific for D-methylmalonyl-CoA and does not act on L-methylmalonyl-CoA (Kovachy et al. 1983)

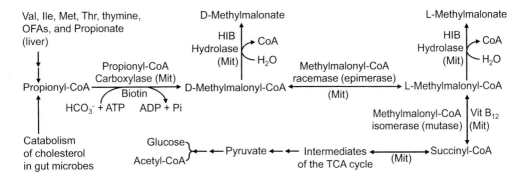

FIGURE 4.12 Catabolism of propionyl-CoA in humans and other animals. The catabolism of L-isoleucine, L-valine, L-methionine, L-threonine, thymine, fatty acids with odd-number carbons, and propionate in the liver generates propionyl-CoA. This 3-carbon metabolite can also be derived from the degradation of the cholesterol side chain by intestinal microbes. In the mitochondria of hepatocytes, propionyl-CoA is carboxylated into D-methylmalonyl-CoA, which undergoes racemization to form L-methylmalonyl-CoA. The latter is isomerized into succinyl-CoA in the mitochondrial matrix. Succinyl-CoA is subsequently metabolized to pyruvate via the mitochondrial Krebs cycle and cytosolic reactions for the production of glucose, acetyl-CoA, or both, depending on nutritional and physiological states. When the catabolism of D-methylmalonyl-CoA is impaired due to a deficiency of vitamin B_{12} or genetic defects in the expression of methylmalonyl-CoA racemase (epimerase) and methylmalonyl-CoA isomerase (mutase), D-methylmalonyl-CoA is accumulated and then hydrolyzed by the mitochondrial D-methylmalonyl-CoA hydrolase, which appears to the same protein as β-hydroxyisobutyryl-CoA hydrolase. D-Methylmalonyl-CoA hydrolase does not act on L-methylmalonyl-CoA. HIB, β-hydroxyisobutyryl-CoA; Ile, L-isoleucine; Met, L-methionine; Mit, mitochondria; OFAs, fatty acids with odd-number carbons; TCA, tricarboxylic acid; Thr, L-threonine; Val, L-valine; Vit, vitamin.

and appears to be the same protein as the mitochondrial β-hydroxyisobutyryl-CoA hydrolase based on their similar biochemical characteristics, such as the molecular weight, K_m for D-methylmalonyl-CoA, pH profiles, specific activity, and substrate-binding properties of the enzyme (Shimomura et al. 2000). The catabolism of L-methylmalonyl-CoA generates succinyl-CoA in the mitochondria and then pyruvate in the cytosol. Depending on nutritional and physiological states, pyruvate is used for either glucose synthesis in the liver and kidneys or ATP and fatty acid production via the formation of acetyl-CoA.

Healthy humans and other animals normally excrete only a small amount of methylmalonate in the urine (Keyfi et al. 2016). However, when the degradation of D-methylmalonyl-CoA is impaired due to a deficiency of vitamin B_{12} or genetic defects in the expression of methylmalonyl-CoA racemase (epimerase) and methylmalonyl-CoA isomerase (mutase), D-methylmalonyl-CoA is accumulated in the liver and then hydrolyzed by the mitochondrial D-methylmalonyl-CoA hydrolase to produce D-methylmalonate. Under these abnormal conditions, the urinary excretion of methylmalonate is markedly increased (Keyfi et al. 2016). L-Methylmalonyl-CoA is hydrolyzed to L-methylmalonate by the mitochondrial β-hydroxyisobutyryl-CoA hydrolase. Note that propionyl-CoA is also produced from: (1) the catabolism of L-methionine, L-threonine, thymine, fatty acids with odd-number carbons, and propionate in the liver of humans and other animals; and (2) the degradation of the cholesterol side chain by intestinal microbes (Griffin et al. 2012). Currently, there is interest in the metabolism of methylmalonate, because its concentration in the plasma increases with aging in humans and may enhance the risk for metastasis in older people by promoting cancer spread (Gomes et al. 2020).

D-Methylmalonyl-CoA   L-Methylmalonyl-CoA   Succinyl-CoA

4.2.4.5 Nutritional and Physiological Regulation of BCAA Catabolism

BCAA catabolism in humans and other animals is influenced by both nutritional and physiological states. For example, in response to exercise (e.g., walking on a treadmill) and high protein intake (1.8 vs. 0.7 g/kg BW/day), the rates of whole-body leucine oxidation in adult humans are increased by approximately 200% and 80%, respectively (Bowtell et al. 2000). Similarly, insulin stimulates leucine uptake and KIC's oxidative decarboxylation in skeletal muscle (Hutson et al. 1980). Thus, the whole-body catabolism of BCAA is impaired and their circulating levels are markedly increased in individuals with insulin resistance (e.g., obese and diabetic patients; Yang et al. 2015). Likewise, short-term (24-h) fasting increases the rates of the net transamination and oxidative decarboxylation of leucine in the skeletal muscle of young chicks by 39% and 43%, respectively (Wu and Thompson 1987). By contrast, short-term (18-h) food deprivation reduces the rate of whole-body leucine flux and leucine oxidation to CO_2 in adult humans by 45% and 65%, respectively (Rennie et al. 1982); these data are summarized in Table 4.15. Similarly, the half-life of leucine in the blood of adults is doubled by 4 days of starvation (Elia et al. 1980), indicating a decrease in whole-body leucine catabolism under the fasting condition. Likewise, the half-life of leucine in the blood of adult patients with insulin-dependent diabetes mellitus is 76% greater than that for healthy adults (Bratusch-Marrain et al. 1980), reflecting the impaired catabolism of BCAAs in the diabetic persons. In addition, there is evidence that consumption of glucose (0.75 g/kg BW/day) reduces the rate of whole-body leucine oxidation during and after exercise by 20% in healthy adult humans previously consuming a high-protein diet (1.8 g/kg BW/day) but has no effect on individuals previously consuming a low-protein diet (0.7 g/kg BW/day) (Bowtell et al. 2000). Note that in humans and other animals, antagonism in both transport and catabolism exists among the three BCAAs. For example, in adult

TABLE 4.15
Rates of Whole-Body Leucine Turnover in Fed and 18-h Fasted Healthy Adult Men[a]

Variable	Fed Men	Fasted Men (18-h fasted)	P-value
		µmol/kg of body weight/h	
Leucine flux (Q)	194 ± 7.6	106 ± 7.2	<0.01
Leucine oxidation (O)	40 ± 3.0	14 ± 1.5	<0.01
Leucine oxidation/Leucine flux, %	20 ± 3.0	13 ± 1.5	<0.05
Leucine used for protein synthesis (S)	154 ± 11	92 ± 6.1	<0.01
Leucine supplied from the diet (D)	55 ± 1.5	0.0	–
Leucine oxidation/Dietary leucine intake, %	73 ± 1.5	0.0	–
Leucine supplied from protein breakdown ($B = Q - D$)	139 ± 7.6	106 ± 7.2	NS
Leucine balance ($S - B$)	$+15 \pm 0.76$	-14 ± 0.76	<0.01

Source: Adapted from Rennie, M.J. et al. 1982. *Clin. Sci.* 63:519–523.

[a] Seven normal healthy men (21–59 years of age; 80.8 ± 7.3 kg of body weight; mean $\pm$ SEM, $n = 7$) were studied under either fed or 18-h fasted conditions. Within 3 days before fasting, the study participants consumed a meat-free diet providing 70–80 g protein and 8,400–13,500 kJ/day. In the morning of the tracer study, the fed individuals consumed meals hourly, which began 3 h before the collection of baseline samples. After L-[1-¹³C] leucine was infused into a forearm vein, blood samples were taken at 0.5-h intervals for 2 h and thereafter at 1-h intervals. Values are means $\pm$ SEM, $n = 7$.

Note: BW, body weight; NS, not significant ($P > 0.05$).

humans, a leucine-deficient diet reduces leucine flux and oxidation but increases valine isoleucine degradation, whereas a valine-deficient diet decreases valine flux and oxidation but has no effect on leucine flux and oxidation (Meguid et al. 1983).

4.2.5 CATABOLISM OF GLYCINE AND SERINE

4.2.5.1 The Glycine Cleavage System (GCS)

Glycine degradation takes place primarily in the liver and kidneys and, to a much lesser extent, in the brain, testes, and small intestine. This AA turns over rapidly in humans (Hahn et al. 1989) and other animals (Wang et al. 2013). Under acidotic conditions, the kidneys are the net consumers of glycine (Lowry et al. 1987). GCS (a mitochondrial enzyme complex) catalyzes the degradation of glycine into ammonia and CO_2, with tetrahydrofolate as the acceptor of the methylene group in this reversible reaction to produce N^5-N^{10}-methylene tetrahydrofolate (Figure 4.13). GCS consists of 4 proteins: a pyridoxal phosphate-dependent glycine dehydrogenase (decarboxylating; P protein), a lipoamide-containing protein (H protein), a tetrahydrofolate-dependent aminomethyltransferase (T protein), and an NAD^+-dependent and FAD-requiring dihydrolipoamide dehydrogenase (L protein) (Kikuchi et al. 2008). The sequence of glycine cleavage is outlined in Figure 4.14. In the absence of tetrahydrofolate, formaldehyde (a potential carcinogen) is produced by aminomethyltransferase.

$$\text{Glycine} + H_4\text{folate} + NAD^+ \rightleftarrows 5,10\text{-methylene-}H_4\text{folate} + CO_2 + NH_3 + NADH + H^+ \quad \text{(GCS)}$$

4.2.5.2 Serine Hydroxymethyltransferase (SHMT)

SHMT (a vitamin B_6-dependent enzyme) catalyzes the reversible conversion of serine and tetrahydrofolate into glycine and N^5-N^{10}-methylene tetrahydrofolate, with glycine serving as the acceptor of the methyl group from serine (Figure 4.13). This enzyme plays an important role in one-carbon metabolism in animals (Bazer et al. 2021; Seo et al. 2021). SHMT has two isoforms in mitochondria-containing animal cells: the cytosolic SHMT1 and the mitochondrial SHMT2, which have

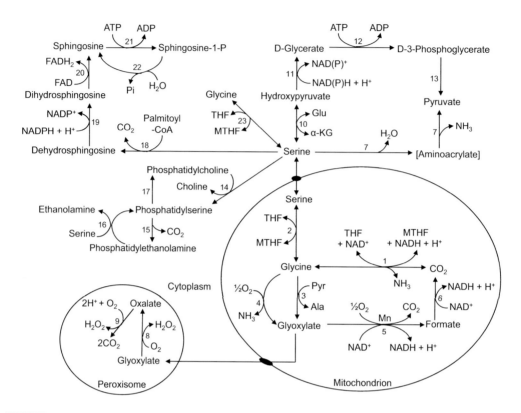

FIGURE 4.13 Catabolism of glycine and serine in humans and other animals. These pathways are active in the liver and kidneys. Some of the reactions occur in other tissues, such as the brain, testes, and small intestine. The enzymes catalyzing the indicated reactions are as follows: (1) glycine cleavage system (also known as glycine synthase, requiring pyridoxal phosphate and FAD in addition to the indicated cofactors); (2) serine hydroxymethyltransferase (the mitochondrial isoform); (3) alanine:glyoxylate transaminase; (4) glycine oxidase; (5) glyoxylate dehydrogenase; (6) formate dehydrogenase; (7) serine dehydratase (requiring pyridoxal phosphate); (8) glyoxylate oxidase; (9) oxalate oxidase; (10) serine transaminase; (11) hydroxypyruvate reductase; (12) D-glycerate kinase; (13) enzymes of glycolysis; (14) phosphatidylserine synthase I; (15) phosphatidylserine decarboxylase; (16) phosphatidylserine synthase I; (17) a series of enzymes with ethanolamine as an initial substrate; (18) dihydrosphingosine synthase; (19) dihydrosphingosine reductase; (20) dihydrosphingosine dehydrogenase; (21) sphingosine kinase; (22) sphingosine-1-phosphate phosphatase; and (23) serine hydroxymethyltransferase (the cytosolic isoform). MTHF, N^5-N^{10}-methylene-tetrahydrofolate; P, phosphate; THF, tetrahydrofolate.

different biochemical properties (Bouzidi et al. 2020; Herbig et al. 2002; MacFarlane et al. 2008; Tramonti et al. 2018) and play different roles in metabolism (Chapter 3). For example, the cytosolic SHMT1 is primarily responsible for the synthesis of glycine from serine, as well as the formation of serine from glycine. Through its conversion into serine, glycine can serve as a substrate for glucose synthesis in mammals and other animals. Hetenyi et al. (1988) reported that of the carbon atoms of glucose in the plasma, 2.9% were derived from glycine in fasted-normal and diabetic rats, whereas 4.5% and 6.8% originated from serine in fasted-normal and diabetic rats, respectively. The mitochondrial SHMT2 contributes to one-carbon metabolism via the interconversion of tetrahydrofolate into glycine and N^5-N^{10}-methylene tetrahydrofolate, as well as the oxidation of glyoxylate to formate and CO_2 by glyoxylate dehydrogenase (Lamarre et al. 2012). SHMT2 also participates in the oxidation of serine and glycine to oxalate in animal cells via glycine oxidase (a mitochondrial enzyme) or alanine:glyoxylate transaminase (located in both the mitochondria and the cytoplasm), as well as the peroxisomal glyoxylate oxidase. Oxalate is either oxidized to CO_2 by oxalate oxidase in the peroxisomes or excreted in the urine.

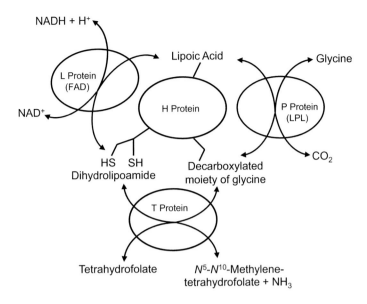

FIGURE 4.14 The glycine cleavage system in humans and other animals. This reaction starts with glycine decarboxylation by glycine dehydrogenase (P protein; a homodimer in humans, animals, and bacteria; ~200kDa) in the presence of a lipoic acid-binding protein (a monomer; ~14kDa; H protein). The decarboxylated moiety of glycine is deaminated by a tetrahydrofolate-dependent enzyme (aminomethyltransferase; a monomer with a molecular weight of ~40kDa; T protein), with the production of dihydrolipoamide. Dihydrolipoamide is reduced by an NAD^+-dependent and FAD-requiring dihydrolipoamide dehydrogenase (L protein; a homodimeric flavoprotein; the molecular weight of each subunit = 50.2kDa), which is the common E3 protein component of the α-ketoacid dehydrogenase complex. The liver is highly active to degrade glycine, followed by the kidneys.

4.2.5.3 Glycine *N*-Methyltransferase (GNMT)

GNMT is another enzyme for the initiation of glycine metabolism in humans and other animals. This cytosolic enzyme transfers a methyl group from SAM to glycine to form *S*-adenosylhomocysteine and sarcosine (Luka et al. 2009). GNMT is present in the liver, prostate, and pancreas's exocrine tissues, as well as proximal kidney tubules, submaxillary glands, the intestinal mucosa, cortical neurons, and the brain's Purkinje cells in animals. The hepatic GNMT is not detected or is present at a very low level during pregnancy, but is strongly expressed immediately after birth possibly due to an induction by glucocorticoids and glucagon.

$$\text{Glycine} + S\text{-Adenosylmethionine} \rightarrow \text{Sarcosine} + S\text{-Adenosylhomocysteine} \quad (\text{GNMT})$$

4.2.5.4 Other Enzymes for the Degradation of Serine

Besides its degradation to glycine by SHMT, serine is dehydrated by serine dehydratase (a cytosolic and pyridoxal phosphate-dependent enzyme) to form pyruvate and ammonia (Figure 4.13). Cystathionine synthetase can also deaminate serine. In addition, serine can be transaminated to form hydroxypyruvate, which is then converted sequentially into D-glycerate, D-3-phosphoglycerate, 3-phosphohydroxypyruvate, and phosphoserine. D-3-phosphoglycerate can be metabolized to pyruvate via the enzymes of glycolysis. Finally, serine reacts with homocysteine to generate cystathionine in the pathway of methionine catabolism. This reaction provides a biochemical basis for dietary supplementation with serine or glycine to ameliorate the toxicity of excess methionine in animals (Regina et al. 1993).

4.2.6 Catabolism of Histidine

Catabolism of histidine in animals is initiated by histidase, histidine decarboxylase, and histidine transaminase in a cell- and tissue-specific manner (Figure 4.15). The elucidation of the histidase pathway spanned almost one century. In 1874, even before histidine was known as a component of protein, M. Jaffe reported that the urine of a dog contained urocanic acid. This finding was independently confirmed by S. Edlbacher in the same year. Several groups of investigators between in 1898 and 1933 consistently observed that the urinary excretion of this metabolite by animals was substantially increased in response to the oral administration of histidine. During this intervening period, H. Raistrick found in 1917 that bacteria could synthesize urocanate from histidine and suggested that microorganisms in the lumen of the intestine might be the source of urocanate produced by the intact animal. However, in 1926, P. György and H. Röthler demonstrated that mammalian liver can cleave the imidazole ring of histidine via histidase to form ammonia, glutamate, and formic acid. The authors proposed that urocanate is an intermediate of histidine degradation in mammals. This hypothesis was supported by Y. Sera and S. Yada in 1939 when they performed a series of elegant studies to identify how liver fractions can convert histidine to urocanic acid and

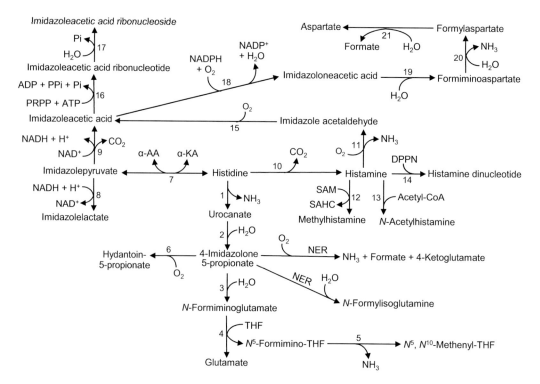

FIGURE 4.15 Catabolism of histidine in humans and other animals. The liver is highly active to degrade glycine. The enzymes that catalyze the indicated reactions are as follows: (1) histidase (histidine ammonia lyase); (2) urocanate hydratase; (3) imidazolone propionase; (4) glutamate formiminotransferase; (5) N^5-formimino-tetrahydrofolate cyclodeaminase; (6) 4-imidazolone 5-propionate oxidase; (7) histidine transaminase; (8) imidazolepyruvate reductase; (9) imidazolepyruvate dehydrogenase; (10) histidine decarboxylase; (11) histaminase (diamine oxidase); (12) histamine methyltransferase; (13) acetylhistamine synthase; (14) imidazoleacetate phosphoribosyltransferase; (15) xanthine oxidase or aldehyde dehydrogenase (in the presence of diphospho-pyridine nucleotide); (16) imidazoleacetic acid ribonucleotide synthase; (17) acid phosphatase; (18) imidazoleacetic acid oxidase; (19) imidazoloneacetic acid ribonucleoside; (20) formiminoaspartate deaminase; and (21) formylaspartate deformylase. α-AA, α-amino acid (e.g., glutamate and alanine); α-KA, α-ketoacid (e.g., α-ketoglutarate and pyruvate); DPPN, diphosphopyridine nucleotide; NER, nonenzymatic reaction; SAHC, S-adenosylhomocysteine; SAM, S-adenosylmethionine; THF, tetrahydrofolate.

glutamate derivatives. These reactions were unequivocally established by the studies of H. Tabor in 1952 that involved specifically labeled histidine. Meanwhile, the conversion of histidine to urocanate was found to be irreversible because urocanic acid could not replace histidine in the diet to support the growth of young rats. Additionally, nutritional studies have revealed that folate-deficient animals excreted N-formiminoglutamate in urine and had a reduced rate of histidine catabolism by the liver. Subsequent work in the mid-1950s led to the recognition that tetrahydrofolate is required for converting N-formiminoglutamate to glutamate. This discovery was supported by the purification in 1959 of glutamate formiminotransferase from the porcine liver. Over the past 60 years, many of the genes involved in histidine catabolism via the histidase pathway have been cloned, sequenced, and characterized (Braeuning et al. 2006; Luu et al. 2017).

Another pathway for histidine catabolism is pyridoxal phosphate-dependent transamination. J. Roche and coworkers discovered in 1954 that histidine undergoes transamination to form imidazolepyruvate in the hepatopancreas of the mussel. In the 1960s, histidine aminotransferase in the liver was reported by several research groups. Two isoforms of histidine aminotransferase in rat liver were shown in the 1970s to differ in substrate requirements, kinetics, and hormonal induction. Isoenzyme I is present only in the liver and is induced by glucagon. By contrast, isoenzyme II is expressed in the liver, kidneys, heart, and skeletal muscle, has catalytic activity with pyruvate but not α-KG, and is not induced by glucagon. The further metabolism of imidazolepyruvate results in the production of imidazoleacetate and imidazoleacetate ribonucleoside. The occurrence of the histidine transamination pathway explains the following: (1) the excretion of these products in the urine of human, rats, and other animals; and (2) the results of nutritional studies that D-histidine can partially replace L-histidine in the diets of animals because the organisms can convert some D-histidine into L-histidine (Chapter 3).

Histidine degradation can also be initiated by histidine decarboxylase (a vitamin B_6-dependent enzyme) to form histamine in animals (Ohtsu 2011). This pathway is quantitatively significant in cells of the immune system and immunologically important. Furthermore, histidine is used for the synthesis of carnosine and homocarnosine in animals. These metabolic pathways will be described in Chapter 5. Collectively, histidine plays an important role in the metabolism and function of histidine in humans and other animals (Moro et al. 2020).

4.2.7 Catabolism of Lysine

4.2.7.1 Lysine Degradation via Saccharopine and Pipecolate Pathways

Lysine is degraded to α-aminoadipate-6-semialdehyde primarily in the liver and, to a much lesser extent, the kidneys of humans and other animals through the saccharopine and pipecolic acid pathways, with the saccharopine pathway being almost the exclusive pathway for lysine degradation in these organs (Pena et al. 2016). These two metabolic pathways are outlined in Figure 4.16, with the chemical structures of some key intermediates being shown in Figure 4.17. The brain has low activities of the initial enzymes involved in the saccharopine and pipecolic acid pathways and, therefore, a very low rate of lysine catabolism, with the saccharopine pathway being the major route of lysine degradation in cultured human brain cells but the pipecolic acid pathway being more predominant in the rodent (rat and mouse) brains (Crowther et al. 2019). α-Aminoadipate-6-semialdehyde is subsequently converted to acetyl-CoA and acetoacetate. The saccharopine pathway is present in mitochondria and primarily responsible for lysine catabolism in animals. This pathway was based on the early suggestion in 1913 by A.I. Ringer and colleagues that lysine is metabolized to glutaric acid in dogs, and subsequently established by H. Borsook and coworkers in 1948. In the pipecolic acid pathway, which was originally proposed by M. Rothstein and L.L. Miller in 1953 from studies with rats, lysine is converted to Δ^1-piperideine-6-carboxylate via three steps in peroxisomes. Using L-[α-^{15}N]lysine or L-[ε-^{15}N]lysine, these authors also noted that the α-amino group rather than the ε-amino group of lysine is removed during the conversion of lysine to pipecolic acid. Oxidation of lysine via the pipecolate pathway occurs in peroxisomes. Increasing dietary intake of lysine or

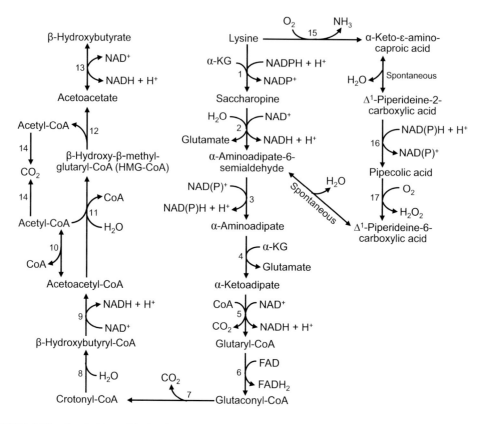

FIGURE 4.16 Catabolism of lysine in humans and other animals. Lysine is degraded via the mitochondrial saccharopine pathway and the peroxisomal pipecolate pathway. These pathways are most active in the liver and may occur at low rates in the brain. The enzymes that catalyze the indicated reactions are as follows: (1) lysine:α-ketoglutarate reductase; (2) saccharopine dehydrogenase (NAD⁺, glutamate-forming); (3) aminoadipate semialdehyde dehydrogenase; (4) aminoadipate aminotransferase; (5) α-ketoacid dehydrogenase; (6) glutaryl-CoA dehydrogenase; (7) glutaconyl-CoA decarboxylase; (8) enol-CoA hydratase; (9) β-hydroxyacyl-CoA dehydrogenase; (10) thiolase; (11) HMG-CoA synthase; (12) HMG-CoA lyase; (13) β-hydroxybutyrate dehydrogenase; (14) enzymes of the Krebs cycle; (15) lysine oxidase (a peroxisomal protein); (16) peperideine-2-carboxylic acid reductase; and (17) pipecolate oxidase (a peroxisomal protein).

protein enhances the hepatic activity of lysine-α-KG reductase activity and lysine oxidation in the liver (Chu and Hegsted 1976). There is evidence that the low uptake of lysine by hepatocytes and their mitochondria limits hepatic lysine oxidation (Blemings et al. 1998).

Oxidation of lysine to CO_2 is absent in most extrahepatic cells and tissues of mammals (e.g., pigs, rats, and sheep) and chickens, including lymphocytes, macrophages, enterocytes, the small-intestinal mucosa, skeletal muscle, heart, lung, pancreas, and spleen. Note that like leucine, the catabolism of lysine in animals produces acetyl-CoA, but no intermediates of the Krebs cycle, and, therefore, is a strictly ketogenic AA (Benevenga and Blemings 2007). There are antagonisms in transport by cells among basic AAs (arginine, lysine, and histidine). Thus, proper ratios of these AAs are crucial for the nutrition and health of humans and other animals.

4.2.7.2   Decarboxylation of Lysine to Cadaverine by ODC in Animal Cells

Animal cells lack lysine decarboxylase. However, there are reports that ODC can use lysine as a substrate, and thus, mammalian tissues (e.g., rat and mouse liver and kidneys) can produce a very small amount of cadaverine (1,6-diamino-pentane; a foul-smelling diamine) from L-lysine

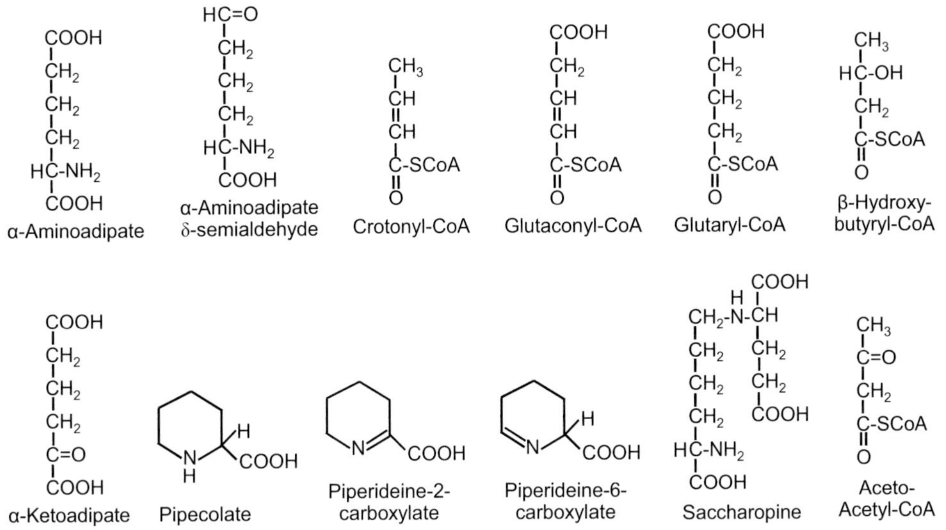

FIGURE 4.17 Chemical structures of some key intermediates of lysine catabolism in humans and other animals. These substances are presented in their non-ionized forms but they occur in their ionized forms under physiological conditions.

(Pegg and McGill 1979; Persson 1977). Because ODC activity is quantitatively very low in animal cells and this enzyme has a much lower affinity for lysine than ornithine, there is very limited or virtually no production of cadaverine from lysine in the tissues of living animals. Similarly, mammalian cells, such as macrophage-like RAW 264 and H36 hepatoma cells, can synthesize and release a very small amount of cadaverine as a product of lysine decarboxylation (Hawel et al. 1994). The V_{max} of the purified ODC for ornithine is about fourfold greater than that for lysine but the K_m of the enzyme for lysine (9 mM) is about 100 times greater than that for ornithine (0.09 mM) (Pegg and McGill 1979). Thus, significant cadaverine production in animal tissues could occur only when their ODC activity is comparatively high and their lysine concentrations substantially exceed those of ornithine. By contrast, bacteria, including gastrointestinal bacteria, express lysine decarboxylase (a vitamin B_6-dependent enzyme) to decarboxylate L-lysine to cadaverine and CO_2 (Dai et al. 2011). Microbial production of cadaverine is enhanced through the putrefaction of tissues after an animal dies.

$$\text{L-Lysine} \rightarrow \text{Cadaverine} + CO_2 \ \left(\text{ornithine decarboxylase; animal cells}\right)$$

$$\text{L-Lysine} \rightarrow \text{Cadaverine} + CO_2 \ \left(\text{lysine decarboxylase; bacteria}\right)$$

4.2.8 Catabolism of Phenylalanine and Tyrosine

Phenylalanine and tyrosine were among the AAs whose catabolic pathways were identified largely due to inborn diseases in humans. As early as 1903, it was noted that homogentisic acid was present in the urine of animals after consuming phenylalanine and tyrosine. In 1904, O. Neubauer and colleagues found that the oral administration of phenylalanine or tyrosine to alkaptonuric patients resulted in the urinary excretion of large amounts of homogentisic acid, suggesting that homogentisic acid is an intermediate of the degradation of these two AAs. In 1909, Neubauer proposed that phenylalanine was converted into tyrosine in animals. This suggestion was supported by G. Embden and K. Baldes who reported in 1913 the formation of tyrosine from phenylalanine in perfused livers. In the same year, the authors also observed the production of acetoacetate from phenylalanine or tyrosine. These results were confirmed by subsequent studies involving isotopes and liver slices in the 1940s. Such work led to the finding that malate and fumarate are products of the degradation of phenylalanine or tyrosine.

A seminal discovery on the BH4-dependent hydroxylation of phenylalanine was made by S. Kaufman in 1957, which provides a biochemical basis for the treatment of phenylketonuria with BH4 in humans who have a deficiency of this cofactor for phenylalanine hydroxylase. The pathway for phenylalanine and tyrosine catabolism to produce CO_2 and water via phenylalanine hydroxylase and tyrosine transaminase is illustrated in Figure 4.18. The K_m values of phenylalanine hydroxylase (a major regulatory enzyme for phenylalanine degradation) for phenylalanine and BH4 are summarized in Table 4.16.

In addition to the major hydroxylation pathway for phenylalanine degradation to generate tyrosine, phenylalanine can be catabolized via a minor transamination pathway. Namely, phenylalanine is transaminated with α-KG to form glutamate and phenylpyruvate. Phenylpyruvate is either decarboxylated to form phenylacetate by PLP-dependent phenylpyruvate decarboxylase (Chapter 5) or converted into phenyllactate by NADH-dependent phenylpyruvate reductase. Among the tissues of animals, the liver is most active in the catabolism of both phenylalanine and tyrosine, followed by the kidneys and pancreas (Parthasarathy et al. 2018). Note that phenylalanine is hydrolyzed into tyrosine but tyrosine is not converted into phenylalanine in humans and other animals. When phenylalanine catabolism is impaired in humans, an inherited disease called phenylketonuria occurs.

Two metabolic pathways are responsible for tyrosine degradation in animals: transamination and hydroxylation. In the former, tyrosine is transaminated with α-KG to form p-hydroxyphenylpyruvate and glutamate (Figure 4.18). p-Hydroxyphenylpyruvate is converted into (1) fumarate and acetoacetate (via the homogentisate, 4-maleylacetoacetate, and 4-fumuraylacetoacetate intermediates) and (2) other phenolic acids, including p-hydroxyphenylacetate, p-hydroxyphenyllactate, phloretate, p-coumarate, and p-hydroxybenzoate, as reported for rats and rabbits (Booth et al. 1960). 4-Fumuraylacetoacetate is reduced to succinylacetoacetate (an inhibitor of p-hydroxyphenylpyruvic acid dioxygenase), which is spontaneously decarboxylated to succinylacetone. The succinylacetone- and phenolic acid-yielding reactions are independent

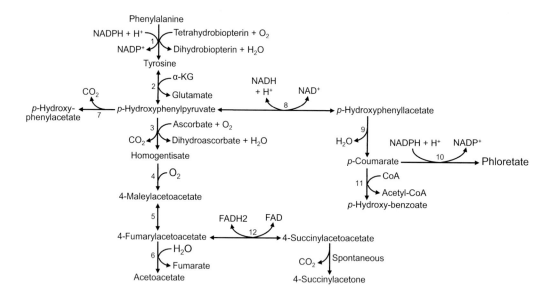

FIGURE 4.18 Catabolism of phenylalanine and tyrosine to fumarate and acetoacetate in humans and other animals. These metabolic pathways are most active in the liver. The enzymes that catalyze the indicated reactions are as follows: (1) phenylalanine hydroxylase; 2) tyrosine aminotransferase; (3) p-hydroxyphenylpyruvate dioxygenase; (4) homogentisate dioxygenase; (5) maleylacetoacetate isomerase; (6) fumarylacetoacetate; (7) p-hydroxyphenylpyruvate decarboxylase (a vitamin B_6-dependent enzyme); (8) p-hydroxyphenylpyruvate dehydrogenase; (9) p-hydroxyphenyllactate dehydratase; (10) p-coumarate reductase; (11) enzymes of the mitochondrial β-oxidation; and (12) succinylacetoacetate dehydrogenase.

TABLE 4.16

K_m **Values of Substrates and Cofactors for Tetrahydrobiopterin-Dependent Enzymes in Mammalian Cells**

		Amino Acid Substrate		BH4 Cofactor	
Enzyme	Substrate	K_m of Enzyme for Substrate (μM)	Substrate Concentration in Cells (μM)	K_m of Enzyme for Cofactor (μM)	Cofactor Concentration in Cells (μM)
Nitric oxide synthase	L-Arginine	3–20	50–2000[a]	0.2–2	1.3–2.8 (EC)
Phenylalanine hydroxylase	L-Phenylalanine	200–300	100–300	15–25	5–10 (liver)
Tryptophan hydroxylase-1	L-Tryptophan	23	30–120	29	0.6 – 1.0 (brain)
Tryptophan hydroxylase-2	L-Tryptophan	40–140	30–120	20–27	0.6–1.0 (brain)
Tyrosine hydroxylase	L-Tyrosine	25–50	150–350	15–20	5–10 (liver)

Source: Kohli, R. et al. 2004. *J. Nutr.* 134:600–608; Li, P. et al. 2008. *Nitric Oxide* 19:259–265; Li, P. et al. 2009. *Amino Acids* 37:709–716; Werner, E.R. et al. 2011. *Biochem. J.* 438:397–414.

[a] The concentrations of arginine are 0.05–0.10 mM in mammalian hepatocytes and 0.5–2 mM in other mammalian cells.

Note: BH4, tetrahydrobiopterin; EC, endothelial cells.

of intestinal microbes and likely occur in the liver and kidneys of animals via dehydrogenation, decarboxylation, hydration, and conjugation reactions (Figure 4.18). In the BH4-dependent hydroxylation pathway, tyrosine is metabolized to DOPA, dopamine, norepinephrine, and epinephrine (Chapter 5). Several inborn errors of metabolism in humans result from a deficiency of one of the enzymes involved in tyrosine catabolism (Chapter 12).

4.2.9 CATABOLISM OF PROLINE, 4-HYDROXYPROLINE, AND 3-HYDROXYPROLINE

The helical region of collagen comprises the repeat of Gly-X-Y, where proline can be in the *X* or *Y* position and hydroxyproline occurs only in the *Y* position. On a per gram basis, the proline requirement for whole-body protein synthesis is the highest among all AAs. The unique ring structure of proline and hydroxyproline distinguishes them from other AAs in terms of rigidity, chemical stability, and biochemical reactions. The discovery of proline oxidase in the 1960s created a new research area in proline biochemistry.

Earlier studies of proline metabolism between the 1910s and 1960s were often conducted along with those of glutamate and arginine. In 1913, H.D. Dakin reported that proline, like glutamate, is metabolized to glucose via succinate as an intermediate in animals. The work of H.A. Krebs in 1935 identified the conversion of proline to glutamate in kidneys. In 1944, M.R. Stetten and R. Schoenheimer reported the incorporation of [¹⁵N] proline into arginine, glutamate, and ornithine in rats. Subsequently, glutamate γ-semialdehyde was known in 1949 as an intermediate of this pathway. Using rat liver mitochondria, A.B. Johnson and H.J. Strecker discovered in 1962 that the initial reaction of this pathway is catalyzed by proline oxidase that requires oxygen and cytochrome C for activity. It is now known that most mammalian tissues, possibly except for mammary tissue, express proline oxidase activity (Figure 4.8), with the highest activity in the mucosa of the small intestine, followed by the kidneys and liver in descending order. In gestating mammals (e.g., pigs and sheep), placentae also possess relatively high proline oxidase activity (Wu et al. 2011b).

4.2.9.1 Proline Oxidase, 4-Hydroxyproline Oxidase, and 3-Hydroxyproline Oxidase

Proline oxidase (a mitochondrial enzyme) is also known as proline dehydrogenase 1, and is encoded by the PRODH1 gene in animals. In humans, the *PRODH1* gene maps to chromosome 22q.11.21. This enzyme uses ferricytochrome C as an electron acceptor to oxidize proline to P5C, which takes a central stage in the metabolism of the arginine family of AAs (Tanner 2019). A byproduct of this reaction is superoxide anion (O_2^-), which can be converted into H_2O_2 and other reactive oxygen species with both physiological and pathological significance (Hu et al. 2007; Krishnan et al. 2008; Phang and Liu 2012). In intact cells, water is likely produced from proline oxidation, as there is no detectable generation of O_2^- and H_2O_2 by non-tumor cells (e.g., enterocytes and placenta). Much evidence shows that the proline-P5C cycle supports ATP production, protein and nucleotide synthesis, anaplerosis, and redox homeostasis in cancer cells (Liu et al. 2012; Phang 1985). In recent years, there has been a suggestion that proline catabolism may be a target for cancer therapy (Tanner et al. 2018).

In the porcine placenta and in the enterocytes of neonatal pigs that do not contain arginase activity, proline oxidase replaces arginase to provide ornithine for supporting the synthesis of polyamines that are required for high rates of protein synthesis and cell proliferation (Wu et al. 2005). This is of enormous importance in both nutrition and physiology because (1) polyamines are key molecules regulating DNA and protein synthesis, as well as cell proliferation, differentiation, and migration; (2) both placentae and the neonatal small intestine grow very rapidly. The low activity of P5C dehydrogenase in these two tissues helps channel ornithine to ODC rather than oxidation into CO_2. As noted previously, ruminant placentae contain both arginase and proline oxidase, which helps to compensate for relatively low concentrations of proline in the maternal blood.

Like proline oxidase, 4-hydroxyproline oxidase (also known as proline dehydrogenase 2, a mitochondrial enzyme encoded by the *PRODH2* gene) is widespread in animal tissues (Wu et al. 2019). In humans, the *PRODH2* gene maps to chromosome 19q13.12. As detailed in Chapter 3, about 95% of the collagen-derived 4-hydroxyproline is oxidized via the 4-hydroxyproline oxidase pathway to generate primarily glycine and, to a much lesser extent, glycolate and oxalate, in humans and other animals. Endogenous synthesis of glycine from 4-hydroxyproline helps to conserve AAs, while providing a large amount of glycine to meet its needs by the body.

At present, little is known about the catabolism of 3-hydroxyproline in mammals, birds, or fish. There is evidence that 3-hydroxyproline is oxidized by 3-hydroxyl-proline oxidase in animals (Risteli et al. 1977; Tryggvason et al. 1979). Adams and Frank (1980) reported that mammals catabolized 3-hydroxyproline as efficiently as 4-hydroxyproline, and rat tissues converted [U-^{14}C] 3-hydroxyproline to [^{14}C] proline, thereby conserving AAs. Thus, it appears to be unlikely that the major pathways for 3-hydroxyproline catabolism in humans and other animals parallel those for 4-hydroxyproline.

4.2.9.2 Metabolism of P5C

While all cells can recycle P5C into proline by P5C reductase (PYCR) and convert P5C into ornithine by OAT, the utilization of P5C for net synthesis of citrulline occurs only in the small intestine (Wu 1998). This indicates a unique role for the small intestine in proline catabolism and is consistent with the finding that proline oxidase activity is the highest in the small intestine among all of the studied tissues in swine, including the liver, pancreas, and kidneys.

Three homologous PYCR isoforms have been reported in animal cells: PYCR1, PYCR2, and PYCR3 (also known as PYCRL). They are encoded for by three separate genes that map to chromosomes 17q25.3 (PYCR1), 1q42.12 (PRCR2), and 8q24.3 (PRCR3), respectively, in humans. PYCR1 and PYCR2, which share 85% sequence similarity, have been reported to be localized to the mitochondria in fibroblasts and tumor cells (Burke et al. 2020). In contrast, PYCR3 (a cytosolic enzyme) shares ~45% sequence similarity with PYCR1 and PYCR2, and is likely the major isoform of PYCR in the liver, intestine, kidneys and other tissues of mammals (e.g., pigs and rats) and birds.

Although the mammalian liver can convert P5C into citrulline and arginine via the urea cycle, there is no net synthesis of these two AAs in this organ because exceedingly high arginase activity rapidly hydrolyzes arginine into ornithine and urea (Wu and Morris 1998). In the liver and kidneys,

P5C can be oxidized completely to CO_2 via the formation of α-KG by P5C dehydrogenase. However, in placentae and enterocytes with limited P5C dehydrogenase activity, oxidation of proline to CO_2 is negligible. This prevents an irreversible loss of proline carbons and maximizes the availability of P5C for the synthesis of polyamines.

4.2.9.3 The "Arginine-Proline Cycle" between Mother and Neonate

A noteworthy metabolic phenomenon is the use of milk-derived proline for the synthesis of citrulline and arginine by the small intestine in suckling neonates (Wu 1997). Arginine is actively utilized to form proline in the lactating mammary gland, resulting in a deficiency of arginine and an abundance of proline in milk (Trottier et al. 1997). Interestingly, milk-derived proline is a major precursor for the synthesis of citrulline (the precursor of arginine) in the enterocytes of postnatal pigs. Thus, there is an "arginine-proline cycle" between mother and neonate. Although intestinal synthesis of citrulline and arginine partially compensates for an arginine deficiency in the milk of most mammals (including humans, cows, and swine), one must wonder why there is extensive catabolism of arginine by the lactating mammary gland. There are several possible answers to this intriguing question. First, the uptake of proline from the maternal blood by the lactating mammary glands may be inadequate for milk protein synthesis. Consequently, arginine catabolism may be necessary to provide sufficient proline for maximizing protein synthesis by the lactating mammary gland. Second, through the NADPH-dependent conversion of P5C into proline, arginine may regulate the cellular redox state and glucose metabolism via the pentose cycle (pentose phosphate pathway). The pentose cycle generates ribose-5-phosphate and most NADPH for a variety of metabolic processes (Wu 2018). For example, NADPH is required for fatty acid synthesis, whereas ribose-5-phosphate is essential for purine synthesis and cell proliferation. This notion is consistent with the finding that dietary arginine supplementation to sows increases production of milk lipids and piglet growth. Third, arginine is the common substrate for both arginase and nitric oxide synthase, and thus, arginase may play an important role in regulating NO and polyamine synthesis by the lactating mammary gland. Although NO is quantitatively a minor product of arginine catabolism, it may play a crucial role in the regulation of mammary gland blood flow and thus the uptake of nutrients from the blood by the lactating mammary glands. Likewise, polyamines produced by mammary tissue regulate lactogenesis and greatly contribute to their relatively high abundance in milk. There is little arginase activity in the small intestine of neonates, and yet polyamines are essential for cell proliferation and differentiation. Thus, milk-borne polyamines are of nutritional and physiological importance for growth and development of the neonatal intestine. Finally, because the neonate has a low capacity to synthesize proline (a nutritionally essential AA), arginine catabolism via the arginase pathway in the lactating mammary gland will ensure an adequate supply of proline to the neonate to support tissue protein synthesis and extracellular matrix formation. Therefore, through the "arginine-proline cycle" between mother and neonate, the mother sustains a capacity for milk synthesis and provides both proline and polyamines to her offspring, whereas the neonate can synthesize arginine and have both exogenous and endogenous polyamines required for protein synthesis and cell growth.

4.2.10 CATABOLISM OF SULFUR-CONTAINING AAs

Nutritional studies in the 1930s revealed that the need of animals for cysteine can be met by dietary methionine and that part of the dietary requirement for methionine can be fulfilled by dietary cysteine. These results indicate that cysteine is formed from methionine and, therefore, can spare some of the dietary methionine by reducing methionine catabolism. In 1939, V. du Vigneaud and coworkers reported that homocysteine can also replace dietary methionine and cysteine in rats fed a diet containing adequate amounts of choline and the vitamin B complex. These authors discovered in 1940 that methionine undergoes transmethylation in animals, with its methyl group being transferred to choline and creatine. A series of papers from the du Vigneaud group in 1942 established that homocysteine and serine are converted to cysteine via cystathionine as an intermediate. In 1947, H.

Borsook found that the transmethylation of methionine involves its reaction with ATP enzymatically to generate an active methionine derivative, which was shown in 1952 by G.L. Cantoni (an Italian chemist) to be SAM. It is now known that SAM is the major donor of methyl groups in animals.

Interest in cysteine catabolism in the early 20th century originated, in part, from the human inborn disease cystinuria. V. du Vigneaud and coworkers reported in 1934 that cystine (cysteine) is oxidized in animals to sulfate, thiosulfate, and sulfite. Catabolism of cysteine occurs primarily in hepatocytes. However, many cell types (including neurons, endothelial cells, and vascular smooth muscle cells) can produce H_2S (a signaling gas) from cysteine (Stipanuk 2004). Additionally, cysteine can be oxidized by formaldehyde to N-formylcysteine, and acetylation of cysteine residue in N-formylcysteine conjugates with electrophiles and physiological metabolites forms mercapturate. Finally, cysteine, along with glutamate and glycine, is used to synthesize GSH and coenzyme A in organisms (Bender 2012).

4.2.10.1 Transsulfuration Pathway for Methionine Catabolism

In the liver of humans and other animals, methionine is degraded to cysteine via the transsulfuration pathway (Figure 4.19). The initial step is the formation of SAM from methionine and ATP by SAM synthase, followed by the hydrolysis of SAM into adenosine and homocysteine. Cystathionine-β-synthase (a vitamin B_6-dependent enzyme) converts homocysteine and serine into cystathionine. The latter is hydrolyzed by cystathionine γ-lyase (a vitamin B_6-dependent enzyme) to ammonia, α-ketobutyrate, and cysteine. The conversion of homocysteine into cysteine is crucial for the health of humans and other animals, because elevated levels of homocysteine modify protein structure, reduce the synthesis and bioavailability of NO, and are toxic to cells (Jakubowski, H. 2019).

There are unique aspects of cysteine metabolism in humans and other animals. First, the amino group and all the carbons of cysteine are derived from the serine molecule, whereas the sulfur atom of cysteine comes from methionine, as indicated in Figure 4.20. Second, the SAM generated via the methionine transsulfuration pathway is quantitatively important for many methylation reactions in animal cells, including the syntheses of (1) creatine by guanidinoacetate methyltransferase,

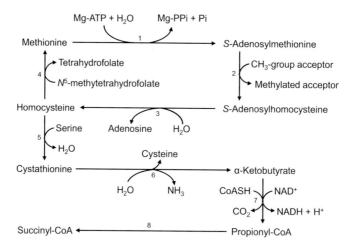

FIGURE 4.19 Catabolism of methionine via the transulfuration pathway in humans and other animals. This metabolic pathway occurs exclusively in the liver. The enzymes that catalyze the indicated reactions are as follows: (1) S-adenosylmethionine synthase (methionine adenosyltransferase); (2) methylase; (3) S-adenosylhomocysteinase; (4) homocysteine methyltransferase (methionine synthase; a vitamin B_{12}-dependent enzyme); (5) cystathionine β-synthase (a pyridoxal phosphate-dependent enzyme); (6) cystathionine γ-lyase (a pyridoxal phosphate-dependent enzyme); (7) α-ketobutyrate dehydrogenase; (8) a series of enzymes [propionyl-CoA carboxylase, methylmalonyl-CoA racemase, and methylmalonyl-CoA mutase (a vitamin B_{12}-dependent enzyme)]. All the carbons of cysteine are derived from serine.

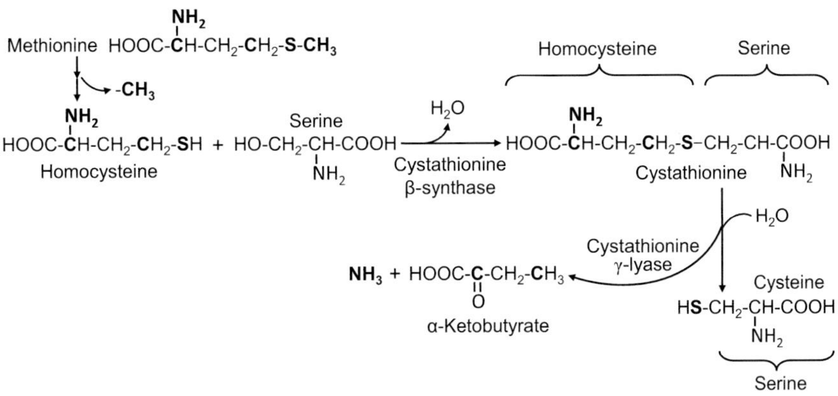

FIGURE 4.20 Requirement for serine in the catabolism of methionine in humans and animals. The methionine-derived homocysteine combines with serine to form cystathionine, which is deaminated and cleaved to generate α-ketobutyrate and cysteine. The amino group and the whole carbon skeleton of cysteine are derived from the serine molecule, whereas the sulfur atom of cysteine comes from methionine. The bold letters denote the common source of the atoms from methionine.

(2) phosphatidylcholine by phosphatidylethanolamine methyltransferase, and (3) sarcosine by glycine N-methyltransferase (Mudd et al. 2007). In mammals and other animals, greater than 90% of SAM is used for methylation reactions by at least 50 different methyltransferases (Luca et al. 2009).

Experimental evidence shows that GNMT plays an important role in regulating the catabolism and intracellular concentrations of methionine and SAM, as well as the ratio of SAM to *S*-adenosylhomocysteine in the liver. For example, compared with wild-type (normal) mice, the hepatic concentrations of methionine and SAM in GNMT-knockout mice increased by about six- and 35-fold, respectively, but the hepatic concentrations of *S*-adenosylhomocysteine in GNMT-knockout mice decreased by 70% and the hepatic ratio of SAM to *S*-adenosylhomocysteine increased by about 100-fold (Luca et al. 2006). Although GNMT-knockout mice had similar growth and reproductive performance to those for wild-type (normal) mice, the absence of hepatic GNMT in the GNMT-knockout mice resulted in the progressive accumulation of fats, as well as the development of fibrosis, steatosis, and hepatocellular carcinoma in their livers at 3 to 8 months of age. This is analogous to the occurrence of fatty livers in rodents that are deficient in methionine, choline, folate, and vitamin B_{12}. Thus, GNMT is essential for methionine catabolism, as well as the structure and function of the liver.

4.2.10.2 Catabolism of Cysteine to Taurine, H_2S, SO_2, and Sulfate

In the liver of humans and other animals, there are multiple pathways for cysteine catabolism to generate taurine, H_2S, pyruvate, and sulfate, as detailed in Chapter 3. H_2S is also produced from cysteine in other tissues, including the brain, kidneys, lung, and vasculature. Sulfate is the major metabolite of the sulfur of cysteine and is quantitatively excreted in the urine (Finkelstein 1990). Furthermore, SO_2 can be generated from (1) the spontaneous degradation of b-sulfinylpyruvate (an intermediate of cysteine degradation); (2) oxidation of H_2S by NADPH oxidase; and (3) oxidation of H_2S through a series of reactions involving the nonenzymatic formation of thiosulfate and its subsequent enzyme-catalyzed reaction with reduced glutathione (Li et al. 2009). Both H_2S and SO_2 are exhaled by the lungs, but sulfite and sulfate are excreted by the kidneys.

In saline, H_2S exists in equilibrium with HS^-, with the ratio of H_2S to HS^- being approximately 1:2. In physiological solutions, SO_2 spontaneously reacts with water to yield sulfurous acid (H_2SO_3) and then sulfite (SO_3^{2-}) through the dissociation of bisulfate (HSO_3^-):

$$SO_2 + H_2O \leftrightarrow H_2SO_3 \leftrightarrow HSO_3^- + H^+ \leftrightarrow SO_3^{2-} + 2H^+.$$

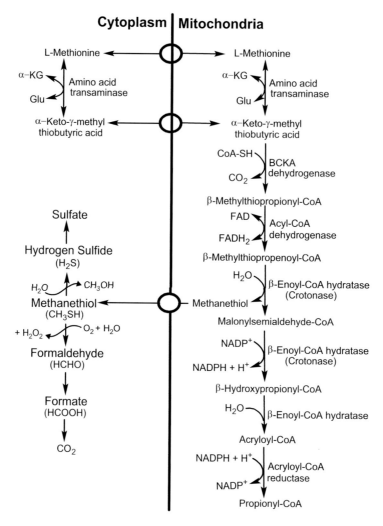

FIGURE 4.21 Catabolism of methionine via the transamination pathway in humans and animals. Many tissues have an ability to transaminate methionine primarily through the action of branched-chain amino acid transaminases. Under physiological conditions (e.g., the presence of all amino acids), this pathway does not play a significant role in methionine degradation in humans or other animals. BCKA, branched-chain α-ketoacids; α-KG, α-ketoglutarate.

4.2.10.3 Transamination Pathway for Methionine Catabolism

N.J. Benevenga proposed in 1978 that an alternative pathway for methionine degradation in animals involved transamination (Figure 4.21). This proposal was based on the detection of methionine transamination in homogenates of rat skeletal muscle, liver, small intestine, and other tissues. However, these studies were performed in the presence of very high concentrations of methionine (10–20 mM) and the absence of other AAs. In 1989, G. Wu and J.R. Thompson found that BCAAs strongly inhibit methionine transamination in rat and chick muscle homogenates. In the absence of BCAAs, rates of transamination of 0.5 mM methionine are very low in intact rat skeletal muscle but relatively high in intact chick skeletal muscle. Physiological levels of BCAAs essentially block methionine transamination in skeletal muscle from both rats and chicks (Wu and Thompson 1989). Thus, methionine transamination may occur in animals with exceeding high concentrations of methionine in the plasma (Scislowski and Pickard 1994), but it is normally a minor pathway for methionine degradation. This conclusion is supported by findings from clinical studies with healthy humans regardless of the oral administration of methionine (Blom et al. 1989).

Tavares et al. (2016) recently reported that mouse hepatocytes cultured in the presence of 0.25 to 4 mM methionine (about 4 to 64 times the physiological concentration of methionine in the plasma) but the absence of all other AAs could degrade methionine via the transamination pathway. Under these physiologically irrelevant conditions, methionine or 2 mM 3-methylthiopropionate (a metabolite of methionine via the transamination pathway; exceedingly high and unphysiological concentration) activated the GCN5 acetyltransferase-induced acetylation of PGC-1α (the transcriptional coactivator) to reduce hepatic gluconeogenesis. This *in vitro* finding is interesting, but should be confirmed by experiments that are conducted with liver slices or hepatocytes in the presence of physiological concentrations of AAs. Furthermore, the authors found that the intraperitoneal administration of methionine (100 mg/kg BW) to 16-h fasted C57BL/6 mice (n = 3) numerically reduced blood glucose concentration by ~ 10% (from ~ 10.4 mM in the phosphate-buffered saline control group to ~ 9.4 mM in the methionine treatment group) at 2 h post-administration. However, the change in blood glucose concentration did not appear to be statistically significant, and the high glucose concentrations in the two groups of mice are not consistent with those in fasted, nondiabetic mice (~ 4.5 to 5 mM). Thus, it remains to be determined whether methionine transamination may play a role in regulating glucose metabolism in cultured hepatocytes or in animals.

4.2.10.4   Catabolism of Taurine in Animal Cells

It was previously thought that taurine is degraded only in microorganisms but not in animal cells. However, this view is incorrect, as there is evidence that inhibition of AA transamination markedly increases concentrations of taurine in the plasma of young pigs (Flynn and Wu 1996). It is now known that taurine undergoes limited catabolism by taurine:pyruvate transaminase or taurine:α-ketoglutarate transaminase in the liver, kidneys, and brain of animals. These enzymes catalyze the transamination of taurine with pyruvate or α-ketoglutarate to form 2-sulfoacetaldehyde (also known as 2-oxoethanesulfonate, 2-hydroxyethanesulfonate, or isethionate) and L-alanine or L-glutamate (Figure 4.22). The 2-sulfoacetaldehyde is metabolized by intestinal bacteria to sulfite, sulfate, H_2S, and acetyl-CoA, as described below. Note that the liver of humans and other animals expresses sulfite oxidase to convert sulfite into sulfate.

4.2.10.5   Catabolism of Taurine in Intestinal Bacteria

In intestinal bacteria, taurine undergoes: (1) transamination to form 2-sulfoacetaldehyde; (2) oxygenation by taurine dehydrogenase in the presence of cytochrome C as the physiological electron acceptor to form 2-sulfoacetaldehyde; and (3) oxidation by α-ketoglutarate-dependent taurine dioxygenase to generate sulfite and 2-aminoacetaldehyde (Brüggemann et al. 2004; Cook and Denger 2006). In these cells, 2-sulfoacetaldehyde is reduced to isethionate by 2-sulfoacetaldehyde reductase or converted into sulfite plus acetyl-phosphate by sulfoacetaldehyde acetyltransferase. Isethionate is cleaved by isethionate sulfite-lyase to sulfite and acetaldehyde (Peck et al. 2019). Subsequently, sulfite is either reduced to hydrogen sulfite (H_2S) by sulfite reductase or oxidized to sulfate by sulfite reductase. Acetyl-phosphate is degraded to acetyl-CoA by phosphate acetyl-CoA transferase, whereas acetaldehyde undergoes oxidation to acetyl-CoA. Sulfite is oxidized to sulfate (SO_4^{2-}) by sulfite dehydrogenase. 2-Aminoacetaldehyde is unstable and undergoes self-condensation with two other molecules of 2-aminoacetaldehyde to form 2-aminoacetaldehyde diethylacetal (Figure 4.22). These metabolites of taurine are excreted primarily in the feces. Among them, sulfate is the major sulfur-containing metabolite. Taurine is strictly a ketogenic AA.

4.2.11   Catabolism of Threonine

There is a rich history of studying threonine catabolism via multiple pathways in animals (Figure 4.23). A.E. Braunshtein and G.Y. Vilenkina reported in 1949 that threonine is cleaved to glycine and acetaldehyde in animals. This reaction was confirmed by H.L. Meltzer and D.B. Sprinson in 1950. The responsible enzyme (a cytosolic protein) was named "threonine aldolase" in 1954 by D.M. Greenberg. Meanwhile, threonine dehydratase [also known as threonine hydrolyase

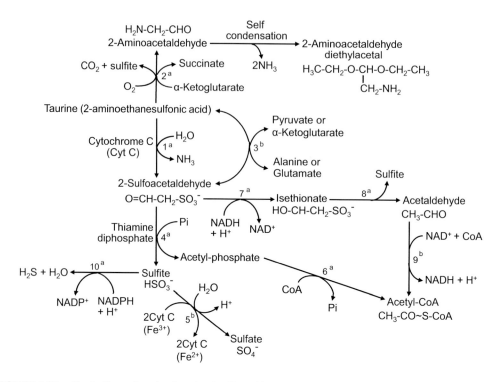

FIGURE 4.22 Catabolism of taurine in animal cells and intestinal microbes. The liver and kidneys of humans and other animals have a low ability to degrade taurine via transamination. Intestinal bacteria catabolize taurine via multiple metabolic pathways initiated via α-ketoglutarate- and cytochrome C-dependent oxidation, as well as dehydrogenation. The enzymes that catalyze the indicated reactions are as follows: (1) taurine dehydrogenase (requiring cytochrome C for electron transfer); (2) taurine dioxygenase; (3) taurine:pyruvate transaminase or taurine:α-ketoglutarate transaminase; (4) 2-sulfoacetaldehyde acetyltransferase; (5) sulfite oxidase (dehydrogenase); (6) phosphate acetyl-CoA transferase; (7) sulfoacetaldehyde reductase; (8) isethionate sulfite-lyase; (9) acetaldehyde dehydrogenase; and (10) sulfite reductase. 2-Aminoacetaldehyde is unstable and undergoes self-condensation with two additional molecules of 2-aminoacetaldehyde to form 2-aminoacetaldehyde diethylacetal. The major metabolic fate of the taurine sulfur is sulfite in strictly anaerobic, facultatively anaerobic, or strictly aerobic bacteria. Sulfite is then oxidized to sulfate. [a] Present in intestinal bacteria; [b] Present in intestinal bacteria, as well as the liver and kidneys of humans and other animals.

(deaminating)] was proposed in 1952 by H.L. Meltzer and D.B. Sprinson to hydrolyze threonine to ammonia and α-ketobutyrate in the cytoplasm of liver. This enzyme was subsequently found to be dependent on pyridoxal phosphate for catalytic activity. Based on earlier reports that threonine was catabolized to form aminoacetone, D.M. Greenberg discovered in 1964 the presence of threonine dehydrogenase in the liver mitochondria of animals. Thus, nutritional and biochemical studies led to identification of three metabolic pathways responsible for the degradation of threonine in the liver of animals (including humans), which are initiated by threonine dehydratase, threonine aldolase, and threonine dehydrogenase.

Catabolism of threonine via the threonine dehydratase pathway produces ammonia, α-ketobutyrate, and propionyl-CoA, but no glycine. By contrast, both the threonine aldolase and the threonine dehydrogenase pathways generate glycine from threonine. In the rat liver, threonine dehydratase and lactate dehydrogenase (or an α-ketoacid-linked NADPH dehydrogenase) may be responsible for threonine aldolase activity (Yeung 1986), but cannot explain the formation of glycine plus acetaldehyde from threonine by threonine aldolase. In animals [e.g., growing pigs (Ballevre et al. 1990; Le Floc'h et al. 1994), rats (Bird and Nunn 1983; Moundras et al. 1992), and chickens (Davis and Austic 1994, 1997)], the threonine dehydrogenase pathway accounts for approximately 80% of threonine catabolism.

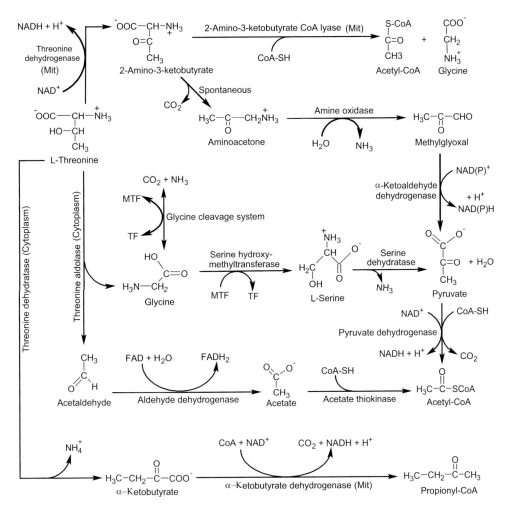

FIGURE 4.23 Catabolism of threonine in humans and other animals. Threonine degradation in the liver is initiated primarily by threonine dehydrogenase (a mitochondrial enzyme) and, to a much lesser extent, threonine dehydratase and threonine aldolase (cytosolic enzymes). Products of threonine catabolism include glycine, pyruvate, and propionyl-CoA.

The rate of whole-body threonine catabolism is influenced by dietary AA intake and balance, as well as age. For example, either high dietary protein intake or dietary threonine imbalance stimulates threonine dehydrogenase activity in rats and chickens, whereas the opposite occurs in the animals fed a low-protein diet containing proper ratios of AAs (Davis and Austic 1994, 1997). Furthermore, in young pigs fed a milk protein-based or corn- and soybean meal-based diet, quantitatively only a small amount of threonine is degraded to form glycine and CO_2, because the threonine supply in the diet is limited and barely meets requirements for tissue protein synthesis (Wang et al. 2013).

In humans, the relative importance of the threonine dehydratase, threonine aldolase, and threonine dehydrogenase pathways in threonine degradation remains largely unknown. Darling et al. (1999, 2000) reported that 44% of threonine oxidation in human infants occurs via the threonine dehydrogenase pathway, but this pathway plays only a minor role (contributing to 7–10% of total threonine degradation) in adult humans as based on the measurement of the flux of threonine to glycine in the plasma. It is possible that the measurement of the flux of threonine to glycine in the plasma may not truly indicate threonine catabolism via the threonine dehydrogenase pathway.

This is because some of the resultant glycine is converted into other molecules (e.g., glutathione, bile salts, hippurate, heme, and serine) and also oxidized to CO_2 in tissues and, therefore, does not appear in the blood during the period of isotope infusion. Thus, the findings from the human studies remain to be confirmed. Nonetheless, there are possibly species differences in threonine catabolism among animals and also developmental differences within the same species. These metabolic differences may be related to the nutritional and physiological needs of the body for glycine.

4.2.12 CATABOLISM OF TRYPTOPHAN

In humans and other animals, three pathways are responsible for degrading tryptophan in a highly cell- and tissue-specific manner: the kynurenine, serotonin, and transamination pathways (Yao et al. 2011). The kynurenine pathway, which involves the deamination and the vitamin B_6-dependent decarboxylation of tryptophan to form kynurenine, occurs primarily in the liver and brain. The serotonin pathway, which requires the BH4-dependent hydroxylation and the vitamin B_6-dependent decarboxylation of tryptophan to generate serotonin (5-hydroxytryptamine), takes place mainly in the gastrointestinal tract and brain (Figure 4.24). The catabolism of kynurenine produces indole-acetic acid, niacin, pyruvate, and acetyl-CoA. Serotonin is a biogenic amine which functions as a neurotransmitter, a gastrointestinal hormone, and an antioxidant.

4.2.12.1 The Kynurenine Pathway

There is a rich history of tryptophan degradation in animals via the kynurenine pathway. In 1925, Z. Matsuoka and N. Yoshimatsu discovered kynurenine in the urine of rabbits fed a large amount of tryptophan. Subsequently, it was found that kynurenine is converted to kynurenic acid (kynurenate), a substance that was discovered by J. von Liebig in 1853. These seminal findings paved the way for elucidation of the major pathway for tryptophan degradation. Thus, tryptophan 2,3-dioxygenase (TDO) was discovered in mammalian liver in 1936 and was first characterized in the rat liver in 1955, whereas indoleamine 2,3-dioxygenase (IDO) was initially found in the rabbit small intestine in 1967. Concentrations of kynurenic acid, which undergoes little catabolism in animals, are relatively high in bile and pancreatic juice (e.g., approximately $1\,\mu M$ in porcine bile and pancreatic juice; Paluszkiewicz et al. 2009). This substance has an antiexcitotoxic and anticonvulsant function mainly through acting as an antagonist at receptors for excitatory AAs. Quantitatively, the kynurenine pathway accounts for the degradation of about 95% of tryptophan in the body (Badawy 2017). At the tissue level, hepatic and extrahepatic kynurenine pathways contribute to 90%–95% and 5%–10% of whole-body tryptophan catabolism under normal physiologic conditions.

The first and rate-controlling step in the kynurenine pathway is catalyzed by either the ubiquitous IDO activity or the highly cell-specific TDO. They are structurally distinct proteins but have evolved separately to catalyze the same reaction (Rafice et al. 2009). TDO is selective for L-tryptophan, whereas IDO uses a broader range of indole-containing substrates (including L-tryptophan, D-tryptophan, tryptamine, 5-hydroxytryptophan, and 5-hydroxytryptamine; Ball et al. 2014). Mammalian TDO and IDO have K_m values of 100–200 and 3–50 μM for arginine, respectively (namely, TDO has a lower affinity for arginine than IDO), but TDO has a higher catalytic capacity than IDO. In addition, glucocorticoids induce the expression of TDO but not IDO in anima tissues (Badawy 2017). Note that both IDO and TDO are heme enzymes and require BH4 as an essential cofactor for catalytic activity.

There are two isoforms of IDO: IDO-1 (a cytosolic enzyme; about 45 kD) and IDO-2 (a perinuclear or nuclear subcellular enzyme as shown in the liver; about 45 kD). Under normal physiologic conditions, IDO activity is relatively low or negligible but is widely distributed in animal tissues. Studies with mice have shown that IDO-1 is expressed at higher levels in the epididymis and the small intestine than those in the spleen, large intestine, and esophagus (Dai and Zhu 2010). IDO-1 expression is noticeable in the skin, brain, stomach, prostate, bladder, and uterus, but is weakly expressed or nearly absent in the pancreas, thymus, lymph nodes, adrenal gland, liver,

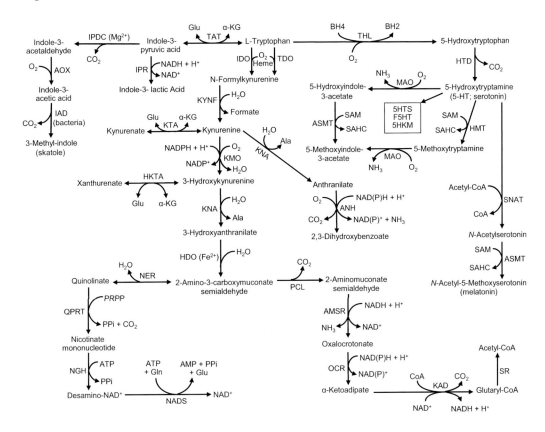

FIGURE 4.24 Catabolism of tryptophan in humans and other animals. Degradation of L-tryptophan is initiated by indoleamine 2,3-dioxygenase (IDO), tryptophan 2,3-dioxygenase (TDO), and tryptophan hydroxylase (THL). These pathways are cell- and tissue-specific. Serotonin, melatonin, and their metabolites can form sulfate and glucuronide conjugates for excretion in urine and feces. Products of tryptophan catabolism include NAD, serotonin, melatonin, kynurenine, indoles, and acetyl-CoA. AMSR, 2-aminomuconate semialdehyde reductase; ANH, anthranilate hydroxylase [also known as Anthranilate 3-monooxygenase (deaminating)]; AOC, aldehyde oxidase; AOX, indole-3-acetaldehyde oxidase; ASMT, *N*-acetylserotonin *O*-methyltransferase; F5HT, formyl 5-hydroxytryptamine; HDO, 3-hydroxyanthranilate dioxygenase (Fe-S); 5HKM, 5-hydroxykynuremine; HKTA, 3-hydroxykynurenine transaminase; HMT: 5-hydroxyindole-*O*-methyltransferase; 5-HT, 5-hydroxytryptamine; HTD, 5-hydroxytryptopohan decarboxylase; 5HTS, 5-hydroxytryptamine sulfate; 5-HTP, 5-hydroxy-l-tryptophan; IAD, indoleacetate decarboxylase (a bacterial enzyme); IPDC, indole-3-pyruvate decarboxylase (a thiamine diphosphate-dependent enzyme); IPR, indole-3-pyruvate reductase; KAD, α-ketoadipate dehydrogenase; KHL, kynurenine hydroxylase; KMO, kynurenine monooxygenase; KNA, kynureninase; KTA, kynurenine transaminase; KYN, kynurenine; KYNF, kynurenine formamidase; MAO, monoamine oxidase; NADS, NAD synthase; NER, nonenzymatic reaction; NGH, NAD glycohydrolase; OCR, oxalocrotonate reductase; PCL, picolinate carboxylase; PLP, pyridoxal phosphate; PRPP, 5-phosphoribosyl-1-pyrophosphate; QPRT, quinolinate phosphoribosyl transferase; SNAT, serotonin-N-acetyltransferase; SAM, *S*-adenosylmethionine; SAHC, *S*-adenosylhomocysteine; SR, a series of reactions for the conversion of glutaryl-CoA to acetyl-CoA; TAT, tryptophan aminotransferase. The following enzymes require pyridoxal phosphate for catalytic activities: HTD, HKTA, KNA, KTA, and TAT. QPRT is inhibited by high concentrations of leucine.

kidneys, brain, ovaries, and testes (Dai and Zhu 2010). IDO-1 appears to play quantitatively only a minor role in whole-body tryptophan degradation under basal conditions, but this enzyme is inducible by inflammatory stimuli to contribute significantly to whole-body tryptophan homeostasis under inflammatory conditions (Mellor et al. 2017). An exciting new development in tryptophan metabolism is that the expression of IDO-1 in dendritic cells, lymphocytes, and macrophages mediates the function of the immune system and is potently induced by inflammatory cytokines (e.g., interferon-γ, interferon-α, and tumor necrosis factor-α) and endotoxin (Ball et al. 2014; Mellor et al. 2017). Thus, under inflammatory conditions, proinflammatory cytokines can induce IDO expression to reduce the concentration of tryptophan in the plasma (Ball et al. 2014; Mellor et al. 2017). Conversely, anti-inflammatory cytokines (interleukin-4, interleukin-10, and transforming growth factor β) inhibit IDO induction by interferon-γ. In contrast to IDO-1, the expression of IDO-2 is more restricted in animal tissues than IDO-1. Studies with mice revealed that IDO-2 is expressed at higher levels in the liver and kidneys than in the epididymis, large intestine, brain, testes, and spermatozoa (Jusof et al. 2017). Under physiological conditions, IDO-2 does not appear to affect tryptophan homeostasis in the liver or the whole body. It remains to be determined whether IDO-2 may contribute significantly to local tryptophan catabolism in cells under certain conditions such as sepsis, infection, and tumorigenesis.

Unlike IDO-1 and IDO-2, TDO is constitutively expressed at high levels in the liver and plays a quantitatively major role in degrading tryptophan in humans and other animals (Ball et al. 2014). In mammals and birds, TDO is predominantly expressed in the liver with a half-life of about 2 h and, to a much lesser extent, also occurs in a few other tissues (e.g., the brain, placenta, endometrium, and skin). The extrahepatic TDO may not be the same protein as the hepatic TDO. For example, the molecular weights of the TDO protein in the rat liver and skin are 167 and 16 kD, respectively (Ishiguro et al. 1993). Additionally, although the intraperitoneal administration of arginine to rats increases TDO activity in both the liver and skin, the intraperitoneal administration of hydrocortisone to rats induces the expression of the hepatic TDO but has no effect on the skin TDO (Ishiguro et al. 1993). TDO activity is increased by tryptophan and its analogues via an allosteric binding site, as well as by the administration of epinephrine and norepinephrine, but is competitively inhibited by some common indoleamines (including tryptamine) and is subject to feedback inhibition by high concentrations of $NAD(P)^+$.

The hepatic catabolism of tryptophan in humans and most of other animals (e.g., dogs, pigs, rats, ruminants, and chickens) via the kynurenine pathway yields niacin (niacin, vitamin B_3). The rates of niacin biosynthesis differ greatly among animal species. This is partially due to a much higher activity of picolinate carboxylase than that of quinolinate phosphoribosyl transferase, thereby diverting 2-amino-3-carboxymuconate semialdehyde into 2-aminomuconate semialdehyde rather than nicotinate mononucleotide. For example, the hepatic activity of picolinate carboxylase (U/mg fresh tissue) is as follows: cats, 50.5; ducks, 17.3; turkeys, 9.23; cows, 8.30; pigs, 7.12; pigeons, 6.95; chickens, 3.20–5.38; humans, 3.18; and rats, 1.57 (Scott 1982). Most species except for postweaning ruminants are not able to synthesize sufficient niacin and, therefore, need dietary niacin for normal metabolism and good health. For example, although young chicks can produce niacin from tryptophan, the amount of endogenously formed niacin is insufficient for their optimum growth. Note that cats, mink, and carnivorous fish have a very low ability to synthesize niacin, compared with omnivores.

4.2.12.2 The Serotonin Pathway

Tryptophan undergoes hydroxylation by BH4-dependent tryptophan hydroxylase (TPH) to form 5-hydroxytryptophan. This enzyme is the rate-controlling step for serotonin synthesis and has two isoforms: TPH1 and TPH2 (Sakowski et al. 2006). TPH1 is expressed mainly in the pineal gland and the enterochromaffin cells of the intestine, whereas TPH2 selectively occurs in neurons of the brain. Other tissues, such as the small intestine, liver, spleen, and thymus, have relatively low levels of TPH1 expression (Hagiwara et al. 2020). 5-Hydroxytryptophan is decarboxylated by vitamin B_6-dependent 5-hydroxytryptophan decarboxylase to generate 5-hydroxytryptamine (serotonin). Serotonin is further metabolized via SAM-dependent reactions to form 5-methoxytryptamine, 5-methoxyindole 3-acetate, and melatonin, as well as SAM-independent reactions to generate 5-hydroxyindole 3-acetate, 5-hydroxytryptamine sulfate, formyl 5-hydroxytryptamine, and 5-hydroxykynuremine (Figure 4.24). Under inflammatory conditions where IDO-1 expression is enhanced in immune cells and tissues, whole-body tryptophan catabolism is augmented to reduce the circulating level of tryptophan for serotonin synthesis.

4.2.12.3 The Transamination Pathway

Tryptophan catabolism can also be initiated by vitamin B_6-dependent transamination to form indolepyruvate in many animal species (including pigs and rats). Indolepyruvate can be further metabolized to indole-3-acetaldehyde and indolelactate by indole-3-pyruvate decarboxylase and indole-3-pyruvate reductase, respectively. Indole-3-acetaldehyde is oxidized by indole-3-acetaldehyde oxidase to form indole-3-acetate. Interestingly, indole-3-acetaldehyde oxidase (an oxidoreductase) requires three 3 cofactors (FAD, heme, and molybdenum) for enzymatic activity. The presence of the transamination pathway for tryptophan catabolism in mammals and birds is supported by the findings of nutritional studies that D-tryptophan can be utilized by animals to replace some or all L-tryptophan in diets (see Chapter 3). In such a series of reactions, D-tryptophan is transaminated with an α-ketoacid (e.g., α-KG) to form indolepyruvate, which is transaminated with an α-AA (e.g., glutamate) to generate L-tryptophan.

4.2.13 CATABOLISM OF SELENOCYSTEINE IN ANIMALS

Selenocysteine is cleaved by the vitamin B_6-dependent selenocysteine lyase into L-alanine and selenide (H_2Se). A [2H] donor (i.e., reduced acceptor; e.g., dithiothreitol or 2-mercaptoethanol) is required for this reaction *in vitro*. Selenide can be recycled for selenocysteine formation during mRNA translation. Selenocysteine lyase is expressed in tissues of mammals, including the cat, cattle, dog, guinea pig, monkey, mouse, pig, rabbit, and rat (Esaki et al. 1982), as well as humans (Collins et al. 2012), and does not act on L-cysteine, L-serine, L-cysteine sulfinate, selenocysteamine, Se-ethyl-DL-selenocysteine, or L-selenohomocysteine. In rats, the activity of this enzyme is the highest in the pancreas, followed by the liver, kidneys, adrenal gland, thymus, spleen, lung, brain, heart, testes, and skeletal muscle in descending order (Esaki et al. 1982).

$$\text{L-Selenocysteine} + \text{Reduced acceptor}\left([2H] \text{ donor}\right) \rightarrow \text{Selenide}\left(H_2Se\right) + \text{L-Alanine} + \text{Acceptor}$$

4.2.14 CATABOLISM OF N-ACETYLATED AAS IN HUMANS AND OTHER ANIMALS

As noted in Chapter 1, humans and other animals synthesize N-acetylated AAs, including N-acetyl-glutamate, N-acetyl-aspartate, N-acetyl-L-histidine, and N-acetyl-1-methylhistidine (N-acetyl-π-methylhistidine) in a species- and tissue-specific manner. These acetylated AAs may play important roles in neurological and osmoregulation functions of humans and other animals and should be maintained at constant concentrations under physiological conditions. This is achieved by not only their synthesis (Chapter 3) but also their catabolism. Specifically, N-acetyl-glutamate is hydrolyzed in the liver, enterocytes, and brain by N-acetyl-glutamate deacylase into acetate and glutamate. N-Acetyl-L-aspartate is hydrolyzed by N-acetyl-L-aspartate amidohydrolase (also known as aspartoacylase) in the brain, the lens of eyes, and kidneys into acetate and L-aspartate, whereas N-acetyl-L-histidine is hydrolyzed by N-acetyl-L-histidine amidohydrolase in the brain of fish, reptiles, and amphibians or the ocular fluid of fish into acetate and L-histidine (Baslow 1997). Of note, N-acetyl-L-histidine amidohydrolase is absent from the mouse and rat brain, as well as the lens of the eyes in fish. In fish, N-acetyl-L-histidine exits the lens of their eyes into ocular fluid, where this AA is hydrolyzed extracellular by N-acetyl-L-histidine amidohydrolase. N-Acetyl-1-methylhistidine is hydrolyzed by N-acetyl-1-methylhistidine amidohydrolase in the brain, liver, and kidneys into acetate and 1-methyl-L-histidine. All of these enzymes responsible for the hydrolysis of acetylated AAs are localized in the cytosol of the specific tissues. The physiological significance of the catabolism of acetylated AAs is indicated by Canavan's disease (an inherited metabolic disorder) in humans, which is characterized by aspartoacylase deficiency with the concomitant accumulation of N-acetyl-L-aspartate in the brain and urine, as well as a spongy degeneration of the brain (Baslow 1997).

$$N\text{-Acetyl-L-glutamate} + H_2O \rightleftharpoons \text{Acetate} + L\text{-Glutamate} \quad \left(N\text{-acetyl-glutamatedeacylase}\right)$$

$$N\text{-Acetyl-L-aspartate} + H_2O \rightleftharpoons \text{Acetate} + L\text{-Aspartate} \quad \left(N\text{-acetyl-L-aspartateamidohydrolase}\right)$$

$$N\text{-Acetyl-L-histidine} + H_2O \rightleftharpoons \text{Acetate} + L\text{-Histidine} \quad \left(N\text{-acetyl-L-histidineamidohydrolase}\right)$$

$$N\text{-Acetyl-1-methylhistidine} + H_2O \rightleftharpoons \text{Acetate} + 1\text{-Methyl-L-histidine}$$

$$\left(N\text{-acetyl-1-methylhistidineamidohydrolase}\right)$$

4.3 CATABOLISM OF D-AAs IN ANIMAL CELLS

4.3.1 D-AA Transporters in Animal Cells

Like L-AAs, the entry of D-AAs into cells is the first step in their catabolism. It appears that some transporters for L-AAs can transport D-AAs across the plasma and other biological membranes although they preferentially transport L-AAs. For example, a Na^+-dependent AA transporter, $ATB^{0,+}$, can transport: (1) D-serine at the same affinity and capacity as L-serine, and (2) some other D-AAs, including D-alanine, D-leucine, D-methionine, and D-tryptophan (Hatanaka et al. 2002). Another Na^+-dependent AA transporter, $ATB^{0,+}$, can transport some D-AAs, including D-serine. In the intestine, both $ATB^{0,+}$ and ATB^0 are localized to the apical membrane of the absorptive epithelial cells and, therefore, are responsible for the absorption of some D-AAs. Interestingly, AA transporters L1 and system ascl, which are facilitative (Na^+-independent) transporters that mediate AA exchange across the plasma membrane, can transport D-AAs to a significant extent (Fukasawa et al. 2000; Kanai et al. 1998). Both L1 and ascl contain, as a common subunit, the heavy chain of the 4F2 cell surface antigen (4F2hc) that is localized exclusively to the basolateral membrane of the absorptive cells of the intestine and kidneys. Thus, these two transporters participate in the efflux of AAs from the intestinal and renal epithelial cells into the blood. Compared with L-AAs, the rate of the transport of many D-AAs is lower and the affinity of the L-AA transporters for most D-AAs is also lower in mammalian cells. In neurons, the L-Glu/L-Asp transporter, which utilizes the Na^+/K^+- electrochemical gradient to move excitatory AAs against their concentration gradient, can transport D-Asp but not D-glutamate (Kanai and Hediger 2003). Interestingly, in *Drosophila*, the invertebrate B^0 system transporter (*D. melanogaster* NAT1), which normally transports a broad range of neutral AAs, can equally or even preferentially transport the D-isomers to support intestinal and neurological functions (Miller et al. 2008). It is possible that the fly has developed a symbiotic relationship with D-AA-producing microbes.

4.3.2 Enzymes for Initiating D-AA Catabolism in Animal Cells

Animal cells do not express D-AA transaminase but contain D-AA racemases (or epimerases), D-AA deaminase, and D-AA oxidase (strategically localized in peroxisomes with peroxidase and catalase) as almost the exclusive enzymes to degrade D-AAs (including D-alanine, D-aspartate, and D-serine). Racemases may convert D-AAs directly to their L-isomers, but this enzymatic activity is quantitatively low or limited for most, if not all, D-AAs, in mammals, birds, and fish (Bada 1984; Ohide et al. 2011). Because the intracellular concentrations of L-AAs are generally greater than those of D-AAs, the equilibrium of the transamination does not favor the formation of L-AAs from D-AAs. However, in the animal kingdom, there is substantial formation of certain D-AAs (e.g., D-serine, D-alanine, and D-aspartate) in a cell-, tissue-, species-, and developmental stage-specific manner (Chapters 1 and 3), because of their biologically significant functions. Excess D-AAs are toxic to animals and must be degraded via multiple pathways.

D-AA deaminase removes the amino group from D-AAs to yield the corresponding α-ketoacid and ammonia. D-AA oxidase (FAD-containing flavoprotein) converts D-AAs into not only α-ketoacids and ammonia but also hydrogen peroxide (see Chapter 3). An overall reaction catalyzed by D-AA oxidase is as follows:

$$D\text{-}AA + O_2 + H_2O \rightarrow \alpha\text{-}Ketoacid + H_2O_2 + NH_4^+ \quad (D\text{-}AA \text{ oxidase})$$

D-AA oxidase generally acts on both neutral and basic D-AAs, whereas D-aspartate oxidase uses only acidic D-AAs (e.g., D-aspartate, D-glutamate, and NMDA) as preferred substrates in mammals (e.g., pigs, rats, and mice) and birds (e.g., chickens and pigeons). D-aspartate oxidase is the sole enzyme which selectively degrades D-aspartate and is inactive toward D-Ser. In contrast to mammals, D-AA oxidase is not expressed in the chicken brain. Rather, D-serine dehydratase (a cytosolic enzyme requiring pyridoxal-5′-phosphate as a cofactor) is responsible for the catabolism of D-serine to form pyruvate and ammonia in the brain, kidney, and liver of chickens. This indicates a cell- and species-specific difference in D-AA oxidation. In all animals, D-AA-derived ketoacids can be oxidized to acetyl-CoA and then to CO_2 plus water (Figure 4.1).

4.4 CATABOLISM OF L-AAs AND D-AAs IN MICROORGANISMS

4.4.1 L-AA Catabolism in Microbes

Microbes degrade L-AAs via the same as, or similar to, the metabolic pathways present in animal cells as detailed in the preceding sections. This can be illustrated by the utilization of L-arginine (Figure 4.25), L-proline (Becker and Thomas 2001), and L-cysteine (Pecka et al. (2019) by bacteria. For example, proline dehydrogenase and P5C dehydrogenase are two different proteins in eukaryotes and certain bacteria, but are fused into a bifunctional enzyme known as proline utilization A (PutA) in some bacteria, such as *Escherichia coli and Salmonella typhimurium*. In contrast to proline oxidase in animal cells, microbial proline dehydrogenase uses FAD as an electron acceptor (Arentson et al. 2012). In addition, microbes possess unique biochemical pathways for AA catabolism (e.g., the acetylation and transamination of nearly all AAs, the coupled deamination of nearly all AAs (possibly except for histidine) via the Stickland reaction, as well as the oxidation and dehydrogenation of taurine) that are absent in animal cells. The Stickland reaction occurs in anaerobic bacteria, where the oxidation of one AA by AA dehydrogenase is coupled with the reduction of another AA by AA hydrogenase (e.g., in the case of glycine and proline) or AA reductase (Nisman 1954). AAs that are hydrogen donors include alanine, valine, leucine, isoleucine, serine, threonine, cysteine, lysine, methionine, and phenylalanine, whereas AAs that are hydrogen acceptors include

Stickland reaction for the coupled deamination of amino acids (AAs) in anaerobic bacteria

glycine, proline, 4-hydroxyproline, and ornithine. Through the Stickland reaction in anaerobic bacteria, either the deamination of ornithine or the reduction of proline generates 5-aminovaleric acid, and the deamination of lysine forms 6-aminocaproic acid (an inducer of blood clotting). Further degradation of 5-aminovaleric acid yields valerate, acetate, and propionate (Huang et al. 2018).

Gastrointestinal microbes play an important role in AA catabolism. In certain ruminants, ruminal bacteria can degrade some toxic AAs (Chapter 2). In addition, Huang et al. (2018) recently reported that anaerobic bacteria (e.g., *Firmicutes* and *Bacteroidetes*) possess 4-hydroxyproline

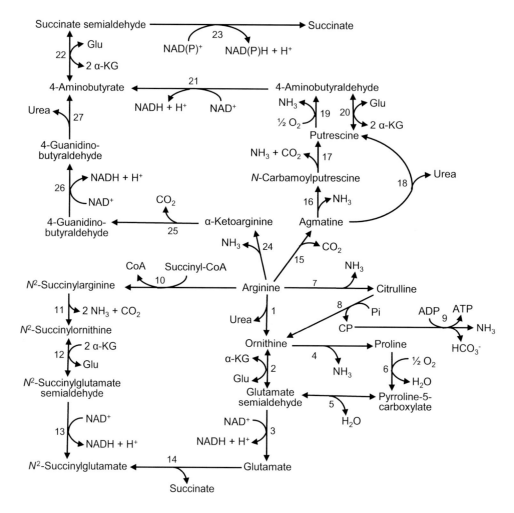

FIGURE 4.25 Catabolism of arginine in bacteria via multiple pathways. The enzymes that catalyze the indicated reactions are as follows: (1) arginase; (2) ornithine aminotransferase; (3) pyrroline-5-carboxylate dehydrogenase; (4) ornithine cyclase; (5) spontaneous reaction; (6) proline dehydrogenase; (7) arginine deiminase; (8) ornithine carbamoyltransferase; (9) carbamate kinase; (10) arginine succinyltransferase; (11) succinylarginine dihydrolase; (12) succinylornithine aminotransferase; (13) succinylglutamate semialdehyde dehydrogenase; (14) succinylglutamate desuccinylase; (15) arginine decarboxylase; (16) agmatine deiminase; (17) N-carbamoylputrescine hydrolase; (18) agmatine ureohydrolase; (19) putrescine oxidase; (20) putrescine transaminase; (21) 4-aminobutyraldehyde dehydrogenase; (22) 4-aminobutyrate transaminase; (23) succinate semialdehyde dehydrogenase; (24) arginine oxidase; (25) α-ketoarginine decarboxylase; (26) 4-guanidinobutyraldehyde oxidoreductase; and (27) 4-guanidinobutyrase.

dehydratase to convert *trans* 4-hydroxyproline into P5C via the removal of one H_2O molecule. At present, the significance of this reaction in the intestinal bacteria of humans and other animals is unknown. Furthermore, intestinal bacteria can convert indoleacetate into 3-methylindole (skatole) through the action of indoleacetate decarboxylase (Whitehead et al. 2008), but this reaction is absent from animal cells (Figure 4.24). Most of the 3-methylindole (a lipid-soluble substance) is excreted in the feces but some of it is stored in the tissues (e.g., adipose tissue, liver, and skeletal muscle) of the host animal. Interestingly, 3-methylindole is a malodorous compound that gives animal feces a characteristic smell and also contributes to boar taint in the pork meat of intact male pigs (another contributing factor being androstenone).

$$trans\text{-}4\text{-Hydroxyproline (Hyp)} \rightarrow \Delta^1\text{-Pyrroline-5-carboxylate (P5C)} + H^+ + H_2O$$

$$(4\text{-hydroxyprolinedehydratase; anaerobic bacteria})$$

Also note that ruminal microbes in cattle and sheep do not degrade extracellular citrulline due to the lack of uptake and have a limited ability to degrade extracellular glutamate due to a negligible uptake (Chapter 2), but mammals and birds actively catabolize extracellular citrulline and glutamate (Chapter 3). It remains to be determined whether ruminal microbes can catabolize extracellular aspartate. These findings have important implications for understanding AA catabolism in the lumen of the large intestine of both humans and other animals.

4.4.2 D-AA Catabolism in Microbes

Catabolism of D-AAs by intestinal bacteria in animals can be substantial. For example, D-lysine is poorly metabolized in animal cells but can be degraded by microorganisms. Ratner and coworkers reported in 1943 that in young rats fed a diet containing D-[^{15}N]lysine, approximately 50% of the D-lysine was excreted unchanged in urine, approximately 20% of the total ^{15}N administered appeared in urinary urea and ammonia, and approximately 20% of the total ^{15}N administered was found in non-lysine AAs in tissue proteins. Like D-lysine, D-threonine is not utilized by animal cells but is extensively oxidized by D-AA oxidase, as noted previously. Much evidence shows that microorganisms contain D-AA transaminases, D-AA oxidases, D-AA deaminases, and D-AA dehydrogenases to degrade D-AAs (Li and Lu 2009). Some bacteria also possess NAD$^+$- or NADP$^+$-linked D-AA dehydrogenase (e.g., D-threonine dehydrogenase in *Pseudomonas cruciviae* and D-arginine dehydrogenase in *Pseudomonas aeruginosa*) to initiate the catabolism of D-AAs. In addition, D-serine dehydratase is expressed in bacteria as another pathway for D-serine utilization. Because the large intestine has a limited ability to absorb L-AAs and D-AAs into the blood circulation, these results indicate a potentially important contribution of bacterial metabolism to the *de novo* synthesis of AAs in the small intestine and to the loss of dietary AAs from the hindgut.

Excessive amounts of some D-AAs can be used by bacteria to support growth and survival. For example, *Pseudomonas aeruginosa* (an opportunistic human pathogen), in which the expression of D-arginine dehydrogenase is inducible by D-arginine, can grow on medium containing D-arginine as the sole source of carbon and nitrogen (Haas et al. 1984). Interestingly, Li and Lu (2009) reported that *Pseudomonas aeruginosa* contains a two-component metabolic pathway for the conversion of D-arginine into L-arginine for catabolism. In this bacterium, DauA (a dehydrogenase) catalyzes the oxidative deamination of D-arginine into α-ketoarginine and ammonia, and DauB (a dehydrogenase) converts α-ketoarginine and ammonia into L-arginine in the presence of NADPH or NADH (Li and Lu 2009). L-Arginine is then degraded via the arginase, arginine succinyltransferase, and arginine transaminase pathways. Thus, although the racemization of most AAs is catalyzed by a single enzyme, some bacteria may be able to coupled dehydrogenases to complete the D-to-L racemization of certain AAs.

$$D\text{-Arginine} + NAD(P)^+ \rightarrow \alpha\text{-Ketoarginine} + Ammonia + NAD(P)H + H^+$$

$$(D\text{-arginine dehydrogenase, DauA})$$

$$\alpha\text{-Ketoarginine} + Ammonia + NAD(P)H + H^+ \rightarrow L\text{-Arginine} + NAD(P)^+$$

$$(L\text{-arginine dehydrogenase, DauB})$$

4.4.3 Metabolites from the Catabolism of L- and D-AAs in Microbes

Nearly all of the pathways for AA catabolism to generate ammonia, other nitrogenous metabolites (e.g., nitrite and nitrate), H_2S, sulfate, indoles, CO_2, and water in animal cells as discussed in the preceding sections are present in microorganisms. Metabolic pathways for AA catabolism are more similar between bacteria and yeast than between the microorganisms and animals, although both yeast and animals are eukaryotes. Different strains of bacteria (e.g., commensal vs. pathogenic) or yeasts [e.g., *Saccharomyces cerevisiae* (a baker's yeast) vs. *Candida albicans* (a highly infectious yeast)] may also have different metabolic patterns (Flynn et al. 2010). For example, glycine is degraded to a much greater extent in *C. albicans* than in *S. cerevisiae*, as are intracellular threonine concentrations. In addition, almost all of the disappearance of glycine from incubation medium can be accounted for by the formation of serine, threonine, and CO_2 in *S. cerevisiae*, whereas these products represent only 50% of the metabolized glycine in *C. albicans*. The unidentified metabolites of glycine in *C. albicans* (e.g., purines) may contribute to its infectious capacity.

Besides odorous products (e.g., cadaverine, skatole, and trimethylamine), microbial catabolism of some AAs may result in the production of toxic substances. An example is the formation of anatoxin (a bicyclic secondary amine is anatoxin) from the catabolism of proline and acetate in blue-green algae (which are actually cyanobacteria, but are not algae) found in freshwater lakes, streams, ponds, and brackish water ecosystems (Kust et al. 2020). Anatoxin is a neurotoxin, which is also known as the very fast death factor. The ingestion of this toxin by humans and other animals (e.g., birds, cattle, and dogs) can be lethal within minutes due to the irreversible binding to nicotinic acetylcholine receptors and the inhibition of acetylcholinesterase.

Anatoxin ($C_{10}H_{15}NO$, M.W. = 165.23 Da)

4.4.4 Differences in AA Catabolism between Bacteria and Animals

There are noteworthy differences in AA catabolism between bacteria and animals. First, rates of AA degradation per protein basis are generally higher in bacteria than in avian and mammalian cells. This is clearly illustrated by Z.L. Dai and colleagues who studied AA catabolism in bacteria from the lumen of the pig small intestine and jejunal enterocytes (Dai et al. 2010, 2011, 2012). Second, pathways for AA catabolism take place within a single bacterium, but the degradation of most AAs involves inter-organ or inter-cellular coordination in animals. For example, in humans, pigs, and rats, BCAAs are transaminated in extrahepatic tissues and their α-ketoacids are oxidized primarily in the liver. Third, some enzyme-catalyzed reactions (e.g., the conversion of glutamate to P5C and proline oxidation) and intermediates of the pathways for AA degradation (e.g., conversion of glutamine to arginine) differ between eukaryotes (e.g., animals) and prokaryotes (e.g., bacteria). Fourth, the metabolic fate of the carbons of AAs and their metabolites differ between bacteria and animals. For example, AAs can be fermented to methane (CH_4) in anaerobic bacteria due to the lack of oxygen, but this pathway is absent from animal cells. Rather, oxidation to CO_2 and H_2O via the Krebs cycle and the mitochondrial electron transport system is the major pathway for the complete catabolism of AA carbons in mammals, birds, and fish (Figure 4.26). Also, indole is metabolized to indican in the liver of animals, but to anthranilic acid and salicylic acid in bacteria. Furthermore, catabolism of arginine is almost the exclusive source of energy for certain bacteria but plays only a minor role in ATP production in animal cells. Fifth, bacteria possess some unique enzymes for degradation of some AAs [e.g., arginine deiminase (Figure 4.25), D-arginine dehydrogenase, L-arginine dehydrogenase, tryptophanase (a pyridoxal phosphate-dependent enzyme), D-homoserine racemase, and tryptophan decarboxylase (a pyridoxal phosphate-dependent enzyme), and β-tyrosinase] and their products (e.g., urease for urea, sulfite reductase for SO_3^{2-}, tryptamine, and nitrate reductase for nitrate), but these enzymes are absent from animal cells. In the hepatic

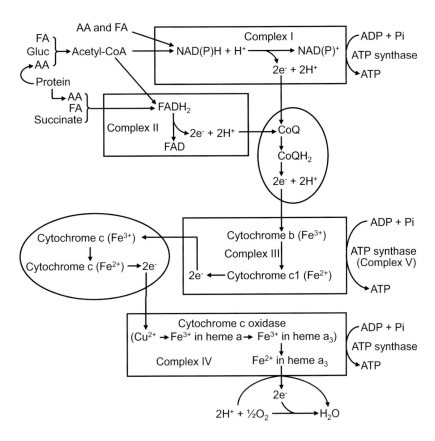

FIGURE 4.26 Oxidation of NAD(P)H and FADH$_2$ via the mitochondrial electron transport system in humans and other animals. This respiratory chain consists of complex I (NADH dehydrogenase) for the transfer of electrons from NADH to coenzyme Q (CoQ, a lipid-soluble mobile carrier); complex II (succinate dehydrogenase) for the transfer of electrons from succinate to coenzyme Q; complex III (cytochrome c reductase) for the transfer of electrons from reduced coenzyme Q to cytochrome c (a water-soluble mobile carrier); complex IV (cytochrome c oxidase) for the transfer of electrons from reduced cytochrome c to O$_2$; and complex V (ATP synthase). Complexes I, III, and IV also act as proton pumps that contribute to generation of the proton-motive force across the inner mitochondrial membrane. In complex IV, O$_2$ serves as the final oxidant of NADH and FADH$_2$, where 1/2 O$_2$ is reduced to 1/2 O$_2^-$ (superoxide anion), which reacts with 2H$^+$ to form H$_2$O. AA, amino acids; FA, fatty acids; Gluc, glucose.

microsomal hydroxylating system, indole is converted to indoxyl, which is conjugated with potassium sulfate to form indican. Some bacteria (e.g., *Escherichia coli* and *Fusobacterium nucleatum*) in the lumen of the intestine can further degrade indole to yield sequentially isatin, formylanthranilic acid, anthranilic acid, and salicylic acid.

1. L-Tryptophan $\rightarrow$ Indole + Pyruvate + NH$_3$ (Tryptophanase)
2. L-Tryptophan $\rightarrow$ Tryptamine + CO$_2$ (Tryptophan decarboxylase)
3. Tyrosine $\rightarrow$ Phenol + Pyruvate + NH$_3$ (β-Tyrosinase)
4. Urea + H$_2$O $\rightarrow$ 2 NH$_3$ + CO$_2$ (Urease)
5. Nitrate + NADPH + H$^+$ $\rightarrow$ Nitrite + NADP$^+$ (Nitrate reductase)

Likewise, some reactions for AA catabolism (e.g., conversion of cysteine to taurine) occur in animals but are virtually absent from microorganisms. An example is that many prokaryotes and lower eukaryotes (including the protozoan parasites) lack, or are severely deficient in, spermine synthase and thus have little or no spermine (Heby et al. 2003), whereas all animal cells normally express this enzyme and contain high concentrations of spermine in the millimolar range (Agostinelli 2020; Wu et al. 2000a, b). Sixth, major nitrogenous products of AA catabolism in animals are urea, uric acid, and ammonia, depending on species and their living environments, but are primarily ammonia and also sulfate (in the case of sulfur-containing AAs) in microorganisms. Detoxification of ammonia as urea and uric acid in animals will be discussed in Chapter 6.

4.5   SUMMARY

Multiple pathways exist for the catabolism of glycine, L-AAs, and D-AAs AAs to CO_2, ammonia, water, and SO_4^{2-} in animals and microorganisms. These pathways are not only species-specific but also depend on cell type and developmental stage. Except for glycine whose catabolism via the glycine cleavage system takes only one step, a series of reactions spanning both the cytoplasm and mitochondria are required for degrading AAs to the above metabolites in mammals, birds, fish, and crustaceans. Based on their metabolic fates, AAs can be classified into three groups: ketogenic, glucogenic, and ketogenic plus glucogenic (Table 4.17). Catabolism of leucine, lysine, and taurine yields only acetyl-CoA (a precursor of either ketone bodies or long-chain fatty acids, depending on nutritional and hormonal status), and therefore, they are strictly ketogenic AAs. However, the degradation of many AAs (e.g., alanine, aspartate, glutamate, glutamine, and arginine) generates pyruvate and 4–5 carbon unit metabolites (e.g., oxaloacetate and α-KG) for glucose synthesis in the liver and kidneys, and they are glucogenic AAs. Catabolism of some AAs results in the formation of both acetyl-CoA and 4–5 carbon metabolites, and they are called ketogenic plus glucogenic AAs. The complete oxidation of most AAs to CO_2 involves the formation of acetyl-CoA, which enters the Krebs cycle for oxidation to CO_2, NADH, and $FADH_2$. NADPH is generated from the catabolism of certain AAs (e.g., arginine, ornithine, and proline). NAD(P)H and $FADH_2$ are oxidized into water via the mitochondrial electron transport system, where ATP is synthesized from ADP plus Pi. Because of the different lengths of carbon skeletons and different numbers of N atoms, the efficiency of oxidation of different AAs for ATP production varies greatly. Microbes degrade AAs via multiple pathways that are either the same as, similar to, or different than those in animals. Substantial catabolism of AAs by animal tissues and bacteria in the gastrointestinal tract of the animal host plays an important role in utilizing AAs (either food- or endogenously-derived), affecting the efficiency of the utilization of dietary protein for intracellular protein synthesis and other metabolic pathways, and regulating AA homeostasis in the body.

TABLE 4.17

Classification of Amino Acids into Ketogenic, Glucogenic, and Ketogenic Plus Glucogenic Groups in the Metabolism of Humans and Other Animals

Group	Amino Acids
Ketogenic	Leucine, lysine, and taurine
Glucogenic	Alanine, γ-aminobutyrate, arginine, asparagine, aspartate, citrulline, cysteine, glutamate, glutamine, glycine, histidine, methionine, ornithine, phosphoarginine, proline, serine, and valine
Ketogenic and glucogenic	Isoleucine, phenylalanine, threonine, tryptophan, and tyrosine

REFERENCES

Adams, E. and L. Frank. 1980. Metabolism of prolline and the hydroxyprolines. *Annu. Rev. Biochem.* 49:1005–1061.

Agostinelli, E. 2020. Biochemical and pathophysiological properties of polyamines. *Amino Acids* 52:111–117.

Alderton, W.K., C.E. Cooper, and R.G. Knowles. 2001. Nitric oxide synthases: structure, function and inhibition. *Biochem. J.* 357:593–615.

Arentson, B.W., N. Sanyal, and D.F. Becker. 2012. Substrate channeling in proline metabolism. *Front. Biosci.* 17:375–388.

Bada, J.L. 1984. *In vivo* racemization in mammalian proteins. *Methods Enzymol.* 106:98–115.

Badawy, A.A. 2017. Kynurenine pathway of tryptophan metabolism: Regulatory and functional aspects. *Int. J. Tryptophan Res.* 10:1178646917691938.

Ball, H.J., F.F. Jusof, S.M. Bakmiwewa, N.H. Hunt, and H.J. Yuasa. 2014. Tryptophan-catabolizing enzymes – party of three. *Front. Immunol.* 5:485.

Ballevre, O., A. Cadenhead, A.G. Calder, W.D. Rees, G.E. Lobley, M.F. Fuller, and P.J. Garlick. 1990. Quantitative partition of threonine oxidation in pigs: effect of dietary threonine. *Am. J. Physiol.* 259:E483–E491.

Baslow, M.H. 1997. A review of phylogenetic and metabolic relationships between the acylamino acids, *N*-acetyl-L-aspartic acid and *N*-acetyl-L-histidine, in the vertebrate nervous system. *J. Neurochem.* 68:1335–1344.

Bazer, FW, H. Seo, G.A. Johnson, and G. Wu. 2021. One-carbon metabolism and development of the conceptus during pregnancy: Lessons from studies with sheep and pigs. *Adv. Exp. Med. Biol.* 1285:1–15.

Beaufrere, B., F.F. Horber, W.F. Schwenk, H.M. Marsh, D. Matthews, J.E. Gerich, and M.W. Haymond. 1989. Glucocorticosteroids increase leucine oxidation and impair leucine balance in humans. *Am. J. Physiol.* 257:E712–E721.

Beaufrere, B., V. Fournier, B. Salle, and G. Putet. 1992. Leucine kinetics in fed low-birth-weight infants: importance of splanchnic tissues. *Am. J. Physiol.* 263:E214–E220.

Becker, D.F. and E.A. Thomas. 2001. Redox properties of the PutA protein from *Escherichia coli* and the influence of the flavin redox state on PutA-D NA interactions. *Biochemistry* 40:4714–4722.

Bender, D.A. 2012. The metabolism of "surplus" amino acids. *Br. J. Nutr.* 108:S113–S121.

Benevenga, N.J. and K.P. Blemings. 2007. Unique aspects of lysine nutrition and metabolism. *J. Nutr.* 137:1610S–1615S.

Bird, M.I. and P.B. Nunn. 1983. Metabolic homeostasis of L-threonine in the normally-fed rat. *Biochem. J.* 214:687–694.

Blachier, F., A.M. Davila, R. Benamouzig, and D. Tome. 2011. Channelling of arginine in NO and polyamine pathways in colonocytes and consequences. *Front. Biosci.* 16:1331–1343.

Blemings, K.P., T.D. Crenshaw, and N.J. Benevenga. 1998. Mitochondrial lysine uptake limits hepatic lysine oxidation in rats fed diets containing 5, 20, or 60% casein. *J. Nutr.* 128:2427–2434.

Blom, H.J., G.H.J. Boers, P.A.M. van den Elzen, W.A. Gahl, and A. Tangerman. 1989. Transamination of methionine in humans. *Clin. Sci.* 76:43–49.

Böger, R.H. and S.M. Bode-Böger. 2001. The clinical pharmacology of L-arginine. *Annu. Rev. Pharmacol. Toxicol.* 41:79–99.

Booth, A.N., M.S. Masri, D.J. Robbins, O.H. Emerson, F.T. Jones, and F. Deeds. 1960. Urinary phenolic acid metabolites of tyrosine. *J. Biol. Chem.* 235:2649–2652.

Borgonha, S., M.M. Regan, S.-H. Oh, M. Condon, and V.R. Young. 2002. Threonine requirement of healthy adults, derived with a 24-h indicator amino acid balance technique. *Am. J. Clin. Nutr.* 75:698–704.

Borsook, H. and J.W. Dubnoff. 1943. The metabolism of proteins and amino acids. *Annu. Rev. Biochem.* 12:183–204.

Bouzidi, A., M.C. Magnifico, A. Paiardini, A. Macone, G. Boumis, G. Giardina et al. 2020. Cytosolic serine hydroxymethyltransferase controls lung adenocarcinoma cells migratory ability by modulating AMP kinase activity. *Cell Death Dis.* 11:1012.

Bowtell, J.L., G.P. Leese, K. Smith, P.W. Watt, A. Nevill, O. Rooyackers et al. 2000. Effect of oral glucose on leucine turnover in human subjects at rest and during exercise at two levels of dietary protein. *J. Physiol.* 525:271–281.

Braeuning, A., C. Ittrich, C. Köhle, S. Hailfinger, M. Bonin, A. Buchmann, and M. Schwarz. 2006. Differential gene expression in periportal and perivenous mouse hepatocytes. *FEBS J.* 273:5051–5061.

Bratusch-Marrain, P., P. Ferenci, and W. Waldhäusl. 1980. Leucine assimilation in patients with diabetes mellitus. *Acta Endocrinol. (Copenhagen)* 93:461–465.

Bröer, S. and A. Bröer. 2017. Amino acid homeostasis and signalling in mammalian cells and organisms. *Biochem. J.* 474:1935–1963.

Broome, J.D. 1981. L-Asparaginase: discovery and development as a tumor-inhibitory agent. *Cancer Treat. Rep.* 65 (Suppl 4):111–114.

Brosnan, J.T. and M.E. Brosnan. 2006. Branched-chain amino acids: enzyme and substrate regulation. *J. Nutr.* 136:207S–211S.

Brüggemann, C., K. Denger, A.M. Cook, and J. Ruff. 2004. Enzymes and genes of taurine and isethionate dissimilation in *Paracoccus denitrificans*. *Microbiology* 150:805–816.

Burke, L., I. Guterman, R.P. Gallego, R.G. Britton, D. Burschowsky, C. Tufarelli, and A. Rufini. 2020. The Janus-like role of proline metabolism in cancer. Cell Death Discov. 6:104.

Camacho, J.A. and N. Rioseco-Camacho. 2009. The human and mouse SLC25A29 mitochondrial transporters rescue the deficient ornithine metabolism in fibroblasts of patients with the hyperornithinemia-hyperammonemia-homocitrullinuria (HHH) syndrome. *Pediatr. Res.* 66:35–41.

Chapman, K.P., R. Elango, R.O. Ball, and P.B. Pencharz. 2013. Splanchnic first pass disappearance of threonine and lysine do not differ in healthy men in the fed state. *J. Nutr.* 143:290–294.

Chen, J.Q., Y.H. Jin, Y. Yang, Z.L. Wu, and G. Wu. 2020. Epithelial dysfunction in lung diseases: effects of amino acids and potential mechanisms. *Adv. Exp. Med. Biol.* 1265:57–70.

Chu, S.W. and D.M. Hegsted. 1976. Adaptive response of lysine and threonine degrading enzymes in adult rats. *J. Nutr.* 106:1089–1096.

Closs, E.I., J.-P. Boissel, A. Habermeier, and A. Rotmann. 2006. Structure and function of cationic amino acid transporters (CATs). *J. Membr. Biol.* 213:67–77.

Collins, R., A.L. Johansson, T. Karlberg, N. Markova, S. van den Berg, K. Olesen et al. 2012. Biochemical discrimination between selenium and sulfur 1: a single residue provides selenium specificity to human selenocysteine lyase. *PLoS One* 7:e30581.

Cook, A.M. and K. Denger. 2006. Metabolism of taurine in microorganisms: a primer in molecular biodiversity? *Adv. Exp. Med. Biol.* 583:3–13.

Coon, C. and R. Balling. 1984. Asparagine and glutamine metabolism in chicks. *Poult. Sci.* 63:717–729.

Cooper, A.J.L. and A. Meister. 1981. Comparative studies of glutamine transaminases from rat tissues. *Comp. Biochem. Physiol.* 69B:137–145.

Cooper, A.J.L., Y.I. Shurubor, T. Dorai, J.T. Pinto, E.P. Isakova, Y.I. Deryabina et al. 2016. ω-Amidase: an underappreciated, but important enzyme in L-glutamine and L-asparagine metabolism; relevance to sulfur and nitrogen metabolism, tumor biology and hyperammonemic diseases. *Amino Acids* 48:1–20.

Cortiella, J., J.S. Marchini, S. Branch, T.E. Chapman, and V.R Young. 1992. Phenylalanine and tyrosine kinetics in relation to altered protein and phenylalanine and tyrosine intakes in healthy young men. *Am. J. Clin. Nutr.* 56:517–525.

Crowther, L.M., D. Mathis, M. Poms, and B. Plecko. 2019. New insights into human lysine degradation pathways with relevance to pyridoxine-dependent epilepsy due to antiquitin deficiency. *J. Inher. Metab. Dis.* 42:620–628.

Curthoys, N.P. and M. Watford. 1995. Regulation of glutaminase activity and glutamine metabolism. *Annu. Rev. Nutr.* 15:133–159.

Dai, X. and B.T. Zhu. 2010. Indoleamine 2,3-dioxygenase tissue distribution and cellular localization in mice: implications for its biological functions. *J. Histochem. Cytochem.* 58:17–28.

Dai, Z.L., J. Zhang, G. Wu, and W.Y. Zhu. 2010. Utilization of amino acids by bacteria from the pig small intestine. *Amino Acids* 39:1201–1215.

Dai, Z.L., G. Wu, and W.Y. Zhu. 2011. Amino acid metabolism in intestinal bacteria: links between gut ecology and host health. *Front. Biosci.* 16:1768–1786.

Dai, Z.L., X.L. Li, P.B. Xi, J. Zhang, G. Wu, and W.Y. Zhu. 2012. Metabolism of select amino acids in bacteria from the pig small intestine. *Amino Acids* 42:1597–1608.

Darling, P.B., M. Dunn, G. Sarwar, S. Brookes, R.O. Ball, and P.B. Pencharz. 1999. Threonine kinetics in preterm infants fed their mothers' milk or formula with various ratios of whey to casein. *Am. J. Clin. Nutr.* 69:105–114.

Darling, P.B., J. Grunow, M. Rafii, S. Brookes, R.O. Ball, and P.B. Pencharz. 2000. Threonine dehydrogenase is a minor degradative pathway of threonine catabolism in adult humans. *Am. J. Physiol.* 278:E877–E884.

Dasarathy, J., L.L. Gruca, C. Bennett, P.S. Parimi, C. Duenas, S. Marczewski et al. 2010. Methionine metabolism in human pregnancy. *Am. J. Clin. Nutr.* 91:357–365.

Davis, A.J. and R.E. Austic. 1994. Dietary threonine imbalance alters threonine dehydrogenase activity in isolated hepatic mitochondria of chicks and rats. *J. Nutr.* 124:1667–1677.

Davis, A.J. and R.E. Austic. 1997. Dietary protein and amino acid levels alter threonine dehydrogenase activity in hepatic mitochondria of *Gallus domesticus*. *J. Nutr.* 127:738–744.

Denne, S.C., E.M. Rossi, and S.C. Kalhan. 1991. Leucine kinetics during feeding in normal newborns. *Pediatr. Res.* 30:23–27.

Deutz, N.E., P.L. Reijven, G. Athanasas, and P.B. Soeters. 1992. Post-operative changes in hepatic, intestinal, splenic and muscle fluxes of amino acids and ammonia in pigs. *Clin. Sci. (London)* 83:607–614.

Dillon, E.L., D.A. Knabe, and G. Wu. 1999. Lactate inhibits citrulline and arginine synthesis from proline in pig enterocytes. *Am. J. Physiol.* 276:G1079–G1086.

Elia, M., R. Farrell, V. Ilic, R. Smith, and D.H. Williamson. 1980. The removal of infused leucine after injury, starvation and other conditions in man. *Clin. Sci. (London)* 59:275–283.

Engineering ToolBox. 2008. Solubility of Gases in Water. https://www.engineeringtoolbox.com/gases-solubility-water-d_1148.html. Accessed September 22, 2020.

Esaki, N., T. Nakamura, H. Tanaka, and K. Soda. 1982. Selenocysteine lyase, a novel enzyme that specifically acts on selenocysteine. Mammalian distribution and purification and properties of pig liver enzyme. *J. Biol. Chem.* 257:4386–4391.

FDA (U.S. Food and Drug Administration). 2004. http://www.accessdata.fda.gov/drugsatfda_docs/label/2004/21677_nutreStore_lbl.pdf. Accessed July 22, 2020.

Felig, P., J. Wahren, and L. Räf. 1973. Evidence of inter-organ amino-acid transport by blood cells in humans. *Proc. Natl. Acad. Sci. USA.* 70:1775–1779.

Field, C.J., I. Johnson, and V.C. Pratt. 2000. Glutamine and arginine: immunonutrients for improved health. *Med. Sci. Sports Exerc.* 32:S377–S388.

Fiermonte, G., V. Dolce, L. David, F.M. Santorelli, C. Dionisi-Vici, F. Palmieri, and J.E. Walker. 2003. The mitochondrial ornithine transporter. Bacterial expression, reconstitution, functional characterization, and tissue distribution of two human isoforms. *J. Biol. Chem.* 278:32778–32783.

Finkelstein, J.D. 1990. Methionine metabolism in mammals. *J. Nutr. Biochem.* 1:228–2377.

Flynn, N.E. and G. Wu. 1996. An important role for endogenous synthesis of arginine in maintaining arginine homeostasis in neonatal pigs. *Am. J. Physiol.* 271:R1149–R1155.

Flynn, N.E., M.E. Patryak, J.B. Seely, and G. Wu. 2010. Glycine oxidation and conversion into amino acids in *Saccharomyces cerevisiae* and *Candida albicans*. *Amino Acids* 39:605–608.

Förstermann, U. and T. Münzel. 2006 Endothelial nitric oxide synthase in vascular disease: from marvel to menace. *Circulation* 113:1708–1714.

Fukagawa, N.K., Y.M. Yu, and V.R. Young. 1998. Methionine and cysteine kinetics at different intakes of methionine and cystine in elderly men and women. *Am. J. Clin. Nutr.* 68:380–388.

Fukasawa, Y., H. Segawa, J.Y. Kim, A. Chairoungdua, D.K. Kim, H. Matsuo et al. 2000. Identification and characterization of a Na+-independent neutral amino acid transporter that associates with the 4F2 heavy chain and exhibits substrate selectivity for small neutral D- and L-amino acids. *J. Biol. Chem.* 275:9690–9698.

Gomes, A.P., D. Ilter, V. Low, J.E. Endress, J. Fernández-García, A. Rosenzweig et al. 2020. Age-induced accumulation of methylmalonic acid promotes tumour progression. *Nature* 585:283–287.

Griffin, J.E., A.K. Pandey, S.A. Gilmore, V. Mizrahi, J.D. Mckinney, C.R. Bertozzi, and C.M. Sassetti. 2012. Cholesterol catabolism by *Mycobacterium tuberculosis* requires transcriptional and metabolic adaptations. *Chem. Biol.* 19:218–227.

Gutiérrez-Aguilar, M. and C.P. Baines. 2013. Physiological and pathological roles of mitochondrial SLC25 carriers. *Biochem. J.* 454:371–386.

Haas, D., H. Matsumoto, P. Moretti, V. Stalon, and A. Mercenier. 1984. Arginine degradation in *Pseudomonas aeruginosa* mutants blocked in two arginine catabolic pathways. *Mol. Gen. Genet.* 193:437–444.

Hagiwara, A., Y. Nakamura, R. Nishimoto, S. Ueno, and Y. Miyagi. 2020. Induction of tryptophan hydroxylase in the liver of s.c. tumor model of prostate cancer. *Cancer Sci.* 111:1218–1227.

Hahn, R.G., H.P. Stalberg, and S.A. Gustafsson. 1989. Intravenous infusion of irrigating fluids containing glycine or mannitol with and without ethanol. *J. Urol.* 142:1102–1105.

Hall, S.E.H., J.T. Braaten, J.B.R. McKendry, T. Bolton, D. Foster, and M. Berman. 1979. Normal alanine-glucose relationships and their changes in diabetic patients before and after insulin treatment. *Diabetes* 28:737–745.

Hämäläinen, J. and W. Helme. 1907. Ein Beitrag zur Kenntnis des Eiweiss-stoffwechsels. *Skand. Arch. Physiol.* 19:182–200.

Hankard, R.G., M.W. Haymond, and D. Darmaun. 2000. Role of glucose in the regulation of glutamine metabolism in health and in type 1 insulin-dependent diabetes. *Am. J. Physiol.* 279:E608–E613.

Hanigan, M.D., J.P. Cant, D.C. Weakley, and J.L. Beckett. 1998. An evaluation of postabsorptive protein and amino acid metabolism in the lactating dairy cow. *J. Dairy Sci.* 81:3385–3401.

Harper, A.E., R.H. Miller, and K.P. Block. 1984. Branched-chain amino acid metabolism. *Annu. Rev. Nutr.* 4:409–454.

Harris, R.A., M. Joshi, and N.H. Jeoung. 2004. Mechanisms responsible for regulation of branched-chain amino acid catabolism. *Biochem. Biophys. Res. Commun.* 313:391–396.

Hatanaka, T., W. Huang, T. Nakanishi, C.C. Bridges, S.B. Smith, P.D. Prasad et al. 2002. Transport of D-serine via the amino acid transporter $ATB^{0,+}$ expressed in the colon. *Biochem. Biophys. Res. Commun.* 291:291–295.

Haussinger, D. 1990. Nitrogen metabolism in liver: structural and functional organization and physiological significance. *Biochem. J.* 267:281–290.

Hawel, L. III, R.R. Tjandrawinata, G.H. Fukumoto, and C.V. Byus. 1994. Biosynthesis and selective export of 1,5-diaminopentane (cadaverine) in mycoplasma-free cultured mammalian cells. *J. Biol. Chem.* 269:7412–7418.

He, W.L. and G. Wu. 2020. Metabolism of amino acids in the brain and their roles in regulating food intake. *Adv. Exp. Med. Biol.* 1265:167–185.

Heby, O., S.C. Roberts, and B. Ullman. 2003. Polyamine biosynthetic enzymes as drug targets in parasitic protozoa. *Biochem. Soc. Trans.* 31:415–419.

Herbig, K., E.-P. Chiang, L.-R. Lee, J. Hills, B. Shane, and P.J. Stover. 2002. Cytoplasmic serine hydroxy-methyltransferase mediates competition between folate-dependent deoxyribonucleotide and S-adenosylmethionine biosynthesis. *J. Biol. Chem.* 277:38381–38389.

Hetenyi, G., P.J. Anderson, M. Raman, and C. Ferrarotto. 1988. Gluconeogenesis from glycine and serine in fasted normal and diabetic rats. *Biochem. J.* 253:27–32.

Hou, Y.Q. and G. Wu. 2018. L-Glutamate nutrition and metabolism in swine. *Amino Acids* 50:1497–1510.

Hou, Y.Q., S.D. Hu, X.Y. Li, W.L. He, and G. Wu. 2020. Amino acid metabolism in the liver: nutritional and physiological significance. *Adv. Exp. Med. Biol.* 1265:21–37.

Hu, C.A., S.P. Donald, J. Yu, W.W. Lin, Z. Liu, G. Steel et al. 2007. Overexpression of proline oxidase induces proline-dependent and mitochondria-mediated apoptosis. *Mol. Cell. Biochem.* 295:85–92.

Huang, Y.Y., A. Martínez-del Campo, and E.P. Balskus. 2018. Anaerobic 4-hydroxyproline utilization: Discovery of a new glycyl radical enzyme in the human gut microbiome uncovers a widespread microbial metabolic activity. *Gut Microbes* 9:437–451.

Hutson, S.M., C. Zapalowski, T.C. Cree, and A.E. Harper. 1980. Regulation of leucine and alpha-ketoisocaproic acid metabolism in skeletal muscle. Effects of starvation and insulin. *J. Biol. Chem.* 255:2418–2426.

Hutson, S.M., A.J. Sweatt, and K.F. LaNoue. 2005. Branched-chain amino acid metabolism: implications for establishing safe intakes. *J. Nutr.* 135:1557S–1564S.

Ishiguro, I., J. Naito, K. Saito, and Y. Nagamura. 1993. Skin L-tryptophan-2,3-dioxygenase and rat hair growth. *FEBS Lett.* 329:178–182.

Islam, M.M., R. Wallin, R.M. Wynn, M. Conway, H. Fujii, J.A. Mobley et al. 2007. A novel branched-chain amino acid metabolon. Protein-protein interactions in a supramolecular complex. *J. Biol. Chem.* 282:11893–11903.

Jakubowski, H. 2019. Homocysteine modification in protein structure/function and human disease. *Physiol. Rev.* 99:555–604.

Jia, S.C., X.Y. Li, S.X. Zheng, and G. Wu. 2017. Amino acids are major energy substrates for tissues of hybrid striped bass and zebrafish. *Amino Acids* 49:2053–2063.

Jungas, R.L., M.L. Halperin, and J.T. Brosnan. 1992. Quantitative analysis of amino acid oxidation and related gluconeogenesis in humans. *Physiol. Rev.* 72:419–448.

Jürss, K. and R. Bastrop. 1995. Amino acid metabolism in fish. In: *Biochemistry and Molecular Biology of Fishes* (Hochachka, P.W. and T.P. Mommsen, eds). Elsevier, New York. Vol. 4, pp. 159–189.

Jusof, F.F., S.M. Bakmiwewa, S. Weiser, L.K. Too, R. Metz, G.C. Prendergast et al. 2017. Investigation of the tissue distribution and physiological roles of indoleamine 2,3-dioxygenase-2. *Int. J. Tryptophan Res.* 10:1–12.

Kalhan, S.C. and D.M. Bier. 2008. Protein and amino acid metabolism in the human newborn. *Annu. Rev. Nutr.* 28:389–410.

Kanai, Y. and M.A. Hediger. 2003. The glutamate and neutral amino acid transporter family: physiological and pharmacological implications. *Eur. J. Pharmacol.* 479:237–247.

Kanai, Y., H. Segawa, K. Miyamoto, H. Uchino, E. Takeda, and H.J. Endou. 1998. Expression cloning and characterization of a transporter for large neutral amino acids activated by the heavy chain of 4F2 antigen (CD98). *J. Biol. Chem.* 273:23629–23632.

Kao, M., D.A. Columbus, A. Suryawan, J. Steinhoff-Wagner, A. Hernandez-Garcia, H.V. Nguyen et al. 2016. Enteral β-hydroxy-β-methylbutyrate supplementation increases protein synthesis in skeletal muscle of neonatal pigs. *Am. J. Physiol.* 310:E1072–E1084.

Kaushik, S.J. and I. Seiliez. 2010. Protein and amino acid nutrition and metabolism in fish: current knowledge and future needs. *Aquac. Res.* 41:322–332.

Kera, Y., H. Aoyama, N. Watanabe, and R.H. Yamada. 1996. Distribution of D-aspartate oxidase and free D-glutamate and D-aspartate in chicken and pigeon tissues. *Comp. Biochem. Physiol. B* 115:121–126.

Keyfi, F., S. Talebi, and A. Varasteh. 2016. Methylmalonic acidemia diagnosis by laboratory methods. *Rep. Biochem. Mol. Biol.* 5:1–14.

Kharitonov, S.A., G. Lubec, B. Lubec, M. Hjelm, and P.J. Barnes. 1995. L-arginine increases exhaled nitric oxide in normal human subjects. *Clin. Sci.* 88:135–139.

Kikuchi, G., Y. Motokawa, T. Yoshida, and K. Hiraga. 2008. Glycine cleavage system: reaction mechanism, physiological significance, and hyperglycinemia. *Proc. Jpn. Acad., Ser. B* 84:246–263.

Kohli, R., C.J. Meininger, T.E. Haynes, W. Yan, J.T. Self, and G. Wu. 2004. Dietary L-arginine supplementation enhances endothelial nitric oxide synthesis in streptozotocin-induced diabetic rats. *J. Nutr.* 134:600–608.

Kovachy, R.J., S.D. Copley, and R.H. Allen. 1983. Recognition, isolation, and characterization of rat liver D-methylmalonyl coenzyme A hydrolase. *J. Biol. Chem.* 258:11415–11421.

Krall, A.S., S. Xu, T.G. Graeber, D. Braas, and H.R. Christofk. 2016. Asparagine promotes cancer cell proliferation through use as an amino acid exchange factor. *Nat. Commun.* 7:11457.

Krebs H.A. 1935. Metabolism of amino acids: IV. The synthesis of glutamine from glutamic acid and ammonia and the enzymic hydrolysis of glutamine in animal tissues. *Biochem. J.* 29:1951–1969.

Krebs, H.A. 1964. The metabolic fate of amino acids. In: *Mammalian Protein Metabolism* (Munro, H.N. and J.B. Allison, eds). Academic Press, New York. pp. 125–176.

Krebs, H.A. 1972. Some aspects of the regulation of fuel supply in omnivorous animals. *Adv. Enzyme Regul.* 10:397–420.

Krishnan, N., M.B. Dickman, and D.F. Becker. 2008. Proline modulates the intracellular redox environment and protects mammalian cells against oxidative stress. *Free Radical Biol. Med.* 44:671–681.

Kuhn, K.S., K. Schuhmann, P. Stehle, D. Darmaun, and P. Fürst. 1999. Determination of glutamine in muscle protein facilitates accurate assessment of proteolysis and de novo synthesis-derived endogenous glutamine production. *Am. J. Clin. Nutr.* 70:484–489.

Kust, A., A. Méjean, and O. Ploux. 2020. Biosynthesis of anatoxins in cyanobacteria: identification of the carboxy-anatoxins as the penultimate biosynthetic intermediates. *J. Nat. Prod.* 83:142–151.

Lamarre, S.G., G. Morrow, L. Macmillan, M.E. Brosnan, and J.T. Brosnan. 2012. Formate: an essential metabolite, a biomarker or more? *Clin. Chem. Lab. Med.* 14:1–8.

Lassala, A., F.W. Bazer, T.A. Cudd, P. Li, X.L. Li, M.C. Satterfield et al. 2009. Intravenous administration of L-citrulline to pregnant ewes is more effective than L-arginine for increasing arginine availability in the fetus. *J. Nutr.* 139:660–665.

Le Floc'h, N., B. Seve, and Y. Henry. 1994. The addition of glutamic acid or protein to a threonine-deficient diet differentially affects growth performance and threonine degydrogenase activity in fattening pigs. *J. Nutr.* 124:1987–1995.

Le Floc'h, N., W. Otten, and E. Merlot. 2011. Tryptophan metabolism, from nutrition to potential therapeutic applications. *Amino Acids* 41:1195–1205.

Li, C. and C.D. Lu. 2009. Arginine racemization by coupled catabolic and anabolic dehydrogenases. *Proc. Natl. Acad. Sci. USA* 106:906–911.

Li, P., S.W. Kim, X.L. Li, S. Datta, W.G. Pond and G. Wu. 2008. Dietary supplementation with cholesterol and docosahexaenoic acid increases the activity of the arginine-nitric oxide pathway in tissues of young pigs. *Nitric Oxide* 19:259–265.

Li, P., D.A. Knabe, S.W. Kim, C.J. Lynch, S.M. Hutson, and G. Wu. 2009a. Lactating porcine mammary tissue catabolizes branched-chain amino acids for glutamine and aspartate synthesis. *J. Nutr.* 139:1502–1509.

Li, P., S.W. Kim, X.L. Li, S. Datta, W.G. Pond, and G. Wu. 2009b. Dietary supplementation with cholesterol and docosahexaenoic acid affects concentrations of amino acids in tissues of young pigs. *Amino Acids* 37:709–716.

Li, X.L., S.X. Zheng, and G. Wu. 2020a. Nutrition and metabolism of glutamate and glutamine in fish. *Amino Acids* 52:671–691.

Li, X.Y., S.X. Zheng, and G. Wu. 2020b. Amino acid metabolism in the kidneys: nutritional and physiological significance. *Adv. Exp. Med. Biol.* 1265:71–95.

Li, X.L., S.X. Zheng, S.C. Jia, F. Song, C.P. Zhou, and G. Wu. 2020c. Oxidation of energy substrates in tissues of largemouth bass (*Micropterus salmoides*). *Amino Acids* 52:1017–1032.

Li, X.Y., S.X. Zheng, and G. Wu. 2021a. Nutrition and functions of amino acids in fish. *Adv. Exp. Med. Biol.* 1285:133–168.

Li, X.Y., T. Han, S.X. Zheng, and G. Wu. 2021b. Nutrition and functions of amino acids in aquatic crustaceans. *Adv. Exp. Med. Biol.* 1285:169–197.

Liu, W., A. Le, C. Hancock, A.N. Lane, C.V. Dang, T.W.M. Fan, and J.M. Phang. 2012. Reprogramming of proline and glutamine metabolism contributes to the proliferative and metabolic responses regulated by oncogenic transcription factor c-MYC. *Proc. Natl. Acad. Sci. USA* 109:8983–8988.

Lowry, M., D.E. Hall, M.S. Hall, and J.T. Brosnan. 1987. Renal metabolism of amino acids *in vivo*: studies on serine and glycine fluxes. *Am. J. Physiol.* 252:F304–F309.

Luiking, Y.C., G.A. Ten Have, R.R. Wolfe, and N.E. Deutz. 2012. Arginine de novo and nitric oxide production in disease states. *Am. J. Physiol.* 303:E1177–E1189.

Luka, Z., A. Capdevila, J.M. Mato, and C. Wagner. 2006. *Transgenic Res.* 15:393–397.

Luka, Z., S.H. Mudd, and C. Wagner. 2009. Glycine N-methyltransferase and regulation of S-adenosylmethionine levels. *J. Biol. Chem.* 284:22507–22511.

Lund, P. and M. Watford. 1976. Glutamine as a precursor of urea. In: *The Urea Cycle* (Grisolia, S., R. Baguena, and F. Mayor. John Wiley and Sons, New York. pp. 479–488.

Lusk, G. 1921. *The Elements of the Science of Nutrition*, 3rd edition. W. B. Saunders Company, London.

Luu, N., L. Fu, K. Fujimoto, and Y.-B. Shi. 2017. Direct regulation of histidine ammonia-lyase 2 gene by thyroid hormone in the developing adult intestinal stem cells. *Endocrinology* 158:1022–1033.

MacFarlane, A.J., X. Liu, C.A. Perry, P. Flodby, R.H. Allen, S.P. Stabler, and P.J. Stover. 2008. Cytoplasmic serine hydroxymethyltransferase regulates the metabolic partitioning of methylenetetrahydrofolate but is not essential in mice. *J. Biol. Chem.* 283:25846–25853.

McGee, M., O. Greengard, and W.E. Knox. 1971. The developmental formation of asparaginase in liver and its distribution in rat tissues. *Enzyme* 12:1–12.

Meguid, M.M., H. Schwarz, D.E. Matthews, I.E. Karl, V.R. Young, and D.M. Bier. 1983. *In vivo* and *in vitro* branched-chain amino acid interactions. In: *Amino Acids: Metabolism and Medical Applications* (Blackburn, G.L., J.P. Grant, and V.R. Young, eds). John Wright Inc., Boston, MA. pp. 147–154.

Meijer, A.J., W.H. Lamers, and R.A.F.M. Chamuleau. 1990. Nitrogen metabolism and ornithine cycle function. *Physiol. Rev.* 70:701–748.

Mellor, A.L., H. Lemos and L. Huang. 2017. Indoleamine 2,3-dioxygenase and tolerance: Where are we now? *Front. Immunol.* 8:1360.

Meredith, C.N., Z.-M. Wen, D.M. Bier, D.E. Matthews, and V.R. Young. 1986. Lysine kinetics at graded lysine intakes in young men. *Am. J. Clin. Nutr.* 43:787–794.

Miller, M.M., L.B. Popova, E.A. Meleshkevitch, P.V. Tran, and D.Y. Boudko. 2008. The invertebrate B(0) system transporter, *D. melanogaster* NAT1, has unique D-amino acid affinity and mediates gut and brain functions. *Insect Biochem. Mol. Biol.* 38:923–931.

Mistry, S.K., T.J. Burwell, R.M. Chambers, L. Rudolph-Owen, F. Spaltmann, W.J. Cook, and S.M. Morris, Jr. 2002. Cloning of human agmatinase. An alternate path for polyamine synthesis induced in liver by hepatitis B virus. *Am. J. Physiol.* 282:G375–G381.

Møller, N., S. Meek, M. Bigelow, J. Andrews, and K.S. Nair. 2000. The kidney is an important site for *in vivo* phenylalanine-to-tyrosine conversion in adult humans: a metabolic role of the kidney. *Proc. Natl. Acad. Sci. USA* 97:1242–1246.

Monné, M., A. Vozza, F.M. Lasorsa, V. Porcelli, and F. Palmieri. 2019. Mitochondrial carriers for aspartate, glutamate and other amino acids: a review. *Int. J. Mol. Sci.* 20:4456.

Moro, J., D. Tomé, P. Schmidely, T.-C. Demersay, and D. Azzout-Marniche. 2020. Histidine: a systematic review on metabolism and physiological effects in human and different animal species. *Nutrients* 12:1414.

Morris, S.M., Jr. 2009. Recent advances in arginine metabolism: roles and regulation of the arginases. *Br. J. Pharmacol.* 157:922–930.

Moundras, C., D. Bercovici, C. Remesy, and C. Demigne. 1992. Influence of glucogenic amino acids on the hepatic metabolism of threonine. *Biochim. Biophys. Acta* 115:212–219.

Mudd, S.H., J.T. Brosnan, M.E. Brosnan, R.L. Jacobs, S.P. Stabler, R.H. Allen et al. 2007. Methyl balance and transmethylation fluxes in humans. *Am. J. Clin. Nutr.* 85:19–25.

Newsholme, E.A., B. Crabtree, and M.S. Ardawi. 1985. Glutamine metabolism in lymphocytes: its biochemical, physiological and clinical importance. *Q. J. Exp. Physiol.* 70:473–489.

Newsholme, P., F. Abdulkader, E. Rebelato, T. Romanatto, C.H.J. Pinheiro, K.F. Vitzel et al. 2011. Amino acids and diabetes: implications for endocrine, metabolic and immune function. *Front. Biosci.* 16:315–339.

Nisman, B. 1954. The Stickland reaction. *Bacteriol. Rev.* 18:16–42.

Ohide, H., Y. Miyoshi, R. Maruyama, K. Hamase, and R. Konno. 2011. D-Amino acid metabolism in mammals: biosynthesis, degradation and analytical aspects of the metabolic study. *J. Chromatogr. B* 879:3162–3168.

Ohtsu, H. 2011. Histamine synthesis and lessons learned from histidine decarboxylase deficient mice. *Adv. Exp. Med. Biol.* 709:21–31.

Parimi, P.S., S. Devapatla, L. Gruca, A.M. O'Brien, R.W. Hanson, and S.C. Kalhan. 2002. Glutamine and leucine nitrogen kinetics and their relation to urea nitrogen in newborn infants. *Am. J. Physiol.* 282:E618–E625.

Parimi, P.S., L.L. Gruca, and S.C. Kalhan. 2005. Metabolism of threonine in newborn infants. *Am. J. Physiol.* 289:E891–E895.

Parimi, P.S., S. Devapatla, L.L. Gruca, S.B. Amini, R.W. Hanson, and S.C. Kalhan. 2004. Effect of enteral glutamine or glycine on whole-body nitrogen kinetics in very-low-birth-weight infants. *Am. J. Clin. Nutr.* 79:402–409.

Parthasarathy, A., P.J. Cross, R.C.J. Dobson, L.E. Adams, M.A. Savka, and A.O. Hudson. 2018. A three-ring circus: metabolism of the three proteogenic aromatic amino acids and their role in the health of plants and animals. *Front. Mol. Biosci.* 5:29.

Paluszkiewicz, P., W. Zgrajka, T. Saran, J. Schabowski, J.L.V. Piedra, O. Fedkiv et al. 2009. High concentration of kynurenic acid in bile and pancreatic juice. *Amino Acids* 37:637–641.

Pecka, S.C., K. Dengerb, A. Burrichterb, S.M. Irwina, E.P. Balskusa, and D. Schleheck. 2019. A glycyl radical enzyme enables hydrogen sulfide production by the human intestinal bacterium *Bilophila wadsworthia*. *Proc. Natl. Acad. Sci. USA* 116:3171–3176.

Pegg, A.E. and S. McGill. 1979. Decarboxylation of ornithine and lysine in rat tissues. *Biochim. Biophys. Acta.* 568:416–427.

Pena, I.A., L.A. Marques, A.B. Laranjeira, J.A. Yunes, M.N. Eberlin, A. MacKenzie, and P. Arruda. 2016. Mouse lysine catabolism to aminoadipate occurs primarily through the saccharopine pathway; implications for pyridoxine dependent epilepsy (PDE). *Biochim. Biophys. Acta* 1863:121–128.

Persson, L. 1977. Evidence of decarboxylation of lysine by mammalian ornithine decarboxylase. *Acta Physiol. Scand.* 100:424–429.

Phang, J.M. 1985. The regulatory functions of proline and pyrroline-5-carboxylic acid. *Curr. Top. Cell Regul.* 25:91–132.

Phang, J.M. and W. Liu. 2012. Proline metabolism and cancer. *Front. Biosci.* 17:1835–1845.

Porcelli, V., G. Fiermonte, A. Longo, and F. Palmieri. 2014. The human gene SLC25A29, of solute carrier family 25, encodes a mitochondrial transporter of basic amino acids. *J. Biol. Chem.* 289:13374–13384.

Rafice, S.A., N. Chauhan, I. Efimov, J. Basran, and E.L. Raven. 2009. Oxidation of L-tryptophan in biology: a comparison between tryptophan 2,3-dioxygenase and indoleamine 2,3-dioxygenase. *Biochem. Soc. Trans.* 37:408–412.

Raguso, C.A., M.M. Regan, and V.R. Young. 2000. Cysteine kinetics and oxidation at different intakes of methionine and cystine in young adults. *Am. J. Clin. Nutr.* 71:491–499.

Reed, L.J., F.H. Pettit, D.M. Bleile, and T.-L. Wu. 1980. Structure, function, and regulation of mammalian pyruvate dehydrogenase complex. In: *Metabolic Interconversion of Enzymes* (Holzer, H., ed.). Springer, New York. pp 124–133.

Regina, M., V.P. Korhonen, T.K. Smith, L. Alakuijala, and T.O. Eloranta. 1993. Methionine toxicity in the rat in relation to hepatic accumulation of S-adenosylmethionine: prevention by dietary stimulation of the hepatic transsulfuration pathway. *Arch. Biochem. Biophys.* 300:598–607.

Rennie, M.J., R.H.T. Edwards, D. Halliday, D.E. Matthews, S.L. Wolman, and D.J. Millward. 1982. Muscle protein synthesis measured by stable isotope techniques in man: the effects of feeding and fasting. *Clin. Sci.* 63:519–523.

Richards, N.G. and M.S. Kilberg. 2006. Asparagine synthetase chemotherapy. *Annu. Rev. Biochem.* 75:629–654.

Risteli, J., K. Tryggvason, and K.I. Kivirikko. 1977. Proyl 3-hydroxylase: partial characterization of the enzyme from rat kidney cortex. *Eur. J Biochem.* 73:485–492.

Sakai, R., Y. Ooba, A. Watanabe, H. Nakamura, Y. Kawamata, T. Shimada et al. 2020. Glutamate metabolism in a human intestinal epithelial cell layer model. *Amino Acids* 52:1505–1519.

Sakowski, S.A., T.J. Geddes, D.M. Thomas, E. Levi, J.S. Hatfield, and D.M. Kuhn. 2006. Differential tissue distribution of tryptophan hydroxylase isoforms 1 and 2 as revealed with monospecific antibodies. *Brain Res.* 1085:11–18.

Sastre, M., E. Galea, D. Feinstein, D.J. Reis, and S. Regunathan. 1998. Metabolism of agmatine in macrophages: modulation by lipopolysaccharide and inhibitory cytokines. *Biochem. J.* 330:1405–1409.

Scislowski, P.W.D. and K. Pickard. 1994. The regulation of transaminative flux of methionine in rat liver mitochondria. *Arch. Biochem. Biophys.* 314:412–416.

Scott, M.L., M.C. Nesheim, and R.J. Young. 1982. *Nutrition of the Chicken*, 4th edition. M.L. Scott & Associates, Ithaca, NY.

Self, J.T., T.E. Spencer, G.A. Johnson, J. Hu, F.W. Bazer, and G. Wu. 2004. Glutamine synthesis in the developing porcine placenta. *Biol. Reprod.* 70:1444–1451.

Seo, H., G.A. Johnson, F.W. Bazer, G. Wu, B.A. McLendon, and A.C. Kramer. 2021. Cell-specific expression of enzymes for serine biosynthesis and glutaminolysis in farm animals. *Adv. Exp. Med. Biol.* 1285:17–28.

Shimomura, Y., T. Murakami, N. Nakai, B. Huang, J.A. Hawes, and R.A. Harris. 2000. 3-Hydroxyisobutyryl-CoA hydrolase. *Methods Enzymol.* 324:229–240.

Squires, E.J. and J.T. Brosnan. 1983. Measurements of the turnover rate of glutamine in normal and acidotic rats. *Biochem. J.* 210:277–280.

Stack, T., P.J. Reeds, T. Preston, S. Hay, D.J. Lloyd, and P.J. Aggett. 1989. ^{15}N tracer studies of protein metabolism in low birth weight preterm infants: a comparison of ^{15}N glycine and^{15}N yeast protein hydrolysate and of human milk- and formula-fed babies. *Pediatr. Res.* 25:167–172.

Staten, M.A., D.M. Bier, and D.E. Matthews. 1984. Regulation of valine metabolism in man: a stable isotope study. *Am. J. Clin. Nutr.* 40:1224–1234.

Stipanuk, M.H. 2004. Sulfur amino acid metabolism: pathways for production and removal of homocysteine and cysteine. *Annu. Rev. Nutr.* 24:539–577.

Stumvoll, M., G. Perriello, N. Nurjhan, S. Welle, J. Gerich, A. Bucci et al. 1996. Glutamine and alanine metabolism in NIDDM. *Diabetes* 45:863–868.

Tanner, J.J. 2019. Structural biology of proline catabolic enzymes. *Antioxid. Redox Signal.* 30:650–673.

Tanner, J.J., F. Sarah-Maria, and D.F. Becker. 2018. The proline cycle as a potential cancer therapy target. *Biochemistry* 57:3433–3444.

Tavares, C.D.J., K. Sharabi, J.E. Dominy, Y.J. Lee, M. Isasa, J.M. Orozco et al. 2016. The methionine transamination pathway controls hepatic glucose metabolism through regulation of the GCN5 acetyltransferase and the PGC-1α transcriptional coactivator. *J. Biol. Chem.* 291:10635–10645.

Thorn, B., R.H. Dunstan, M.M. Macdonald, N. Borges, and T.K. Roberts. 2020. Evidence that human and equine erythrocytes could have significant roles in the transport and delivery of amino acids to organs and tissues. *Amino Acids* 52:711–724.

Tomlinson, C., M. Rafii, M. Sgro, R.O. Ball, and P. Pencharz. 2011. Arginine is synthesized from proline, not glutamate, in enterally fed human preterm neonates. *Pediatr. Res.* 69:46–50.

Tramonti, A., C. Nardella, M.L. di Salvo, A. Barile, F. Cutruzzolà, and R. Contestabile. 2018. Human cytosolic and mitochondrial serine hydroxymethyltransferase isoforms in comparison: Full kinetic characterization and substrate inhibition properties. *Biochemistry* 57:6984–6996.

Trottier, N.L., C.F. Shipley, and R.A. Easter. 1997. Plasma amino acid uptake by the mammary gland of the lactating sow. *J. Anim. Sci.* 75:1266–1278.

Tryggvason, K., K. Majamaa, and K.I. Kivirikko. 1979. Prolyl 3-hydroxylase and 4-hydroxylase activities in certain rat and chick-embryo tissues and age-related changes in their activities in the rat. *Biochem. J.* 178:127–131.

Van Der Schoor, S.R., P.J. Reeds, B. Stoll, J.F. Henry, J.R. Rosenberger, D.G. Burrin, and J.B. Van Goudoever. 2002. The high metabolic cost of a functional gut. *Gastroenterology* 123:1931–1940.

Van Der Schoor, S.R.D., D.L. Wattimena, J. Huijmans, A. Vermes, and J.B. van Goudoever. 2007. The gut takes nearly all: threonine kinetics in infants. *Am. J. Clin. Nutr.* 86:1132–1138.

Van Der Schoor, S.R.D., H. Schierbeek, P.M. Bet, M.J. Vermeulen, H.N. Lafeber, J.B. van Goudoever, and R.M. van Elburg. 2010. Majority of dietary glutamine is utilized in first pass in preterm infants. *Pediatr. Res.* 67:194–199.

Wang, W.W., Z.L. Wu, Z.L. Dai, Y. Yang, J.J. Wang, and G. Wu. 2013. Glycine metabolism in animals and humans: implications for nutrition and health. *Amino Acids* 45:463–477.

Wang, X.Q., W. Ying, K.A. Dunlap, G. Lin, M.C. Satterfield, R.C. Burghardt et al. 2014. Arginine decarboxylase and agmatinase: an alternative pathway for de novo biosynthesis of polyamines for development of mammalian conceptuses. *Biol. Reprod.* 90:84.

Watford, M. 1985. Gluconeogenesis in the chicken: regulation of phosphoenolpyruvate carboxykinase gene expression. *Fed. Proc.* 44:2469–2474.

Watford, M. 2015. Glutamine and glutamate: non-essential or essential amino acids? *Anim. Nutr.* 1:119–122.

Watford, M., Y. Hod, Y.B. Chiao, M.F. Utter, and R.W. Hanson. 1981. The unique role of the kidney in gluconeogenesis in the chicken. The significance of a cytosolic form of phosphoenolpyruvate carboxykinase. *J. Biol. Chem.* 256:10023–10027.

Werner, E.R., N. Blau, and B. Thöny. 2011. Tetrahydrobiopterin: biochemistry and pathophysiology. *Biochem. J.* 438:397–414.

Wester, T.J., G. Kraft, D. Dardevet, S. Polakof, I. Ortigues-Marty, D. Rémond, and I. Savary-Auzeloux. 2015. Nutritional regulation of the anabolic fate of amino acids within the liver in mammals: concepts arising from *in vivo* studies. *Nutr. Res. Rev.* 28:22–41.

Whitehead, T.R., N.P. Price, H.L. Drake, and M.A. Cotta. 2008. Catabolic Pathway for the production of skatole and indoleacetic acid by the acetogen *Clostridium drakei, Clostridium scatologenes,* and swine manure. *Appl. Environ. Microbiol.* 74:1950–1953.

Windmueller, H.G. and A.E. Spaeth. 1975. Intestinal metabolism of glutamine and glutamate from the lumen as compared to glutamine from blood. *Arch. Biochem. Biophys.* 171:662–672.

Windmueller, H.G. and A.E. Spaeth. 1976. Metabolism of absorbed aspartate, asparagine, and arginine by rat small intestine *in vivo. Arch. Biochem. Biophys.* 175:670–676.

Wu, G. 1997. Synthesis of citrulline and arginine from proline in enterocytes of postnatal pigs. *Am. J. Physiol.* 272:G1382–G1390.

Wu, G. 1998. Intestinal mucosal amino acid catabolism. *J. Nutr.* 128:1249–1252.

Wu, G. 2009. Amino acids: metabolism, functions, and nutrition. *Amino Acids* 37:1–17.

Wu, G. 2018. *Principles of Animal Nutrition.* CRC Press, Boca Raton, FL.

Wu, G. 2020a. Metabolism and functions of amino acids in sense organs. *Adv. Exp. Med. Biol.* 1265:201–217.

Wu, G. 2020b. Management of metabolic disorders (including metabolic diseases) in ruminant and nonruminant animals. In: *Animal Agriculture: Challenges, Innovations, and Sustainability* (Bazer, F.W., G.C. Lamb, and G. Wu, eds). Elsevier, New York. pp. 471–492.

Wu, G. 2020c. Important roles of dietary taurine, creatine, carnosine, anserine and hydroxyproline in human nutrition and health. *Amino Acids* 52:329–360.

Wu, G. and J.R. Thompson. 1987. The effect of fasting on leucine degradation in chick skeletal muscle. *Can. J. Anim. Sci.* 67:179–186.

Wu, G., and J.R. Thompson. 1989. Methionine transamination and glutamine transaminases in skeletal muscle. *Biochem. J.* 262:690–691.

Wu, G., and J.R. Thompson. 1990. The effect of glutamine on protein turnover in chick skeletal muscle *in vitro. Biochem. J.* 265:593–598.

Wu, G., and S.M. Morris, Jr. 1998. Arginine metabolism: nitric oxide and beyond. *Biochem. J.* 336:1–17.

Wu, G., D.A. Knabe, N.E. Flynn, W. Yan, and S.P. Flynn. 1996. Arginine degradation in developing porcine enterocytes. *Am. J. Physiol.* 271:G913–G919.

Wu, G., M. Chung-Bok, N. Vincent, T.J. Kowalski, Y.H. Choi, and M. Watford. 1998. Distribution of phosphate-activated glutaminase isozymes in the chicken: absence from liver but presence of high activity in pectoralis muscle. *Comp. Biochem. Physiol. B* 120:285–290.

Wu, G., N.E. Flynn, and D.A. Knabe. 2000a. Enhanced intestinal synthesis of polyamines from proline in cortisol-treated piglets. *Am. J. Physiol.* 279:E395–E402.

Wu, G., N.E. Flynn, D.A. Knabe, and L.A. Jaeger. 2000b. A cortisol surge mediates the enhanced polyamine synthesis in porcine enterocytes during weaning. *Am. J. Physiol.* 279:R554–R559.

Wu, G., T.E. Haynes, W. Yan, and C.J. Meininger. 2001. Presence of glutamine: fructose-6-phosphate amidotransferase for glucosamine-6-phosphate synthesis in endothelial cells: effects of hyperglycaemia and glutamine. *Diabetologia* 44:196–202.

Wu, G., K.A. Kelly, K. Hatakeyama, and C.J. Meininger. 2004. Regulation of endothelial tetrahydrobiopterin synthesis by L-arginine. In: *Pterins, Folates, and Neurotransmitters in Molecular Medicine* (Thony, B. and N. Blau, eds). SPS Verlagsgesellschaft mbh, Heilbronn. pp. 54–59.

Wu, G., F.W. Bazer, J. Hu, G.A. Johnson, and T.E. Spencer. 2005. Polyamine synthesis from proline in the developing porcine placenta. *Biol. Reprod.* 72:842–850.

Wu, G., F.W. Bazer, T.A. Cudd, W.S. Jobgen, S.W. Kim, A. Lassala et al. 2007. Pharmacokinetics and safety of arginine supplementation in animals. *J. Nutr.* 137:1673S–1680S.

Wu, G., F.W. Bazer, R.C. Burghardt, G.A. Johnson, S.W. Kim, D.A. Knabe et al. 2010. Functional amino acids in swine nutrition and production. In: *Dynamics in Animal Nutrition* (Doppenberg, J. and P. van der Aar, ed.), Wageningen Academic Publishers, Wageningen. pp. 69–98.

Wu, G., F.W. Bazer, G.A. Johnson, D.A. Knabe, R.C. Burghardt, T.E. Spencer et al. 2011a. Important roles for L-glutamine in swine nutrition and production. *J. Anim. Sci.* 89:2017–2030.

Wu, G., F.W. Bazer, R.C. Burghardt, G.A. Johnson, S.W. Kim, D.A. Knabe et al. 2011b. Proline and hydroxyproline metabolism: implications for animal and human nutrition. *Amino Acids* 40:1053–1063.

Wu, Z.L., Y.Q. Hou, S.D. Hu, F.W. Bazer, C.J. Meininger, C.J. McNeal, and G. Wu. 2016. Catabolism and safety of supplemental L-arginine in animals. *Amino Acids* 48:1541–1552.

Yang, Y., Z.L. Wu, C.J. Meininger, and G. Wu. 2015. L-Leucine and NO-mediated cardiovascular function. *Amino Acids* 47:435–447.

Yao, K., Y.L. Yin, Z.M. Feng, Z.R. Tang, J. Fang, and G. Wu. 2011. Tryptophan metabolism in animals: important roles in nutrition and health. *Front. Biosci.* S3:286–297.

Yao, K., Y.L. Yin, X.L. Li, P.B. Xi, J.J. Wang, J. Lei et al. Alpha-ketoglutarate inhibits glutamine degradation and enhances protein synthesis in intestinal porcine epithelial cells. *Amino Acids* 42:2491–2500.

Yeung, Y.G. 1986. L-threonine aldolase is not a genuine enzyme in rat liver. *Biochem. J.* 237:187–190.

Yoshida, S., S. Lanza-Jacoby, and T.P. Stein. 1991. Leucine and glutamine metabolism in septic rats. *Biochem. J.* 276:405–409.

Zhang, H., Y.J. Liu, X.Q. Nie, L.X. Liu, Q. Hua, G.P. Zhao, and C. Yang. 2018. The cyanobacterial ornithine-ammonia cycle involves an arginine dihydrolase. *Nature Chem. Biol.* 14:575–581.

Zhang, Q., Y.Q. Hou, F.W. Bazer, W.L. He, E.H. Posey, and G. Wu. 2021. Amino acids in swine nutrition and production. *Adv. Exp. Med. Biol.* 1285:81–107.

Zhao, X.-H., Z.M. Wen, C.N. Meredith, D.E. Matthews, D.M. Bier, and V.R. Young. 1986. Threonine kinetics at graded threonine intakes in young men. *Am. J. Clin. Nutr.* 43:795–802.

5 Synthesis and Catabolism of Special Substances from Amino Acids

Most of the metabolic products arising from amino acid (AA) catabolism in organisms are described in Chapter 4. However, multiple AAs (two or three) or a single AA also serve as substrates for syntheses of other biologically important metabolites (e.g., betaine, bilirubin, carnosine and related dipeptides, carnitine, catecholamines, choline, creatine, glucosamine, glutathione (GSH), γ-aminobutyrate (GABA), heme, histamine, homoarginine, polyamines, purines, pyrimidines, and serotonin) in a cell- and tissue-specific manner (Agostinelli et al. 2020; Fernstrom and Wurtman 1971; Krebs 1964; Lubec and Rosenthal 1990; Meister 1973; Yamada et al. 2005). Structures and chemical properties of some of these special nitrogenous substances are illustrated in Figure 5.1 and Table 5.1, respectively. Their synthetic pathways share one or more of the following characteristics. First, AAs are utilized to produce unique compounds without undergoing extensive oxidation. Second, histidine and its methylated derivatives are used to form major dipeptides in the skeletal muscle, brain, and other tissues. Third, methionine plays a critical role in the formation of polyamines, creatine, and carnitine by providing the necessary methyl group via *S*-adenosylmethionine (SAM). Fourth, most of the synthetic pathways for utilizing multiple AAs involve the cooperation of several organs, such as the liver, kidney, and skeletal muscle, where glutamine [or its metabolites (e.g., arginine, proline, and glutamate)] and glycine are essential precursors. Fifth, cysteine and tyrosine play important roles in the synthesis of antioxidant and neuromodulatory molecules, respectively.

As a mechanism responsible for the maintenance of their homeostasis in the body, the special nitrogenous products of AAs undergo continuous catabolism, yielding unique substances with both physiological and pathological significance. Some of these metabolites are useful indicators of the nutritional status and the progression of certain genetic or metabolic diseases in humans and other animals (Scriver et al. 2001; Valman et al. 1971). In addition, the conjugation with glucuronic acid or bile acid is an important pathway for removing many nitrogenous products. Furthermore, as shown below, some AA metabolites spontaneously undergo keto-enol (e.g., uric acid) or amino-imino (e.g., creatinine) tautomerization, or both (e.g., guanine) in physiological fluids (Chapter 1) to alter their chemical (e.g., ionic charges) and biochemical (e.g., transcellular transport and metabolism) properties. To expand our knowledge of AA metabolism, the pathways for the synthesis and catabolism of nitrogenous products beyond those described for animals in the preceding chapters are highlighted here in this chapter.

5.1 PRODUCTION OF DIPEPTIDES CONSISTING OF HISTIDINE OR ITS METHYLATED DERIVATIVES

5.1.1 History of Research on Carnosine and Related Dipeptides in Animal Tissues

Animals contain dipeptides consisting of histidine or its methylated derivatives as well as β-alanine or GABA in a species- and tissue-specific manner (Table 5.2). Discoveries of most of these peptides date back to the early 20th century. In 1900, the Russian biochemist W. Gulewitsch found that the total nitrogen content in minced beef muscle was greater than the sum of the total nitrogen accounted for by protein and nonprotein substances known to be present in skeletal muscle

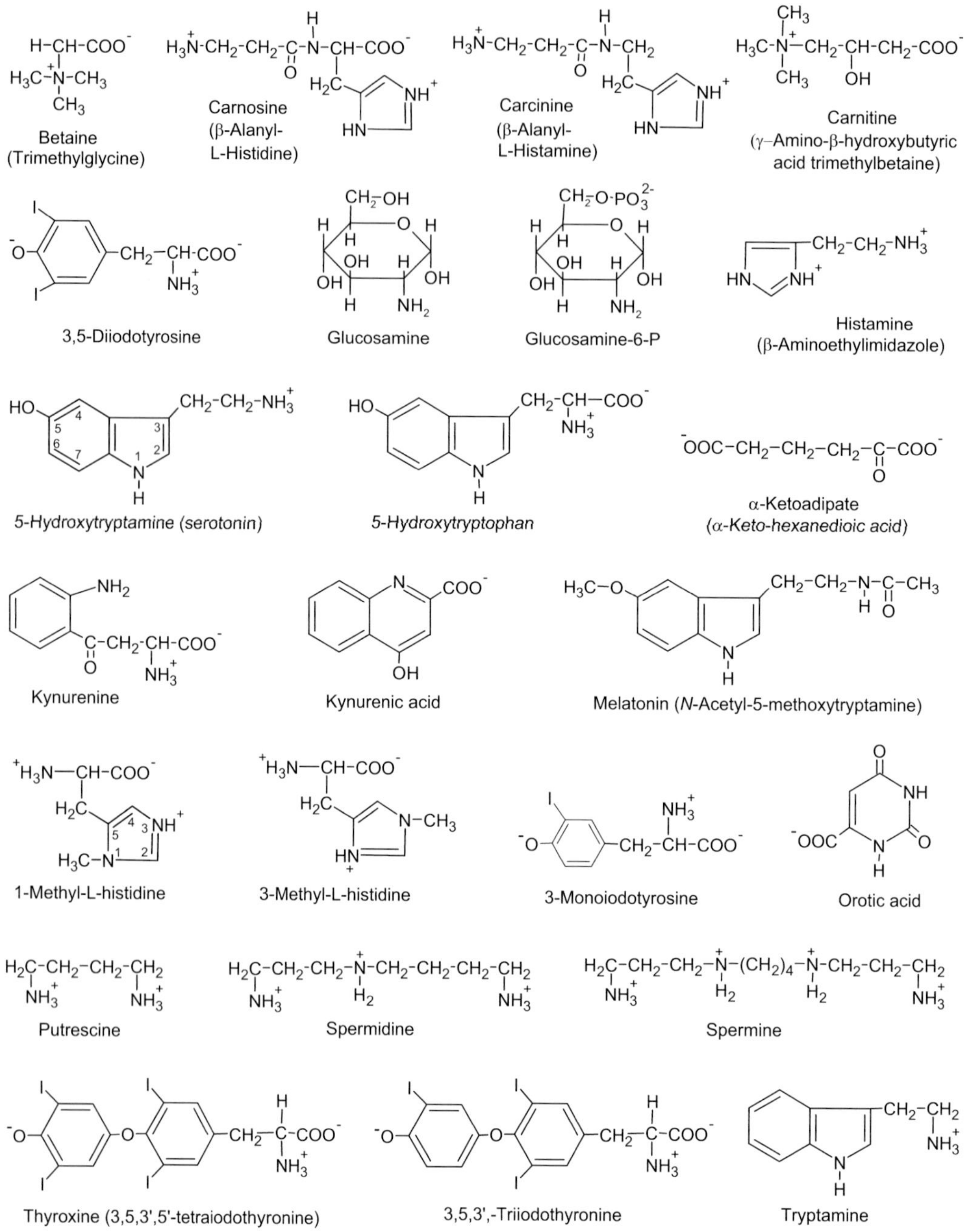

Betaine (Trimethylglycine)

Carnosine (β-Alanyl-L-Histidine)

Carcinine (β-Alanyl-L-Histamine)

Carnitine (γ–Amino-β-hydroxybutyric acid trimethylbetaine)

3,5-Diiodotyrosine

Glucosamine

Glucosamine-6-P

Histamine (β-Aminoethylimidazole)

5-Hydroxytryptamine (serotonin)

5-Hydroxytryptophan

α-Ketoadipate (α-Keto-hexanedioic acid)

Kynurenine

Kynurenic acid

Melatonin (N-Acetyl-5-methoxytryptamine)

1-Methyl-L-histidine

3-Methyl-L-histidine

3-Monoiodotyrosine

Orotic acid

Putrescine

Spermidine

Spermine

Thyroxine (3,5,3′,5′-tetraiodothyronine)

3,5,3′,-Triiodothyronine

Tryptamine

FIGURE 5.1 Chemical structures of some special metabolites of amino acids found in humans and other animals. Glucosamine and polyamines (putrescine, spermidine, and spermine) are synthesized from their respective substrates in all cell types. Generation of 1-methyl-L-histidine is very limited in animal cells. Other substances are formed in a cell- and tissue-specific manner.

at that time. He demonstrated that this difference was attributed to an abundant molecule named *carnosine* (meaning "meat" in Latin). Eleven years later, W. Gulewitsch reported that β-alanine is a constituent of carnosine. In 1918, through chemical synthesis, two American scientists, L. Baumann and T. Ingvaldsen, identified carnosine to be β-alanyl-L-histidine. Synthesis of the dipeptide is

TABLE 5.1
Molecular Weights, Number of Nitrogen (N) Atoms, N Content, and Chemical Properties of Amino Acid Metabolites

Amino Acid Metabolite	MW (Da)	Number of N Atoms	N Content (%)	MP (°C)	Solub[a] in H_2O	pK_1	pK_2	pK_3	pI
N-Acetyl Asp ($C_6H_9NO_5$)	175.14	1	8.00	139	2.11	3.09	4.52	---	3.81
N-Acetyl Glu ($C_7H_{11}NO_5$)	189.17	1	7.40	199	3.60	3.43	5.41	---	4.42
N-Acetylhistidine ($C_8H_{11}N_3O_3$)	197.19	3	21.31	187	0.609	3.53	7.20	7.55	7.38
N-Acetyl serotonin ($C_{12}H_{14}N_2O_2$)	218.25	2	12.84	121	0.057	9.56	---	---	9.56
Agmatine ($C_5H_{14}N_4$)	130.19	4	43.03	231	3.61	9.78	12.6	---	11.2
Allantoin ($C_4H_6N_4O_3$)	158.12	4	35.43	238	0.57	8.96	---	---	8.96
Ammonia (NH_3, gas)	17.03	1	82.25	−77.7	31.0	9.20	---	---	9.20
Anserine ($C_{10}H_{16}N_4O_3$)	240.26	4	23.32	227	0.401	2.64	9.49	7.04	8.27
Anthranilic acid ($C_7H_7NO_2$)	137.14	1	12.21	147	0.572	2.17	7.53	---	4.85
Balenine ($C_{10}H_{16}N_4O_3$)	240.26	4	23.32	225	0.411	2.71	9.32	7.0	8.16
N-Bromotaurine ($C_2H_6BrNO_3S$)	204.05	1	6.86	---	High	<1.5	---	---	<1.5
Cadaverine ($C_5H_{14}N_2$)	102.18	2	27.42	9.0	8.91	10.25	9.13	---	9.69
Carnitine ($C_7H_{15}NO_3$)	161.20	1	8.69	197	100	3.79	9.40	---	6.60
Carnosine ($C_9H_{14}N_4O_3$)	226.23	4	24.77	253	1.11	2.77	9.66	6.83	8.25
Choline ($C_5H_{14}NO$)	104.17	1	13.45	302[c]	14.0[c]	13.9	---	---	13.9
N-Chlorotaurine ($C_2H_6ClNO_3S$)	159.59	1	8.77	138	2.83	−0.30	---	---	−0.30
Creatine ($C_4H_9N_3O_2$)	131.13	3	32.04	255	1.33	2.67	11.02	---	6.85
Creatinine ($C_4H_7N_3O$)	113.12	3	37.15	303	8.01	4.84	9.20	---	7.02
Creatine-P ($C_4H_{10}N_3O_5P$)	211.11	3	19.90	195	3.52	2.70	4.50	13.57	3.60
Dopamine ($C_8H_{11}NO_2$)	153.18	1	9.14	128	0.535	8.86	10.5	---	9.68
Epinephrine ($C_9H_{13}NO_3$)	183.20	1	7.65	212	1.86	8.91	9.69	---	9.30
Formate (CH_2O_2)	46.03	0	0	8.4	97.2	3.77	---	---	3.77
Glucosamine-6-P ($C_6H_{14}NO_8P$)	259.15	1	5.40	>127	3.48	6.0	8.2	---	7.10
Glutathione ($C_{10}H_{17}N_3O_6S$)	307.32	3	13.67	191	29.25	2.12	3.53	8.66, 9.12	2.83
GSSG ($C_{20}H_{32}N_6O_{12}S_2$)	612.63	6	13.72	178	4.06	2.0, 2.6	3.3, 4.0	8.7, 9.6	2.98
Guanine ($C_5H_5N_5O$)	151.13	5	46.34	360	3.84×10^{-4}	3.3	9.2	12.3	10.8
Hippurate ($C_9H_9NO_3$)	179.17	1	7.82	187	0.375	3.62	---	---	3.62
Histamine ($C_5H_9N_3$)	111.15	3	37.80	83.5	3.40	6.04	9.75	---	7.90
Homoanserine ($C_{11}H_{18}N_4O_3$)	254.29	4	22.03	203	0.319	3.52	9.99	6.80	8.40
Homocarnosine ($C_{10}H_{16}N_4O_3$)	240.26	4	23.32	243	0.737	2.95	8.16	6.86	7.51
Hyaluronic acid ($C_{14}H_{21}NO_{11}$)$_n$	(379.32)n	1(n)	3.69	244	High[d]	~3.0	---	---	~3.0
Kynurenic acid ($C_{10}H_7NO_3$)	189.17	1	7.40	283	0.0095	2.50	11.6	---	7.05
Kynurenine ($C_{10}H_{12}N_2O_3$)	208.22	2	13.5	191	0.167	2.38	9.39	---	5.89
Melanin ($C_{18}H_{10}N_2O_4$)	318.29	2	8.80	−20	0.031	1.34	12.65	---	7.00
Melatonin ($C_{13}H_{16}N_2O_2$)	232.28	2	12.06	117	0.2	12.5	---	---	12.5
3-Methylhistidine ($C_7H_{11}N_3O_2$)	169.18	3	24.84	254	0.693	1.96	9.25	6.47	7.86
1-Methylhistidine ($C_7H_{11}N_3O_2$)	169.18	3	24.84	247	0.693	1.69	8.85	6.48	7.67
Norepinephrine ($C_8H_{11}NO_3$)	169.18	1	8.28	217	1.25	8.55	10.32	---	9.44
Phenylacetyl-Gln ($C_{13}H_{16}N_2O_4$)	264.28	2	10.60	117	0.039	3.9	---	---	3.9
Putrescine ($C_4H_{12}N_2$)	88.15	2	31.78	27.5	23.6	9.35	10.8	---	10.1
Sarcosine ($C_3H_7NO_2$)	89.09	1	15.72	208	30.8	2.23	10.01	---	6.12
Serotonin ($C_{10}H_{12}N_2O$)	176.22	2	15.90	168	0.25	9.31	10.0	---	9.66
Spermidine ($C_7H_{19}N_3$)	145.25	3	28.93	23.5	14.5	8.40	10.81	9.94	10.4

(Continued)

TABLE 5.1 (*Continued*)

Molecular Weights, Number of Nitrogen (N) Atoms, N Content, and Chemical Properties of Amino Acid Metabolites

Amino Acid Metabolite	MW (Da)	Number of N Atoms	N Content (%)	MP (°C)	Solub[a] in H_2O	pK$_1$	pK$_2$	pK$_3$	pI
Spermine ($C_{10}H_{26}N_4$)	202.34	4	27.69	29.0	10.0	10.8	10.0	8.9, 8.0	10.4
Triiodothyronine ($C_{15}H_{12}I_3NO_4$)	650.97	1	2.15	230	0.4×10^{-3}	2.08	9.48	8.5	5.78
Thyroxine (T_4; $C_{15}H_{11}I_4NO_4$)	776.87	1	1.80	236	0.47×10^{-3}	2.40	10.1	6.87	6.25
Trimethylhistidine ($C_9H_{16}N_3O_2$)[b]	198.24	3	21.20	238	0.221	1.69	6.48	8.85	7.67
Tryptamine ($C_{10}H_{12}N_2$)	160.22	2	17.49	118	0.134	10.2	---	---	10.2
Tyramine ($C_8H_{11}NO$)	137.18	1	10.21	165	1.05	9.74	10.52	---	10.1
Urea (CH_4N_2O)	60.06	2	46.64	133	54.5	---	---	---	---
Uric acid ($C_5H_4N_4O_3$)	168.11	4	33.33	300	0.006	5.75	---	---	5.75
Urocanic acid ($C_6H_6N_2O_2$)	138.12	2	20.28	225	4.25	3.85	6.13	---	4.99

Source: Bégué, J.-P. and D. Bonnet-Delpon. 2008. *Bioorganic and Medicinal Chemistry of Fluorine*, Wiley, Hoboken, NJ. p. 271; Berfield, J.L. et al. 1999. *J. Biol. Chem.* 274:4876–4882; Boldyrev, A.A. et al. 2013. *Physiol. Rev.* 93:1803–1845; Crovetto, L. et al. 2004. *J. Phys. Chem.* 108:6082–6092; Deutsch, A. and P. Eggleton. 1938. *Biochem. J.* 32:209–211; Gottardi, W. and M. Nagl. 2010. *J. Antimicrob. Chemother.* 65:399–409; Matsuo, H. et al. 1972. *J. Biochem.* 72:1057–1060; Nollet, L.M.L. and F. Toldra. 2015. *Handbook of Food Analysis*. CRC Press, Boca Raton. p. 303; Paiva, A.C., L. Juliano and P. Boschcov. 1976. *J. Am. Chem. Soc.* 98:7645–7648; Steglich, W. et al. 2000. *RÖMPP Encyclopedia: Natural Products*. Thieme, New York; Tredwell, G.D. et al. 2016. *Metabolomics* 12:151; Williams, R. 2011. pK_a *Data Compiled by R. Williams*. http://www.chem.wisc.edu/areas/organic/index-chem.htm; Xin, Y. and D. Hamelberg. 2010. *RNA* 16:2455–2463; Zelentsova, E.A. et al. 2013. *Photochem. Photobiol. Sci.* 12:546–558; American Society of Chemistry. 2020. https://www.acs.org/content/acs/en/molecule-of-the-week/archive.html?archiv.

Note: Asp, aspartic acid; Da, Daltons; Gln, glutamine; Glu, glutamic acid; GSSG, glutathione disulfide (oxidized glutathione); Insol, insoluble; MP, melting point; MW, molecular weight; and P, phosphate.

[a] Solubility (Solub); g/100 mL of water at 25°C unless otherwise indicated.

[b] Also known as hercynine.

[c] As choline chloride.

[d] 1 g of hyaluronic acid can be mixed with 108 g of water to form a gel.

catalyzed by ATP-dependent carnosine synthetase primarily found in skeletal muscle. Although both acid and base hydrolysis can decompose carnosine, intestinal proteases (e.g., pepsin or trypsin) or intestinal bacteria cannot hydrolyze this dipeptide. In 1949, an enzyme in intestinal juice, named carnosinase, was discovered to convert β-alanyl-L-histidine to β-alanine and L-histidine. A relatively high activity of carnosinase has been demonstrated in the mammalian brain, explaining the very low level of carnosine in this tissue. By contrast, carnosinase activity in muscle is low and varies with species. This accounts for the relatively high concentration of carnosine in mammalian skeletal muscle, which contains high concentrations (in the mM range) of carnosine in a species-dependent manner. Note that carnosine is also present at high concentrations in some avian tissues [e.g., 1.64 μmol/mL of the whole blood of fed adult chickens (predominantly in red blood cells)] (Tinker et al. 1986).

Intensive efforts were made in the 1920s to determine the carnosine content of animal tissues. In 1921, W.M. Clifford concluded that chicken skeletal muscle contains a substance that is similar to carnosine but is not carnosine. In 1929, N. Tolkatschevskaya and D. Ackermann independently identified this carnosine-like compound in chicken skeletal muscle to be a dipeptide (methyl carnosine; β-alanyl-*N*-methyl-L-histidine), which was named *anserine* after the taxonomic name for

TABLE 5.2
Histidine-Related Dipeptides and Glycine-Related Tripeptides in Animals

Common Name	Composition	Storage in Major Tissues
(1) Dipeptides		
N-Acetylcarnosine	N-Acetyl-β-alanyl-L-histidine	Brain, skeletal muscle, and heart (excitable tissues) of mammals (including humans, rats, pigs, and cattle)
N-Acetylhomoanserine	N-Acetyl-γ-aminobutyryl-L-1-methylhistidine	Brain and skeletal muscle of many nonprimate mammals, and fish
N-Acetylhomocarnosine	N-Acetyl-γ-aminobutyryl- L-histidine	Brain and heart of many mammals (including humans and rats)
Anserine[a]	β-Alanyl-L-1-methylhistidine	Skeletal muscle and brain of birds (including chickens and geese), many nonprimate mammals (including cattle and pigs), and fish (including salmon and tuna); red blood cells of nonprimate mammals and birds; absent from humans and other primates
N-Acetyl-anserine	N-Acetyl-β-alanyl-L-1-methylhistidine	Brain, skeletal muscle, and heart of many nonprimate mammals, and fish
Balenine (ophidine)[b]	β-Alanyl-L-3-methylhistidine	Skeletal muscle and brain of many animal species (including cat, cattle, chicken, dog, dolphin; human, pig, snake, sheep, and whale); highly abundant in the skeletal muscles of whales and dolphins
Carcinine	β-Alanyl-histamine	Brain and heart of vertebrates; abundant in crab muscles; present in some tissues (e.g., the heart, kidneys, intestine, and stomach of many mammals (including humans))
Carnosine[c]	β-Alanyl-L-histidine	Skeletal muscle and brain (olfactory neurons) of mammals (e.g., humans, cattle, and pigs), birds, and fish; highly abundant in human, bovine, ovine, porcine, and rat skeletal muscles; red blood cells of mammals and birds
Homocarnosine[d]	γ-Aminobutyryl-L-histidine	Mammalian brain; abundant in the human brain (0.3–1.6 mM); ≤0.07 mM in the brain of other mammals
Homoanserine	γ-Aminobutyryl-L-1-methylhistidine	Brain of most vertebrates; absent from human tissues
(2) Tripeptides		
Glutathione	γ-Glu-Cys-Gly	Animal cells, bile acid, pancreatic juice, and uterine fluid
Collagen peptide	Gly-Pro-4-hydroxyproline	Milk, plasma, and connective tissue

[a] Also known as methyl-carnosine. Anserine is the major histidine-containing dipeptide in the skeletal muscles of birds, dog, cat, lion, rabbit, agouti, mouse, kangaroo, wallaby, opossum, cod, smelt, marlin, whiting, croaker, tuna, Japanese char, salmon, and trout. This dipeptide is also abundant in the skeletal muscles of cattle and pigs, as well as the red blood cells of mammals and birds.

[b] Highly abundant in the skeletal muscle of whale (~45 mmol/kg wet weight), relatively low in swine (~0.7–1 mmol/kg wet weight or 5%–8% of carnosine content), very low in cattle, chickens, and sheep (~0.05–0.1 mmol/kg wet weight), and barely detectable in human and rat skeletal muscles.

[c] Abundant in the skeletal muscles of mammals (e.g., 5–10 mM in humans, 20–30 mM in pigs, and 28–48 mM in cattle) and the red blood cells of mammals and birds.

[d] In the human brain, this dipeptide is more abundant than carnosine.

the goose. Anserine is also abundant in the retina and the whole blood of birds [e.g., 0.60 μmol/mL of the whole blood of fed adult chickens (predominantly in red blood cells)] (Tinker et al. 1986). In 1909, U. Suzuki was the first to report the presence of a carnosine-like substance in fish skeletal muscle. This substance was likely anserine. In 1957, R.W. Cargill and B. Freeburgh demonstrated that anserine was synthesized from either β-alanine plus L-1-methylhistidine by an ATP-dependent synthase or carnosine plus SAM by carnosine-N-methyltransferase in avian skeletal muscle. By contrast, invertebrates contain little carnosine or anserine.

The 1960s witnessed the discovery of homocarnosine (γ-aminobutyryl-L-histidine) and homoanserine (γ-aminobutyryl-L-1-methylhistidine) in the mammalian brain and of balenine in mammalian skeletal muscle. They are derivatives of GABA and histidine. Specifically, the concentrations of homocarnosine in the mammalian brain range from 0.05–0.07 mM (nonprimate mammals) to 0.3–1.6 mM (humans), depending on species and developmental stage, and the values in the human brain are much greater than those of carnosine. The highest concentrations of homocarnosine are found in the substantia nigra, dentate gyrus, and olfactory bulb, as well as the cerebrospinal fluid. In 1963, A. Carisano and F. Cara discovered balenine (β-alanyl-L-3-methylhistidine) in meat extracts. This compound was subsequently found to be present in the skeletal muscles of many animal species (including the cat, cattle, chicken, dog, human, pig, snake, sheep, and whale). Meanwhile, a substance (N-acetyl-histidine or neurosine, a major osmolyte in the lens of fish, such as the Atlantic salmon, rainbow trout, and skipjack tuna; up to 32 mM), structurally similar to carnosine, was found in the brain, retina, and lens of amphibians, reptiles, and fish where both neurosine and carnosine are synthesized (Baslow 1965; Togashi et al. 1998). Acetylated derivatives of anserine, carnosine, and homocarnosine were discovered in the 1970s and 1980s in the mammalian brain and cardiac muscle. In 1985, carcinine (β-alanyl-histamine) was identified in crab muscle and in vertebrate nervous tissue and cardiac muscle. Human heart, kidneys, small intestine, and stomach all contain carcinine, which can be derived from both diet and endogenous synthesis in these tissues.

5.1.2 Synthesis of Carnosine and Related Dipeptides

Based on (1) the k_d (fractional turnover rate) value of 0.0133/day for the loss of intramuscular carnosine at the physiological steady state, (2) the intramuscular concentrations of carnosine in women and men (17.5 and 21.3 mmol/kg dry weight, respectively), (3) skeletal muscle mass (45% of BW), and (4) its dry matter content (30%), it can be estimated that a 60-kg woman and a 70-kg man synthesize 427 and 606 mg carnosine per day, respectively (Spelnikov and Harris 2019). The pathways for the cytosolic syntheses of dipeptides are illustrated in Figure 5.2. The sources of histidine are diets and the degradation of hemoglobin (which is very rich in histidine), actin, myosin, and other proteins in the body. Methylated histidines (3-methylhistidine and 1-methylhistidine) are produced from the hydrolysis of proteins (e.g., myofibrillar proteins) containing 3-methylhistidine and 1-methylhistidine residues. These residues are derived from the posttranslational methylation of histidine residues in polypeptides by SAM-dependent protein methylases. 1-Methylhistidine is not formed in animal cells and occurs at a very low concentration in some plants. β-Alanine is formed from aspartate decarboxylation, as well as the catabolism of pyrimidines, polyamines, and coenzyme A (Chapter 3).

The enzymes that catalyze the synthesis of carnosine and related dipeptides are anserine synthetase, carnosine-N-methyltransferase, carnosine synthetase, carnosine decarboxylase, homocarnosine synthetase, homoserine synthetase, and balenine synthetase. All of these enzymes are localized in the cytoplasm. Carnosine synthetase occurs primarily in the skeletal muscle, heart, and certain regions of the brain (e.g., the olfactory bulb; Drozak et al. 2010). As indicated previously, their expression is species- and tissue-specific. For example, anserine is synthesized in the skeletal muscle and brain of birds, cattle, pigs, and rats but not in some mammals (e.g., humans and

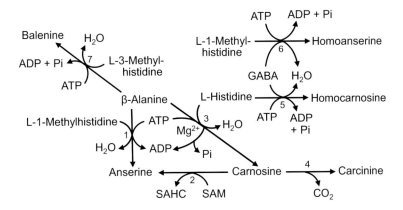

FIGURE 5.2 Synthesis of dipeptides consisting of L-histidine or its methylated derivatives in animals. The enzymes that catalyze the indicated reactions are (1) anserine synthetase; (2) carnosine-N-methyltransferase; (3) carnosine synthetase; (4) carnosine decarboxylase; (5) homocarnosine synthetase; (6) homoserine synthetase; and (7) balenine synthetase. Expression of these enzymes is species- and tissue-specific. GABA, γ-aminobutyrate.

monkeys), whereas carnosine is actively synthesized in the skeletal muscle of mammals (including humans, cattle, pigs, and rats) but not in birds. It is possible that red blood cells, which contain a large amount of carnosine and anserine as reported for chickens, may be capable of synthesizing these two dipeptides. Of note, mammalian and avian livers lack the ability to synthesize anserine and carnosine.

5.1.3 REGULATION OF CARNOSINE SYNTHESIS IN SKELETAL MUSCLE

5.1.3.1 Availability of Substrates

The K_M values of carnosine synthetase for β-alanine and histidine are 1.0–2.3 mM and 16.8 μM, respectively (Horinishi et al. 1978). These values are much greater than or comparable to the intracellular concentration of β-alanine in the brain (0.09 mM) or skeletal muscle (1.0 mM). By contrast, the value of carnosine synthetase for histidine is much lower than the intracellular concentration of histidine in the brain (~140 μM) and skeletal muscle (~400 μM), respectively. As reported for nitric oxide (NO) synthase whose K_M value for arginine is much greater in cells than that in assay tubes (Wu and Meininger 2000), it is possible that the K_M of carnosine synthetase for histidine *in vivo* is much greater than that (i.e., 16.8 μM) reported for the purified enzyme under *in vitro* assay conditions, due to complex protein–protein and enzyme–substrate interactions *in vivo*.

Availability of β-alanine primarily limits carnosine synthesis by carnosine synthetase in human skeletal muscle and the olfactory bulb, but adequate provision of histidine in diets is also critical for maximal production of carnosine because histidine is not synthesized de novo (Hill et al. 2007; Sale et al. 2010). For example, supplementation with β-alanine to humans (e.g., 2–6 g/day) dose-dependently increases the concentrations of carnosine in skeletal muscle by 20%–80%, but dietary supplementation with 3.5 g histidine/day for 23 days has no effect on intramuscular carnosine concentrations in nonvegetarian adults (Blancquaert et al. 2017; Culbertson et al. 2010). Furthermore, dietary supplementation with 3.2 or 6.4 g β-alanine per day (as multiple doses of 400 or 800 mg) or with L-carnosine (isomolar to 6.4 g β-alanine) per day for 4 weeks augmented intramuscular carnosine concentrations by 42%, 64%, and 66%, respectively (Harris et al. 2006). These results reveal that histidine is not a limiting factor in carnosine synthesis in adults consuming adequate histidine from animal-source foods. Thus, in nonvegetarian humans, consumption of an equal amount of β-alanine and carnosine effectively increases intramuscular carnosine concentrations to the same extent. It is unknown whether dietary intake of histidine limits carnosine synthesis in vegetarians with or without β-alanine supplementation.

There is evidence that dietary supplementation with β-alanine (6 g/day for 23 days) to adult humans reduces the concentrations of histidine in their plasma and skeletal muscle by 31% and 32%, respectively, possibly due to reduced intestinal absorption of histidine and increased utilization of histidine for carnosine synthesis by skeletal muscle (Blancquaert et al. 2017). Such a finding is an interesting nutritional phenomenon in mammals. Whether this reduction in histidine with β-alanine supplementation has a long-term adverse effect on human health is unknown, but it is prudent to ensure that dietary intake of histidine via supplementation or consumption of histidine-rich foods (e.g., meat) is sufficient. By contrast, the oral administration of carnosine increases the concentration of not only β-alanine but also histidine in the plasma of humans (Asatoor et al. 1970), indicating an advantage of the consumption of synthetic carnosine or carnosine-rich foods (e.g., beef) over the consumption of β-alanine alone.

5.1.3.2 Age, Sex, Muscle Fiber Type, and Physical Activity

Within a mammalian species, the synthesis of carnosine is also affected by multiple factors, including age, sex, muscle fiber type, muscular activity, and diet (Harris et al. 2012). For example, a study with 9- to 83-year-old humans has shown that the concentration of carnosine in skeletal muscle increases between 9 and 18 years of age but decreases thereafter with advanced ages (Baguet et al. 2012). Likewise, the content of carnosine in the soleus muscle declines with age in 17- to 47-year-old persons (Everaert et al. 2011). In adult humans, white muscle fibers contain 30%–100% more carnosine than red muscle fibers, and men have 22%–82% greater concentrations of carnosine in skeletal muscle than women (Everaert et al. 2011; Mannion et al. 1992). Compared to age-matched women, men have 36%, 28%, and 82% greater concentrations of carnosine in the soleus, gastrocnemius, and tibialis anterior muscles, respectively (Everaert et al. 2011). It is possible that androgens enhance carnosine synthesis in skeletal muscle, but the circulating levels of testosterone in healthy adult men do not appear to be related to their intramuscular carnosine concentrations (Everaert et al. 2011). Finally, long-term exercise (e.g., 2 days per week for 8 weeks for sprinters) increases intramuscular carnosine levels in male participants by 113%, which is associated with a 9% increase in the mean power (e.g., during 30-s maximal cycle ergometer sprinting) following training (Suzuki et al. 2004). Similarly, there is a 100% increase in intramuscular carnosine levels in resistance-trained bodybuilders (Tallon et al. 2005). Finally, because plant-source foods contain much lower concentrations of β-alanine and histidine (Hou et al. 2019) than animal products (Wu et al. 2016) and because the formation of β-alanine in vegans is limited (Harris et al. 2012), the synthesis of carnosine in vegans is inadequate and its concentrations in the soleus and gastrocnemius muscles are 17% and 26%, respectively, lower than those in individuals who consume some meat, an excellent source of both β-alanine and histidine (Everaert et al. 2011; Harris et al. 2012).

5.1.4 REGULATION OF ANSERINE SYNTHESIS IN THE SKELETAL MUSCLE OF NONPRIMATES

Nonprimate animals can synthesize anserine via (1) anserine synthetase and (2) carnosine synthetase plus carnosine 1-methyltransferase (Figure 5.2). The anserine synthetase pathway is likely a minor one because 1-methylhistidine is limited in animal tissues. The carnosine N-methyltransferase is quantitatively important and physiologically active for anserine synthesis in skeletal muscle. Because carnosine 1-methyltransferase and guanidinoacetate methyltransferase (the enzyme that converts guanidinoacetate into creatine) compete for SAM, there may be a close metabolic relationship between anserine and creatine syntheses in nonprimate animals. Like carnosine, the homeostasis of anserine in skeletal muscle is also controlled by the availability of β-alanine or its degradation via transamination.

5.1.5 CATABOLISM OF CARNOSINE AND RELATED DIPEPTIDES

5.1.5.1 Carnosinase

Carnosinase [a Xaa-His dipeptidase (EC 3.4.13.3); also known as carnosine dipeptidase; a metallopeptidase] catalyzes the hydrolysis of carnosine and the dipeptides that are structurally similar to carnosine (Sauerhöfer et al. 2007). Two isoforms of the enzyme have been reported for animal tissues (e.g., liver and kidney), but are virtually absent from skeletal muscle. Carnosinase 1 (CN1, a cytosolic enzyme and a Mn^{2+}-dependent extracellular enzyme) has substrate specificity for carnosine and homocarnosine, whereas carnosinase 2 (a Zn^{2+}-dependent cytosolic enzyme in tissues) can hydrolyze carnosine and related dipeptides. Expression of these two isoforms of carnosinase occurs in a tissue-specific manner. Specifically, carnosinase 1 is expressed in the liver, brain, and kidneys and occurs in human serum (with the source of the enzyme being derived from the liver) at a very high activity, but is absent from the skeletal muscle and gastrointestinal mucosae of mammals (including humans, pigs, cattle, and rats), as well as the serum of healthy nonprimate mammals (except for the Syrian golden hamster) and birds. By contrast, carnosinase 2 (CN2) is more widely expressed in mammalian tissues (including skeletal muscle and the small-intestinal mucosae of some species), but is absent from the serum or cerebrospinal fluid of mammals or birds, as well as the gastric and colonic mucosae of mammals (including humans, pigs, cattle and rats) (Boldyrev et al. 2013). Thus, carnosine is stable in the plasma of rats and farm animals but not humans.

Besides using carnosine as a substrate, carnosinase also acts on anserine and related dipeptides, but its enzymatic activity is lower for anserine and related dipeptides than for carnosine (Boldyrev et al. 2013). The resultant products of the dipeptide hydrolysis by carnosinase include histidine, 3-methylhistidine, 1-methylhistidine, and β-alanine. Histidine is degraded as described in Chapter 4, whereas 3-methylhistidine and 1-methylhistidine are excreted in the urine if they are not reutilized for dipeptide synthesis in the body. Finally, β-alanine is catabolized to acetyl-CoA plus CO_2 in animal tissues through a series of enzymes. These enzymes include (1) β-alanine:pyruvate transaminase, forming malonate semialdehyde and alanine; (2) β-alanine:α-ketoglutarate transaminase, yielding malonate semialdehyde and glutamate; (3) alanine aminotransferase, glutamate dehydrogenase, and malonate semialdehyde dehydrogenase (catalyzing the dehydrogenation and decarboxylation of malonate semialdehyde to form acetaldehyde); and (4) aldehyde dehydrogenase, generating acetyl-CoA. Acetyl-CoA is then oxidized to CO_2 and water through the Krebs cycle and electron transport system in the mitochondria.

5.1.5.2 Anserinase

N.R. Jones (1956) reported the presence of anserinase [a Xaa-methyl-His dipeptidase (EC 3.4.13.5), a metallopeptidase] in the skeletal muscle of codling (*Gadus callarias*; an Atlantic cod fish). This enzyme is also present in the brain, retina, and vitreous body of poikilothermic vertebrates (bony fishes, amphibians, and reptiles; Yamada et al. 2005). Anserinase hydrolyzes anserine into β-alanine and 1-methyl-histidine, has broad specificity for substrates (including dipeptides containing *N*-acetylated histidine and *N*-acetylated methionine, carnosine, homocarnosine, alanyl-histidine, glycyl-leucine, and leucyl-glycine), but cannot hydrolyze tripeptides. Available evidence shows that anserinase is expressed only in ectothermic jawed vertebrates (e.g., ray-finned fishes, amphibians, and reptiles) and is absent from endothermic vertebrates (e.g., mammals and birds), including humans and chickens (Oku et al. 2011).

5.1.6 SPECIES-SPECIFIC TISSUE DISTRIBUTION OF CARNOSINE, ANSERINE, AND BALENINE

5.1.6.1 Carnosine

Concentrations of carnosine in the skeletal muscle of humans without carnosine or β-alanine supplementation range from 5 to 10 mM (16.7 to 33.3 mmol/kg dry weight of muscle; Boldyrev et al. 2013). The soleus and gastrocnemius muscles of adult males contain 8 and 10 mM carnosine, respectively (26.7 and 33.3 mmol/kg dry weight of muscle, respectively; Derave et al. 2007). These values are approximately 2, 10, and 20 times greater than those in the skeletal muscle of pigs, rats, and mice, respectively. Bodybuilders can have carnosine concentrations as high as 15.3 mM (51 mmol/kg dry weight), with an average value of 13 mM (43 mmol/kg dry weight; Tallon et al. 2005). The concentrations of carnosine in the olfactory bulb of the brain and the cardiac muscle are comparable to those in skeletal muscle, but the concentrations in other tissues (e.g., ~0.1 mM in the kidneys and white adipose tissue) are only 0.1%–10% of those in skeletal muscle. Based on the mean concentrations of carnosine in the skeletal muscles of women and men (17.5 and 21.3 mmol/kg dry weight, respectively), a 60-kg woman and a 70-kg man have 32 and 45 g of carnosine, respectively (Mannion et al. 1992). In mammals (including humans), about 99% of carnosine is present in skeletal muscle (Sale et al. 2010). Carnosine is more abundant in the white muscle of humans than in their red muscle, as a type II muscle fiber has 66% more carnosine than a type I muscle fiber (Hill et al. 2007). Elite athletes can have up to 80% of either type I or type II muscle fibers, depending on the category of their sport (speed vs endurance). The amount and percentage of these muscle fibers are a determinant of their success in competition. In addition, adequate availability of carnosine in skeletal muscle will be beneficial for healthy aging.

Carnosine is highly abundant in the skeletal muscles of mammals other than humans. For example, the chuck (serratus ventralis, rhomboideus, and splenius muscles), round (semimembranosus muscle), and loin (longissimus lumborum muscle) cuts of cattle contain 28.4, 38.6, and 47.6 mM carnosine, respectively (Wu et al. 2016). Likewise, the skeletal muscles of pigs contain 20–30 mM carnosine, depending on the type of muscle fiber (Carnegie et al. 1982). The intramuscular concentrations of carnosine in cattle and pigs are about 4.5 and 2 times those of taurine, respectively.

As noted previously, whole blood of fed adult chickens contains a large amount of carnosine, but food deprivation for 6 days does not affect the concentration of this dipeptide (Tinker et al. 1986). The avian skeletal muscle and liver do not appear to take up carnosine from the blood under either fed or starved conditions (Tinker et al. 1986). Interestingly, the kidneys of starved chickens take up a large amount of carnosine from the whole blood, although there is no renal uptake of this dipeptide under the fed condition (Tinker et al. 1986).

5.1.6.2 Anserine in Nonprimates

Anserine is abundant in the skeletal muscles of birds, certain fish [e.g., salmon, tuna, and trout (Boldyrev et al. 2013)], and beef (Wu et al. 2016), but is absent from human tissues (including skeletal muscle, heart, and brain) (Mannion et al. 1992). Among the animal kingdom, anserine is the major histidine-containing dipeptide in the skeletal muscles of the bird, dog, cat, lion, rabbit, agouti, mouse, kangaroo, wallaby, opossum, cod, smelt, marlin, whiting, croaker, tuna, Japanese char, salmon, and trout (Boldyrev et al. 2013). Intramuscular concentrations of anserine in these nonprimate species range from 2 mM for opossum to 21 mM for marlin. High concentrations of anserine in the mM range are also present in the skeletal muscles of cattle [e.g., 4.9, 5.5, and 6.8 mM in the chuck (serratus ventralis, rhomboideus, and splenius muscles), round (semimembranosus muscle), and loin (longissimus lumborum muscle) cuts of cattle, respectively (Wu et al. 2016)], as well as the brains of nonprimate animals. By contrast, the concentration of anserine in the plasma of nonprimate animals is exceedingly low, ranging from 2 to 10 µM, depending on species (Boldyrev et al. 2013).

Intramuscular and cardiac concentrations of anserine are affected by a number of factors, including muscle fiber type, muscular contractility, and health status. For example, white muscle fibers contain much more anserine than red muscle fibers, as the concentrations of anserine and carnosine were 2.2- and 2.8-fold higher, respectively, in breast versus thigh muscle (Barbaresi et al. 2019). In rat skeletal muscles (longissimus dorsi and quadriceps femoris), the concentrations of carnosine and anserine decrease by 35%–50% during senescence and are 35%–45% lower in hypertensive animals than in normotensive ones (Johnson and Hammer 1992). Similarly, in rat cardiac muscle, the concentrations of total histidine dipeptides decline by 22% during senescence and are 35% lower in hypertensive animals than in normotensive ones.

As noted previously, the whole blood of fed adult chickens also contains a large amount of anserine, and, as with carnosine, food deprivation for 6 days did not affect the concentration of this dipeptide (Tinker et al. 1986). Avian tissues (e.g., skeletal muscle, kidney, and liver) do not appear to take up anserine from the blood under either fed or starved conditions (Tinker et al. 1986).

5.1.6.3 Balenine

The concentrations of balenine (β-alanyl-L-3-methylhistidine, an antioxidant and a buffering substance) in skeletal muscle are particularly high in whale (~45 mmol/kg wet weight; ~65 mM), relatively low in swine (~0.7–1 mmol/kg wet weight; 1–1.43 mM; or 5%–8% of carnosine concentration), and very low in cattle, chickens, and sheep (~0.05–0.1 mmol/kg wet weight; 0.07–0.143 mM) (Boldyrev et al. 2013; Carnegie et al. 1982; Harris and Milne 1986). This dipeptide is barely detectable in human and rat muscles (Boldyrev et al. 2013).

5.2 SYNTHESIS AND DEGRADATION OF GSH

5.2.1 HISTORY OF GSH RESEARCH

GSH was discovered by J. de Rey-Paihade in 1888 from extracts of yeast, many different animal tissues (beef skeletal muscle and liver, fish skeletal muscle, lamb small intestine, and sheep brain), and fresh egg white. de Rey-Paihade named this substance "*philothion*" meaning love and sulfur in Greek. In 1921, F. Gowland Hopkins suggested that the *philothion* isolated from the liver, skeletal muscle, and yeast is a dipeptide consisting of cysteine and glutamate. However, these authors overlooked the presence of glycine in *philothion* possibly due to a misinterpretation of the Van Slyke amino nitrogen data. Honoring the history of the discovery of *philothion*, Hopkins named the substance "glutathione". Based on the content of nitrogen and sulfur in GSH isolated from yeast, the blood, and the liver, G. Hunter and B.A. Eagles indicated in 1927 that GSH is not a dipeptide containing Glu-Cys but is a tripeptide consisting of Glu-Cys and an additional low-molecular-weight AA (possibly serine). Using an acid hydrolysate of GSH, Hopkins proposed in 1929 that GSH is a tripeptide formed from cysteine, glutamate, and glycine. This proposal was supported by the independent work of E.C. Kendall and coworkers in 1929 and 1930. Based on the titration of GSH in water and formaldehyde as well as the observed pK_a values, N.W. Pirie and K.G. Pinhey reported in 1929 that the structure of GSH is γ-Glu-Cys-Gly and it is an acidic peptide. The structure of GSH was confirmed by C.R. Harington and T.H. Mead in 1935 through its chemical synthesis from N-carbobenzoxycystine and glycine ethyl ester. One year later, another chemical synthesis of GSH was performed by V. du Vigneaud and G.L. Miller using S-benzylcysteinylglycine methyl ester and the acid chloride of N-carbobenzoxyglutamate-α-methyl ester. Over the past half-century, GSH has been found in all cells. Related substances reported to date include γ-Glu-Cys-Gly-spermidine in *E. coli* and (γ-Glu-Cys)$_n$-Gly in plants.

5.2.2 CONCENTRATIONS OF GSH IN PHYSIOLOGICAL FLUIDS AND TISSUES OF HUMANS AND OTHER ANIMALS

GSH is the predominant low-molecular-weight thiol in animal cells, ranging from 0.5 to 10 mM. Most of the cellular GSH (85–90%) is present in the cytosol, with the remainder in many organelles (including the mitochondria, nuclear matrix, and peroxisomes; Wu et al. 2004). With the exception of bile acids, which may contain up to 10 mM GSH, extracellular concentrations of GSH are relatively low (e.g., 2–20 µM in the plasma). Because of the cysteine residue, GSH is readily oxidized nonenzymatically to glutathione disulfide (GSSG) by electrophilic substances (e.g., free radicals and reactive oxygen/nitrogen species; Sies 1999). GSSG efflux from cells contributes to a net loss of intracellular GSH. Cellular GSH concentrations are reduced markedly in response to protein malnutrition, oxidative stress, and many pathological conditions. Like other sulfur-containing AA metabolites, GSH plus 2 GSSG represents total glutathione in cells, a significant amount of which, up to 15%, may be bound to protein. The ratio of [GSH] to [GSSG], which is often used as an indicator of the cellular redox state, is >10 under normal physiological conditions (Sies 1999). GSH/GSSG is the major redox couple that determines the antioxidative capacity of cells, but its value can be affected by other redox couples, including NADPH/NADP$^+$ and thioredoxin$_{red}$/thioredoxin$_{ox}$.

$$2 \text{ Glutathione (reduced, GSH)} + \tfrac{1}{2}O_2 \rightarrow \text{Glutathione (oxidized, GS-SG)} + H_2O$$

5.2.3   GSH SYNTHESIS

GSH is synthesized from cysteine, glutamate, and glycine sequentially by two cytosolic enzymes, γ-glutamylcysteine synthetase and GSH synthetase (Figure 5.3). Virtually all cell types can synthesize GSH, with the liver being the major producer and exporter of this tripeptide (Lu 2013). In the γ-glutamylcysteine synthetase reaction, the γ-carboxyl group of glutamate reacts with the amino group of cysteine to form a peptidic γ-linkage, which protects GSH from hydrolysis by intracellular peptidases. Although γ-glutamyl-cysteine can be a substrate for γ-glutamylcyclotransferase, GSH synthesis is favored in animal cells because of the much higher affinity and activity of GSH synthetase. Mammalian γ-glutamylcysteine synthetase is a heterodimer consisting of a catalytically active heavy subunit (73 kDa) and a light (regulatory) subunit (31 kDa). The heavy subunit contains all the substrate-binding sites, whereas the light subunit modulates the affinity of the heavy subunit for substrates and inhibitors. The K_M values of mammalian γ-glutamylcysteine synthetase for glutamate and cysteine are 1.7 and 0.15 mM, respectively, which are similar to intracellular concentrations of glutamate (2–4 mM) and cysteine (0.15–0.25 mM) in the rat liver (Griffith 1999). Mammalian GSH synthetase is a homodimer (52 kDa/subunit) and is an allosteric enzyme with cooperative binding for its γ-glutamyl substrate. The K_M values of mammalian GSH synthetase for ATP and glycine are ~0.04 and 0.9 mM, respectively, which are lower than intracellular concentrations of ATP (2–4 mM) and glycine (1.5–2 mM) in the liver of healthy rats. Thus, GSH synthetase is saturated with its substrates (ATP and glycine) in animal cells under normal physiological conditions.

5.2.4   REGULATION OF GSH SYNTHESIS

Both biochemical and metabolic studies have established that γ-glutamylcysteine synthetase is the rate-controlling enzyme in the *de novo* synthesis of GSH (Lu 2013). Among the substrates, cysteine is a major limiting AA for GSH synthesis. Cysteine is readily oxidized to cystine in oxygenated extracellular solutions. Thus, cysteine concentrations in the plasma are low (10–25 μM), compared with cystine (50–150 μM). Cysteine and cystine are transported by distinct membrane carriers, and cells typically transport one more efficiently than the other. Interestingly, some cell types (e.g., hepatocytes) have little or no capacity for direct transport of extracellular cystine. However, the GSH that effluxes from the liver can reduce cystine to cysteine on the outer cell membrane, and the resulting cysteine is taken up by hepatocytes (Griffith 1999). Other cell types (e.g., endothelial cells) can take up cystine and reduce it intracellularly to cysteine because cellular reducing conditions normally favor the presence of cysteine. Compelling evidence shows that increasing the provision of cysteine or its precursors (e.g., cystine, *N*-acetylcysteine, L-2-oxothiazolidine-4-carboxylate) via oral or intravenous administration enhances GSH synthesis and prevents GSH deficiency in humans and other animals under various nutritional and pathological conditions, including protein malnutrition, adult respiratory distress syndrome, HIV, and AIDS. Dietary methionine can also replace cysteine to support GSH synthesis in individuals with a functional liver (Wu et al. 2004).

Extracellular and intracellularly generated glutamate can be used for GSH synthesis. Besides its function as a substrate for γ-glutamylcysteine synthetase, glutamate plays a regulatory role in

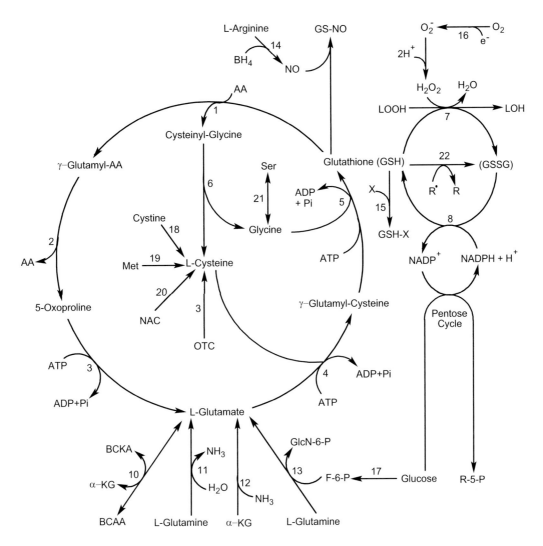

FIGURE 5.3 Glutathione synthesis and utilization in humans and other animals. The enzymes that catalyze the indicated reactions are (1) γ-glutamyl transpeptidase; (2) γ-glutamyl cyclotransferase; (3) 5-oxoprolinase; (4) γ-glutamyl-cysteine synthetase; (5) glutathione synthetase; (6) dipeptidase; (7) glutathione peroxidase; (8) glutathione reductase; (9) superoxide dismutase; (10) branched-chain amino acid transaminase (cytosolic and mitochondrial); (11) glutaminase; (12) glutamate dehydrogenase; (13) glutamine:fructose-6-phosphate transaminase (cytosolic); (14) nitric oxide synthase; (15) glutathione *S*-transferase; (16) NADPH oxidase and mitochondrial respiratory complexes; (17) glycolysis; (18) glutathione-dependent thiol-disulfide or thioltransferase; (19) transsulfuration pathway; (20) deacylase (cytosolic); (21) serine hydroxymethyltransferase (cytosolic and mitochondrial); and (22) nonenzymatic reaction. AA, amino acid; BCAA, branched-chain amino acid (primarily providing an amino group for glutamate synthesis); BCKA, branched-chain α-ketoacid; BH4, (6*R*)-5,6,7,8-tetrahydro-L-biopterin; GlcN-6-P, glucosamine-6-phosphate; GS-NO, glutathione-NO adduct; GSSG, glutathione disulfide; KG, α-ketoglutarate; LOO•, lipid peroxyl radical; LOOH, lipid hydroperoxide; NAC, N-acetylcysteine; OTC, L-2-oxothiazolidine-4-carboxylate; R•, radicals; R, nonradicals; R-5-P, ribulose-5-phosphate; and X, electrophilic xenobiotics.

GSH synthesis through two mechanisms: (1) uptake of cystine and (2) prevention of GSH inhibition of γ-glutamylcysteine synthetase (Lu 2013). Glutamate and cystine share the System X_c^- AA transporter. When extracellular glutamate concentrations are high, as in patients with advanced cancer, HIV infection, and spinal cord or brain injury as well as in cultured cells (e.g., endothelial cells), cystine uptake is competitively inhibited by glutamate, resulting in reduced GSH synthesis. GSH is a nonallosteric feedback inhibitor of γ-glutamylcysteine synthetase, but glutamate competes with GSH for the binding to the enzyme. Thus, when intracellular glutamate concentrations are unusually high, as in canine erythrocytes, GSH synthesis is enhanced and its concentration is particularly high (Griffith 1999). Interestingly, rat erythrocytes do not take up or release glutamate. Glutamine, leucine, valine, and isoleucine are the precursors of glutamate in these cells. Also, as noted in Chapter 4, the branched-chain AAs donate their amino group for glutamate synthesis. Therefore, glutamine is an effective precursor of glutamate for GSH synthesis in many cell types, including enterocytes, neural cells, hepatocytes, and lymphocytes. Thus, supplementing glutamine to patients receiving total parenteral nutrition maintains tissue GSH concentrations and improves survival after reperfusion injury, ischemia, acetaminophen toxicity, chemotherapy, inflammatory stress, and bone marrow transplantation (Gould and Pazdro 2019). Similarly, dietary supplementation with glutamate or glutamine increases GSH concentration in the small-intestinal mucosae of neonates.

Glycine may become a limiting AA for GSH synthesis under conditions such as protein malnutrition, sepsis, inflammatory stimuli, weaning, obesity, and diabetes (Fan et al. 2019; McCarty et al. 2018). For example, glycine availability limits erythrocyte GSH synthesis in burn patients (Yu et al. 2002) and in children recovering from severe malnutrition (Persaud et al. 1996). Also, dietary glycine supplementation increases hepatic GSH concentration in protein-deficient rats challenged with tumor necrosis factor-α (Grimble et al. 1992). At present, it is not known how concentrations of glycine are reduced in the plasma of obese animals, but the underlying mechanisms may include a reduction in glycine synthesis and an increase in glycine catabolism. A deficiency of this AA may contribute to oxidative stress in these individuals.

5.2.5 Transport and Degradation of GSH

GSH can be transported out of the cell. In the plasma, most GSH originates primarily from the liver, but some dietary GSH can enter the portal circulation. GSH is transported out of the sinusoidal and canalicular membranes of the liver via a carrier-dependent facilitative mechanism. GSH molecules exit the liver either intact or as γ-Glu-(Cys)$_2$ due to γ-glutamyl transpeptidase activity on the outer plasma membrane (Figure 5.4). Because of the rapid degradation of GSH by γ-glutamyl transpeptidase (Meister 1973), the concentrations of GSH plus GSSG in the plasma are usually very low, ranging from 5 to 50 μM, depending on the animal species, physiological state, and sampling sites. This is in striking contrast to intracellular concentrations of GSH ranging from 0.5 to 10 mM in animal tissues. Such an extremely high concentration gradient across the plasma membrane makes the transport of extracellular GSH or GSSG into the cell thermodynamically unfavorable. However, γ-Glu-(Cys)$_2$ and Cys-Gly, which are derived from GSH and (Cys)$_2$, are readily taken up by extrahepatic cells and tissues, including the kidneys, brain, heart, skeletal muscle, and adipose tissue (Griffith 1999). In these cells, γ-Glu-(Cys)$_2$ and Cys-Gly are utilized for GSH synthesis (Figure 5.3). Thus, the interorgan metabolism of GSH serves to transport cysteine in a nontoxic form between tissues and also helps maintain intracellular concentrations of GSH and the cellular redox state.

5.3 PRODUCTION OF GLY-PRO-4-HYDROXYPROLINE

5.3.1 Abundance of Gly-Pro-4-Hydroxyproline in the Milk and Plasma

Results of recent studies identify the presence of the neutral tripeptide Gly-Pro-4-hydroxyproline (a tripeptide) in physiological fluids (e.g., the plasma and milk; Wu et al. 2019). Collagen proteins in connective tissue turn over in animals to release its repeat constituent, glycine-proline-hydroxyproline. The rate of collagen degradation is greater in neonates than in adults. Studies with young pigs (7- to 21-day-old) indicate that concentrations of this tripeptide in the plasma range from 6 to 10 mM.

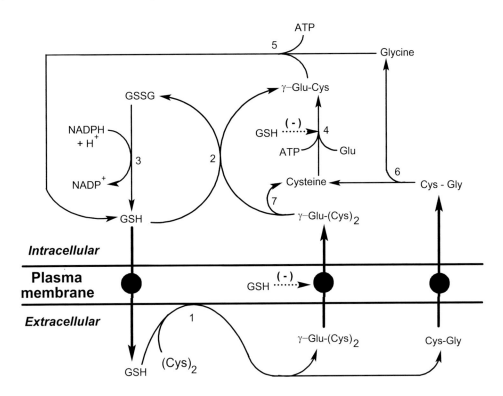

FIGURE 5.4 Transport and catabolism of glutathione in humans and other animals. Transport of glutathione occurs in most cell types. The liver is the major site for glutathione synthesis in the body. Glutathione is transported out of the hepatocyte by a specific transporter for utilization in extrahepatic tissues. Glutathione is the major vehicle for interorgan transport of cysteine in a nontoxic form. The enzymes that catalyze the indicated reactions are (1) γ-glutamyl transpeptidase; (2) transhydrogenase; (3) glutathione disulfide reductase; (4) γ-glutamyl-cysteine synthetase; (5) glutathione synthetase; and (6) dipeptidase. GSH is an inhibitor of γ-Glu-(Cys)$_2$ transport and γ-glutamyl-cysteine synthetase. Cys, cysteine; (Cys)$_2$, cystine (Cys-Cys); GSH, reduced glutathione; and GSSG, glutathione disulfide (oxidized glutathione).

Sow's milk also contains relatively high concentrations of the peptide (in the range of 2–3 mM). Based on a kilogram of body weight (BW), larger amounts of glycine-proline-4-hydroxyproline are produced from collagen degradation in the connective tissue (e.g., the bone, joints, and skin) of young animals compared with older ones.

5.3.2 Utilization of Gly-Pro-4-Hydroxyproline by Animals

The utilization of Gly-Pro-4-hydroxyproline requires interorgan cooperation in the body. The small peptide is readily transported from the lumen of the small intestine into enterocytes via PepT-1. Some of this tripeptide is hydrolyzed by peptidases inside the enterocytes, and the remaining tripeptide enters the systemic blood circulation. Besides glycine and proline, which are utilized in multiple pathways (Chapter 4), 4-hydroxyproline (a posttranslational product of proline) may be a precursor for glycine generation in the kidneys via 4-hydroxyproline oxidase (Chapter 3). The quantitative contribution of this pathway to endogenous glycine provision in all animal species is unknown but is substantial in both humans and pigs (Chapter 4). It is likely that the synthesis of glycine from 4-hydroxyproline will compensate, in part, for the severe glycine deficiency in milk and also allow the efficient utilization of proline by piglets and possibly the newborns of other animal species (including humans). Thus, Gly-Pro-4-hydroxyproline may play an important role in the

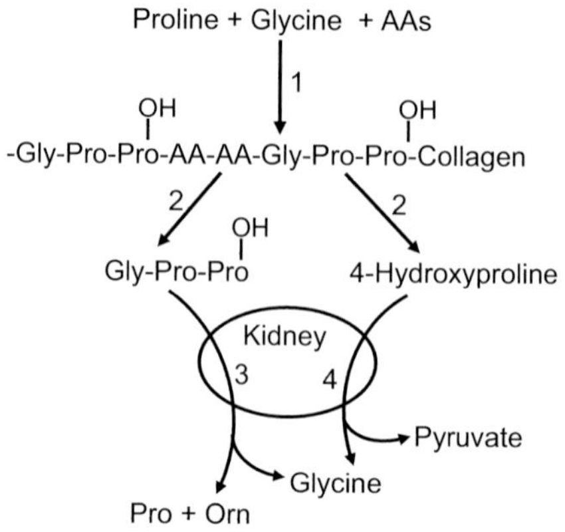

Proline + Glycine + AAs

|
1
↓

OH   OH
| |
-Gly-Pro-Pro-AA-AA-Gly-Pro-Pro-Collagen

2 ╱   ╲ 2
OH
|
Gly-Pro-Pro   4-Hydroxyproline

Kidney
3   4

→ Pyruvate

→ Glycine

Pro + Orn

FIGURE 5.5 Metabolism of Gly-Pro-4-hydroxyproline in humans and other animals. Most tissues, including the skeletal muscle, heart, kidney, liver, and small intestine, can degrade this tripeptide. Through protein synthesis, proline is incorporated into collagen proteins in the connective tissue (Step 1). Degradation of collagen by collagenase in animals results in the release of relatively large amounts of 4-hydroxy-proline and the tripeptide Gly-Pro-4-hydroxyproline (Step 2). The kidneys take up both 4-hydroxy-proline and Gly-Pro-4-hydroxyproline from the circulation where the tripeptide is hydrolyzed into free 4-hydroxyproline by peptidases (Steps 3 and 4). In the kidneys, as in other tissues, a dipeptide containing proline or 4-hydroxy-proline is hydrolyzed by a special dipeptidase, prolidase. 4-Hydroxyproline is converted to glycine in the kidneys via a series of reactions involving 4-hydroxyproline oxidase. Proline oxidase oxidizes proline to form pyrroline-5-carboxylate, which reacts with glutamate to generate ornithine by ornithine aminotransferase. AAs, amino acids; Orn, ornithine; and Pro, proline.

interorgan metabolism of glycine and proline (Figure 5.5). Because arginine, glutamine, and glutamate are substrates for the formation of proline in most mammals (Chapter 4), these AAs can indirectly contribute to glycine synthesis through the posttranslational generation of 4-hydroxyproline in collagens. Much work on the physiology and nutrition of this tripeptide remains to be done.

5.4 ENDOGENOUS AND FOOD-DERIVED OLIGOPEPTIDES CONSISTING OF 3–20 OR MORE AA RESIDUES

5.4.1 ENDOGENOUS SYNTHESIS OF OPIOID PEPTIDES IN HUMANS AND OTHER ANIMALS

Endogenous opioid peptides are small molecules produced from the degradation of precursor proteins by the central nervous system (e.g., neurons) and various glands (e.g., pituitary and adrenal glands) in the body. They are oligopeptides usually consisting of 3–20 AA residues, but some peptides may contain more than 20 AA residues. Since the first report of John Hughes and Hans Kosterlitz in 1975 that enkephalins were present as endogenous opioid peptides in brain extracts and could inhibit the release of acetylcholine from nerves in the guinea pig ileum, more than 20 opioid peptides have been identified to date. They include many classes: enkephalins, endorphins, dynorphins, nociceptin, and endomorphins, with members in each class sharing similar AA sequences (Stein 2016). Examples of endogenous opioid peptides in humans and other animals are shown in Table 5.3.

Endogenous opioid peptides bind to specific receptors on the plasma membranes of their target cells. These receptors (μ, δ, and κ) differ in their functions, binding characteristics, and tissue distribution [e.g., the receptor μ mainly in the central nervous system, the receptor δ in both the central nervous system and spinal cord, and the receptor κ primarily in the spinal cord] (Stein 2016). An opioid peptide can interact with more than one type of opioid receptor. For example, enkephalins bind to and activate opioid receptors μ and δ. Upon binding to an opioid receptor, the opioid receptor

TABLE 5.3

Endogenous Opioid Peptides in Humans and Other Animals

Endogenous Opioid Peptides	Amino Acid Sequence
(1) Enkephalins	
Leu-enkephalin	Tyr-Gly-Gly-Phe-Leu
Met-enkephalin	Tyr-Gly-Gly-Phe-Met
Metorphamide[a]	Tyr-Gly-Gly-Phe-Met-Arg-Arg-Val-NH$_2$
(2) Endorphins	
α-Endorphin	Tyr-Gly-Gly-Phe-Met-Thr-Ser-Glu-Lys-Ser-Gln-Thr-Pro-Leu-Val-Thr
β-Endorphin	[α-Endorphin]-Leu-Phe-Lys-Asn-Ala-Ile-Ile-Lys-Asn-Ala-Tyr-Lys-Lys-Gly-Glu
γ-Endorphin	[α-Endorphin]-Leu
(3) Dynorphins	
Dynorphin A	Tyr-Gly-Gly-Phe-Leu-Arg-Arg-Ile-Arg-Pro-Lys-Leu-Lys-Trp-Asp-Asn-Gln
Dynorphin A (1–8)	Tyr-Gly-Gly-Phe-Leu-Arg-Arg-Ile
Dynorphin B	Tyr-Gly-Gly-Phe-Leu-Arg-Arg-Gln-Phe-Lys-Val-Val-Thr
Big dynorphin	[Dynorphin A]-Lys-Arg-Tyr-Gly-Gly-Phe-Leu-Arg-Arg-Gln-Phe-Lys-Val-Val-Thr
α-Neoendorphin	Tyr-Gly-Gly-Phe-Leu-Arg-Lys-Tyr-Pro-Lys
β-Neoendorphin	Tyr-Gly-Gly-Phe-Leu-Arg-Lys-Tyr-Pro
(4) Endomorphins	
Endomorphin-1	Tyr-Pro-Trp-Phe-NH$_2$
Endomorphin-2	Tyr-Pro-Phe-Phe-NH$_2$

[a] Produced from the proteolytic cleavage of proenkephalin A.

couples to (1) G proteins, causing the dissociation of the Gα and Gβγ subunits, the direct interaction of the Gα subunit with inwardly rectifying K$^+$ channels (resulting in cell membrane hyperpolarization), an inhibition of adenylyl cyclase by the Gα subunit, a decrease in the conductance of voltage-gated Ca^{2+} channels, and a reduction in the cAMP-dependent Ca^{2+} influx (Childers 1991); and (2) other cell signaling systems, such as the mitogen-activated protein kinases and the phospholipase C-mediated cascade, resulting in their activation and the formation of inositol-1,4,5-triphosphate and diacylglycerol (Akil et al. 1997). The opioid peptides elicit the same effects as the classic alkaloid opiates (e.g., morphine and heroin), including analgesia and euphoria. For example, enkephalins and endomorphins are natural opioid neurotransmitters that contribute to pain relief and a sense of well-being (Bodnar 2018). Thus, the endogenous opioid peptides act as both hormones and neuromodulators.

5.4.2 Bioactive Peptides in Protein Hydrolysates for Improving Human Nutrition and Health

Enzymatic hydrolysis and microbial fermentation of food proteins are the two common methods for the industrial production of protein hydrolysates (containing bioactive peptides) for human consumption (Barati et al. 2020; Chakrabarti et al. 2018). The sources of animal, plant, and microbial food proteins include (1) eggs, milk (casein and whey), cheese, pork, poultry, and beef; (2) rice, corn, soy and soy products, oat, pulses (chickpea, beans, peas, and lentils), canola, wheat, flaxseed, hemp seed, and broccoli; (3) fish, squid, salmon, sea urchin, oyster, seahorse, and snow crabs; and (4) microalgae (*Chlorella vulgaris*), and fungi (*Fusarium venenatum*), mushroom, and Brewer's yeast. The food-grade products consist of many bioactive peptides, which can be defined as the fragments of AA sequences in a protein that confer biological functions beyond their nutritional value. Furthermore, the gastrointestinal tract of humans produces some bioactive peptides from ingested proteins (Table 5.4–5.7). For example, β-casomorphins (opioid peptides) and soymorphin (opioid peptides) are released during the gastrointestinal digestion of the β-casein of milk and soybean proteins, respectively.

Most of the cell-free enzymes for producing protein hydrolysates are obtained from animal, plant, and microbial sources. Enzymes of animal sources (particularly pigs) for protein hydrolysis are pancreatin, trypsin, pepsin, carboxylpeptidases, and aminopeptidases; enzymes of plant sources are papain and bromelain; and enzymes of bacterial and fungal sources are many kinds of proteases with a broad spectrum of optimal temperatures, pH, and ion concentrations. The enzymes from commercial sources may be purified, semipurified, or crude from the biological sources. The hydrolysis of proteins can be achieved by a single enzyme (e.g., trypsin) or multiple enzymes (e.g., a mixture of proteases known as Pronase, pepsin, and prolidase). The choice of enzymes depends on the protein source and the degree of hydrolysis. For example, if the protein has a high content of hydrophobic AAs, the enzyme of choice would be the one that preferentially breaks down the peptide bonds formed from these AAs. Fractionation of protein hydrolysates is often performed to isolate specific peptides or remove undesired peptides. Compared to acid and alkaline hydrolysis of proteins, the main advantages of enzyme hydrolysis of proteins include that (1) the hydrolysis conditions (e.g., like temperature and pH) are mild and do not result in any loss of AAs; (2) proteases are more specific and precise to control the degree of peptide-bond hydrolysis; and (3) the small amounts of enzymes can be easily deactivated after the hydrolysis (e.g., 85°C for 3 min) to facilitate the isolation of the protein hydrolysates.

TABLE 5.4
Opioid Peptides Generated from the Enzymatic Hydrolysis of Animal and Plant Proteins in the Gastrointestinal Tract

Source	Name of Opioid Peptide	Amino Acid Sequence
Milk casein	Bovine β-casomorphin 1-3	Tyr-Pro-Phe-OH
	Bovine β-casomorphin 1-4	Tyr-Pro-Phe-Pro-OH
	Bovine β-casomorphin 1-4, amide	Tyr-Pro-Phe-Pro-NH$_2$
	Bovine β-casomorphin 5	Tyr-Pro-Phe-Pro-Gly-OH
	Bovine β-casomorphin 7	Tyr-Pro-Phe-Pro-Gly-Pro-Ile-OH
	Bovine β-casomorphin 8	Tyr-Pro-Phe-Pro-Gly-Pro-Ile-Pro-OH[a]
Gluten protein	Gluten exorphin A5	Gly-Tyr-Tyr-Pro-Thr-OH
	Gluten exorphin B4	Tyr-Gly-Gly-Trp-OH
	Gluten exorphin C	Tyr-Pro-Ile-Ser-Leu-OH
	Gliadorphin	Tyr-Pro-Gln-Pro-Gln-Pro-Phe-OH
Soybean protein	Soymorphin-5[b]	Tyr-Pro-Phe-Val-Val-OH
	Soymorphin-5, amide	Tyr-Pro-Phe-Val-Val-NH2
	Soymorphin-6	Tyr-Pro-Phe-Val-Val-Asn-OH
	Soymorphin-7	Tyr-Pro-Phe-Val-Val-Asn-Ala-OH
Spinach protein	Rubiscolin-5	Gly-Tyr-Tyr-Pro-OH
	Rubiscolin-6	Gly-Tyr-Tyr-Pro-Thr-OH

Source: Hou, Y.Q. et al. 2017. *J. Anim. Sci. Biotechnol.* 8:24.

[a] Another form of bovine β-casomorphin 8 has histidine instead of proline in position 8, depending on whether the peptide is derived from A1 or A2 beta-casein.

[b] Derived from β-conglycinin β-subunit

TABLE 5.5

Antihypertensive Peptides Generated from the Hydrolysis of Animal Products

Source	Protease(s)	Amino Acid Sequence	IC$_{50}$ (μM)[a]
Pig muscle myosin	Thermolysin	Ile-Thr-Thr-Asn-Pro	549
Pig muscle myosin	Pepsin	Lys-Arg-Val-Ile-Thr-Tyr	6.1
Pig muscle actin	Pepsin	Val-Lys-Arg-Gly-Phe	20.3
Pig muscle troponin	Pepsin	Lys-Arg-Gln-Lys-Tyr-Asp-Ile	26.2
Pig muscle	Pepsin+Pancreatin	Lys-Leu-Pro	500
Pig muscle	Pepsin+Pancreatin	Arg-Pro-Arg	382
Chicken muscle	Thermolysin	Leu-Ala-Pro	3.2
Chicken muscle myosin	Thermolysin	Phe-Gln-Lys-Pro-Lys-Arg	14
Chicken muscle	Thermolysin	Ile-Lys-Trp	0.21
Chicken collagen	*Aspergillus* proteases+Proteases FP, A, G, and N	Gly-Ala-X-Gly-Leu-X-Gly-Pro	29.4
Cow muscle	Thermolysin+Proteinase A	Val-Leu-Ala-Gln-Tyr-Lys	32.1
Cow muscle	Thermolysin+Proteinase A	Phe-His-Gly	52.9
Cow muscle	Proteinase K	Gly-Phe-His-Ile	64.3
Cow skin gelatin	Alcalase+Pronase E+Collagenase	Gly-Pro-Val	4.67
Cow skin gelatin	Alcalase+Pronase E+Collagenase	Gly-Pro-Leu	2.55
Bonito (fish) muscle	Thermolysin	Leu-Lys-Pro-Asn-Met	2.4
Bonito (fish) muscle	Thermolysin	Leu-Lys-Pro	0.32
Bonito (fish) muscle	Thermolysin	Ile-Lys-Pro	6.9
Salmon muscle	Thermolysin	Val-Trp	2.5
Salmon muscle	Thermolysin	Met-Trp	9.9
Salmon muscle	Thermolysin	Ile-Trp	4.7
Sardine muscle	Alcalase	Ile-Tyr	10.5
Sardine muscle	Alcalase	Ala-Lys-Lys	3.13
Sardine muscle	Alcalase	Gly-Trp-Ala-Pro	3.86
Sardine muscle	Alcalase	Lys-Tyr	1.63
Alaska pollack skin	Alcalase+Pronase+Collagenase	Gly-Pro-Leu	2.65
Alaska pollack skin	Alcalase+Pronase+Collagenase	Gly-Pro-Met	17.1
Shark muscle	Protease SM98011	Glu-Tyr	1.98
Shark muscle	Protease SM98012	Phe-Glu	2.68
Shark muscle	Protease SM98013	Cys-Phe	1.45
Egg yolk	Pepsin	Tyr-Ile-Glu-Ala-Val-Asn-Lys-Val-Ser-Pro-Arg-Ala-Gly-Gln-Phe	9.4[b]
Egg yolk	Pepsin	Tyr-Ile-Asn-Gln-Met-Pro-Gln-Lys-Ser-Arg-Glu	10.1[b]

Source: Hou, Y.Q. et al. 2017. *J. Anim. Sci. Biotechnol.* 8:24.

"X" = hydroxyproline.

[a] Inhibition of angiotensin I-converting enzyme (ACE) activity. All values are expressed as μM, except for egg yolk-derived peptides (μg/mL) as indicated by a superscript "b".

Microorganisms release proteases to hydrolyze extracellular proteins into large peptides, small peptides, and free AAs. Small peptides can be taken up by the microbes to undergo intracellular hydrolysis, yielding free AAs. Microorganisms also produce enzymes other than proteases to degrade complex carbohydrates and lipids. Microbial protein fermentation is classified into a liquid- or solid-state type. Liquid-state fermentation is performed with protein substrates under high-moisture fermentation conditions, whereas the solid-state fermentation is carried out under

TABLE 5.6

Antioxidative Peptides Generated from the Hydrolysis of Animal Proteins

Source	Protease(s)	Amino Acid Sequence
Pig muscle actin	Papain+Actinase E	Asp-Ser-Gly-Val-Thr
Pig muscle	Papain+Actinase E	Ile-Glu-Ala-Glu-Gly-Glu
Pig muscle tropomyosin	Papain+Actinase E	Asp-Ala-Gln-Glu-Lys-Leu-Glu
Pig muscle tropomyosin	Papain+Actinase E	Glu-Glu-Leu-Asp-Asn-Ala-Leu-Asn
Pig muscle myosin	Papain+Actinase E	Val-Pro-Ser-Ile-Asp-Asp-Gln-Glu-Glu-Leu-Met
Pig collagen	Pepsin+Papain+others[a]	Gln-Gly-Ala-Arg
Pig blood plasma	Alcalase	His-Asn-Gly-Asn
Chicken muscle	---	His-Val-Thr-Glu-Glu
Chicken muscle	---	Pro-Val-Pro-Val-Glu-Gly-Val
Deer muscle	Papain	Met-Gln-Ile-Phe-Val-Lys-Thr-Leu-Thr-Gly
Deer muscle	Papain	Asp-Leu-Ser-Asp-Gly-Glu-Gln-Gly-Val-Leu
Bovine milk casein	Pepsin, pH 2, 24 h	Tyr-Phe-Tyr-Pro-Glu-Leu
Bovine milk casein	Pepsin, pH 2, 24 h	Phe-Tyr-Pro-Glu-Leu
Bovine milk casein	Pepsin, pH 2, 24 h	Tyr-Pro-Glu-Leu
Bovine milk casein	Pepsin, pH 2, 24 h	Pro-Glu-Leu
Bovine milk casein	Pepsin, pH 2, 24 h	Glu-Leu
Bovine milk casein	Trypsin, pH 7.8, 24–28 h	Val-Lys-Glu-Ala-Met-Pro-Lys
Bovine milk casein	Trypsin, pH 7.8, 24–28 h	Ala-Val-Pro-Tyr-Pro-Gln-Arg
Bovine milk casein	Trypsin, pH 7.8, 24–28 h	Lys-Val-Leu-Pro-Val-Pro-Glu-Lys
Bovine milk casein	Trypsin, pH 7.8, 24–28 h	Val-Leu-Pro-Val-Pro-Glu-Lys
Bovine whey protein	Thermolysin, 80°C, 8 h	Leu-Gln-Lys-Trp
Bovine whey protein	Thermolysin, 80°C, 8 h	Leu-Asp-Thr-Asp-Tyr-Lys-Lys
Bovine β-lactoglobulin	Corolase PP, 37°C, 24 h	Trp-Tyr-Ser-Leu-Ala-Met-Ala-Ala-Ser-Asp-Ile
Bovine β-lactoglobulin	Corolase PP, 37°C, 24 h	Met-His-Ile-Arg-Leu
Bovine β-lactoglobulin	Corolase PP, 37°C, 24 h	Try-Val-Glu-Glu-Leu
Egg yolk	Pepsin	Tyr-Ile-Glu-Ala-Val-Asn-Lys-Val-Ser-Pro-Arg-Ala-Gly-Gln-Phe
Egg yolk	Pepsin	Tyr-Ile-Asn-Gln-Met-Pro-Gln-Lys-Ser-Arg-Glu

Source: Hou, Y.Q. et al. 2017. *J. Anim. Sci. Biotechnol.* 8:24.

[a] Bovine pancreatic proteases plus bacterial proteases from *Streptomyces bacillus*.

low-moisture fermentation conditions. The low moisture level of the solid-state fermentation can help to reduce the drying time for protein hydrolysates. Soy sauce (also called soya sauce), which originated in China in the 2nd century AD, was perhaps the earliest product of protein fermentation by microorganisms. The raw materials were boiled soybeans, roasted grain, brine, and *Aspergillus oryzae* or *Aspergillus sojae* (a genus of fungus). In Koji culturing, an equal amount of boiled soybeans and roasted wheat is cultured with Aspergillus oryzae, A. sojae, and A. tamari; Saccharomyces cerevisiae (yeasts), and bacteria, such as *Bacillus* and *Lactobacillus* species. Over the past two decades, various microorganisms have been used to hydrolyze plant-source proteins, such as *Lactobacillus rhamnosus* BGT10 and *Lactobacillus zeae* LMG17315 for pea proteins, *Bacillus natto* or *B. subtilis* for soybean, and fungi *A. oryzae* or *R. oryzae* for soybean. Lactic acid bacteria, such as *Lactobacillus* and *Lactococcus* species, are commonly used to ferment milk products. The major advantages of fermentation are that the appropriately used microorganisms can not only break down proteins into peptides and free AAs, but can also remove hyperallergic or antinutritional factors present in the matrix of the ingredients (e.g., trypsin inhibitors, glycinin, β-conglycinin, phytate, oligosaccharides raffinose and stachyose, saponins in soybeans).

TABLE 5.7

Antimicrobial Peptides Generated from the Hydrolysis of Animal Proteins or Synthesized by Intestinal Mucosal Cells

Source	Amino Acid Sequence	Gram-Positive Bacteria	Gram-Negative Bacteria
Bovine meat	Gly-Leu-Ser-Asp-Gly-Glu-Trp-Gln	*Bacillus cereus*	*Salmonella typhimurium*
		Listeria monocytogenes	*Escherichia coli*
	Gly-Phe-His-Ile	No effect	*Pseudomonas aeruginosa*
	Phe-His-Gly	No effect	*Pseudomonas aeruginosa*
Bovine collagen	Peptides <2 kDa (by collagenase)[a]	*Staphylococcus aureus*	*Escherichia coli*
Goat whey	GWH (730 Da) and SEC-F3 (1,183 Da) (hydrolysis by Alcalase)	*Bacillus cereus*	*Salmonella typhimurium*
		Staphylococcus aureus	*Escherichia coli*
Red blood cells	Various peptides (24-h hydrolysis by fungal proteases)	*Staphylococcus aureus*	*Escherichia coli*
			Pseudomonas aeruginosa
Hen egg white lysozyme	Asn-Thr-Asp-Gly-Ser-Thr-Asp-Tyr-Gly-Ile-Leu-Gln-Ile-Asn-Ser-Arg (hydrolysis by papain and trypsin)[b]	*Leuconostoc mesenteroides*	*Escherichia coli*
Trout by-products	Various peptides (20%–30% of hydrolysis) (hydrolysis by trout pepsin)	*Renibacterium salmoninarum*	*Flavobacterium psychrophilum*
Small intestine (Paneth cells)	α-Defensins, lysozyme C, angiogenin-4, and cryptdin-related sequence peptides	Gram-positive bacteria (broad-spectrum)	Gram-negative bacteria (broad-spectrum)
	Phospholipid-*sn*-2 esterase and C-type lectin	Gram-positive bacteria (broad-spectrum)	No effect

Source: Hou, Y.Q. et al. 2017. *J. Anim. Sci. Biotechnol.* 8:24.

Note: GWH = goat whey hydrolysates; SEC-F3 = size exclusion chromatography fraction 3

[a] minimal inhibition concentrations = 0.6–5 mg/mL.

[b] minimal inhibition concentrations = 0.36–0.44 μg/mL.

There is much evidence that the consumption of bioactive peptides in foods improves the functions of the digestive, cardiovascular, immune, nervous, skeletal, and muscular systems in humans (Barati et al. 2020; Chakrabarti et al. 2018; Moughan et al. 2007; Power et al. 2013). Examples include (1) an inhibition of angiotensin-converting enzyme and the amelioration of hypertension; (2) the improvement of insulin secretion and sensitivity, as well as metabolic profiles; (3) the alleviation of stress, pain, and sleeping disorders; (4) the stimulation of appetite in children and elderly persons to increase nutrient intakes; (5) antimicrobial, immunomodulatory, anti-inflammatory responses; (6) enhancements in gastrointestinal motility, digestibility, absorptive capacity, mucin production, and intestinal mucosal barrier; (7) reductions of inflammations and abnormalities in bones; and (8) the promotion of wound healing and recovery from injuries in animals. These beneficial effects result from direct and indirect effects of functional peptides.

5.4.3 Bioactive Peptides in Protein Hydrolysates for Improving Animal Nutrition and Health

In animal nutrition, high-quality protein is not hydrolyzed as feed additives. Only animal by-products, brewer's by-products, and plant ingredients containing antinutritional factors are hydrolyzed to produce peptides for animal feeds (Etemadian et al. 2021; Hou et al. 2017). The method of choice for the hydrolysis of proteins depends on their sources. For example, proteins from feathers, bristles, horns, beaks, or wool contain the keratin structure and, therefore, are usually hydrolyzed by acidic or alkaline treatment, or by bacterial keratinases. By contrast, animal products (e.g., casein, whey, intestine, and meat) and plant ingredients (e.g., soy, wheat, rice, pea, and cottonseed proteins) are often subject to general enzymatic or microbial hydrolysis, as described previously.

Peptides generated by the chemical, enzymatic, or microbial hydrolysis of proteins in the feed industry play important roles in animal nutrition (Table 5.3–5.6). These products not only provide balanced AAs in diets but also have both nutritional and physiological functions in livestock, poultry, and fish. In addition, the gastrointestinal tract of livestock, poultry, fish, and crustaceans may also generate bioactive peptides from the ingested protein hydrolysates and animal by-products (e.g., poultry by-products, ruminant meat and bone meal, and hydrolyzed feather meal). Some peptides of plant or animal sources also have antimicrobial, antioxidant, antihypertensive, and immunomodulatory activities. Those peptides that confer biological functions beyond their nutritional value are called bioactive peptides. They are usually 3–20 AA residues in length. Inclusion of some (e.g., 2%–8%) animal-protein hydrolysates (e.g., porcine intestine, porcine mucosa, salmon viscera, or poultry tissue hydrolysates) or soybean protein hydrolysates in practical corn- and soybean meal-based diets enhances feed intake, nutrient digestibility, lean tissue gain, growth performance, and feed efficiency in weanling pigs, young calves, posthatching poultry, and fish, while improving their intestinal development, behavior, immunity, health (including intestinal health), well-being, and survival (Hou et al. 2017; Khosravi et al. 2015; Kim et al. 2010; Lindemann et al. 2000; Opheim et al. 2016).

Recent studies have shown the potential economic value for the global large-scale production and use of animal and plant protein hydrolysates in animal feeding (Etemadian et al. 2021; Hou et al. 2017). Industrial processing of domestic farm animals generates large amounts of tissues (30%–40% of BW) not consumed by humans, including viscera, carcass-trimmings, bone (20%–30% of BW), fat, skin, feet, small-intestinal tissue (2% of BW), feather (up to 10% of BW), and collectible blood (5% of BW), with the global human-inedible livestock and poultry by-products being ~54 billion kg/year. Likewise, fish processing industries produce large amounts of wastes (up to 55% of BW), such as muscle-trimmings (15%–20%), skin and fins (1%–3%), bones (9%–15%), heads (9%–12%), viscera (12%–18%), and scales, with the global human-inedible fish by-products being ~6 billion kg/year. Thus, the global annual volume of total animal by-products generated by the processing industries is approximately 60 billion kg annually. Assuming that only 5% of the animal by-products and plant products for feed are used for protein hydrolysis, and based on the current average prices of animal, soybean, and wheat protein hydrolysates, their yields are 3, 6.75, and 12.75 billion kg/year, respectively, and their economic values are 4.5, 3.88, and 20.02 billion US $/year (Hou et al. 2017). Thus, protein hydrolysates from the by-products of pigs or poultry and from plant ingredients hold great promise in sustaining the animal agriculture and managing companion animals worldwide.

5.5   SYNTHESIS AND CATABOLISM OF POLYAMINES

5.5.1   History of Polyamine Research

The history of polyamines began in 1678 when A. Van Leeuwenhoek used a primitive microscope to observe spermine [N, N'-bis(3-aminopropyl)-1,4-butane-diamine] as a crystalline substance in human semen after several days of standing at room temperature. Such a crystal was described in 1791 by L.N. Vauquelin as a phosphate derivative, which was identified in 1878 by P. Schreiner to be an organic base and named *spermine* (meaning an amine from semen) in 1888 by two German chemists, A. Ladenburg and J. Abel. Putrescine (1,4-butanediamine or propane-1,3-diamine), like cadaverine (1,5-pentanediamine or pentane-1,5-diamine), was first isolated from putrefying meat (decomposing animal material) in 1885 by Ludwig Brieger and its structure was established through the chemical synthesis in 1886 by A. Ladenburg. Putrescine was named because of its origin and the foul smell of putrefaction. A biological function of polyamines was first demonstrated in 1898 by A. Von Poehl who reported that high concentrations of spermine inhibit the growth of Gram-positive bacteria. The structure of spermine was established in 1924 by O. Rosenheim through chemical synthesis. In 1927, O. Rosenheim discovered spermidine [*N*-(3-aminopropyl)-1,4-butane-diamine] in animal tissues (including ox pancreas, liver, kidney, spleen, lung, and brain) and established its structure through its chemical synthesis. Spermidine was named because of its association with and structural similarity to spermine in animal tissues. All polyamines are water-soluble basic molecules and contain no nitrogen atom (Bégué and Bonnet-Delpon. 2008).

Research on the metabolism of polyamines started in 1938 when E. Zeller discovered diamine oxidase as an enzyme responsible for their catabolism in animals. After R. Hämäläinen reported high concentrations of polyamines in animal tissues in 1941, intensive interest arose in metabolic pathways for polyamine biosynthesis, as well as in their physiological functions and pathological roles in disease. In 1958, H. Tabor reported that methionine was required to provide SAM for the synthesis of spermidine and spermine from putrescine in *E. coli* (discovered by H. Tabor in 1958). Meanwhile, other researchers demonstrated that physiological concentrations of polyamines stimulated the growth of many species of Gram-negative bacteria. With these findings, the 1950s and 1960s witnessed the rapid expansion of polyamine research. In exploring the underlying mechanisms for the actions of polyamines, A.M. Liquori observed in 1967 their secondary structures and close association with DNA and RNA (including tRNA and ribosomal RNA) in solution. A crucial role of ornithine in putrescine synthesis in animal tissues was established in 1968 when A.E. Pegg and H.G. Williams-Ashman discovered ornithine decarboxylase (ODC) in the rat prostate gland, whereas D.H. Russell and S.H. Snyder identified ODC in the rat liver, chick embryo, and tumors (including rat hepatomas and fibrosarcomas). At the First International Congress on Polyamines in 1970, there were landmark reports of polyamine accumulation in the regenerating rat liver and brain, in the chick embryo and brain, as well as in mammalian cells and *Drosophila melanogaster* during growth and development. A role for polyamines in disease was proposed in 1971 when D.H. Russell found that concentrations of polyamines in the blood and urine were markedly elevated in cancer patients. Similar results were observed in patients with parasitic diseases. In 1976, E.S. Canellakis and colleagues discovered the 26-kDa protein, antizyme, in the rat liver and in H-35 hepatoma cells exposed to high levels of putrescine. These authors found that antizyme was a non-competitive protein inhibitor of ODC. Antizyme acts by specifically binding to ODC, thereby inhibiting its catalytic activity. Capitalizing on these new findings, B.W. Metcalf synthesized an ornithine analogue, α-difluoromethylornithine (DFMO), as a suicidal inhibitor of ODC in 1978. These seminal studies have greatly advanced the field of polyamine biochemistry and pathophysiology. Due to its effects on inhibiting putrescine production and depleting polyamines in pathogens, DFMO is now used to effectively treat patients suffering from the African Sleeping Sickness caused by the eukaryotic parasite *Trypanosoma brucei* (Willert and Phillips 2011). Thus, there is a rich history of polyamine research over the past 4 centuries.

5.5.2 Polyamine Synthesis

5.5.2.1 Pathways of Polyamine Synthesis

The metabolic pathway for polyamine synthesis is illustrated in Figure 5.6. The source of ornithine can be either the mitochondria, cytoplasm, or diet, depending on cell type. As noted previously, decarboxylated SAM serves as an essential precursor for the conversion of putrescine into spermidine and spermine. All the enzymes required for converting ornithine to spermine are present in the cytoplasm. Additionally, arginine, proline, glutamine, and glutamate are all potential sources of putrescine in animals, depending on cell types and developmental stages (Wu and Morris 1998). Although glutamine and glutamate play a role in providing ornithine via pyrroline-5-carboxylate production in enterocytes, most of the glutamine- and glutamate-derived ornithine is channeled into ornithine carbamoyltransferase for citrulline formation rather than to ODC for putrescine production. It should be borne in mind that arginine is not a precursor of ornithine in all animal

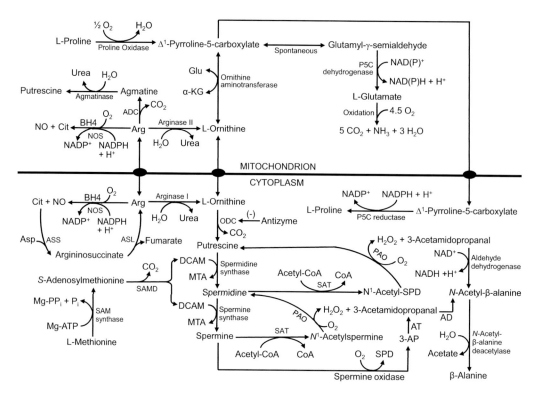

FIGURE 5.6 Synthesis of polyamines and their catabolism via *N*-acetylpolyamine formation in cells of humans and other animals. The enzymes that compete for arginine include arginase I, arginase II, constitutive and inducible nitric oxide synthase (NOS), and arginine decarboxylase (ADC). Arginine is hydrolyzed to ornithine plus urea by arginase I and arginase II in many cell types. Synthesis of putrescine from ornithine is catalyzed by ornithine decarboxylase (ODC) in all cell types. In certain tissues, arginine may be decarboxylated to form agmatine by ADC and agmatine is then converted into putrescine by agmatinase. Argininosuccinate synthase (ASS) and argininosuccinate lyase (ASL) regenerate arginine from citrulline in the presence of aspartate and ATP. Catabolism of polyamines is initiated by polyamine oxidase, spermine oxidase, and spermidine/spermine *N*¹-acetyltransferase (SAT) to produce 3-acetamidopropanal and β-alanine in the cytoplasm. AD, 3-acetamidopropanal dehydrogenase; 3-AP, 3-aminopropanal; AT, 3-aminopropanal *N*¹-acetyltransferase; BH4, (6*R*)-5,6,7,8-tetrahydro-L-biopterin; DCAM, decarboxylated 5-adenosylmethionine; α-KG, α-ketoglutarate; MTA, methylthioadenosine; OAT, ornithine aminotransferase; PAO, *N*¹-acetylpolyamine oxidase; P5C, pyrroline-5-carboxylate; SAM, *S*-adenosylmethionine; SAMD, *S*-adenosylmethionine decarboxylase; and SPD, spermidine.

cells. For example, because there is little expression of arginase in porcine placentae at all stages of gestation or in the enterocytes of neonates (e.g., piglets, lambs, calves, rats, and mice), these cells cannot convert arginine into ornithine. In search of alternative precursors of ornithine, G. Wu and coworkers discovered in the 2000s that proline catabolism via proline oxidase is the exclusive intracellular source of ornithine for polyamine synthesis in the enterocytes of neonatal pigs and in the porcine placentae, both of which share the common feature of rapid cell growth (Wu et al. 2005, 2000a, b).

Microbes possess lysine decarboxylase to decarboxylate lysine to CO_2 and cadaverine (1,5-diaminopentane). The latter is also found in plants. Cadaverine emanates from decaying animal tissues due to bacterial contamination and is a strong repulsive odor to humans. Interestingly, this amine is a feeding attractant for some animals, such as rats and goldfish.

The work of Wang et al. (2014) showing that about 50% of ovine embryos survived in response to *in vivo* translational knockdown of the ODC1 mRNA led to the discovery that agmatine

[1-(4-aminobutyl)guanidine] is a precursor of polyamines in ovine conceptuses. In this alternative pathway for polyamine synthesis, arginine is decarboxylated by mitochondrial arginine decarboxylase to agmatine [also known as argamine; 1-(4-aminobutyl)guanidine]. The latter is hydrolyzed by mitochondrial agmatinase to putrescine. Note that porcine conceptuses lack arginine decarboxylase and, therefore, cannot produce agmatine from arginine.

5.5.2.2 Regulation of Polyamine Synthesis

Reduced availabilities of substrates (e.g., ornithine, arginine, proline, and methionine) and vitamin B_6 can limit polyamine synthesis in mammalian cells. Evidence shows that arginase activity is a limiting factor for polyamine synthesis and cell proliferation in many cell types, including endothelial cells, macrophages, and smooth muscle cells (Ignarro et al. 2001; Kepka-Lenhart et al. 2000; Li et al. 2001; Wei et al. 2001). Arginase, which can be released from cells and tissues, is present in extracellular fluid (e.g., the plasma, intestinal lumen, and ovine allantoic fluid) and in wounds to degrade arginine to ornithine plus urea. Indeed, under conditions of inflammation and injury (particularly liver disease), a high activity of arginase in the plasma results in a severe deficiency of arginine and, therefore, impaired synthesis of polyamines by stressed cells (Reid et al. 2007).

ODC, a pyridoxal phosphate-dependent enzyme, plays a key role in the regulation of polyamine synthesis in animal cells (Agostinelli 2020). Active mammalian ODC is a homodimer, with each monomer containing 461 AA residues (~51 kDa). ODC has a short half-life of approximately 10 min, allowing for a rapid response of the cell to a variety of stimuli to regulate polyamine synthesis. The activity of ODC is increased by elevated physiological levels of cAMP and NO but inhibited by high concentrations of putrescine, spermidine, and spermine. ODC is a rate-controlling enzyme in polyamine synthesis and is subject to inhibition by antizyme, which has several isoforms (i.e., antizymes 1, 2, 3, and 4). Antizyme 1 is induced after the addition of putrescine to the culture medium of tumor cells (e.g., hepatoma cells and neuroblastoma cells; Fong et al. 1976). Immediately following this report, antizyme 1 was found to be present in several other cell lines (e.g., IEC-6 intestinal cells and prostate cancer cells) and to be induced by spermidine and spermine, which have a greater effect than putrescine on stimulating antizyme 1 expression. It is now known that antizyme 1 is ubiquitous in animal tissues and cells (Kahana 2018). Antizyme 2 is also ubiquitous but is less abundant than antizyme 1. Antizyme 3 is present only in male germ cells in the postmeiotic stage of their differentiation to mature sperm. Antizyme 4 is structurally most closely related to antizyme 1 but has not been well characterized. Antizyme has a high affinity for the monomer of ODC. Upon binding ODC, antizyme inactivates the enzyme and also tags it for degradation by the proteasome. Antizyme also inhibits the transport of polyamines by cells via yet unknown mechanisms. Results of recent studies indicate that asparagine and glutamine, which increase ODC activity in diverse cell types, inhibit antizyme 1 expression at both mRNA and protein levels (Ray et al. 2012).

5.5.3 Polyamine Degradation

5.5.3.1 Diamine Oxidase and Polyamine Oxidase

Polyamine uptake by animal cells is mediated by caveolin-1-dependent endocytosis, whereas the Na^+-dependent AA transporter SLC3A2 acts as an exporter of polyamines from the cells. Catabolism of polyamines occurs in both the cytoplasm and peroxisomes. In 1953, a diamine oxidase, first designated as spermine oxidase, was reported to be present in ovine and bovine sera. This enzyme could oxidize putrescine, spermine, and spermidine at the terminal primary amino group to their respective aminoaldehydes (RCHO), NH_3, and H_2O_2 (Lee and Sayre 1998). Subsequently, more specific polyamine oxidases (including putrescine oxidase, spermidine oxidase, and spermine oxidase) for individual polyamines were identified in animal cells and tissues to catalyze the oxidative deamination of polyamines at the secondary amino group (Lee and Sayre 1998; Tabor and Tabor 1984). In 2002, an inducible flavin-containing spermine oxidase (SMO/PAOh1; a cytosolic protein) was found in mammalian cells to selectively oxidize spermine to produce H_2O_2, spermidine, and the aldehyde 3-aminopropanal (Vujcic et al. 2002). In contrast to the previously reported "spermine oxidase", SMO/PAOh1 does not use spermidine as a substrate. The discovery of SMO/PAOh1 adds a new enzyme-catalyzed reaction to the complexity of the polyamine catabolic pathways.

$$\text{Polyamine} + 2\,H_2O + O_2 \rightarrow 2\,H_2O_2 + NH_3 + \text{Aminoaldehyde (diamine oxidase; polyamine oxidase)}$$

Both diamine oxidase (a copper-containing protein) and polyamine oxidase (a FAD-dependent enzyme) are responsible for the degradation of polyamines in humans and other animals (Figure 5.7). Both enzymes are widespread in animal cells, tissues, and physiological fluids (e.g., the blood and seminal plasma) and are physiologically relevant for polyamine catabolism. Of particular note, diamine oxidase is highly active in the mucosa of the small intestine and the placenta (Kim et al. 1969; Tabor and Tabor 1984). Note that diamine oxidase is different from the mitochondrial flavin-dependent amine oxidases present in mammalian cells that mainly degrade primary amines but can also dehydrogenate some secondary and tertiary amines (Ding et al. 1993). The labile (unstable) aldehyde intermediate of the oxidation of spermidine by diamine oxidase undergoes either spontaneous (nonenzymatic) β-elimination to acrolein and putrescine or spontaneous cyclization to 1-(3-aminopropyl)-2-pyrroline. Likewise, the labile (unstable) aldehyde intermediate of the oxidation of spermine by diamine oxidase undergoes spontaneous β-elimination to spermidine and putrescine. The products of diamine oxidase and polyamine oxidase are further metabolized to smaller molecules via enzymatic and spontaneous reactions. Specifically, γ-aminobutyraldehyde (also known as 4-aminobutanal) undergoes (1) dehydrogenation by γ-aminobutyraldehyde dehydrogenase to γ-aminobutyrate (4-aminobutanoate) and (2) spontaneous cyclization to Δ^1-pyrroline. In addition, β-aminopropionaldehyde (also known as 3-aminopropanal) undergoes (1) dehydrogenation by β-aminopropionaldehyde dehydrogenase to β-alanine and (2) spontaneous cyclization to acrolein and ammonia.

Elevated levels of the products of polyamine catabolism by diamine oxidase and polyamine oxidases, particularly acrolein, are toxic to animal cells. Thus, the physiological concentrations of putrescine, spermidine, and spermine in the plasma of humans and other animals are usually about

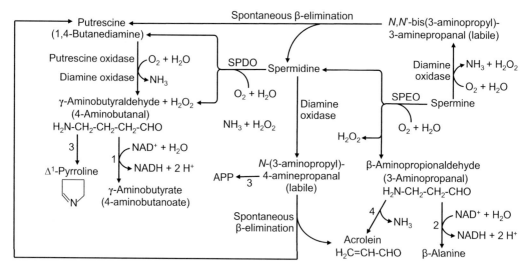

FIGURE 5.7 Catabolism of polyamines via diamine oxidase and polyamine oxidase in humans and other animals. Diamine oxidase is a copper-containing protein, whereas polyamine oxidase is a FAD-dependent enzyme. Elevated levels of polyamine metabolites are cytotoxic. The enzymes that catalyze the indicated reactions are (1) γ-aminobutyraldehyde dehydrogenase; (2) β-aminopropionaldehyde dehydrogenase; (3) spontaneous (nonenzymatic) cyclization; and (4) spontaneous (nonenzymatic) cleavage. APP, 1-(3-aminopropyl)-2-pyrroline; SPDO, spermidine oxidase; and SPEO, spermine oxidase.

2–5 μM. Increasing extracellular concentrations of polyamines (e.g., >50 μM putrescine) inhibits the growth of animal cells and also induces apoptosis. The underlying mechanism may involve polyamine-induced oxidative stress and the destruction of the outer layer of the plasma membrane.

5.5.3.2 Spermidine/Spermine N^1-Acetyltransferase and N^1-Acetylpolyamine Oxidase

Spermidine and spermine can be oxidized by acetyl-CoA:spermidine-N^1-acetyltransferase (spermidine/spermine N^1-acetyltransferase, SAT) to N^1-acetyl-spermidine and N^1-acetyl-spermine, respectively (Figure 5.6). N^1-acetyl-spermidine is then oxidized by N^1-acetylpolyamine oxidase (PAO) to putrescine, H_2O_2, and 3-acetamidopropanal. Similarly, N^1-acetyl-spermine is oxidized by PAO to spermidine, H_2O_2, and 3-acetamidopropanal. Spermine is also oxidized by spermine oxidase to 3-aminopropanal, which is acetylated to 3-acetamidopropanal. Thus, 3-acetamidopropanal is produced via three metabolic pathways.

3-Acetamidopropanal undergoes oxidation by 3-acetamidopropanal dehydrogenase (NAD^+-linked) to generate N-acetyl-β-alanine. The latter is deacetylated by N-acetyl-β-alanine deacetylase to form β-alanine. PAO and SMO/PAOh1 may play key roles in regulating intracellular polyamine homeostasis under various conditions (e.g., changes in cellular signals, drug treatment, oxidative stress, and other environmental and/or cellular stressors). Both PAO and SMO/PAOh1 generate toxic aldehydes and H_2O_2 (an oxidant) and are strongly induced by antitumor polyamine analogues (Stewart et al. 2018). This explains, in part, why excess polyamines are cytotoxins. Depending on the concentrations and cell types, these products can be either antineoplastic drugs or carcinogens.

5.6 SYNTHESIS AND UTILIZATION OF CREATINE

5.6.1 History of Creatine Research

Creatine (N-[aminoiminomethyl]-N-methylglycine), "*kreas*" in Greek meaning meat, was discovered by the French chemist, M.E. Chevreul, in 1832 as a water-soluble component of skeletal muscle in cattle. In the analysis of urine from humans and other animals, J. von Liebig discovered creatinine in 1847. Both creatine and creatinine are neutral substances. In 1925, G. Edgar and H.E. Shiver found that, at physiological temperatures (e.g., 37°C in humans and 40°C in chickens), creatine is in chemical equilibrium with creatinine in aqueous solution. Both creatine and creatinine have no net charge at neutral pH. In 1927, two British biochemists at University College, London, P. Eggleton and G. Eggleton, reported a labile form of organic phosphate "*phosphagen*" in the frog gastrocnemius muscle. Immediately thereafter, C. Fiske and Y. Subbarow at Harvard Medical School identified this new compound as creatine phosphate (also known as phosphocreatine), in which phosphate is linked to creatine via a phosphoamide bond. A few years later, D. Nachmansohn discovered an important role of phosphocreatine in energy metabolism in the skeletal muscle and the nervous system. The mechanism responsible for the production of phosphocreatine was elucidated in 1934 when K. Lohmann discovered creatine kinase. Multiple molecular forms of creatine kinase were first reported by A. Burger and coworkers in 1964. Since then, many isoforms of the enzyme have been cloned, sequenced, and characterized. Interestingly, recent studies by J.T. Brosnan and colleagues have identified nutritionally significant amounts of creatine in milk (e.g., porcine, bovine, and human milk) to support neonatal growth and development (Brosnan et al. 2009; Edison et al. 2013). Note that creatine contains a guanidino group and a carboxyl group but no amino group and, therefore, is not an AA. Likewise, creatine phosphate and creatinine do not contain an amino group and, therefore, are not AAs.

5.6.2 Creatine Synthesis Through Interorgan Cooperation

Creatine synthesis is a quantitatively important pathway for arginine catabolism via interorgan cooperation in mammals and birds. This pathway is initiated by arginine:glycine amidinotransferase (a mitochondrial enzyme), which transfers the guanidino group from arginine to glycine to form guanidinoacetate and ornithine (Figure 5.8). In these terrestrial animals, arginine:glycine amidinotransferase is expressed primarily in the renal tubules, pancreas, and to a much lesser extent in the liver and other organs. Thus, the kidneys are the major site of guanidinoacetate formation in the body. The guanidinoacetate released by the kidneys is methylated by guanidinoacetate *N*-methyltransferase (a cytosolic SAM-dependent enzyme), which is located predominantly in the liver, pancreas, and, to a much lesser extent, in the kidneys to produce creatine. The SAM required by guanidinoacetate *N*-methyltransferase is generated from methionine and ATP by SAM synthetase (a cytosolic enzyme). Creatine in the arterial blood is actively taken up by many tissues, including the skeletal muscle, heart, and brain. Approximately 95% of creatine in the body is present in skeletal muscle. A small amount of creatine and phosphocreatine (1.7%/day) is spontaneously converted into creatinine. Note that guanidinoacetate, creatine, phosphocreatine, and creatinine have no *asymmetric* carbon and, therefore, have no D- or L-isoform.

To date, little is known about creatine synthesis in aquatic animals. In fish, this metabolic pathway may occur primarily, if not exclusively, in skeletal muscle. There are reports that mRNA transcripts for creatine-synthetic enzymes are present in the kidney and liver of zebrafish, and also

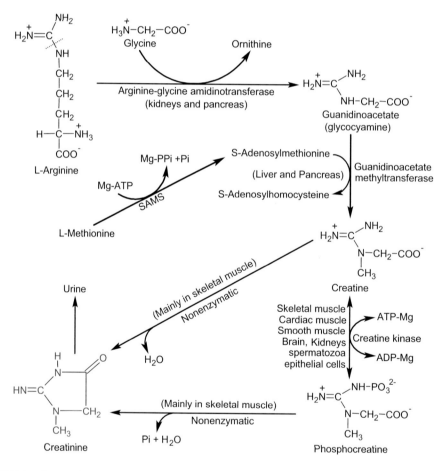

FIGURE 5.8 Synthesis and catabolism of creatine in humans and other animals. Creatine is synthesized from arginine, glycine, and methionine in mammals and birds via interorgan cooperation involving the kidneys, liver, and pancreas. In fish, the synthesis of creatine occurs primarily in skeletal muscle. In all animals, skeletal muscle is the major site for the conversion of creatine to creatinine in the body. Creatine and phosphocreatine (also known as creatine phosphate) are not highly stable in an aqueous solution and are spontaneously converted into creatinine at 1.7% per day. SAMS, SAM synthetase.

in skeletal muscle of four fish species including pikes, rainbow trout, zebra mbuna, and tilapia (Borchel et al. 2019). Based on mRNA expression, Borchel et al. (2019) suggested that skeletal muscle may be a major site for creatine synthesis in teleost. However, there is a paucity of data on the activities and tissue distribution of creatine-synthetic enzymes or creatine synthesis in fish tissues. In fish species (e.g., largemouth bass) with a low concentration of arginine (25–40 μM) in the plasma (Li et al. 2021), creatine synthesis may not be highly active. In support of this notion, the concentration of creatine in the skeletal muscle of largemouth bass is only 0.26 mM (Li and Wu 2020), in comparison with ~20 mM in human skeletal muscle.

A 70-kg healthy adult synthesizes 1.7 g creatine per day from 2.3 g arginine, 1.0 g glycine, and 2.0 g methionine (Wu and Morris 1998), which represent 46%, 36%, and 87%, respectively, of their daily dietary intakes. This amount of creatine is necessary to replace its daily irreversible loss (1.7 g/day) as creatinine from the subject through the excretion of the urine. A greater loss of creatine from the body occurs in response to enhanced muscular activity (Kreider et al. 2017), and this amount of creatine should be replenished through enhanced endogenous synthesis and dietary supplementation. For example, cycle ergometer exercise (approximately 45% of maximum O_2 consumption for 90 min) increases the loss of creatine (as indicated by urinary creatinine excretion) by 52% above pre- and postexercise values (Calles-Escandon et al. 1984). Based on the urinary excretion of creatine and creatinine, the concentrations of creatine and creatine phosphate in skeletal muscle, the accumulation of creatine plus phosphocreatine in porcine (Wu et al. 2018) and ovine (Baharom et al. 2017; Xue et al. 1988) conceptuses, the ruminal synthesis and the true digestibility of microbial protein (Wu 2018), and arginine content in microbial protein (Gilbreath et al. 2021), it can be estimated that creatine synthesis represents 52% and 43% of arginine utilization in gestating swine and sheep fed a ~12%-crude protein diet, respectively.

5.6.3 Regulation of Creatine Synthesis

5.6.3.1 Expression of Arginine: Glycine Amidinotransferase

Creatine synthesis is regulated primarily through changes in the expression of renal arginine: glycine amidinotransferase in both rats and humans. Dietary intake of creatine and circulating levels of growth hormone are major factors affecting *de novo* synthesis of creatine. Activities and mRNA levels for arginine:glycine amidinotransferase in rat kidney are greatly reduced by hypophysectomy or by feeding a diet containing creatine. By contrast, the administration of growth hormone to hypophysectomized rats induces the expression of arginine:glycine amidinotransferase, but this induction is largely blunted when the animals are simultaneously fed a creatine-supplemented diet. The mechanisms responsible for the effects of growth hormone or creatine on the expression of renal arginine:glycine amidinotransferase remain unknown. Neither creatine supplementation nor growth hormone influences the hepatic activity of guanidinoacetate *N*-methyltransferase in animals.

5.6.3.2 Availability of Substrates

In addition to the expression of arginine:glycine amidinotransferase, the availability of substrates (arginine, glycine, and methionine) can also limit creatine synthesis in humans and other animals. This view is supported by the findings that (1) vegan athletes, who generally have low intake of creatine and its precursor AAs, are at high risk for creatine deficiency (Rogerson 2017); and (2) an arginine deficiency decreases the concentrations of arginine, guanidinoacetate, and creatine in mouse tissues (brain, skeletal muscle, liver, and kidneys). Because the methylation of guanidinoacetate to form creatine consumes more methyl groups than all other methylation reactions in the body combined, creatine synthesis from arginine regulates the availability of the methyl group donor for other methylation reactions, such as the synthesis of methionine from homocysteine. Thus, arginine can indirectly affect one-carbon unit metabolism in the whole body.

5.6.4 METABOLISM OF CREATINE AND THE URINARY EXCRETION OF CREATININE

Creatine undergoes limited irreversible catabolism in animals. However, after the newly synthesized creatine is released from the liver and pancreas, the creatine in the blood, the circulating creatine is actively taken up by the skeletal muscle and nerves, as well as other tissues. In all of these tissues, creatine is phosphorylated by ATP-dependent creatine kinase to form phosphocreatine. The energy of the γ-phosphate bond (51.6 kJ/mol or 12.3 kcal/mol) in one mole of ATP is transferred to one mole of creatine for storage *in vivo*. Creatine kinase exists in the cytosolic and mitochondrial isoforms. This enzyme is most abundant in the skeletal muscle and brain, but also occurs in many other tissues and cell types. In addition, creatine is spontaneously and irreversibly cyclized into creatinine through the loss of one molecule of water. Furthermore, creatine phosphate is also spontaneously converted into creatinine, with the losses of phosphate and one molecule of water (Figure 5.8).

$$\text{Creatine} + \text{ATP}^{4-} \leftrightarrow \text{Creatine phosphate}^{2-} + \text{ADP}^{3-} + \text{H}^{+} \quad \left(\text{creatine kinase, Mg}^{2+}\right)$$

Creatinine has complex chemical properties. It spontaneously undergoes both amino-imino and keto-enol tautomerization reactions in aqueous solutions at physiological pH values (Gao et al. 2013; Valadbeigi et al. 2015), yielding imino-enol, imino-keto, amino-keto, and amino-enol forms (Figure 5.9). The enol form of creatinine can be deprotonated to the corresponding anionic form. Both the enol- and keto-forms of creatinine can be protonated to the corresponding cationic form.

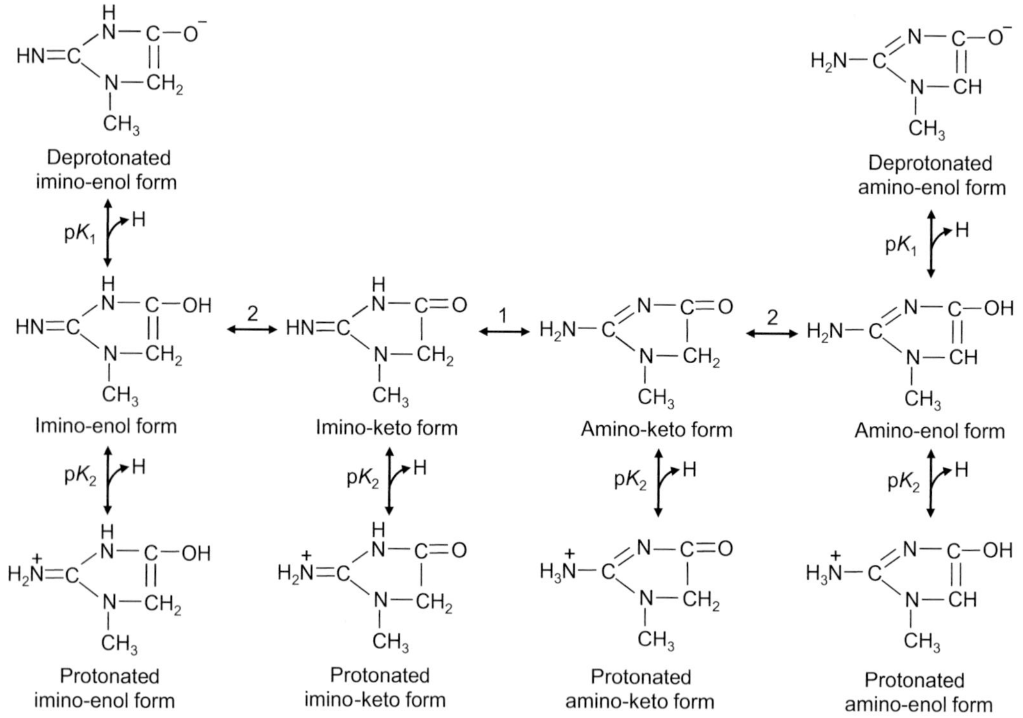

FIGURE 5.9 Spontaneous tautomerization of creatinine in the physiological fluids of humans and other animals. Creatinine occurs (1) only in the protonated form at pH 2–5, (2) in both protonated and deprotonated forms at pH 6, and (3) predominantly in the protonated form and, to a lesser extent, in the deprotonated form at pH 7. Thus, creatinine exists as both anions and cations in the blood, cells, and urine of animals. The indicated reactions are (1) amino-imino tautomerization and (2) keto-enol tautomerization. The pK$_1$ refers to the dissociation of the enol form of creatinine to its anion form, and pK$_2$ refers to the dissociation of the cationic (protonated) enol or keto form of creatinine.

The amino form of creatinine is much more stable and abundant than its imino form in physiological fluids. Creatinine occurs (1) in the protonated form only at pH 2–5, (2) in both protonated and deprotonated forms at pH 6, and (3) predominantly in the protonated form and, to a lesser extent, in the deprotonated form at pH 7 (Gao et al. 2013). Thus, creatinine exists as both anions and cations in the blood and in cells.

The creatine- and creatine phosphate-derived creatinine (mainly a charged molecule) in the blood crosses the basolateral membrane of the epithelial cells of renal proximal tubules via select transporters [organic cation transporters (OCTs) 2 and 3, as well as organic anion transporters (OATs) 2 and 3] into the cells and exits the cells through their apical membrane via multidrug and toxin extrusion (MATE) transporters 1 and 2-K into the lumen (urine) of the renal proximal tubules (Lepist et al. 2014; Tredwell et al. 2016). The OCTs play a role in the transport of creatine because some of it exists in the anion forms, as noted previously.

Creatine is not a source of cellular energy, but rather helps to store energy as phosphocreatine in animal tissues, particularly the brain and skeletal muscle. Creatine homeostasis in humans and other animals primarily involves three major organs: the kidneys, liver, and skeletal muscle. When healthy adult humans consume 4.4 g creatine monohydrate once, plasma creatine peaks (762 μM; an 18-fold increase over the 0-min baseline value of about 40 μM) in 60 min and its half-life in the plasma is 30 min (Jäger et al. 2007). Thus, creatine is rapidly cleared from the plasma. Urinary excretion of creatinine is the most widely used clinical marker of renal function in humans and other animals and is also a useful indicator of skeletal muscle mass.

$$\text{Creatine} + \text{ATP} \leftrightarrow \text{Creatine phosphate} + \text{ADP} \qquad \left(\text{creatine kinase, } Mg^{2+}\right)$$

5.6.5 Tissue Distribution of Creatine

Creatine is abundant in skeletal muscle, heart, brain, and pancreas. A 70-kg adult has about 120 g of total creatine (creatine phosphate plus free creatine), with about 95% of it being in skeletal muscle (Casey and Greenhaff 2000). Total creatine is about 45% more abundant in white (fast-twitch fibers, type II) muscle than in red (slow-twitch fibers, type I) muscle (Murphy et al. 2001). In skeletal muscle and brain, creatine stores energy primarily as creatine phosphate through the action of creatine kinase. In a resting state, about two-third and one-third of total creatine exist as creatine phosphate and creatine, respectively, in human skeletal muscle (McGilvery and Murray 1974). The irreversible loss of whole-body creatine and creatine phosphate as creatinine is 1.7%/day, as noted previously. This means that each day, 98.3% of the total creatine in the whole body is continuously recycled to store ATP energy via creatine kinase. In human skeletal muscle, the concentration of creatine phosphate is about 3 to 4 times that of ATP.

5.7 SYNTHESIS AND CATABOLISM OF L-CARNITINE

5.7.1 History of Carnitine Research

L-carnitine (a quaternary ammonium compound; the betaine derivative of β-hydroxybutyrate) was discovered by two Russian scientists, W. Gulewitsch and R. Krimberg, in 1905 as a nitrogenous substance of meat. The word "*carnitine*" is derived from the Latin word *carno* or *carnis*, which means flesh or *meat*. The structure of carnitine was established by two Japanese chemists, M. Tomita and Y. Sendju, in 1927. The role of L-carnitine (the biologically active isomer of carnitine) as an essential growth factor for mealworm larvae (*Tenebrio molitor*) was reported by G. Fraenkel and S. Friedman in 1957. I.B. Fritz discovered in 1961 that carnitine stimulates the oxidation of long-chain fatty acids in animal tissues and further demonstrated in 1965 that carnitine is an essential substrate for carnitine palmitoyltransferase I on the outer mitochondrial membrane to convert acyl-CoA into acylcarnitine. Acyl-carnitine is transported across the inner mitochondrial membrane by carnitine acylcarnitine translocase into the mitochondrial matrix where acylcarnitine is hydrolyzed by carnitine palmitoyltransferase II to release acyl-CoA and carnitine. Thus, carnitine plays an essential role in the transport of long-chain fatty acids from the cytoplasm into mitochondria for β-oxidation, a major mechanism for ATP production in insulin-sensitive tissues, including the skeletal muscle, heart, liver, and adipose tissue. In 1973, A.G. Engel and C. Angelini reported that carnitine deficiency in human skeletal muscle results in a rare disease of lipid storage myopathy that is prevented by dietary supplementation with carnitine. It is now known that carnitine plays additional important roles in (1) protecting organisms from oxidative stress, (2) promoting substrate oxidation in brown adipose tissue, and (3) regulating energy partitioning in the body.

5.7.2 Carnitine Synthesis Through Interorgan Cooperation in Humans and Other Animals

Mammals and birds express enzymes for de novo synthesis of carnitine, but there is no report for de novo synthesis of carnitine in any bacterial species (Fennerna et al. 2016). The pathway for carnitine synthesis in humans and other animals (e.g., rats, pigs, and chickens) is illustrated

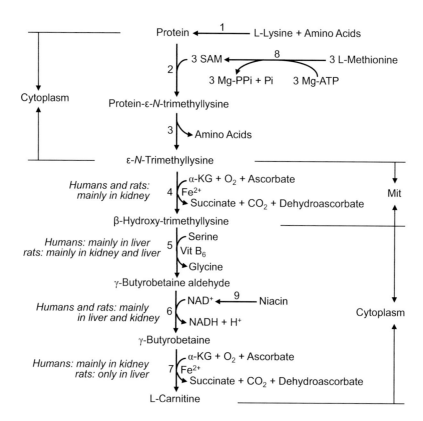

FIGURE 5.10 Synthesis of L-carnitine from lysine and methionine in humans and other animals via interorgan cooperation. The enzymes that catalyze the indicated reactions are (1) protein synthesis; (2) S-adenosylmethionine-dependent protein methyltransferase; (3) protein degradation; (4) ε-N-L-trimethyllysine dioxygenase (a mitochondrial enzyme); (5) β-hydroxy-trimethyllysine aldolase (possibly identical to the cytosolic isoform of serine hydroxymethyl transferase); (6) γ-butyrobetaine aldehyde dehydrogenase (also known as ε-N-trimethylaminobutyraldehyde dehydrogenase); and (7) γ-butyrobetaine dioxygenase (also known as γ-butyrobetaine hydroxylase). The conversion of β-hydroxy-trimethyllysine to L-carnitine occurs in the cytoplasm. Amino acids, glycine plus L-amino acids; α-KG, α-ketoglutarate; Mit, mitochondrion; SAM, S-adenosylmethionine; and Vit B_6, vitamin B_6.

in Figure 5.10. Although free lysine can be methylated by ε-*N*-L-lysine methyltransferase to form trimethyllysine in *Neurospora crassa*, this enzyme is not present in animal tissues. Rather, in animals, protein-bound lysine residues are methylated by SAM-dependent protein methyltransferase to form ε-*N*-L-trimethyllysine residues (Strijbis et al. 2010). Partially methylated protein-bound lysines are not precursors for carnitine synthesis in animals. The degradation of proteins by proteases releases ε-*N*-L-trimethyllysine, which serves as a substrate for carnitine synthesis via the sequential formation of β-hydroxy-trimethyllysine, γ-butyrobetaine aldehyde (ε-*N*-trimethylaminobutyraldehyde), and γ-butyrobetaine. SAM (a metabolite of L-methionine) was known to be the donor of the three methyl groups on the nitrogen of carnitine in the 1960s, and the source of the carbon backbone (chain) of the carnitine molecule was identified to be lysine in the early 1970s. Three vitamins [ascorbate (vitamin C), niacin (the precursor of NAD$^+$), and vitamin B$_6$ (the precursor of pyridoxal 5'-phosphate)] and serine are also required for carnitine synthesis (Figure 5.10). A healthy adult human synthesizes 1.2 μmol carnitine/kg BW/day (Rebouche 1992).

The enzymes responsible for carnitine synthesis are expressed in a species- and tissue-specific manner. In rats and humans, the highest activity of ε-*N*-L-trimethyllysine dioxygenase (a mitochondrial enzyme) occurs in the kidney, and this enzyme is also expressed in the liver, skeletal muscle, heart, and brain. ε-*N*-L-trimethyllysine dioxygenase is a rate-controlling enzyme in carnitine synthesis. β-hydroxy-trimethyllysine aldolase (a pyridoxal 5'-phosphate-dependent cytosolic enzyme) is present at high activity in both the kidneys and liver of rats, but predominantly in the liver of humans. There is evidence that β-hydroxy-trimethyllysine aldolase may be identical to the cytosolic isoform of serine hydromethyl transferase. In humans, cattle, and rats, γ-butyrobetaine aldehyde dehydrogenase (an NAD$^+$-dependent cytosolic enzyme) is expressed primarily in the liver and kidneys and, to a much lesser extent, in brain, heart, and skeletal muscle. In animals, no activity of this enzyme is found in either mitochondria or microsomes. In both rats and humans, the conversion of trimethyllysine to γ-butyrobetaine takes place primarily in the kidney and, to a lesser extent, in the liver, skeletal muscle, heart, and brain. Studies with rats show that the testes and epididymis can also produce γ-butyrobetaine from trimethyllysine. In rats, dogs, guinea pigs, and mice, only the liver can convert γ-butyrobetaine to L-carnitine via the action of γ-butyrobetaine dioxygenase (also known as γ-butyrobetaine hydroxylase; a cytosolic enzyme), and this reaction is absent from the kidneys. In humans, the activity of γ-butyrobetaine dioxygenase in the kidneys is 3- to 16-fold and 6- to 32-fold greater than that in the liver and brain, respectively; therefore, the hydroxylation of γ-butyrobetaine to carnitine occurs primarily in the kidneys and to a lesser extent in the liver and brain. The kidneys of cats, hamsters, rabbits, and pigs have levels of γ-butyrobetaine dioxygenase activity equal to or exceeding those in their livers; in these species, the kidney and liver are important sites for hydroxylating γ-butyrobetaine to carnitine.

5.7.3 Contribution of Diet and Endogenous Synthesis to Carnitine in Humans and Other Animals

About 75% and 25% of the total carnitine in meat-consuming humans are derived from diet and endogenous synthesis, respectively (Bremer 1983; Rebouche 1992). Carnitine is taken up by cells and tissues through the Na$^+$-dependent organic cation transporter 2 (OCTN2, SLC22A5). Endogenous synthesis of carnitine is important for strict vegetarians because this nutrient is present primarily in foods of animal origin and occurs at very low concentrations in plants (Bourdin et al. 2007). In these individuals, carnitine comes almost exclusively from its endogenous synthesis. This is analogous to chickens and pigs that are typically fed plant-based diets. Such diets do not appear to meet the requirements of (1) laying hens either fed the rations containing high levels of pro-oxidants or with advanced age (Ringseis et al. 2018) and (2) gestating swine because dietary supplementation with carnitine enhances their fetal growth (Ramanau et al. 2006; Waylan et al. 2005).

5.7.4 Regulation of Carnitine Synthesis in Humans and Other Animals

Carnitine synthesis in humans and other animals is regulated by diet, age, hormones, and disease states (Vaz and Wanders 2002). First, a deficiency of dietary protein, lysine, methionine, vitamin C, niacin, or vitamin B_6 impairs carnitine synthesis in animals. In adult rats, dietary supplementation with 1% carnitine decreases the hepatic activity of γ-butyrobetaine hydroxylase by approximately 40%, whereas dietary supplementation with 1% γ-butyrobetaine increases the enzyme activity by approximately 60%. By contrast, supplementation with either 1% carnitine or 1% γ-butyrobetaine does not affect the renal activity of trimethyllysine dioxygenase. During starvation, the carnitine content of the liver is markedly elevated, possibly as a result of increases in protein degradation and the expression of key enzymes for carnitine synthesis. Under such a condition, enhanced synthesis of carnitine is of physiological significance as the oxidation of long-chain fatty acids promotes keto-genesis to provide ketone bodies to the brain as metabolic fuels. Similarly, the intravenous admin-istration of lipids reduces the concentration of carnitine in the plasma and the urinary excretion of carnitine possibly due to enhanced uptake by the liver and skeletal muscle to facilitate the oxidation of long-chain fatty acids.

Second, there are developmental changes in carnitine synthesis in mammals (Lin et al. 2020; Ling et al. 2012). In rats, the hepatic activity of γ-butyrobetaine dioxygenase is low in the fetus despite rapid development during late gestation and rises to adult levels on Day 8 after birth. In humans, the hepatic activity of γ-butyrobetaine dioxygenase in infants is only 12% of the value for adults but increases to the adult level at 15 years of age. Similarly, in pigs, the activity of γ-butyrobetaine dioxygenase (also known as γ-butyrobetaine hydroxylase) in the kidney and liver is low at birth and increases progressively within the subsequent 7 weeks of life. However, the activity of this enzyme in the liver and kidneys of pigs does not differ between 56 and 210 days of age.

Third, hormones (e.g., high levels of glucagon, glucocorticoids, and thyroid hormones) that can stimulate protein degradation to supply trimethyllysine can enhance carnitine synthesis (Vaz and Wanders 2002). Additionally, the administration of thyroxine to rats enhances the hepatic activity of trimethyllysine dioxygenase twofold, as well as concentrations of carnitine in both the plasma and the liver by nearly 100%. Sex hormones and pituitary hormones increase carnitine content in tissues likely through augmenting carnitine synthesis.

Fourth, pathological conditions greatly affect carnitine synthesis and availability in humans and other animals (Flanagan et al. 2010; Strijbis et al. 2010). For example, within the first 10 days after injury, concentrations of carnitine are reduced in the plasma due to elevation of its urinary excretion but are enhanced in the liver and skeletal muscle partly because of enhanced whole-body proteolysis and carnitine synthesis. Similar results have been reported for burn patients, who exhibit a reduction of circulating levels of carnitine and an increase of urinary excretion. Interestingly, concentrations of carnitine in the plasma are substantially lower in obese mice compared with lean mice, which may contribute, in part, to reduced oxidation of fatty acids in the insulin-sensitive tissues of obese persons. Accordingly, the administration of clofibrate (a peroxisome proliferator and ligand for the nuclear receptor peroxisome proliferator-activated receptor α) to rats increases hepatic carnitine and acylcarnitine concentrations by 6- and 5-fold, respectively, primarily due to enhanced synthesis of carnitine in the liver. There is also evidence that denervation in rats causes a pronounced decline in the intramuscular levels of carnitine, with the change being greater in red than in white fibers. Thus, carnitine synthesis is precisely regulated at multiple steps to meet the physiological and nutritional needs of animals.

5.7.5 Catabolism of Carnitine in Humans and Other Animals

Eukaryotes (e.g., mammals, birds, fish, and crustaceans) have no enzymes to degrade carnitine (Strijbis et al. 2010). The catabolism of carnitine in humans and other animals takes place only in the gut microorganisms. Carnitine is taken up by bacteria via (1) an ATP-binding cassette (ABC) transport system (utilizing a transmembrane domain, an ATPase, and a periplasmic binding protein); and (2) a betaine/choline/carnitine transporter (BCCT) that is driven by the sodium or proton motive force and a carnitine:γ-butyrobetaine antiporter. Inside the bacteria, carnitine degradation is initiated by (1) carnitine decarboxylase to form β-methylcholine; (2) carnitine dehydrogenase to yield 3-dehydrocarnitine; (3) crotonobetainyl-CoA reductase and γ-butyrobetainyl-CoA:carnitine CoA-transferase to generate γ-butyrobetaine (4-*N*-trimethylaminobutyrate); and (4) the carnitine oxygenase-carnitine reductase system to produce trimethylamine and malate semialdehyde (Figure 5.11). β-Methylcholine can be acetylated to generate acetyl-β-methylcholine (methacholine,

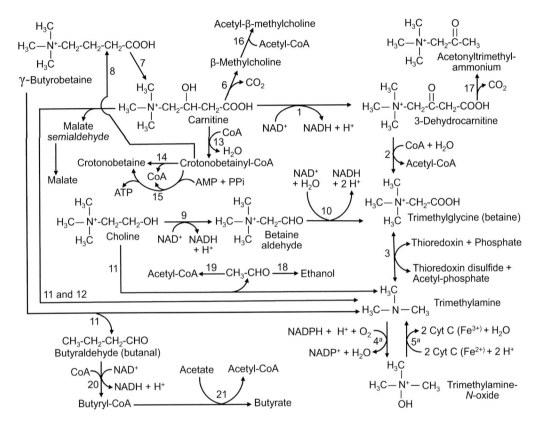

FIGURE 5.11 Catabolism of carnitine and choline in intestinal microbes and the conversion of trimethylamine (TMA) to trimethylamine *N*-oxide (TMAO) in the liver of humans and other animals. The enzymes that catalyze the indicated reactions are (1) carnitine dehydrogenase; (2) 3-ketoacid CoA-transferase; (3) betaine reductase; (4) TMA monooxygenase; (5) TMAO reductase; (6) carnitine decarboxylase; (7) γ-butyrobetaine hydroxylase (γ-butyrobetaine+α-ketoglutarate+O_2 → carnitine+succinate+CO_2); (8) two enzymes [crotonobetainyl-CoA reductase (crotonobetainyl-CoA+reduced electron acceptor → γ-butyrobetainyl-CoA+oxidized electron acceptor); γ-butyrobetainyl-CoA:carnitine CoA-transferase (γ-butyrobetainyl-CoA+carnitine → γ-butyrobetaine+carnitinyl-CoA)]; (9) choline dehydrogenase; (10) betaine aldehyde dehydrogenase; (11) choline:TMA lyase; (12) a two-enzyme system consisting of carnitine oxygenase and carnitine reductase; (13) two enzymes [carnitine-CoA ligase (carnitine CoA+ATP → carnitinyl-CoA+AMP+PPi); carnitinyl-CoA dehydratase (carnitinyl-CoA → crotonobetainyl-CoA+H_2O)]; (14) crotonobetainyl-CoA:carnitine CoA-transferase (carnitine+crotonobetainyl-CoA → carnitinyl-CoA+crotonobetaine); (15) crotonobetaine-CoA ligase (crotonobetaine-CoA+AMP+diphosphate → crotonobetaine-CoA+ATP); (16) acetyl-β-methylcholine synthase; (17) spontaneous (nonenzymatic) reaction; (18) acetaldehyde (CH_3-CHO) reductase (acetaldehyde+NADPH+H^+ → ethanol+NAD^+); (19) acetaldehyde dehydrogenase; (20) butyraldehyde dehydrogenase; and (21) butyryl-CoA:acetate transferase. [a] The enzyme activity is present in the liver of humans and other animals. The kidneys and liver express TMA monooxygenases 1 and 3, respectively.

an analogue of acetylcholine), whereas 3-dehydrocarnitine can be either spontaneously converted into acetonyltrimethylammonium or deacetylated by 3-ketoacid CoA-transferase to produce betaine (N, N, N-trimethylglycine). Betaine is further metabolized to the odorous trimethylamine and the nonodorous trimethylamine N-oxide by betaine reductase and trimethylamine monooxygenase, respectively. The oxygen required by γ-butyrobetaine hydrolase and trimethylamine monooxygenase can come from drinking water. In addition, carnitine is converted into crotonobetaine via a series of enzymes (carnitine-CoA ligase, carnitinyl-CoA dehydratase, and crotonobetainyl-CoA:carnitine CoA-transferase/crotonobetaine-CoA ligase). Furthermore, trimethylamine, dimethylamine, monomethylamine, and trimethylamine N-oxide can be oxidized to formaldehyde, with ammonia being a product of monomethylamine catabolism. Thus, carnitine is metabolized to ammonia, formaldehyde, trimethylamine, trimethylamine N-oxide, butyrobetaine, crotonobetaine, and trimethylaminoacetone in the gastrointestinal bacteria. Note that gut bacteria contain trimethylamine N-oxide reductase, which converts trimethylamine N-oxide (an abundant substance in fish and related products such as fishmeal) into trimethylamine. Trimethylamine and trimethylamine N-oxide may affect gene expression and nutrient metabolism in humans and other animals (Fennema et al. 2016).

Trimethylamine-oxide → Dimethylamine + Formaldehyde   (trimethylamine-oxide aldolase)

Trimethylamine + NAD^+ → Dimethylamine + Formaldehyde + NADH + H^+

(trimethylamine dehydrogenase)

Dimethylamine + NAD^+ → Monomethylamine + Formaldehyde + NADH + H^+

(dimethylamine dehydrogenase)

Monomethylamine + NAD^+ → Ammonia + Formaldehyde + NADH + H^+

(monomethylamine dehydrogenase)

After trimethylamine and trimethylamine N-oxide are generated by the intestinal microbes, these two metabolites are rapidly absorbed into the portal circulation and taken up by the liver through the Na^+-dependent OCT-2. In this organ, trimethylamine is oxidized to trimethylamine N-oxide by flavin-containing monooxygenase 3. The kidneys express flavin-containing monooxygenase 1 to oxidize a relatively small proportion of trimethylamine to trimethylamine N-oxide. In humans, the major metabolites of the orally administered carnitine are trimethylamine (excreted primarily in the urine) and γ-butyrobetaine (excreted primarily in the feces) (Rebouche 1991). Trimethylamine N-oxide is a metabolite of both the intestinal microbes and the host.

β-Methylcholine   Acetyl-β-methylcholine   Crotonobetaine   Crotonobetainyl-CoA

5.8 SYNTHESIS AND CATABOLISM OF PURINE AND PYRIMIDINE NUCLEOTIDES

5.8.1 HISTORY OF PURINE AND PYRIMIDINE RESEARCH

Purines and pyrimidines are nitrogen-containing heterocyclic substances. A purine consists of a pyrimidine ring fused to an imidazole ring. The history of both chemical and biochemical research

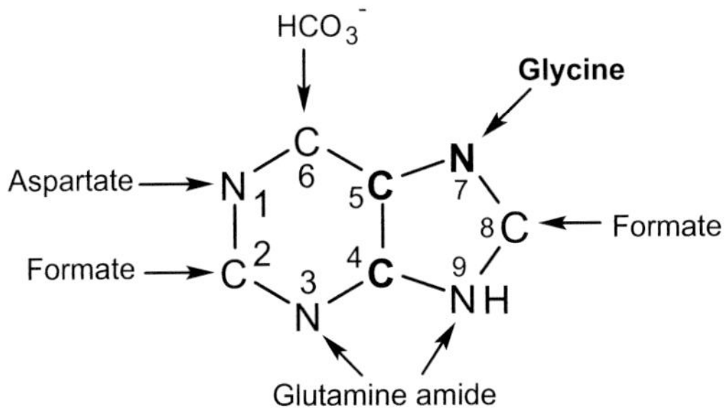

Origins of purine ring atoms

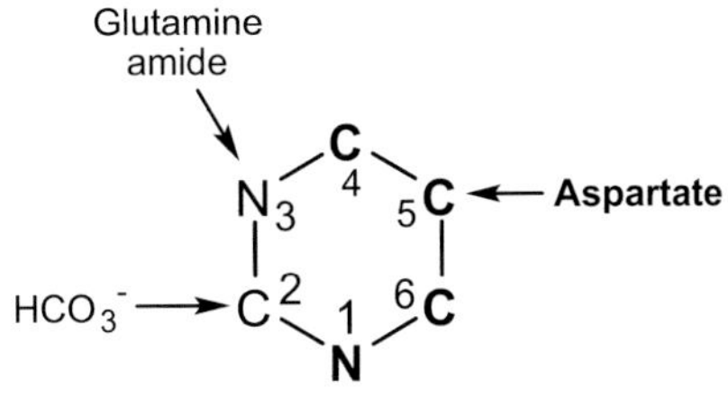

Origins of pyrimidine ring atoms

FIGURE 5.12 Sources of carbon and nitrogen in purine and pyrimidine rings in cells of humans and other animals. Glutamine, aspartate, ribose-5-phosphate, HCO_3^-, and tetrahydrofolate are common substrates for the ATP-dependent synthesis of purine and pyrimidine nucleotides in animal cells. Glycine is also required for the formation of purines (C_4, C_5, and N_7).

on purines and pyrimidines includes many groundbreaking discoveries (Olsson 2003). The terms *purine* and *pyrimidine* were coined, respectively, by E. Fischer and A. Pinner in 1884. The term *pyrimidine* was derived from a combination of the words *pyridine* and *amidine*. The research on purines and pyrimidines dates back to 1868 when the young Swiss physician, J.F. Miescher, isolated *nuclein* (now known as nucleic acids) from the nuclei of white blood cells. In search of the chemical composition of *nuclein*, A. Kossel discovered and named adenine in 1886, cytosine in 1894, guanine in 1882, thymine in 1893, and uracil in 1900. E. Fischer first synthesized purine from uric acid in 1899, and his work on purines brought him the 1902 Nobel Prize in Chemistry. Meanwhile, A. Kossel synthesized cytosine in 1903 and won the 1910 Nobel Prize in Chemistry for this work. In 1906, H. Steudel reported that nucleic acids contain 2 purine and 2 pyrimidine bases in approximately the same molar proportion. While working at the Rockefeller Institute of Medical Research, P.A. Levene found in 1911 that adenosine monophosphate (AMP) contains adenine and ribose-5-phosphate. He went on to identify the structure of deoxynucleic acids in 1929. In the same year, K. Lohmann, A.N. Drury, and A. Szent-Györgyi discovered ATP. Using pigeon liver and isotopes, J.M. Buchanan and colleagues elucidated the pathways for purine and pyrimidine syntheses during the 1940s and 1950s that require glutamine, aspartate, ribose-5-P, ATP, HCO_3^-, and tetrahydrofolate as common substrates. In addition, glycine and formate were found to be needed for purine synthesis. The precursors of the carbon and nitrogen atoms in the purine and pyrimidine rings are illustrated in Figure 5.12.

5.8.2 Purine and Pyrimidine Bases in Nucleotides

Purine (adenine and guanine) and pyrimidine (cytosine, uracil, and thymine) bases are components of nucleosides and nucleotides (phosphorylated nucleosides) in all cell types (Table 5.8). Nucleoside triphosphates are the monomer unit precursors of ribonucleic acid, which has two types: deoxyribonucleic acid (DNA) and ribonucleic acid (RNA). DNA, which contains the genetic information, consists of four deoxynucleotides: deoxyadenylate, deoxyguanylate, deoxycytidylate, and thymidylate (methylated deoxyuridylate). These monomeric units of DNA are held together by 3′, 5′-phosphodiester bridges to constitute a single strand. Two complementary strands of DNA are paired through hydrogen bonding between adenine and thymidine, as well as between guanosine and cytidine to form a double-stranded helical molecule (Blanco and Blanco 2017). By contrast, RNA is a polymer of purine (adenine and guanine) and pyrimidine (cytosine and uracil)

TABLE 5.8
Purines, Pyrimidines, Nucleosides, Nucleotides, and Nucleic Acids

Heterocyclic Compound	Base	Nucleoside (Base + Ribose or Deoxyribose)	Nucleotide (Base + Ribose 5-Phosphate)	Nucleic Acid
Purine	Adenine	Adenosine	Adenosine monophosphate	DNA and RNA
Purine	Guanine	Guanosine	Guanosine monophosphate	DNA and RNA
Pyrimidine	Cytosine	Cytidine	Cytidine monophosphate	DNA and RNA
Pyrimidine	Uracil	Uridine	Uridine monophosphate	RNA
Pyrimidine	Thymine	Thymidine	Thymidine monophosphate	DNA

Note: DNA, deoxyribonucleic acid; RNA, ribonucleic acid.

ribonucleotides linked by 3′, 5′-phosphodiester bridges as a single-strand molecule. At present, little is known about the content of purines and pyrimidines in foodstuffs for humans and other animals.

5.8.3 Synthesis of Purine Nucleotides

In animal and bacterial cells, purine nucleotides are synthesized by *de novo* and salvage pathways via enzyme-catalyzed reactions in the cytoplasm (Lane and Fan 2015). The *de novo* pathway requires, as starting materials, glutamine, glycine, aspartate, ribose-5-P (a product of glucose metabolism via the pentose cycle), ATP, HCO_3^-, and tetrahydrofolate (Figure 5.13). Intermediates of this pathway include 5-phosphoribosyl-1-pyrophosphate (PRPP), glycinamide ribosyl-5-P, formylglycinamidine ribosyl-5-P, and 5-aminoimidazole-4-carboxamide ribosyl-5-P. In the salvage pathway, purine bases, released from the hydrolysis of nucleic acids and nucleotides, can be salvaged and recycled into purine nucleotides. Adenine phosphoribosyltransferase catalyzes the formation of AMP from PRPP and adenosine. Furthermore, hypoxanthine-guanine phosphoribosyltransferase catalyzes the formation of guanosine monophosphate (GMP) or inosine monophosphate (IMP) from PRPP and guanine or hypoxanthine, respectively. The enzymes in both the *de novo* and salvage pathways are present as a macromolecular aggregate to increase the efficiency of purine nucleotide synthesis in cells.

Control of purine nucleotide synthesis occurs primarily at three steps (Kim et al. 1992; Pedley and Benkovic 2017). The first regulatory step is the production of PRPP by PRPP synthetase, which is activated by inorganic phosphate and inactivated by purine ribonucleotides. The second controlled step in purine nucleotide synthesis is catalyzed by amidophosphoribosyltransferase (APRT). Specifically, APRT is under allosteric control by feedback inhibition. AMP, GMP, or IMP alone can inhibit this enzyme, while either AMP plus GMP or AMP plus IMP acts synergistically as inhibitors. The nucleotides inhibit APRT by causing the enzyme to aggregate to a larger inactive complex. PRPP can also regulate APRT activity, because intracellular concentrations of PRPP are normally below the K_M of APRT for PRPP. Of particular note, very high concentrations of PRPP can overcome the nucleotide feedback inhibition by converting a large, inactive aggregate of APRT into a small active enzyme. The third controlled step in purine nucleotide synthesis involves the maintenance of an appropriate balance between intracellular concentrations of ATP and GTP. This is because (1) each of these two purine nucleotides stimulates the synthesis of the other by providing energy, (2) ATP and GTP are required for GMP and AMP syntheses, respectively, and (3) GMP inhibits the conversion of IMP to xanthine monophosphate, whereas AMP inhibits the conversion of IMP to adenylosuccinate. It is now known that in response to high demands for purines, the *de novo* purine biosynthetic enzymes cluster near mitochondria and microtubules to form dynamic multienzyme complexes (purinosomes). The generation of the purinosomes maximizes the rates of purine production.

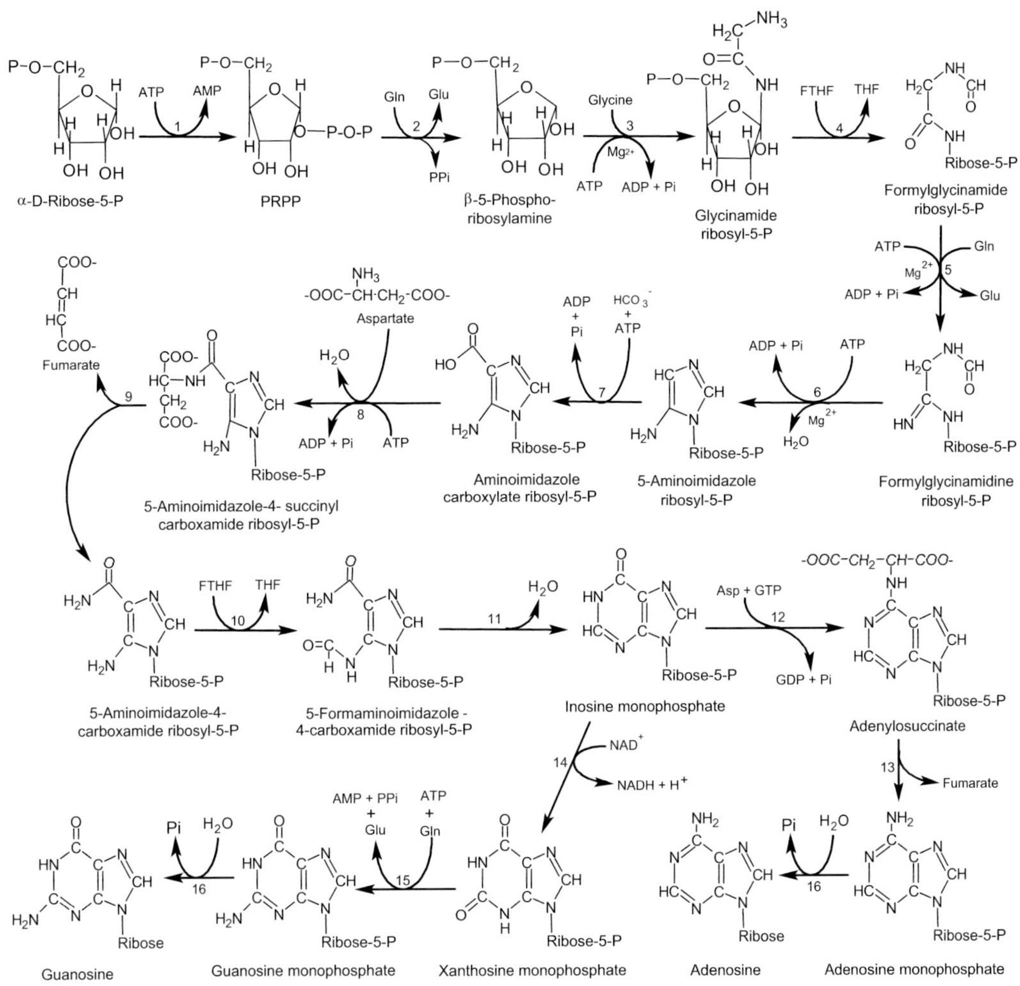

FIGURE 5.13 The pathway for *de novo* synthesis of purine nucleosides from ribose-5-phosphate, glutamine, glycine, aspartate, bicarbonate, and formate in humans and other animals. The enzymes that catalyze the indicated reactions are (1) ribose phosphate pyrophosphokinase (5-phosphoribosyl-1-pyrophosphate synthetase); (2) amidophosphoribosyltransferase (glutamine PRPP amidotransferase); (3) glycinamide ribosyl-5-P (also known as glycinamide ribotide or glycinamide ribonucleotide) synthetase; (4) glycinamide transformylase; (5) formylglycinamidine ribosyl-5-P synthetase; (6) 5-aminoimidazole ribosyl-5-P synthetase; (7) 5-aminoimidazole ribosyl-5-P carboxylase; (8) 5-aminoimidazole-4-succinylocarboxamide ribosyl-5-P synthetase; (9) adenylosuccinate lyase; (10) 5-aminoimidazole-4-carboxamide ribosyl-5-P (AICAR) transformylase; (11) inosine monophosphate cyclohydrolase; (12) adenylosuccinate synthetase; (13) adenylosuccinate lyase; (14) inosine monophosphate dehydrogenase; (15) guanosine monophosphate synthase; and (16) 5'-nucleotidase. FTHF, N^{10}-formyl-tetrahydrofolate; PRPP, 5-phosphoribosyl-1-pyrophosphate; and THF, tetrahydrofolate.

5.8.4 SYNTHESIS OF PYRIMIDINE NUCLEOTIDES

In animal and bacterial cells, pyrimidine nucleotides are synthesized by *de novo* and salvage pathways (Lane and Fan 2015). The *de novo* synthesis of pyrimidine nucleotides depends on the availability of glutamine, aspartate, ribose-5-P, ATP, HCO_3^-, and tetrahydrofolate (Figure 5.14). In animals, this synthetic pathway spans both the cytoplasm and mitochondria, with high activities in tissues possessing rapid rates of protein synthesis such as the gastrointestinal tract, liver, spleen, testis, and thymus. In bacteria, pyrimidine nucleotides are synthesized *de novo* in the cytoplasm.

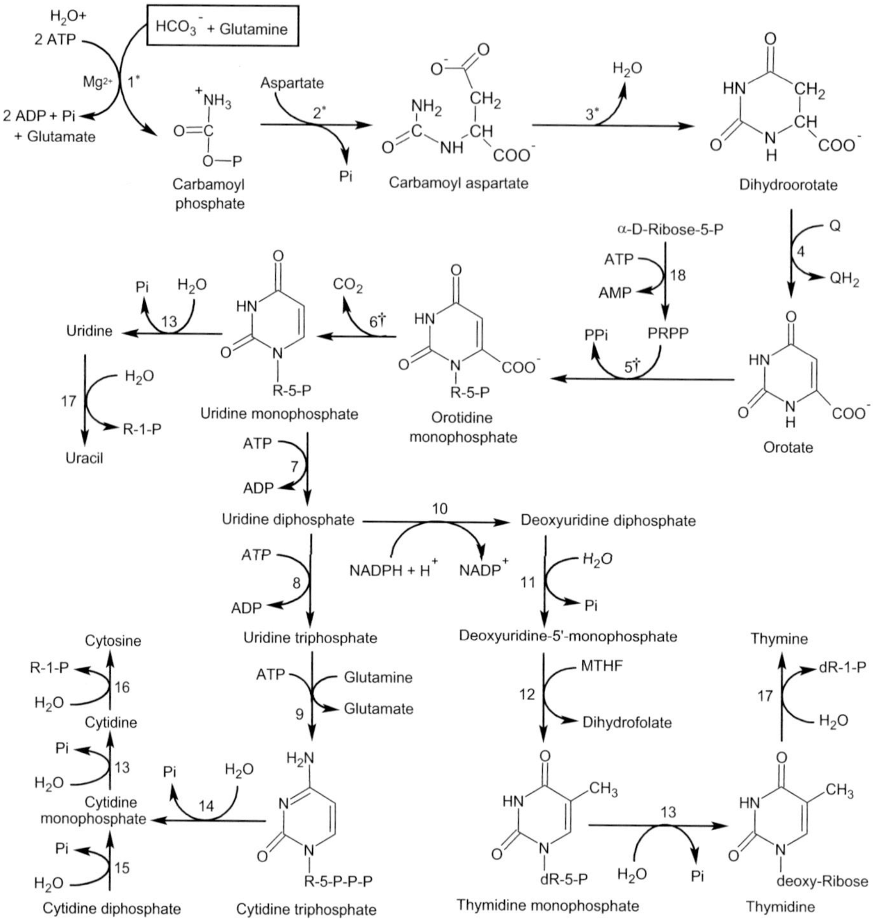

FIGURE 5.14 The pathway for *de novo* synthesis of pyrimidine nucleotides from glutamine, aspartate, and bicarbonate in humans and other animals. The enzymes that catalyze the indicated reactions are (1) carbamoylphosphate synthetase II; (2) aspartate transcarbamylase; (3) dihydroorotase; (4) dihydroorotate dehydrogenase (a mitochondrial enzyme); (5) orotate phosphoribosyltransferase; (6) orotidine monophosphate decarboxylase; (7) uridine monophosphate kinase; (8) uridine diphosphate kinase; (9) cytidine triphosphate synthetase; (10) ribonucleotide reductase (thioredoxin is required for the activity of this enzyme); (11) nucleotide phosphatase; and (12) thymidylate synthetase. Note that (a) in animals, the catalytic activities of carbamoylphosphate synthetase II, aspartate transcarbamylase, and dihydroorotase are carried out by a trifunctional protein (known as CAD protein); (b) the catalytic activities of orotate phosphoribosyltransferase and orotidine monophosphate decarboxylase are carried out by a bifunctional enzyme (known as uridine monophosphate synthase) in animals and other multicellular organisms, but are separate proteins encoded by two different genes in bacteria and yeast; and (c) in animal cells, pyrimidine nucleotide synthesis involves the cytoplasm and mitochondria, as dihydroorotate is transported from the cytoplasm to the mitochondria for conversion into orotate by dihydroorotate dehydrogenase. The latter is located in the inner mitochondrial membrane, with its substrate-binding site facing the mitochondrial intermembrane space, and requires quinone as an electron acceptor. Orotate is then transported out of the mitochondria into the cytoplasm for further metabolism. dR-5-P, deoxyribose-5-phosphate; MTHF, N^5-N-^{10}-methylenetetrahydrofolate; Q, quinone; QH_2, reduced quinone; PRPP, 5-phosphoribosyl-1-pyrophosphate; R-1-P, ribose-1-phosphate; R-5-P-P-P, ribose-5-triphosphate; and THF, tetrahydrofolate; * In animals, these three enzymatic activities are possessed in one trifunctional protein, called CAD protein (consisting of carbamoylphosphate synthetase II, aspartate transcarbamylase, and dihydroorotase); [†], In animals, these two enzymatic activities are possessed in one bifunctional protein, designated as UMPS (uridine monophosphate synthase). Both CAD protein and UMPS are cytosolic proteins that are considered to be closely associated with each other outside the outer mitochondrial membrane in proximity to dihydroorotate dehydrogenase on the inner mitochondrial membrane.

Like purines, the sugar phosphate portion of the pyrimidine molecule is supplied by PRPP. However, in contrast to *de novo* purine synthesis in which a nucleotide is formed first (Figure 5.13), pyrimidines are first synthesized as free bases before their attachment to ribose-5-P and there is no branch in the pyrimidine synthesis pathway. In both animal and bacterial cells, pyrimidine bases and ribonucleosides are salvaged to nucleotides by the following reactions:

Cytosine + $H_2O \rightarrow$ Uracil + NH_3 (spontaneously or cytosine deaminase)

Cytidine + ATP $\rightarrow$ Cytidine monophosphate + ADP   (uridine/cytidine kinase)

Deoxycytidine + ATP $\rightarrow$ Deoxycytidine monophosphate + ADP   (deoxycytidine kinase)

Uracil + Ribose-1-P $\rightarrow$ Uridine + Pi   (uridine phosphorylase)

Uridine + ATP $\rightarrow$ Uridine monophosphate + ADP   (uridine/cytidine kinase)

Deoxyuridine + ATP $\rightarrow$ Deoxyuridine monophosphate + ADP   (thymidine kinase)

Thymine + Deoxyribose-1-P $\rightarrow$ Thymidine + Pi   (thymine phosphorylase)

Thymidine + ATP $\rightarrow$ Thymidine monophosphate + ADP   (thymidine kinase)

The control of pyrimidine nucleotide synthesis is exerted primarily at the level of carbamoylphosphate synthase II, which is part of a trifunctional protein known as CAD protein (made up of carbamoylphosphate synthetase II, aspartate transcarbamylase, and dihydroorotase) found in animals (Evans and Guy 2004). This enzyme is inhibited by UTP (acting competitively with ATP) but activated by PRPP. Unlike the mitochondrial carbamoylphosphate synthase I, the cytosolic carbamoylphosphate synthase II is not activated by *N*-acetylglutamate synthase. Secondary sites of control are the inhibition of orotate monophosphate decarboxylase (part of the bifunctional UMP synthase) by uridine monophosphate and cytidine monophosphate. A frequent inborn error of pyrimidine nucleotide synthesis is a mutation of the UMP synthase, preventing the conversion of orotate into UMP and the accumulation of orotate in the plasma and urine (Brosnan and Brosnan 2007). In bacteria, aspartate transcarbamylase is a key regulatory enzyme in pyrimidine synthesis, where carbamoyl phosphate participates in the synthesis of either pyrimidine nucleotides or arginine in the cytoplasm.

5.8.5 CATABOLISM OF PURINES AND PYRIMIDINES

Concentrations of purines and pyrimidines in cells depend on the rates of their synthesis and degradation (Lane and Fan 2015). The catabolism of these nucleotides occurs primarily in the liver, although other cell types contain some of the enzymes in the degradation pathways. Figure 5.15 illustrates the pathways for the conversion of AMP, IMP, xanthosine monophosphate, and GMP by 5-nucleotidase to adenosine, inosine, xanthosine, and guanosine, respectively. Xanthosine is converted into xanthine through the action of purine nucleoside phosphorylase. The further catabolism of adenosine, inosine, and guanosine to uric acid and allantoin will be described in Chapter 6.

In contrast to purines, catabolism of pyrimidines in the liver produces water-soluble metabolites, including CO_2, ammonia, β-alanine, and β-aminoisobutyrate (Figure 5.16). Some of the β-aminoisobutyrate is transaminated to form methylmalonate semialdehyde, which is subsequently metabolized to succinyl-CoA. The remaining β-aminoisobutyrate is excreted in the urine. Interestingly, approximately 25% of human adults of Chinese or Japanese ancestry routinely excrete large amounts of β-aminoisobutyrate in the urine, indicating individual differences in pyrimidine metabolism (Blanco and Blanco 2017; Yanai et al. 1969). This is a genetically transmitted metabolic characteristic and does not result in any clinical disorders.

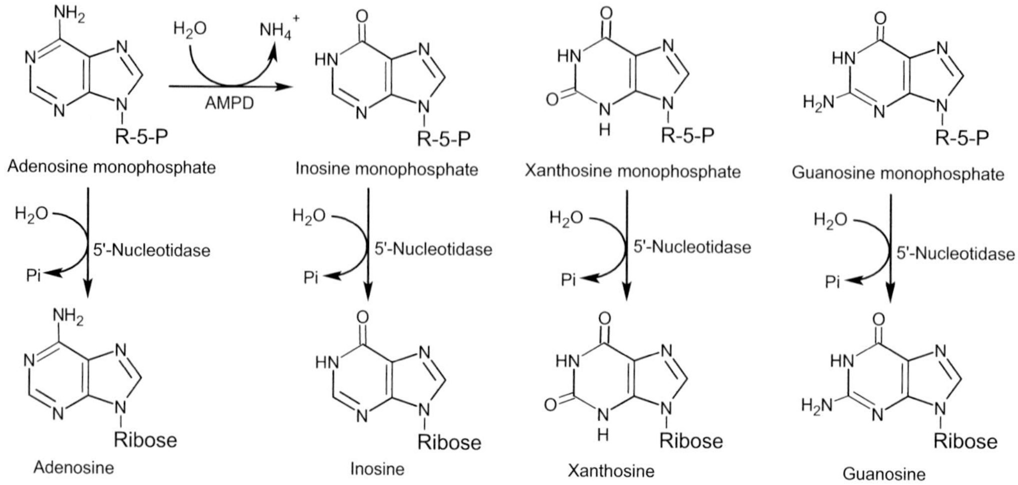

FIGURE 5.15 Catabolism of purine nucleotides to purine nucleosides in animals. These reactions occur virtually in all cell types, with hepatocytes being the most active. Adenosine, inosine, and guanosine are degraded to uric acid in humans and other animals. AMPD, adenosine monophosphate (AMP) deaminase; R-5-P, ribose-5-phosphate.

5.9 HEME SYNTHESIS AND CATABOLISM

5.9.1 History of Heme Research

Heme (MW, 616.5 Da) is a highly lipophilic iron-porphyrin. The history of its discovery dates back to 1747 when the Italian physician V.A. Menghini found that the blood contains iron. Almost one century later, in 1840, F.L. Hünefeld discovered hemoglobin, which accounts for 97% of the dry matter content in red blood cells. Hemoglobin was described then as a protein, but its actual composition was unknown. In 1841, during the course of investigating the nature of the blood, H. Scherer discovered porphyrin (a dark red substance) after treating the dried blood with concentrated sulfuric acid followed by the sequential removal of precipitated iron and then protein through alcohol treatment. In 1844, G.J. Mulder determined the composition of this iron-free substance (named *hematin*) derived from the blood and found that hematin can take up molecular oxygen. In 1853, L.K. Teichmann discovered hemin (also known as Teichmann's crystals) in the blood, which was later found to be the hydrochloride of heme. Following the coining of the term "porphyrin" (a Greek word, meaning reddish-purple) by F. Hoppe-Seyler in 1864, J.L.W. Thudichum prepared the first porphyrin (a red porphyrin with a unique spectrum and fluorescence properties) from hemoglobin through treatment with concentrated acid in 1867. In 1871, E.F. Hoppe-Seyler crystallized hematin and reported its physiological property of reversibly binding molecular oxygen. Between 1874 and 1889, human diseases associated with abnormal porphyrin metabolism and reddish urine were described. Meanwhile, C.A. MacMunn discovered heme-containing pigments (now known as cytochromes) in animal tissues in 1884. The chemical composition of heme was identified by H. Bertin-Sans and J. de Moitessier in 1892.

In the early 1900s, H. Fisher began his groundbreaking research on porphyrin chemistry. By 1915, he had shown that uroporphyrins differ from coproporphyrins and hematoporphyrins. Subsequently, he synthesized porphyrins in 1925, hemin in 1929 (for which he won the 1930 Nobel Prize in Chemistry), and bilirubin (which was previously found by him to be a product of hemin degradation) in 1944. Among the first biochemists to use [15]N- and ^{14}C-labeled substrates and metabolites, D. Shemin and D. Rittenberg elucidated the metabolic pathways for mammalian heme synthesis in 1945. Using X-ray crystallography, M. Perutz determined in 1959 the molecular

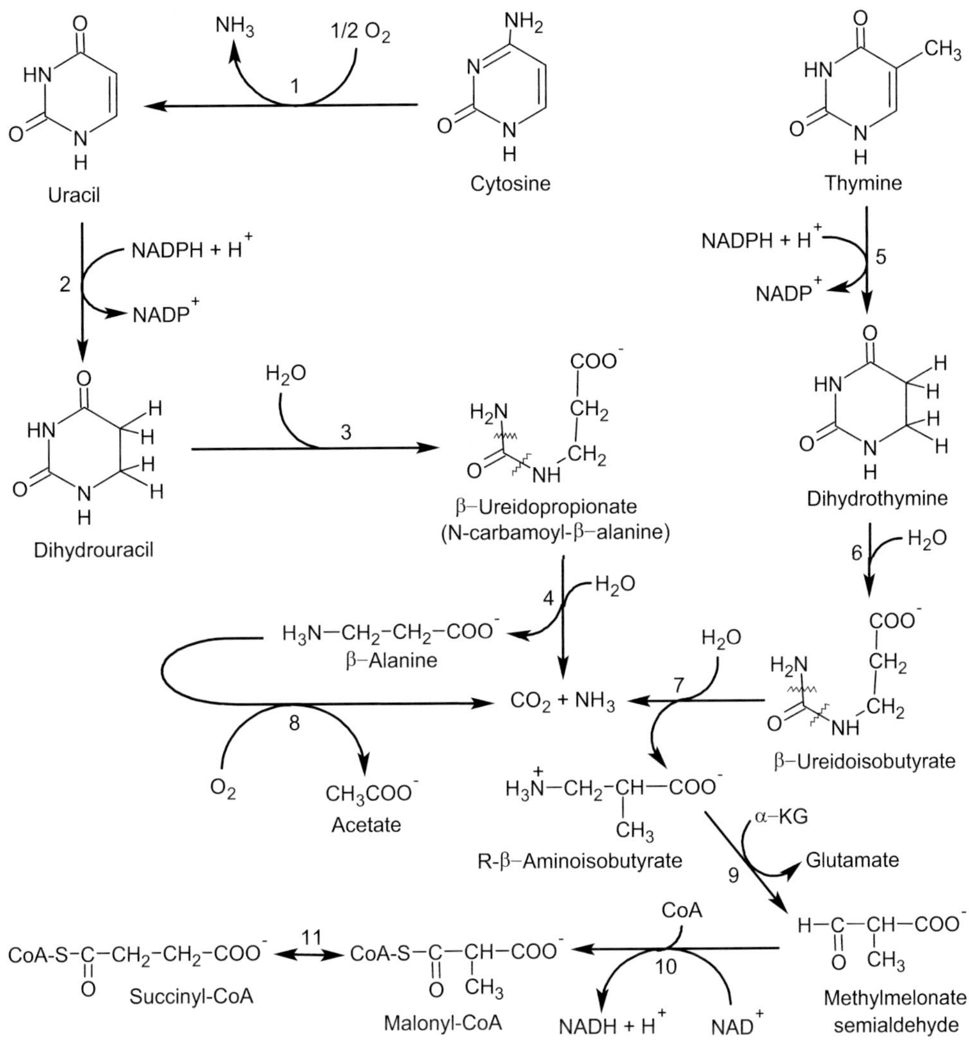

FIGURE 5.16 Catabolism of pyrimidine nucleosides in humans and other animals. The enzymes that catalyze the indicated reactions are (1) cytosine deaminase; (2) uracil reductase (also known as dihydropyrimidine dehydrogenase); (3) dihydrouracil hydratase; (4) β-ureidopropionase; (5) thymine reductase (also known as dihydropyrimidine dehydrogenase); (6) dihydrothymine hydratase; (7) β-ureidoisobutyrate hydratase; (8) a series of enzymes, which includes β-alanine:pyruvate transaminase (forming malonic semialdehyde and alanine), β-alanine:α-ketoglutarate transaminase (forming malonic semialdehyde and glutamate), alanine aminotransferase, glutamate dehydrogenase, malonate semialdehyde dehydrogenase (catalyzing both dehydrogenation and decarboxylation of malonate semialdehyde to form acetaldehyde), and aldehyde dehydrogenase (forming acetyl-CoA); (9) β-aminoisobutyrate:α-ketoglutarate transaminase; (10) methylmalonate semialdehyde dehydrogenase; and (11) methylmalonyl-CoA isomerase. These reactions occur in virtually all cell types, with hepatocytes being the most active. α-KG, α-ketoglutarate.

structure of hemoglobin, which contains both four heme molecules and four globin polypeptides (2 α-subunits and 2 β-subunits) as a tetramer. This work resulted in his winning the 1962 Nobel Prize in Chemistry.

Heme is a component of hemoglobin (a heterotetrameric oxygen-transporting protein), myoglobin (a monomeric oxygen-storing protein), and other heme-containing proteins (including enzymes). Hemoglobin accounts for 85% of the total heme in humans (Ferreira 2013). The concentrations of hemoglobin in the blood of healthy adult men and women are 13.5-17.5 and 12.0-15.5 g per 100 mL, respectively. By weight, 1 g of hemoglobin contains 38.2 mg of heme and 3.46 mg of iron. Heme constitutes 95% of iron in the human body and about two-thirds of dietary iron intake by humans in developed nations.

5.9.2 PATHWAYS OF HEME SYNTHESIS IN ANIMAL CELLS

Heme is synthesized from glycine and succinyl-CoA (a metabolite of glucose and glucogenic AAs) by virtually all cell types in aerobic organisms (Ajioka et al. 2006). In humans, approximately 85% of heme is synthesized in immature red blood cells (erythroid cells) in the bone marrow during their development from proerythroblasts to reticulocytes, and the remaining 15% is synthesized primarily in the liver (mainly hepatocytes) and to a much lesser extent in other organs (Blanco and Blanco 2017). Similar tissue distributions of heme synthesis occur in *birds*, amphibians, and reptiles. In fish, which lack bone marrow, lymph nodes, and adrenal glands, their head kidney is the adult hematopoietic organ functionally analogous to the mammalian bone marrow [including its ability to synthesize heme and produce red blood cells (erythropoiesis)] (Li et al. 2020). In fish and amphibians, the earliest erythropoiesis takes place in the yolk sac, followed by internal organs, such as the kidneys, spleen, and liver.

In erythroid cells and hepatocytes, as well as the fish's head kidney, the metabolic pathway for heme synthesis can be divided into three phases: (1) condensation of succinyl-CoA with glycine to form δ-aminolevulinic acid (ALA) in mitochondria, (2) conversion of ALA into coproporphyrinogen III in the cytoplasm, and (3) synthesis of heme from coproporphyrinogen III in the mitochondria (Figure 5.17). Four mitochondrial enzymes involved in heme synthesis are localized within the mitochondrial inner membrane, with the active site of ferrochelatase being on the matrix-facing side of the membrane. Such strategic metabolic channeling ensures a high efficiency for this metabolic pathway. Stoichiometrically, the synthesis of 1 mol of heme requires 2 mol of glycine and 2 mol of succinyl-CoA. Heme synthesis does not occur in mature erythrocytes that contain neither nuclei nor mitochondria, or in some other cells at the very end of their differentiation pathways.

5.9.3 REGULATION OF HEME SYNTHESIS IN ANIMAL CELLS

Heme synthesis depends on not only the amounts of the enzymes but also on the availabilities of AAs, glucose, iron, vitamin B_6, and vitamin C (Ajioka et al. 2006). Thus, nutrition, including the transport of nutrients, plays a crucial role in this synthetic event in both the bone marrow and liver. Common to heme synthesis in both bone marrow and the liver is the inhibition of porphobilinogen synthase and ferrochelatase by lead, which is the biochemical basis for the toxicity of the heavy metal (Layer et al. 2010). However, heme synthesis is regulated differently in erythroid cells compared to hepatocytes, at molecular levels, reflecting the different functions of heme in these two cell types. In the liver, heme is the prosthetic group of many proteins involved in cellular respiration and antioxidation reactions. In differentiating erythroid cells, the additional function of heme is to serve as a component of hemoglobin. There are tissue-specific mechanisms for the regulation of heme synthesis (Ponka 1997).

5.9.3.1 Regulation of Heme Synthesis in Hepatocytes

In the liver, the major control target in heme synthesis is δ-aminolevulinic acid synthase (ALAS), which has a relatively short half-life (approximately 60 min). Heme, hemin, or metalloporphyrins suppress hepatic heme synthesis through (1) the direct feedback inhibition of ALAS activity, (2) the inhibition of ALAS synthesis, and (3) the inhibition of the transport of ALAS from its site of synthesis in the cytoplasm to its site of action in mitochondria (Ajioka et al. 2006). The molecular mechanisms responsible for these effects of heme involve the binding of heme to the cysteine-proline

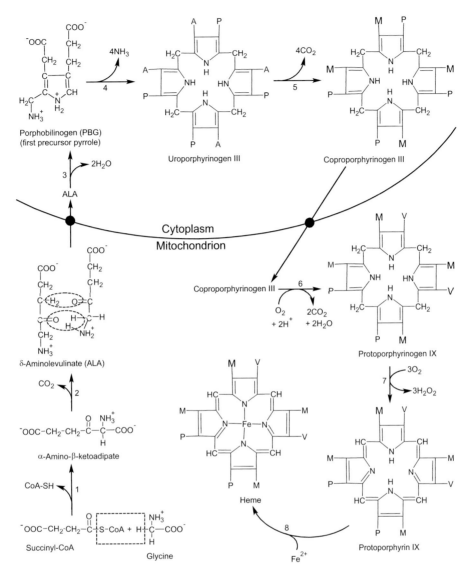

FIGURE 5.17 Synthesis of heme from glycine, succinyl-CoA, and iron in humans and other animals. This synthetic pathway consists of a series of eight enzymatic reactions that originate in the mitochondria, continue in the cytosol, and complete in the mitochondria. The enzymes that catalyze the indicated reactions are (1) and (2) δ-aminolevulinic acid synthase (ALAS, a pyridoxal phosphate-dependent enzyme localized in the matrix side of the inner mitochondrial membrane); (3) porphobilinogen synthase (a Zn-requiring enzyme; also known as ALA dehydratase); (4) uroporphyrinogen synthase (also known as porphobilinogen deaminase or hydroxymethylbilane synthase) and uroporphyrinogen III cosynthase; (5) uroporphyrinogen decarboxylase; (6) coproporphyrinogen oxidase; (7) protoporphyrinogen oxidase (an FAD-dependent enzyme); and (8) ferrochelatase. Note that (a) there are two forms of the ALAS, with ALAS-1 expressed in all cell types and ALAS-2 specifically in erythroid cells and fetal liver; (b) the CO_2 lost in the ALAS-catalyzed reaction originates from the carboxyl group of glycine; (c) ALA exits from the mitochondria to the cytoplasm, where two molecules of ALA are linked to yield the pyrrole ring compound porphobilinogen; (d) coproporphyrinogen III in the cytoplasm is transported into mitochondria for its decarboxylation by coproporphyrinogen oxidase to form protoporphyrinogen IX; (e) coproporphyrinogen oxidase requires molecular oxygen and is inactive under anaerobic conditions, and this enzyme is not affected by NAD(P)+, NAD(P)H, FAD, FMN, riboflavin, or ATP; and (f) ferrochelatase inserts Fe^{2+} into the tetrapyrrole nucleus of protoporphyrin IX to produce heme in the presence of ascorbic acid and cysteine or reduced glutathione.

motifs of *ALAS-1* and those of the transcriptional repressor Bach1, thereby repressing the expression of the genes for ALAS-1 and the ALAS-1 transporter. This results in the inhibition of the translocation of the ALAS-1 protein from the cytoplasm to mitochondria where the functionally active ALAS acts (Figure 5.17).

Fasting increases, while elevated levels of glucose suppress, expression of ALAS-1 in hepatocytes, whereas nonheme iron (including dietary supplementation with iron) has no effect. Additionally, phospholipids (e.g., phosphatidylethanolamine and L-α-lysophosphatidylcholine) increase hepatic ALAS activity (Blanco and Blanco 2017). Results of recent studies have shown that the expression of the peroxisome proliferator-activated receptor coactivator 1 *(PGC-1α)* gene mediates the stimulating effect of fasting on the expression of hepatic ALAS-1. Specifically, through coactivating nuclear respiratory factor 1 (NRF-1) and forkhead box protein O1 (FOXO1), both of which directly bind to the *ALAS-1* promoter, PGC-1α enhances ALAS-1 expression. Thus, knockout of the liver-specific *PGC-1α* gene in mice prevents a fasting-induced increase in hepatic ALAS activity (Handschin et al. 2005). In animals, glucose reduces ALAS-1 expression in hepatocytes through increased secretion of insulin and decreased secretion of glucagon. Insulin can activate the protein kinase Akt, which then phosphorylates FOXO1. This results in impaired binding of FOXO1 to PGC-1α and its export from the nucleus, thereby inhibiting the action of PGC-1α on ALAS-1 expression.

Peroxisome proliferator-activated receptor-α (PPAR-α) increases the expression of ALAS-1 in hepatocytes (Degenhardt et al. 2009). This effect of PPAR-α is mediated by two functional PPAR-binding sites at positions −9 and −2.3 kb relative to the *ALAS1* transcription start site. Additionally, PPAR-α enhances the expression of ALA dehydratase, uroporphyrinogen III synthase, uroporphyrinogen decarboxylase, coproporphyrinogen oxidase, and protoporphyrinogen oxidase in hepatocytes, resulting in increased synthesis of heme. Thus, PPAR-α may beneficially improve heme homeostasis in the liver. By contrast, hypoxia reduces heme synthesis in hepatocytes by decreasing the transcription of the genes for uroporphyrinogen synthase and uroporphyrinogen III cosynthase without affecting the half-lives (approximately 9–10 h) of their mRNAs. These results suggest that transcription plays an important role in regulating the expression of the heme-synthetic genes in the liver.

5.9.3.2 Regulation of Heme Synthesis in Erythroid Cells

Erythropoiesis drives heme synthesis in immature erythroid cells. In reticulocytes, major factors limiting heme synthesis include not only ALAS-2, but also uroporphyrinogen synthase and ferrochelatase, as well as the transport of iron in the plasma by transferrin and the uptake of the iron-transferrin complex by cells via receptor-mediated endocytosis (Chiabrando et al. 2014). At the transcriptional level, expression of the transferrin receptor 1 and ferrochelatase genes, like many other genes, is controlled by their methylation status. For example, 5-aza-2′-deoxycytidine (5-aza-CdR; a hypomethylating agent) and its derivatives can stimulate heme synthesis by inducing erythroid cell differentiation and increasing the expression of transferrin receptor 1 and ferrochelatase. Recent studies have identified new regulatory E-boxes outside of CpG islands in the transferrin receptor 1 and ferrochelatase promoters and have shown that the methylation status of these sites is altered by 5-aza-CdR. Nuclear translocation of the transcription factor c-myc and its subsequent binding to these promoter elements results in increased expression of the transferrin receptor 1 and ferrochelatase genes.

In contrast to hepatocytes, physiological levels of heme or hemin stimulate the synthesis of proteins in erythroid cells, such as globin and the enzymes involved in heme synthesis (including ALAS-2, ferrochelatase, and the receptor for the iron-transferrin complex) (Beuzard et al. 1973). The global increase in protein synthesis brought about by elevated levels of heme results from an inhibition of eFI-2α kinase activity, leading to reduced phosphorylation of eFI-2α, a key factor in the initiation of polypeptide synthesis. The coordinated increases in the synthesis of both heme and globin ensure the correct ratio of these two components for assembly into hemoglobin. In explaining the different mechanisms in the control of heme synthesis between erythroid and nonerythroid cells, emerging evidence shows that ALAS-1 and ALAS-2 differ in their gene structure (including the DNA sequence encoding the heme regulatory motif) and transcription patterns (Chiabrando et al. 2014). For example, results from studies with mouse reticulocytes indicate that over 90% of the total ferrochelatase mRNA is present as the 2.2 kb transcript, a characteristic phenomenon not found for hepatocytes. This 2.2 kb transcript is produced due to the preferential utilization of the upstream polyadenylation signal in the erythrocyte ferrochelatase gene.

5.9.4 Catabolism of Heme in Animal Cells

Depending on cell type, the intracellular degradation of heme-containing proteins in the cytoplasm (e.g., NOS, hemoglobin, and myoglobin), mitochondria (e.g., cytochromes), peroxisomes (e.g., catalase), and other organelles (e.g., nucleus) releases their heme into membrane-bound vesicles of the endo-lysosomal system. Red blood cells (with a life span of approximately 120 days in humans) contain approximately 85% of the heme in the body (Blanco and Blanco 2017). When these cells are aged or injured and when hemorrhage occurs, they release large amounts of heme into the circulation. Other cell types, including hepatocytes, skeletal muscle, cardiac myocytes, and macrophages, contain about 15% of the heme in the organism. Recently, a heme transporter HRG-1 was identified in the endolysosomal system to transport heme from the site of its release to the site of its degradation (White et al. 2013). While red blood cells were known in the 19th century to be a source of color compounds, including biliverdin and bilirubin, it was only in 1968 when R. Tenhunen discovered heme oxygenase (HO) that the metabolic pathways for heme catabolism via interorgan cooperation began to be unraveled (Figure 5.18).

$$\text{Heme} + [O] \rightarrow \text{CO (carbon monoxide)} + Fe^{3+} + \text{Biliverdin} \qquad \text{(heme oxygenase)}$$

Cleavage of the heme methene bridge is initiated by membrane-bound HO to form equimolar amounts of CO, Fe^{3+}, and biliverdin (a green, lipophilic, and linear tetrapyrrole). The HO system depends on NADPH-cytochrome 450 for its catalytic activity. There are three isoforms of HO, namely HO1 (also known as heat-shock protein 32), HO2, and HO3 with different intracellular trafficking patterns (Kikuchi et al. 2005). HO1 is a highly inducible protein (e.g., induced by heme and other agents) and its activity can increase up to 100-fold when cells are treated with oxidants, endotoxins, or inflammatory cytokines. By contrast, HO2 is constitutively expressed and its activity is not altered by these compounds. HO1 and HO2 proteins are encoded by two different genes. In 1997, the HO3 cDNA was isolated from the rat brain and its protein was purified. Recent work shows that white adipose tissue expresses HO3 and its mRNA levels are markedly increased by L-arginine (Fu et al. 2005). The predicted AA sequence of HO3 differs from that of HO1, but has ~90% identity with HO2. Many cell types (including the liver, spleen, brain, heart, and macrophages) express HO1 and HO2. Erythroid precursor cells lack a significant level of HO1 and exhibit progressive reduction in HO2 expression during differentiation. Mature erythrocytes have little HO activity. Thus, heme released from these cells is taken up by other cell types for degradation by the various isoforms of HO.

Biliverdin is reduced to bilirubin (a highly lipophilic antioxidant; red-orange color) by biliverdin reductase, which is a soluble cytosolic enzyme (O'Brien et al. 2015). In the liver, some of the bilirubin is esterified with glucuronic acid (a metabolite of glucose) to form a more hydrophilic substance, bilirubin diglucuronide. This reaction is catalyzed by bilirubin glucuronyl transferase, whose low activity in the liver of infants (particularly preterm infants) causes the accumulation of bilirubin in the blood, skin, and the tissues surrounding the eyes, leading to jaundice (Maisels 2015). In

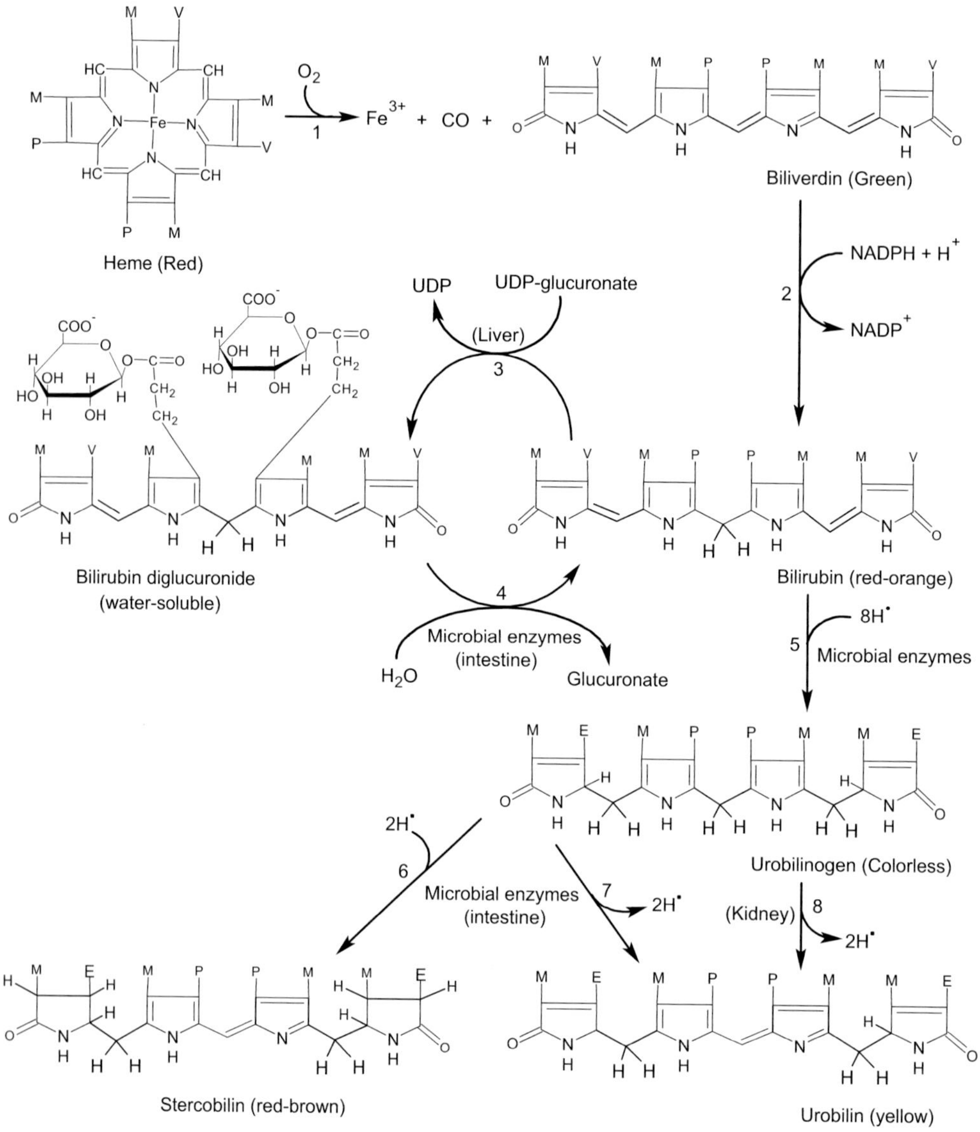

FIGURE 5.18 Catabolism of heme via interorgan cooperation in humans and other animals. The enzymes that catalyze the indicated reactions are (1) heme oxygenase; (2) biliverdin reductase; (3) bilirubin glucuronyl transferase (a microsomal enzyme); (4) β-glucuronidases; (5) intestinal microbial enzymes (bilirubin reductases); (6) intestinal microbial enzymes (urobilinogen oxidases and urobilinogen reductases); (7) intestinal microbial enzymes (urobilinogen dehydrogenases); and (8) urobilinogen dehydrogenase (kidneys). Note that this series of reactions releases iron from heme and generates some colored metabolites (e.g., green, yellow, or red-brown).

healthy individuals, bilirubin diglucuronide is secreted into the bile. In the lumen of the intestines, microbial enzymes convert bilirubin and bilirubin diglucuronide to urobilinogen. Most of the urobilinogen is further reduced by microbial enzymes to generate stercobilin (red-brown color), which is then excreted in feces. Some of the urobilinogen is taken up by the kidneys where it is oxidized to urobilin (yellow color), which is excreted in the urine. Thus, the color of feces and urine is a useful indicator of heme degradation in the body and the development of certain diseases (e.g., hepatitis, liver cancer, and colorectal cancer).

5.10 SYNTHESIS AND CATABOLISM OF HISTAMINE

5.10.1 SYNTHESIS OF HISTAMINE

Histamine (formerly known as β-iminazolylethylamine) was the second AA-derived amine to be isolated, following tyramine. Work on histamine began in 1907 when it was first chemically synthesized by A. Windaus and W. Vogt. In 1910, this substance was obtained for the first time by D. Ackermann from putrefactive organisms treated with histidine. In the same year, G. Barger and H. Dale and F. Kutscher simultaneously announced the isolation of histamine from ergot extracts. In 1936, W. Bloch and H. Pinösch reported that administrating large amounts of histidine to guinea pigs resulted in increases in urinary excretion of histamine and in the concentration of histamine in the lungs. One year later, E. Werle and H. Herrmann identified the presence of histidine decarboxylase (a cytosolic enzyme) in animal tissues, including the small intestine, stomach, lungs, and brain. Using [^{14}C]histidine, R.W. Schayer demonstrated the mammalian biosynthesis of histamine from histidine in 1952. Bacterial histidine decarboxylase was characterized by H.M. Epps in 1945. In both eukaryotic and prokaryotic cells, histidine decarboxylase requires pyridoxal phosphate for its catalytic activity (Moya-Garcia et al. 2005). In response to allergens, the production and release of histamine by mast cells are markedly increased. This enzyme is inhibited by synthetic histidine analogues. In addition, it is possible that histidine decarboxylase is potently inhibited and/or the actions of histamine on cells are effectively blocked by heat-stable catechin-like phytochemicals [e.g., those in the soup (water-soluble extracts plus the solid portion) of green mung beans *Vigna radiata*, which is prepared through boiling the beans in water for about 30 min, followed by the addition of a small amount of brown sugar for flavor]. Thus, the consumption of the soup by humans after its cooling down to a room temperature (e.g., 25°C–30°C) can rapidly alleviate allergic reactions [e.g., hives (red bumps) on the skin] within minutes. Despite the physiological and immunological importance of histamine, the transcriptional regulation of the expression of the histidine decarboxylase gene in humans and other animals remains poorly understood (Huang et al. 2018).

5.10.2 CATABOLISM OF HISTAMINE

In the 1940s, there were extensive studies to characterize histamine catabolism in humans and other animals. Histamine was found in 1949 to be converted to acetylhistamine by an acetyl-CoA-dependent enzyme. H. Tabor observed in 1951 that animals metabolize histamine via histaminase (also known as diamine oxidase) to imidazoleacetaldehyde, which is further oxidized to imidazoleacetate and imidazoleacetic acid ribonucleoside. In 1956, methylhistamine was reported to be formed from histamine by imidazole *N*-methyltransferase in animals via an SAM-dependent mechanism. Interestingly, there are tissue- and species-specific differences in the activities of this enzyme in animals (e.g., high in the small intestine but negligible in the stomach of rats; high in guinea pigs but low in rats) that are associated with their different biological responses to histamine (e.g., low sensitivity in rats; Kim et al. 1969; Yoshikawa et al. 2019). Imidazole *N*-methyltransferase is widely distributed in tissues, including the small intestine, placenta, large intestine, kidneys, liver, brain, lung, and skin. The K_M values of the human, rat, and mouse histaminase for histamine are 19, 7.1, and 5.3 μM, respectively (Yoshikawa et al. 2019). Activity of this enzyme is inhibited by histamine analogues [e.g., metoprine (a derivative of 2,4-diaminopyrimidine), etoprine, and chloroquine]. The pathways for histamine catabolism are summarized in Figure 4.14 of Chapter 4.

Histamine + [O] → Imidazole acetaldehyde   (histaminase, a diamine oxidase)

Histamine + SAM → Methylhistamine + SAHC   (histamine methyltransferase)

Histamine + Acetyl-CoA → *N*-Acetylhistamine   (acetylhistamine synthase)

Histamine + Diphosphopyridine nucleotide → Histamine dinucleotide

(imidazoleacetate phosphoribosyltransferase)

5.11 SYNTHESIS AND CATABOLISM OF CATECHOLAMINES, THYROID HORMONES, AND MELANIN

Tyrosine is utilized for the synthesis of dopamine (4-(2-aminoethyl)benzene-1,2-diol), epinephrine (4-[(1R)-1-hydroxy-2-(methylamino)ethyl]-1,2-benzenediol), norepinephrine (4-[(1R)-2-amino-1-hydroxyethyl]benzene-1,2-diol), thyroid hormones, and melanin in animals (Kopin 1985). The initial step for the synthesis of these molecules is commonly catalyzed by tyrosine hydroxylase, an enzyme dependent on (6R)-5,6,7,8-tetrahydro-L-biopterin (BH4) for catalytic activity (see Chapter 4). In the brain, this enzyme prefers to use tyrosine as its substrate but can also act on phenylalanine at a much lower activity (Fernstrom and Fernstrom 2007). However, phenylalanine is converted into tyrosine primarily in the liver and kidneys by phenylalanine hydroxylase, another enzyme that requires BH4 for catalytic activity. Both tyrosine hydroxylase and phenylalanine hydroxylase (nonheme iron-dependent monooxygenases) catalyze the insertion of one atom of molecular oxygen onto the aromatic ring of their AA substrates, using a BH4 molecule as a two-electron donor to reduce the second oxygen atom to water (Roberts and Fitzpatrick 2013). Phenylalanine hydroxylase activity is present in the small intestine but is not detected in the brain (He and Wu 2020). Tyrosine hydroxylase and phenylalanine hydroxylase are absent from many other tissues, including the heart, skeletal muscle, and adipose tissue.

5.11.1 SYNTHESIS AND CATABOLISM OF CATECHOLAMINES

Catecholamines include dopamine, norepinephrine, and epinephrine. Epinephrine (also known as adrenaline) is both a hormone and a neurotransmitter. It was discovered in the adrenal gland by the Japanese chemist, J. Takamine in 1900. Using [²H]- or [³H]-labeled phenylalanine, S. Gurin and A.M. Delluva reported, in 1947, that epinephrine is formed from tyrosine via a series of enzyme-catalyzed reactions, with norepinephrine as an intermediate (Figure 5.19). Methylation of nor-epinephrine by SAM-dependent phenylethanolamine N-methyltransferase (a cytosolic enzyme) generates epinephrine. This synthetic pathway occurs in the chromaffin cells of the adrenal medulla,

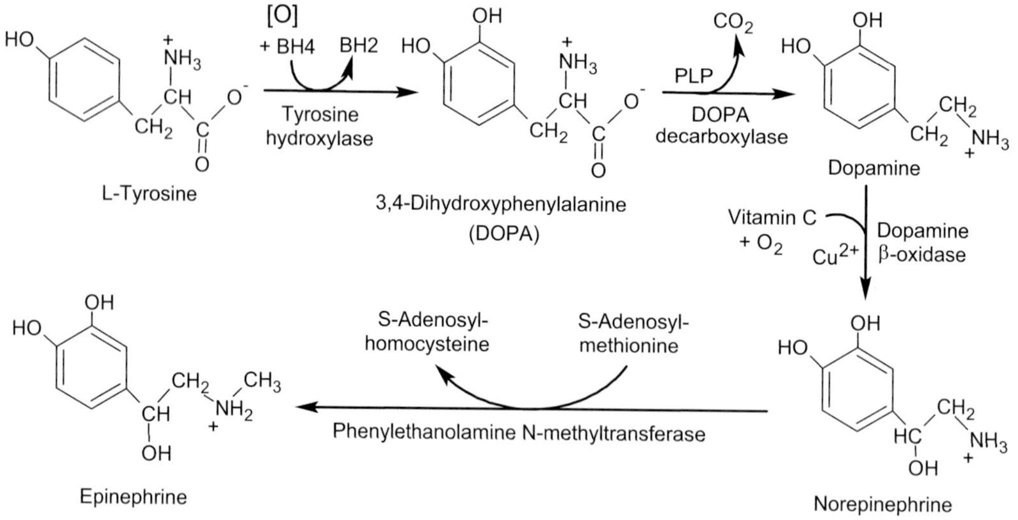

FIGURE 5.19 Conversion of tyrosine to catecholamines in humans and other animals. A series of enzyme-catalyzed reactions converts tyrosine into DOPA, dopamine, norepinephrine, and epinephrine, which are collectively referred to as catecholamines. Tetrahydrobiopterin (BH4) and S-adenosylmethionine are essential cofactors for catecholamine synthesis. BH2, dihydrobiopterin; PLP, pyridoxal phosphate.

some neurons of the central nervous system, and human epidermis keratinocytes (Fernstrom and Fernstrom 2007; Schallreuter et al. 1992).

In animals, the circulating catecholamines have a half-life of only a few minutes, reflecting the high rates of their uptake and catabolism by cells and tissues (King et al. 2000). Catecholamines are degraded through (1) O-methylation by Mg^{2+}-dependent catechol-O-methyltransferases, (2) deamination by FAD-dependent monoamine oxidases, and (3) sulfoconjugation by phenolsulfotransferase in all animals, as well as the formation of glucuronide conjugates by UDP-glucuronosyltransferases in most species (e.g., humans, dogs, pigs, sheep, cattle, and rats) (Figure 5.20).

Catechol-O-methyltransferase, which has both membrane-bound and cytoplasmic forms, is expressed in most animal tissues, including the brain and liver (Du et al. 2008; Schendzielorz et al. 2011). This enzyme introduces a methyl group from SAM to a catecholamine, generating a methylated derivative. Such a reaction is essential for auditory function in mammals, including humans and mice (Du et al. 2008). Monoamine oxidase, which exists in two distinct types in mitochondria, oxidizes catecholamine to generate the corresponding aldehyde and ammonia. Note that because epinephrine has no amino group, this catecholamine is not a substrate for monoamine oxidase or diamine oxidase. Phenolsulfotransferase, which has both cytosolic and membrane-bound isoforms, catalyzes the production of the sulfate derivatives of catecholamines. In mammals (including humans), the activity of this enzyme is relatively higher in the liver than in other tissues (Weinshilboum 1986). Inorganic sulfate, derived from food, the catabolism of sulfur-containing AAs, or degradation of highly sulfated glycosaminoglycans, is activated in an ATP-dependent enzymatic reaction to form phosphoadenosinephosphosulfate, which is the sulfate donor for the sulfation catalyzed by phenolsulfotransferase. Finally, glucuronide formation (glucuronidation) plays an important role in metabolizing a variety of foreign and endogenous compounds. Such a reaction is performed by UDP-glucuronosyltransferases (a cytosolic and membrane-bound enzyme) primarily in the liver and, to a lesser extent, in the gastrointestinal tract, kidneys, skin, and possibly other tissues (King et al. 2000). This enzyme catalyzes the transfer of the glucuronic acid

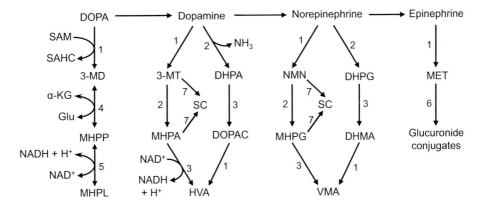

FIGURE 5.20 Catabolism of catecholamines in humans and other animals. The enzymes that catalyze the indicated reactions are (1) catechol-O-methyltransferases (Mg^{2+}-dependent enzyme); (2) monoamine oxidases (FAD-dependent enzymes); (3) aldehyde dehydrogenase; (4) 3-O-methyldopa transaminase (possibly tyrosine aminotransferase); (5) 3-methoxy-4-hydroxyphenylpyruvate reductase; (6) formation of glucuronide conjugates by uridine diphosphoglucuronyl transferase; and (7) phenolsulfotransferase. DHMA, 3,4-dihydroxymandelic acid; DHPA, 3,4-dihydroxyphenylacetaldehyde; DHPG, dihydroxyphenylglycol; DOPAC, 3,4-dihydroxyphenylacetic acid; Glu, glutamate; HVA, homovanillic acid; α-KG, α-ketoglutarate; 3-MD, 3-methoxydopa; MET, metanephrine; MHPA, 3-methoxy-4-hydroxyphenylacetaldehyde; MHPG, 3-methoxy-4-hydroxyphenylglycol; MHPL, 3-methoxy-4-hydroxyphenyllactate (vanillactate); MHPP, 3-methoxy-4-hydroxyphenylpyruvate; 3-MT, 3-methoxytyramine; NMN, normetanephrine; SAHC, S-adenosylhomocysteine; SAM, S-adenosylmethionine; SC, sulfate conjugates; and VMA, vanillylmandelic acid.

(glucose metabolite) component of UDP-glucuronic acid to the phenolic hydroxide of catechol-amine metabolites. Catecholamine metabolites (including sulfate and glucuronic acid conjugates) are water-soluble and excreted in the urine.

5.11.2 Synthesis and Catabolism of Thyroid Hormones

Thyroid hormones include thyroxine (T_4, the predominant form) and triiodothyronine (T_3). They are formed in vertebrates from tyrosine and iodine by thyroid gland follicular cells. These substances are poorly soluble in water (Table 5.1) but are readily soluble in lipids. T_4 was first isolated in a pure form from extracts of porcine thyroid glands in 1914 at the Mayo Clinic by the American biochemist E. Kendall and then chemically synthesized in 1926 by the British chemist C.R. Harington. Due to the availability of chromatographic techniques and ^{125}I-labeled compounds, T_3 was isolated from enzymatic hydrolysates of thyroglobulin (a glycoprotein) in 1952. Studies in the 1960s and 1970s led to the recognition that the iodination of tyrosyl residues in thyroglobulin (a tyrosine-rich protein) as mono- and diiodotyrosyl residues is essential to the formation of thyroid hormones (Figure 5.21). In thyroglobulin, T_4 residues can be converted into T_3 by a deiodinase (5′-iodinase; Bianco and Kim 2006). Proteolysis of thyroglobulin results in the release of free T_4 and T_3. In the plasma, both T_4 (the main form of thyroid hormone circulating in the blood) and T_3 are transported in the protein (thyroid hormone-binding globulin or albumin)-bound form (Pardridge and Mietus 1980). The physiological effects of thyroid hormones are mediated by nuclear thyroid hormone receptors that have their highest affinity for T_3, ultimately inducing the expression of many genes related to energy metabolism and cell development in various tissues (Brent 2012). Thus, thyroid signaling defects contribute to a variety of pathological conditions, including mental retardation, obesity, metabolic disorders, and cancers (Krashin et al. 2019).

T_4 is converted to either the more active form T_3 by 5′-deiodination of its outer phenolic ring or inactive reverse-T_3 by 5-deiodination of its inner tyrosyl ring. Likewise, T_3 can be metabolized to an inactive diiodotyrosine. Deiodination of thyroid hormones is catalyzed by hepatic phase II sulfotransferases and glucuronosyltransferases. Outer ring deiodination is inhibited, while inner ring deiodination is stimulated by sulfation of the phenolic hydroxyl group of T_4 (McNabb 1995). Glucuronidation of T_3 and T_4 by UDP-glucuronosyltransferases generates inactive, water-soluble products that are excreted into bile (ultimately feces) and urine. Thyroid hormone degradation can be enhanced by treatment with phenobarbital or other antiepileptic drugs through a nuclear receptor CAR-dependent induction of phase II enzymes of xenobiotic metabolism (Ortiga-Carvalho et al. 2014). Additionally, PPARα agonists synergize with phenobarbital to induce another prototypical CAR target gene, CYP2B1, to stimulate the breakdown of thyroid hormones.

5.11.3 Synthesis of Melanin

In 1887, K. Mörner discovered a dark substance, melanin, in the urine of patients with melanotic tumors. Subsequently, J.J. Abel and W.S. Davis identified melanin in the black hair and skin of humans in 1896. Similarly, in 1903, E. Spiegler reported melanin in the wool from black sheep and in the hair of black horses. Based on the suggestion in 1901 by V. Fürth that an aromatic AA is the precursor of melanin, the work of H.S. Raper in the 1920s and 1930s led to the elucidation of the synthetic pathway via DOPA as an intermediate (Figure 5.22). Melanin is chemically very similar to lignin (a major constituent of wood) and is insoluble in water. There are three types of melanin: eumelanin, pheomelanin, and neuromelanin, with the most common type being eumelanin. Eumelanin has two subtypes: brown eumelanin and black eumelanin.

In the skin of mammals and birds, melanocytes are the site of melanin synthesis. The initial step of this metabolic pathway is catalyzed by BH4-dependent tyrosinase to form DOPA from tyrosine. This enzyme is a type I membrane protein found in melanosomes, which are lysosomal-like organelles and specific for pigment cells (Sitaram and Marks 2012). Note that cysteine and glutathione participate in melanin synthesis. The enzymes involved in melanin synthesis occur exclusively in

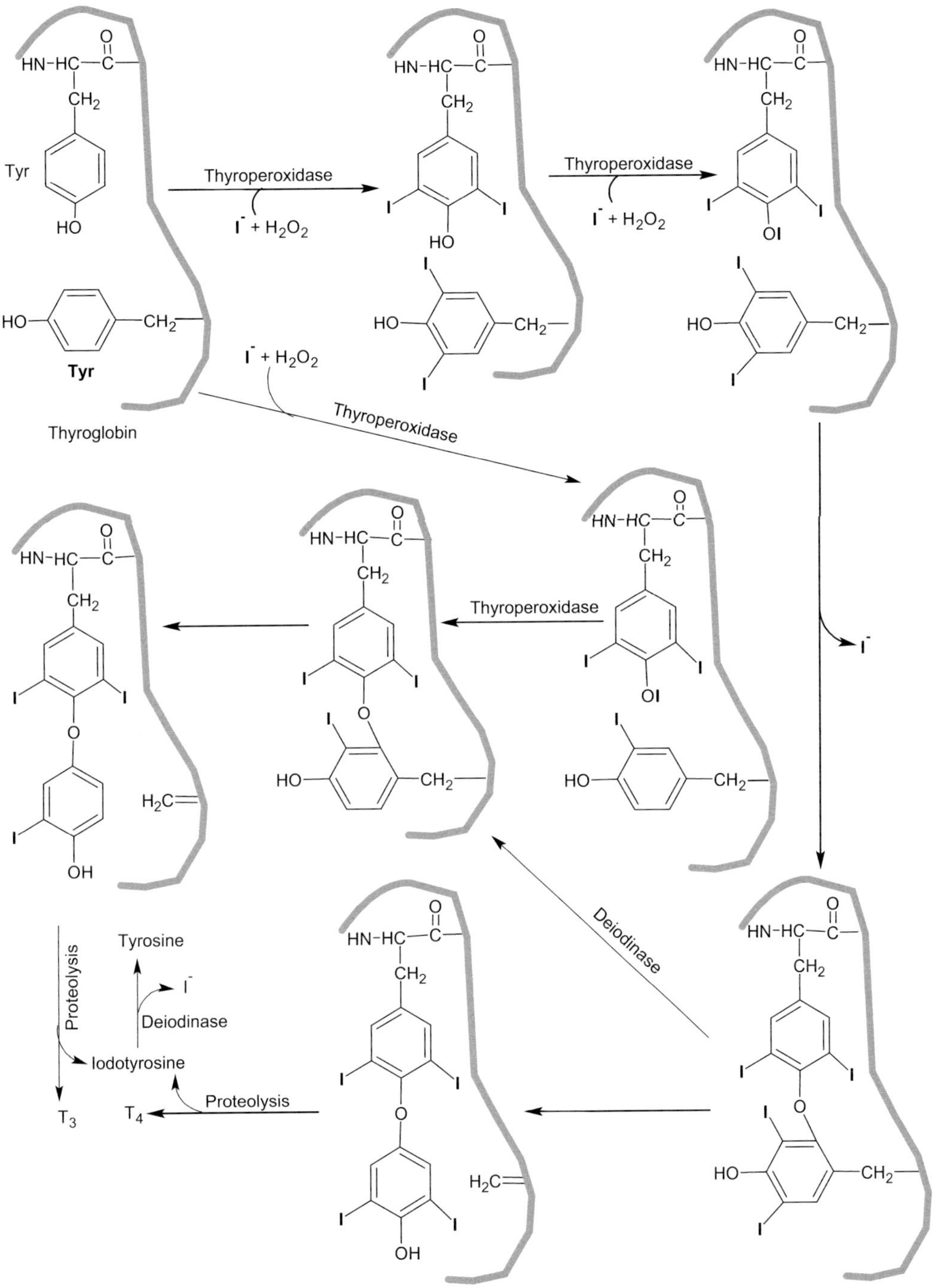

FIGURE 5.21 Synthesis of triiodothyronine (T_3) and thyroxine (T_4) on thyroglobulin in the thyroid gland of humans and other animals. This synthetic process involves the following steps: (1) formation of the tyrosine-rich thyroglobulin protein in the thyroid gland; (2) uptake of iodide (I^-) by the thyroid gland; (3) the (3) oxidation of I^- to iodine, followed by the iodination of the tyrosyl residues of thyroglobulin by thyroid peroxidase (also known as thyroperoxidase) to generate mono- and diiodotyrosyl residues; (4) coupling of iodotyrosyl to iodothyronyl residues; (5) proteolysis of thyroglobulin to release free T_3 and T_4, as well as free iodotyrosines; and (6) free iodotyrosines are deiodinated to tyrosine and iodide, thereby allowing their recycling for T_3 and T_4 synthesis within the thyroid gland.

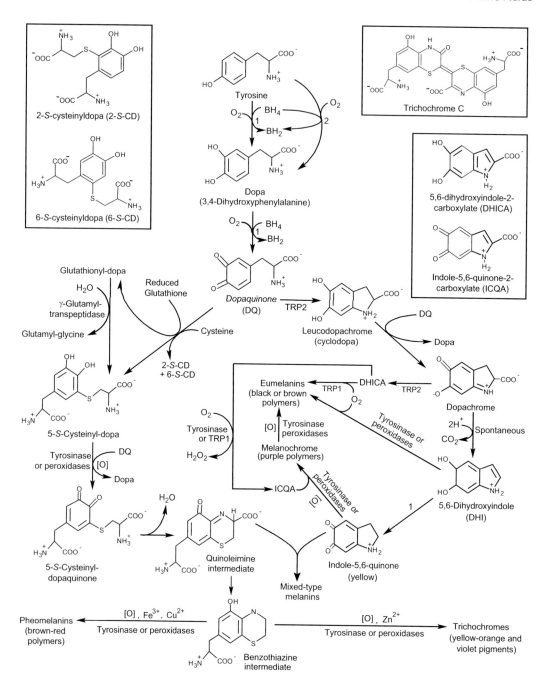

FIGURE 5.22 Conversion of tyrosine to the melanin polymers, eumelanins and pheomelanins, in humans and other animals. These reactions occur primarily in the skin. Both eumelanins and pheomelanins are colored polymers. Their production leads to pigmentation in the skin and hair. The enzymes that catalyze the indicated reactions are (1) tyrosinase and (2) tyrosine hydroxylase. TRP1, tyrosinase-related protein 1; TRP2, tyrosinase-related protein 2 (also known as dopachrome tautomerase). DHICA, 5,6-dihydroxy-indole-2-carboxylic acid.

melanosomes. It is now known that melanin is ubiquitously synthesized from tyrosine in melano-cytes of the skin and in select cell types [e.g., retinal pigment epithelial cells (see below), the mela-nocytes of hair follicles, and ovine placentome] of most organisms (including humans, cattle, sheep, goats, birds, pigs, cats, and insects) (Slominski et al. 2005; Sugumaran and Barek 2016).

In addition to the skin, melanin synthesis in eye melanocytes is responsible for the eye color of humans and other animals (Sitiwin et al. 2019). Specifically, choroidal melanocytes are the melanin-producing cells in the vascular uvea (iris, ciliary body, and choroid) of the eyes. The choroid is a pigmented, vascularized layer between the neural retina and outer protective sclera of the eye. As the largest component of the uveal tract, the choroid is essential for supplying oxygen and nutrients to, and removing metabolic wastes from, the adjacent outer retinal layers, the retinal pigment epithelium, and photoreceptors. Thus, melanin plays important physiological roles, including photoprotection, as well as the regulation of oxidative damage and immune responses in the eyes.

As noted previously, the most common form of melanin in humans and other animals is eumelanin, which is a black or brown polymer of dihydroxyindole carboxylic acids. The other form of melanin is pheomelanin, which is a brown-red or yellow-orange and violet polymer. A combination of these melanin types is responsible for hair color. For example, in humans, black hair contains 99% eumelanin and 1% pheomelanin, brown hair and blond hair contain 95% eumelanin and 5% pheomelanin, and red hair contains 67% eumelanin and 33% pheomelanin (Serre et al. 2018). In the eyes, the major melanins are eumelanin and pheomelanin (Sitiwin et al. 2019). The type of melanin synthesized by melanocytes is regulated by genetic, hormonal, and environmental factors.

In contrast to mammals and birds, insects possess enzymes for melanin synthesis in the exoskeleton and some other tissues (including hemolymph) of the body (Sugumaran and Barek 2016). In general, the metabolic pathway for melanin synthesis in insects is very similar to the classic Raper–Mason pathway described for mammals. However, there are differences in the enzymes and their regulation. For example, the dopachrome-decarboxylating enzyme in insects is also a tautomerase, and this bifunctional protein exhibits wide substrate specificity and attacks a number of L-dopachrome derivatives but not D-dopachromes. Mammalian dopachrome-decarboxylating enzyme and tautomerase are two different proteins. In addition, mammalian tyrosinase performs both the oxidation of tyrosine and DOPA to dopaquinone, but insect phenoloxidases do not seem to possess much "tyrosine hydroxylase" activity. Thus, insects mainly use a specific tyrosine hydroxylase for DOPA production. Furthermore, the stage of the dopachrome conversion reaction differs between mammals and insects, as mammalian dopachrome tautomerase converts dopachrome to 5,6-dihydroxyindole-2-carboxylic acid but insect dopachrome decarboxylase/tautomerase generates 5,6-dihydroxyindole. Eumelanin appears to be the dominant melanin in many insect species although they also contain a smaller amount of pheomelanin, just like mammalian skin and hair. Interestingly, Polidori et al. (2017) recently reported that eumelanin and pheomelanin are major pigments in bumblebee pubescence, just like mammalian eyes.

5.11.4   ELIMINATION AND CATABOLISM OF MELANIN

As a component of the epidermis, intact melanin is gradually sloughed off the skin and hair. This is the major mechanism for the elimination of melanin from the body. At present, there is a paucity of information about melanin degradation in humans and other animals. Limited evidence shows that the hair does not appear to degrade melanin. However, human keratinocytes have lysosomal enzymes to degrade melanin (Mammone et al. 2004). These enzymes include manganese-dependent and independent peroxidases in mammals and birds, as well as copper-dependent laccase in certain animals such as insects and sponges (Sakurai and Kataoka 2007). Macrophages in tissues (e.g., the retinal pigmented epithelium) can engulf melanin and then degrade it through the action of lysosomal hydrolases (Takematsu and Seiji 1983). Furthermore, autophagy regulates the degradation of melanosomes in keratinocytes and, therefore, skin color (Murase et al. 2013). Likewise, bacteria in the lumen of the intestinal tract can also break down melanin through the actions of manganese-dependent and independent peroxidases, as well as the heme-containing lignin peroxidase and the copper-dependent laccase. Specifically, microbial laccase degrades melanin to generate, as a product, hydrogen peroxide, which elicits a synergistic effect with peroxidases. The activity of the laccase-peroxidase complex is about 6-fold greater than that of laccase alone (Sakurai and

Kataoka 2007). In either mammalian cells or microorganisms, the products of melanin degradation have not been identified but may include pyrrole-2,3-dicarboxylic acid, pyrrole-2,3,5-tricarboxylic acid, 3-aminotyrosine, and 4-amino-3-hydroxyphenylalanine (Borges et al. 2001).

5.12 SYNTHESIS AND CATABOLISM OF SEROTONIN AND MELATONIN

5.12.1 SYNTHESIS OF SEROTONIN AND MELATONIN

Tryptophan catabolism via the hydroxylation and decarboxylation pathway generates serotonin, *N*-acetylserotonin, melatonin, anthranilic acid, and ammonia, as indicated in Figure 4.20 of Chapter 4. This pathway originated from the initial observation in 1935 by the Italian scientist V. Erspamer that a substance in an extract from enterochromaffin cells can make the intestine contract. Two years later, Erspamer recognized this unknown substance to be an amine and named it "enteramine". In 1948, M. Rapport and colleagues at the Cleveland Clinic found a vasoconstrictor molecule in serum that could affect vascular tone and named it "serotonin". In 1952, enteramine was shown to be identical to serotonin. J.D. Fernstrom and R.J. Wurtman reported in 1971 that concentrations of serotonin in the brain depend on the circulating levels of tryptophan. It is now known that two isoforms of tryptophan hydroxylase (TPH) catalyze serotonin synthesis from tryptophan in mammals (Roberts and Fitzpatrick 2013). This enzyme critically depends on BH4 for catalytic activity (Table 4.8 of Chapter 4) and acts like tyrosine hydroxylase. TPH1 generates serotonin in the enterochromaffin cells of the intestine and in the pineal gland of the brain. TPH2 produces serotonin in the neurons of the raphe nuclei (the major site for the synthesis of this hormone in the brain) and in the myenteric plexus. Consistent with the site of its synthesis, serotonin is present predominantly in the gastrointestinal tract (80%–90% of body stores; Sanger 2008). This neurotransmitter is involved in the regulation of gastrointestinal secretion, motility, and sensation. There is also evidence that an increase in serotonin synthesis can be a sensitive biomarker of oxidative stress and the generation of reactive oxygen/nitrogen species (Schiavone et al. 2013).

In serotonergic or serotoninergic neurons of the central nervous system and peripheral cells (including the retina, the gastrointestinal tract, bone marrow cells, epithelial cells, and lymphocytes), serotonin can be transformed into melatonin (Tordjman et al. 2017). This indoleamine was first discovered in the pineal gland of cows in 1917 and isolated from urine in 1958. In the metabolic pathway of its synthesis, *N*-acetyltransferase transfers an acetyl group from acetyl-CoA to the amino group of serotonin to form *N*-acetylserotonin, which is the precursor for the synthesis of melatonin primarily in the pineal gland (Chapter 4). This tissue exhibits a diurnal rhythm in *N*-acetyltransferase activity, with low and high values in the light and dark periods, respectively (Abe et al. 2000). Exposure to constant light reduces *N*-acetyltransferase activity in the pineal gland and suppresses the circadian rhythm of this enzyme. By contrast, the synthesis or concentrations of melatonin in peripheral cells do not appear to be regulated by the photoperiod (Reiter 1991).

5.12.2 CATABOLISM OF SEROTONIN AND MELATONIN

Catabolism of serotonin in animals takes place primarily in the cytoplasm of the brain, liver, and neurons of the gastrointestinal tract, and, to a lesser extent, in other tissues and cell types (including kidneys and cells of the immune system; Höglund et al. 2019). Serotonin is degraded to 5-hydroxyindole-3-acetate and 5-methoxytryptamine by monoamine oxidase and SAM-dependent methyltransferase, respectively. 5-hydroxyindole-3-acetate and 5-methoxytryptamine are converted to 5-methoxyindole-3-acetate by *N*-acetylserotonin *O*-methyltransferase and monoamine oxidase, respectively. Serotonin can also be metabolized in the cytoplasm to other derivatives, including formyl 5-hydroxytryptamine, 5-hydroxykynurenine, and 5-hydroxytryptamine sulfate (Chapter 4). Furthermore, results of recent studies indicate that serotonin-derived 5-hydroxyindoleacetaldehyde may be condensed with cysteine to form 5-hydroxyindole thiazolidine carboxylic acid in the mitochondria of the rodent brain and small intestine (Squires et al. 2006). In contrast to tryptophan, serotonin is not a substrate for indoleamine 2,3-dioxygenase. Melatonin is enzymatically oxidized in a different manner than tryptophan (Ferry et al. 2005). Catabolism of melatonin involves conjugation and oxidative cleavage of its indole moiety. Approximately 70% of melatonin (either diet-derived or endogenously synthesized) is catabolized in animals by sulfoconjugation and glucuronoconjugation pathways, which have been described previously (Leone et al. 1987). Some melatonin (~15%) is excreted in the untransformed form in the urine. About 15% of melatonin is degraded in the presence of H_2O_2 through oxidation by two cytosolic enzymes myeloperoxidase and indoleamine 2,3-dioxygenase. Both enzymes have similar K_M values (in the micromolar range) for melatonin. In addition, the metabolism of melatonin may result in the production of an acetylated kynurenine derivative (N^1-acetyl-N^5-methoxykynurenamine) by kynurenine formamidase (a cytosolic enzyme) and of N-formyl-N-acetyl-5-methoxy kynurenamine by indole 2,3-dioxygenase (Höglund et al. 2019).

Like melanin, melatonin results in skin darkening. Because the liver plays an important role in the degradation of both melanin and melatonin, black skin syndrome may appear when metabolic defects occur in the liver (Li et al. 2021). For example, humans and other animals (including fish) with hepatic dysfunction because of viral, bacterial, and parasite infections or inadequate nutrition have an impaired ability to degrade or remove (1) the black-color products (e.g., melanin and homogentisate) of phenylalanine and tyrosine catabolism by melanocytes and the liver and (2) melatonin (a product of tryptophan) generated primarily by the pineal gland. The tyrosine metabolites are accumulated in the skin, directly resulting in black skin syndrome (Hou et al. 2020; Li et al. 2021).

5.13 SYNTHESIS AND CATABOLISM OF D-GLUCOSAMINE AND GLYCOSAMINOGLYCANS

5.13.1 HISTORICAL PERSPECTIVES

D-Glucosamine was first prepared from the hydrolysis of chitin by G. Ledderhose in 1876 using concentrated hydrochloric acid. The structure of D-glucosamine was established by W. Haworth in 1939. C.E. Becker and H.G. Day reported in 1953 that D-[^{14}C]glucose was converted into hexosamine in rats, indicating a role for glucose or its metabolite in the synthetic pathway. In the same year, L.F. Leloir and C.E. Cardini found that extracts from *Neurospora crassa* produced D-glucosamine-6-phosphate and L-glutamate from L-glutamine and hexose phosphate. The enzyme that catalyzed this reaction was identified in 1960 by S. Ghosh and colleagues. The pathway for the biosynthesis of amino sugars was elucidated thereafter in the 1960s.

5.13.2 SYNTHESIS AND CATABOLISM OF D-GLUCOSAMINE

5.13.2.1 Synthesis of D-Glucosamine

Glutamine:fructose-6-phosphate transaminase (a cytosolic enzyme; GFAT) catalyzes the formation of glucosamine-6-phosphate and glutamate from fructose-6-phosphate and L-glutamine in all cell types. Results from studies with endothelial cells indicate that GFAT is activated by elevated levels of glucose, glutamine, and leucine (Wu et al. 2001; Yang et al. 2015). Glutamine donates the amide group ($-NH_2$) for the synthesis of glucosamine-6-phosphate (Figure 5.23). This reaction may be the major source of glutamate in red blood cells that do not take up extracellular glutamate. It is noteworthy that (1) GFAT is particularly abundant in red blood cells, endothelial cells, placental cells (early gestation), and the small intestine; and (2) fructose and glutamine are also unusually abundant in the fetal fluids of ruminants and other mammals. For example, in sheep and pigs, there are high concentrations of fructose (e.g., up to 30 mM in ovine allantoic fluid) and glutamine (e.g., up to 25 mM in ovine allantoic fluid) in the conceptus during early- and mid-gestation (Wu et al. 2006).

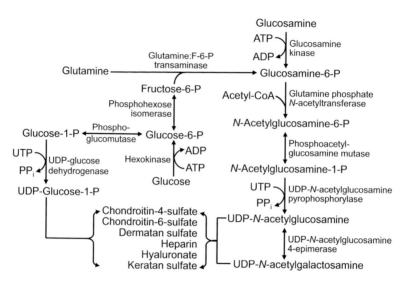

FIGURE 5.23 Synthesis of hexosamine from glutamine and fructose-6-phosphate in humans and other animals. All enzymes for D-glucosamine synthesis are present in the cytoplasm. Fructose-6-phosphate is generated from glucose by hexokinase. D-Hexosamine is required for the production of all glycoproteins. P, phosphate; PPi, pyrophosphate.

Both fructose and glutamine promote glucosamine-6-phosphate synthesis, placental growth, and fetal development (Kim et al. 2012; Wang et al. 2016). In humans, GFAT may compete, for the glutamine substrate, with other glutamine-utilizing enzymes [including glutamine N-phenylacetyltransferase (Figure 5.24)] in the cytoplasm.

5.13.2.2 Catabolism of Glucosamine-6-Phosphate

Glucosamine-6-phosphate deaminase (GNPDA) catalyzes the conversion of glucosamine-6-phosphate to fructose-6-phosphate plus NH_3 (Figure 5.25). This cytosolic enzyme was first identified in mammalian tissues by D.G. Comb and S. Roseman in 1958 and was cloned by H. Wolosker and colleagues in 1998. GNPDA is selectively localized to (1) tissues with high energy requirements, including the apical zone of transporting epithelia in the proximal convoluted tubules of the kidney and the small intestine, as well as the placenta, uterus, testis, and skin; (2) neurons (but not glia) and especially nerve terminals in the brain; and (3) motile sperm cells. Like the bacterial enzyme, mammalian GNPDA is allosterically activated by N-acetyl-D-glucosamine-6-phosphate (Arreola et al. 2003). Products of GNPDA enter glycolysis and nitrogen-utilizing pathways.

5.13.3 Synthesis and Catabolism of Glycosaminoglycans

5.13.3.1 Synthesis of Glycosaminoglycans

Glycosaminoglycans are heteropolysaccharides composed of repeating disaccharide units that consist of either sulfated or nonsulfated monosaccharides (Pomin and Mulloy 2018). These macromolecules are based on different carbohydrates in the backbone structures, such as glucose residues in hyaluronic acid (HA, also known as hyaluronan); galactose and uronic sugars (e.g., glucuronic acid or iduronic acid) in chondroitin and dermatan (formed from the epimerization and sulfation of chondroitins); and glucose residues and uronic sugars in heparan and heparin (formed from the epimerization and sulfation of heparin). Their molecular size and the sulfation type vary with the tissue and their state (e.g., part of proteoglycan or free chains). All animals synthesize glycosaminoglycans from glucosamine-6-phosphate, a product of glutamine and fructose-6-phosphate.

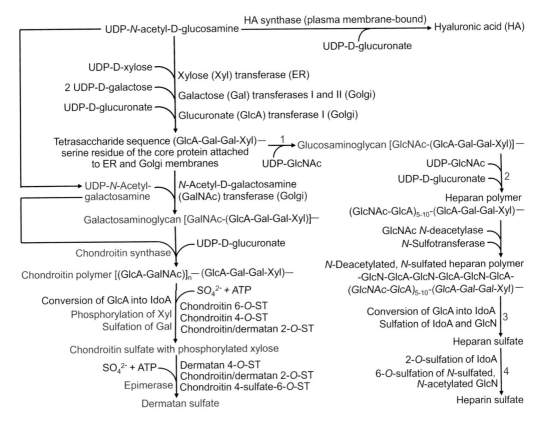

FIGURE 5.24 Synthesis of glycosaminoglycans (hyaluronic acid, chondroitin sulfate, dermatan sulfate, heparin sulfate, and heparin sulfate) in humans and other animals. The enzymes that catalyze the indicated reactions are (1) N-acetyl-D-glucosamine (GlcNAc) transferase; (2) a series of enzymes (heparan sulfate transferase II, GlcNAc transferase, and glucuronate transferase); (3) a series of enzymes (uronyl C5-epimerase, 2-O-sulfotransferase, 6-O-sulfotransferase, and 3-O-sulfotransferase); and (4) a series of enzymes (C-5 epimerase, heparin 2-O-sulfotransferase, and heparin 6-O-sulfotransferase). ER, endoplasmic reticulum; GlcN, glucosamine; and UDP-GlcNAc, UDP-N-acetylglucosamine.

Glucosamine-6-phosphate is converted, via a series of reactions, into UDP-N-acetylglucosamine and UDP-N-acetylgalactosamine (Figure 5.23). These acetylated molecules, along with UDP-D-glucuronate, a product of UDP-D-glucose dehydrogenation, are utilized for the formation of all macromolecules containing amino sugars (including membrane hormone receptors, intracellular glycoproteins, cell membrane-associated mucins in the intestinal mucosa, and extracellular matrix proteins). All enzymes required for their synthesis are expressed in specific cell types present in the connective tissue, placenta, gastrointestinal mucosa, and other tissues. Heparin (an anticoagulant) and heparan are synthesized mainly in mast cells, whereas HA, chondroitin, and dermatan are generated in almost all cell types.

5.13.3.1.1 Synthesis of HA
Hyaluronan synthase generates HA from UDP-N-acetyl-D-glucosamine and UDP-D-glucuronate. It belongs to a class of plasma membrane-bound proteins (Stern 2004). To date, 3 isoforms of HA synthase have been reported for vertebrates. HA is a nonsulfated member of the glycosaminoglycan family and is a critical component of the extracellular matrix in the tissues of animals. In HA, D-glucuronic acid and N-acetyl-D-glucosamine (also known as N-acetylglucosamine) are linked via alternating β-1,4 and β-1,3 glycosidic bonds (Stern 2004). HA can be 250–25,000 disaccharide

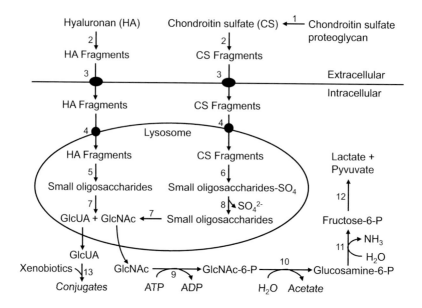

FIGURE 5.25 Catabolism of glycosaminoglycans in humans and other animals. Hyaluronan (HA) and chondroitin sulfate (CS) proteoglycan are degraded in multiple cell types (e.g., keratocytes, synovial fibroblasts, endothelial cells, sinusoidal cells, placental trophoblasts, and tumors) through a series of reactions that involve extracellular and lysosomal hyaluronidases, as well as exoglycosidases. Entry of HA and CS into the cell occurs through cell-surface receptors, including CD44, RHAMM (receptor for HA-mediated motility), and ICAM1 (intercellular adhesion molecule 1). The internalized glycosaminoglycans enter the lysosome for degradation to N-acetyl-D-glucosamine (GlcNAc) and D-glucuronic acid (GlcUA), which subsequently exit the lysosome and enter the cytoplasm for further catabolism. The enzymes that catalyze the indicated reactions are (1) extracellular proteases; (2) extracellular hyaluronidases [HYAL (e.g., HYAL2)]; (3) cell-surface receptors; (4) endocytosis; (5) endoglycosidases (e.g., HYAL 1 and 3); (6) endoglycosidases (e.g., HYAL 1 and 4); (7) exoglycosidases; (8) arylsulfatase B and N-acetylgalactosamine-6-sulfatase; (9) N-acetyl-D-glucosamine kinase; (10) N-acetylglucosamine-6-phosphate deacetylase; (11) glucosamine-6-phosphate deaminase; (12) enzymes of glycolysis; and (13) enzymes for glucuronidation. 6-P, 6-phosphate.

repeats in length, and its molecular weight often reaches the million Dalton range. All vertebrates (e.g., mammals, birds, and fish) synthesize and contain HA (Messner and Gillquist 1996). Of note, it is a primary glycosaminoglycan that is synthesized by placental cells and present in the placental stroma and supports embryonic survival, growth, and development.

The average healthy 70-kg adult person contains ~15 g of HA, with one-third of the whole-body HA being turned over (i.e., ~5 g of HA being degraded and ~5 g of HA being synthesized) per day (Stern 2004). Both glucose and fructose activate the synthesis of glucosamine-6-phosphate and HA in placental cells via the mechanistic target of rapamycin (MTOR) pathway to support their growth and development during gestation (Kim et al. 2012). Note that the HA molecules synthesized by cells are exported to the extracellular matrix. HA production is essential for (1) lubrication of the joints; (2) angiogenesis (the formation of new blood vessels from existing ones); (3) the structure and function of the extracellular matrix in connective tissue present in the skin, blood vessels, and bones; and (4) cell proliferation and migration, wound repair, and skin healing.

5.13.3.1.2 Synthesis of Chondroitin and Dermatan Sulfates

The synthesis of chondroitin in the endoplasmic reticulum/Golgi vesicles involves several steps: (1) the synthesis of the core protein from AAs in the cytosol; (2) the formation of precursors from glutamine and glucose; (3) the generation of a tetrasaccharide sequence (glucuronate-galactose-galactose-xylose) that is linked (via xylose) to a serine residue in the core protein; (4) the production of chondroitin polymer through the alternate addition of D-glucuronate and galactosamine to form the repeating disaccharide units (GlcA-GalNAc); and (5) the modification of chondroitin through the sulfation of the galactose residue and the phosphorylation of the xylose residue in the nascent chondroitin. Note that (1) the transfer of galactosamine from *N*-acetylgalactosamine to the oligo-saccharide sequence linkage to form galactosaminoglycan directs the synthesis of chondroitin and dermatan; (2) chondroitin synthase has both glucuronate transferase and *N*-acetylgalactosamine transferase activities; (3) sulfation of the chondroitin polymer by specific sulfotransferases occurs as it is being formed; (4) chondroitin sulfate is a major component of the connective tissue matrix (e.g., skin and cartilage); and (5) this sulfated glycosaminoglycan is composed of alternating units of *N*-acetyl-β-D-galactosamine(β1,3)β-D-glucuronate linked to each other by a β(1,4) linkage and is usually attached to proteins as part of a proteoglycan. Dermatan is derived from chondroitin through the epimerization of varying amounts of D-glucuronate residues into L-iduronic acid resi-dues during or subsequent to the formation of chondroitin and concomitant with its 2-*O*-, 4-*O*-, and 6-*O*-sulfation (Silbert and Sugumaran. 2002). These synthetic pathways, along with the necessary enzymes, are illustrated in Figure 5.24.

5.13.3.1.3 *Synthesis of Heparan and Heparin*

The initial steps of heparin synthesis for the generation of a tetrasaccharide sequence (glucuronate-galactose-galactose-xylose) linked (via xylose) to a serine residue in the core protein are the same as those for chondroitin synthesis (Sugahara and Kitagawa 2002). The subsequent reactions of heparin synthesis are analogous to those for chondroitin synthesis, except that (1) UDP-*N*-acetylglucosamine, rather than UDP-*N*-acetylgalactosamine, is transferred to the oligosaccharide sequence; (2) UDP-*N*-acetylgalactosamine directs the synthesis of heparin; (3) the glucosaminoglycan chain under-goes elongation through the alternate addition of glucuronate and *N*-acetylglucosamine; and (4) the 5-epimerization of D-glucuronic acid residues on heparan sulfate to L-iduronic acid by a C-5 epimerase. The formation of L-iduronic acid, the 2-O-sulfation of L-iduronic acid, and the 6-O-sulfation of *N*-sulfated, *N*-acetylated glucosamine together convert heparan sulfate into hepa-rin sulfate. The latter is released from mast cells into the blood as an important anticoagulant. Heparan sulfate has the most common repeating disaccharide unit of glucuronic acid linked to sulfated *N*-acetylglucosamine via β-1,4 bonds in a linear chain and occurs in all animal tissues. By contrast, heparin sulfate is characterized by a repeating disaccharide unit of 2-*O*-sulfated L-iduronic acid and 6-*O*-sulfated, *N*-sulfated *N*-acetylglucosamine in α-1,4 glycosidic linkages and is present in tissues such as the heart, blood, intestine, lungs, and skin.

5.13.3.1.4 *Synthesis of Chitin*

Chitin (β-(1–4)-poly-*N*-acetyl D-glucosamine) is a species-specific long-chain polymer of *N*-acetylglucosamine. This glycosaminoglycan is the major component of the cell walls of bacteria and fungi (e.g., mushrooms), as well as in the microfilarial sheath of parasitic nema-todes. Chitin also constitutes the exoskeletons of crustaceans (e.g., crabs, lobsters, and shrimps), worms and insects, the lining of the digestive tracts of many insects, the radulas of mol-lusks, the scales of fish, and the beaks of cephalopods (including squid and octopuses; Peter 2005). In all of these lower organisms, chitin is synthesized from UDP-*N*-acetylglucosamine by chitin synthase (a cytosolic enzyme). UDP-*N*-acetylglucosamine is formed from glutamine and fructose-6-phosphate, as described in Figure 5.23. Vertebrates lack chitin synthase and, therefore, do not synthesize or contain chitin.

5.13.3.2 Catabolism of Glycosaminoglycans

5.13.3.2.1 *Digestion of Dietary Glycosaminoglycans in the Gastrointestinal Tract*

The gastrointestinal mucosae release enzymes (e.g., exoglycosidases, endoglycosidases, sulfohy-drolase, and hyaluronidase-like enzymes) to the lumen of the small intestine to degrade dietary glycosaminoglycans. These enzymes include heparanases (endoglycosidase) that cleave the heparan sulfate glycosaminoglycans from proteoglycan core proteins and degrade them to small oligosaccharides. Exoglycosidases are glycoside hydrolases that cleave specific terminal-monosaccharides from glycans. Dietary glycosaminoglycans are also hydrolyzed by bacterial enzymes in the lumen of the small intestine, including polysaccharide lyases (e.g., heparin lyase and chondroitin sulfate lyase), heparanases, chondroitinases, and chitinases in the cytoplasm (Ahn et al. 1998). The resulting products [e.g., uronic acids (L-iduronic acid and D-glucuronic acid) and low-molecular-weight amino sugars (D-galactosamine and D-glucosamine)] are absorbed into the portal circulation or enter the lumen of the large intestine. Glycosaminoglycans that escape the small intestine undergo degradation by the same bacterial enzymes.

5.13.3.2.2 *Degradation of Extracellular Glycosaminoglycans by Animal Cells*

Available evidence shows that degradation of extracellular HA and chondroitin sulfate occurs in certain cell types, which include (1) keratocytes in the skin; (2) synovial fibroblasts; (3) endothelial cells; (4) sinusoidal cells in the lymph nodes, liver, and spleen; (5) placental cells (including trophoblasts); (6) macrophages; and (7) tumors. These cell types take up the fragments of extracellularly hydrolyzed HA and chondroitin, and their lysosomes are the major site for initiating and completing the intracellular degradation of HA and chondroitin sulfate (Boonen et al. 2014; Gushulak et al. 2012; McKee et al. 1996). Interestingly, hyaluronidases are highly active in the venom of various animals, such as snakes, scorpions, and spiders. Chitin can be degraded by chitinases (cytosolic enzymes) in some animals (including mammals, birds, and insects; Boot et al. 2001).

The current model for HA degradation includes the actions of extracellular (the interstitial matrix) and lysosomal hyaluronidases (also known as hyaluronoglucosaminidases) as well as exoglycosidases (Figure 5.25). According to this model, the degradation of HA begins with the cleavage of low- to high-molecular-weight HA by an extracellular hyaluronidase (HYAL2), which is a glycosylphosphatidylinositol-anchored, lipid raft-associated hyaluronidase (Stern 2004). The resulting HA fragments, which include those with specific biological activities (e.g., mediating inflammation, ovulation, and angiogenesis), may be internalized through interactions with a cell-surface receptor into the lysosome, where other hyaluronidases (including the endoglycosidases HYAL1 and HYAL3) break down HA to form small oligosaccharides that serve as substrates for lysosomal exoglycosidases [β-glucuronidase and β-hexosaminidase (*N*-acetyl-β-D-glucosaminidase)]. Results of recent studies indicate that both HYAL1 and β-hexosaminidase (lysosomal acid hydrolases) can degrade HA. This function of β-hexosaminidase explains the absence of the accumulation of HA in multiple tissues in transgenic mice deficient in any hyaluronidase. The *N*-acetylglucosamine released from HA hydrolysis enters the cytoplasm where it is converted by *N*-acetylglucosamine kinase to form *N*-acetylglucosamine-6-phosphate (Jadin et al. 2012). The latter is deacetylated by a deacetylase to glucosamine-6-P, which is a substrate of GNPDA for further catabolism (Figure 5.25).

Catabolism of extracellular chondroitin sulfate proteoglycan in a tissue involves the cleavage of its core proteins by extracellular proteinases and the subsequent entry, through endocytosis, of the proteolytic products (chondroitin sulfate and proteins) into the target cell (Garantziotis and Savani 2019; Stern 2003). The degradation of chondroitin sulfate in the lysosome requires a family of enzymes known as hyaluronidases [e.g., HYAL4 (a dedicated chondroitinase) and HYAL1] that catalyze the hydrolysis of the large chondroitin sulfate polymer to small oligosaccharides (e.g., hexa- and tetrasaccharides) and eventually into chondroitin sulfate disaccharides. Because the sugars in the chondroitin sulfate molecule are sulfated, specific enzymes (e.g., arylsulfatase B and *N*-acetylgalactosamine-6-sulfatase) remove the sulfate groups, resulting in regular disaccharide molecules that are further hydrolyzed into monomers (Figure 5.25).

Chitinases are hydrolytic enzymes that break down glycosidic bonds in chitin. Macrophages and epithelial cells of the lung and digestive tracts in animals (including mammals) express two functional chitinases (chitotriosidase and acidic mammalian chitinase) in their cytoplasm to degrade chitin (Boot et al. 2001; Garantziotis and Savani 2019). These enzymes cleave chitin polymers into oligosaccharides (e.g., chitotriose) of varying sizes (endochitinase activity) and release glucosamine monosaccharides (e.g., *N*-acetyl-D-glucosamine) from the end of a chitin polymer (exochitinase activity). The presence of chitinases in such strategic sites may be the body's first line of defense against exogenous agents including chitin-containing pathogens. Additionally, mammals and insects contain β-*N*-acetyl-D-hexosaminidase (a cytosolic enzyme) to degrade chitin, releasing *N*-acetylglucosamine.

5.13.3.2.3 *Degradation of Intracellular Glycosaminoglycans by Animal Cells*

Many cell types (e.g., endothelial cells, skin fibroblasts, chondrocytes, vascular smooth muscle cells, and retinal pigment epithelial cells) synthesize glycosaminoglycans, including chondroitin 4-sulfate, chondroitin 6-sulfate, dermatan sulfate, heparan sulfate, and small amounts of keratan sulfate (Garantziotis and Savani 2019). These molecules are degraded by various isoforms of HYAL, arylsulfatase B, *N*-acetylgalactosamine-6-sulfatase, and lysosomal exoglycosidases, as described previously. In humans and other animals, the half-life of intracellular glycosaminoglycans is shorter than extracellular glycosaminoglycans (Bleckmann and Kresse 1980; Gamse et al. 1978).

5.14 SYNTHESIS AND CATABOLISM OF CHOLINE

5.14.1 HISTORY OF CHOLINE RESEARCH

A French chemist, T. Gobley, isolated a substance termed "lecithine" from brain tissue and carp (fish) eggs in 1850, which was named after the Greek "lekithos" for egg yolk. A German chemist, A. Strecker, found in 1862 that a new nitrogenous substance was generated after the lecithin from the bile of pigs and cattle was heated, and he named this biochemical "choline". Three years later, a German pharmacologist, O. Liebreich, identified lecithin as a component of phosphatidylcholine and synthesized choline (a trimethyl quaternary nitrogen) in the laboratory. The name "choline" was derived from the Greek word for bile – "chole". The work by O. Loewi and H. Dale in the 1910s and the early 1920s established the role for choline as part of acetylcholine, a neurotransmitter.

5.14.2 SYNTHESIS OF CHOLINE IN HUMANS AND OTHER ANIMALS

5.14.2.1 Synthesis of Choline in Humans

In 1932, C. Best identified an important role of choline in regulating mammalian lipid metabolism by demonstrating that fatty liver in dogs could be prevented by dietary supplementation with either raw pancreas or lecithin. Three years later, C. Best confirmed this seminal finding from studies of rats with a fatty liver. The underlying mechanisms involve the incorporation of choline into phosphatidylcholine through reactions with (1) cytidine 5-dihphosphocholine (discovered by E. Kennedy in 1954) and (2) phosphatidylethanolamine (identified by J. Bremer and D. Greenberg in 1960). Extensive research in the 1940s resulted in the following salient observations: (1) dietary choline could prevent the bone disease "perosis" in developing chickens; (2) a deficiency of dietary choline was associated with atheromatous changes in the aorta, carotid, and coronary arteries of rats; (3) hemorrhagic kidneys and intraocular hemorrhages developed in young rats deprived of choline; and (4) syndromes of choline deficiency could be manifested in the rabbit, calf, guinea pig, hamster, and baboon fed choline-deficient diets. Interestingly, work in the 1950s led to the recognition that choline-deficient animals had high risk for developing liver cancers. Furthermore, in the 1970s, R. Wurtman and D. Haubrich independently found that the rate of acetylcholine synthesis in both rats and guinea pigs was modulated by dietary choline intake. In the 1980s, several groups noted that the dietary availability of choline to fetal and infant rats greatly influenced their neurological function as assessed by spatial maze tests (see Zeisel 2012 for review). The results of these nutritional investigations led to an important suggestion that endogenous synthesis of choline may be limited in humans and other animals.

A series of papers from the group of S.H. Zeisel in the 1990s to 2010s indicated that humans synthesize choline in a sex-dependent manner. For example, men consuming defined, low-choline diets developed fatty liver and liver damage that resolved after choline was added to their diets (Zeisel et al. 1991). By contrast, premenopausal women who were deprived of dietary choline often did not develop the metabolic problem (Fischer et al. 2007), because estrogen induces the expression of the key gene (phosphatidylethanolamine N-methyltransferase) for the de novo biosynthesis of phosphatidylcholine in the liver as a source for choline (Resseguie et al. 2011). The subpopulation of premenopausal women who did develop choline deficiency when fed a low choline diet usually had a genetic variation in phosphatidylethanolamine N-methyltransferase that abrogated the estrogen responsiveness of this gene. Despite the resistance to choline deficiency seen in young women, almost all men and postmenopausal women developed fatty liver, liver damage, and/or muscle damage when fed a low choline diet (<50 mg choline/70 kg BW/day) for a prolonged period (42 days), and the metabolic defects resolved when choline was supplemented to the diets (Fischer et al. 2007). Collectively, these clinical findings indicate that humans have a limited ability to synthesize de novo choline. This notion is supported by the reports that (1) patients fed choline-free total parenteral nutrition solutions developed fatty liver and liver dysfunction in association with reduced concentrations of choline in the plasma (Tayek et al. 1990); and (2) administering choline to patients fed by total parenteral nutrition prevented the development of fatty liver (Buchman et al. 1995). Clearly, choline is a nutritionally essential nutrient for men and postmenopausal women, and for some premenopausal women. Abundant dietary sources of choline include eggs, meat, poultry, dairy products, fish, crustaceans, cruciferous vegetables, and peanuts.

5.14.2.2 Synthesis of Choline in Farm and Laboratory Animals

Chickens, pigs, and rats can synthesize choline from methionine, serine, and palmitate via the formation of phosphatidylethanolamine in the liver and brain (Wu 2018). The synthesis of phosphatidylcholine and other phospholipids occurs in both axons and cell bodies. In the rat liver, the cytidine 5-diphosphocholine and phosphatidylethanolamine pathways contribute to about 70% and 30% of phosphatidylcholine synthesis, respectively (Li and Vance 2008). In addition, gastrointestinal microbes possess this metabolic pathway and are also capable of forming choline via the generation of phosphatidylserine (Figure 5.26). However, the rate of the de novo synthesis of choline in the whole body is insufficient to meet the nutritional requirements of all these species under both normal and diseased conditions. Similar observations have been reported for fish and crustaceans (NRC 2011). Thus, the diets of all farm and laboratory animals must contain adequate choline to support their growth, development, and health.

5.14.3 Catabolism of Choline in Animal Cells and in Microbes

5.14.3.1 Catabolism of Choline in Cells of Humans and Other Animals

In mammals and birds, choline is oxidized to betaine and then to glycine in the liver and kidneys (Chapter 3) and is also converted into acetylcholine by choline acetyltransferase in the nervous system. Glycine is degraded in animal cells as described in Chapter 4. Acetylcholine is hydrolyzed by acetylcholine esterase into choline and acetate. For clearance from the body, choline is taken up by the liver to be reincorporated into phosphatidylcholine, phosphatidylethanolamine, very low-density lipoproteins, and high-density lipoproteins. Phosphatidylcholine, phosphatidylethanolamine, and free choline are secreted via the bile into the duodenum. Approximately 95% of the biliary choline is reabsorbed at the terminal ileum into the portal circulation, about 40% and 60% of this choline are returned to the liver and extrahepatic tissues, respectively (Li and Vance 2008). The 5% of secreted biliary choline is excreted from the body via the feces.

Choline + Acetyl-CoA → Acetylcholine + CoA   (choline acetyltransferase; liver and kidneys)

Acetylcholine + H_2O → Choline + Acetate   (acetylcholine esterase; the nervous system)

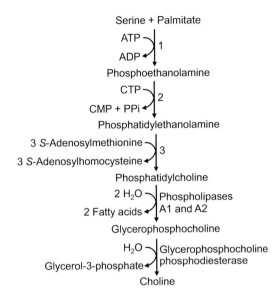

FIGURE 5.26 Synthesis of choline in the liver and brain of humans and other animals. The enzymes that catalyze the indicated reactions are (1) a series of enzymes [serine palmitoyl transferase (vitamin B_6), keto-sphinganine reductase, ceramide, synthase, dihydroceramide desaturase, ceramidase, sphingosine kinase, and sphingosine-1-phosphate lyase]; (2) two enzymes (CTP:phosphoethanolamine cytidylyltransferase and CDP-ethanolamine:1,2-diacylglycerol ethanolamine-phosphotransferase); and (3) a phosphatidylethanolamine *N*-methyltransferase.

5.14.3.2 Catabolism of Choline in Microbes

Choline is catabolized into trimethylamine and acetaldehyde in the anaerobic microbes, including those in the intestine of humans and other animals. The responsible enzymes are choline:trimethylamine lyase, as well as choline dehydrogenase and betaine aldehyde dehydrogenase (Craciun and Balskus 2012). Trimethylamine is oxidized to trimethylamine N-oxide as described previously (Figure 5.11) and is also an important substrate for methanogenesis in both the gastrointestinal tracts of ruminants and marine sediments. In the intestinal bacteria, acetaldehyde is oxidized by (1) acetaldehyde dehydrogenase to yield acetyl-CoA and (2) acetaldehyde reductase to generate ethanol (Figure 5.11). In adult ruminants, choline is extensively degraded in the rumen and, therefore, dietary choline contributes insignificantly to the choline pool in the body. Supplemental choline must be protected to ensure its availability for absorption by the small intestine.

5.15 SYNTHESIS AND CATABOLISM OF FORMATE

5.15.1 Historic Perspectives

Formic acid [HCOOH; formate (HCOO⁻) in the deionized form] occurs widely in animals, microbes, and plants. It was first described in 1670 by John Wray in his letter to the *Philosophical Transactions of the Royal Society* that was based on the information sent to him from fellow scientists. Interestingly, in contrast to birds, most mammals, and stomached fish that generate HCl as gastric acid, the stomach of the giant anteater (also known as the ant bear, an insectivorous mammal native to Central and South America) does not produce HCl. The giant anteater depends on the *formic acid* of its prey to acidify the gastric juice and digest food (Macdonald 2001). It is now known that the liver and kidneys of humans and other animals synthesize formate for one-carbon metabolism. The concentration of this substance in the plasma of nonpregnant mammals is about 30 μM, which is much greater than that of tetrahydrofolate (THF, another key molecule in one-carbon metabolism) and can reach up to 200 µM in the fetal plasma (Washburn et al. 2015), indicating an important role for folate in cell growth and development.

5.15.2 Synthesis and Catabolism of Formate in Animals

5.15.2.1 Synthesis of Formate in Humans and Other Animals

Diet is a source of formate for humans and other animals. In addition, mammals, birds, fish, and crustaceans produce formate from (1) the catabolism of AAs (including serine, glycine, histidine, and tryptophan) in the mitochondria and cytosol; (2) the α-oxidation of branched-chain fatty acids (e.g., phytanic acid and branched-chain α-ketoacids) in the peroxisome; (3) cytochrome P450-catalyzed demethylation reactions (e.g., the demethylation of lanosterol to cholestatrienol by lanosterol 14α-demethylase during cholesterol synthesis in the liver, the demethylation of testosterone to estradiol by aromatase); and (4) the oxidation of formaldehyde via formaldehyde dehydrogenase in the mitochondria and a cytochrome-P450 (CYP2E1)-catalyzed reaction in the endoplasmic reticulum (Brosnan and Brosnan 2016). These THF-dependent and THF-independent metabolic pathways are illustrated in Figure 5.27. Choline and methanol are sources of formaldehyde in animals. Serine appears to be the major source of formate in mammals. This is consistent with the previous report that serine itself accounts for about 60% of total α-AAs in the allantoic fluid of fetal lambs on Day

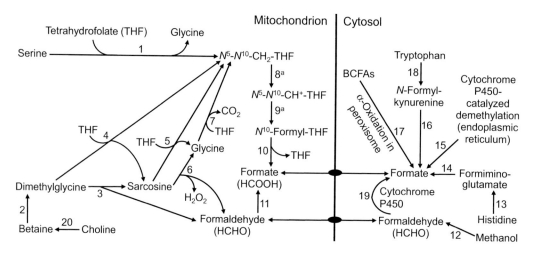

FIGURE 5.27 Formation of formate via tetrahydrofolate (THF)-dependent and THF-independent pathways in humans and other animals. The enzymes that catalyze the indicated reactions are (1) serine hydroxymethyltransferase; (2) betaine transmethylase; (3) dimethylglycine oxidase; (4) dimethylglycine dehydrogenase; (5) sarcosine dehydrogenase; (6) sarcosine oxidase; (7) glycine dehydrogenase; (8) N^5,N^{10}-methylene-THF dehydrogenase; (9) N^5,N^{10}-methenyl-THF cyclohydrolase; (10) N^{10}-formyl-THF dehydrogenase; (11) formaldehyde dehydrogenase (NAD+-dependent); (12) methanol dehydrogenase (NAD+-dependent); (13) a series of enzymes (histidase, urocanate hydratase, and imidazole propionase); (14) a series of enzymes (glutamate formiminotransferase, N^5-formimo-tetrahydrofolate cyclodeaminase, N^5,N^{10}-methylene-THF dehydrogenase, N^5,N^{10}-methenyl-THF cyclohydrolase, and N^{10}-formyl-THF dehydrogenase); (15) cytochrome P450-catalyzed demethylation in the endoplasmic reticulum (e.g., the demethylation of lanosterol to cholestatrienol by lanosterol 14α-demethylase during cholesterol synthesis in the liver, the demethylation of testosterone to estradiol by aromatase); (16) kynurenine formamidase; (17) the α-oxidation of branched-chain fatty acids (e.g., phytanic acid and branched-chain α-ketoacids) in the peroxisome; (18) indoleamine-2,3-dioxygenase and tryptophan 2,3-dioxygenase; (19) oxidation of formaldehyde by a cytochrome-P450 (CYP2E1)-catalyzed reaction in the endoplasmic reticulum; and (20) two enzymes (choline oxidase and betaine aldehyde dehydrogenase). BCFAs, branched-chain fatty acids. [a] bifunctional protein in mammalian mitochondria.

140 of gestation, when their absolute growth is very rapid (Kwon et al. 2003). Knockout of the mitochondrial serine hydroxymethyltransferase in mice leads to neural tube defects of fetuses (Momb et al. 2013), further highlighting the key role of serine and one-carbon metabolism in embryonic survival, growth, and development.

5.15.2.2 Catabolism of Formate in Humans and Other Animals

In mammals and birds, formate is oxidized to CO_2 through (1) mitochondrial NAD^+-dependent formate dehydrogenase; (2) catalase in the peroxisome; and (3) the oxidation of the formyl group of N^{10}-formyl-THF by N^{10}-formyl-THF dehydrogenase to CO_2 in the cytosol. The catalase-catalyzed oxidation of formate depends on the availability of H_2O_2, and this reaction may be limited by the production of the oxidant (Waydhas et al. 1978). The formyl group of N^{10}-formyl-THF is derived from formate, and this incorporation reaction is catalyzed by N^{10}-formyl-THF synthase, a cytosolic, ATP-driven trifunctional protein that also possesses N^5,N^{10}-methenyl-THF cyclohydrolase and N^5,N^{10}-methylene-THF dehydrogenase activities in mammalian cells.

$$HCOOH + NAD^+ \rightarrow CO_2 + NADH + H^+ \quad \text{(formate dehydrogenase; mitochondria)}$$

$$HCOOH + H_2O_2 \rightarrow CO_2 + 2H_2O \quad \text{(formate dehydrogenase; mitochondria)}$$

$$HCOOH + THF \rightarrow N^{10}\text{-formyl-THF} \quad \left(N^{10}\text{-formyl-THF synthase, trifunctional protein; cytosol}\right)$$

$$N^{10}\text{-formyl-THF} + NAD^+ \rightarrow CO_2 + THF + NADH + H^+ \quad (N^{10}\text{-formyl-THF dehydrogenase;}$$
$$\text{mitochondrial and cytosol)}$$

5.15.3 Synthesis and Catabolism of Formate in Microbes

Fermentation of AAs, carbohydrates, and fatty acids by anaerobic microbes produces formate via complex metabolic pathways (Wu 2018). Some of these reactions are similar to those described for animal cells. Microbes degrade formate to CO_2 via reactions similar to those described for animal cells, except that N^5,N^{10}-methenyl-THF cyclohydrolase and N^5,N^{10}-methylene-THF dehydrogenase is a bifunctional protein (one protein with two different enzymatic activities) in bacteria, and N^{10}-formyl-THF synthase is a monofunctional protein. In the ruminal bacteria of ruminants, formate is further used to produce methane via a series of complex reactions (Wu 2018).

5.16 CONJUGATION PRODUCTS FOR URINARY EXCRETION

5.16.1 Formation of Hippurate from Glycine

A pathway for glycine utilization is the synthesis of hippurate, which shares a long history with AA metabolism. In 1829, J. von Liebig identified a difference between hippuric acid and benzoic acid and in 1839 determined the composition of hippuric acid. The structure of hippuric acid was established by its chemical synthesis from benzoyl chloride and the zinc salt of glycine in 1873 by V. Dessaignes. In humans and other animals, benzoic acid reacts with glycine to form hippurate in the mitochondria of hepatocytes (Figure 5.28). Hippurate is excreted in the urine (1–2.5 g per day by the average healthy adult man; Stein et al. 1954). This pathway is physiologically important for herbivores and omnivores who consume significant amounts of benzoic acid that naturally occurs in plants, particularly berries and fruits. Because ammonia is incorporated into glycine via the glycine cleavage system and the formation of serine (Figure 5.28), the formation of hippurate irreversibly removes ammonia from the circulation. Thus, sodium benzoate is often used to treat patients with hyperammonemia in clinical practice. In healthy humans, their urine contains only a small amount of hippurate. Interestingly, concentrations of hippurate are relatively high in the urine of healthy herbivores.

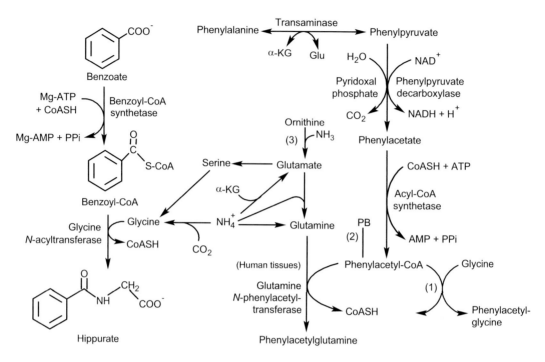

FIGURE 5.28 Formation of hippurate and phenylacetylglutamine in the mitochondria of the liver and kidneys of humans and other select animals. Hippurate is produced from glycine and benzoate in all animals (including humans), whereas phenylacetylglutamine is synthesized from phenylalanine and glutamine in select species (e.g., humans and swine). As reported for swine, phenylacetate-derived phenylacetyl-CoA reacts with glycine to generate phenylacetylglycine. In some animal species (e.g., rats) that normally do not produce phenylacetylglutamine, exogenous phenylbutyrate is converted into phenylacetyl-CoA, which then reacts with glutamine to generate phenylacetylglutamine. These reactions play an important role in the removal of ammonia after it is incorporated into glycine, serine, glutamate, and glutamine through the metabolism of amino acids. Thus, ornithine phenylacetate or ornithine phenylbutyrate can be used to reduce the concentration of ammonia in humans and other animals with hyperammonemia. The enzymes that catalyze the indicated reactions are (1) glycine *N*-phenylacetyltransferase; (2) enzymes of the mitochondrial β-oxidation; and (3) ornithine aminotransferase and pyrroline-5-carboxylate dehydrogenase. PB, phenylbutyrate.

5.16.2 Species-Specific Formation of Phenylacetylglutamine from Phenylalanine and Glutamine

Phenylacetylglutamine was originally described in 1914 by H. Thierfelder and C.P. Sherwin as a normal constituent of human urine. This substance was present in large amounts in the plasma of humans after the oral or intravenous administration of phenylacetate (Thibault et al. (1994) and in patients with renal insufficiency (Jankowski et al. 2003). A pathway for the utilization of phenylalanine and glutamine is the synthesis of phenylacetylglutamine occurring in a species-specific manner. In the liver and kidneys of humans, phenylalanine is transaminated to yield phenylpyruvate, which is decarboxylated to form phenylacetate (Figure 5.28). Phenylacetate is activated by an acylating enzyme (e.g., acyl-CoA synthetase) to become phenylacetyl-CoA. The latter reacts with glutamine to produce phenylacetylglutamine, and this reaction is catalyzed by glutamine *N*-phenylacetyltransferase. Phenylacetylglutamine is excreted in the urine (250–500 mg per day by the average healthy adult man; Stein et al. 1954). The urinary concentration of phenylacetylglutamine increases markedly in patients who have elevated levels of phenylalanine in the circulation. Because glutamine is synthesized from ammonia and α-ketoglutarate, phenylacetate (sodium salt) is often used to treat human patients with hyperammonemia (Chapter 12).

In addition to humans, pigs are also capable of synthesizing phenylacetylglutamine from phenylacetate and glutamine (Ytrebø et al. 2009). Furthermore, the exogenous administration of phenylacetate into pigs increases the synthesis and urinary excretion of phenylacetylglycine as another route for ammonia removal (Ytrebø et al. 2009). Interestingly, the amount of phenylacetylglycine excreted in the urine is greater than that of phenylacetylglutamine in this species (Kristiansen et al. 2014). It is possible that the activity of glycine *N*-phenylacetyltransferase in the porcine liver and kidneys is greater than that of glutamine *N*-phenylacetyltransferase.

Some animal species, including the cat, dog, horse, monkey, rabbit, rat, and sheep, do not appear to convert phenylalanine and glutamine into phenylacetylglutamine under normal physiological conditions (Moldave and Meister 1957). Thus, the exogenous administration of phenylacetate into rats does not result in detectable phenylacetylglutamine in their blood or urine (Dadsetan et al. 2013). This suggests that phenylacetate is not metabolized to phenylacetyl-CoA in the rat liver and kidneys possibly due to the absence or negligible activity of acyl-CoA synthetase for phenylacetate. Such an explanation may also apply to cats, dogs, horses, monkeys, rabbits, and sheep. Of note, preclinical studies have also shown that the exogenous administration of phenylbutyrate into rats increases the synthesis and urinary excretion of phenylacetylglutamine (Davies et al. 2009). Phenylbutyrate can be converted, via the mitochondrial β-oxidation, into phenylacetyl-CoA, which then reacts with glutamine to generate phenylacetylglutamine (Figure 5.28). These findings further support the view that a lack of acyl-CoA synthetase activity for phenylacetate is the biochemical basis for the inability of rats and possibly some other species (e.g., cats, dogs, horses, monkeys, rabbits, and sheep) to synthesize phenylacetylglutamine.

5.17 SUMMARY

In humans and other animals, AAs are utilized in many synthetic pathways to produce amino sugars, carnitine, catecholamines, choline, creatine, dipeptides, formate, glutathione, glycine-proline-hydroxyproline, heme, hexosamine, hippurate, imidazoles, melanin, melatonin, phenylacetylglutamine (species-specific), polyamines, purines, pyrimidines, serotonin, and thyroid hormones. Physiologically significant imidazoles include anserine (in many species but absent in humans), acetylhistidine, carcinine, carnosine, histamine, homoanserine, homocarnosine, and urocanic acid, which are all derivatives of methylhistidine. Syntheses of most of these imidazoles and nonimidazoles require (1) BH4, SAM, and pyridoxal phosphate; (2) glutamine, glutamate, glycine, histidine, and tyrosine; (3) either interorgan metabolism of multiple AAs involving skeletal muscle, brain, kidney and liver (e.g., creatine and carnitine), ubiquitous expression of enzymes in all cell types (purines and pyrimidines), or specific endocrine glands (e.g., pineal gland and thyroid); and (4) intracellular compartmentation involving the mitochondria and the cytoplasm. Mammalian liver and skeletal muscle have particularly high concentrations of glutathione and carnosine, respectively, whereas creatine is very abundant in both the central nervous system and skeletal muscle. Hippurate, creatinine, carnitine, phenylacetylglutamine, as well as the sulfate and glucuronide conjugates of catecholamines, melatonin, melanin, and foreign compounds are nontoxic substances for urinary nitrogen excretion from the body. It is expected that the rich history for the synthesis of the AA derivatives described in this chapter will guide the future discovery of new AA metabolites, dipeptides, and tripeptides with biological importance.

REFERENCES

Abe, M., M.T. Itoh, M. Miyata, K. Shimizu, and Y. Sumi. 2000. Circadian rhythm of serotonin N-acetyltransferase activity in rat lens. *Exp. Eye Res.* 70:805–808.

Agostinelli, E. 2020. Biochemical and pathophysiological properties of polyamines. *Amino Acids* 52:111–117.

Ahn, M.Y., K.H. Shin, D.H. Kim, E.A. Jung, T. Toida, R.J. Linhardt, and Y.S. Kim. 1998. Characterization of a *Bacteroides* species from human intestine that degrades glycosaminoglycans. *Can. J. Microbiol.* 44:423–429.

Ajioka, R.S., J.D. Phillips, and J.P. Kushner. 2006. Biosynthesis of heme in mammals. *Biochim. Biophys. Acta* 1763:723–736.

Akil, H., F. Meng, D.P. Devine, and S.J. Watson. 1997. Molecular and neuroanatomical properties of the endogenous opioid system: implications for the treatment of opiate addiction. *Semin. Neurosci.* 9:70–83.

Arreola, R., B. Valderrama, M.L. Morante, and E. Horjales. 2003. Two mammalian glucosamine-6-phosphate deaminase: a structural and genetic study. *FEBS Lett.* 551:63–70.

Asatoor, A.M., J.K. Bandoh, A.F. Lant, M.D. Milne, and F. Navab. 1970. Intestinal absorption of carnosine and its constituent amino acids in man. *Gut* 11:250–254.

Baguet, A, I. Everaert, E. Achten, M. Thomis, and W. Derave. 2012. The influence of sex, age and heritability on human skeletal muscle carnosine content. *Amino Acids* 43:13–20.

Baharom, S., R. De Matteo, S. Ellery, P. Della Gatta, C.R. Bruce, G.M. Kowalski et al. 2017. Does maternal-fetal transfer of creatine occur in pregnant sheep? *Am. J. Physiol.* 313:E75–83.

Barati, M., F. Javanmardi, S.M.H.M. Jazayeri, M. Jabbari, and J. Rahmani. 2020. Techniques, perspectives, and challenges of bioactive peptide generation: a comprehensive systematic review. *Comprehensive Rev. Food Sci. Food Safety* 19:1488–1520.

Barbaresi, S., L. Maertens, E. Claeys, W. Derave, and S. De Smet. 2019. Differences in muscle histidine-containing dipeptides in broilers. *J. Sci. Food Agric.* 99:5680–5686.

Baslow, M.H. 1965. Neurosine, its identification with *N*-acetyl-L-histidine and distribution in aquatic vertebrates. *Zoologica* 50:63–66.

Bégué, J.-P. and D. Bonnet-Delpon. 2008. *Bioorganic and Medicinal Chemistry of Fluorine,* Wiley, Hoboken, NJ. p. 271.

Beuzard, Y., R. Rodvien, and I.M. London. 1973. Effect of hemin on the synthesis of hemoglobin and other proteins in mammalian cells. *Proc. Nat. Acad. Sci. USA.* 70:1022–1026.

Bianco, A.C. and B.W. Kim. 2006. Deiodinases: implications of the local control of thyroid hormone action. *J. Clin. Invest.* 116:2571–2579.

Blanco, A. and G. Blanco. 2017. *Medical Biochemistry.* Academic Press, San Diego, CA.

Blancquaert, L., I. Everaert, M. Missinne, A. Baguet, S. Stegen, A. Volkaert et al. 2017. Effects of histidine and β-alanine supplementation on human muscle carnosine storage. *Med. Sci. Sports Exerc.* 49:602–609.

Bleckmann, H. and H. Kresse. 1980. Glycosaminoglycan metabolism of cultured cornea cells derived from bovine and human stroma and from bovine epithelium. *Exp. Eye Res.* 30:469–479.

Boldyrev, A.A., G. Aldini, and W. Derave. 2013. Physiology and pathophysiology of carnosine. *Physiol. Rev.* 93:1803–45.

Bodnar, R.J. 2018. Endogenous opiates and behavior: 2016. *Peptides* 101:167–212.

Boonen, M., E. Puissant, F. Gilis, B. Flamion, and M. Jadot. 2014. Mouse liver lysosomes contain enzymatically active processed forms of Hyal-1. *Biochem. Biophys. Res. Commun.* 446:1155–1160.

Boot, R.G., E.F.C. Blommaart, E. Swart, K. Ghauharali-van der Vlugt, N. Bijl, C. Moe et al. 2001. Identification of a novel acidic mammalian chitinase distinct from chitotriosidase. *J. Biol. Chem.* 276:670–6778.

Borges, C.R., J.C. Roberts, D.G. Wilkins, and D.E. Rollins. 2001. Relationship of melanin degradation products to actual melanin content: application to human hair. *Anal. Biochem.* 290:116–125.

Bourdin, B., H. Adenier, and Y. Perrin. 2007. Carnitine is associated with fatty acid metabolism in plants. *Plant Physiol. Biochem.* 45:926–931.

Bremer, J. 1983. Carnitine – metabolism and functions. *Physiol. Rev.* 63:1420–1480.

Brent, G.A. 2012. Mechanisms of thyroid hormone action. *J. Clin. Invest.* 122:3035–3043.

Brosnan, M.E. and J.T. Brosnan. 2007. Orotic acid excretion and arginine metabolism. *J. Nutr.* 137:1656S–1661S.

Brosnan, M.E. and J.T. Brosnan. 2016. Formate: the neglected member of one-carbon metabolism. *Annu. Rev. Nutr.* 36:369–388.

Brosnan, J.T., E.P. Wijekoon, L. Warford-Woolgar, N.L. Trottier, M.E. Brosnan, J.A. Brunton, and R.F.P. Bertolo. 2009. Creatine synthesis is a major metabolic process in neonatal piglets and has important implications for amino acid metabolism and methyl balance. *J. Nutr.* 139:1292–1297.

Buchman, A., M. Dubin, A. Moukarzel, D. Jenden, M. Roch, K. Rice, J. Gornbein, and M. Ament. 1995. Choline deficiency: a cause of hepatic steatosis during parenteral nutrition that can be reversed with intravenous choline supplementation. *Hepatology* 22:1399–1403.

Calles-Escandon, J., J.J. Cunningham, P. Snyder, R. Jacob, G. Huszar, J. Lake, and P. Felig. 1984. Influence of exercise on urea, creatinine, and 3-methylhistidine excretion in normal human subjects. *Am. J. Physiol.* 246:E334–338.

Carnegie, P.R., K.P. Hee, and A.W. Bell. 1982. Ophidine (β-alanyl-L-3-methylhistidine, 'balenine') and other histidine dipeptides in pig muscles and tinned hams. *J. Sci. Food Agric.* 33:795–801.

Casey, A. and P.L. Greenhaff. 2000. Does dietary creatine supplementation play a role in skeletal muscle metabolism and performance? *Am. J. Clin. Nutr.* 72:607S–617S.

Chakrabarti, S., S. Guha, and K. Majumder. 2018. Food-derived bioactive peptides in human health: challenges and opportunities. *Nutrients* 10:1738.

Chiabrando, D., S. Mercurio, and E. Tolosano. 2014. Heme and erythropoieis: more than a structural role. *Haematologica* 99:973–983.

Childers, S.R. 1991. Opioid receptor-coupled second messenger systems. *Life Sci.* 48:1991–2003.

Craciun, S. and E.P. Balskus. 2012. Microbial conversion of choline to trimethylamine requires a glycyl radical enzyme. *Proc. Natl. Acad. Sci. USA.* 109:21307–21312.

Culbertson, J.Y., R.B. Kreider, M. Greenwood, and M. Cooke. 2010. Effects of beta-alanine on muscle carnosine and exercise performance: a review of the current literature. *Nutrients* 2:75–98.

Dadsetan, S., M. Sørensen, L.K. Bak, H. Vilstrup, P. Ott, A. Schousboe et al. 2013. Interorgan metabolism of ornithine phenylacetate (OP)-A novel strategy for treatment of hyperammonemia. *Biochem. Pharmacol.* 85:115–123.

Davies, N.A., G. Wright, L.M. Ytrebø, V. Stadlbauer, O.-M. Fuskevåg, C. Zwingmann et al. 2009. L-Ornithine and phenylacetate synergistically produce sustained reduction in ammonia and brain water in cirrhotic rats. *Hepatology* 50:155–164.

Degenhardt, T., S. Väisänen, M. Rakhshandehroo, S. Kersten, and C. Carlberg. 2009. Peroxisome proliferator-activated receptor alpha controls hepatic heme biosynthesis through ALAS. *J. Mol. Biol.* 388:225–238.

Derave, W., M.S. Ozdemir, R.C. Harris, A. Pottier, H. Reyngout, K. Koppo, J.A. Wise, and E. Achten. 2007. Beta-alanine supplementation augments muscle carnosine content and attenuates fatigue during repeated isokinetic contraction bouts in trained sprinters. *J. Appl. Physiol.* 103:1736–1743.

Ding, C.Z., X. Lu, K. Nishimura, and R.B. Silverman. 1993. Transformation of monoamine oxidase-B primary amine substrates into time-dependent inhibitors. Tertiary amine homologs of primary amine substrates. *J. Med. Chem.* 36:1711–1715.

Drozak, J., M. Veiga-da-Cunha, D. Vertommen, V. Stroobant, and E. Van Schaftingen. 2010. Molecular identification of carnosine synthase as ATP-grasp domain-containing protein 1 (ATPGD1). *J. Biol. Chem.* 285:9346–9356.

Du, X., M. Schwander, E.M.Y. Moresco, P. Viviani, C. Haller, M.S. Hildebrand et al. 2008. A catechol-*O*-methyltransferase that is essential for auditory function in mice and humans. *Proc. Natl. Acad. Sci. USA.* 105:14609–14614.

Edison, E.E., M.E. Brosnan, K. Aziz, and J.T. Brosnan. 2013. Creatine and guanidinoacetate content of human milk and infant formulas: implications for creatine deficiency syndromes and amino acid metabolism. *Br. J. Nutr.* 110:1075–1078.

Etemadian, Y., V. Ghaemi, A.R. Shaviklo, P. Pourashouri, A.R.S. Mahoonak, and F. Rafipour. 2021. Development of animal/ plant-based protein hydrolysate and its application in food, feed and nutraceutical industries: state of the art. *J. Cleaner Prod.* 278:123219.

Evans, D.R. and H.I. Guy. 2004. Mammalian pyrimidine biosynthesis: fresh insights into an ancient pathway. *J. Biol. Chem.* 279:33035–33038.

Everaert, I., A. Mooyaart, A. Baguet, A. Zutininc, H. Baelde, E. Achten et al. 2011. Vegetarianism, female gender and increasing age, but not CNDP1 genotype, are associated with reduced muscle carnosine levels in humans. *Amino Acids* 40:1221–1229.

Fan, X.X., S. Li, Z.L. Wu, Z.L. Dai, J. Li, X.L. Wang, and G. Wu. 2019. Glycine supplementation to breast-fed piglets attenuates postweaning jejunal epithelial apoptosis: a functional role of CHOP signaling. *Amino Acids* 51:463–473.

Fennema, D., I.R. Phillips, and E.A. Shephard. 2016. Trimethylamine and trimethylamine N-oxide, a flavin-containing monooxygenase 3 (FMO3)-mediated host-microbiome metabolic axis implicated in health and disease. *Drug Metab. Dispos.* 44:1839–1850.

Fernstrom, J.D. and M.H. Fernstrom. 2007. Tyrosine, phenylalanine, and catecholamine synthesis and function in the brain. *J. Nutr.* 137:1539S–1547S.

Fernstrom, J.D. and R.J. Wurtman. 1971. Brain serotonin content: physiological dependence on plasma tryptophan levels. *Science* 173:149–152.

Ferreira, G.C. 2013. Heme synthesis. In: *Encyclopedia of Biological Chemistry* (Lennarz, W.J. and M.D. Lane, eds). Academic Press, San Diego, CA. pp. 539–542.

Ferry, G., C. Ubeaud, P. Lambert, S. Bertin, F. Cogé, P. Chomarat et al. 2005. Molecular evidence that melatonin is enzymatically oxidized in a different manner than tryptophan: investigations with both indoleamine 2,3-dioxygenase and myeloperoxidase. *Biochem. J.* 388:205–215.

Fischer, L.M., K. daCosta, L. Kwock, P. Stewart, T. Lu, S. Stabler, R. Allen, and S. Zeisel. 2007. Sex and menopausal status influence human dietary requirements for the nutrient choline. *Am. J. Clin. Nutr.* 85:1275–1285.

Flanagan, J.L., P.A. Simmons, J. Vehige, M.D.P. Willcox, and Q. Garrett. 2010. Role of carnitine in disease. *Nutr. Metab.* (Lond) 7:30.

Fong, W.F., J.S. Heller, and E.S. Canellakis. 1976. The appearance of an ornithine decarboxylase inhibitory protein upon the addition of putrescine to cell cultures. *Biochim. Biophys. Acta* 428:456–465.

Fu, W.J., T.E. Haynes, R. Kohli, J. Hu, W. Shi, T.E. Spencer et al. 2005. Dietary L-arginine supplementation reduces fat mass in Zucker diabetic fatty rats. *J. Nutr.* 135:714–721.

Gamse, G., H.G. Fromme, and H. Kresse. 1978. Metabolism of sulfated glycosaminoglycans in cultured endothelial cells and smooth muscle cells from bovine aorta. *Biochim. Biophys. Acta* 544:514–528.

Gao, J., Y. Hu, S. Li, Y. Zhang, and X. Chen. 2013. Tautomeric equilibrium of creatinine and creatininium cation in aqueous solutions explore by Raman spectroscopy and density functional theory calculations. *Chem. Phys.* 410:81–89.

Garantziotis, S. and R.C. Savani. 2019. Hyaluronan biology: a complex balancing act of structure, function, location and context. *Matrix Biol.* 78–79:1–10.

Gilbreath, K.R., F.W. Bazer, M.C. Satterfield, and G. Wu. 2021. Amino acid nutrition and reproductive performance in ruminants. *Adv. Exp. Med. Biol.* 1285:43–61.

Gould, R.L. and R. Pazdro. 2019. Impact of supplementary amino acids, micronutrients, and overall diet on glutathione homeostasis. *Nutrients* 11:1056.

Griffith, O.W. 1999. Biologic and pharmacologic regulation of mammalian glutathione synthesis. *Free Radical Biol. Med.* 27:922–935.

Grimble, R.F., A.A. Jackson, C. Persaud, M.J. Wride, F. Delers, and R. Engler. 1992. Cysteine and glycine supplementation modulate the metabolic response to tumor necrosis factor alpha in rats fed a low protein diet. *J. Nutr.* 122:2066–2073.

Gushulak, L., R. Hemming, D. Martin, V. Seyrantepe, A. Pshezhetsky, and B. Triggs-Raine. 2012. Hyaluronidase 1 and β-hexosaminidase have redundant functions in hyaluronan and chondroitin sulfate degradation. *J. Biol. Chem.* 287:16689–16697.

Handschin, C., J. Lin, J. Rhee, A. Peyer, S. Chin, P. Wu, U.A. Meyer, and B.M. Spiegelman. 2005. Nutritional regulation of hepatic heme biosynthesis and porphyria through PGC-1α. *Cell* 122:505–515.

Harris, C.I. and G. Milne. 1986. The identification of the N tau-methyl histidine-containing dipeptide, balenine, in muscle extracts from various mammals and the chicken. *Comp. Biochem. Physiol.* B 86:273–279.

Harris, R.C., M.J. Tallon, M. Dunnett, L. Boobis, J. Coakley, H.J. Kim et al. 2006. The absorption of orally supplied beta-alanine and its effect on muscle carnosine synthesis in human vastus lateralis. *Amino Acids* 30:279–289.

Harris, R.C., J.A. Wise, K.A. Price, H.J. Kim, C.K. Kim, and C. Sale. 2012. Determinants of muscle carnosine content. *Amino Acids* 43:5–12.

He, W.L. and G. Wu. 2020. Metabolism of amino acids in the brain and their roles in regulating food intake. *Adv. Exp. Med. Biol.* 1265:167–185.

Hill, C.A., R.C. Harris, H.J. Kim, B.D. Harris, C. Sale, L.H. Boobis, C.K. Kim, and J.A. Wise. 2007. Influence of beta-alanine supplementation on skeletal muscle carnosine concentrations and high intensity cycling capacity. *Amino Acids* 32:225–233.

Höglund, E., Ø. Øverli, and S. Winberg. 2019. Tryptophan metabolic pathways and brain serotonergic activity: a comparative review. *Front. Endocrinol.* 10:158.

Horinishi, H., M. Grillo, and F.L. Margolis. 1978. Purification and characterization of carnosine synthetase from mouse olfactory bulbs. *J. Neurochem.* 31:909–919.

Hou, Y.Q., Z.L. Wu, Z.L. Dai, G.H. Wang, and G. Wu. 2017. Protein hydrolysates in animal nutrition: industrial production, bioactive peptides, and functional significance. *J. Anim. Sci. Biotechnol.* 8:24.

Hou, Y.Q., W.L. He, S.D. Hu, and G. Wu. 2019. Composition of polyamines and amino acids in plant-source foods for human consumption. *Amino Acids* 51:1153–1165.

Hou, Y.Q., S.D. Hu, X.Y. Li, W.L. He, and G. Wu. 2020. Amino acid metabolism in the liver: nutritional and physiological significance. *Adv. Exp. Med. Biol.* 1265:21–37.

Huang, H., Y. Li, J. Liang, and F.D. Finkelman. 2018. Molecular regulation of histamine synthesis. *Front. Immunol.* 9:1392.

Ignarro, L.J., G.M. Buga, L.H. Wei, P.M. Bauer, G. Wu, and P. del Soldato. 2001. Role of the arginine-nitric oxide pathway in the regulation of vascular smooth muscle cell proliferation. *Proc. Natl. Acad. Sci. USA.* 98:4202–4208.

Jadin, L., L.H. Bookbinder, and G.I. Frost. 2012. A comprehensive model of hyaluronan turnover in the mouse. *Matrix Biol.* 31:81–89.

Jäger, R., R.C. Harris, M. Purpura, and M. Francaux. 2007. Comparison of new forms of creatine in raising plasma creatine levels. *J. Int. Soc. Sports Nutr.* 4:17.

Jankowski, J., M. van der Giet, V. Jankowski, S. Schmidt, M. Hemeier, B. Mahn et al. 2003. Increased plasma phenylacetic acid in patients with end-stage renal failure inhibits iNOS expression. *J. Clin. Invest.* 112:256–264.

Johnson, P. and J.L. Hammer. 1992. Histidine dipeptide levels in ageing and hypertensive rat skeletal and cardiac muscles. *Comp. Biochem. Physiol.* B 103:981–984.

Jones, N.R. 1956. Anserinase and other dipeptidase activity in skeletal muscle of codling (*Gadus callarias*). *Biochem. J.* 64:20.

Kahana, C. 2018. The antizyme family for regulating polyamines. *J. Biol. Chem.* 293:18730–18735.

Kepka-Lenhart, D., S.K. Mistry, G. Wu, and S.M. Morris, Jr. 2000. Arginase I: a limiting factor for nitric oxide and polyamine synthesis by activated macrophages? *Am. J. Physiol.* 279:R2237–2242.

Khosravi, S., S. Rahimnejad, M. Herault, V. Fournier, C.R. Lee, H.T. Dio Bui et al. 2015. Effects of protein hydrolysates supplementation in low fish meal diets on growth performance, innate immunity and disease resistance of red sea bream Pagrus major. *Fish Shellfish Immunol.* 45:858–868.

Kikuchi, G, T. Yoshida, and M. Noguchi. 2005. Heme oxygenase and heme degradation. *Biochem. Biophys. Res. Commun.* 338:558–567.

Kim, K.S., B. Backus, M. Harris, and P. Rourke. 1969. Distribution of diamine oxidase and imidazole-*N*-methyltransferase along the gastrointestinal tract. *Comp. Biochem. Physiol.* 31:137–145.

Kim, Y., M.T. King, W.E. Teague, G.A. Rufo, Jr., R.L. Veech, and J.V. Passonneau. 1992. Regulation of the purine salvage pathway in rat liver. *Am. J. Physiol.* 262:E344–E352.

Kim, S.W., E. van Heugten, F. Ji, C.H. Lee, and R.D. Mateo. 2010. Fermented soybean meal as a vegetable protein source for nursery pigs: I. Effects on growth performance of nursery pigs. *J. Anim. Sci.* 88:214–224.

Kim, J.Y., G.W. Song, G. Wu, and F.W. Bazer. 2012. Functional roles of fructose. *Proc. Natl. Acad. Sci. USA.* 109:E1619–1628.

King, C., G. Rios, M. Green, and T. Tephly. 2000. UDP-glucuronosyltransferases. *Curr. Drug Metab.* 1:143–161.

Kopin, I.J. 1985. Catecholamine metabolism: basic aspects and clinical significance. *Pharmacol Rev.* 37:333–364.

Krashin, E., A. Piekiełko-Witkowska, M. Ellis, and O. Ashur-Fabian. 2019. Thyroid hormones and cancer: a comprehensive review of preclinical and clinical studies. *Front. Endocrinol.* 10:59.

Krebs, H.A. 1964. The metabolic fate of amino acids. In: *Mammalian Protein Metabolism* (Munro, H.N. and Allison, J.B., ed). Academic Press, New York. pp. 125–176.

Kreider, R.B., D.S. Kalman, J. Antonio, T.N. Ziegenfuss, R. Wildman, R. Collins et al. 2017. International Society of Sports Nutrition position stand: safety and efficacy of creatine supplementation in exercise, sport, and medicine. *J. Int. Soc. Sports Nutr.* 14:18.

Kristiansen, R.G., C.F. Rose, O.-M. Fuskevåg, H. Mæhre, A. Revhaug, R. Jalan, and L.M. Ytrebø. 2014. L-Ornithine phenylacetate reduces ammonia in pigs with acute liver failure through phenylacetylglycine formation: a novel ammonia-lowering pathway. *Am. J. Physiol.* 307:G1024–G1031.

Kwon, H., T.E. Spencer, F.W. Bazer, and G. Wu. 2003. Developmental changes of amino acids in ovine fetal fluids. *Biol. Reprod.* 68:1813–1820.

Lane, A.N. and T.W. Fan. 2015. Regulation of mammalian nucleotide metabolism and biosynthesis. *Nucleic Acids Res.* 43:2466–2485.

Layer, G., J. Reichelt, D. Jahn, and D.W. Heinz. 2010. Structure and function of enzymes in heme biosynthesis. *Protein Sci.* 19:1137–1161.

Lee, Y. and L.M. Sayre. 1998. Reaffirmation that metabolism of polyamines by bovine plasma amine oxidase occurs strictly at the primary amino termini. *J. Biol. Chem.* 273:19490–19494.

Leone, A.M., P.L. Francis, and R.E. Silma. 1987. The isolation, purification, and characterisation of the principal urinary metabolites of melatonin. *J. Pineal Res.* 4:253–266.

Lepist, E., X. Zhang, J. Hao, J. Huang, A. Kosaka, G. Birkus et al. 2014. Contribution of the organic anion transporter OAT2 to the renal active tubular secretion of creatinine and mechanism for serum creatinine elevations caused by cobicistat. *Kidney Int.* 86:350–357.

Li, P. and G. Wu. 2020. Composition of amino acids and related nitrogenous nutrients in feedstuffs for animal diets. *Amino Acids* 52:523–542.

Li, Z. and D.E. Vance. 2008. Phosphatidylcholine and choline homeostasis. *J. Lipid Res.* 49:1187–1194.

Li, H., C.J. Meininger, J.R. Hawker, Jr., T.E. Haynes, D. Kepka-Lenhart, S.K. Mistry, S.M. Morris, Jr., and G. Wu. 2001. Regulatory role of arginase I and II in nitric oxide, polyamine, and proline syntheses in endothelial cells. *Am. J. Physiol.* 280:E75–E82.

Li, X.Y., S.X. Zheng, and G. Wu. 2020. Amino acid metabolism in the kidneys: nutritional and physiological significance. *Adv. Exp. Med. Biol.* 1265:71–95.

Li, X.Y., S.X. Zheng, and G. Wu. 2021. Nutrition and functions of amino acids in fish. *Adv. Exp. Med. Biol.* 1285:133–168.

Lin, X., P.A. Lyvers Peffer, J. Woodworth, and J. Odle. 2020. Ontogeny of carnitine biosynthesis in *Sus scrofa domesticus*, inferred from γ-butyrobetaine hydroxylase (dioxygenase) activity and substrate inhibition. *Am. J. Physiol.* 319:R43–R49.

Lindemann, M.D., G.L. Cromwell, H.J. Monegue, H. Cook, K.T. Soltwedel, S. Thomas et al. 2000. Feeding value of an enzymatically digested protein for early-weaned pigs. *J. Anim. Sci.* 78:318–327.

Ling, B., C. Aziz, and J. Alcorn. 2012. Systematic evaluation of key L-carnitine homeostasis mechanisms during postnatal development in rat. *Nutr. Metab.* 9:66.

Lu, S.C. 2013. Glutathione synthesis. *Biochim. Biophys. Acta* 1830:3143–3153.

Lubec, G. and G.A. Rosenthal (eds.) 1990. *Amino acids: Chemistry, Biology and Medicine.* ESCOM Science Publisher B.V., Leiden, The Netherlands.

Macdonald, D.W. 2001. *The New Encyclopedia of Mammals.* Oxford University Press, Oxford, UK.

Maisels, M.J. 2015. Managing the jaundiced newborn: a persistent challenge. *CMAJ.* 187:335–343.

Mammone, T., K. Marenus, N. Muizzuddin, and D. Maes. 2004. Evidence and utility of melanin degrading enzymes. *J. Cosmet. Sci.* 55:116–117.

Mannion, A.F., P.M. Jakeman, M. Dunnett, R.C. Harris, and P.L.T. Willan. 1992. Carnosine and anserine concentrations in the quadriceps femoris muscle of healthy humans. *Eur. J. Appl. Physiol. Occup. Physiol.* 64:47–50.

McCarty, M.F., J.H. O'Keefe, and J.J. DiNicolantonio. 2018. Dietary glycine is rate-limiting for glutathione synthesis and may have broad potential for health protection. *Ochsner J.* 18:81–87.

McGilvery, R.W. and T.W. Murray. 1974. Calculated equilibria of phosphocreatine and adenosine phosphates during utilization of high energy phosphate by muscle. *J. Biol. Chem.* 249:5845–5850.

McKee, C.M., M.B. Penno, M. Cowman, M.D. Burdick, R.M. Strieter, C. Bao et al. 1996. Hyaluronan (HA) fragments induce chemokine gene expression in alveolar macrophages. The role of HA size and CD44. *J. Clin. Invest.* 98:2403–2413.

McNabb, F.M. 1995. Thyroid hormones, their activation, degradation and effects on metabolism. *J. Nutr.* 125:1773S–1776S.

Meister, A. 1973. On the enzymology of amino acid transport. *Science* 180:33–39.

Messner, K. and J. Gillquist. 1996. Cartilage repair: a critical review. *Acta Orthop Scand.* 67:523–529.

Moldave, K. and A. Meister 1957. Synthesis of phenylacetylglutamine by human tissues. *J. Biol. Chem.* 229:463–476.

Momb, J., J.P. Lewandowski, J.D. Bryant, R. Fitch, D.R. Surman, S.A. Vokes, and D.R. Appling. 2013. Deletion of Mthfd1l causes embryonic lethality and neural tube and craniofacial defects in mice. *Proc. Natl. Acad. Sci. USA.* 110:549–554.

Moughan, P.J., M.F. Fuller, K.S. Han, A.K. Kies, and W. Miner-Williams. 2007. Food-derived bioactive peptides influence gut function. *Int. J. Sport Nutr. Exerc. Metab.* 17:S5–S22.

Moya-Garcia, A.A., M.A. Medina, and F. Sánchez-Jiménez. 2005. Mammalian histidine decarboxylase: from structure to function. *BioEssays* 27:57–63.

Murase, D., A. Hachiya, K. Takano, R. Hicks, M.O. Visscher, T. Kitahara et al. 2013. Autophagy has a significant role in determining skin color by regulating melanosome degradation in keratinocytes. *J. Invest. Dermatol.* 133:2416–2424.

Murphy, R., G. McConell, D. Cameron-Smith, K. Watt, L. Ackland, B. Walzel et al. 2001. Creatine transporter protein content, localization, and gene expression in rat skeletal muscle. *Am. J. Physiol.* 280:C415–C422.

National Research Council (NRC). 2011. *Nutrient Requirements of Fish.* National Academy Press, Washington, DC.

O'Brien, L., P.A. Hosick, K. John, D.E. Stec, and T.D. Hinds, Jr. 2015. Biliverdin reductase isozymes in metabolism. *Trends Endocrinol. Metab.* 26:212–220.

Oku, T., S. Ando, T. Hayakawa, K. Baba, R. Nishi, K. Shiozaki, and S. Yamada. 2011. Purification and identification of a novel primitive secretory enzyme catalyzing the hydrolysis of imidazole-related dipeptides in the jawless vertebrate *Lethenteron reissneri. Peptides* 32:648–655.

Olsson, R.A. 2003. Robert Berne: his place in the history of purine research. *Drug Dev. Res.* 58:296–301.

Opheim, M., H. Sterten, M. Øverland, and N.P. Kjos. 2016. Atlantic salmon (*Salmo salar*) protein hydrolysate – Effect on growth performance and intestinal morphometry in broiler chickens. *Livest. Sci.* 187:138–145.

Ortiga-Carvalho, T.M., A.R. Sidhaye, and F.E. Wondisford. 2014. Thyroid hormone receptors and resistance to thyroid hormone disorders. *Nat. Rev. Endocrinol.* 10:582–591.

Pardridge, W.M. and L.J. Mietus. 1980. Influx of thyroid hormones into rat liver in vivo: differential availability of thyroxine and triiodothyronine bound by plasma proteins. *J. Clin. Invest.* 66:367–374.

Pedley, A.M. and S.J. Benkovic. 2017. A New view into the regulation of purine metabolism – the purinosome. *Trends Biochem. Sci.* 42:141–154.

Persaud, C., T. Forrester, and A. Jackson. 1996. Urinary excretion of 5-L-oxoproline (pyroglutamic acid) is increased during recovery from severe childhood malnutrition and responds to supplemental glycine. *J. Nutr.* 126:2823–2830.

Peter, M.G. 2005. Chitin and chitosan from animal sources. In: *Biopolymers* (Steinbüchel, A., ed). Wiley-VCH Verlag, Weinheim. pp. 481–574.

Polidori, C., A. Jorge, and C. Ornosa. 2017. Eumelanin and pheomelanin are predominant pigments in bumblebee (Apidae: *Bombus*) pubescence. *Peer J.* 5:e3300.

Pomin, V.H. and B. Mulloy. 2018. *Pharmaceuticals* (Basel) 11:27.

Ponka, P. 1997. Tissue-specific regulation of iron metabolism and heme synthesis: distinct control mechanisms in erythroid cells. *Blood* 89:1–25.

Power, O., P. Jakeman, and R.J. FitzGerald. 2013. Antioxidative peptides: enzymatic production, in vitro and in vivo antioxidant activity and potential applications of milk-derived antioxidative peptides. *Amino Acids* 44:797–820.

Ramanau, A., R. Schmidt, H. Kluge, and K. Eder. 2006. Body composition, muscle fibre characteristics and postnatal growth capacity of pigs born from sows supplemented with L-carnitine. *Arch. Anim. Nutr.* 60:110–118.

Ray, R.M., M.J. Viar, and L.R. Johnson. 2012. Amino acids regulate expression of antizyme-1 to modulate ornithine decarboxylase activity. *J. Biol. Chem.* 287:3674–3690.

Rebouche, C.J. 1991. Quantitative estimation of absorption and degradation of a carnitine supplement by human adults. *Metabolism* 40:1305–1310.

Rebouche, C.J. 1992. Carnitine function and requirements during the life cycle. *FASEB J.* 6:3379–3386.

Reid, K.M., A. Tsung, T. Kaizu, G. Jeyabalan, A. Ikeda, L. Shao et al. 2007. Liver I/R Injury is improved by the arginase inhibitor, N-ω-hydroxy-nor-L-arginine (Nor-NOHA). *Am. J. Physiol.* 292:G512–517.

Reiter, R.J. 1991. Pineal melatonin: cell biology of its synthesis and of its physiological interactions. *Endocr. Rev.* 12:151–180.

Resseguie, M.E., K.A. da Costa, J.A. Galanko, M. Patel, I.J. Davis, and S.H. Zeisel. 2011. Aberrant estrogen regulation of PEMT results in choline deficiency-associated liver dysfunction. *J. Biol. Chem.* 286:1649–1658.

Ringseis, R., J. Keller, and K. Eder. 2018. Basic mechanisms of the regulation of L-carnitine status in monogastrics and efficacy of L-carnitine as a feed additive in pigs and poultry. *J. Anim. Physiol. Anim. Nutr.* 102:1686–1719.

Roberts, K.M. and P.F. Fitzpatrick. 2013. Mechanisms of tryptophan and tyrosine hydroxylase. *IUBMB Life* 65:350–357.

Rogerson, D. 2017. Vegan diets: practical advice for athletes and exercisers. *J. Int. Soc. Sports Nutr.* 14:36.

Ryter, S.W., J. Alam, and A.M. Choi. 2006. Heme oxygenase-1/carbon monoxide: from basic science to therapeutic applications. *Physiol. Rev.* 86:583–650.

Sakurai, T. and K. Kataoka. 2007. Basic and applied features of multicopper oxidases, CueO, bilirubin oxidase, and laccase. *Chem. Rec.* 7:220–229.

Sale, C., B. Saunders, and R.C. Harris. 2010. Effect of beta-alanine supplementation on muscle carnosine concentrations and exercise performance. *Amino Acids* 39:321–333.

Sanger, G.J. 2008. 5-Hydroxytryptamine and the gastrointestinal tract: where next? *Trends Pharmacol. Sci.* 29:465–471.

Sauerhöfer, S., G. Yuan, G.S. Braun, M. Deinzer, M. Neumaier, N. Gretz et al. 2007. L-Carnosine, a substrate of carnosinase-1, influences glucose metabolism. *Diabetes* 56:2425–2432.

Schallreuter, K.U., J.M. Wood, R. Lemke, C. LePoole, P. Das, W. Westerhof et al. 1992. Production of catecholamines in the human epidermis. *Biochem. Biophys. Res. Commun.* 189:72–78.

Schendzielorz, N., A. Rysa, I. Reenila, A. Raasmaja, and P.T. Mannisto. 2011. Complex estrogenic regulation of catechol-O-methyltransferase (COMT) in rats. *J. Physiol. Pharmacol.* 62:483–490.

Schiavone, S., V. Jaquet, L. Trabace, and K. Krause. 2013. Severe life stress and oxidative stress in the brain: from animal models to human pathology. *Antioxid. Redox. Signal.* 18:1475–1490.

Scriver, C.R., W.S. Sly, A.L. Beaudet, W.S. Sly, D. Valle, B. Childs, K.W. Kinzler, and B. Vogelstein. 2001. *The Metabolic and Molecular Bases of Inherited Disease*, 8th Edition. McGraw-Hill, New York.

Serre, C., V. Busuttil and J.-M. Botto. 2018. Intrinsic and extrinsic regulation of human skin melanogenesis and pigmentation. *Int. J. Cosmetic Sci.* 40:328–347.

Sies, H. 1999. Glutathione and its cellular functions. *Free Radical Biol. Med.* 27:916–921.

Silbert, J.E. and G. Sugumaran. 2002. Biosynthesis of chondroitin/dermatan sulfate. *IUBMB Life* 54:177–186.

Sitaram, A. and M.S. Marks. 2012. Mechanisms of protein delivery to melanosomes in pigment cells. *Physiology (Bethesda).* 27:85–99.

Sitiwin, E., M.C. Madigan, E. Gratton, S. Cherepanoff, R.M. Conway, R. Whan, and A. Macmillan. 2019. Shedding light on melanins within *in situ* human eye melanocytes using 2-photon microscopy profiling techniques. *Sci. Rep.* 9:18585.

Slominski, A., J. Wortsman, P.M. Plonka, K.U. Schallreuter, R. Paus, and D.J. Tobin. 2005. Hair follicle pigmentation. *J. Invest. Dermatol.* 124:13–21.

Spelnikov, D. and R.C. Harris. 2019. A kinetic model of carnosine synthesis in human skeletal muscle. *Amino Acids* 51:115–121.

Squires, L.N., J.A. Jakubowski, J.N. Stuart, S.S. Rubakhin, N.G. Hatcher, W.S. Kim et al. 2006. Serotonin catabolism and the formation and fate of 5-hydroxyindole thiazolidine carboxylic acid. *J. Biol. Chem.* 281:13463–13470.

Stein, C. 2016. Opioid receptors. *Annu. Rev. Med.* 67:433–451.

Stein, W.H., A.C. Paladini, C.H.W. Hirs, and S. Moore. 1954. Phenylacetylglutamine as a constituent of normal human urine. *J. Am. Chem. Soc.* 76:2848–2849.

Stern, R. 2003. Devising a pathway for hyaluronan catabolism: are we there yet? *Glycobiology* 13:105R–115R.

Stern, R. 2004. Hyaluronan catabolism: a new metabolic pathway. *Eur. J. Cell Biol.* 83:317–325.

Stewart, T.M., T.T. Dunston, P.M. Woster, and R.A. Casero, Jr. 2018. Polyamine catabolism and oxidative damage. *J. Biol. Chem.* 293:18736–18745.

Strijbis, K., F.M. Vaz, and B. Distel. 2010. Enzymology of the carnitine biosynthesis pathway. *IUBMB Life* 62:357–362.

Sugahara, K. and H. Kitagawa. 2002. Heparin and heparan sulfate biosynthesis. *IUBMB Life* 54:163–175.

Sugumaran, M. and H. Barek. 2016. Critical analysis of the melanogenic pathway in insects and higher animals. *Int. J. Mol. Sci.* 17:1753.

Suzuki, Y., O. Ito, H. Takahashi, and K. Takamatsu. 2004. The effect of sprint training on skeletal muscle carnosine in humans. *Int. J. Sport. Health Sci.* 2:105–110.

Tabor, C.W. and H. Tabor. 1984. Polyamines. *Annu. Rev. Biochem.* 53:749–790.

Tallon, M.J., R.C. Harris, L.H. Boobis, J.L. Fallowfield, and J.A. Wise. 2005. The carnosine content of vastus lateralis is elevated in resistance-trained bodybuilders. *J. Strength Cond. Res.* 19:725–729.

Takematsu, H. and M. Seiji. 1983. Effect of macrophages on elimination of dermal melanin from the dermis. *Arch. Dermatol. Res.* 31:276:96–98.

Tayek, J.A., B. Bistrian, N.F. Sheard, S.H. Zeisel, and G.L. Blackburn. 1990. Abnormal liver function in malnourished patients receiving total parenteral nutrition: a prospective randomized study. *J. Am. Coll. Nutr.* 9:76–83.

Thibault, A., M.R. Cooper, W.D. Figg, D.J. Venzon, A.O. Sarton, A.C. Tompkins et al. 1994. A phase I and pharmacokinetic study of intravenous phenylacetate in patients with cancer. *Cancer Res.* 54:1690–1694.

Tinker, D.A., J.T. Brosnan, and G.R. Herzberg. 1986. Interorgan metabolism of amino acids, glucose, lactate, glycerol and uric acid in the domestic fowl (*Gallus domesticus*). *Biochem. J.* 240:829–836.

Togashi, M., E. Okuma, and H. Abe. 1998. HPLC determination of N-acetyl-L-histidine and its related compounds in fish tissues. *Fish. Sci.* 64:174–175.

Tordjman, S., S. Chokron, R. Delorme, A. Charrier, E. Bellissant, N. Jaafari, and C. Fougerou. 2017. Melatonin: pharmacology, functions and therapeutic benefits. *Curr. Neuropharmacol.* 15:434–443.

Tredwell, G.D., J.G. Bundy, M. De Lorio, and T.M.D. Ebbels. 2016. Modelling the acid/base ^{1}H NMR chemical shift limits of metabolites in human urine. *Metabolomics* 12:151.

Valadbeigi, Y., V. Ilbeigi, and M. Tabrizchi. 2015. Effetc of mono- and di-hydration on the stability and tautomerisms of different tautomers of creatinine: a thermodynamic and mechanistic study. *Comput. Theor. Chem.* 1061:27–35.

Valman, H.B., R.J.K. Brown, T. Palmer, V.G. Oberholzer, and B. Levin. 1971. Protein intake and plasma amino acids of infants of low birth weight. *Br. Med. J.* 4:789–791.

Vaz, F.M. and R.A. Wanders. 2002. Carnitine biosynthesis in mammals. *Biochem. J.* 361:417–429.

Vujcic, S., P. Diegelman, C.J. Bacchi, D.L. Kramer, and C.W. Porter. 2002. Identification and characterization of a novel flavin-containing spermine oxidase of mammalian cell origin. *Biochem. J.* 367:665–675.

Wang, X.Q., W. Ying, K.A. Dunlap, G. Lin, M.C. Satterfield, R.C. Burghardt et al. 2014. Arginine decarboxylase and agmatinase: an alternative pathway for de novo biosynthesis of polyamines for development of mammalian conceptuses. *Biol. Reprod.* 90:84.

Wang, X.Q., D.F. Li, G. Wu, and F.W. Bazer. 2016. Functional roles of fructose: crosstalk between *O*-linked glycosylation and phosphorylation of Akt-TSC2-MTOR cell signaling cascade in ovine trophectoderm cells. *Biol. Reprod.* 95:102.

Washburn, S.E., M.A. Caudill, O. Malysheva, A.J. MacFarlane, N.A. Behan, B. Harnett et al. 2015. Formate metabolism in fetal and neonatal sheep. *Am. J. Physiol.* 308:E921–927.

Waydhas, C., K. Weigl, and H. Sies. 1978. The disposition of formaldehyde and formate arising from drug N-demethylations dependent on cytochrome P-450 in hepatocytes and in perfused rat liver. *Eur. J. Biochem.* 89:143–150.

Waylan, A.T., J.P. Kayser, D.P. Gnad, J.J. Higgins, J.D. Starkey, E.K. Sissom et al. 2005. Effects of L-carnitine on fetal growth and the IGF system in pigs. *J. Anim. Sci.* 83:1824–1831.

Wei, L.H., G. Wu, S.M. Morris, Jr., and L.J. Ignarro. 2001. Elevated arginase I expression in rat aortic smooth muscle cells increases cell proliferation. *Proc. Natl. Acad. Sci. USA.* 98:9260–9264.

Weinshilboum, R.M. 1986. Phenol sulfotransferase in humans: properties, regulation, and function. *Fed. Proc.* 45:2223–2228.

White, C., X.J. Yuan, and P.J. Schmidt. 2013. HRG1 is essential for heme transport from the phagolysosome of macrophages during erythrophagocytosis. *Cell Metab.* 17:261–270.

Willert, E. and M.A. Phillips. 2011. Regulation and function of polyamines in African trypanosomes. *Trends Parasitol.* 28:66–72.

Wu, G. 2018. *Principles of Animal Nutrition.* CRC Press, Boca Raton, FL.

Wu, G. and S.M. Morris, Jr. 1998. Arginine metabolism: nitric oxide and beyond. *Biochem. J.* 336:1–17.

Wu, G. and C.J. Meininger. 2000. Arginine nutrition and cardiovascular function. *J. Nutr.* 130:2626–2629.

Wu, G., N.E. Flynn, and D.A. Knabe. 2000a. Enhanced intestinal synthesis of polyamines from proline in cortisol-treated piglets. *Am. J. Physiol.* 279:E395–402.

Wu, G., N.E. Flynn, D.A. Knabe, and L.A. Jaeger. 2000b. A cortisol surge mediates the enhanced polyamine synthesis in porcine enterocytes during weaning. *Am. J. Physiol.* 279:R554–559.

Wu, G., T.E. Haynes, W. Yan, and C.J. Meininger. 2001. Presence of glutamine:fructose-6-phosphate amidotransferase for glucosamine-6-phosphate synthesis in endothelial cells: effects of hyperglycaemia and glutamine. *Diabetologia* 44:196–202.

Wu, G., Y.Z. Fang, S. Yang, J.R. Lupton, and N.D. Turner. 2004. Glutathione metabolism and its implications for health. *J. Nutr.* 134:489–492.

Wu, G., F.W. Bazer, J. Hu, G.A. Johnson, and T.E. Spencer. 2005. Polyamine synthesis from proline in the developing porcine placenta. *Biol. Reprod.* 72:842–850.

Wu, G., F.W. Bazer, J.M. Wallace, and T.E. Spencer. 2006. Intrauterine growth retardation: implications for the animal sciences. *J. Anim. Sci.* 84:2316–2337.

Wu, G., H.R. Cross, K.B. Gehring, J.W. Savell, A.N. Arnold, and S.H. McNeill. 2016. Composition of free and peptide-bound amino acids in beef chuck, loin, and round cuts. *J. Anim. Sci.* 94:2603–2613.

Wu, G., F.W. Bazer, G.A. Johnson, and Y.Q. Hou. 2018. Arginine nutrition and metabolism in growing, gestating and lactating swine. *J. Anim. Sci.* 96:5035–5051.

Wu, Z.L., Y.Q. Hou, Z.L. Dai, C.A. Hu, and G. Wu. 2019. Metabolism, nutrition and redox signaling of hydroxyproline. *Antioxid. Redox Signal.* 30:674–682.

Xue, G.P., A.M. Snoswell, and R.C. Fishlock. 1988. Quantitative study on creatine metabolism in sheep tissues. *Biochem. Int.* 16:623–628.

Yamada, S., Y. Tanaka, and S. Ando. 2005. Purification and sequence identification of anserinase. *FEBS J.* 272:6001–6013.

Yanai, Y., Y. Kakimoto, T. Tsujio, and I. Sano. 1969. Genetic study of beta-aminoisobutyric acid excretion by Japanese. *Am. J. Hum. Genet.* 21:115–132.

Yang, Y., Z.L. Wu, C.J. Meininger, and G. Wu. 2015. L-Leucine and NO-mediated cardiovascular function. *Amino Acids* 47:435–447.

Yoshikawa, T., T. Nakamura, and K. Yanai. 2019. Histamine *N*-methyltransferase in the brain. *Int. J. Mol. Sci.* 20:737.

Ytrebø, L.M., R.G. Kristiansen, H. Maehre, O.M. Fuskevag, T. Kalstad, A. Revhaug et al. 2009. L-Ornithine phenylacetate attenuates increased arterial and extracellular brain ammonia and prevents intracranial hypertension in pigs with acute liver failure. *Hepatology* 50:165–174.

Yu, Y.M., C.M. Ryan, Z. Fei, X.M. Lu, L. Castillo, J.T. Schultz et al. 2002. Plasma L-5-oxoproline kinetics and whole blood glutathione synthesis rates in severely burned adult humans. *Am J. Physiol.* 282:E247–E258.

Zeisel, S.H. 2012. A brief history of choline. *Ann. Nutr. Metab.* 61:254–258.

Zeisel, S.H., K.A. daCosta, P.D. Franklin, E.A. Alexander, J.T. Lamont, N.F. Sheard, and A. Beiser. 1991. Choline, an essential nutrient for humans. *FASEB J.* 5:2093–2098.

6 Synthesis of Urea and Uric Acid

During the 18th century, urea and uric acid were first obtained from urine and urine stones, respectively. These two metabolites have since become a focus of researchers studying protein metabolism and nutrition. During the following century, it was established that urea and uric acid are the major nitrogenous end products of protein catabolism in mammals and birds, respectively. At the beginning of the 20th century, ammonia and purines were known to be the precursors of urea and uric acid, respectively; however, the underlying biochemical processes had yet to be elucidated. In 1932, H.A. Krebs and K. Henseleit studied nitrogen metabolism in incubated liver slices and proposed the urea cycle (ornithine cycle) in the rat liver for the conversion of ammonia into urea. The urea cycle was the first metabolic cycle discovered in animals and this concept has led to major advances in biochemistry, medicine, nutrition, and physiology. Using the same technique for preparing liver slices, H.A. Krebs and coworkers identified the biochemical pathway for uric acid synthesis from purine via xanthine oxidase in 1936. It turned out that ammonia is a substrate for the production of purines via the formation of glutamine in animal cells.

The urea cycle and uric acid synthesis are the major metabolic pathways for the removal of ammonia (a neurotoxic substance at elevated concentrations) in mammals and birds, respectively (Schmidt-Nielsen 1952; Singer 2003). The elucidation of the hepatic urea cycle resulted in another landmark discovery of the citric acid (tricarboxylic acid) cycle. Specifically, guided by the concept of cyclic metabolic pathways, H.A. Krebs used pigeon breast muscle homogenates as a model system to study substrate metabolism and discovered the citric acid cycle in 1937 (Chapter 4). This metabolic cycle is responsible for the oxidation of acetyl-CoA produced from the catabolism of amino acids (AAs), glucose, and fatty acids in mitochondria-containing eukaryotic cells (Jungas et al. 1992). The landmark discovery of the citric acid cycle also helps to explain how proteins, carbohydrates, and lipids from ingested food are converted into CO_2, water, and biological energy in the body (Krebs 1981 and 1982). Notably, AAs bridge the ornithine cycle with the citric acid cycle, indicating the central role of nitrogenous and non-nitrogenous nutrients in intermediary metabolism and their interactions to influence ammonia detoxification in mammals (including humans, pigs, dogs, cats, and rats) (Meijer et al. 1990; Watford 2020). In birds and other animals without the urea cycle, the oxidation of AAs into uric acid is regulated by dietary intakes of lipids, carbohydrates, vitamins, and minerals, just like the urea cycle in mammals (Wu 2018). This chapter highlights the biochemical pathways for the syntheses of urea and uric acid in animals.

6.1 AMMONIA PRODUCTION AND TOXICITY IN HUMANS AND OTHER ANIMALS

6.1.1 HISTORICAL OBSERVATIONS ON THE PRODUCTION OF AMMONIA BY HUMANS AND OTHER ANIMALS

For over 16 centuries, it has been known that ammonia (a colorless alkaline gas with a very pungent odor) is a physiologically significant substance in the urine of humans and other animals. The term ammonia was derived from Ammon, the Sun God of ancient Egypt, because Romans found ammonium chloride deposits near Amun (Ammon in Greek), the Temple of Jupiter. During the Middle Ages, ammonia was obtained from the distillation of stale urine. Gaseous ammonia was first obtained in 1774 by J. Priestley (a British chemist) and its composition was determined in 1780 by the

French scientist, C.L. Berthollet. In 1893, C. van Caulaert and coworkers reported that dogs that had a shunt placed between the portal system and the peripheral venous system to bypass the liver developed characteristic symptoms, including dizziness, anorexia, and death when fed high-protein diets. Meanwhile, these investigators observed the toxic effects of intravenous infusion of ammonium salts into patients with cirrhosis of the liver and suggested that high levels of ammonia in the blood contributed to neurological disorders and mortality. By the end of the 19th century, it was known that ammonia is present in the blood of healthy individuals at low concentrations and that urinary ammonia is a by-product of protein and AA catabolism in humans and other animals. However, the major organs or AA precursors that contributed to urinary ammonia remained unclear. In 1909, F. Haber and C. Bosch produced ammonia from nitrogen in the air, further supporting the notion that metabolites in the body can be produced through organic synthesis, paving the way for ammonia analysis and developments in research on AA metabolism. Based on the reports of biological deamination of AAs in the early 1900s, H.A. Krebs discovered the degradation of glutamine by phosphate-activated glutaminase in animal tissues, including the kidneys, in 1935 (Chapter 4). In a classic study, D.D. Van Slyke and colleagues reported in 1943 that glutamine degradation by the kidneys is the major source of ammonia in dog's urine, particularly under acidotic conditions. This seminal observation was confirmed by subsequent studies in the 1950s–1980s, involving humans, rats, sheep, and other species (Bergen 2021; Gougeon-Reyburn and Marliss 1989). All of these findings have established that ammonia is produced from AA oxidation in all animals.

6.1.2 REMOVAL OF AMMONIA IN HUMANS AND OTHER ANIMALS UNDER PHYSIOLOGICAL CONDITIONS

In vertebrates, glutamate dehydrogenase and glutamine synthetase play significant roles in the removal of ammonia from the blood circulation and tissues (Chapters 3 and 4). Other means of clearing ammonia from the body depend on species. Specifically, ammonotelic fish directly release ammonia as the major nitrogenous metabolite through their gills into the aqueous environment, uricotelic animals (e.g., birds, most terrestrial reptiles, and most insects) excrete uric acid as the primary product of nitrogen metabolism, and ureotelic species (e.g., mammals) generate urea from ammonia and bicarbonate for excretion in their urine (Table 6.1). By weight, NH_3, urea, and uric acid contain 82.25%, 46.64%, and 33.33% of nitrogen, respectively. The species differences in ammonia disposal may be related to the animal's living environment, the solubility of end nitrogenous products, and physiological adaptations to evolution. For example, the aqueous niche of the teleostean fish compels them to excrete water, therefore facilitating the continuous excretion of water-soluble ammonia. Note that some of the teleostean fish can convert a physiologically significant proportion of ammonia into urea to eliminate the need for ammonium transporters (Singer 2003). Urea, which is highly water-soluble and non-toxic, is a desirable form to dispose of ammonia in mammals that periodically excrete water primarily as the major component of urine. By contrast, uric acid has low solubility in water (Chapter 5) and is excreted as a concentrated salt, therefore allowing birds to conserve water and maintain a low body weight during flights (Gerson and Guglielmo 2011). Accordingly, chelonian reptiles (e.g., turtles) excrete ammonia, uric acid, or urea, depending on whether they are primarily aquatic or on land.

As indicated previously, the most important pathways for the removal of ammonia in mammals and birds are the hepatic urea cycle and uric acid synthesis, respectively (Singer 2003; Watford 2020). Some individual enzymes of the urea cycle are present in various animal tissues, including macrophages, endothelial cells, smooth muscle cells, enterocytes, brain, and kidneys, but these cell types are not capable of synthesizing urea from ammonia. Urea can also be produced from arginine by extrahepatic arginase in birds, and their urinary excretion increases with increasing the dietary intake of protein or arginine. Uric acid is the major end product of nitrogen metabolism in avian species in which urea synthesis from ammonia does not occur because of the absence of carbamoylphosphate synthetase-I (CPS-I), *N*-acetylglutamate synthase (NAGS), and ornithine

TABLE 6.1

Species Differences in the Excretion of Major Nitrogenous Metabolites by Animals

Metabolites	Animal species	Examples
Urea	Ureotelic	Mammals, most terrestrial amphibians beyond the larval and tadpole stages[a] (e.g., frogs and toads), some aquatic amphibians in water (e.g., newts[b]), some aquatic reptiles [e.g., aquatic turtles (chelonians)], marine elasmobranchs (sharks, rays, and skates), most freshwater elasmobranchs, and a few teleost fish (e.g., the Lake Magadi tilapia)
Uric acid	Uricotelic	Birds, most terrestrial reptiles [such as lizards, snakes, terrestrial turtles, and desert tortoises], freshwater reptiles (crocodiles[c] and alligators[c]), terrestrial snails, Dalmatian dogs, mollusks, some terrestrial crustaceans (e.g., certain land crabs such as Gecarcinid, Ocypodid, and Birgus latro), most insects (e.g., mosquitoes and drosophila fries), and a few arid amphibians (e.g., tree frogs, waxy monkey frogs, and reed frogs)
Urea and uric acid	Both ureotelic and uricotelic	Some terrestrial reptiles (e.g., tortoises and *Sphenodon punctatus*)
Ammonia	Ammonotelic	Most fish (including most teleost fish[d] and dipnoans), and some aquatic amphibians (e.g., aquatic frogs), larvae and tadpoles of amphibians, earthworms, some insects (e.g., American cockroaches), aquatic crustaceans, some terrestrial crustaceans [e.g., certain crabs (such as *Geograpsus grayi*[e]), and woodlice[e]], and all protozoans
Allantoin	Uricotelic	Most mammals (except for primates), earthworms, lizards, aquatic turtles (chelonians), and various insects
Allantoic acid	Uricotelic	Various insects
Guanine	Guanotelic	Spiders, scorpions, and mites

[a] Beyond the larval and tadpole stages, most terrestrial amphibians also produce a large amount of ammonia when they are in water. Excretion of urea and ammonia in the presence of adequate water can save the metabolic energy from being expended on uric acid synthesis.

[b] The newt is a member of the family Salamandridae. Unlike other members of the family Salamandridae, newts are semiaquatic, alternating between aquatic and terrestrial habitats.

[c] These animals also produce a large amount of ammonia.

[d] Most teleost fish release a significant proportion of their total excreted nitrogen as urea (5%–20%), depending on age and nutrient intake. Interestingly, a teleost fish, the marine gulf toadfish, *Opsanus beta*, can rapidly switch between ammonotelism in the native environment and ureotelism via a hepatic urea cycle under laboratory conditions; in this species, the synthesis of urea from ammonia is induced under such stressful conditions as crowding, confinement, elevated environmental ammonia, or air exposure, and urea is eliminated across the gills.

[e] These animals release ammonia primarily as gas to conserve water.

carbamoyltransferase (OCT) from their tissues. Uric acid is also a product of purine nucleoside metabolism in both mammalian and avian species. Thus, all animals can produce urea and uric acid, with the amounts of these two nitrogenous metabolites differing markedly among mammals, birds, insects, reptiles, amphibians, fish, and crustaceans. Finally, at physiological concentrations, uric acid is a scavenger of oxygen free radicals and can protect cells and tissues from oxidative damage.

6.1.3 NORMAL AND ABNORMAL CONCENTRATIONS OF AMMONIA IN HUMANS AND OTHER ANIMALS

Ammonia is produced from AA catabolism in both animal cells and the microorganisms of the gastrointestinal tract. Concentrations of ammonia in the lumen of the small intestine are relatively high (e.g., 0.20–0.28 mM in preweaning pigs at 2 h after their consumption of milk) without causing damage to the mucosal cells (Wu 2020). Similarly, intracellular concentrations of ammonia in tissues (e.g., liver and skeletal muscle) can range from 0.3 to 0.5 mM without causing adverse effects

(Davis and Wu 1998; Graham and MacLean 1992; Meijer et al. 1990; Meyer et al. 1980). Intensive exercise markedly increases the concentration of ammonia in the skeletal muscle of both humans and other animals, ranging from 0.48 to 2.3 mM in rats (Meyer et al. 1980) or from 0.45 to 1.3 mM in adult humans (Graham and MacLean 1992).

The circulating levels of ammonia are very low in healthy humans due to its rapid removal via the synthesis of urea, glutamate, and glutamine (Table 6.2). For example, concentrations of ammonia ($NH_3 + NH_4^+$) in the plasma of healthy children and adults are usually $\leq 35\,\mu M$ (Raina et al. 2020) and $\leq 30\,\mu M$ (Sakusic et al. 2018), respectively. Hyperammonemia, which is generally defined as a concentration of ammonia ($NH_3 + NH_4^+$) in plasma being $\geq 50\,\mu M$ in infants, children, and adolescents (Raina et al. 2020) or $>30\,\mu M$ in adults (Sakusic et al. 2018), frequently occurs under various nutritional and pathological conditions. Infants (particularly preterm neonates) fed a total parenteral nutrition (TPN) solution without adequate arginine have very low concentrations of arginine in plasma (25–40 μM), compared with the mean concentration of arginine in the plasma of breast-fed term infants (~95 μM) (Wu et al. 2004). Consequently, the TPN-fed compromised neonates

TABLE 6.2

Concentrations of Ammonia ($NH_3 + NH_4^+$) in the Plasma of Humans and Other Animals in the Postabsorptive State or after Feeding

Species	Age	Feeding	Ammonia concentration in plasma			Definition of hyperammonemia (μM)	Comment
			Normal (μM)	Intensive exercise (μM)	Disease (μM)		
Humans	Term infants	Breast-fed	<35	–	>50	>50	Postabsorptive state
	Preterm infants	TPN	–	–	271–371	>50	Without arginine treatment
		TPN	25	–	>50	>50	After treatment with arginine[a]
	Adults	Enteral	<30	–	>30	>30	Postabsorptive state
		Enteral	<30	Up to 110	–	>30	At the end of a 2 h 70% of $VO_{2\,Max}$ exercise
Cats	Near-adult	Enteral	82	–	821	>250	Postabsorptive state
Cattle	Adult	Enteral	86	–	>150	>150	Postabsorptive state
Chicken	Adult	Enteral	145	–	>250	>250	Postabsorptive state
Dogs	Adult	Enteral	<150	–	>300	>250	Postabsorptive state
Ferrets	Adults	Enteral	141	–	2547[b]	>250	Postabsorptive state
Horse	Adult	Enteral	<20	Up to 200	>150	≥60	Postabsorptive state
Mice	Adult	Enteral	45	Up to 150	>150	>100	Postabsorptive state
Pigs	7 days of age	TPN or IG	74	–	>150	>150	Monitored for up to 8 h
Sheep	Adult	Enteral	90	–	>150	>150	Postabsorptive state
Rats	Adults	Enteral	<100	Up to 550	>150	>150	Postabsorptive state

Source: Brunton, J.A. et al. 1999. *Am. J. Physiol.* 277:E223–E231; Chen et al. 2020. *Sci. Rep.* 10:6065; Gilbreath, K.R. et al. 2020a. *J. Anim. Sci.* 98:skz370; Gilbreath, K.R. et al. 2020b. *J. Anim. Sci.* 98:skaa164; Graham, T.E. and D.A. MacLean. 1992. *Can. J. Physiol. Pharmacol.* 70:132–141; Harris, R.C. et al. 1999. *Equine Vet. J.* 30(Suppl.):546–551; Heird, W.C. et al. *J. Pediatr.* 81:162–165; Meyer, R.A. et al. 1980. *J. Appl. Physiol.* 49:1037–1041; Morris, J.G. 1985. *J. Nutr.* 115:524–531; Morris, J.G. and Q.R. Rogers. 1978. *J. Nutr.* 108:1944-1953; Raina, R. et al. 2020. *Nat. Rev. Nephrol.* 16:471-482; Sakusic, A. et al. 2018. *Crit. Care Med.* 46:e897–e903; Wu et al. 2014. *J. Nutr. Biochem.* 15:442–451.

[a] Intravenous administration of 1 mmol arginine–glutamate/kg BW/day.
[b] Fed a diet containing no arginine.
Note: IG, intragastric; TPN, total parenteral nutrition.

have very high concentrations of blood ammonia (e.g., 107–371 μM), and the values are reduced to 25–60 μM after the intravenous administration of 0.5–1 mmol arginine–glutamate (a mixture of arginine and glutamate)/kg BW/day (Johnson et al. 1972; Heird et al. 1972). Poorly managed infants with a urea cycle defect have plasma ammonia concentrations of >300 μM and often as high as 500–1,500 μM (Wijburg and Nassogne 2012). Major factors responsible for hyperammonemia in humans include arginine deficiency, liver failure, inherited metabolic diseases (a defect in a urea cycle enzyme or fatty acid oxidation), an excessive AA load, and intensive exercise.

Like humans, companion (Che et al. 2021; Oberbauer and Larsen 2021), zoo (Herring et al. 2021), and farm (Gilbreath et al. 2021; Zhang et al. 2021) animals are also at high risks for hyperammonemia when fed either high-protein or arginine-deficient diets. Of particular note, overnight-fasted cats rapidly develop hyperammonemia within 45 min after consuming an arginine-free purified diet with proper amounts of other AAs (Table 6.3), with the concentration of ammonia in plasma increasing from 0.16 mM immediately before feeding to 1.4 mM at 2 h after the meal. Likewise, hyperammonemia occurs rapidly in neonatal pigs within 8 h after receiving an arginine-free diet via intragastric or intravenous feeding (Brunton et al. 1999). These findings indicate that dietary arginine is essential for the detoxification of ammonia produced from AA oxidation and for the health of animals.

6.1.4 Toxicity of Ammonia to Humans and Other Animals

As noted above, hyperammonemia results in multiple organ dysfunctions and death in humans and other animals, particularly preterm neonates (Adeva et al. 2011; Lee et al. 2016; Ozanne et al. 2012). For example, elevating the concentrations of ammonia in plasma from 30 to 80 μM can generally result in vomiting, nausea, and seizures in humans (particularly infants), contributing to high rates of morbidity and mortality (Walker 2012). Similar syndromes occur in other mammals (e.g., cats, dogs, and pigs) with hyperammonemia [e.g., the plasma concentration of ammonia being >150 μM in piglets (Table 6.2)]. Interestingly, hyperammonemia (the median concentration of ammonia in serum being 43.5 μM, ranging from 35 to 58 μM) unrelated to hepatic dysfunction appears to be a biomarker for a poor prognosis and deaths in adults hospitalized in the intensive care unit (Sakusic et al. 2018).

TABLE 6.3

Time Course in Concentrations of Ammonia ($NH_3 + NH_4^+$) in the Plasma of Overnight Fasted Cats Fed Diets with Arginine, without Arginine, or with Ornithine but without Arginine[a]

Diet	Time after the consumption of diet (min)						
	0	**45**	**90**	**120**	**150**	**210**	**300**
	Experiment "D"						
Basal ($n = 8$ cats except for $n = 7$ at time 300 min)	174	169	–	135	–	–	129
Basal – arginine ($n = 8$ cats)	156	344	–	1,396	–	–	335
	Experiment "E"						
Basal – arginine ($n = 1$ cat)	91	311	1,085	–	1,337	969	135
Basal – arginine + 1.52% ornithine ($n = 5$ cats)	111	154	141	–	129	179	93

Source: Morris, J.G. and Q.R. Rogers. 1978. *J. Nutr.* 108:1944–1953.

[a] Values, expressed as μM. The basal diet contains the following (% of diet): L-Arg·HCl, 2.0; L-His-HCl·H₂O, 1.2; L-Ile, 1.8; L-Leu, 2.4; L-Lys·HCl, 2.8; L-Met, 1.1; L-Cys-Cys, 0.80; L-Phe, 1.5; L-Tyr, 1.4; L-Thr, 1.4; L-Trp, 0.40; L-Val, 1.8; L-Asn, 2.0; L-Ser, 1.0; L-Pro, 2.0; Gly, 2.0; L-Glu, 6.0; L-Ala, 1.0; sodium acetate, 2.5. Crude protein content in the basal diet is 27.2% and represents 23% of total calories.

Birds are also negatively affected by elevated levels of ammonia in the blood, as indicated by their reduced growth, impaired behavior, and abnormal metabolic profiles (Baker 2009). In both mammals and birds, hyperammonemia causes severe neurologic impairment, cerebral edema, coma, and death, indicating the potential for extremely toxic effects of ammonia on the central nervous system.

Ammonia exists as both NH_3 and NH_4^+ ion in physiological fluids (Chapter 4). Elevated levels of atmospheric ammonia have an irritating effect on the respiratory system, eyes, and skin of humans and other animals (particularly poultry and pigs, housed indoors), while compromising their immune response, health, growth, and development. These problems also occur in fish and crustaceans living in water with high concentrations of ammonia and are exacerbated in a hot environment. Note that the ammonia in the housing facilities of farm animals comes from both endogenous (e.g., AA catabolism) and exogenous (e.g., the microbial fermentation of manure and the outside air) production.

6.1.5 BIOCHEMICAL MECHANISMS RESPONSIBLE FOR AMMONIA TOXICITY TO THE NERVOUS SYSTEM

It had long been thought that high levels of ammonia drain α-ketoglutarate (α-KG) from the Krebs cycle, thereby reducing the production of ATP by cells and reducing intracellular ATP concentrations (Krebs 1964). This, in turn, causes dysfunction of cells in the central nervous system. However, such an effect of ammonia on ATP depletion can potentially also occur in other cell types (e.g., enterocytes and lymphocytes), and yet they do not exhibit an accelerated rate of apoptosis when extracellular concentrations increase from 0.05 to 0.5 mM in culture medium (Haynes et al. 2009; Wu 1995; Wu et al. 1994). Thus, in the presence of adequate buffering mechanisms, ammonia itself is not toxic to cells. Interestingly, hyperammonemia in humans and other animals is often associated with elevated levels of glutamine in plasma (up to ≥2 mM) due to the enhanced synthesis of glutamine by multiple tissues (Chapter 3). Thus, the plasma concentrations of both ammonia (>40 μM in humans) and glutamine (>900 μM in humans) in an overnight fasting state are often used as biomarkers of disease control in patients with urea cycle disorders (Lee et al. 2015). Patients with inborn urea cycle disorders frequently have >2 mM glutamine in their plasma, compared with the values of 0.5–0.6 mM in the normal, postabsorptive adults (Wijburg and Nassogne 2012). However, the culture medium of cells and tissues usually contains 2–4 mM glutamine to maintain their metabolism, growth, and survival, and these levels of glutamine are not cytotoxic at all (Meininger et al. 1988).

Warren and Schenker (1964) reported that the administration of methionine sulfoximine (an inhibitor of glutamine synthetase) improved the survival of rats acutely exposed to toxic concentrations of ammonia. Subsequent works showed that inhibition of brain glutamine accumulation by methionine sulfoximine also prevented cerebral edema in hyperammonemic rats (Takahashi et al. 1991). Interestingly, the beneficial effect of methionine sulfoximine occurs despite a concomitant increase in brain ammonia levels. Emerging evidence from animal studies shows that hyperammonemia *per se* does not result in coma or death when glutamine synthesis is inhibited *in vivo* (Albrecht and Norenberg 2006; Fries et al. 2014). However, high extracellular concentrations of glutamine (e.g., ≥1 mM) inhibit nitric oxide (NO) synthesis by vascular endothelial cells *in vitro* and *in vivo* (Arnal et al. 1995; Lee et al. 1996; Okada et al. 2000), whereas an increase in endothelial NO synthesis can ameliorate the adverse effects of hyperammonemia on rats (Kawaguchi et al. 2005). These results indicate that prolonged elevation of glutamine in plasma is potentially harmful to organisms in an NO-dependent manner. A possible mechanism is that high concentrations of glutamine (e.g., >2 mM) inhibit NO synthesis via NO synthase (NOS) in endothelial cells through its catabolism to glucosamine-6-phosphate (Wu et al. 2001). This hexosamine, an analog of glucose-6-phosphate, competitively inhibits the generation of NADPH (an essential cofactor for NOS) via the pentose cycle, thereby reducing blood flow and the supply of oxygen and nutrients to the brain, as well as ATP production by neuronal cells (Figure 6.1).

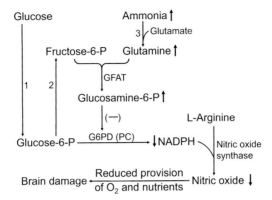

FIGURE 6.1 Inhibition of endothelial nitric oxide (NO) synthesis by glutamine as a possible mechanism to mediate hyperammonemia-induced toxicity to the brain in humans and other animals. The concentrations of glutamine in plasma are increased in patients with high levels of ammonia due to the synthesis of glutamine. Glutamine is metabolized to glucosamine-6-phosphate, which competitively inhibits the activity of glucose-6-phosphate dehydrogenase, a key enzyme of the pentose cycle to generate NADPH. The latter is an essential cofactor of NO synthase for converting arginine into NO (a major vasodilator). Thus, in individuals with hyperammonemia, the supply of oxygen and nutrients (including glucose) from the blood to the brain is impaired possibly due, in part, to a glutamine-induced deficiency of NO, leading to tissue damage in the central nervous system. Enzymes that catalyze the indicated reactions are: (1) hexokinase; (2) phosphohexose isomerase; and (3) glutamine synthetase. GFAT, glutamine:fructose-6-phosphate transaminase; G6PD, glucose-6-phosphate dehydrogenase; P, phosphate; ↑, increase; ↓, decrease.

6.1.6 Treatment of Hyperammonemia

Effective strategies for the treatment of hyperammonemia depend on its underlying causes (Cooper 2012; Enns et al. 2007). For example, in neonates and adults, ammonia toxicity induced by arginine deficiency can be successfully prevented by oral or intravenous administration of arginine, citrulline, or ornithine (Heird et al. 1972; Meijer et al. 1990; Morris 2002). Oral administration of proline is also effective to ameliorate neonatal death brought about by diet-induced hypoargininemia (Brunton et al. 1999). In patients who have defects in enzymes of the hepatic urea cycle and elevated levels of ammonia in the circulation, the intravenous administration of sodium benzoate is often used to prevent death (Chapter 5). This method can also apply to birds and other animal species. In the case of N-acetylglutamate (NAG) deficiency due to low mitochondrial NAG synthase-I activity, the oral or intravenous administration of N-carbamoylglutamate (a metabolically stable analog of NAG) can specifically reduce high concentrations of ammonia in the blood of both humans and other mammals (e.g., pigs) by the allosteric activation of CPS-I (Wu et al. 2004). In ruminants, vinegar (consisting mainly of acetic acid and water) is often used to treat ammonia toxicity because H^+ from this acid rapidly combines with free NH_3 to form NH_4^+, which is then quantitatively excreted with an anion (e.g., Cl^-) in urine (Bates and Payne 2017). Additionally, acetic acid can help to normalize blood pH, while providing the energy required for the liver to convert ammonia into urea (Wu 2018).

6.2 UREA PRODUCTION IN MAMMALS

6.2.1 Historical Perspectives

The Dutch physician-chemist H. Boerhaave discovered urea in urine in 1727. Indeed, urea was the first animal metabolite to be isolated in crystalline form. In 1773, H. Rouelle (a French chemist) prepared urea from dog's urine and, in 1816, the British physician-chemist W. Prout reported the presence of urea in the blood plasma. With the improved method, urea composition was first determined accurately in 1817 by Prout. By the late 19th century, it was known that urea is the major nitrogenous product of protein and AA catabolism in mammals. Research on urea metabolism was greatly facilitated when F. Wöhler (a German chemist) first synthesized urea from silver isocyanate and ammonium chloride in 1828. In search of the origin of urinary urea, A. Clementi reported in 1913 that the mammalian liver can convert ammonia and AAs into urea. The pathway for urea biosynthesis had been elusive until H.A. Krebs and K. Henseleit proposed the urea (ornithine) cycle in 1932. Extensive research from the 1950s to the 1980s greatly expanded our knowledge of the metabolic control of the urea cycle by substrates, cofactors, protein turnover, allosteric regulators, and hormones (Meijer et al. 1990).

6.2.2   The Hepatic Urea Cycle in Mammals

6.2.2.1   Discovery of the Urea Cycle

In the early 1930s, H.A. Krebs observed that either ornithine or arginine stimulated the conversion of ammonia to urea in rat liver slices incubated in the presence of physiological concentrations of major cations and anions (including sodium and bicarbonate). Interestingly, there was no change in the amount of ornithine in the medium or tissue. In his 1981 book entitled "Reminiscences and Reflections", Krebs wrote that "The interpretation of this finding was not at once obvious. It took a full month to find the correct interpretation. At first, we were skeptical about the correctness of the observations. Was the ornithine perhaps contaminated with arginine? The answer was no. Then it occurred to us that the effect of ornithine might be related to the presence of arginase in the liver, the enzyme which converts arginine into ornithine and urea, known since the work of Kossel and Dakin in 1904". Based on this consideration, Krebs and Henseleit proposed the following sequential reactions:

$$\text{Ornithine} + NH_3 + CO_2 \rightarrow \text{Citrulline} \rightarrow \text{Arginine} \rightarrow \text{Urea} + \text{Ornithine}$$

After H.A. Krebs published his paper on the urea cycle, he was congratulated on this important discovery by some biochemists, but he also received severe criticisms from other scientists who could not reproduce his findings from studies with perfused rat livers. In his reminiscence of the discovery of the ornithine cycle, Krebs (1981) wrote the following comments. "Luck, it is true, is necessary, but the more experiments are carried out, the greater is the probability of meeting with luck. The story also shows that adverse criticisms are liable to be raised on the grounds that either the observations are not confirmed or that some other observations do not fit in with the interpretation of the findings. Almost every major development in science meets with criticisms of this kind". The basic concept of the originally proposed cycle has stood the test of time over the past 90 years. The kinetics, activators, and substrate concentrations of the urea cycle enzymes are summarized in Tables 6.4, 6.5, and 6.6, respectively. Based on decreases in NAGS and N-acetylglutamate deacetylase activities in the rat liver over a 3-day period of fasting (Gomez et al. 1983), the half-lives of these two hepatic proteins are estimated to be 2.3 and 2.7 min, respectively. The mammalian liver releases urea to the bloodstream via a urea transporter (UT), UT-A (Sands and Blount 2014).

6.2.2.2   Characteristics of the Urea Cycle

One of the most remarkable features of the urea cycle is its compartmentation (Figure 6.2). Namely, urea synthesis involves both the cytoplasm and mitochondria in the liver. Note that NH_3 (rather than NH_4^+) and HCO_3^- (rather than CO_2) are substrates for CPS-I. However, NH_3 is in chemical equilibrium with NH_4^+, whereas HCO_3^- is produced from CO_2 and H_2O by the mitochondrial carbonic anhydrase. Both NH_3 and HCO_3^- are formed from the catabolism of AAs (including glutamate, glutamine, and glycine) in the mitochondria. Glutamate dehydrogenase is the major intramitochondrial source of ammonia for urea production in mammals (Meijer et al. 1990). Once ammonia is generated within the mitochondria or the blood ammonia enters this organelle, it reacts with HCO_3^- to generate carbamoyl phosphate by CPS-I, with the hydrolysis of ATP to ADP and Pi

TABLE 6.4

Kinetics of Urea Cycle Enzymes in the Liver and Enterocytes

Enzyme	Reactant or activator	Rat liver[a]		Pig liver[b]		Pig enterocytes[b]	
		V_{max}	K_m (mM)	V_{max}	K_m (mM)	V_{max}	K_m (mM)
CPS-I	Ammonia	21	1–2 (0.6)	18.6	1.2	6.68	1.34
	HCO_3^-	21	4–5 (2)	18.6	5.77	6.68	58.6
	Mg-ATP	21	0.5–3 (1.2)	18.6	1.69	6.68	15.2
	Mg^{2+}	21	0.17–2 (<1)	18.6	ND	6.68	ND
	NAG (free)	21	0.04–0.1 (0.1)	18.6	0.13	6.68	0.82
	NAG (total)	21	(0.8)	18.6	0.96	6.68	ND
OCT	Ornithine	799	0.2–1.8	921	1.58	706	5.13
	CP	799	0.02–0.4 (>0.15)	921	0.46	706	17.1
ASS	Citrulline	7.4	0.04 (>0.2)	8.45	0.068	1.89	0.15
	Aspartate	7.4	0.02	8.45	0.031	1.89	0.054
	Mg-ATP	7.4	0.15	8.45	0.24	1.89	2.86
ASL	AS	13.3	0.04–0.13 (>0.03)	17.7	0.12	3.50	0.63
Arginase-I	Arginine	5,143	3.5 (>0.06)	3,072	3.38	7.13	7.46
NAGS	Glutamate	0.22	3	0.28	3.56	0.064	4.25
	Acetyl-CoA	0.22	0.7	0.28	0.84	0.064	1.02
	Arginine	0.22	0.01 (0.05)	0.28	0.061	0.064	0.11

Source: Meijer, A.J., W.H. Lamers, and R.A. Chamuleau. 1990. *Physiol. Rev.* 70:701–748; and Davis, P.K. and G. Wu. 1998. *Comp. Biochem. Physiol. B* 119:527–537.

[a] Values in parentheses are K_m values for enzymes *in situ*, either in permeabilized mitochondria (CPS-I), intact mitochondria (OCT), or intact hepatocytes (ASS, ASL, arginase, and NAGS). V_{max} is expressed as µmol/min/g of dry weight (adult rats).

[b] V_{max} is expressed as µmol/min/g of tissue protein (60-day-old growing pigs).

Note: ND, Not determined. Ammonia is the sum of NH_4^+ and NH_3

(PO_4^{3-}). The carbamoyl phosphate combines with ornithine to yield citrulline by OCT. The source of ornithine for OCT is the diet, blood, or cytosolic arginase. In either case, ornithine is transported by ORNT1 (mitochondrial ornithine transporter 1) from the cytoplasm to the mitochondrial matrix in the mammalian hepatocyte (Monné et al. 2015). ORNT1 is an antiporter whereby mitochondrial citrulline is exchanged for cytosolic ornithine across the inner mitochondrial membrane to exit into the cytoplasm. In the cytosol of the hepatocytes, citrulline is rapidly metabolized to arginine and then to urea plus ornithine.

Argininosuccinate synthase [ASS (a cytosolic enzyme)] converts citrulline and aspartate into argininosuccinate, and a major source of this aspartate is the mitochondrial aspartate through the action of citrin (a transporter in the mitochondrial membrane). Citrin exchanges the cytosolic glutamate for the mitochondrial aspartate (Monné et al. 2015). The mitochondrial aspartate can be derived from ammonia and oxaloacetate via glutamate dehydrogenase and glutamate–oxaloacetate transaminase (Figure 6.3). Glutamate is required for the synthesis of NAG (an allosteric activator of CPS-I) in the mitochondria, whereas aspartate is essential for the conversion of citrulline into argininosuccinate by ASS in the cytosol. The fumarate (derived from the mitochondrial oxaloacetate) is generated from argininosuccinate by argininosuccinate lyase (ASL) and converted into L-malate by cytosolic fumarase (Tuboi et al. 1986), with the cytosolic L-malate entering the mitochondria for the conversion into oxaloacetate. In support of this view, there is evidence for the transport of the urea cycle–derived L-malate from the cytosol into the mitochondria (Pesi et al. 2018). The formation of L-malate from fumarate in the cytosol as an intermediate allows regeneration of oxaloacetate in the mitochondria for the incorporation of ammonia into aspartate for another turn of the urea cycle.

TABLE 6.5

Subunits, Cofactors, and Allosteric Activator of Urea Cycle Enzymes in the Mammalian Liver[a]

Enzyme	Half-life (days; means)	Structure	Subunit molecular mass (kDa)	Total molecular mass (kDa)	Cofactor or allosteric factor
NAGS	2.3[b]	Homotrimer	57	171	Arginine[c]
CPS-I	7.7	Homodimer	155	310	N-Acetylglutamate[d]
OCT	7.5	Homotrimer	36	108	None
ASS	7.9	Homotetramer	46.25	185	Mg^{2+}
ASL	7.8	Homotetramer	51.7	206.8	None
Arginase-I	5.0	Homotrimer	35	105	Mn^{2+}

Source: Das, T.K. and J.C. Waterlow. 1974. *Br. J. Nutr.* 32:353–373; Jackson, M.J. et al. 1986. *Annu. Rev. Genet.* 20:431–464; Morris, S.M. Jr. 2002. *Annu. Rev. Nutr.* 22:87–105; Schmike, R.T. 1973. *Adv. Enzymol.* 37:135–187; Wallace, R. et al. 1986. *FEBS Lett.* 208:427–430.

[a] The half-life of *N*-acetylglutamate in the mitochondria of rat liver is 45 min. For comparison, the half-lives of glutamate dehydrogenase, alanine transaminase, aspartate transaminase, cytosolic fumarase, and mitochondrial fumarase in the rat liver are 10.1, 8.8, 8.2, 4.8, and 9.7 days, respectively.

[b] Estimated on the basis of a decline in *N*-acetylglutamate synthase activity in the rat liver over a 3-day period of fasting (Gomez et al. 1983).

[c] Allosteric activator of *N*-acetylglutamate synthase.

[d] Allosteric activator of carbamoyl phosphate synthetase-I.

Notes: ASL, argininosuccinate lyase; ASS, argininosuccinate synthase; NAGS, *N*-acetylglutamate synthase; CPS-I, carbamoyl phosphate synthetase-I; OCT, ornithine carbamoyltransferase.

TABLE 6.6

Concentrations of Urea Cycle Enzyme Substrates or Activators in the Pig Liver and Enterocytes[a]

Substrate	Pig liver		Pig enterocytes	
	Cytoplasm	Mitochondria	Cytoplasm	Mitochondria
Ammonia ($NH_4^+ + NH_3$)	0.35	0.52	0.45	1.18
ATP	5.97	12.6	4.28	8.56
Aspartate	2.26	2.50	5.56	2.41
Citrulline	0.10	0.12	0.36	0.52
Arginine	0.13	0.14	0.84	0.75
Ornithine	0.65	0.82	0.30	0.61
Argininosuccinate	0.078	ND	0.042	ND
Carbamoyl phosphate	1.63	0.50	2.26	0.59
N-Acetylglutamate	ND	1.08	ND	0.64

Source: Davis, P.K. and G. Wu. 1998. *Comp. Biochem. Physiol. B* 119:527–537.

[a] Values are expressed as mM. The liver and enterocytes were obtained from 60-day-old fed pigs.

Note: ND, not detectable.

The detailed steps of the urea cycle and its associated reactions in the liver are:

$$NH_3 + HCO_3^- \rightarrow \text{Carbamoyl phosphate (mitochondria)} \tag{6.1}$$

$$\text{Ornithine} + \text{Carbamoyl phosphate} \rightarrow \text{Citrulline (mitochondria)} \tag{6.2}$$

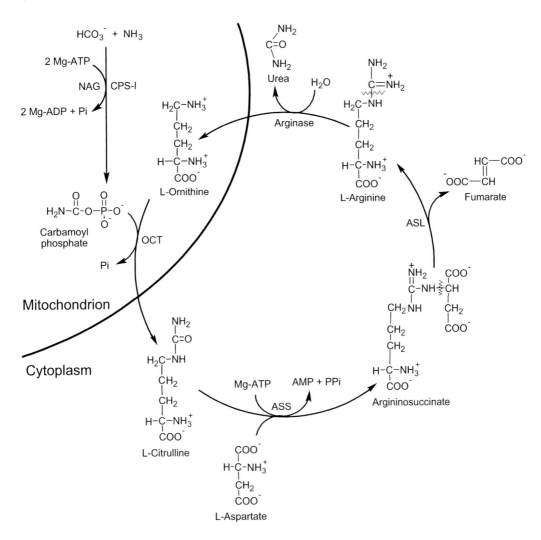

FIGURE 6.2 The urea cycle in mammals. The synthesis of urea from ammonia and bicarbonate involves both the mitochondrion and the cytoplasm. Citrulline exits the mitochondrion into the cytoplasm where it is converted into arginine, which is rapidly hydrolyzed by arginase into urea plus ornithine. Ornithine is then reused for another turnover of the cycle. ASL, argininosuccinate lyase; ASS, argininosuccinate synthase; CPS-I, carbamoyl phosphate synthetase -I; NAG, N-acetylglutamate.

$$NH_3 + \alpha\text{-Ketoglutarate} \rightarrow \text{Glutamate (mitochondria)} \qquad (6.3)$$

$$\text{Glutamate} + \text{Oxaloacetate} \rightarrow \alpha\text{-Ketoglutarate} + \text{Aspartate (mitochondria)} \qquad (6.4)$$

The net reaction of (6.3) and (6.4): $NH_3 + \text{Oxaloacetate} \rightarrow \text{Aspartate}$

$$\text{Citrulline} + \text{Aspartate} \rightarrow \text{Argininosuccinate (cytosol)} \qquad (6.5)$$

$$\text{Argininosuccinate} \rightarrow \text{Arginine} + \text{Fumarate (cytosol)} \qquad (6.6)$$

$$\text{Arginine} + H_2O \rightarrow \text{Ornithine} + \text{Urea (cytosol)} \qquad (6.7)$$

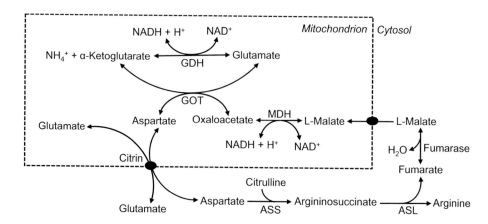

FIGURE 6.3 The source of aspartate required for and the fate of fumarate produced in the hepatic urea cycle. Ammonia (either produced from the mitochondrial oxidation of AAs or derived from the blood) and oxaloacetate are the ultimate sources of aspartate for ASS in the cytosol. The mitochondrial aspartate is transported by citrin into the cytosol in exchange for the cytosolic glutamate. ASL generates fumarate in the cytosol, which is converted into L-malate by the cytosolic fumarase. After the L-malate enters the mitochondria via the malate shuttle, this intermediate is oxidized to oxaloacetate for the regeneration of oxaloacetate to allow another turn of the urea cycle. ASL, argininosuccinate lyase; ASS, argininosuccinate synthase; GDH, glutamate dehydrogenase; GOT, glutamate–oxaloacetate transaminase; MDH, NAD^+-linked malate dehydrogenase.

$$Fumarate + H_2O \rightarrow L\text{-}Malate \qquad (cytosol) \qquad (6.8)$$

$$L\text{-}Malate \rightarrow Oxaloacetate \qquad (mitochondria) \qquad (6.9)$$

Thus, the two nitrogen atoms of the urea molecule are ultimately derived from ammonia. The net reaction of the urea cycle in terms of nitrogen and carbon balances is:

$$2NH_3 + HCO_3^- \rightarrow Urea \qquad (H_2N\text{--}CO\text{--}NH_2)$$

Another important feature of the urea cycle is metabolic channeling, which can be defined as the restricted flow of substrates and products in a series of enzyme-catalyzed reactions (Srere 1987). Studies of the urea cycle in the 1980s involving the use of labeled substrates or intermediates led to the development of this concept in cell metabolism. Interestingly, the hepatic pool of arginine in the cytosol involved in the urea cycle seems to be metabolically sequestered and is not in equilibrium with, or rapidly exchangeable with, arginine in plasma or other hepatic arginine pools (Yang et al. 2000). Metabolic channeling facilitates the immediate transfer of intermediates between enzymes and helps maintain relatively high concentrations of substrates in catalytic sites. This ensures the rapid and efficient formation of end products via a series of biochemical reactions. Available evidence shows that metabolic channeling in the hepatic urea cycle occurs in both the cytoplasm and mitochondria (Cheung et al. 1989).

6.2.2.3 Coupling of the Urea Cycle with Gluconeogenesis in the Liver

Under physiological conditions, the mammalian liver does not completely oxidize the carbon skeletons of AAs to CO_2 due to the constraints of oxygen consumption and ATP turnover (Jungas et al. 1992). Some of the carbons of AAs are metabolized to glucose (for glucogenic AAs), ketone bodies (for ketogenic AAs), both glucose and ketone bodies (for glucogenic plus ketogenic AAs), and fatty acids and cholesterol (for all AAs), depending on the physiological needs (Watford 2020). In the fed state, some of the glucose and fatty acids are converted into glycogen and triacylglycerols, respectively, in the liver and other tissues, whereas some of the AA carbons can also be used for cholesterol synthesis. When the catabolism of AAs generates ammonia, oxygen- and hydrogen-containing carbon skeletons, NADH, and ATP in the mammalian liver, most of the carbon skeletons (except for those from ketogenic AAs) in the form of C_3 units, NADH, and ATP are used for the synthesis of glucose to account for carbon, nitrogen, oxygen, and hydrogen balances in the biochemical reactions (Watford 2020). The regeneration of NAD^+ and ADP is essential for AA catabolism to continue in the liver. Thus, the urea cycle for the removal of AA-derived ammonia is always coupled with gluconeogenesis in mammalian hepatocytes under both fed and fasting conditions (Figure 6.4). This is analogous to glutamine degradation in the kidneys, where the resulting ammonia and α-KG are used for NH_4^+ and glucose production, respectively (Watford 2020).

6.2.3 SYNTHESIS OF UREA FROM AMMONIA IN THE EXTRAHEPATIC CELLS OF MAMMALS

In studying intestinal AA metabolism, G. Wu found in 1995 that enterocytes in postweaning mammals (e.g., pigs and rats) contain all the enzymes required for the synthesis of urea from either ammonia and CO_2 or glutamine. These cells synthesize urea from either the extracellular ammonia or the ammonia generated from the catabolism of AAs (e.g., glutamine) within the mitochondria in a concentration-dependent manner (Table 6.7). This physiologically relevant pathway was established by measuring the formation of urea in enterocytes from these nitrogenous substrates at concentrations present in the lumen of the small intestines of pigs and rats. Results from studies with postweaning pigs indicate that, at the same concentrations of substrates, the rate of ureagenesis from extracellular ammonia or glutamine in enterocytes is approximately 5% of that in hepatocytes (Wu 1995). Thus, enterocytes are capable of producing significant amounts of urea from extracellular- and intramitochondrially-derived ammonia. Urea is also formed from arginine via arginase in the enterocytes of weaned mammals. Urea synthesis by enterocytes in postweaning mammals is the first line of defense against the potential toxicity of ammonia that is: (1) produced by extensive intestinal degradation of dietary and blood-derived glutamine (a major fuel for enterocytes) and (2) derived from diets and luminal microorganisms. Additionally, F. Blachier and B.J. Bequette reported, respectively, that colonocytes of the rat's large intestine (Mouille et al. 1999) and the

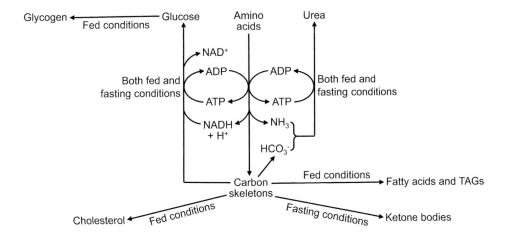

FIGURE 6.4 Coupling of the urea cycle with gluconeogenesis in the mammalian liver. When the catabolism of AAs is the source of ammonia in the mitochondria, their α-ketoacids (for glucogenic AAs) undergo partial oxidation to CO_2 and are converted into glucose in the liver under both fed and fasting conditions, and also serve as substrates for fatty acid/cholesterol synthesis and ketogenesis in the liver under fed and fasting conditions, respectively. In the fed state, glucose can be converted into glycogen in periportal hepatocytes. Carbon, nitrogen, NAD^+, and ATP must be balanced in all reactions. TAGs, triacylglycerols.

TABLE 6.7

Synthesis of Urea from Ammonia and Glutamine in the Enterocytes of Pigs[a]

Age of pigs (days)	Urea Synthesis (nmol/mg protein/30 min)				
	No substrate	1 mM glutamine	5 mM glutamine	0.5 mM NH$_4$Cl + 2 mM ornithine + 2 mM aspartate	2 mM NH$_4$Cl + 2 mM ornithine + 2 mM aspartate
0–21	ND	ND	ND	ND	ND
29	ND	6.27 ± 0.74[b]	15.2 ± 1.28[c]	13.4 ± 1.56[c]	21.6 ± 2.07[d]
58	ND	7.91 ± 0.82[b]	16.5 ± 1.43[c]	14.6 ± 1.28[c]	23.4 ± 3.26[d]

Source: Wu, G. 1995. *Biochem. J.* 312:717–723.

[a] Values are means ± SEM, $n = 8$. Pigs were weaned at 21 days of age to a corn- and soybean meal–based diet. Jejunal enterocytes were incubated at 37°C for 0 to 30 min in Krebs–Henseleit buffer (pH 7.4), containing 5 mM D-glucose and the substrate(s) as indicated.

[b–d] Within a row, means not sharing the same superscript letter differs ($P < 0.05$).

Note: ND, not detected.

epithelial cells lining the ovine rumen (Oba et al. 2004) can synthesize urea from ammonia and bicarbonate. In the epithelial cells of the mammalian gastrointestinal tract which do not possess gluconeogenesis, ureagenesis is closely linked with the synthesis of AAs (e.g., alanine, aspartate, citrulline, and proline). Although the liver is undoubtedly the major site of ureagenesis in mammals, the hepatocyte is not the only cell type that can convert ammonia into urea. Thus, the traditional textbook view that the urea cycle occurs only in the mammalian liver must be corrected. Furthermore, it would be more informative and accurate if urea synthesis in the gastrointestinal epithelial cells is considered to model urea recycling in mammals, including ruminants.

6.2.4 Calculation of Urea Production by Mammals

Urea is the major nitrogenous metabolite of AAs in mammals, including humans (Diem 1962; Sands et al. 1987). Based on the reactions of the urea cycle, the production of urea by healthy adult mammals fed a protein-containing diet can be accurately estimated. The chemical composition, by weight, of the average protein is as follows:

N   13%–19% (16%)
C   51%–55% (53%)
O   20%–24% (22%)
H   6.5%–7.3% (7%)
S   0.5%–2% (1.2%)
P   0%–1.5% (0.8%)

When an individual consumes 100 g protein/day, the dietary intake of nitrogen and carbon can be calculated as follows:

100 g protein × 16 g N/100 g protein = 16 g N
16 g N/14 g N/ mol N = 1.14 mol N
100 g protein × 53 g C/100 g protein = 53 g C
53 g C/12 g C/mol C = 4.42 mol C

Assuming that an adult man (70 kg) consumes 100 g protein per day and the true digestibility of protein is 90%, then 1.026 mol N (1.14 × 0.9 = 1.026) and 3.978 mol C (4.42 × 0.9 = 3.978) would be available for utilization by the small intestine and extraintestinal tissues. Based on the ratio of N to C in urea (2:1), namely,

$$2 \text{ mol } NH_3 + 1 \text{ mol } HCO_3^- \rightarrow 1 \text{ mol Urea}$$

the following equation is obtained.

$$1.026 \text{ mol N} + 0.513 \text{ mol } HCO_3^- \rightarrow 0.513 \text{ mol Urea}$$

Assuming that the daily production of urea by an adult is 0.513 mol, this would leave 3.465 mol C ($3.978 - 0.513 = 3.465$) available for the oxidation to CO_2 or the synthesis of glucose and lipids. Therefore, it is evident that AA oxidation in the liver is sufficient to provide bicarbonate for urea production and that the urea cycle itself does not necessarily depend on bicarbonate in the blood plasma or affect the acid–base balance in the body (Nissim et al. 1996). This notion can also be explained by the following examples of the oxidation of alanine, glutamate, and glutamine to form urea and provide additional C, H, and O atoms for other metabolic pathways in mammals. Respiratory quotients (CO_2/O_2) differ among these AAs when they are completely oxidized to CO_2 and H_2O in the body.

(1) Alanine oxidation

$$C_3H_7NO_2\,(\text{Alanine}) - 0.5CH_4N_2O\,(\text{Urea}) \rightarrow C_{2.5}H_5O_{1.5}$$

$$C_{2.5}H_5O_{1.5} + 3O_2 \rightarrow 2.5CO_2 + 2.5H_2O;\ RQ = 2.5/3 = 0.833$$

(2) Glutamate oxidation

$$C_5H_9NO_4\,(\text{Glutamate}) - 0.5CH_4N_2O\,(\text{Urea}) \rightarrow C_{4.5}H_7O_{3.5}$$

$$C_{4.5}H_7O_{3.5} + 4.5O_2 \rightarrow 4.5CO_2 + 3.5H_2O;\ RQ = 4.5/4.5 = 1.00$$

(3) Glutamine oxidation

$$C_5H_{10}N_2O_3\,(\text{Glutamine}) - CH_4N_2O\,(\text{Urea}) \rightarrow C_4H_6O_2$$

$$C_4H_6O_2 + 4.5O_2 \rightarrow 4CO_2 + 3H_2O;\ RQ = 4/4.5 = 0.889$$

For growing mammals, urea production can be estimated when the intake of dietary protein, the digestibility of dietary protein, and the growth rate (protein deposition) are known. When the enzymes of the urea cycle are functioning normally, concentrations of its cofactors (e.g., Mg^{2+} and Mn^{2+}) are adequate, and the AA composition in the diet is optimal, the urinary excretion of ammonia and urea can be used to determine an animal's dietary protein and AA requirements. Likewise, concentrations of ammonia and urea in plasma and urine (when its volume is known) may be useful indicators of whole-body AA oxidation in animals.

6.2.5 NUTRITIONAL AND METABOLIC IMPLICATIONS OF UREA SYNTHESIS IN MAMMALS

The synthesis of urea from ammonia is the major route of ammonia removal in mammals and also provides a metabolic pathway to scavenge AA and non-AA nitrogen for reutilization. In healthy humans and other mammalian species (including ruminants, swine, rodents, cats, and dogs), the whole-body urea production is generally proportionate to the dietary intake of nitrogen so as to minimize the concentration of ammonia in the blood. A failure to compensate for an excessive flow of ammonia into the portal vein via hepatic ureagenesis can rapidly lead to ammonia toxicity in humans and other animals. This is particularly important for ruminants because a large amount of ammonia enters from their rumen into their portal circulation. For example, in dairy cows and beef cattle, the net absorption of ammonia nitrogen into the portal-drained viscera represents about 30%–42% of dietary nitrogen intake (Lapierre et al. 2005; Firkins and Reynolds 2005). Such a high load of ammonia must be immediately converted into urea by the liver at the expense of energy to prevent an accumulation of ammonia in the blood. Additionally, as discussed in the following section on urea recycling, a significant proportion of urea in the blood returns to the lumen of the gastrointestinal tract. Subsequently, the urea is hydrolyzed by microbial urease into ammonia and CO_2, with both the metabolites being used for the synthesis of AAs (e.g., glutamate, glutamine, citrulline, and arginine), bicarbonate (a buffer), and urea in the epithelial cells of the gut. Thus, the liver, enterocytes, and gastrointestinal microbes act in concert to regulate the efficiency of nitrogen utilization by animals.

6.2.6 REGULATION OF THE UREA CYCLE IN MAMMALS

Regulation of the urea cycle under physiological conditions is complex and is still not fully understood (Watford 2020). The activity of the urea cycle is controlled by nutritional, physiological, and pathological factors. First, energy supply, dietary protein intake, as well as the availability of substrates (e.g., AAs and ammonia) and cofactors [e.g., Mn^{2+} (the cofactor for arginase; Ash 2004) and Mg^{2+} (the cofactor for ASS)] in plasma and cells are key nutritional factors influencing ureagenesis in the mammalian liver (Beaumier et al. 1995; Brosnan and Brosnan 2007; Caldovic et al. 2010; Curis et al. 2005; Eklou-Lawson et al. 2009). In most mammals (including cattle, dogs, humans, pigs, and rats), the expression and activities of hepatic urea cycle enzymes are gradually enhanced by the high intake of dietary protein and AAs to facilitate the removal of AA-derived ammonia from the body but are markedly reduced in response to the low intake of dietary protein or AAs as an adaptation mechanism to conserve both energy and nitrogen (Das and Waterlow 1974; Morris 2002). Interestingly, in adult cats, the hepatic activities of transaminases (e.g., alanine and aspartate aminotransferases) and the enzymes of the urea cycle do not adapt to a low or high intake of dietary protein (Rogers et al. 1977), indicating a unique aspect of nitrogen metabolism in this species.

Second, a change in the hepatic activities of most enzymes of the urea cycle requires a prolonged period of time. For example, because the half-lives of urea cycle enzymes are 5–8 days (Table 6.5), restoration of their levels in the liver of mammals with prior long-term protein deficiency will take a considerable amount of time (e.g., 5–8 days in the case of a 50% reduction in enzyme levels) after the individuals resume to consume protein-adequate diets (Schmike 1973). Therefore, a substantial increase in the consumption of dietary protein immediately after a prolonged period of severe protein malnutrition may result in hyperammonemia, vomiting, and even sudden death. These are some cases of refeeding syndrome in humans and other animals (Mehanna et al. 2008). During long-term fasting, urea synthesis is reduced in order to: (1) conserve AA nitrogen and ultimately body protein; (2) maintain a relatively constant concentration of HCO_3^- in the circulation (because the source of CO_2 is limited due to decreased AA oxidation); and (3) minimize energy expenditure.

Third, the extracellular pH can modulate ureagenesis at substrate transport and enzyme expression levels. For example, reducing the extracellular pH from 7.4 to 7.1 inhibits the uptake of AAs by hepatocytes and, therefore, inhibits urea production (Meijer et al. 1990). This allows more glutamine in the blood to be channeled into the kidneys for ammoniagenesis and the buffering of excess H^+. In response to the low extracellular pH, the liver diverts more glutamate into glutamine synthesis and reduces the conversion of glutamate into ammonia and α-KG, thereby increasing the release of glutamine. By contrast, increasing the extracellular pH from 7.4 to 7.6 stimulates urea synthesis from glutamine by enhancing the flux of glutamine through phosphate-activated glutaminase and, therefore, the generation of ammonia and glutamate (a precursor of NAG). A higher pH (e.g., 7.6) can precipitate Ca^{2+}, leading to an impairment of Ca^{2+}-dependent signaling pathways (including those involved in AA metabolism) in cells.

Fourth, compelling evidence shows that CPS-I and ASS are two key regulatory enzymes in hepatic urea synthesis from ammonia (Table 6.4). In hepatocytes, K_m values of the urea cycle enzymes for their substrates and activators (Table 6.5) are similar to the concentrations of the substrates and activators in mitochondria and the cytoplasm (Table 6.6). Studies in the 1970s and 1980s by A.J. Meijer and colleagues led to the identification of arginine as the allosteric activator of NAG. This enzyme converts acetyl-CoA and glutamate to NAG, which is the allosteric activator of CPS-I. Thus, when arginine is deficient, ammonia exits the mitochondria into the cytoplasm, where it is utilized for the synthesis of purines and then orotate and uric acid (Figure 6.5). When OCT is deficient, carbamoyl phosphate is accumulated in the mitochondria, exits into the cytosol, and enters the trifunctional CAD protein beyond the control step (CPS-II) for pyrimidine nucleotide synthesis (Wendler et al. 1983). This results in the loss of a feedback inhibition of CPS-II activity by uridine triphosphate and the accumulation of orotate in the plasma. High concentrations of orotate (which was first discovered in ruminant milk) and uric acid potentially result in a fatty liver and gout, respectively (Visek 1984).

Fifth, some hormones also regulate urea synthesis. For example, growth hormone reduces the activities of CPS-I, ASS, ASL, arginase, and glutaminase in the liver, thereby contributing to the conservation of AAs for protein synthesis (Table 6.8). Insulin reduces the circulating levels of AAs by stimulating whole-body protein synthesis and suppressing proteolysis, thereby decreasing the availability of the AA substrates for urea synthesis (Bush et al. 2002). By contrast, high concentrations of glucocorticoids (stress hormones), glucagon, and cAMP upregulate the expression of urea cycle enzymes and also enhance the degradation of some AAs (e.g., arginine, glutamine, and glycine), but the effects of glucocorticoids are not entirely identical to those of glucagon and cAMP (Morris 2002). It is now known that glucocorticoids act via both genomic (either activation or inhibition of the expression of genes in a cell-specific manner) and non-genomic (e.g., Ca^{2+} influx and cAMP production) mechanisms (Nuñez et al. 2020). This helps to explain, in part, the increased excretion of ammonia and urea under catabolic conditions.

At present, little is known about the nutritional or hormonal regulation of the urea cycle in the enterocytes of the small intestine. Increasing the extracellular concentrations of ammonia or glutamine from 0 to 5 mM enhances ureagenesis in these cells in a concentration-dependent manner (Table 6.7). Thus, substrate availability is a key factor affecting urea production by the intestinal mucosa. Like in hepatocytes, ASS is likely the major rate-controlling enzyme for intestinal ureagenesis and NAG also activates CPS-I. In most mammals (e.g., pigs, humans, and rats), the relatively low activity of arginase-I in enterocytes allows the small intestine to release citrulline and arginine. In contrast to hepatocytes, intestinal CPS-I has a particularly high requirement for bicarbonate (Davis and Wu 1998). Its concentration in the lumen of the small intestine (75–100 mM) is two- to three-fold greater than that in plasma (25 mM). Studies with young pigs have shown that, as reported for the rat liver (Morris 2002), glucocorticoids stimulate the intestinal expression of arginase-II, ASS, and ASL primarily at transcriptional and translational levels and, therefore, the conversion of ammonia to urea in the gut (Flynn et al. 1999; Wu et al. 2000). However, in contrast to the liver, growth hormone does not regulate the activity of any urea cycle enzymes in the small intestine (Table 6.8). At present, the mechanisms responsible for the tissue-specific effect of growth hormone on urea synthesis are largely unknown.

6.2.7 ENERGY REQUIREMENT OF UREAGENESIS IN MAMMALS

A relatively large proportion of dietary energy is required to maintain the urea cycle in an active state. The ATP requirements for urea synthesis are calculated as follows:

1. Formation of 1 mol urea from 1 mol each of ammonia, aspartate, and HCO_3^-:

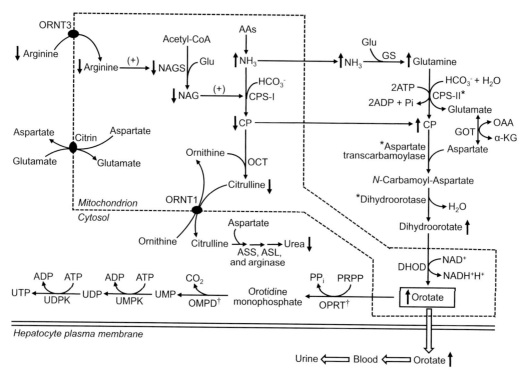

FIGURE 6.5 Biochemical mechanisms responsible for arginine deficiency to impair ammonia detoxification and enhance orotate production in mammals. Arginine in the cytosol enters the mitochondria primarily via ORNT3, although ORNT (an exchanger of ornithine and citrulline) can also transport arginine across the mitochondrial membrane. A deficiency of arginine (an allosteric activator of NAG synthase) impairs the conversion of ammonia into carbamoyl phosphate in the mitochondria, leading to the exit of ammonia into the cytoplasm for the production of dihydroorotate by CAD protein. Dihydroorotate enters the mitochondria for conversion into orotate by dihydroorotate dehydrogenase. Orotate enters the blood for excretion in the urine. Abbreviations: AAs, amino acids; α-KG, α-ketoglutarate; Asp, aspartate; Citrin, mitochondrial aspartate/glutamate antiporter (an exchanger of cytosolic glutamate for mitochondrial aspartate); CP, carbamoyl phosphate; CPS-I, carbamoyl phosphate synthetase-I (ammonia); CPS-II, carbamoyl phosphate synthetase-II (glutamine); DHOD, dihydroorotate dehydrogenase (a mitochondrial enzyme); Glu, glutamate; GOT, glutamate–oxaloacetate transaminase; GS, glutamine synthetase; NAG, N-acetylglutamate; NAGS, N-acetylglutamate synthase; OAA, oxaloacetate; OCT, ornithine carbamoyltransferase; OMPD, orotidine monophosphate decarboxylase; ORNT1, mitochondrial ornithine/citrulline antiporter (an exchanger of cytosolic ornithine for mitochondrial citrulline); ORNT3, mitochondrial basic amino acid carrier; OPRT, orotate phosphoribosyl transferase; PRPP, 5-phosphoribosyl-1-pyrophosphate; UDP, uridine diphosphate; UDPK, uridine diphosphate kinase; UMPK, uridine monophosphate kinase; UMP, uridine monophosphate; UTP, uridine triphosphate; $\uparrow$, Increase; $\downarrow$, Decrease; * In animals, these three enzymatic activities are possessed in one trifunctional protein, designated as CAD protein (CPS-II, aspartate transcarbamylase, and dihydroorotase); †, In animals, these two enzymatic activities are possessed in one bifunctional protein, designated as UMPS (uridine monophosphate synthase).

This process requires 4 mol ATP, as calculated below.

$$NH_3 + HCO_3^- + 2Mg\text{-}ATP \rightarrow \text{Carbamoyl phosphate} \left(NH_2CO_2PO_3^{2-}\right) + 2Mg\text{-}ADP + Pi\,(CPS\text{-}I)$$

$$\text{Citrulline} + \text{Aspartate} + Mg\text{-}ATP \rightarrow \text{Argininosuccinate} + AMP + PPi\;(ASS)$$

Note that when ATP is converted to AMP + PPi in the ASS-catalyzed reaction, two high-energy phosphate bonds are hydrolyzed to provide energy, which is equivalent to the use of 2 moles of ATP (ATP $\rightarrow$ ADP + Pi; ADP $\rightarrow$ AMP + Pi).

TABLE 6.8

Effects of Somatotropin (Growth Hormone) Treatment on the Activities of Urea Cycle Enzymes as well as Related Enzymes and Metabolites in the Liver and Jejunum of Young Pigs[a]

Enzyme	Control	Somatotropin	Metabolites	Control	Somatotropin
	Liver (nmol/mg protein/min)			Liver (nmol/mg tissue)	
Carbamoyl phosphate synthetase-I	16.7 ± 0.7	$9.1 \pm 1.4^*$	N-Acetylglutamate	16.9 ± 1.2	$12.5 \pm 1.2^*$
Ornithine carbamoyltransferase	391 ± 32	367 ± 30	Carbamoyl phosphate	385 ± 46	$307 \pm 33^*$
Argininosuccinate synthase	12.9 ± 0.8	$8.1 \pm 0.9^*$			
Argininosuccinate lyase	16.9 ± 0.8	$13.0 \pm 1.7^*$		Blood (mM)	
Arginase	$16,93 \pm 108$	$1,223 \pm 135^*$			
Ornithine aminotransferase	3.2 ± 0.3	2.9 ± 0.4	Urea	3.25 ± 0.45	$1.75 \pm 0.40^*$
Phosphate-activated glutaminase	38.3 ± 2.8	$31.4 \pm 2.4^*$	Ammonia	0.111 ± 0.025	$0.061 \pm 0.006^*$
Glutamate dehydrogenase	385 ± 18	371 ± 31	Bicarbonate	24.7 ± 1.3	23.3 ± 0.8
	Jejunum (nmol/mg protein/min)			Jejunum (nmol/mg tissue)	
Carbamoyl phosphate synthetase-I	1.3 ± 0.2	1.4 ± 0.1	N-Acetylglutamate	10.8 ± 1.4	$13.9 \pm 1.0^*$
Ornithine carbamoyltransferase	296 ± 40	325 ± 47	Carbamoyl phosphate	124 ± 15	$159 \pm 17^*$
Argininosuccinate synthase	1.2 ± 0.1	1.2 ± 0.1			
Argininosuccinate lyase	2.1 ± 0.3	2.1 ± 0.2			
Arginase	4.9 ± 0.4	5.0 ± 0.5			
Ornithine aminotransferase	31.4 ± 2.4	28.6 ± 3.1			
Phosphate-activated glutaminase	32.4 ± 2.2	$35.6 \pm 2.4^*$			
Glutamate dehydrogenase	8.0 ± 1.3	7.4 ± 1.2			

Source: Bush, J.A. et al. 2002. *J. Nutr.* 132:59–67.

[a] Growing pigs with a mean body weight of 16.4 kg were fed a corn- and soybean meal–based diet and received the intramuscular administration of either saline (control) or recombinant porcine somatotropin (150 µg/kg BW, once daily) for 7 days. Values are means ± SD, $n = 7$ for the control group and $n = 9$ for the somatotropin group.

* $P < 0.05$ vs. the control group.

2. Incorporation of 1 mol ammonia into 1 mol aspartate:

$$NH_4^+ + \alpha\text{-Ketoglutarate} + NADH + H^+ \rightarrow Glutamate + NAD^+ \left(\text{equivalent to 2.5 mol ATP}\right)$$

(This reaction is catalyzed by the mitochondrial glutamate dehydrogenase.)

$$Glutamate + Oxaloacetate \leftrightarrow \alpha\text{-Ketoglutarate} + Aspartate$$

(This reaction is catalyzed by the mitochondrial glutamate–oxaloacetate transaminases.)
The mitochondrial aspartate is transported by citrin into the cytosol in exchange for the entry of cytosolic glutamate into the mitochondria.

3. Conversion of fumarate back into oxaloacetate
The fumarate released from argininosuccinate by ASL is derived from oxaloacetate in the mitochondria. The fumarate is converted into L-malate by the cytosolic fumarase (Tuboi et al. 1986), as noted previously. After entering the mitochondria via the malate shuttle, L-malate undergoes oxidation to generate oxaloacetate and NADH (equivalent to 2.5 mol ATP) by the NAD^+-linked malate dehydrogenase (Figure 6.3). This offsets the NADH consumed for the conversion of ammonia into glutamate by glutamate dehydrogenase.

Thus, a total of net 4 mol ATP (4 + 2.5 − 2.5 = 4) are required to convert 2 mol ammonia to 1 mol urea in the mammalian liver. This is equivalent to 2 mol ATP per mol ammonia (or 2.4 mol ATP for the oxidation of 100 g meat protein). Depending on the AA, the detoxification of protein-derived ammonia as urea consumes approximately 6%–22% of ATP produced from AA oxidation. Optimizing the quality and quantity of dietary AA requirements by mammals can reduce urea production, thereby improving the efficiency of protein and energy utilization. Compared with mammals, aquatic animals, which excrete ammonia directly into the environment (water), have a higher efficiency of the utilization of dietary AAs for protein synthesis.

When the rate of the formation of carbamoyl phosphate from ammonia, CO_2, and ATP exceeds the rate of conversion of carbamoyl phosphate plus ornithine into citrulline in the mitochondria, carbamoyl phosphate exits into the cytoplasm for the synthesis of orotic acid. This can occur when (1) OCT or ORNT1 is deficient and (2) the dietary intake of protein or ammonia concentrations in plasma is very high. Elevated production of orotic acid is associated with the development of a fatty liver in experimental animals (Visek 1984) and also with an increased incidence of colon and liver cancers in susceptible individuals who chronically consume high quantities of dietary protein (Visek 1992).

6.2.8 Urea Recycling in Ruminants

In ruminants, urea in the circulation enters the lumen of the rumen through saliva and uptake from the arterial blood across rumen epithelium via facilitative UTs, such as UT-B1 and UT-B2 (Lu et al. 2014). Within the rumen, urease, which is produced by bacteria, rapidly hydrolyzes urea to form ammonia and CO_2. A large proportion of urea-derived ammonia is utilized for the synthesis of free AAs, small peptides, and proteins by ruminal bacteria, archaea, and fungi, and protozoa consume those microbes to obtain AAs (Chapter 2). These nitrogenous products of ammonia flow into the lumen of the abomasum and thence into the lumen of the small intestine for digestion and absorption. Once absorbed, free AAs and small peptide–derived AAs are used for protein synthesis or undergo metabolism in tissues, and their nitrogen is ultimately transformed into urea in the liver (Firkins et al. 2007). Some of this urea nitrogen is again recycled into the gastrointestinal tract via saliva and from the arterial blood into the rumen, as described in Chapter 2. The transport of urea across the ruminal epithelium into the rumen is stimulated by ruminal short-chain fatty acids and CO_2 with the maximum rate of urea flux at ruminal pH of 5.8, but is inhibited by elevated ruminal ammonia (with saturation at 5 mM) and reduced ruminal pH below 5.8 (Lu et al. 2014). In addition, a substantial proportion of the ammonia derived from ruminal urea hydrolysis is directly absorbed through the ruminal epithelium into the blood for hepatic urea synthesis (Reynolds and Kristensen 2008). Collectively, these events are referred to as urea recycling. Urea kinetics in the whole animal can be measured with a ^{15}N-tracer technique, which involves the constant intravenous administration of $[^{15}N, {}^{15}N]$ urea and the measurement of the enrichment of $[^{15}N, {}^{14}N]$ urea and $[^{15}N, {}^{15}N]$ urea in the urine and feces, as well as bacterial and plasma ^{15}N or bacterial and duodenal ^{15}N to include the microbial capture of the recycled urea nitrogen (Lobley et al. 2000; Marini et al. 2004; Wickersham et al. 2009).

The proportion of urea transferred from the liver to the gastrointestinal tract ranges from 10% to 80% in ruminants and is affected by species and diet (Batista et al. 2017; Bergen 2021; Li et al. 2019). Under normal feeding conditions, the ratio of hepatic urea synthesis (g of urea N) to digestible nitrogen intake from the diet (g of N) is 1.15 for bulls, 1.07 for steers, 0.87 for dairy cows, 1.42 for sheep fed forage diets, 2.34 for sheep fed hay/barley diets, 1.05–1.21 for growing goats, 2.83–4.86 for wapiti, 0.54–1.32 for white-tailed deer, and 0.82–1.79 for reindeer/caribou (NRC 2006). Thus, an extensive recycling of urea to the rumen for microbial synthesis of AAs and proteins provides a metabolic basis for: (1) reindeer/caribou to meet maintenance requirements in winter; and (2) bulls, sheep, wapiti, and deer to support maintenance requirements plus weight

TABLE 6.9
Urea–Nitrogen Recycling in Growing Ewe Lambs[a]

	Crude protein levels in diet (%, DM basis)		
	9.7	**17.8**	**25.8**
Nitrogen content in diet, g/kg DM	15.5	28.4	41.3
DM intake, g/day	575	705	630
Nitrogen (N) intake, g/day	8.9	20.3	25.9
Weight gain, g/day	40	144	122
Plasma urea, mM	1.5	7.2	9.9
Urinary excretion of N, g/day	2.4	10.0	16.5
Urinary excretion of urea, g N/day	0.7	7.0	13.4
Fecal excretion of N, g/day	5.0	5.2	4.9
N balance, g/day	1.5	5.1	4.4
Urea production in the whole body, g N/day	2.4	11.8	19.2
Urea recycled to the GI tract, g N/day	1.8	4.8	5.8
Percentage of urea produced in the body recycled to the GI tract, %	75	41	30

Source: Marini, J.C. et al. 2004. *J. Anim. Sci.* 82:1157–1164.

[a] Ewe lambs with a mean body weight of 21 kg were individually fed three isocaloric diets (2.75 Mcal metabolizable energy/kg dry matter) for 25 days before the measurements of urea recycling were made.

Note: DM, dry matter; GI, gastrointestinal tract.

gain as tissue protein (meat and wool) or milk protein. The magnitude of urea recycling in ruminants is affected greatly by their dietary intake of protein and nitrogen (NRC 2006; Reynolds and Kristensen 2008) and the concentration of ammonia in the rumen (Firkins et al. 2007; Kennedy and Milligan 1980). The proportions of urea synthesized in the liver that is returned to the gastrointestinal tract are high and low, respectively, at low and high intakes of dietary nitrogen (Table 6.9). In ewe lambs fed diets containing 9.7%, 17.8%, and 25.8% crude protein, 75%, 41%, and 30% of the urea produced in the liver is reutilized each day, respectively, via urea recycling. This involves both microbial protein synthesis and hepatic urea resynthesis. In beef cattle fed diets with 5% and 15% crude protein, 53% and 21% of the recycled urea nitrogen are assimilated by ruminal microbes, respectively (Batista et al. 2017). Similarly, about 15%–20% of the recycled urea nitrogen is captured as microbial protein in dairy cows fed diets containing 15–18% crude protein (Reynolds and Kristensen 2008). Urea recycling in ruminants serves to spare dietary and endogenous nitrogen for protein synthesis and other metabolic functions and carries nitrogen in a non-toxic form (i.e., urea rather than toxic ammonia) for interorgan metabolism. This is very important for ruminants that generally consume relatively low-protein (e.g., 10% crude protein) diets, particularly when compared with non-ruminant herbivores grazing the same low-protein pasture. Thus, urea recycling is an evolutionary advantage in ruminant nutrition and physiology.

6.2.9 EXCRETION OF UREA BY THE KIDNEYS

6.2.9.1 Excretion of Urea in the Urine

Studies with adult humans and growing pigs have shown that about 20%–25% of the urea newly synthesized in the liver is taken by the small and large intestines, where urea is hydrolyzed into ammonia and CO_2 (Bergen and Wu 2009; Walser and Bondelos 1959). As indicated previously, some of the ammonia is used for urea synthesis by the enterocytes of the small intestine and the colonocytes of the large intestine, with the intestine-derived urea returning to the blood circulation. Blood urea is filtered by the renal glomerulus into the proximal renal tubules. Some of the filtered urea is reabsorbed into the blood by the proximal renal tubules and the distal renal tubules, with the amounts being affected by nutritional and physiological factors. In 1962, K. Diem provided the following data (g N/day) showing the composition of nitrogen-containing compounds in the urine of healthy adult humans consuming 100 g of highly digestible protein per day (~16 g N/day).

Urea	12.8
Ammonia	0.7
Amino acids	0.7
Creatinine	0.7
Uric acid	0.3
Hippuric acid	0.1
Total	15.3

The amount of nitrogen in urinary phenylacetylglutamine (0.04 g N/day) could have been included as a metabolite of AAs in the above list. Thus, the total amount of urinary nitrogen is 15.34 g/day. In contrast to most renal solutes, the majority (~97%) of renal ammonia excreted by humans derives from intrarenal production (e.g., degradation of glutamine, glycine, and other AAs), but not from glomerular filtration (which accounts for only ~3% of renal ammonia excretion) (Weiner and Verlander 2013). Assuming that the digestibility of the dietary protein is 95%, the amount of dietary AAs available for metabolism in an adult human is 15.2 g N/day (i.e., 16 g N×0.95). Some of the dietary protein that is not digested in the small intestine is catabolized in the large intestine to generate ammonia and AAs, and a proportion of these nitrogenous metabolites (possibly 0.5 g N/day; equivalent to 3.1% of the dietary nitrogen intake) is absorbed into the portal circulation for utilization. Based on the urinary excretion of urea and ammonia, it can be estimated that: (1) urea excretion accounts for 83.4% of total nitrogen in the urine, and (2) nearly all (99.8%) of the net amount of urea produced in humans [i.e., $(12.8 \times 100)/(12.8 + 0.7 \times 0.03)$] is eventually excreted by the kidneys within 24 h.

6.2.9.2 Important Roles of Renal Transporters of Urea in Its Urinary Excretion

Until about 60 years ago, it was thought that urea in the blood was filtered and reabsorbed passively into the proximal renal tubules. However, this simplistic view was challenged by B. Schmidt-Nielsen who reported in 1952 that urea clearance in desert kangaroo rats fed a high-protein diet can exceed the filtered load. Based on her subsequent extensive studies, she proposed that urea clearance and glomerular filtration by the kidneys must be independently regulated in response to the intakes of different amounts of dietary protein (Kokko and Sands 2006; Schmidt-Nielsen et al. 1985). In other words, renal tubules likely express specific transporters to transport urea across their plasma membrane and their expression is influenced by AA intake. Therefore, it was surmised that UTs in the kidneys would play an important role in both the salvaging of urea nitrogen and its urinary concentration.

In support of the notion of B. Schmidt-Nielsen (1952), J.M. Sands and coworkers proposed, for the first time in 1987, that urea is transported by a facilitated or carrier-mediated transporter in the mammalian collecting duct. Subsequently, Beyer and Gelarden (1988) reported Na⁺-dependent active transport of urea by the mammalian kidneys. Five years later, M.A. Hediger and colleagues identified and cloned the first facilitative UT, now named UT-A2 1993 (You et al. 1993). To date, evidence shows that humans and other mammals have two types of urea transport proteins, UT-A and UT-B, which are encoded by two distinct genes, *SLC14A2* (UT-A) and *SLC14A1* (UT-B), respectively (Sands and Blount 2014).

The UT-A proteins are important for the renal handling of urea and are produced by alternative splicing of the *SLC14A2* gene under the control of alternative promoters. There are six protein isoforms of UT-A (UT-A1 through UT-A6), with a distinct pattern of expression in various cell

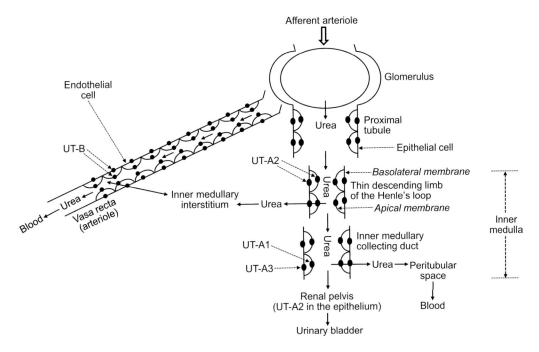

FIGURE 6.6 Scheme for the distribution of key UTs (UT-A and UT-B) and urea reabsorption along the nephron and the vasa recta (arteriole) of kidneys. Nephron is the functional unit of kidneys and consists of glomerulus and its associated tubules. Not all structural components of the kidneys are shown in this figure. UT-A1 is located in the apical membrane of the inner medullary collecting duct, UT-A3 in the basolateral membrane of the inner medullary collecting duct, UT-A2 in the apical and basolateral membranes of the descending thin limb of Henle's loops, and UT-B in the basolateral and apical membranes of the endothelial cells of the descending vasa recta (arteriole). Urea in the blood is filtered by the renal glomerulus into the lumen of the proximal tubule. Urea flows along the nephron, including the thin descending limb of the Henle's loop, the inner medullary collecting duct, and the outer medullary collecting duct before entering the renal pelvis and the urinary bladder. UT-A1 and UT-A3 reabsorb urea from the tubular lumen to the peritubular space followed by entry into the blood. UT-A2 and UT-B contribute to urea recycling across the renal tubules, the inner medullary interstitium, and the vasculature in the inner medulla.

types. UT-A1 is located in the apical plasma membrane of the inner medullary collecting duct of the kidneys, UT-A3 in the basolateral membrane of the inner medullary collecting duct of the kidneys, UT-A2 in the apical and basolateral membranes of the descending thin limb of Henle's loops of the kidneys (Figure 6.6), UT-A4 in low abundance in the renal medulla, UT-A5 in the testis, and UT-A6 in the colon. Both UT-A5 and UT-A6 are absent from the kidneys. The single isoform of UT-B protein is encoded by the SLC14A1 gene. UT-B is widely expressed in the kidneys, erythrocytes, small intestine, large intestine, blood–brain barrier, and skin. Renal UT-B is located in the basolateral and apical membranes of the endothelial cells of the descending vasa recta (capillary-sized microvessels that supply the blood to the renal medulla). There are two forms of UT-B protein: 32-kDa (non-glycosylated form) and 47-kDa (N-glycosylated form). Another facilitative UT, UT-C, has been reported to be present in the proximal tubules of the seawater eel (Mistry et al. 2005). Based on the localization of UTs in the kidneys, UT-A1 and UT-A3 reabsorb urea from the tubular lumen to the blood, whereas UT-A2 and UT-B are involved in the recycling of urea across the tubular lumen, the interstitium, and the vasculature in the outer medullary compartment (Figure 6.6). Thus, the formation of concentrated urine for urea excretion requires interactions between UTs in the renal tubules and the vasculature in the renal medulla.

6.2.9.3   Regulation of the Expression of Renal Urea Transporters

Expression of UTs, UT-A1 and UT-A2, in the kidneys is increased by vasopressin (also known as antidiuretic hormone or arginine vasopressin; a peptide hormone synthesized in the posterior pituitary gland), whereas the expression of renal UT-A1 and UT-A3 is stimulated by hypertonicity (Sands and Blount 2014). In addition, vasopressin activates cAMP-dependent protein kinase A, which phosphorylates UT-A1 at serines 486 and 499. Increased UT-A expression and activity promote the reabsorption of water and urea from the renal tubules to the inner medullary interstitium (and then into the blood), thereby reducing the excretion of water and urea in the urine. By contrast, the abundance of UT-A1 is reduced by glucocorticoids, aldosterone, glucagon, and lithium, as well as in aging animals, type 2 diabetes mellitus (e.g., obese Zucker diabetic rats), and the early stage of type 1 diabetes (e.g., within 5 days after the onset of diabetes in rats), leading to a reduction in urea reabsorption by renal tubules into the blood and an increase in urinary urea excretion (Klein et al. 2012). Interestingly, renal UT-A1 mRNA and protein abundances are increased at 10–21 days of type 1 diabetes mellitus in rats via a vasopressin-dependent mechanism to reabsorb urea from the renal tubules to the blood so as to regulate blood urea concentration and osmolality in the face of increased excretion of metabolites (e.g., urea, glucose, ketone bodies, and potassium) in the urine. There may be species differences in the response of renal UT-A expression to dietary protein intake. For example, compared with the control diet with 20% protein, feeding a low (10%) protein or a high (40%) protein for 1 week does not affect the mRNA levels of UT-A1, UT-A2, and UT-B1 in the kidneys of normal Sprague-Dawley rats, although the renal UT-A1 level is reduced by the low-protein diet in Brattleboro rats (an animal model without vasopressin) (Hu et al. 1999). However, compared with a diet with 8.6% crude protein (on a dry matter basis), feeding adult sheep with a low-protein diet (5.4% crude protein, dry matter basis) for 5 weeks reduces the mRNA level of UT-A2 in the epithelium of the kidney's pelvis by 58% in association with reduced urea excretion in the urine (Artagaveytia et al. 2005). Interpretation of this result could be facilitated by the availability of data on the expression of other UTs (such as UT-A1 and UT-A3) in the ovine kidneys.

By contrast to UT-A, UT-B abundance is not affected by vasopressin (Klein et al. 2012). The abundance of the UT-B protein in the outer medulla, but not the inner medulla, of young rats is increased by 25% in response to the consumption of a low (14%)-protein diet for 12 days, when compared with the control diet containing 23% protein (Inoue et al. 2005). This may enhance the recycling of urea to preserve adequate urea concentration and osmolality in the medullary interstitium when the whole-body production of urea is reduced. By contrast, in rats fed a high (43%)-protein diet for 2 weeks, the abundance of the UT-B protein is decreased in the outer medulla and inner medulla by 50% and 54%, respectively, despite a 100% increase in its mRNA level in the outer medulla and no change in its mRNA level in the inner medulla, when compared with the control diet containing 23% protein. Hu et al. (1999) reported that feeding a low-protein (10% casein) or a high-protein (40% casein) diet for 1 week did not affect the mRNA level of UT-B in the kidneys of adult Sprague-Dawley rats, in comparison with the control diet containing 20% casein. The dismatch between the protein and mRNA abundances of UT-B suggests complex mechanisms for the regulation of UT-B expression at transcriptional and translational levels in the renal tubules. Nonetheless, with an increase in the renal UT-B protein, the reabsorption of urea from the outer medulla of the kidneys into the blood and the recycling of urea within the medulla are reduced to promote urea excretion in the urine. As with UT-A, there may also be species differences in the response of renal UT-B expression to dietary protein intake. For example, Ludden et al. (2009) reported that supplementing protein to low-quality forage to achieve 7%, 10% and 13% crude protein in the diets for 28 days did not affect the abundance of the UT-B protein in the kidneys of lambs.

6.2.10   Urea Synthesis from Ammonia in Certain Teleost Fish and in the Elasmobranchs

The urea cycle is present in: (1) certain teleost fish (e.g., the Lake Magadi tilapia that has adapted to living in waters with a pH of 10.5, the marine gulf toadfish that are managed under laboratory conditions, and Indian freshwater air-breathing teleosts that have adapted to living in waters with pH 8.5–10), as well as marine and freshwater elasmobranchs (sharks, rays, and skates) (Anderson 2001; Saha and Ratha 2007; Wright 1995). In these fishes, glutamine and bicarbonate are substrates for the synthesis of carbamoyl phosphate by the mitochondrial CPS-III (the first enzyme of the urea cycle). This enzyme differs from the mammalian CPS-I, which uses ammonia as the nitrogenous donor of carbamoyl phosphate. Interestingly, in the Lake Magadi tilapia, hepatic CPS-III activity is too low to account for the high rate of urea production from ammonia, but CPS-III and other enzymes of the urea cycle are present in the skeletal muscles at sufficiently high levels to catalyze the synthesis of a large amount of urea (Lindley et al. 1999). The use of blood bicarbonate for urea synthesis from ammonia in the muscles can help to reduce pH in fish. By contrast, high levels of urea cycle enzymes occur in the liver of the marine gulf toadfish when they switch from ammonotelic and ureotelic producers in response to crowding or confinement stress (Laberge et al. 2009), although the skeletal muscles of this fish also express a lower level of CPS-III (Kong et al. 2000). Likewise, the liver and kidneys of four species of Indian freshwater air-breathing teleosts, the singhi catfish (*Heteropneustes fossilis*), walking catfish (*Clarias batrachus*), mud eel (*Amphipnous cuchia*), and the climbing perch (*Anabas testudineus*) express high levels of urea cycle enzymes possibly as an adaptation to a high alkaline environment (pH 8.5–10) (Saha and Ratha 2007). In elasmobranchs, such as the dogfish shark, all urea cycle enzymes are expressed in the liver and skeletal muscle, but the skeletal muscle appears to make a greater contribution to ureagenesis than the liver (Kajimura et al. 2006). Thus, there are species differences in tissue-specific ureagenesis among the ureotelic fish. The subcellular localization of urea cycle enzymes in all these aquatic animals are the same as those in the mammalian liver. Expression of urea cycle enzymes in the ureotelic fishes is upregulated by glucocorticoids, protein feeding, and environmental salinity (Laberge et al. 2009; Saha and Ratha 2007).

$$\text{Glutamine} + H_2O + HCO_3^- + 2\text{Mg-ATP} \rightarrow \text{Carbamoyl phosphate} \left(NH_2CO_2PO_3^{2-}\right) + \text{Glutamate}$$

$$+ 2\text{Mg-ADP} + \text{Pi} \left(\text{CPS-III, NAG; mitochondria}\right)$$

Ureagenesis in certain teleost fish functions in nitrogen excretion, but urea is the major osmolyte in elasmobranchs (Anderson 2001). For example, concentrations of urea in the plasma of marine elasmobranchs are about 300–600 mM, as their gill epithelia have a very low permeability to urea and therefore prevent its release from the blood into the living environment (Anderson 2001; Ballantyne and Robinson 2010; Goldstein and Forster 1971; Pärt et al. 1998). Lower plasma concentrations of urea (70–220 mM) are present in most freshwater elasmobranchs (except for potamytrygonid rays) as a significant or major osmolyte, but the values are still exceedingly high in comparison with terrestrial mammals (2–5 mM). Thus, the urea cycle is of nutritional and physiological importance in ureotelic fishes.

6.3 URIC ACID SYNTHESIS

6.3.1 HISTORICAL PERSPECTIVES

Uric acid is a heterocyclic organic compound consisting of carbon, nitrogen, oxygen, and hydrogen. It was first isolated from kidney stones by the Swedish chemist, K. Wilheim Scheele, in 1776. One century later, W. von Kninerem reported in 1877 that AAs or ammonium salts were converted into uric acid in birds, which was confirmed by I. von Schroeder in 1878. The chemical synthesis of uric acid was first achieved in 1882 by E. Hoffmann, who used trichlorolactimide as the starting material. In the same year, the Ukrainian medical chemist, Ivan Horbaczewski, synthesized uric acid from urea and glycine while working at the University of Vienna, Austria. By 1890, it was known that uric acid was the major metabolite of nitrogen metabolism in birds, serpents, insects, and a great majority of invertebrate species. The structure of uric acid was established by Emil Fischer in

1902. In 1936, 4 years after the discovery of the urea cycle, H.A. Krebs and coworkers elucidated the biochemical pathway for uric acid synthesis from purines in the avian liver, kidneys, and pancreas, with hypoxanthine as an intermediate. This metabolic pathway for uric acid synthesis was subsequently confirmed in mammals, other vertebrates, and invertebrates (Schmidt-Nielsen 1988). It is now known that degradation of purines (adenosine and guanosine) to uric acid is common to all animal species (including humans, pigs, cattle, sheep, dogs, cats, and insects). Thus, uric acid is produced in mammals, birds, fish, and crustaceans.

6.3.2 Chemistry of Uric Acid

Uric acid (lactam form) undergoes spontaneously keto–enol tautomerization to its lactim form, which deprotonates to form the negatively charged urate ion in the blood. Thus, uric acid, which has a pK_a of 5.75, is a weak organic acid at physiological pH values (e.g., 7.0 and 7.4). At pH 7.4 (blood pH) and pH 7.0 (cytosolic pH in the cell), about 98% and 95% of uric acid occur in an ionized form as urate, respectively (Grassi et al. 2013). The major form of urate in the blood is monosodium urate (Grassi et al. 2013). When the pH of urine is 5.7 (e.g., in healthy humans), about 50% of uric acid is present in a non-ionized form and 50% in an ionized form as urate (mainly as potassium, ammonium, and calcium urate).

Tautomers of Uric acid and Urate ion at Neutral pH

6.3.3 Conversion of Ammonia and Bicarbonate to Purine Nucleosides

Purine nucleosides (adenosine and guanosine) are nitrogenous substrates for uric acid synthesis. As described in Chapter 5, the use of isotopes by J.M. Buchanan and coworkers in their experiments led to the discovery of purine synthesis from HCO_3^-, aspartate, glutamine, glycine, and N^{10}-formyl-tetrahydrofolate in animals. The nitrogen atoms in these AAs are ultimately derived from NH_4^+ (Figure 6.7). Carbons other than those from glycine are derived from HCO_3^- and formate. Formate is converted into N^{10}-formyl-tetrahydrofolate before its incorporation into purines. Thus, knowledge of AA metabolism and purine synthesis is essential for our understanding of uric acid production.

The synthesis of purines occurs in all avian and mammalian tissues and is most active in the liver of all animal species (Chapter 5). Hepatic purine synthesis is regulated not only by the availability of substrates (ammonia and AAs) and nucleotides, but also by the activities of key enzymes, including adenylosuccinate synthetase, adenosine kinase, 5′-nucleotidase, and adenylate deaminase (Pedley and Benkovic 2016). Interestingly, the purine synthetic enzymes cluster near the mitochondria and microtubules of the cells to form dynamic multienzyme complexes (known as purinosomes) to facilitate metabolic flux. Additionally, energy supply is a key factor influencing the synthesis of purines and, therefore, uric acid.

6.3.4 Uric Acid Synthesis from Purine Nucleosides

In mammals, fish, shrimp, aquatic crabs, and uricotelic species (e.g., birds), the synthesis of uric acid from purines (adenosine and guanosine) takes place primarily in the liver and, to a lesser extent in other tissues, including the kidneys, pancreas, and mucosa of the gastrointestinal tract (Cheng et al. 2005; Chin and Quebbemann 1978; Lallier and Walsh 1991; Moriwaki et al. 1999; Tinker et al. 1986). This metabolic pathway is outlined in Figure 6.7. Xanthine oxidase (a homodimer and

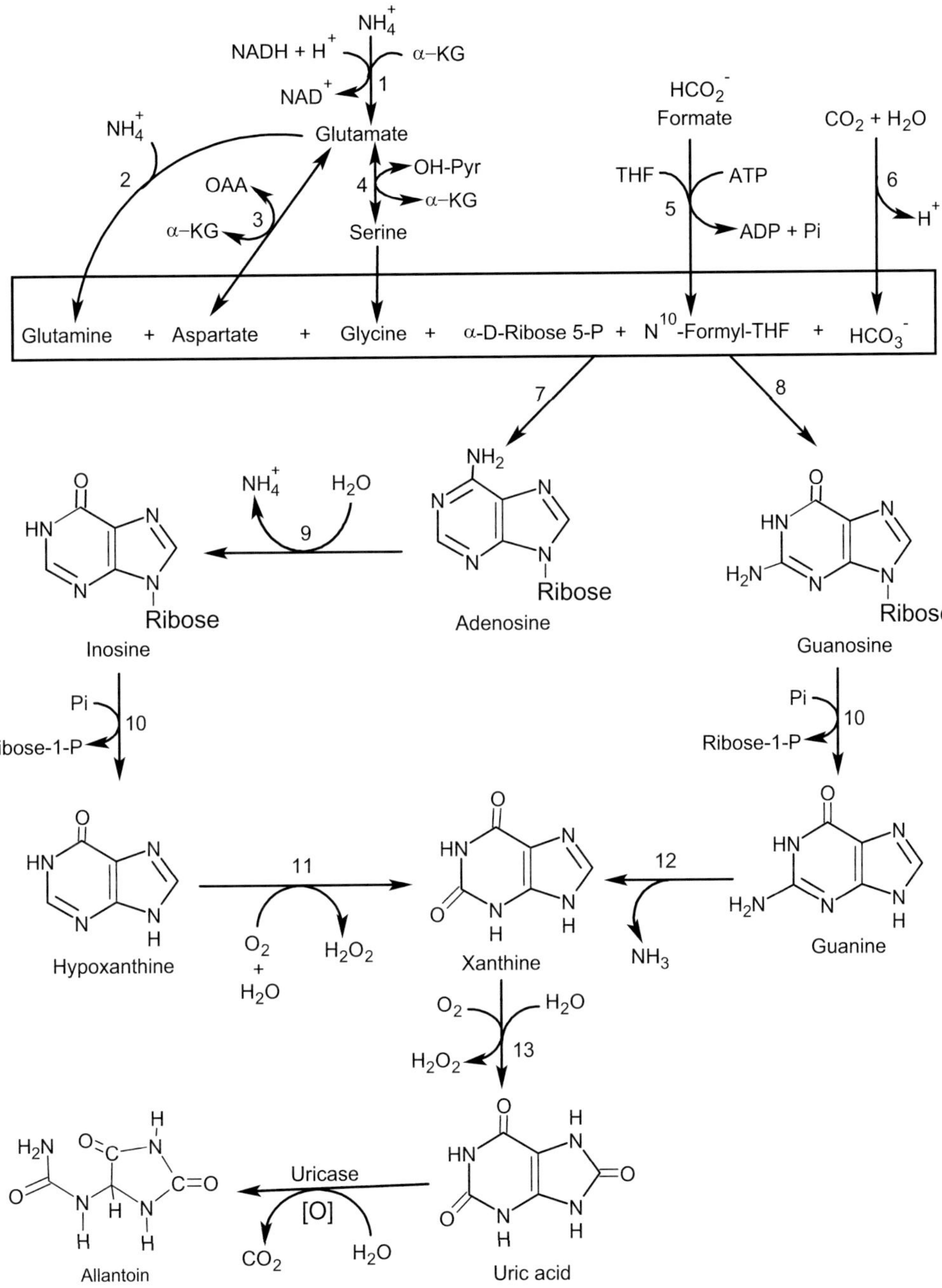

FIGURE 6.7 Uric acid synthesis. The enzymes that catalyze the indicated pathways are: (1) glutamate dehydrogenase; (2) glutamine synthetase; (3) glutamate–oxaloacetate transaminase; (4) glutamate–hydroxypyruvate transaminase; (5) N^{10}-formyl-tetrahydrofolate synthetase; (6) carbonic anhydrase; (7) a series of enzymes for adenosine synthesis; (8) a series of enzymes for guanosine synthesis; (9) adenosine deaminase; (10) purine nucleoside phosphorylase; (11) xanthine oxidase; (12) guanine deaminase (guanase); and (13) xanthine oxidase.

a molybdenum-dependent enzyme), the last enzyme in the uric acid synthetic pathway, possesses xanthine dehydrogenase activity which requires NAD^+ as a cofactor to form uric acid and NADH. In humans, the catalytic activities of xanthine oxidase and xanthine dehydrogenase are carried out by the same bifunctional protein encoded by the same gene *XDH*. In other animals, xanthine dehydrogenase (a homodimer and a molybdenum-dependent enzyme) is converted into xanthine oxidase by reversible sulfhydryl oxidation or limited proteolysis.

The liver, kidneys, pancreas, the mucosa of the gastrointestinal tract, heart, skeletal muscle, and lymphoid organs of birds (e.g., chickens, parrots, and penguins) and mammals (e.g., humans, rats, pigs, and cattle) can release hypoxanthine (Moriwaki et al. 1999). In pigeons, whose liver has a low xanthine oxidase/xanthine dehydrogenase activity, hypoxanthine released by the liver is taken up by the kidneys for conversion into uric acid by xanthine oxidase/xanthine dehydrogenase (Nagahara et al. 1987). Likewise, in chickens, skeletal muscle may take up hypoxanthine from the circulation and convert this purine metabolite into uric acid (Moriwaki et al. 1999; Tinker et al. 1986). Some of the enzymes involved in purine metabolism, such as adenosine deaminase and purine nucleoside phosphorylase, are particularly abundant in lymphocytes (e.g., thymocytes, lymph node lymphocytes, and splenic lymphocytes) and can degrade adenosine to hypoxanthine. Because the accumulation of adenosine is deleterious to cells (particularly lymphocytes), a deficiency of one or both of these two enzymes can result in cytotoxicity to lymphocytes and lymphopenia. Thus, rates of purine synthesis and degradation must be precisely controlled in organisms.

Note that in spiders, scorpions, and mites, guanine produced from guanosine does not undergo further metabolism due to the lack of guanine deaminase and is released from the body (Grishin et al. 2020). This is an adaptation to life in arid habitats that are generally without water. These animals excrete guanine as the primary nitrogenous metabolite and are called guanotelic species. Like uric acid, guanine is nearly insoluble in pure water. The solubility of guanine in water at 25°C and pH 5.0–7.5 does not differ and is 25.4 µM (Darvishzad et al. 2018). However, in the physiological solutions of animals that contain sodium and other cationic minerals, the solubility of guanine is likely greater, as found for uric acid.

6.3.5 Regulation of Uric Acid Synthesis

Uric acid synthesis is regulated by a number of factors in response to physiological needs: (1) dietary intakes of protein and AAs; (2) energy supply in cells; (3) concentrations of ammonia, AAs, and tetrahydrofolate in plasma; (4) rates of the incorporation of ammonia into glutamine and then purines; and (5) activities of adenosine deaminase, purine nucleoside phosphorylase, and xanthine oxidase/xanthine dehydrogenase. One-carbon metabolism serves a crucial role in modulating the production of uric acid via the synthesis of purine nucleosides (Pedley and Benkovic 2016). Increasing the dietary intake of purines can stimulate the hepatic expression and enzymatic activity of urate oxidase in allantoin-synthesizing species, such as the Atlantic salmon (Andersen et al. 2006). In addition, as reported for the chicken liver, the ratio of adenine nucleotides to guanine nucleotides, as well as the interaction between substrates and purine nucleotides, also contribute to the regulation of urate synthesis (Burns and Buttery 1984). Furthermore, elevated concentrations of AMP (an indicator of low intracellular energy status) inhibit the activities of both amidophosphoribosyltransferase and aminoimidazole ribonucleotide synthetase (key enzymes for purine synthesis, Chapter 5) in the pigeon liver (Rowe et al. 1978). Thus, in chickens, starvation reduces uric acid synthesis by the liver (Table 6.10). Tumor necrosis factor-α, interferon-γ, interleukin-1, interleukin-6, and dexamethasone all increase the expression of xanthine dehydrogenase/xanthine oxidase at both mRNA and protein levels in the renal epithelial cells (Battelli et al. 2014; Pfeffer et al. 1994), thereby stimulating urate production under inflammatory and stressful conditions.

TABLE 6.10
Arteriovenous Differences for Uric Acid and Related Metabolites across the Liver, Kidney, and Hindquarter of Fed and Starved Adult Chicken[a]

| Metabolite | Concentration in Whole arterial blood (nmol/mL) | | Arteriovenous difference (nmol/mL of Whole Blood) | | | | | |
| | | | Liver | | Kidney | | Hindquarter | |
	Fed	Starved	Fed	Starved	Fed	Starved	Fed	Starved
Glucose	10,360	11,670	−940	−1,450	−44	−307	792	199
Glutamine	444	370	ND	121	62	ND	−48	−109
Ammonia	−	−	ND	ND	ND	−123	ND	41
Uric acid	212	230	−100	−76	84	83	−72	−50

Source: Tinker, D.A., J.T. Brosnan, and G.R. Herzberg. 1986. *Biochem. J.* 240:829–836.

[a] Eight-week-old adult male white Leghorn chickens, which were either fed a regular diet or starved for 6 days, were used in the study. Rates of hepatic blood flow were 59 and 36 mL/min/kg BW in fed and 6-day-starved chickens, respectively. Thus, based on the arteriovenous difference, the release of uric acid by the liver and hindquarter (skeletal muscle) is markedly reduced in the starved than in the fed chickens. It is unlikely that *de novo* synthesis of uric acid occurs in skeletal muscle. However, the muscle can take up hypoxanthine from the arterial blood and convert this purine metabolite to uric acid.

Note: ND, not detected; "−", release; "+", uptake.

6.3.6 ENERGY REQUIREMENT FOR URIC ACID SYNTHESIS FROM AMMONIA

The ATP requirements for the synthesis of uric acid from ammonia are determined by the rates of three events: (1) the formation of adenosine or guanosine from glutamine, aspartate, glycine, ribose-5-P, bicarbonate, and N^{10}-formyltetrahydrofolate; (2) the incorporation of ammonia into glutamine, aspartate, and glycine; and (3) the formation of N^{10}-formyl-tetrahydrofolate from formate and tetrahydrofolate. One mole of ammonia is generated from 1 mol adenosine by adenosine deaminase in the pathway for uric acid synthesis from adenosine. This ammonia molecule subsequently participates in another round of purine and uric acid synthesis. Thus, 4 mol NH_4^+ are incorporated into 1 mol uric acid. As indicated by the following calculations, 46% more ATP is required to detoxify 1 mol ammonia via uric acid synthesis than via urea synthesis. Note that the conversion of adenosine or guanosine into uric acid does not require energy.

6.3.6.1 Energy Required for the Synthesis of Uric Acid from Ammonia via Adenosine

The amount of energy needed to convert ammonia into uric acid via the formation of adenosine can be calculated as follows. This calculation applies to all birds.

1. As illustrated in Chapter 5, the synthesis of 1 mol adenosine requires 8 mol ATP.
2. Incorporation of 5 mol ammonia into 2 mol glutamine, 2 mol aspartate, and 1 mol glycine requires 9.5 mol ATP.
   a. Net 2 mol of ATP are required to incorporate 2 mol ammonia into 2 mol glutamine.

$$2NH_4^+ + 2\alpha\text{-Ketoglutarate} + 2NADH + 2H^+ \rightarrow 2Glutamate + 2NAD^+$$

$$2Glutamate + 2NH_4^+ + 2ATP \rightarrow 2Glutamine + 2ADP$$

In the metabolic pathway of adenosine synthesis:

$$2Glutamine + 2H_2O \rightarrow 2Glutamate + 2NH_4^+$$

$$2\text{Glutamate} + 2\text{NAD}^+ \rightarrow 2\text{NH}_4^+ + 2\alpha\text{-Ketoglutarate} + 2\text{NADH} + 2\text{H}^+$$

$$\text{Net reaction: } 2\text{Glutamate} + 2\text{NH}_4^+ + 2\text{ATP} \rightarrow 2\text{Glutamine} + 2\text{ADP}$$

b. 5 mol ATP are required to convert 2 mol ammonia and 2 mol oxaloacetate to 2 mol aspartate.

$$2\text{NH}_4^+ + 2\alpha\text{-Ketoglutarate} + 2\text{NADH} + 2\text{H}^+ \rightarrow 2\text{Glutamate} + 2\text{NAD}^+$$

$$2\text{Glutamate} + 2\text{Oxaloacetate} \leftrightarrow 2\alpha\text{-Ketoglutarate} + 2\text{Aspartate}$$

c. 2.5 mol ATP are required to convert 1 mol ammonia and 1 mol CO_2 to 1 mol glycine (via the glycine cleavage system or serine synthesis).

$$\text{NH}_4^+ + \text{CO}_2 + \text{NADH} + \text{H}^+ \rightarrow \text{Glycine} + \text{NAD}^+ \left(\text{equivalent to 2.5 mol ATP}\right)$$

or

$$\text{NH}_4^+ + \alpha\text{-Ketoglutarate} + \text{NADH} + \text{H}^+ \rightarrow \text{Glutamate} + \text{NAD}^+$$

$$\text{Glutamate} + \text{Hydroxypyruvate} \leftrightarrow \alpha\text{-Ketoglutarate} + \text{Serine}$$

$$\text{Serine} + \text{Tetrahydrofolate} \leftrightarrow \text{Glycine} + N^5, N^{10} - \text{Methylene-tetrahydrofolate}$$

3. 2 mol ATP are required for the formation of 2 mol N^{10}-formyl-tetrahydrofolate from 2 mol formate and 2 mol tetrahydrofolate.

$$2\text{Formate} + 2\text{Tetrahydrofolate} + 2\text{ATP} \leftrightarrow 2N^{10}\text{-formyl-tetrahydrofolate} + 2\text{ADP} + 2\text{Pi}$$

4. 1 mol ammonia is produced from adenosine by adenosine deaminase in the pathway of uric acid synthesis.

$$\text{Adenosine} + \text{H}_2\text{O} \rightarrow \text{Inosine} + \text{NH}_4^+$$

Thus, 4 mol ammonia (the net amount) are converted to 1 mol uric acid via adenosine as an intermediate. Overall, this pathway for uric acid synthesis requires 19.5 mol ATP.

6.3.6.2 Energy Required for the Synthesis of Uric Acid from Ammonia via Guanosine

The amount of energy needed to convert ammonia into uric acid via the formation of guanosine can be calculated as follows. This calculation applies to all birds.

1. As illustrated in Chapter 5, the synthesis of 1 mol guanosine requires 8.5 mol ATP.
2. Incorporation of 5 mol ammonia into 3 mol glutamine, 1 mol aspartate, and 1 mol glycine requires:

a. Net 3 mol ATP are required to incorporate 3 mol ammonia for the formation of 3 mol glutamine.

$$3NH_4^+ + 3\alpha\text{-Ketoglutarate} + 3NADH + 3H^+ \rightarrow 3Glutamate + 3NAD^+$$

$$3Glutamate + 3NH_4^+ + 3ATP \rightarrow 3Glutamine + 3ADP$$

In the metabolic pathway of adenosine synthesis:

$$3Glutamine + 3H_2O \rightarrow 3Glutamate + 3NH_4^+$$

$$3Glutamate + 3NH_4^+ + 3ATP \rightarrow 3Glutamine + 3ADP$$

Net reaction: $3Glutamate + 3NH_4^+ + 3ATP \rightarrow 3Glutamine + 3ADP$

b. 2.5 mol ATP are required to convert 1 mol ammonia and 1 mol oxaloacetate to 1 mol aspartate.

$$NH_4^+ + \alpha\text{-Ketoglutarate} + NADH + H^+ \rightarrow Glutamate + NAD^+$$

$$Glutamate + Oxaloacetate \leftrightarrow \alpha\text{-Ketoglutarate} + Aspartate$$

c. 2.5 mol ATP are required to convert 1 mol ammonia and 1 mol CO_2 to 1 mol glycine (via the glycine cleavage system or serine synthesis).

$$NH_4^+ + CO_2 + NADH + H^+ \rightarrow Glycine + NAD^+ \left(\text{equivalent to 2.5 mol ATP}\right)$$

or

$$NH_4^+ + \alpha\text{-Ketoglutarate} + NADH + H^+ \rightarrow Glutamate + NAD^+$$

$$Glutamate + Hydroxypyruvate \leftrightarrow \alpha\text{-Ketoglutarate} + Serine$$

$$Serine + Tetrahydrofolate \leftrightarrow Glycine + N^5, N^{10}\text{-Methylene-tetrahydrofolate}$$

3. 2 mol ATP are required for the formation of 2 mol N^{10}-formyl-tetrahydrofolate from 2 mol formate and 2 mol tetrahydrofolate.

$$2Formate + 2Tetrahydrofolate + 2ATP \leftrightarrow 2N^{10}\text{-formyl-tetrahydrofolate} + 2ADP + 2Pi$$

4. 1 mol ammonia and 1 mol of xanthine are produced from guanosine-derived guanine by guanase in the pathway of uric acid synthesis. This reaction does not require ATP or GTP.

$$Guanine \rightarrow Xanthine + NH_3$$

Thus, 4 mol ammonia are incorporated into 1 mol uric acid via guanosine as an intermediate. Overall, this pathway for uric acid synthesis requires 18.5 mol ATP.

6.3.6.3 Energy Required for the Overall Synthesis of Uric Acid from Ammonia

Assuming that equal amounts of ammonia are converted into uric acid through the adenosine and guanosine pathways, the entire process for uric acid synthesis from 4 mol ammonia requires, on average, 19 mol ATP. This is equivalent to 4.75 mol ATP per mol of ammonia.

6.3.7 NUTRITIONAL AND METABOLIC SIGNIFICANCE OF URIC ACID SYNTHESIS

In birds, uric acid is the major nitrogenous end product of protein catabolism and the predominant nitrogen-containing metabolite in urine. The high requirements for both glycine and glutamine by avian species to synthesize uric acid place high demands for the provision of these two AAs from diets and endogenous synthesis. The higher ATP requirement for hepatic uric acid synthesis in birds than for ureagenesis in mammals may contribute to the higher body temperature in birds (e.g., 40°C in chickens and ducks) than mammals (e.g., 37°C in humans and pigs and 38.5°C in cattle). Despite the nutritional and metabolic burdens on animals, the production of uric acid and its physiological concentrations (e.g., 0.2 mM in chicken plasma) can confer benefits. For example, because uric acid is relatively water insoluble, its excretion through urine is associated with little loss of water. This certainly has physiological significance for birds, particularly when there is a need to fly for long distances, during which drinking water is not available. In addition, uric acid is an antioxidant, protecting cells from oxidative stress (Ames et al. 1981; Fang et al. 2002). However, it should be borne in mind that elevated levels of uric acid in tissues (including the blood) are associated with various metabolic diseases, including diabetes, obesity, renal disease, and cardiovascular disorders (Soltani et al. 2013). An elevated concentration of uric acid in plasma is a useful biomarker for metabolic syndrome in humans and other animals (Ali et al. 2020; Kanbay et al. 2016). Also, as noted previously, in mammals (e.g., humans), high levels of uric acid in the blood (uricaciduria) and other tissues result in gout, urolithiasis, as well as acute and chronic nephropathy due to the deposition of urate crystals in the joints and the urinary tract (Visek 1984).

6.3.8 SPECIES-SPECIFIC DEGRADATION OF URIC ACID TO ALLANTOIN, ALLANTOIC ACID, UREA, AND GLYOXYLATE

Birds, humans, higher apes (e.g., such as chimpanzee, gorilla, and orangutan), and many reptiles lack urate oxidase (also known as uricase), which is a copper-containing enzyme that oxidizes uric acid into allantoin (also known as 5-ureidohydantoin or glyoxyldiureide) (Keebaugh and Thomas 2010; Moriwaki et al. 1999). Thus, these animals excrete uric acid as the major metabolite of purines. By contrast, urate oxidase is present in the liver of: (1) many mammals, including cattle, cats, dogs, pigs, rats, and sheep (Hayashi et al. 2000); (2) many fish species, including Atlantic salmon (*Salmo salar*), Atlantic cod (*Gadus morhua*), Atlantic halibut (*Hippoglossus hippoglossus*), African lungfish (*Protopterus annectens*), pufferfish (*Takifugu rubripes*), zebrafish (*Danio rerio*), and medaka (*Oryzias latipes*) (Andersen et al. 2006); (3) many species of shrimp and aquatic crabs (Hayashi et al. 2000; Lallier and Walsh 1991; (4) some insect species, such as adult *Aedes aegypti* mosquitoes (Scaraffia et al. 2008) and drosophila (Friedman and Johnson 1977); and (5) some amphibians, such as frogs (Usuda et al. 1994). The kidneys of amphibians can also oxidize uric acid into allantoin.

Mammals do not express allantoinase or allantoicase, whereas these two enzymes occur in many species of fish, crustaceans (e.g., shrimp and aquatic crabs), amphibians, and reptiles (Keebaugh and Thomas 2010; Moriwaki et al. 1999). Allantoinase hydrolyzes allantoic into allantoic acid, and allantoicase degrades allantoic acid into ureidoglycolate and urea. Ureidoglycolate lyase, which cleaves ureidoglycolate into glyoxylate (the ionized form of glyoxylic acid) and urea, is expressed in the liver of most animal species, including mammals (e.g., rats, cattle, and monkeys), birds, fish, shrimp, aquatic crabs, amphibians, reptiles, and some insects (Fujiwara and Noguchi 1995; Yeldani et al. 1995). Interestingly, the adrenal gland, brain, heart, intestine, kidneys, lung, pancreas,

TABLE 6.11
Distribution of Uric Acid-Degrading Enzymes in Animal Species

Enzyme	Mammals	Birds	Fish	Shrimp	Aquatic crabs	Amphibians	Insects	Reptiles
Urate oxidase	+[a]; −[b]	−	+[a]	+[a]	+[a]	+[a]	+[c]	−[d]
Allantoinase	−	−	+[a]	+[a]	+[a]	+[a]	+[c]	+[c]
Allantoicase	−	−	+[a]	+[a]	+[a]	+[a]	+[c]	+[c]
Ureidoglycolate lyase	+ (Mit)	+ (Mit)	+ (PO)	+ (PO)	+ (PO)	+ (Mit)	+, ?	+, ?

Source: Hayashi, S. et al. 2000. *Cell Biochem. Biophys.* 32:123–129; Keebaugh, A.C. and J.W. Thomas. 2010. *Mol. Biol. Evol.* 27:1359–1369; Moriwaki, Y. et al. 1999. *Histol. Histopathol.* 14:1321–1340; Usuda, N. et al. 1994. *J. Cell Sci.* 107:1073–1081; Yeldandi, A.V. et al. 1995. *Acta Histochem. Cytochem.* 28:173–180.

[a] Expressed in the liver peroxisomes of many species.
[b] Absent from humans and other primates.
[c] Expressed in some species.
[d] Absent from many species.
Note: Mit, mitochondria; PO, peroxisomes; "?", the subcellular localization of the enzyme is unknown; "+", present; "−", absent.

skeletal muscle, spleen, and submandibular gland of rats also possess ureidoglycolate lyase activity (Fujiwara and Noguchi 1995). The species-specific expression of the uric acid–degrading enzymes in the liver is summarized in Table 6.11. Thus, under normal physiological conditions, mammals (including humans and higher apes), birds, and many reptiles excrete uric acid as the primary product of purine catabolism and possess little or low concentrations of allantoin in their plasma and urine. By contrast, many species of fish, crustaceans, amphibians, and some insects have all the enzymes in the liver to convert uric acid into glyoxylate and urea.

Note that intestinal microbes in humans and other animals contain urate oxidase, allantoinase, allantoicase, and ureidoglycolate lyase activity and, therefore, can produce glyoxylate and urea from uric acid, and can further hydrolyze urea into ammonia and CO_2 through the action of urease (Vogels and van der Drift 1976). Urease is present in microbes but absent from animal cells. The species-dependent degradation of uric acid to allantoin, allantoic acid, urea, and glyoxylate is illustrated in Figure 6.8.

In all the animal species that possess urate oxidase, allantoinase, and allantoicase, these enzymes are localized in the peroxisomes of their liver (Keebaugh and Thomas 2010; Moriwaki et al. 1999). In amphibians, the peroxisomes of their kidneys also contain urate oxidase. In the adult salmon, urate oxidase is also expressed in several non-hepatic organs (including brain, gills, gonads, intestine, spleen, and tongue) but not in skeletal muscle and kidneys (Andersen et al. 2006). Interestingly, the intracellular localization of ureidoglycolate lyase in animals is species-specific. It is a mitochondrial enzyme in mammals, birds, and amphibians, but a peroxisomal protein in fish, shrimp, and aquatic crabs. At present, it is unknown about the intracellular compartmentation of ureidoglycolate lyase in reptiles. The subcellular localization of the uric acid–degrading enzymes in the liver may be related to purine catabolism, as well as the functions of uric acid and its metabolites in animals (Mapes and Krebs 1978).

6.3.9 Oxidation of Uric Acid by Reactive Oxygen and Nitrogen Species into Allantoin

Uric acid can be oxidized by reactive oxygen species (ROS) and reactive nitrogen species (RNS) to form allantoin (Ames et al. 1981). In humans and other animals, the whole-body production of ROS and RNS is enhanced during exercise, under the conditions of oxidative stress, and in response to inflammation (Black et al. 2008; Fang et al. 2002; Ji 1999). Thus, allantoin is present in the plasma of chickens and turkey as a result of its non-enzymatic formation from uric acid (Simoyi et al. 2003), and exercise results in the release of allantoin from the skeletal muscle of humans (Hellsten et al.

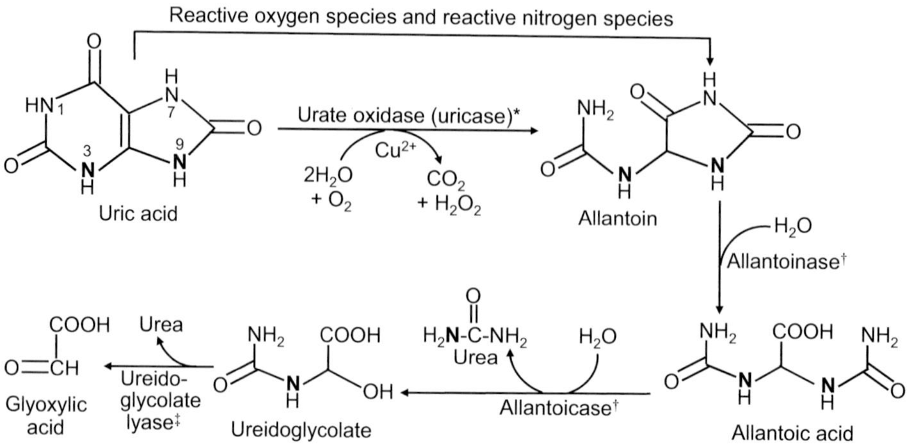

FIGURE 6.8 Oxidation of uric acid to allantoin and related metabolites in animals. The oxidation of uric acid into allantoin and related metabolites via enzyme reactions in animals is species-dependent. By contrast, the *reactive oxygen or nitrogen species mediate the non-enzymatic oxidation of uric acid into allantoin in all animal species.* * Urate oxidase is present in the liver peroxisomes of most mammals (including cattle, cats, dogs, pigs, rats, and sheep), many fish and crustacean species (shrimp and aquatic crabs), many amphibians, and some insects, but is absent from primates (humans and higher apes), birds, and many reptiles. [†]Allantoinase and allantoicase are present in the liver peroxisomes of many species of fish, crustaceans (shrimp and aquatic crabs), amphibians, and reptiles and in the liver peroxisomes of some insects, but are absent from mammals and birds. [‡] Ureidoglycolate lyase is expressed in the liver mitochondria of mammals, birds, and amphibians, but in the liver peroxisomes of fish and crustacean species (shrimp and aquatic crabs). Ureidoglycolate lyase is also present in some species of insects and reptiles, but its subcellular location in these animals is unknown.

1997), even though these species lack uric acid oxidase. There are suggestions that the concentrations of allantoin in the plasma and urine may be a useful indicator of oxidative stress in humans (Grootveld and Halliwell 1987) and other animals, including birds (Tsahar et al. 2006).

6.3.10 EXCRETION OF URIC ACID BY THE KIDNEYS

In humans, approximately 70% and 30% of uric acid in the arterial circulation is excreted by the kidneys (via urine) and intestine (via feces), respectively (Grassi et al. 2013). In birds, because of their anatomy, uric acid is found collectively in the urine plus feces. In the kidneys, the elimination of uric acid involves glomerular filtration followed by reabsorptive and secretory processes in the renal tubules (Lipkowitz 2012). The relative importance of the reabsorption and secretion of uric acid by the kidneys differs quantitatively among species. Humans, mice, and rats predominantly reabsorb uric acid, whereas birds, pigs, rabbits, and reptiles have more active secretory mechanisms (So and Thorens 2010). Reabsorption of uric acid takes place in the proximal tubules in humans but in both proximal and distal convoluted tubules in mice. The urate transport systems in the tubules are complicated because of their bidirectional transport and species differences.

In 2002, A. Enomoto and colleagues identified the urate/anion exchanger URAT1 (a protein consisting of 12 transmembrane domains) through a search for organic anion transporter–like molecules in gene databases and expression/functional studies in *Xenopus* oocytes. URAT1 is encoded by the *SLC22A12* gene and expressed in the apical membrane of proximal tubule epithelial cells (Enomoto et al. 2002). This protein transports urate in exchange for Cl^- or organic anions. Urate reabsorption by kidney epithelial cells on the apical membrane involves URAT1, as well as organic anion transporters (OAT) 4 and 10, and intracellular urate is released through Glut9 (an isoform of the family of glucose transporters) (Matsuo et al. 2008). Glut9 is localized to both the apical and basolateral membranes of distal convoluted tubules for urate transport (reabsorption into the blood).

Expression of Glut9 in the liver and kidneys is a major determinant of uric acid concentrations in plasma. Most recently, Toyoda et al. (2020) have shown that GLUT12 (an isoform of the family of glucose transporters) is present in the renal tubules of mice as a urate transporter for the urinary excretion of urate and that the dysfunction of GLUT12 increases the concentration of urate in the blood. In addition to URAT1, GLUT9, GLUT12, and OAT 4 and 10, OAT1 and OAT3 can exchange intracellular urate with extracellular dicarboxylates (So and Thorens 2010). The urate transport systems exist in the proximal tubules but they are complicated because of their bidirectional transport and species differences. An anti-uricosuric agent (e.g., lactate, pyrazinoate, and nicotinate) can serve as a substrate for the antiporter activity of URAT1 to increase urate reabsorption. By contrast, URAT1 is inhibited by classical uricosuric agents, such as benzbromarone, probenecid, and losartan. At present, little is known about the nutritional and physiological regulation of renal GLUT9 and GLUT12 expression.

6.4 COMPARISONS BETWEEN URIC ACID AND UREA SYNTHESES

6.4.1 SIMILARITIES BETWEEN UREA AND URIC ACID SYNTHESES

The pathways of uric acid and urea syntheses share some common features. First, both pathways are catalyzed by a series of well-organized enzymes, utilize ammonia as a substrate in the initial reaction, and involve mitochondrial and cytoplasmic compartments. The conversion of ammonia to glutamine in the avian liver (uric acid synthesis) and citrulline in the mammalian liver (urea synthesis) occurs within the mitochondria. Both glutamine and citrulline are nitrogen-rich neutral AAs, which exit the mitochondria into the cytoplasm for subsequent metabolism in their respective pathways for uric acid and urea syntheses. Second, HCO_3^-, aspartate, and ATP are required for both uric acid and urea syntheses. These three substrates can be sufficiently produced from the transamination and oxidation of AAs (e.g., glutamate and glutamine) in the mitochondria. Third, interorgan cooperation is required for both ureagenesis and uricogenesis in that the ammonia produced in the extrahepatic tissues and cells is transported via alanine and glutamine shuttles to the liver for detoxification. Importantly, the liver is the most active organ for the synthesis of urea and uric acid from ammonia, whereas these two pathways occur in the small intestinal mucosae of postweaning mammals as well, but to a much lesser extent. Fourth, the physiological concentrations of urea and uric acid have no feedback inhibitory effects on their respective synthetic pathways from ammonia. Both urea and uric acid are excreted primarily in urine via the kidneys and, to a small extent, via the feces.

6.4.2 DIFFERENCES BETWEEN UREA AND URIC ACID SYNTHESES

There are many differences between uric acid and urea syntheses. First, as indicated previously, uric acid synthesis (4.75 mol ATP/mol ammonia) requires 138% more energy than ureagenesis (2 mol ATP/mol ammonia). This can contribute to a higher heat increment and a lower energetic efficiency of AA utilization in birds, as compared with mammals. Second, urea and uric acid synthesis requires AAs and purines, respectively, as intermediates. Thus, urea is highly soluble in water (545 mg/mL at 25°C). By contrast, uric acid is largely hydrophobic and its solubility in water is very limited (0.06 mg/mL at 25°C). Third, the enzymes and the regulation of their activities differ between urea and uric acid syntheses. As noted previously, feedback inhibition by intermediates or products is an important mechanism for the regulation of purine synthesis, but such a mechanism is apparently absent from the metabolic control of ureagenesis. Fourth, large amounts of glycine are required as a direct substrate for uric acid synthesis, whereas glycine participates in urea production only as a precursor of ammonia. Fifth, urea synthesis from ammonia is species-dependent and takes place in mammals, certain teleost fish, and elasmobranchs as the primary end product of ammonia detoxification (Table 6.1). By contrast, uric acid is produced by all animal species as a major metabolite of purine catabolism. Sixth, ureagenesis is cell-specific and takes place only in periportal hepatocytes and enterocytes, whereas virtually all cell types can synthesize uric acid albeit at different rates. Finally, the products of urea cycle and purine degradation have very different physiological functions. Physiological concentrations of uric acid have a potent antioxidative action in the body and allantoin may promote wound healing (Araújo et al. 2010), whereas physiological concentrations of urea do not have an antioxidative action.

6.5 SUMMARY

All mammals possess the hepatic urea cycle to convert ammonia into water-soluble non-toxic urea. This pathway requires CPS-I, OCT, ASS, ASL, arginase, as well as ATP, bicarbonate, and NAG (synthesized from glutamate and acetyl-CoA by NAGS). CPS-I, OCT, and NAGS localize in the mitochondrion to generate citrulline (a neutral AA) from ammonia, bicarbonate, and ornithine, whereas ASS, ASL, and arginase are cytosolic enzymes to convert citrulline to arginine and then urea plus ornithine. Enterocytes of the small intestine in postweaning mammals, as well as colonocytes and ruminal epithelial cells, also have a functional urea cycle to generate urea from extracellularly and intramitochondrially derived ammonia. Urea synthesis in the small intestine is the first line of defense against the potential toxicity of ammonia that is: (1) produced by extensive intestinal degradation of glutamine (a major fuel for enterocytes) and (2) derived from the diet and luminal microorganisms. In contrast to mammals, uric acid is the major end product of AA catabolism via purine formation in avian species, which virtually lack CPS-I, OCT, and arginase in their liver and enterocytes. Uric acid synthesis occurs primarily in the liver and involves the conversion of ammonia into glutamine (a neutral AA) by glutamine synthetase (a mitochondrial enzyme in avian hepatocytes), followed by the production of adenosine and guanosine in the cytoplasm. The catabolism of uric acid to allantoin, ureidoglycolate, glyoxylate, and urea via the urate oxidase pathway in animals is species-specific and is absent in primates (humans and higher apes), birds, and many reptiles. However, reactive oxygen or nitrogen species can non-enzymatically oxidize uric acid into allantoin in all animals. In both mammals and birds, ammonia detoxification requires large amounts of ATP and is essential to survival, growth, and development. Interestingly, some fish synthesize urea from ammonia in their skeletal muscles as a mechanism for consuming bicarbonate and reducing body pH if the fish live in an alkaline environment, but directly excrete ammonia if the fish live in fresh water. Despite major species differences in the removal of ammonia from tissues, the biochemical processes are highly compartmentalized in animals and span both the mitochondrion and the cytoplasm. Such highly orchestrated metabolic pathways function to efficiently detoxify ammonia in organisms via facilitative urea and uric transporters without disturbing the acid–base balance. Although ureagenesis from ammonia is limited to mammals, all animals can produce uric acid from ammonia and possess arginase to hydrolyze arginine into urea plus ornithine.

REFERENCES

Adeva, M.M., G. Souto, N. Blanco, and C. Donapetry. 2012. Ammonium metabolism in humans. *Metabolism* 61:1495–1511.

Albrecht, J. and M.D. Norenberg. 2006. Glutamine: a trojan horse in ammonia neurotoxicity. *Hepatology* 44:788–794.

Ali, N., R. Miah, M. Hasan, Z. Barman, A.D. Mou, J.M. Hafsa et al. 2020. Association between serum uric acid and metabolic syndrome: a cross-sectional study in Bangladeshi adults. *Sci. Rep.* 10:7841.

Ames, B.N., R. Cathcart, E. Schwiers, and P. Hochstein. 1981. Uric acid provides an antioxidant defense in humans against oxidant- and radical-caused aging and cancer: a hypothesis. *Proc. Natl. Acad. Sci. USA* 78:6858–6862.

Andersen, Ø., T.S. Aas, S. Skugor, H. Takle, S. van Nes, B. Grisdale-Helland et al. 2006. Purine-induced expression of *urate oxidase* and enzyme activity in Atlantic salmon (*Salmo salar*): cloning of urate oxidase liver cDNA from three teleost species and the African lungfish *Protopterus annectens*. *FEBS Lett.* 273:2839–2850.

Anderson, P.M. 2001. Urea and glutamine synthesis: environmental influences on nitrogen excretion. *Fish Physiol.* 20:239–277.

Araújo, L.U., A. Grabe-Guimarães, V.C.F. Mosqueira, C.M. Carneiro, and N.M. Silva-Barcellos. 2010. Profile of wound healing process induced by allantoin. *Acta Cir. Bras.* 25:460–466.

Arnal, J.F., T. Munzel, R.C. Venema, N.L. James, C.I. Bai, W.E. Mitch, and D.G. Harrison. 1995. Interactions between L-arginine and L-glutamine change endothelial NO production. *J. Clin. Invest.* 95:2565–2572.

Artagaveytia, N., J. Elalouf, C. de Rouffignac, R. Boivin, and A. Cirio. 2005. Expression of urea transporter (UT-A) mRNA in papilla and pelvic epithelium of kidney in normal and low protein fed sheep. *Comp. Biochem. Physiol. B* 140:279–285.

Ash, D.E. 2004. Structure and functions of arginases. *J. Nutr.* 134:2760S–2764S.

Baker, D.H. 2009. Advances in protein-amino acid nutrition of poultry. *Amino Acids* 37:29–41.

Ballantyne, J.S. and J.W. Robinson. 2010. Freshwater elasmobranchs: a review of their physiology and biochemistry. *J. Comp. Physiol. B* 180:475–493.

Bates, N. and J. Payne. 2017. Common farm poisons: Part 1. *Livestock* 22:258–263.

Batista, E.D., E. Detmann, S.C.V. Filho, E.C. Titgemeyer, and R.F.D. Valadares. 2017. The effect of CP concentration in the diet on urea kinetics and microbial usage of recycled urea in cattle: a meta-analysis. *Animal* 11:1303–1311.

Battelli, M.G., A. Bolognesi, and L. Polito. 2014. Pathophysiology of circulating xanthine oxidoreductase: new emerging roles for a multi-tasking enzyme. *Biochim. Biophys. Acta* 1842:1502–1517.

Beaumier, L., L. Castillo, A.M. Ajami, and V.R. Young. 1995. Urea cycle intermediate kinetics and nitrate excretion at normal and "therapeutic" intakes of arginine in humans. *Am. J. Physiol.* 269:E884–E896.

Bergen, W.G. 2021. Amino acids in beef cattle nutrition and production. *Adv. Exp. Med Biol.* 1285:29–42.

Bergen, W.G. and G. Wu. 2009. Intestinal nitrogen recycling and utilization in health and disease. *J. Nutr.* 139:821–825.

Beyer, K.H. Jr and R.T. Gelarden. 1988. Active transport of urea by mammalian kidney. *Proc. Natl. Acad. Sci. USA* 85:4030–4031.

Black, M.A., D.J. Green, and N.T. Cable. 2008. Exercise prevents age-related decline in nitric-oxide-mediated vasodilator function in cutaneous microvessels. *J. Physiol.* 586:3511–3524.

Brosnan, M.E. and J.T. Brosnan. 2007. Orotic acid excretion and arginine metabolism. *J. Nutr.* 137:1656S–1661S.

Brunton, J.A., R.F.P. Bertolo, P.B. Pencharz, and R.O. Ball. 1999. Proline ameliorates arginine deficiency during enteral but not parenteral feeding in neonatal piglets. *Am. J. Physiol.* 277:E223–E231.

Burns, R.A. and P.J. Buttery. 1984. Purine metabolism and urate biosynthesis in isolated chicken hepatocytes. *Arch. Biochem. Biophys.* 233:507–514.

Bush, J.A., G. Wu, A. Suryawan, H.V. Nguyen, and T.A. Davis. 2002. Somatotropin-induced amino acid conservation in pigs involves differential regulation of liver and gut urea cycle enzyme activity. *J. Nutr.* 132:59–67.

Caldovic, L., N. Ah Mew, D. Shi, H. Morizono, M. Yudkoff, and M. Tuchman. 2010. *N*-acetylglutamate synthase: structure, function and defects. *Mol. Genet. Metab.* 100(Suppl 1):S13–S19.

Che, D., P.S. Nyingwa, K.M. Ralinala, G.M.T. Maswanganye, and G. Wu. 2021. Amino acids in the nutrition, metabolism, and health of domestic cats. *Adv. Exp. Med. Biol.* 1285:217–231.

Chen, S., Y. Minegishi, T. Hasumura, A. Shimotoyodome, and N. Ota. 2020. Involvement of ammonia metabolism in the improvement of endurance performance by tea catechins in mice. *Sci. Rep.* 10:6065.

Cheng, S.-Y., W.-C. Lee, and J.-C. Chen. 2005. An increase of uricogenesis in the Kuruma shrimp *Marsupenaeus japonicus* under nitrite stress. *J. Exp. Zool. A* 303:308–318.

Cheung, C.W., N.S. Cohen, and L. Raijman. 1989. Channeling of urea cycle intermediates *in situ* in permeabilized hepatocytes. *J. Biol. Chem.* 264:4038–4044.

Chin, T.Y. and A.J. Quebbemann. 1978. Quantitation of renal uric acid synthesis in the chicken. *Am. J. Physiol.* 234:F446–F451.

Cooper, A.J. 2012. The role of glutamine synthetase and glutamate dehydrogenase in cerebral ammonia homeostasis. *Neurochem. Res.* 37:2439–2455.

Curis, E., I. Nicolis, C. Moinard, S. Osowska, N. Zerrouk, S. Bénazeth, and L. Cynober. 2005. Almost all about citrulline in mammals. *Amino Acids* 29:177–205.

Darvishzad, T., T. Lubera, and S.S. Kurek. 2018. Puzzling aqueous solubility of guanine Obscured by the formation of nanoparticles. *J. Phys. Chem. B* 122:7497–7502.

Das, T.K. and J.C. Waterlow. 1974. The rate of adaptation of urea cycle enzymes, aminotransferases and glutamic dehydrogenase to changes in dietary protein intake. *Br. J. Nutr.* 32:353–373.

Davis, P.K. and G. Wu. 1998. Compartmentation and kinetics of urea cycle enzymes in porcine enterocytes. *Comp. Biochem. Physiol. B* 119:527–537.

Diem, K. 1962. *Documenta Geigy Scientific Tables*, 6th edition. Geigy Pharmaceutical Co. Ltd, Manchester.

Eklou-Lawson, M., F. Bernard, N. Neveux, C. Chaumontet, C. Bos, A.M. Davila-Gay et al. 2009. Colonic luminal ammonia and portal blood L-glutamine and L-arginine concentrations: a possible link between colon mucosa and liver ureagenesis. *Amino Acids* 37:751–760.

Enns, G.M., S.A. Berry, G.T. Berry, W.J. Rhead, S.W. Brusilow, and A. Hamosh. 2007. Survival after treatment with phenylacetate and benzoate for urea-cycle disorders. *N. Engl. J. Med.* 356:2282–2292.

Enomoto, A., H. Kimura, A. Chairoungdua, Y. Shigeta, P. Jutabha, S.H. Cha et al. 2002. Molecular identification of a renal urate anion exchanger that regulates blood urate levels. *Nature* 417:447–452.

Fang, Y.Z., S. Yang, and G. Wu. 2002. Free radicals, antioxidants, and nutrition. *Nutrition* 18:872–879.

Firkins, J. and C. Reynolds. 2005. Whole animal nitrogen balance in cattle. In: *Nitrogen and Phosphorus Nutrition of Cattle: Reducing the Environmental Impact of Cattle Operations* (Pfeffer, E. and A. Hristov, eds). CAB International, Wallingford, UK. pp. 167–186.

Firkins, J.L., Z. Yu, and M. Morrison. 2007. Ruminal nitrogen metabolism: perspectives for integration of microbiology and nutrition for dairy. *J. Dairy Sci.* 90(Suppl. 1):E1–16.

Flynn, N.E., C.J. Meininger, K. Kelly, N.H. Ing, S.M. Morris Jr., and G. Wu. 1999. Glucocorticoids mediate the enhanced expression of intestinal type II arginase and argininosuccinate synthase in postweaning pigs. *J. Nutr.* 129:799–803.

Flynn, N.E., C.J. Meininger, T.E. Haynes, and G. Wu. 2002. The metabolic basis of arginine nutrition and pharmacotherapy. *Biomed. Pharmacother.* 56:427–438.

Friedman, T.B. and D.H. Johnson. 1977. Temporal control of urate oxidase activity in Drosophila: evidence of an autonomous timer in malpighian tubules. *Science* 197:477–479.

Fries, A.W., S. Dadsetan, S. Keiding, L.K. Bak, A. Schousboe, H.S. Waagepetersen et al. 2014. Effect of glutamine synthetase inhibition on brain and interorgan ammonia metabolism in bile duct ligated rats. *J. Cereb. Blood Flow Metab.* 34: 460–466.

Fujiwara, S. and T. Noguchi. 1995. Degradation of purines: only ureidoglycollate lyase out of four allantoin-degrading enzymes is present in mammals. *Biochem J.* 312: 315–318.

Gerson, A.R. and C.G. Guglielmo. 2011. Flight at low ambient humidity increases protein catabolism in migratory birds. *Science* 333:1434–1436.

Gilbreath, K.R., G.I. Nawaratna, T.A. Wickersham, M.C. Satterfield, F.W. Bazer, and G. Wu. 2020a. Metabolic studies reveal that ruminal microbes of adult steers do not degrade rumen-protected or unprotected L-citrulline. *J. Anim. Sci.* 98:skz370.

Gilbreath, K.R., F.W. Bazer, M.C. Satterfield, J.J. Cleere, and G. Wu. 2020b. Ruminal microbes of adult sheep do not degrade extracellular L-citrulline. *J. Anim. Sci.* 98:skaa164.

Gilbreath, K.R., F.W. Bazer, M.C. Satterfield, and G. Wu. 2021. Amino acid nutrition and reproductive performance in ruminants. *Adv. Exp. Med. Biol.* 1285:43–61.

Goldstein, L. and R.P. Forster. 1971. Urea biosynthesis and excretion in fresh-water and marine elasmobranchs. *Comp. Biochem. Physiol. B* 39:415–421.

Gomez, M., A. Jordá, J. Cabo, and S. Grisolía. 1983. Effect of starvation on the *N*-acetylglutamate system of rat liver. *FEBS Lett.* 156:119–122.

Gougeon-Reyburn, R. and E.B. Marliss. 1989. Effects of sodium bicarbonate on nitrogen metabolism and ketone bodies during very low energy protein diets in obese subjects. *Metabolism* 38:1222–1230.

Graham, T.E. and D.A. MacLean. 1992. Ammonia and amino acid metabolism in human skeletal muscle during exercise. *Can. J. Physiol. Pharmacol.* 70:132–141.

Grassi, D., L. Ferri, G. Desideri, P.D. Giosia, P. Cheli, R.D. Pinto, G. Properzi, and C. Ferri. 2013. Chronic hyperuricemia, uric acid deposit and cardiovascular risk. *Curr. Pharm. Des.* 19:2432–2438.

Grishin, D.V., E.Y. Kasap, A.A. Izotov, and A.V. Lisitsa. 2020. Multifaceted ammonia transporters. *All Life* 13:486–497.

Grootveld, M. and B. Halliwell. 1987. Measurement of allantoin and uric acid in human body fluids: a potential index of free-radical reactions *in vivo*? *Biochem. J.* 243:803–808.

Harris, R.C., D.B. Harris, M. Dunett, P.A. Harris, J. Fallowfield, and J.R.J. Naylor. 1999. Plasma ammonia and lactate responses using incremental and constant speed exercise tests. *Equine Vet. J.* 31 (Suppl. 30):546–551.

Hayashi, S., S. Fujiwara, and T. Noguchi. 2000. Evolution of urate-degrading enzymes in animal peroxisomes. *Cell Biochem. Biophys.* 32:123–129.

Haynes, T.E., P. Li, X.L. Li, K. Shimotori, H. Sato, N.E. Flynn et al. 2009. L-Glutamine or L-alanyl-L-glutamine prevents oxidant- or endotoxin-induced death of neonatal enterocytes. *Amino Acids* 37:131–142.

Heird, W.C., J.F. Nicholson, J.M. Driscoll, J.N. Schullinger, and R.W. Winters. 1972. Hyperammonemia resulting from intravenous alimentation using a mixture of synthetic L-amino acids: a preliminary report. *J. Pediatr.* 81:162–165.

Hellsten, Y., P.C. Tullson, E.A. Richter, and J. Bangsbo. 1997. Oxidation of urate in human skeletal muscle during exercise. *Free Radic. Biol. Med.* 22:169–174.

Herring, C.M., F.W. Bazer, and G. Wu. 2021. Amino acid nutrition for optimum growth, development, reproduction, and health of zoo animals. *Adv. Exp. Med. Biol.* 1285:233–253.

Hu, M.C., L. Bankir, and M.M. Trinh-Trang. 1999. mRNA expression of renal urea transporters in normal and Brattleboro rats: effect of dietary protein intake. *Exp. Nephrol.* 7:44–51.

Inoue, H., S.D. Kozlowski, J.D. Klein, J.L. Bailey, J.M. Sands, and S.M. Bagnasco. 2005. Regulated expression of renal and intestinal UT-B urea transporter in response to varying urea load. *Am. J. Physiol.* 289:F451–458.

Jackson, M.J., A.L. Beaudet, and W.E. O'Brien. 1986. Mammalian urea cycle enzymes. *Annu. Rev. Genet.* 20:431–64.

Ji, L.L. 1999. Antioxidant and oxidative stress in exercise. *Proc. Soc. Exp. Biol. Med.* 222:283–292.

Johnson, J.D., W.C. Albritton, and P. Sunshine. 1972. Hyperammonemia accompanying parenteral nutrition in newborn infants. *J. Pediatr.* 81:152–161.

Jungas, R.L., M.L. Halperin, and J.T. Brosnan. 1992. Quantitative analysis of amino acid oxidation and related gluconeogenesis in humans. *Physiol. Rev.* 72:419–448.

Kajimura, M., P.J. Walsh, T.P. Mommsen, and C.M. Wood. 2006. The dogfish shark (*Squalus acanthias*) increases both hepatic and extrahepatic ornithine urea cycle enzyme activities for nitrogen conservation after feeding. *Physiol. Biochem. Zool.* 79:602–613.

Kanbay, M., T. Jensen, Y. Solak, M. Le, C. Roncal-Jimenez, C. Rivard et al. 2016. Uric acid in metabolic syndrome: from an innocent bystander to a central player. *Eur. J. Intern. Med.* 29:3–8.

Kawaguchi, T., S.W. Brusilow, R.J. Traystman, and R.C. Koehler. 2005. Glutamine-dependent inhibition of pial arteriolar dilation to acetylcholine with and without hyperammonemia in the rat. *Am. J. Physiol.* 288:R1612–R1619.

Keebaugh, A.C. and J.W. Thomas. 2010. The Evolutionary fate of the genes encoding the purine catabolic enzymes in hominoids, birds, and reptiles. *Mol. Biol. Evol.* 27:1359–1369.

Kennedy, P.M. and L.P. Milligan. 1980. The degradation and utilization of endogenous urea in the gastrointestinal tract of ruminants: a review. *Can. J. Anim. Sci.* 60:205–221.

Klein, J.D., M.A. Blount, and J.M. Sands. 2012. Molecular mechanisms of urea transport in health and disease. *Pflugers Arch.* 464:561–572.

Kokko, J.P. and J.M. Sands. 2006. Significance of urea transport: the pioneering studies of Bodil Schmidt-Nielsen. *Am. J. Physiol.* 291:F1109–F1112.

Kong, H., N. Kahatapitiya, K. Kingsley, W.L. Salo, P.M. Anderson, Y. Wang, and P.J. Walsh. 2000. Induction of carbamoyl-phosphate synthetase III and glutamine synthetase mRNA during confinement stress in the gulf toadfish (*Opsanus beta*). *J. Exp. Biol.* 203:311–320.

Krebs, H.A. 1964. The metabolic fate of amino acids. In: *Mammalian Protein Metabolism* (Munro, H.N. and J.B. Allison, eds). Academic Press, New York. pp. 125–176.

Krebs, H.A. 1981. *Reminiscences and Reflections*. Oxford University Press, Oxford, UK.

Krebs, H.A. 1982. The discovery of the ornithine cycle of urea synthesis. *Trends Biochem. Sci.* 7:76–78.

Laberge, T., P.J. Walsh, and M.D. McDonald. 2009. Effects of crowding on ornithine-urea cycle enzyme mRNA expression and activity in gulf toadfish (*Opsanus beta*). *J. Exp. Biol.* 212:2394–2402.

Lallier, F.H. and P.J. Walsh. 1991. Activities of uricase, xanthine oxidase, and xanthine dehydrogenase in the hepatopancreas of aquatic and terrestrial crabs. *J. Crustacean Biol.* 11:506–512.

Lapierre, H., R. Berthiaume, G. Raggio, M. Thivierge, L. Doepel, D. Pacheco et al. 2005. The route of absorbed nitrogen into milk protein. *Anim. Sci.* 80:11–22.

Lee, T.J.F., S. Sarwinski, T. Ishine, C.C. Lai, and F.Y. Chen. 1996. Inhibition of cerebral neurogenic vasodilation by L-glutamine and nitric oxide synthase inhibitors and its reversal by L-citrulline. *J. Pharmacol. Exp. Ther.* 276:353–358.

Lee, B., G.A. Diaz, W. Rhead, U. Lichter-Konecki, A. Feigenbaum, S.A. Berry et al. 2015. Blood ammonia and glutamine as predictors of hyperammonemic crises in patients with urea cycle disorder. *Genet. Med.* 17:561–568.

Lee, B., G.A. Diaz, W. Rhead, U. Lichter-Konecki, A. Feigenbaum, S.A. Berry et al. 2016. Glutamine and hyperammonemic crises in patients with urea cycle disorders. *Mol. Genet. Metab.* 117: 27–32.

Li, M.M., E.C. Titgemeyer, and M.D. Hanigan. 2019. A revised representation of urea and ammonia nitrogen recycling and use in the Molly cow model. *J Dairy Sci.* 102:5109–5129.

Lindley, T.E., C.L. Scheiderer, P.J. Walsh, C.M. Wood, H.L. Bergmani, A.L. Bergmani et al. 1999. Muscle as the primary site of urea cycle enzyme activity in an alkaline lake-adapted tilapia, *Oreochromis alcalicus graham. J. Biol. Chem.* 274:29858–29861.

Lipkowitz, M.S. 2012. Regulation of uric acid excretion by the kidney. *Curr. Rheumatol. Rep.* 14:179–188.

Lobley, G.E., D.M. Bremner, and G. Zuur. 2000. Effects of diet quality on urea fates in sheep assessed by a refined, non-invasive [^{15}N^{15}N]-urea kinetics. *Br. J. Nutr.* 84:459–468.

Lu, Z., F. Stumpff, C. Deiner, J. Rosendahl, H. Braun, K. Abdoun et al. 2014. Modulation of sheep ruminal urea transport by ammonia and pH. *Am. J. Physiol.* 307:R558–R570.

Ludden, P.A., R.M. Stohrer, K.J. Austin, R.L. Atkinson, E.L. Belden, and H.J. Harlow. 2009. Effect of protein supplementation on expression and distribution of urea transporter-B in lambs fed low-quality forage. *J. Anim. Sci.* 87:1354–1365.

Mapes, J.P. and H.A. Krebs. 1978. Rate-limiting factors in urate synthesis and gluconeogenesis in avian liver. *Biochem. J.* 172:193–203.

Marini, J.C., J.D. Klein, J.M. Sands, and M.E. Van Amburgh. 2004. Effect of nitrogen intake on nitrogen recycling and urea transporter abundance in lambs. *J. Anim. Sci.* 82:1157–1164.

Matsuo, H., T. Chiba, S. Nagamori, A. Nakayama, H. Domoto, K. Phetdee et al. 2008. Mutations in glucose transporter 9 gene SLC2A9 cause renal hypouricemia. *Am. J. Hum. Genet.* 83:744–751.

Mehanna, H., J. Moledina, and J. Travis. 2008. Refeeding syndrome: what it is, and how to prevent and treat it. *Br. Med. J.* 336:1495–1498.

Meijer, A.J., W.H. Lamers, and R.A. Chamuleau. 1990. Nitrogen metabolism and ornithine cycle function. *Physiol. Rev.* 70:701–748.

Meininger, C.J., M.E. Schelling, and H.J. Granger. 1988. Adenosine and hypoxia stimulate proliferation and migration of endothelial cells. *Am. J. Physiol.* 255:H554–H562.

Meyer, R.A., G.A. Dudley, and R.L. Terjung. 1980. Ammonia and IMP in different skeletal muscle fibers after exercise in rats. *J. Appl. Physiol.* 49:1037–1041.

Mistry, A.C., G. Chen, A. Kato, K. Nag, J.M. Sands, and S. Hirose. 2005. A novel type of urea transporter, UT-C, is highly expressed in proximal tubule of seawater eel kidney. *Am. J. Physiol.* 288:F455–F465.

Monné, M., D.V. Miniero, L. Daddabbo, L. Palmieri, V. Porcelli, and F. Palmieri. 2015. Mitochondrial transporters for ornithine and related amino acids: a review. *Amino Acids* 47:1763–1777.

Moriwaki, Y., T. Yamamoto, and K. Higashino. 1999. Enzymes involved in purine metabolism – a review of histochemical localization and functional implications. *Histol. Histopathol.* 14:1321–1340.

Morris, J.G. 1985. Nutritional and metabolic responses to arginine deficiency in carnivores. *J. Nutr.* 115:524–531.

Morris, S.M. Jr. 2002. Regulation of enzymes of the urea cycle and arginine metabolism. *Annu. Rev. Nutr.* 22:87–105.

Morris, J.G. and Q.R. Rogers. 1978. Arginine: an essential amino acid for the cat. *J. Nutr.* 108:1944–1953.

Mouille, B., E. Morel, V. Robert, G. Guihot-Joubrel, and F. Blachier. 1999. Metabolic capacity for L-citrulline synthesis from ammonia in rat isolated colonocytes. *Biochim. Biophys. Acta* 1427:401–407.

Nagahara, N., T. Nishino, M. Kanisawa, and K. Tsushima. 1987. Effect of dietary protein on purine nucleoside phosphorylase and xanthine dehydrogenase activities of liver and kidney in chicken and pigeon. *Comp. Biochem. Physiol. B* 88:589–593.

NRC (National Research Council). 2006. *Nutrient Requirements of Small Ruminants.* National Academy Press, Washington, DC.

Nissim, I., M. Yudkoff, and J.T. Brosnan. 1996. Regulation of [^{15}N] urea synthesis from [5-^{15}N] glutamine. Role of pH, hormones, and pyruvate. *J. Biol. Chem.* 271:31234–31242.

Nuñez, F.J., T.B. Johnstone, M.L. Corpuz, A.G. Kazarian, N.N. Mohajer, O. Tliba et al. 2020. Glucocorticoids rapidly activate cAMP production via $G_{\alpha s}$ to initiate non-genomic signaling that contributes to one-third of their canonical genomic effects. *FASEB J.* 34: 2882–2895.

Oba, M., R.L. Baldwin VI, S.L. Owens, and B.J. Bequette. 2004. Urea synthesis by ruminal epithelial and duodenal mucosal cells from growing sheep. *J. Dairy Sci.* 87:1803–1805.

Oba, M., R.L. Baldwin VI, S.L. Owens, and B.J. Bequette. 2005. Metabolic fates of ammonia-N in ruminal epithelial and duodenal mucosal cells isolated from growing sheep. *J. Dairy Sci.* 88:3963–3970.

Oberbauer, A.M. and J.A. Larsen. 2021. Amino acids in dog nutrition and health. *Adv. Exp. Med. Biol.* 1285:199–216.

Okada, T., Y. Watanabe, S.W. Brusilow, R.J. Traystman, and R.C. Koehler. 2000. Interaction of glutamine and arginine on cerebrovascular reactivity to hypercapnia. *Am. J. Physiol.* 278:H1577–H1584.

Ozanne, B., J. Nelson, J. Cousineau, M. Lambert, V. Phan, G. Mitchell et al. 2012. Threshold for toxicity from hyperammonemia in critically ill children. *J. Hepatol.* 56:123–128.

Pärt, P., P.A. Wright, and C.M. Wood. 1998. Urea and water permeability in dogfish (*Squalus acanthias*) gills. *Comp. Biochem. Physiol. A* 119:117–123.

Pedley, A.M. and S.J. Benkovic. 2016. A new view into the regulation of purine metabolism – the purinosome. *Trends Biochem. Sci.* 42:141–154.

Pesi, R., F. Balestri, and P.L. Ipata. 2018. Metabolic interaction between urea cycle and citric acid cycle shunt: a guided approach. *Biochem. Mol. Biol. Ed.* 46:182–185.

Pfeffer, K.D., T.P. Huecksteadt, and J.R. Hoidal. 1994. Xanthine dehydrogenase and xanthine oxidase activity and gene expression in renal epithelial cells. Cytokine and steroid regulation. *J. Immunol.* 153:1789–1797.

Raina, R., J.K. Bedoyan, U. Lichter-Konecki, P. Jouvet, S. Picca, N.A. Mew et al. 2020. Consensus guidelines for management of hyperammonaemia in paediatric patients receiving continuous kidney replacement therapy. *Nat. Rev. Nephrol.* 16:471–482.

Reynolds, C.K. and N.B. Kristensen. 2008. Nitrogen recycling through the gut and the nitrogen economy of ruminants: an asynchronous symbiosis. *J. Anim. Sci.* 86:E293–E305.

Rogers, Q.R., J.G. Morris, and R.A. Freedland. 1977. Lack of hepatic enzymatic adaptation to low and high levels of dietary protein in the adult cat. *Enzyme* 22:348–356.

Rowe, P.B., E. McCairns, G. Madsen, D. Sauer, and H. Elliott. 1978. De novo purine synthesis in avian liver. *J. Biol. Chem.* 253:7711–7721.

Saha, N. and B.K. Ratha. 2007. Functional ureogenesis and adaptation to ammonia metabolism in Indian freshwater air-breathing catfishes. *Fish Physiol. Biochem.* 33:283–295.

Sakusic, A., M. Sabov, A.J. McCambridge, A.A. Rabinstein, T.D. Singh, K. Mukesh et al. 2018. Features of adult hyperammonemia not due to liver failure in the intensive care unit. *Crit. Care Med.* 46:e897–e903.

Sands, J.M. and M.A. Blount. 2014. Genes and proteins of urea transporters. *Subcell. Biochem.* 73:45–63.

Sands, J.M., H. Nonoguchi, and M.A. Knepper. 1987. Vasopressin effects on urea and H_2O transport in inner medullary collecting duct subsegments. *Am. J. Physiol.* 253:F823–F832.

Scaraffia, P.Y., G. Tan, J. Isoe, V.H. Wysocki, M.A. Wells, and R.L. Miesfeld. 2008. Discovery of an alternate metabolic pathway for urea synthesis in adult *Aedes aegypti* mosquitoes. *Proc. Natl. Acad. Sci. USA* 105:518–523.

Schmidt-Nielsen, B. 1952. Renal tubular excretion of urea in kangaroo rats. *Am. J. Physiol.* 170:45–56.

Schmidt-Nielsen, B. 1988. Excretory mechanisms in the animal kingdom: examples of the principle "the whole is greater than the sum of its parts". *Physiol. Zool.* 61:312–321.

Schmidt-Nielsen, B., J.M. Barrett, B. Graves, and B. Crossley. 1985. Physiological and morphological responses of the rat kidney to reduced dietary protein. *Am. J. Physiol.* 248:F31–F42.

Schmike, R.T. 1973. Control of enzyme levels in mammalian tissues. *Adv. Enzymol.* 37:135–187.

Simoyi, M.F., E. Falkenstein, K. Van Dyke, K.P. Blemings, and H. Klandorf. 2003. Allantoin, the oxidation product of uric acid is present in chicken and turkey plasma. *Comp. Biochem. Physiol. B* 135:325–335.

Singer, M.A. 2003. Do mammals, birds, reptiles and fish have similar nitrogen conserving systems? *Comp. Biochem. Physiol. B* 134:543–558.

So, A. and B. Thorens. 2010. Uric acid transport and disease. *J. Clin. Invest.* 120:1791–1799.

Soltani, Z., K. Rasheed, D.R. Kapusta, and E. Reisin. 2013. Potential role of uric acid in metabolic syndrome, hypertension, kidney injury, and cardiovascular diseases: is it time for reappraisal? *Curr. Hypertens. Rep.* 15:175–181.

Srere P.A. 1987. Complexes of sequential metabolic enzymes. *Annu. Rev. Biochem.* 56:89–124.

Stewart, G. 2011. The emerging physiological roles of the SLC14A family of urea transporters. *Br. J. Pharmacol.* 164:1780–1792.

Takahashi, H., R.C. Koehler, S.W. Brusilow, and R.J. Traystman. 1991. Inhibition of brain glutamine accumulation prevents cerebral edema in hyperammonemic rats. *Am. J. Physiol.* 261:H825–H829.

Tinker, D.A., J.T. Brosnan, and G.R. Herzberg. 1986. Interorgan metabolism of amino acids, glucose, lactate, glycerol and uric acid in the domestic fowl (*Gallus domesticus*). *Biochem. J.* 240:829–836.

Toyoda, Y., T. Takada, H. Miyata, H. Matsuo, H. Kassai, K. Nakao et al. 2020. Identification of GLUT12/SLC2A12 as a urate transporter that regulates the blood urate level in hyperuricemia model mice. *Proc. Natl. Acad. Sci. USA* 117:18175–18177.

Tsahar, E., Z. Arad, I. Izhaki, and C.G. Guglielmo. 2006. The relationship between uric acid and its oxidative product allantoin: a potential indicator for the evaluation of oxidative stress in birds. *J. Comp. Physiol. B* 176:653–661.

Tuboi, S., M. Sato, H. Ono, K. Kobayashi, and K. Hiraga. 1986. Mechanism of synthesis and localization of mitochondrial and cytosolic fumarases in rat liver. *Adv. Enzyme Regul.* 25:461–484.

Usuda, N., S. Hayashi, S. Fujiwara, T. Noguchi, T. Nagata, M.S. Rao et al. 1994. Uric acid degrading enzymes, urate oxidase and allantoinase, are associated with different subcellular organelles in frog liver and kidney. *J. Cell Sci.* 107: 1073–1081.

Visek, W.J. 1984. An update of concepts of essential amino acids. *Annu. Rev. Nutr.* 4:137–55.

Visek, W.J. 1992. Nitrogen-stimulated orotic acid synthesis and nucleotide imbalance. *Cancer Res.* 52:2082s–2084s.

Vogels, G.D. and C. van der Drift. 1976. Degradation of purines and pyrimidines by microorganisms. *Bacteriol. Rev.* 40:403–468.

Walker, V. 2012. Severe hyperammonaemia in adults not explained by liver disease. *Ann. Clin. Biochem.* 49:214–228.

Wallace, R., E. Knecht, and S. Grisolía. 1986. Turnover of rat liver ornithine transcarbamylase. *FEBS Lett.* 208:427–430.

Walser, M. and L.J. Bondelos. 1959. Urea metabolism in man. *J. Clin. Invest.* 38:1617–1626.

Warren, K.S. and S. Schenker. 1964. Effect of an inhibitor of glutamine synthesis (methionine sulfoximine) on ammonia toxicity and metabolism. *J. Lab. Clin. Med.* 64:442–449.

Watford, M. 2020. Ornithine cycle. In: *The Encyclopedia of Biochemistry*, 3rd edition. Elsevier, New York. doi: 10.1016/B978-0-12-819460-7.00062-1.

Weiner, I.D. and J.W. Verlander. 2013. Renal ammonia metabolism and transport. *Compr. Physiol.* 3: 201–220.

Wendler, P.A., J.H. Blanding, and G.C. Tremblay. 1983. Interaction between the urea cycle and the orotate pathway: studies with isolated hepatocytes. *Arch. Biochem. Biophys.* 224:36–48.

Wickersham, T.A., E.C. Titgemeyer, and R.C. Cochran. 2009. Methodology for concurrent determination of urea kinetics and the capture of recycled urea nitrogen by ruminal microbes in cattle. *Animal* 3:372–379.

Wijburg, F.A. and M. Nassogne. 2012. Disorders of the urea cycle and related enzymes. In: *Inborn Metabolic Diseases* (Saudubray, J.M., G. Van den Berghe, and J.H. Walter, eds). Springer, Berlin. pp. 298–310.

Wright, P.A. 1995. Nitrogen excretion: three end products, many physiological roles. *J. Exp. Biol.* 198:273–281.

Wu, G. 1995. Urea synthesis in enterocytes of developing pigs. *Biochem. J.* 312:717–723.

Wu, G. 2018. *Principles of Animal Nutrition*. CRC Press, Boca Raton, FL.

Wu, G. 2020. Metabolism and functions of amino acids in sense organs. *Adv. Exp. Med. Biol.* 1265:201–217.

Wu, G., D.A. Knabe, and N.E. Flynn. 1994. Synthesis of citrulline from glutamine in pig enterocytes. *Biochem. J.* 299:115–121.

Wu, G., C.J. Meininger, K. Kelly, M. Watford, and S.M. Morris Jr. 2000. A cortisol surge mediates the enhanced expression of pig intestinal pyrroline-5-carboxylate synthase during weaning. *J. Nutr.* 130:1914–1919.

Wu, G., T.E. Haynes, H. Li, W. Yan, and C.J. Meininger. 2001. Glutamine metabolism to glucosamine is necessary for glutamine inhibition of endothelial nitric oxide synthesis. *Biochem. J.* 353:245–252.

Wu, G., L.A. Jaeger, F.W. Bazer, and J.M. Rhoads. 2004. Arginine deficiency in premature infants: biochemical mechanisms and nutritional implications. *J. Nutr. Biochem.* 15:442–451.

Yang, D., J.W. Hazey, F. David, J. Singh, R. Rivchum, J.M. Streem et al. 2000. Integrative physiology of splanchnic glutamine and ammonium metabolism. *Am. J. Physiol.* 278:E469–E476.

Yeldandi, A.V., N. Usuda, R. Chu, F. Erfurth, and V.V. Yeldandi. 1995. Molecular analysis, subcellular localization and tissue distribution of enzymes involved in uric acid degradation. *Acta Histochem. Cytochem.* 28:173–180.

You, C., G.P. Smith, Y. Kanai, W.S. Lee, M. Stelznrr, and M.A. Hediger. 1993. Cloning and characterization of the vasopressin-regulated urea transporter. *Nature* 365:844–847.

Zhang, Q., Y.Q. Hou, F.W. Bazer, W.L. He, E.H. Posey, and G. Wu. 2021. Amino acids in swine nutrition and production. *Adv. Exp. Med. Biol.* 1285:81–107.

7 Use of Isotopes for Studying Amino Acid Metabolism

Physics and chemistry are two major scientific fields driving the development of biochemical research over the past century. This is exemplified by the use of radioactive and stable isotopes for studying the biochemistry, physiology, and nutrition of amino acids (AAs) (Brosnan 1982; Brunengraber et al. 1997; Castillo et al. 1993; Darmaun et al. 1986; Marliss et al. 2006; Schoenheimer and Rittenberg 1938; Ten Have et al. 2017; Wijayasinghe et al. 1983; Wolfe 1993; Wu 1997). The history of isotopes dates back to November 8, 1895 when X-rays (emitted by electrons outside the nucleus) were discovered by the British chemist Wilhelm Conrad Roentgen. Two and a half months later, Henri Becquerel (a French physicist) discovered on January 20, 1896 radioactivity (a term coined by Marie Curie in 1899). The existence of isotopes was first suggested in 1912 by the British chemist Frederick Soddy and the term "isotope" was coined in 1914 by the Scottish physician Margaret Todd. Recognizing that isotopes have nearly identical chemical behaviors, George de Hevesy employed radioactive tracers to investigate metabolic processes in plants in 1923. All of these pioneers were awarded the Nobel Prize in Chemistry or Physics for their work.

In the late 1930s, an AA labeled with the stable isotope ^{15}N (e.g., ^{15}N-alanine or ^{15}N-leucine) was employed by R. Schoenheimer et al. (1938) to study protein turnover in humans and laboratory animals. During the 1940s, radioisotopes (^{14}C and ^{3}H) received much attention from biochemists attempting to identify the precursors, intermediates, and products of metabolic pathways. The tracer approaches were extensively utilized in the 1950s through the 1960s as relatively low-cost radioactive and stable isotopes became available at universities and national laboratories that had reactors, cyclotrons, or other accelerators. Publications in the current Web of Science database indicate that radioactive and stable isotopes continue to play an important role in both *in vitro* and *in vivo* studies in life sciences (Allen and Young 2020). To date, the widespread use of radioactive and stable isotopes has greatly advanced research on all aspects of nitrogen-containing compounds, including AA synthesis and catabolism, as well as protein synthesis and degradation in humans (Wilkinson 2018) and other animals, including cattle, chickens, sheep, swine, fish, and shrimp (Frank et al. 2007; Houlihan et al. 1988; Lobley 2003; Maharjan et al. 2020; Watford and Wu 2005). It is necessary to have a basic knowledge about both isotopes and metabolism to design meaningful biological experiments involving the use of isotopes. This chapter, which aims at achieving such a goal, consists of two parts: (1) tracer methodologies, and (2) the interpretation of data from isotope experiments.

7.1 BASIC CONCEPTS ABOUT ISOTOPES

7.1.1 WHAT ARE ISOTOPES?

Before we define "isotopes", let us review the fundamental knowledge of an element. A chemical element is a pure substance consisting of one type of atom [e.g., carbon (C), chlorine (Cl), hydrogen (H), nitrogen (N), oxygen (O), phosphorus (P), and sulfur (S)], as shown in a periodic table of elements. The term "atom" is derived from the Greek word "*atomos*", meaning individual or uncuttable. Atoms are composed of protons, neutrons, and electrons. Elements are made of atoms with the same number of protons. For example, the elements hydrogen, carbon, nitrogen, oxygen, and sulfur are made of atoms containing 1, 6, 7, 8, and 16 protons in the nucleus, respectively. An element is categorized based on its atomic number (also known as the number of protons). Thus, each element contains a unique number of protons referred to as the element's atomic number (Z), an equal number of orbital electrons (e⁻), and neutrons. Protons and neutrons are located in the nucleus. The atom is neutral with respect to electrical charge, because protons are positively charged and electrons are negatively charged. The mass of the electrons is negligible. The outer electrons of atoms govern the chemical properties of the element. Neutrons are uncharged with mass similar to the mass of protons. Neutrons are held together with protons by the nuclear force. Each element has a unique mass number (A; the sum of the number of protons plus the number of neutrons), which is approximately equal to the atomic mass of its constituent atom.

$$A \text{ (Mass Number)} = N \text{ (Neutron Number)} + Z \text{ (Proton Number or Atomic Number)}$$

The term "isotope" is derived from the Greek words "*isos* and *topos*", meaning "the same place". Atoms that contain the same number of protons (i.e., the same atomic number) but different numbers of neutrons are called isotopes of the element. For example, ^{12}C, ^{13}C, and ^{14}C are isotopes of the element carbon. Some isotopes commonly used in metabolic research are listed in Figure 7.1. Thus, isotopes (e.g., ^{2}H and ^{3}H; ^{13}C and ^{14}C; ^{14}N and ^{15}N) have the same atomic number but different mass numbers. Normally, the mass number, but not the atomic number, is shown in a chemical formula. Because of an imbalance between the number of protons and neutrons in the nucleus, some isotopes are not stable and spontaneously disintegrate or decay, emitting electrons, X-rays, or other particles to achieve a stable nuclear composition. These isotopes are called radioactive isotopes (also known as radioisotopes or radionuclides). Examples of radioactive isotopes are ^{3}H (tritium), ^{14}C, ^{32}P, ^{35}S, ^{125}I, and ^{238}U (uranium). Radioactive tracers are often used to study AA metabolism in cultured cells and tissues, as well as small animals. By contrast, some isotopes are stable and do not emit any particle or radiation, and they are referred to as stable isotopes. Examples of stable isotopes are vs.^{1}H, ^{2}H, ^{12}C, ^{13}C, ^{14}N, ^{15}N, ^{16}O, and ^{18}O. Because of the concerns over the adverse effects of radiation in humans and animals, as well as the high cost of disposing of radioactive wastes, stable isotopes are now commonly used to study AA metabolism in humans and other animals (Bequette et al. 2006; Lapierre et al. 2008; Pereira et al. 2008; Stoll et al. 1999; Wilkinson 2018).

Because some stable isotopes (e.g., ^{1}H, ^{12}C, ^{14}N, ^{16}O, ^{31}P, and ^{32}S) have a high abundance in nature, they are not used as tracers in metabolic studies. For example, ^{1}H (protium) and ^{2}H (deuterium) have the natural occurrence of 99.985% and 0.015% of the hydrogen element, respectively, whereas ^{12}C and ^{13}C have the natural occurrence of approximately 98.9% and 1.1% of the carbon element,

$$^{A}_{Z}X_{N}$$

$^{1}_{1}H_{0}$	$^{2}_{1}H_{1}$	$^{3}_{1}H_{2}$
$^{12}_{6}C_{6}$	$^{13}_{6}C_{7}$	$^{14}_{6}C_{8}$
$^{13}_{7}N_{6}$	$^{14}_{7}N_{7}$	$^{15}_{7}N_{8}$
$^{16}_{8}O_{8}$	$^{17}_{8}O_{9}$	$^{18}_{8}O_{10}$
$^{31}_{15}P_{16}$	$^{32}_{15}P_{17}$	$^{33}_{15}P_{18}$
$^{32}_{16}S_{16}$	$^{34}_{16}S_{18}$	$^{35}_{16}S_{19}$
$^{125}_{53}I_{72}$	$^{126}_{53}I_{73}$	$^{131}_{53}I_{78}$

FIGURE 7.1 Relationship among mass number, proton number, and neutron number for isotopes. Isotopes are defined as one of the two or more chemical elements that contain the same number of protons (Z) but different numbers of neutrons (*N*) and, therefore, different mass numbers (*A*).

TABLE 7.1

Natural Abundances of the Common Stable Isotopes Used in Amino Acid (AA) Research

Element	Stable Isotope	Natural Abundance (%)	Examples for Use in Nutritional and Metabolic Research
Hydrogen	^1H	99.985	Not used as a tracer
	^2H	0.0150	Measurements of water production from substrate oxidation, protein synthesis, protein degradation, glycolysis, fatty acid synthesis, biohydrogenation
Carbon	^{12}C	98.893	Not used as a tracer
	^{13}C	1.107	Measurements of CO_2 production from substrate oxidation, protein synthesis, protein degradation, AA synthesis, gluconeogenesis, fatty acid synthesis, carbon recycling, and metabolic channeling
Nitrogen	^{14}N	99.634	Not used as a tracer
	^{15}N	0.366	Measurements of urea synthesis from ammonia, protein synthesis, protein degradation, AA synthesis, nitrogen recycling, and metabolic channeling
Oxygen	^{16}O	99.759	Not used as a tracer
	^{18}O	0.204	Measurements of water production from substrate oxidation, hydroxylation, protein synthesis, protein degradation, AA synthesis
Sulfur	^{32}S	95.02	Not used as a tracer
	^{34}S	4.22	Measurements of the synthesis and metabolic fates of sulfur-containing AAs

Source: http://www.chem.ucla.edu/~harding/IGOC/N/natural_abundance.html.

respectively (Table 7.1). Likewise, radioactive isotopes with a relatively short half-life ($T_{1/2}$) [e.g., ^{11}C ($T_{1/2}=20.4\,min$); ^{13}N ($T_{1/2}=9.97\,min$); ^{15}O ($T_{1/2}=2.04\,min$); ^{30}P ($T_{1/2}=2.50\,min$); and ^{31}S ($T_{1/2}=2.57\,s$)] have limited value in biological research. The half-life of a radioactive isotope is defined as the time required for its disintegration by half (Marshall and Fairbridge 1999). By contrast, those with a low natural abundance and a relatively long half-life [e.g., radioactive isotopes (^3H, ^{14}C, ^{32}P, and ^{35}S) and stable isotopes (^2H, ^{13}C, ^{15}N, and ^{18}O)] are often used.

7.1.2 DECAY OF RADIOISOTOPES

As noted above, radioisotopes undergo spontaneous decay or disintegration. The disintegration of radioisotopes is an exponential process and the rate (disintegration per unit time) is proportional to the number of radioactive atoms present at any time. The half-life and decay constant of a given radioisotope are its unique physicochemical properties that are not affected by the environment. Table 7.2 lists the half-lives and types of disintegration of the radioisotopes commonly employed in AA metabolism and related studies. The following equations relate the number of nuclei, number of radionuclei, decay constant, and $T_{1/2}$.

$$N_t = N_0 \times e^{-\lambda t} \quad \left(N_t, \text{number of nuclei at time } t; N_0, \text{number of nuclei at time } 0\right)$$

$$A_t = A_0 \times e^{-\lambda t} \quad \left(A_t, \text{radioactivity at time } t; A_0, \text{radioactivity at time } 0\right)$$

$$T_{1/2} = 0.693 / \lambda \quad \left(T_{1/2}, \text{half-life}; \lambda, \text{decay constant, which is characteristic of the isotope}\right)$$

TABLE 7.2

Half-Lives and Types of Decay for Some Radioactive Isotopes

Radioisotope	Half-Life	Type of Decay
Hydrogen-3 (^{3}H)	12.32 years	β-emission
Carbon-14 (^{14}C)	5.730 years	β-emission
Sodium-22 (^{22}Na)	2.602 years	γ-Rays
Phosphorus-32 (^{32}P)	14.29 days	β-emission
Sulfur-35 (^{35}S)	87.44 days	β-emission
Chromium-51 (^{51}Cr)	27.70 days	γ-Rays
Iron-59 (^{59}Fe)	44.53 days	β-emission
Cobalt-60 (^{60}Co)	5.271 year	β-emission
Zinc-65 (^{65}Zn)	243.9 days	γ-Rays[a]
Selenium-75 (^{75}Se)	119.8 days	γ-Rays
Iodine-125 (^{125}I)	60.14 days	γ-Rays

[a] Zinc-65 decays primarily via the emission of γ-rays (97.8%) and to a much lesser extent via positron emission (2.2%).

Radioactive isotopes emit β-, α-, or γ-particles, and their decay is known as β-, α-, or γ-decay, respectively (Figure 7.2). During β-decay, a neutron (n) is converted to a proton (p) with the release of a β-particle and an antineutrino. A β-particle is an electron derived from the conversion of a proton to a neutron in the nucleus of a radioactive element, but not from its orbital electrons. Some β-particles have relatively high energy (e.g., those emitted by ^{14}C and ^{32}P), whereas others have relatively low energy (e.g., those emitted by ^{3}H). Thus, β-particles from each radioisotope have very different energy spectra, which provide the basis for their detection using liquid scintillation spectrometry. In α-decay [e.g., the decomposition of ^{238}Uranium to yield ^{234}Th (thorium)], the radio-isotope emits an α-particle (consisting of 2 protons and 2 neutrons bound together) which is identical to the nucleus of a helium atom. α-Particles are usually measured by a Geiger-Mueller counter. In γ-decay [e.g., the decay of ^{125}I (often used to study tyrosine iodization) to form ^{125}Te (tellurium)],

$$\beta\text{-Decay: } n \longrightarrow p + \beta^- + \bar{v}_e$$

$$^3_1H_2 \longrightarrow {}^3_2He_1 + \beta^- + \bar{v}_e$$

$$^{14}_6C_8 \longrightarrow {}^{14}_7N_7 + \beta^- + \bar{v}_e$$

$$^{32}_{15}P_{17} \longrightarrow {}^{32}_{16}S_{16} + \beta^- + \bar{v}_e$$

$$^{35}_{16}S_{19} \longrightarrow {}^{35}_{17}Cl_{18} + \beta^- + \bar{v}_e$$

$$\alpha\text{-Decay: } n + p \longrightarrow \alpha$$

$$^{238}_{92}U_{146} \longrightarrow {}^{234}_{90}Th_{144} + {}^4_2He$$

$$\gamma\text{-Decay: } p \longrightarrow n + \text{Neutrino} + \gamma\text{-Rays}$$

$$^{125}_{53}I_{72} \longrightarrow {}^{125}_{52}Te_{73} + \text{Neutrino} + \gamma\text{-Rays} + \text{X-Rays}$$

FIGURE 7.2 Type of radioisotope decay. Radioisotopes have unstable nuclei and decompose spontaneously by emission of a nuclear electron (β-decay), helium nucleus (α-decay), or γ-rays (γ-decay), thereby achieving a stable nuclear composition.

neither the atomic number nor the mass number of the element is changed and the γ-particles emitted from the nucleus are high energy photons which are usually measured by a γ-counter. In some radioisotopes (e.g., Zinc-65), emission of γ-rays is accompanied with other types of emission (e.g., positron emission).

The rate of disintegration of a radioisotope (radioactivity) is expressed in curies (Ci) in honor of Marie Curie, who made seminal contributions to radiochemistry and discovered radium (a radioactive metallic element). The amount of radioactivity is measured in a liquid scintillation counter, which normally generates a readout in disintegrations per minute (dpm). The relationships among Ci, dpm, and disintegrations per second [dps; also known as Becquerel (Bq); 1 dps = 1 Bq] are as follows:

$$1 \text{ Ci} = 2.22 \times 10^{12} \text{ dpm} = 3.7 \times 10^{10} \text{ dps}$$

In determining the decay of radioisotopes by a liquid scintillation counter, the values measured are normally counts of atomic disintegrations per minute (cpm) recorded by the instrument. This value is then corrected for the counting efficiency of the instrument to provide true numbers of atomic disintegrations per minute (dpm) [namely, dpm = cpm ÷ counting efficiency (%)]. Because efficiency in the detection of radioactive decays is always less than 100%, not all radioactive decays can be registered as cpm. In practice, the counting efficiency is approximately 90% and 40%, respectively, for ^{14}C and ^{3}H in a biological sample that is mixed well with a scintillation cocktail. While measuring radioactivity in some biological samples (e.g., solubilized tissue or $^{14}CO_2$ collected from the oxidation of a ^{14}C-labeled AA), chemiluminescence should be avoided by appropriately setting special parameters in the liquid scintillation counter and placing the vials (containing a mixture of a sample and liquid scintillation fluid known) overnight at room temperature before counting.

7.1.3 EXPRESSION OF RADIOACTIVE AND STABLE ISOTOPES

The nomenclature of a radiolabeled or stable isotope-labeled substance is based on the position of the label in the molecule (Figure 7.3). The numbering of carbon atoms in AAs or related metabolites is based on the conventional method used in organic chemistry. Let us use some radioactive and stable isotopes to illustrate this nomenclature. For example, L-[1-^{14}C]leucine denotes that only the carbon-1 of L-leucine is labeled with ^{14}C. L-[U-^{14}C]leucine means that all the carbons of L-leucine are uniformly labeled with ^{14}C and that all the labeled carbons have the same specific radioactivity. Furthermore, L-[G-^{14}C]leucine or L-[G-^{13}C]leucine means that all the carbons of L-leucine are labeled with ^{14}C or ^{13}C, but their specific radioactivity or isotopic enrichment may differ. The position of a carbon attached to a labeled isotope is specified by a regular non-superscript number, e.g., 1, 2, and 3. For example, L-[ring-2,6-^{3}H]phenylalanine indicates that the hydrogens attached to the carbons 2 and 6 in the ring of L-phenylalanine are labeled with ^{3}H, whereas [6,6-^{2}H]glucose means that two ^{2}H are attached to the carbon-6 of glucose. In some formulas, the number of carbons with an attached labeled isotope is shown by a subscript number next to the labeled isotope. For example, L-[ring-$^{3}H_5$]phenylalanine means that the five carbons of the ring structure in L-phenylalanine are bonded with ^{3}H, and L-[ring-$^{13}C_6$]phenylalanine defines that all the six carbons of the ring structure in L-phenylalanine are labeled with ^{13}C. Likewise, the nitrogen atom of L-leucine that is labeled with ^{15}N is represented by L-[^{15}N]leucine, and the two nitrogen atoms in the guanidino group of L-arginine are designated as L-[guanidino-$^{15}N_2$]arginine. Finally, [ε-^{15}N]lysine denotes that the nitrogen atom in the ε-NH2 group of lysine is labeled with ^{15}N.

It is possible to include two or more differently labeled isotopes in one molecule. Examples are [3-^{13}C,^{15}N]β-alanine, L-[U-^{13}C,^{15}N]aspartate, [1-^{13}C,^{15}N]glycine. Such a labeled substance can be added to a medium for cell incubation or administered into animals. Mass spectrometry can detect more than one labeled molecule at a time. Likewise, D-[5-^{3}H]glucose and L-[U-^{14}C]glutamine can be present simultaneously in the same biological system (e.g., cell culture or perfused organ) to

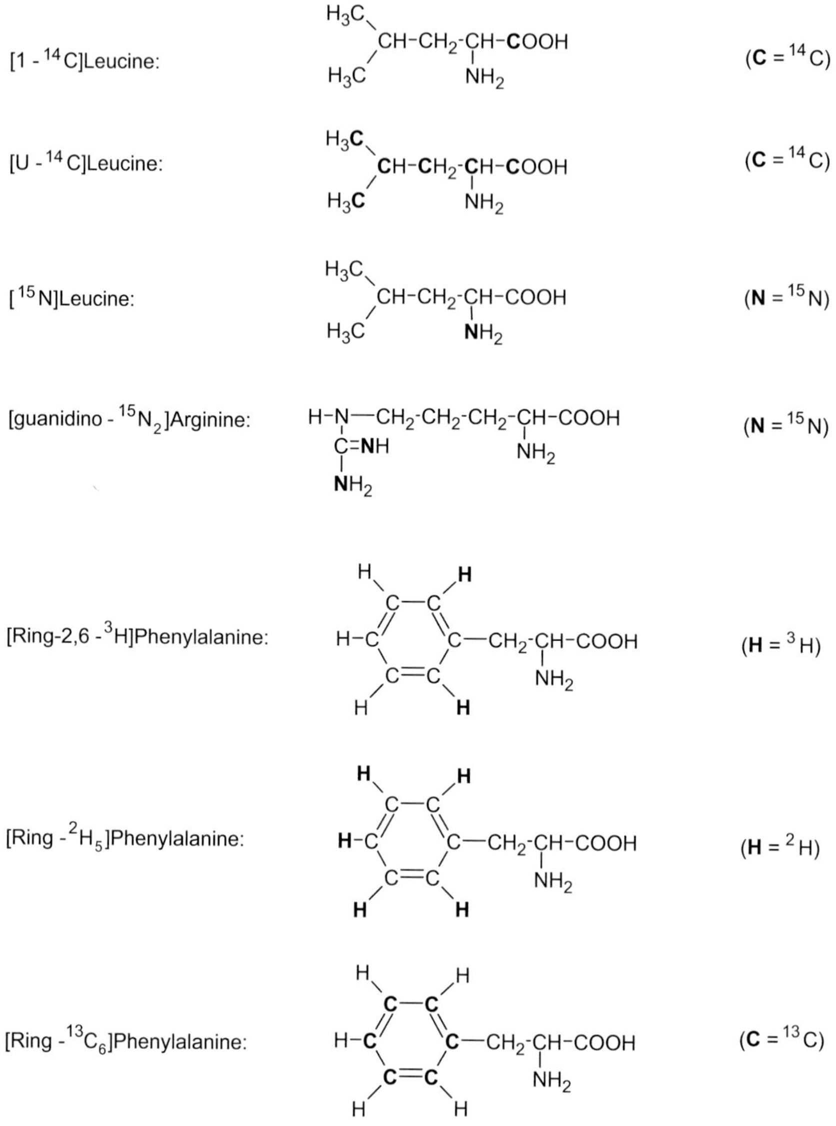

[1 - ^{14}C]Leucine:

$$\begin{array}{c} \text{H}_3\text{C} \\ \\ \text{H}_3\text{C} \end{array} \!\!\! \diagdown\!\!\!\diagup \text{CH-CH}_2\text{-CH-}\textbf{COOH} \\ \underset{\text{NH}_2}{|}$$

(**C** = ^{14}C)

[U - ^{14}C]Leucine:

$$\begin{array}{c} \textbf{H}_3\textbf{C} \\ \\ \textbf{H}_3\textbf{C} \end{array} \!\!\! \diagdown\!\!\!\diagup \textbf{CH-CH}_2\text{-}\textbf{CH-COOH} \\ \underset{\text{NH}_2}{|}$$

(**C** = ^{14}C)

[^{15}N]Leucine:

$$\begin{array}{c} \text{H}_3\text{C} \\ \\ \text{H}_3\text{C} \end{array} \!\!\! \diagdown\!\!\!\diagup \text{CH-CH}_2\text{-CH-COOH} \\ \underset{\textbf{NH}_2}{|}$$

(**N** = ^{15}N)

[guanidino - ^{15}N$_2$]Arginine:

$$\text{H-N}\!-\!\text{CH}_2\text{-CH}_2\text{-CH}_2\text{-CH-COOH} \\ \underset{|}{\text{C=NH}} \underset{\text{NH}_2}{|} \\ \textbf{NH}_2$$

(**N** = ^{15}N)

[Ring-2,6 - ^{3}H]Phenylalanine:

(**H** = ^{3}H)

[Ring - ^{2}H$_5$]Phenylalanine:

(**H** = ^{2}H)

[Ring - ^{13}C$_6$]Phenylalanine:

(**C** = ^{13}C)

FIGURE 7.3 Nomenclature for some common isotopes showing the positions of labeled atoms. Examples are provided for ^{13}C-, ^{14}C-, ^{3}H-, ^{2}H-, or ^{15}N-labeled leucine, arginine, or phenylalanine. The bold letter denotes a labeled atom (either radioactive or stable). Amino acids are shown in the nonionized form.

quantify glycolysis and glutamine oxidation, because a liquid scintillation counter can analyze both ^{14}C and^{3}H in a sample via a dual-label counting program.

The lowest mass of a molecule (e.g., glucose) that is the most abundant form of the element (e.g., ^{12}C, ^{1}H, and ^{16}O) is expressed as M+0 (e.g., 180 Da for glucose). M+0 is sometimes written simply as M, M$_0$, or M0. When a molecule contains 1, 2, 3, 4, 5, and 6 stable isotopes of the same element with a higher mass number (e.g., ^{13}C), the mass of such a molecule is M+1, M+2, M+3, M+4, M+5, and M+6, respectively. The M+1, M+2, M+3, M+4, M+5, and M+6 molecules can be detected by a mass spectrometer and their individual peaks appear in their mass spectrometry spectra. In some publications, M+1, M+2, M+3, M+4, M+5, and M+6 are written as M$_1$, M$_2$, M$_3$, M$_4$, M$_5$, and M$_6$, respectively (Hellerstein 1991), or as M1, M2, M3, M4, M5, and M6, respectively (Brunengraber et al. 1997).

Isomers that have the same composition but differ in the position of heavy atoms are called positional isotopomers. Examples of positional isotopomers are [1-^{13}C]glucose and [2-^{13}C]glucose, as well as [1,2-^{13}C]glucose and [2,3-^{13}C]glucose. Positional isotopomers, which have the same mass, could be detected by mass spectrometry but could not be distinguished by the instrument. Positional information of the isotope could be obtained through either the chemical degradation of glucose into specific carbon units or analyses by gas chromatography-mass spectrometry or tandem liquid chromatography-mass spectrometry. Isomers that have the same heavy atom but differ in its number are designated as mass isotopomers. Examples of mass isotopomers are [1-^{13}C]glucose and [1,2-^{13}C] glucose, as well as [^{14}N,^{14}N]urea, [^{14}N-^{15}N]urea, and [^{15}N,^{15}N]urea. Because the lightest atoms in a molecule are usually not specified, these nitrogen-containing isotopomers are often written as urea, [^{15}N$_1$]urea, and [^{15}N$_2$]urea, respectively. Mass isotopomers have different masses and can be distinguished by a mass spectrometer. Note that: (1) isotopomers may contain two or more different heavy atoms, such as [^{12}C,^{14}N]urea and [^{13}C,^{15}N]urea; and (2) both [^{13}C,^{15}N]urea and [^{15}N$_2$]urea are M+2 isotopomers.

7.1.4 Tracer and Tracee

A radioisotope (e.g., ^{14}C in L-[U-^{14}C]leucine) or a stable isotope (e.g., ^{15}N in L-[^{15}N]leucine) can be used as a tracer. A tracer is used to trace the corresponding atom in an unlabeled molecule (e.g., ^{12}C and ^{14}N in leucine), which is called a tracee. When a specific atom in a compound is labeled (e.g., carbon-1 in L-[1-^{14}C]leucine or L-[1-^{13}C]leucine), it can be used to trace the fate of the specific atom in the unlabeled molecule (e.g., carbon-1 in leucine in this case). Because a liquid scintillation counter or mass spectrometry instrument can detect very low levels of a radioisotope or a stable isotope, respectively, their use as tracers provides a highly sensitive means to study the metabolic fate of the tracee in cells and in the body.

The principle behind the use of isotopes in metabolic studies is that the tracer and its tracee normally have similar biochemical behaviors in cells and in the body. This is likely true for many isotopes, including ^{32}S and ^{35}S, ^{31}P and ^{32}P, ^{16}O and ^{18}O, ^{14}N and ^{15}N, as well as ^{12}C and ^{14}C. However, an isotope effect may occur in cell metabolism due to the different masses of labeled and non-labeled atoms. For example, tritium (^{3}H), which has a mass three times that of hydrogen (^{1}H), can behave differently from ^{1}H. An isotope effect may affect the rate of a biochemical reaction, but still can allow for the tracing of the metabolic fate of a substance in cells and in the body. Potential adverse effects of radioactive isotopes on human health and the high costs for their disposal have limited their use in nutrition research involving humans and other large animals (Kim et al. 2016).

7.1.5 Concepts of Specific Radioactivity and Isotopic Enrichment

The amount of a radioisotope or a stable isotope relative to the unlabeled isotope is expressed as specific radioactivity (SR, sometimes written as SA) or isotope enrichment (IE), respectively. The SR of a radioactive compound is normally expressed as dpm (or Ci) per unit of the amount of substance (e.g., dpm/nmol and mCi/mol). The IE of a stable isotope is defined as the relative abundance of the labeled isotope in a mixture containing both labeled and non-labeled isotopes. Because mass spectrometry does not distinguish the M+1 of a tracer (e.g., ^{13}C-alanine) from the M+1 of the identical tracee (e.g., ^{13}C-alanine) naturally present in a biological sample (e.g., the plasma), true IE values in the sample are calculated by subtracting the natural background IE from the measured sample IE. Information on the SR or IE of a tracer in the precursor pool must be available for the mathematical calculation of product formation and metabolic flux. For example, in experiments involving the constant intravenous infusion of a radioisotope or stable isotope to an animal, SR or IE at an isotopic steady state is needed to calculate product formation and metabolic flux. The flux is defined as the quantity of a substrate or a product that passes through a pathway or enters a metabolic pool per unit time and mass. In cell incubation or culture, relatively high extracellular concentrations of substrates (e.g., 1 mM phenylalanine) are often needed to rapidly attain an intracellular isotopic steady state. In studies involving whole animals, a priming dose of the tracer is usually administered intravenously, followed by the constant infusion of the labeled tracer (Boelens et al. 2005). An appropriate priming dose of a tracer can be determined from published studies and the results of preliminary experiments in the investigator's laboratory.

7.1.5.1 SR of Radioactive Isotopes

The SR of any radioactive isotope can be calculated on the basis of the amount of radioactivity and the mass of the tracee isotope. Blank radioactivity values (dpm) should be subtracted from the sample radioactivity values (dpm) to obtain the corrected sample radioactivity values (dpm). In practice, this can be described by the following equation, with a ^{14}C-labeled isotope as an example:

$$\text{Specific radioactivity (dpm / nmol)} = \frac{\text{Radioactivity of tracer (dpm)}}{\text{Mass of tracer + tracee (μmol)}}$$

$$= \frac{^{14}\text{C (dpm)}}{^{14}\text{C (μmol)} + {}^{12}\text{C plus }{}^{13}\text{C (μmol)}} = \frac{^{14}\text{C (dpm)}}{^{12}\text{C} + {}^{13}\text{C (μmol)}}$$

The mass amount of the radioactive tracer (e.g., ^{14}C or ^{3}H) is negligible, as compared to the amount of the tracee (e.g., ^{12}C plus ^{13}C or ^{1}H). Thus, the mass of the tracer (e.g., ^{14}C or ^{3}H) can be ignored in the calculation, and the SR equals dpm of tracer/μmol of tracee. Let's use alanine as an example to calculate the SR of a radioisotope. If 6×10^3 dpm [3-^{14}C]alanine is mixed with 2 μmol of unlabeled natural alanine in a solution (i.e., the sum of ^{12}C-alanine plus ^{13}C-alanine as analyzed by high-performance liquid chromatography), the SR of [3-^{14}C]alanine is calculated as follows:

$$\text{SR of } \left[3\text{-}^{14}\text{C} \right] \text{alanine} = 6 \times 10^3 \text{ dpm / 2 μmol alanine}$$

$$= 3 \times 10^3 \text{ dpm / μmol alanine}$$

$$= 3 \times 10^3 \text{ dpm/μmol carbon-3 of alanine}$$

Because only carbon-3 of alanine is labeled with ^{14}C, we can say that, in the above example, the SR of [3-^{14}C]alanine is 3×10^3 dpm per μmol of alanine or 3×10^3 dpm per μmol of carbon-3 of alanine.

If 6×10^3 dpm [U-^{14}C]alanine is mixed with 2 μmol alanine, the SR of [U-^{14}C]alanine is calculated as follows:

$$\text{SR of } \left[\text{U-}^{14}\text{C} \right] \text{alanine} = 6 \times 10^3 \text{ dpm / 2 μmol alanine}$$

$$= 3 \times 10^3 \text{ dpm / μmol alanine}$$

$$= 3 \times 10^3 \text{ dpm / 3 carbons in alanine}$$

$$= 1 \times 10^3 \text{ dpm / μmol carbon of alanine}$$

Because all the carbons of alanine are uniformly labeled with ^{14}C, we can say that, in the above example, the SR of [U-^{14}C]alanine is 3×10^3 dpm per μmol of alanine, or 1×10^3 dpm per μmol carbon of alanine.

The expression of the SR of ^{14}C-alanine assumes importance when the rate of the oxidation of an AA to CO_2 in cells or the body is calculated. For example, if the SR of [3-^{14}C]alanine is expressed as dpm/nmol alanine, the rate of CO_2 production from alanine should be multiplied by 3 because alanine has 3 carbons. However, if the SR of [3-^{14}C]alanine is expressed as dpm/nmol carbon-3 of alanine, the rate of CO_2 production from alanine should not be multiplied by a factor. Likewise, if the SR of [U-^{14}C]alanine is expressed as dpm/nmol alanine, the rate of CO_2 production from alanine should be multiplied by 3. However, if the SR of [U-^{14}C]alanine is expressed as dpm/nmol carbon of alanine, the rate of CO_2 production from alanine should not be multiplied by a factor.

7.1.5.2 Isotopic Enrichment of Stable Isotopes

The addition of a stable isotope to an incubation medium or whole-body infusion system enriches the concentration of the isotope above that of natural abundance. The isotope enrichment (IE) of a stable tracer can be expressed as molar percent excess (MPE, %), atom percent excess (APE, %), or tracer to tracee ratio (TTR, mol/mol), and calculated on the basis of the mass of the stable isotope tracer and the mass of the stable isotope tracee. This can be described by the following equations, with a ^{13}C-labled isotope as an example:

$$\text{Molar percent excess (MPE, \%)} = \frac{\text{Mass of stable isotope tracer}}{\text{Mass of stable isotope tracer} + \text{Mass of stable isotope tracee}} \times 100$$

$$= \frac{^{13}\text{C tracer molecule (\mu mol)}}{^{13}\text{C tracer molecule (\mu mol)} + ^{12}\text{C tracee molecule (\mu mol)}} \times 100$$

$$\text{Atom percent excess (APE, \%)} = \frac{\text{Mass of stable isotope (SI) tracer atom}}{\text{Mass of SI tracer atom} + \text{Mass of SI tracee atom}} \times 100$$

$$= \frac{^{13}\text{C (\mu mol)}}{^{13}\text{C (\mu mol)} + ^{12}\text{C (\mu mol)}} \times 100$$

$$\text{Tracer to tracee ratio (TTR, mol / mol)} = \frac{\text{Mass of stable isotope tracer}}{\text{Mass of stable isotope tracee}}$$

$$= \frac{^{13}\text{C (\mu mol)}}{^{12}\text{C (\mu mol)}}$$

$$\text{Molar percent excess (MPE, \%)} = \frac{\text{TTR}}{1 + \text{TTR}} \times 100$$

Because the amount of a stable isotope tracer (e.g., ^{13}C or ^{2}H) is significant as compared to the tracee (e.g., unlabeled ^{12}C- or ^{1}H-substance), the mass of the tracer (e.g., ^{13}C- or ^{2}H-labeled substances) must be included in the calculation of the MPE. Let's use alanine again as an example to calculate TTR, MPE, and APE of ^{13}C-alanine as a stable isotope tracer. When 0.20 μmol [3–^{13}C]alanine (tracer) is mixed with 1.8 μmol unlabeled ^{12}C-alanine plus 0.02 μmol ^{13}C-alanine naturally present in the unlabeled alanine solution (as analyzed by mass spectrometry), the TTR of alanine and the MPE of [3-^{13}C]alanine are 0.111% and 9.901%, respectively, as calculated below. The APE of [3-^{13}C] alanine is 9.901%.

$$\text{TTR (\mu mol / \mu mol)} = \frac{\text{Tracer (\mu mol)}}{\text{Tracee (\mu mol)}} = \frac{[M+1]\text{alanine}\left(\text{i.e.,} \left[3\text{-}^{13}\text{C}\right]\text{alanine}\right), \mu mol}{[M+0]\text{alanine}\left(\text{i.e.,} \left[^{12}\text{C}\right]\text{alanine}\right), \mu mol} = \frac{0.20}{1.8} = 0.111$$

$$\text{MPE (\%)} = \frac{\text{Tracer (\mu mol)}}{\text{Tracer} + \text{Tracee (\mu mol)}} \times 100 = \frac{[M+1]\text{alanine (\mu mol)}}{[M+1]\text{alanine} + [M+0]\text{alanine (\mu mol)}}$$

$$= \frac{0.20}{0.2 + 0.02 + 1.8} \times 100 = 9.901\%$$

If 0.20 μmol [U-^{13}C]alanine is mixed with 1.8 μmol unlabeled ^{12}C-alanine plus 0.02 μmol ^{13}C-alanine naturally present in the unlabeled alanine solution (as analyzed by mass spectrometry), the TTR of alanine and the MPE of [U-^{13}C]alanine are 0.111% and 9.901%, respectively, as calculated above. The APE of [U-^{13}C]alanine is 9.901%.

$$\text{TTR (μmol / μmol)} = \frac{\text{Tracer (μmol)}}{\text{Tracee (μmol)}} = \frac{[M+3]\text{alanine}\left(\text{i.e.,}\left[U\text{-}^{13}C\right]\text{alanine}\right),\text{μmol}}{[M+0]\text{alanine}\left(\text{i.e.,}\left[^{12}C\right]\text{alanine}\right),\text{μmol}} = \frac{0.20}{1.8} = 0.111$$

$$\text{MPE (\%)} = \frac{\text{Tracer (μmol)}}{\text{Tracer + Tracee (μmol)}} \times 100 = \frac{[M+3]\text{alanine (μmol)}}{[M+3]\text{alanine} + [M+0]\text{alanine (μmol)}}$$

$$= \frac{0.20}{0.2 + 0.02 + 1.8} \times 100 = 9.901\%$$

MPE, APE, and TTR are commonly used to study nutrient metabolism in humans and other animals (Kim et al. 2016). Because plasma or tissue samples contain both the tracer (e.g., ^{13}C-glucose or ^{2}H-glucose) and tracee (e.g., ^{12}C-glucose or ^{1}H-glucose) before the tracer (e.g., ^{13}C-glucose) is administered into animals, which are referred to as background (baseline) values, the IE of the stable isotope (expressed as MPE, APE, or TTR) in plasma or tissue samples collected at any time after the tracer is infused should be corrected for the background (baseline) IE of the stable isotope through subtraction. An example for the calculation of the TTR of ^{2}H-glucose in the plasma of humans is illustrated in Table 7.3. In the calculation of the rate of CO_2 production from the oxidation of a ^{13}C-AA, the number of its total carbons and labeled carbons must be considered, as noted previously for studies involving ^{14}C-labeled alanine.

$$\text{Corrected APE} = \text{APE of sample} - \text{APE of background (baseline)}$$

$$\text{Corrected MPE} = \text{MPE of sample} - \text{MPE of background (baseline)}$$

TABLE 7.3

Calculations of the Tracer/Tracer Ratio (TTR) for Stable Isotopes in the Plasma of Humans Receiving Constant Intravenous Infusion of [6,6-^{2}H$_2$]Glucose

	Abundance of [6,6-^{2}H$_2$] Glucose (Tracer) M+2 (m/z, 333)[a]	Abundance of [6,6-^{1}H$_2$]Glucose (Tracee) M+0 (m/z, 331)[b]	TTR
	(A)	(B)	(A/B)
Plasma before infusion of [6,6-^{2}H$_2$]glucose (Background value)	67,498	2,213,121	0.0305
Plasma at isotopic steady state after the constant intravenous infusion of [6,6-^{2}H$_2$]glucose (Sample)	204,673	2,783,834	0.0735
Plasma TTR corrected for background value	---	---	0.0430

Source: Kim, I. et al. 2016. *Exp. Mol. Med.* 48:e203.

Note: [6,6-^{2}H$_2$]glucose=two ^{2}H are attached to the carbon-6 of glucose; m/z=mass-to-charge ratio (the ratio of the mass number of an ion to its charge number).

[a] Adult humans received the constant intravenous infusion of [6,6-^{2}H$_2$]glucose. Blood samples were obtained before the isotope administration and at the isotopic steady state after the isotope administration. Glucose in the plasma was derivatized with pentaacetate, and the derivative had an m/z value that was much higher than 180 for glucose. The M+0 and M+1 of glucose in the plasma were analyzed by a mass spectrometer. M+2 and M+0 refer to molecular ion peaks on the mass spectrometry spectrum for the [6,6-^{2}H$_2$]glucose and [6,6-^{1}H$_2$]glucose derivatives, respectively.

[b] The m/z value for the tracee is 2 less than that for the tracer.

TABLE 7.4

Calculations of the Appearance (Synthesis) and Disappearance (Utilization) of Glucose in Humans Receiving Constant Intravenous Infusion of [1-^{13}C]Glucose[a]

	Molar Percent Enrichment in Plasma (MPE, %)	Glucose Appearance in Plasma (Plasma Flux, R_a)	Glucose Disappearance from Plasma (R_d)
Background value before the infusion of [1-^{13}C]glucose	6.123	---	---
Plasma samples at isotopic steady state (plateau) after the constant infusion of [1-^{13}C]glucose	8.201	---	---
Background-corrected plasma sample at plateau (MPEp)	2.102	---	---
Plasma glucose kinetics (μmol/kg BW/min)	---	10.47[b]	10.47[c]

Source: Kim, I. et al. 2016. *Exp. Mol. Med.* 48:e203.

Note: BW, body weight; [1-^{13}C]glucose=one ^{13}C is attached to the carbon-1 of glucose; MPEp, background-corrected molar percent enrichment of the tracer in the plasma at plateau.

[a] Adult humans received the primed constant intravenous infusion of [1-^{13}C]glucose [prime: 17 μmol/kg BW; the rate of constant infusion (F): 0.22 μmol/kg BW/min]. Blood samples were obtained before the isotope administration and at the isotopic steady state after the isotope administration. The plasma samples were analyzed by a mass spectrometer for the molar percent enrichment of the glucose tracer.

[b] R_a (appearance)=F/MPEp=0.22 μmol/kg BW/min / 2.102%=10.47 μmol/kg BW/min.

[c] R_d (disappearance)=R_a in a physiological steady state.

$$\text{Corrected TTR} = \text{TTR of sample} - \text{TTR of background (baseline)}$$

MPE or APE must be used when both tracer and tracee participate in the biochemical pathways under study, such as protein synthesis, plasma glucose flux (Table 7.4), glucose utilization, AA synthesis, net AA balance, and substrate oxidation. By contrast, *TTR* must be used when only tracee is involved in the biochemical pathways under study, such as (1) protein degradation to release phenylalanine [because the tracee (an AA that is not synthesized de novo in animals), but not tracer, is derived from intracellular protein degradation]; (2) the appearance of palmitate and glycerol from lipolysis [because the tracee, but not the tracer, is derived from intracellular hydrolysis of triacylglycerols (Table 7.5)]; and (3) the flux of an AA that is not synthesized de novo in animals.

7.1.6 SIGNIFICANCE OF SR AND IE OF A TRACER

Accurate values for SR or IE of metabolic substrates at their site of metabolism are required for meaningful calculations of the rates of product formation and metabolic flux in cells, tissues, or the whole body. Intracellular SR or IE of a tracer at a steady state must be measured at steady state when the substrate SR or IE remains constant to avoid the complex problems associated with tracer experiments (see the following sections). If the intracellular SR or IE of a tracer at the location of the metabolic event cannot be measured due to practical problems (e.g., obtaining a sample from an internal organ), the SR or IE of a surrogate metabolite (e.g., [^{14}C]isocaproate or [^{13}C]isocaproate in the venous plasma of individuals infused with L-[1-^{14}C]leucine or L-[1-^{13}C]leucine, respectively) can be used to represent the SR or IE of the substrate (e.g., L-[1-^{14}C]leucine or L-[1-^{13}C]leucine) at the site of metabolism under study. The principle for calculating product formation from the substrate is the same for radioactive or stable isotopes. In either case, the SR or IE should be preferably at an isotopic steady-state (namely, a constant value or plateau throughout the study or sampling period). In the following sections, practical examples will illustrate how radioactive and stable tracers can be used to determine the rates of product formation *in vitro* and *in vivo*, the fluxes of nutrients in the plasma of animals, and the turnover rates of nutrients in the whole body.

TABLE 7.5

Calculations of the Rates of Lipolysis and Palmitate Recycling in Humans Simultaneously Receiving Constant Intravenous Infusion of [1-^{13}C]Palmitate and [1,1,2,3,3-^{2}H]Glycerol[a]

	Background-Corrected Plasma TTR (TTRp)	Appearance (R_a), Lipolysis, and Fatty Acid Recycling (µmol/kg BW per min)				
		R_a in Plasma (Plasma Flux)	Intracellular Recycling (A)	Oxidation to CO_2 (B)	Extracellular Recycling (C=A − B)	Total Recycling (A+C)
Palmitate	0.035	1.143[b]	2.757[c]	0.606[g]	0.537[i]	3.294
Glycerol	0.040	2.00[c]	0.0	ND	ND	ND
Total FAAs	---	1.758[d]	4.242[f]	0.932[h]	0.826[j]	5.068

Source: Kim, I. et al. 2016. *Exp. Mol. Med.* 48:e203.

Note: BW, body weight; FFAs = free fatty acids; [1,1,2,3,3-^{2}H]glycerol = two ^{2}H, one ^{2}H, and two ^{2}H are attached to the carbon-1, carbon-2, and carbon-3 of glycerol, respectively; ND, not determined; [1-^{13}C]palmitate = one ^{13}C is attached to the carbon-1 of palmitate; TTRp, background-corrected tracer-to-tracee ratio in the plasma at plateau.

[a] *Adult humans in the post-absorptive state simultaneously received the constant intravenous infusion of [1-^{13}C]palmitate* [the rate of infusion (F) = 0.04 µmol/kg BW/min] and the primed constant intravenous infusion of [1,1,2,3,3-^{2}H]glycerol [a priming dose = 1.2 µmol/kg BW; the rate of constant infusion (F) = 0.08 µmol/kg BW/min]. A priming dose of [1-^{13}C] palmitate was not used because its plasma pool mixed and turned over rapidly. Blood samples were obtained before the isotope administration and at the isotopic steady state after the isotope administration. The plasma samples were analyzed by a mass spectrometer for the molar percent enrichment of the stable isotopes.

[b] R_a (appearance) of palmitate = F/TTRp = 0.04 µmol/kg BW/min / 0.035 = 1.143 µmol/kg BW/min.

[c] R_a (appearance) of glycerol (an indicator of glycolysis) = F/TTRp = 0.04 µmol/kg BW/min / 0.035 = 1.143 µmol/kg BW/min.

[d] R_a of total FAAs = R_a of palmitate/fractional contribution of palmitate to total FFAs at rest = 1.143/0.65 = 1.758 µmol/kg BW/min.

[e] Intracellular recycling (re-esterification) of palmitate = Intracellular recycling (re-esterification) of total FAAs × fractional contribution of palmitate to total FFAs at rest) = 4.242 × 0.65 = 2.757 µmol/kg BW/min.

[f] Intracellular recycling (re-esterification) of total FAAs = R_a of glycerol × 3 − R_a of total FAAs = 2.00 × 3 − 1.758 = 4.242 µmol/kg BW/min.

[g] Measured from another experiment (0.606 µmol palmitate/kg BW/min; Table 7.6).

[h] Rate of the oxidation of total FAAs = Rate of the oxidation of palmitate/fractional contribution of palmitate to total FFAs at rest = 0.606/0.65 = 0.932 µmol of total FAAs/kg BW/min.

[i] Extracellular recycling of palmitate (i.e., re-use of extracellular palmitate by tissues) = R_a of palmitate in the plasma − Oxidation of palmitate = 1.143 − 0.606 = 0.537 µmol/kg BW/min.

[j] Extracellular recycling of total FAAs (i.e., re-use of extracellular total FFAs) = R_a of total FAAs in the plasma − Oxidation of total FAAs = 1.758 − 0.932 = 0.826 µmol/kg BW/min.

7.1.6.1　Calculations of Rates of Nutrient Metabolism *In Vitro* and *In Vivo* Using Radioisotopes

7.1.6.1.1　Calculations of Substrate Oxidation and Product Formation Using Radioisotopes

In radioisotope-based *in vitro* metabolic studies, one or more radioactive tracers plus their tracees are added to the culture and incubation medium, and the extracellular concentration of the tracee is relatively high (e.g., 1 mM L-phenylalanine for quantifying protein turnover) to achieve a steady-state SR of the intracellular tracee within a relatively short period of time (e.g., 5– to 15 min). *In vivo*, tracer experiments require either a single administration or the constant infusion of one or more radioactive tracers. In the *in vivo* studies involving the constant infusion of a tracer, a priming dose of a tracer is usually administered into the body before the initiation of its constant infusion, so as to achieve a steady-state SR in the plasma within a relatively short period of time (e.g., 30– to

60 min). This method is called the primed constant infusion. The dose of an administered radioactive isotope is normally expressed as dpm/kg body weight (BW) per unit time (e.g., min or h). In both *in vitro* and *in vivo* studies, the doses of tracers must be sufficient for detection by analytical instruments and must not affect normal metabolic or physiological processes. The SR of the labeled substrate at plateau at the site of its metabolism is required to calculate the rate of product formation from the substrate in incubated cells, perfused organ, and the whole body. The equation is given as follows:

$$\text{Product formation (nmol)} = \frac{\text{Amount of radioactivity in product (dpm)}}{\text{Specific radioactivity of tracer at plateau (dpm / nmol)}}$$

Let us use the oxidation of alanine to CO_2 as an example to illustrate the calculation of product formation in a radioactive tracer experiment. Hepatocytes (5×10^6 cells) are incubated at 37°C for 1 h in 2 mL of the Krebs bicarbonate buffer containing 1.5 mM (i.e., 1,500 nmol/mL) alanine plus 300,000 dpm [1-^{14}C]alanine. The SR of the tracer reaches a plateau very rapidly within 5 min after its addition to the incubation medium. At the end of the 1-h incubation, total $^{14}CO_2$ (900 dpm) is collected in 0.2 mL Soluene with an efficiency of 90% for $^{14}CO_2$ trapping. The background (blank, cell-free incubation) radioactivity of ^{14}C in the solution is 50 dpm. How much CO_2 is produced from alanine oxidation by the cells? In this reaction, alanine is the precursor and CO_2 is the product.

$$\text{The SR of } \left[1\text{-}^{14}C \right] \text{alanine} = 300,000 \text{ dpm} \div (1,500 \text{ nmol / mL} \times 2 \text{ mL})$$

$$= 100 \text{ dpm / nmol C-1 of alanine}$$

$$\text{Radioactivity in the product} \left(^{14}CO_2 \right) = \left(900 \text{ dpm} - 50 \text{ dpm} \right) \div 90\% = 944 \text{ dpm}$$

$$\text{Production of } CO_2 = 944 \text{ dpm} \div 100 \text{ dpm / nmol C-1 of alanine}$$

$$= 9.44 \text{ nmol for the total number of } 5 \times 10^6 \text{ cells per hour}$$

$$= 9.44 \text{ nmol} \div \left(5 \times 10^6 \text{ cells} \times 1 \text{ h} \right)$$

$$= 1.89 \text{ nmol / } 10^6 \text{ cells / h}$$

Based on the above example, we can state that the oxidation of carbon-1 of alanine to CO_2 in the hepatocytes is 1.9 nmol/10^6 cells per h. However, if the same amount of ^{14}C was in [U-^{14}C]alanine instead of [1-^{14}C]alanine, the SR of [U-^{14}C]alanine would be 33.3 dpm/nmol alanine carbon (i.e., 100 dpm/nmol alanine ÷ 3) and the rate of CO_2 production would be 5.67 nmol/10^6 cells per h [i.e., 944 dpm ÷ 33.3 dpm/nmol C of alanine ÷ (5×10^6 cells × 1 h)].

7.1.6.1.2 Calculations of the Plasma Fluxes of Nutrients In Vivo Using Radioisotopes

The SR of the labeled substrate at plateau in the plasma, along with the rate of intravenous infusion of the tracer (e.g., dpm/kg BW/min) is required to calculate the flux of the substrate or the rate of production of a metabolite in the whole body. For example, the flux of arginine in the plasma of piglets can be determined using L-[U-^{14}C]arginine or L-[guanidino-^{14}C]arginine, and whole-body production of CO_2 can be measured using [^{14}C]NaHCO$_3$ (Bertolo et al. 2003). In these cases, it is not necessary to know the substrate SR at the site of metabolism. An equation for calculating metabolic fluxes *in vivo* using a radioisotope is as follows. In the calculation of the fractional conversion rate, the SR of the product and its precursor may be measured in the plasma or cells, depending on experimental objectives, and the flux may be the plasma or intracellular flux.

Plasma flux of tracee $(Q, \text{nmol} / \text{kg body weight per min})$

$$= \frac{\text{Rate of the constant infusion of tracer (dpm / kg body weight per min)}}{\text{Specific radioactivity of tracer in plasma at plateau (dpm / nmol)}}$$

Non-oxidative flux = Plasma flux (Q) − Oxidative flux

Fractional conversion rate (nmol / kg body weight per min) =

$$\text{Flux (nmol / kg body weight per min)} \times \frac{\text{Specific radioactivity of product at plateau (dpm / nmol)}}{\text{Specific radioactivity of precursor at plateau (dpm / nmol)}}$$

7.1.6.2 Calculations of Rates of Nutrient Metabolism *In Vitro* and *In Vivo* Using Stable Isotopes

7.1.6.2.1 Calculations of Substrate Oxidation and Product Formation Using Stable Isotopes
Stable isotopes can be used to determine the rate of product formation, as described previously for radioactive isotopes. This can be illustrated by the whole-body production of $^{13}CO_2$ from the oxidation of ^{13}C-palmitate (Table 7.6) and a ^{13}C-AA (Raguso et al. 1999) in humans receiving the

TABLE 7.6
Calculations of the Rates of Palmitate Oxidation in Humans Receiving the Constant Intravenous Infusion of [1-^{13}C]Palmitate[a]

	Background-Corrected APE (APEp, %)	Background-Corrected MPE (MPEp, %)	Percent (%) of Uptake Palmitate Oxidized to CO_2	Disappearance of Palmitate from Plasma, R_d (µmol/kg BW/min)	Palmitate Oxidation Rate (µmol/kg BW/min)	Percent (%) of Expired CO_2 from Palmitate Oxidation
$^{13}CO_2$ in breath	0.012	---	---	---	---	---
Palmitate in plasma	---	3.30	50.0[b]	1.212[c]	0.606[d]	9.696[e]

Source: Kim, I. et al. 2016. *Exp. Mol. Med.* 48:e203.

Note: BW, body weight; APEp, background-corrected atom percent excess at plateau; MPEp, background-corrected molar percent excess at plateau.

[a] Adult humans in the post-absorptive state received the constant intravenous infusion of [1-^{13}C]palmitate [the rate of infusion $(F) = 0.04$ µmol/kg BW/min]. A priming dose of [1-^{13}C]palmitate was not used because its plasma pool mixed and turned over rapidly. Expired CO_2 and blood samples were obtained before the isotope administration and at the isotopic steady state after the isotope administration. The expired CO_2 and plasma samples were analyzed by a mass spectrometer for the atom and molar percent enrichments of the stable isotopes. The rate of total CO_2 production, as determined using indirect calorimetry, was 100 µmol/kg BW/min. The appearance of palmitate (R_a) in the plasma was equal to the disappearance of palmitate (R_d) from the plasma in a post-absorptive, physiological steady state.

[b] % of uptake palmitate oxidized to CO_2 = (APEp of breath $^{13}CO_2 \times$ Total CO_2 produced $\times 100$) / (Rate of ^{13}C-palmitate infusion $\times$ Acetate correction factor) = (0.012% $\times$ 100 µmol/kg BW/min) / (0.04 µmol/kg BW/min $\times$ 0.6) = 50.0%.

[c] R_d (disappearance) of palmitate = F/MPEp = 0.04 µmol/kg BW/min / 3.3% = 1.212 µmol/kg BW/min.

[d] Palmitate oxidation rate = R_d of palmitate $\times$ % of uptake palmitate oxidized to CO_2 = 1.212 $\times$ 0.606 = 0.606 µmol palmitate/kg BW/min.

[e] % of expired CO_2 from palmitate oxidation = (Palmitate oxidation rate $\times$ the number of carbon in palmitate $\times$ 100) / (total CO_2 production) = (0.606 µmol/kg BW/min $\times$ 16 $\times$ 100) / 100 µmol/kg BW/min = 9.696%.

constant intravenous infusion of [1-^{13}C]palmitate and a [1-^{13}C]AA, respectively. Expired $^{13}CO_2$ was collected before the isotope administration (as baseline values) and at the isotopic steady state after the isotope administration.

To determine the rate of whole-body oxidation of an organic nutrient using a ^{13}C-labeled tracer, the rate of whole-body CO_2 production, the IE (APE, %) of expired $^{13}CO_2$ in breath at plateau during the constant infusion of a ^{13}C-labeled AA, and the IE (APE, %) of the ^{13}C-labeled AA in the plasma at plateau must be measured. For example, Bush et al. (2002) used L-[1-^{13}C]phenylalanine to determine its oxidation in young pigs treated with or without growth hormone. Of course, this will provide information only about the oxidation of the carbon-1 of phenylalanine.

$$\text{Rate of whole-body phenylalanine oxidation (μmol / kg body weight per h)} = \frac{\text{IE}_{b2} \times \text{CO}_2\,\text{PR}}{\text{IE}_p}$$

where CO_2 PR is the rate of whole-body CO_2 production (μmol/kg BW/h) estimated using the intravenous infusion of [^{13}C]NaHCO$_3$, IE$_{b2}$ is the IE (APE, %) of expired $^{13}CO_2$ at plateau during the constant infusion of L-[1-^{13}C]phenylalanine, and IE$_p$ is the IE (APE, %) of L-[1-^{13}C]phenylalanine in the plasma at plateau during the last 2 h of L-[1-^{13}C]phenylalanine infusion (Bush et al. 2002). Note that in this case, two separate measurements are required: total CO_2 production from the study participants and the production of CO_2 from phenylalanine in the individuals.

The rate of the recovery of $^{13}CO_2$ produced from the oxidation of a ^{13}C-labeled AA, glucose, and fatty acid in animals can be estimated using the intravenous infusion of [^{13}C]NaHCO$_3$. In the plasma, [^{13}C]NaHCO$_3$ is dissociated to form [^{13}C]HCO$_3^-$, which is in chemical equilibrium with $^{13}CO_2$. It is practically difficult to intravenously administer this gas into humans and other animals, because a constant dose of $^{13}CO_2$ can readily evolve from the infusion solution and becomes irreversibly lost. Thus, [^{13}C]NaHCO$_3$ is often used to estimate the whole-body production of CO_2 from the oxidation of all substrates (namely, the flux of CO_2 into the plasma pool), as described below. This information is useful to assess the relative contribution of AAs to the whole body oxygen consumption.

When the oxidation of long-chain fatty acids to acetyl-CoA and then to CO_2 is measured, a correction for the rate of $^{13}CO_2$ loss should be made (Kim et al. 2016). This is because: (1) losses of labeled ^{13}C occur via isotope exchanges in the Krebs cycle; (2) some $^{13}CO_2$ is retained in the body via biochemical reactions; and (3) not all the $^{13}CO_2$ produced at the cellular level appears in the circulation, and a proportion of ^{13}C can be excreted in the urine and feces. Such a correction for the loss of $^{13}CO_2$ (e.g., 40%) is usually performed by using ^{13}C-acetate as a tracer.

$$\text{Rate of whole-body CO}_2\,\text{prodution (μmol / kg body weight per h)} = \left(\frac{\text{IE}_i}{\text{IE}_{b1}} - 1 \right) \times \text{IR}$$

where IEi is the IE (APE, %) of intravenously infused [^{13}C]NaHCO$_3$, IE$_{b1}$ is the IE (APE, %) of expired $^{13}CO_2$ at plateau during the infusion of [^{13}C]NaHCO$_3$, and IR is the rate of [^{13}C]NaHCO$_3$ infusion (μmol/kg BW/h).

Now let us use, as another example of AA metabolism, the primed constant infusion of L-[ring-^{2}H$_5$]phenylalanine, L-[ring-^{2}H$_2$]tyrosine, and L-[ring-^{2}H$_4$]tyrosine to determine the conversion of phenylalanine into tyrosine, as well as whole-body protein synthesis and degradation in adult humans (Table 7.7). The calculations are based on the principles that: (1) the appearance of phenylalanine (an AA that is not synthesized de novo in animals) in the plasma (R_a) reflects protein degradation in the post-absorptive state; (2) the disappearance of phenylalanine from the plasma (R_d) reflects the use of this AA for protein synthesis and hydroxylation to tyrosine; (3) the R_a of phenylalanine is equal to the R_d of phenylalanine at a physiological steady state; and (4) the whole-body pool size of proteins (e.g., muscle proteins) with slow turnover rates is generally constant in healthy individuals during the time period of the tracer study ($\leq$8 h).

TABLE 7.7

Calculations of the Rates of Whole-Body Phenylalanine (Phe) Catabolism, Production of Tyrosine (Tyr), and Protein Turnover in Humans in the Post-Absorptive State[a]

	Background-Corrected Plasma		R_a of Phe	R_a of Tyr	Fractional R_a of Tyr from Phe	Phe Hydro-xylation Rate	Protein Synthesis rate	Protein Breakdown Rate
	TTR (TTRp)	MPE (MPEp, %)	(μmol/kg BW per min)	(μmol/kg BW per min)	(%)	(μmol/kg BW per min)	(μmol/kg BW per min)	(μmol/kg BW per min)
L-[ring-^{2}H$_5$]Phe	0.0941	8.6007	0.8927[b]	---	---	0.2133[e]	19.085[f]	22.32[g]
L-[ring-^{2}H$_4$]Tyr	0.0241	2.3533	---	---	27.36[d]	---	---	---
L-[ring-^{2}H$_2$]Tyr	0.0442	4.2329	---	0.7796[c]	---	---	---	---

Source: Kim, I. et al. 2016. *Exp. Mol. Med.* 48:e203.

Note: BW, body weight; MPEp, background-corrected molar percent enrichment in the plasma at plateau; TTRp, background-corrected tracer-to-tracee ratio in the plasma at plateau.

[a] *Adult humans simultaneously received the primed constant intravenous infusion of L-[ring-^{2}H$_5$]phenylalanine [prime: 3.07 μmol/kg BW; the rate of constant infusion (F)=0.084 μmol/kg BW per min], L-[ring-^{2}H$_2$]tyrosine (prime, 3.07 μmol/kg BW; the rate of constant infusion=0.033 μmol/kg/min), and L-[ring-^{2}H$_4$]tyrosine (prime, 0.30 μmol/kg BW). Blood samples were obtained before the isotope administration and at the isotopic steady state after the isotope administration. The plasma samples were analyzed by a mass spectrometer for the tracers and tracees. The rate of net protein balance in the whole body=protein synthesis rate−protein breakdown rate=19.085−22.318=−3.233 μmol protein/kg BW per min.*

[b] R_a (appearance) of Phe=F/TTRp=0.084 μmol/kg BW per min / 0.0941=0.8927 μmol/kg BW per min. When MPEp is used for calculation, R_a of Phe=0.084/8.6007=0.9767 μmol/kg BW per min.

[c] R_a (appearance) of Tyr=F/MPEp=0.033 μmol/kg BW per min / 4.2329%=0.7796 μmol/kg BW per min. When TTRp is used for calculation, R_a of Tyr=0.033/0.0442=0.7466 μmol/kg BW per min.

[d] Fractional R_a of Tyr from Phe=MPEp of Tyr/MPEp of Phe×100=2.3533/8.6007×100=27.36%.

[e] Phe hydroxylation rate=Fractional R_a of Tyr from Phe×R_a of Tyr=27.36%×0.7796=0.2133 μmol/kg BW per min.

[f] Protein synthesis rate=(R_a of Phe−Phe hydroxylation rate)/Fractional contribution of Phe to protein=(0.9767−0.2133)/0.04=19.085 μmol/kg BW per min.

[g] Protein breakdown rate=R_a of Phe/ Fractional contribution of Phe to protein=0.8927/0.04=22.32 μmol/kg BW per min.

As noted previously, the MPE must be used to calculate all the components of protein synthesis because both the tracer and the tracee participate in this process, whereas the TTR must be used to assess the R_a of phenylalanine in the plasma because the tracee, but not the tracer, is derived from protein breakdown. In recent years, the stable-tracer bolus pulse technique has been used to determine the rates of whole-body protein synthesis and degradation, as well as metabolic inter-conversions of AAs in post-absorptive humans because of easy applicability and low tracer costs (Deutz et al. 2018; Engelen et al. 2019). Similar methods are also feasible and useful for studies involving laboratory and farm animals (Reeds 1974; Zak et al. 1979). In both the constant infusion and single bolus methods for the use of a stable isotope tracer to quantify whole-body protein turnover and AA metabolism, it is not necessary to co-administer its tracee (Granados et al. 2020; Engelen et al. 2019; Ten Have et al. 2019).

7.1.6.2.2 Calculations of the Plasma Fluxes of Nutrients In Vivo Using Stable Isotopes

Stable isotopes can be used to determine the rate of product formation, as described previously for radioactive isotopes. This can be illustrated by the quantification of phenylalanine flux in adult humans (Table 7.7) and whole-body glucose synthesis in humans (Table 7.4). In the latter case, the study participants received a priming dose of [1-^{13}C]glucose and then the constant intravenous infusion of [1-^{13}C]glucose (Kim et al. 2016). The rate of glucose appearance in the plasma (R_a) can be calculated by the following equation. Note that the choice of the tracer is important to minimize isotope recycling through glucose metabolism.

Rate of the appearance of glucose in plasma (µmol / kg body weight per min) =

$$\frac{\text{Rate of the constant infusion of} \left[1\text{-}^{13}\text{C} \right] \text{glucose (µmol / kg body weight per min)}}{\text{Background-corrected MPE}_\text{p} \text{ of } \left[1\text{-}^{13}\text{C} \right] \text{glucose in plasma (\%)}}$$

where MPEp is the background-corrected molar percent enrichment of the tracer in the plasma at plateau (isotopic steady state). The background MPE in the plasma is measured immediately before the stable tracer is administered to study participants (humans or other animals).

As another example for the application of stable tracers to metabolic research, the simultaneous infusion of palmitate and glycerol can be used to determine the rates of the appearance (flux) of palmitate and glycerol in the plasma (Table 7.5). This is based on the principles that: (1) the hydrolysis of triacylglycerol (containing one mole of the glycerol backbone and 3 moles of long-chain fatty acids) in tissues (primarily white adipose tissue) generates long-chain fatty acids (including palmitate) and glycerol; (2) the triacylglycerol-derived palmitate can be re-esterified into triacylglycerol, oxidized within the tissues, or released into the blood; (3) the triacylglycerol-derived glycerol is not reused for re-esterification in white adipose tissue and skeletal muscle and is released from the tissues into the blood (Figure 7.4). The rates of the appearance of total free fatty acids, as well as the intracellular and extracellular recycling of total fatty acids can be calculated on the basis of the kinetics of palmitate and glycerol. This shows the unique advantage of the use of tracers to assess the complex metabolism of nutrients in the whole body.

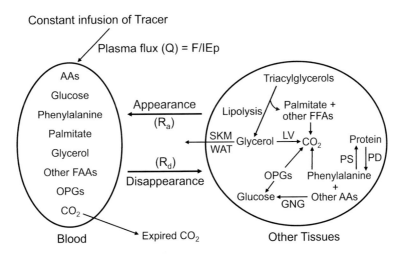

FIGURE 7.4 Scheme for protein, fat, and glucose metabolism in humans and other animals, as well as the appearance (R_a) and the disappearance (R_d) of metabolites in the plasma of their blood. The plasma flux (Q) of a nutrient can be determined by dividing the rate of the constant infusion of an appropriate tracer (F) by its corrected isotopic enrichment in the plasma (IEp) at plateau. In addition, the rates of protein synthesis (PS), protein degradation (PD), gluconeogenesis (GNG), lipolysis, R_a, and R_d can be assessed by using appropriate tracers. Recycling of glucose, amino acids, fatty acids, and glycerol occurs via inter-organ metabolism in the body. Note that glycerol released from triacylglycerol in white adipose tissue and skeletal muscle is released from the tissues due to their lack of glycerol kinase. In healthy post-absorptive individuals, the pool size of each metabolite in the plasma is generally constant, with $R_a=R_d$ and PS=PD. AAs, amino acids; FFAs, free fatty acids; LV, liver; OPGs, other precursors of glucose; SKM, skeletal muscle; WAT, white adipose tissue.

7.1.6.3 Assessments of Product-Precursor Relationships in Metabolism Using Radioactive or Stable Tracers

In humans and other animals, a product (e.g., glucose) can be synthesized from AAs and other substrates (e.g., lactate, propionate, and glycerol). The ratio of the SR (or the MPE) in a product to the SR (or the MPE) in its precursor at the isotopic steady state can be used to determine a product-precursor relationship or the percentage of the contribution of the precursor to product formation (Zak et al. 1979). For example, if the steady-state SR of ^{14}C-glucose in the plasma of an animal infused constantly with ^{14}C-alanine is 50 dpm/nmol and the steady-state SR of ^{14}C-alanine in the plasma is 100 dpm/nmol, we can state that 50% of the newly synthesized glucose is derived from alanine. When a stable isotope tracer (e.g., ^{13}C-alanine) is used, the SR values of ^{14}C-glucose and ^{14}C-alanine in the plasma at plateau are measured to calculate the contribution of alanine to glucose production. The use of MPE or TTR in the calculation depends on whether the tracer plus its tracee or only the tracee participates in the metabolic process under study. A similar approach is used to determine the fraction of protein that has been newly synthesized from AAs (e.g., ^{14}C-Phe or ^{13}C-Phe as a tracer) in cells or the whole body, but the expression of IE (either MPE or TTR) must be consistent.

$$\text{Percentage of product from precursor } (\%) =$$

$$\frac{\text{Specific radioactivity of product at plateau (dpm / nmol)}}{\text{Specific radioactivity of precursor at plateau (dpm / nmol)}} \times 100$$

$$\text{Percentage of product from precursor } (\%) =$$

$$\frac{\text{Isotopic enrichment of product at plateau (MPE or TTR)}}{\text{Isotopic enrichment of precursor at plateau (MPE or TTR)}} \times 100$$

7.1.7 WHY ARE ISOTOPES USED IN METABOLIC RESEARCH?

Radioactive or stable isotopes are extensively used in research involving AA metabolism. The choice of a tracer depends on experimental design or biological questions to be asked. Isotopes offer the following unique advantages over studies that involve no tracers.

7.1.7.1 Tracing Metabolic Pathways

Radioisotopes or stable isotopes allow for the tracing of specific atoms in an AA or other substances in metabolic pathways (Fukagawa et al. 1989; Garlick et al. 1975; Gasier et al. 2009; Wu and Thompson 1987). For example, L-[1-^{14}C]leucine and L-[U-^{14}C]leucine are used to determine (1) the oxidative decarboxylation of leucine plus the net release of its α-ketoacid (α-ketoisocaproate); and (2) the oxidation of all leucine carbons to CO_2, respectively (Table 7.8). Additionally, data on $^{14}CO_2$ production from L-[1-^{14}C]leucine and L-[U-^{14}C]leucine can provide the necessary basis to calculate: (1) the oxidation of leucine carbons 2–6 via the Krebs cycle; (2) the net transamination of leucine; (3) the percentage of transaminated leucine released as its α-ketoacid; and (4) the percentage of decarboxylated leucine oxidized to CO_2. Thus, the metabolic fate of leucine can be identified in response to nutritional, physiological, and pathological changes. In many cases, tracer experiments provide unequivocal evidence to indicate the presence or absence of a metabolic pathway in cells or tissues (e.g., the syntheses of putrescine, spermidine, and spermine from proline in enterocytes and the placenta).

Isotopes also have other important applications in biochemical studies. For example, ^{32}P-ATP is employed to quantify protein phosphorylation as a mechanism that may regulate AA metabolism. L-[2-^{15}N]glutamine is useful to trace the metabolic fate of its α-amino group nitrogen,

TABLE 7.8
Effects of DL-β-Hydroxybutyrate (HB) and Acetoacetate (AcAc) on Leucine (Leu) Degradation in Skeletal Muscle from 10-Day-Old Fed Chicks[a]

Ketone Body	CO_2 Production from Total Leu Oxidation[†] (A)	CO_2 Production from Leu Decarboxylation[‡] (B)	CO_2 Production from the Oxidation of Leu Carbons 2–6 ($C = A - B$)	Net Production of α-Keto-isocaproate from Leu (D)	Net Trans-amination of Leu ($E = B + D$)	Percentage of Trans-aminated Leu Released as KIC, % ($D \times 100)/E$	Percentage of Decarboxylated Leu Oxidized to CO_2, % ($C \times 100)/5B$
0 mM HB	1.33±0.14	0.44±0.05	0.88±0.08	0.09±0.01	0.53±0.05	17.1±1.8	40.1±2.9
1 mM HB	1.16±0.08	0.31±0.03[b]	0.85±0.05	0.10±0.01	0.42±0.04	24.4±2.8	57.4±5.1[c]
4 mM HB	1.16±0.06	0.33±0.02[b]	0.83±0.05	0.38±0.04[c,e]	0.71±0.03[c,e]	52.5±3.9[c,e]	51.4±4.5
1 mM AcAs	0.91±0.12[b]	0.32±0.02[b]	0.59±0.11[b]	0.27±0.03[c]	0.59±0.03	44.6±3.8[c,d]	35.5±5.1
4 mM AcAc	0.59±0.05[c,d]	0.23±0.01[c]	0.36±0.06[c,d]	0.38±0.04[c,d]	0.61±0.04	61.5±2.0[c,e]	31.1±5.1

Source: Wu, G. and J.R. Thompson. 1987. *Int. J. Biochem.* 19:937–943.

[a] Values, expressed as nmol/mg fresh tissue per h, are means±SEM, $n=6$ chicks. The extensor digitorum communis muscle was isolated from 10-day-old fed chicks, inserted into a stainless wire support, and incubated for 2h at 37°C in 3.5 mL of oxygenated (95% O_2/5% CO_2) Krebs bicarbonate buffer (pH 7.4) containing 2 mM HEPES, 5 mM D-glucose, insulin (0.01 U/mL), 0.5 mM L-leucine, and all other amino acids at concentrations found in the plasma of fed young chicks. The incubation medium also contained either L-[U-^{14}C]leucine (300 dpm/nmol leucine) or L-[1-^{14}C]leucine (300 dpm/nmol leucine) to measure the rates of leucine degradation in the muscle. $^{14}CO_2$ produced from ^{14}C-leucine degradation was collected in Hyamine hydroxide. Parallel incubations with the same amount of L-[U-^{14}C]leucine or L-[1-^{14}C]leucine but without muscle were performed as blanks to provide background values for $^{14}CO_2$. Data were statistically analyzed by one-way analysis of variance and the Student-Newman-Keuls multiple comparison test.

[b] $P<0.05$ and [c] $P<0.01$: significantly different from the control group, respectively.

[d] $P<0.05$ and [e] $P<0.01$: significantly different from the corresponding 1 mM ketone body group, respectively.

[†] Determined with L-[U-^{14}C]leucine. All the 6 carbons of leucine were uniformly labeled with ^{14}C. The measured intracellular specific radioactivity of L-[U-^{14}C]leucine was 248 dpm/nmol leucine or 41.35 dpm/nmol carbon of leucine.

[‡] Determined with L-[1-^{14}C]leucine. The carbon-1 (carboxyl carbon) of leucine was labeled with ^{14}C. The measured intracellular specific radioactivity of L-[1-^{14}C]leucine was 248 dpm/nmol leucine or 248 dpm/nmol carbon-1 of leucine.

while distinguishing this nitrogen from the amide group of glutamine. In addition, the generation of ^3H_2O from [5-^{3}H]glucose during glycolysis in cells (e.g., lymphocytes) or tissues (e.g., skeletal muscle) incubated in the presence or absence of 2 mM glutamine is a valid indicator of the effect of this AA on glycolysis. Furthermore, the production of ^{15}NO from L-[guanidino-$^{15}N_2$]arginine provides the definitive proof that one of the two identical nitrogen atoms in the guanidino group of arginine serves as the physiological source of NO synthesized by mammalian cells (e.g., macrophages and endothelial cells). Similarly, L-[ring-2,6-^{3}H]phenylalanine, L-[ring-$^2H_5$]phenylalanine, or L-[ring-$^{13}C_6$]phenylalanine is often used as a tracer to measure protein synthesis and degradation *in vitro* and *in vivo*.

7.1.7.2 High Sensitivity of Detection of Tracers

Radioisotopes and stable isotopes are readily detected with very high sensitivity by liquid scintillation spectrometry and mass spectrometry, respectively. Radiotracer methods are normally much more sensitive than methods using stable isotopes. Among all routine chemical analyses, liquid scintillation spectrometry is the most sensitive technique. With an appropriately managed environment, background values are usually very low (e.g., <20 dpm for ^{14}C and ^{3}H). These instruments offer the most sensitive analytical methods to quantify the rates of many biochemical reactions in cells and organisms. For example, when incubated in the presence of 1 mM L-glutamine, 1×10^6 lymphocytes produce only approximately 3 nmol CO_2 from oxidation of this AA per h. If ^{14}C-glutamine was not included in cell incubation or culture medium, such a very small amount of CO_2 would not have been detected by a CO_2 analyzer. Likewise, in *in vitro* experiments, skeletal muscle from young rats incorporates only about 0.2 nmol phenylalanine into protein per mg tissue within 2 h. Such a small change in protein synthesis relative to the amount of total protein in the tissue cannot be detected by measuring the amount of tissue protein before and after a period of 2-h incubation. However, this seemingly impossible task can be easily accomplished by the administration of a flooding dose of L-phenylalanine plus L-[ring-2,6-^{3}H]phenylalanine to the incubation or culture medium or to the whole body to subsequently quantify the amount of peptide-bound L-[^{3}H]phenylalanine in tissue proteins.

7.2 INTERPRETATION OF DATA FROM ISOTOPE EXPERIMENTS

In tracer experiments, a radioisotope or a stable isotope is administered to an animal, or added to tissue or cell incubation medium, followed by the measurement of labeled products as well as SR (for a radioactive tracer) or IE (for a stable isotope) of the tracer at plateau in cells or a compartment of interest. Based on these data, the rate of the metabolism of a substrate or the rate of product formation is calculated, as detailed in the preceding sections. This means that an investigator obtains data from a black box.

Radioisotope or stable isotope in substrates → BLACK BOX → Radioactivity or stable isotope in products.

To interpret data from tracer studies, it is very important to have adequate knowledge of the metabolic pathways in this black box and to take necessary caution when interpreting the data obtained. For example, if $^{14}CO_2$ is provided to plants or animals, newly formed ^{14}C-glucose is found in both experimental organisms (Figure 7.5). Does this mean that glucose is synthesized from CO_2 in both plants and animals? During the process of photosynthesis, there is a net synthesis of glucose from CO_2 and H_2O in plants, with sunlight as the source of energy. However, there are no known metabolic pathways by which a net synthesis of glucose from CO_2 and H_2O occurs in any animal species, including cattle, chickens, dogs, humans, pigs, rats, and sheep. How does ^{14}C from $^{14}CO_2$ appear in glucose produced in these animals? This question illustrates some of the problems associated with tracer experiments, which will be discussed in the following sections.

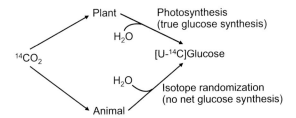

FIGURE 7.5 Appearance of ^{14}C from $^{14}CO_2$ in glucose when the tracer is administered to either plants or animals. Plants can convert CO_2 and H_2O to glucose through photosynthesis. However, this metabolic pathway is absent from animals. The appearance of ^{14}C from $^{14}CO_2$ in the plasma glucose should not be taken to indicate a net synthesis of glucose from CO_2 and H_2O in animals (e.g., cows, pigs, and humans).

7.2.1 CHANGES IN THE SR OR IE OF THE INTRACELLULAR LABELED PRECURSOR POOL

7.2.1.1 Increased Dilution of Labeled Isotopes in Cells

In a radiotracer study, the amount of radioactivity in a product is influenced by the SR of the precursor, which is affected by the dilution of the labeled precursor. Similarly, in an experiment involving a stable isotope, the mass of the stable isotope in a product is influenced by the IE of the precursor, which is affected by the dilution of the labeled precursor. Of particular note, many AAs (including glutamate, glutamine, aspartate, proline, ornithine, and arginine) are metabolized to form intermediates of the Krebs cycle within mitochondria (Chapter 3). The carbons of these AAs do not pass directly through citrate. Rather, a portion of the molecule is converted into citrate and returned to α-ketoglutarate. Because of the enzyme-catalyzed reactions involving both asymmetric and symmetric carbons, the labeled carbons derived from these AAs can be diluted within the Krebs cycle to a different extent. The greater the fraction of mitochondrial oxaloacetate that is recycled within the Krebs cycle, the greater is the differential dilution of substrate's carbon atoms. This phenomenon is known as differential dilution of the isotope within the Krebs cycle, which results in underestimations of both oxidation and glucogenic capacity of AAs in cells and in the whole body.

Isotope dilution may potentially lead to an underestimation of product formation if the intracellular SR of the labeled substrate at the site of its metabolism is not accurately determined. Let's assume that the production of $^{14}CO_2$ from the oxidation of L-[U-^{14}C]arginine in the presence of 0.5 mM L-arginine is decreased by 50% in hepatocytes incubated with 2 mM L-glutamate compared with the absence of L-glutamate. Does this mean that less L-arginine is oxidized in the presence of L-glutamate than in the absence of L-glutamate? The answer is not necessarily so. Why? This is because the oxidation of both arginine and glutamate to form CO_2 occurs via the formation of α-ketoglutarate as a common intermediate. [U-^{14}C]α-Ketoglutarate produced from L-[U-^{14}C]arginine is diluted by unlabeled α-ketoglutarate generated from unlabeled L-glutamate. Therefore, the SR of intracellular L-[U-^{14}C]α-ketoglutarate at the site of oxidation is lower in the presence of 5 mM L-glutamate than in its absence, leading to the reduced production of $^{14}CO_2$ from L-[U-^{14}C]arginine. Note that it is $^{14}CO_2$, but not CO_2, that is analyzed by liquid scintillation spectrometry. However, our ultimate interest is the production of CO_2, but not $^{14}CO_2$, by cells or the body. To determine whether oxidation of L-arginine to CO_2 in hepatocytes is suppressed by exogenous L-glutamate, the SR of [^{14}C]α-ketoglutarate in the mitochondria of hepatocytes incubated in the presence or absence of the added glutamate must be determined for the accurate calculation of CO_2 production.

Now, let us look at another example of isotope dilution. Liver slices are incubated with [1-^{14}C] alanine plus 1 mM alanine in the presence or absence of 5 mM glucose. Addition of 5 mM glucose to the basal incubation medium results in decreased production of $^{14}CO_2$. Does this mean that glucose decreases oxidation of carbon-1 of alanine? The answer is "not necessarily so". The addition of 5 mM glucose to the medium will produce more pyruvate via glycolysis, resulting in the dilution

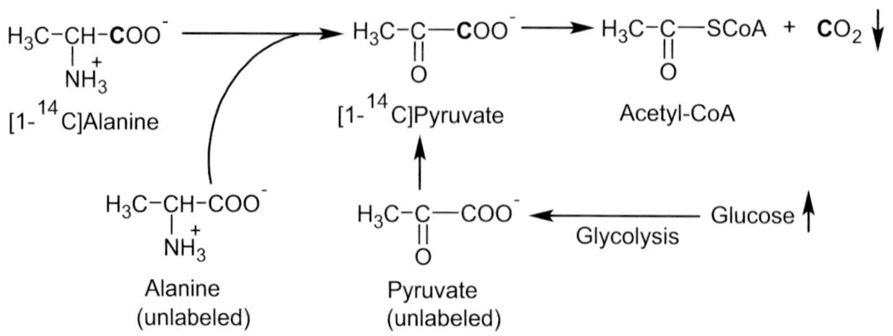

FIGURE 7.6 Dilution of the labeled precursor by the unlabeled substrate in liver. Liver slices are incubated at 37°C for 2 h in the Krebs bicarbonate buffer containing L-[1-^{14}C]alanine plus 1 mM L-alanine. L-[1-^{14}C]Alanine-derived [1-^{14}C]pyruvate is diluted by unlabeled pyruvate produced from glucose. This results in decreased production of $^{14}CO_2$ from L-[1-^{14}C]alanine in the presence of glucose. Under this experimental condition, the specific radioactivity of intracellular [1-^{14}C]pyruvate should be determined to calculate the rate of CO_2 production from alanine. The bold letter represents ^{14}C.

of [1–^{14}C]alanine-derived [1–^{14}C]pyruvate and, consequently, leading to the reduced production of $^{14}CO_2$ (Figure 7.6). In this case, the SR of intracellular [1–^{14}C]pyruvate must be determined to account for isotope dilution so that the researcher could accurately calculate the rate of alanine carbon-1 oxidation.

7.2.1.2 Decreased Dilution of Labeled Isotopes in Cells

While an increase in isotope dilution (namely a decrease in the SR or IE of the labeled precursor) frequently occurs in tracer studies, the opposite may also take place. In response to a treatment, a decrease in isotope dilution leading to a greater value of the SR or IE of the labeled precursor as compared to the control group can result, in part, from a reduction in the formation of an unlabeled intermediate from metabolic pathways (e.g., protein degradation as well as the synthesis and catabolism of AAs) other than the pathway being studied. Let us use the oxidation of L-[1-^{14}C]glutamate in chick skeletal muscle as an example. In this case, a graduate student wanted to use L-cycloserine (an inhibitor of transaminases) to suppress glutamate oxidation by inhibiting glutamate transaminase in skeletal muscle incubated in the presence of L-[1-^{14}C]glutamate plus 1 mM L-glutamate and physiological concentrations of other AAs. However, the student observed that $^{14}CO_2$ production from L-[1-^{14}C]glutamate was actually increased in the presence of 1.5 mM L-cycloserine rather than in its absence. It turned out that a large amount of glutamate was produced from BCAA transamination in chick skeletal muscle. Because L-cycloserine inhibited BCAA transamination, it decreased L-glutamate production from BCAAs in the tissue. This means that, compared with the absence of L-cycloserine, intracellular ^{14}C-glutamate is less diluted in the presence of L-cycloserine, leading to a greater value of the SR of intracellular ^{14}C-glutamate and, therefore, $^{14}CO_2$ production from L-[1-^{14}C]glutamate (Figure 7.7). Again, this example illustrates the fundamental importance of measuring the SR of the substrate at the site where it is metabolized.

7.2.2 Isotope Randomization

In a preceding section of this chapter, we asked the question of why does ^{14}C from the $^{14}CO_2$ infused into animals appear in glucose? The answer to this question is "isotope randomization", which refers to random distribution of a labeled isotope among chemically indistinguishable atoms in a molecule. For example, in succinate, which is a symmetric molecule, its carbon-1 and carbon-4 are identical, and so are its carbon-2 and carbon-3. Thus, when carbon-1 and carbon-2 of succinate in the Krebs cycle are labeled with ^{14}C, all four carbons of this molecule become labeled with ^{14}C

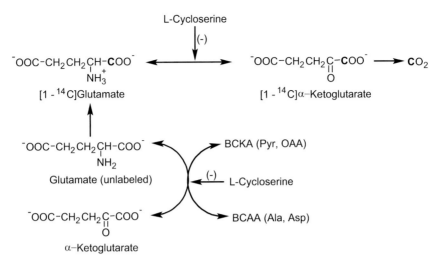

FIGURE 7.7 A reduction in the dilution of the labeled precursor due to decreased formation of the unlabeled intermediate in skeletal muscle. Chick skeletal muscle is incubated at 37°C for 2h in Krebs bicarbonate buffer containing L-[1-14C]glutamate plus 1mM L-glutamate and physiological concentrations of other AAs found in the plasma. Addition of 1.5mM L-cycloserine inhibits the production of unlabeled glutamate from BCAAs, thereby reducing the dilution of L-[1-14C]glutamate when compared with the absence of L-cycloserine. Consequently, the production of 14CO_2 from L-[1-14C]glutamate is higher in the presence of 1.5mM L-cycloserine than in its absence. Under this experimental condition, the specific activity of intracellular [1-14C]glutamate should be determined to calculate the rate of CO_2 production from glutamate. The bold letter represents 14C.

due to isotope randomization. The radioactivity of carbon-1 and carbon-4 each shares 50% of the original radioactivity in carbon-1, whereas the radioactivity of carbon-2 and carbon-3 each shares 50% of the original radioactivity in carbon-2. This means that the SR of carbon-1 and carbon-2 of the succinate molecule is reduced by 50%.

When 14CO_2 is introduced to hepatocytes, 14CO_2 and pyruvate are converted into [4-14C]oxaloacetate by pyruvate carboxylase in the mitochondrion, where [4-14C]oxaloacetate is further metabolized to [4-14C]malate by NAD+-linked malate dehydrogenase (Figure 7.8). Subsequently, [4-14C] malate is converted into [4-14C]fumarate by fumarase and then to [4-14C]succinate by succinate dehydrogenase (Chapter 4, Figure 4.2). Isotope randomization of [4-14C]succinate results in the formation of [1,4-14C]succinate, which is converted back into [1,4-14C]fumarate by succinate dehydrogenase (Brosnan 1982). Because fumarase catalyzes a reversible reaction, [1,4-14C]malate is formed from [1,4-14C]fumarate. The [1,4-14C]malate exits the mitochondrion into the cytoplasm, where it is converted by the NAD+-linked malate dehydrogenase to generate [1,4-14C]oxaloacetate, which is subsequently decarboxylated by phosphoenolpyruvate carboxykinase to produce 14CO_2 and [1-14C] phosphoenolpyruvate. Through the pathway of gluconeogenesis, two molecules of [1-14C]phosphoenolpyruvate form one molecule of [3,4-14C]glucose. In these biochemical reactions, there is a net loss of 1mol CO_2, the same amount of CO_2 that is incorporated into oxaloacetate by pyruvate carboxylase. However, isotope randomization in the Krebs cycle results in the appearance of 14C from the administered 14CO_2 in glucose, without a contribution of CO_2 to a net synthesis of glucose (Figure 7.8).

7.2.3 ISOTOPE EXCHANGE

Interconversion of metabolites results in the transfer of a labeled isotope (either radioisotope or stable isotope) from one molecule to another in cells or the body. This event is known as isotope

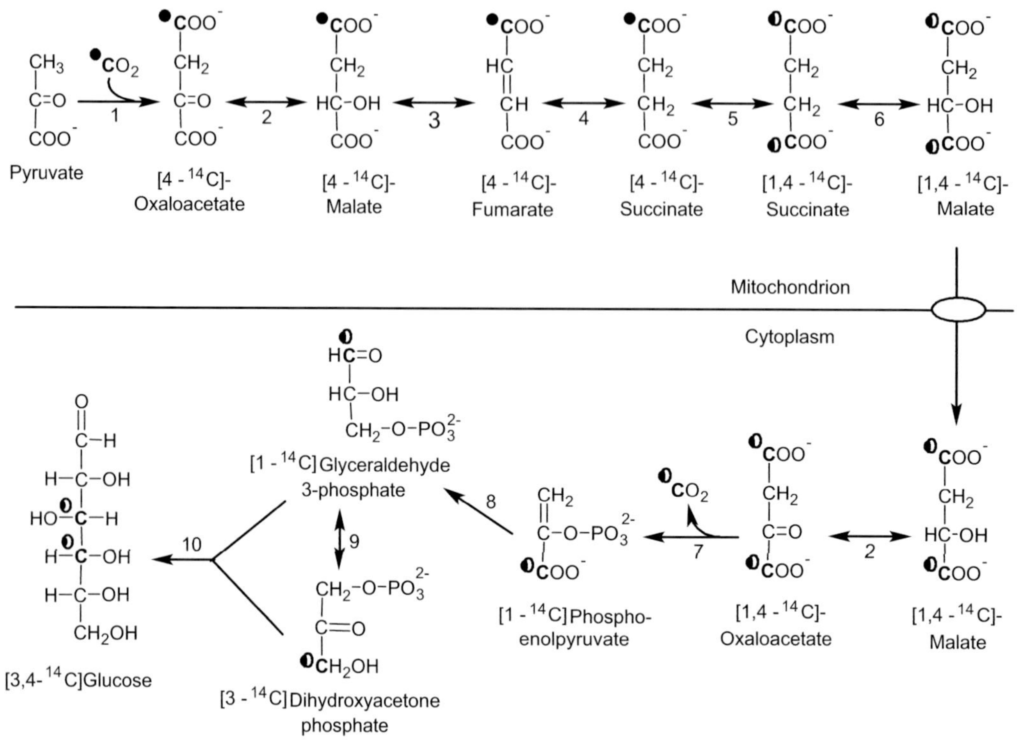

FIGURE 7.8 Isotope randomization. Because succinate is a symmetrical molecule, succinate dehydrogenase cannot distinguish carbon-1 from carbon 4 or carbon-2 from carbon-3 of its substrate, resulting in isotope randomization in the Krebs cycle. The enzymes catalyzing the indicated reactions are: (1) pyruvate carboxylase; (2) malate dehydrogenase; (3) fumarase; (4) succinate dehydrogenase; (5) isotope randomization; (6) succinate dehydrogenase and fumarase; (7) phosphoenolpyruvate carboxykinase; (8) enzymes for glycolysis; (9) phosphotriose isomerase; and (10) enzymes for gluconeogenesis. Isotope randomization results in the appearance of ^{14}C from $^{14}CO_2$ in glucose when the tracer is administered to animals, without an actual net synthesis of glucose from CO_2 and H_2O. The bold letter represents ^{14}C.

exchange (Fink et al. 1988). Let's use [3,4-^{14}C]acetoacetate as an example. When this labeled substance is introduced into skeletal muscle, [3,4-^{14}C]β-hydroxybutyrate, [3,4-^{14}C]acetoacetyl-CoA, and [1,2-^{14}C]acetyl-CoA are formed. In muscle, the oxidation of fatty acids generates unlabeled acetoacetyl-CoA and acetyl-coA. Acetyl-CoA is also produced from the catabolism of glucose, pyruvate, and AAs. Thus, [3,4-^{14}C]acetoacetate undergoes extensive exchange with the unlabeled products (acetyl-CoA and acetoacetyl-CoA) produced from glucose, AAs, and fatty acids regardless of the presence or absence of ketogenesis, resulting in the dilution of the labeled tracer (Figure 7.9). Unfortunately, the dilution of ^{14}C-acetoacetate was previously used by some investigators to estimate the production of acetoacetate and β-hydroxybutyrate by skeletal muscle. This was based on the unsubstantiated assumption that if the tissue produced acetoacetate, the SR of ^{14}C-acetoacetate would be reduced. However, Henry Brunengraber and his coworkers reported in 1988 that, in dog liver with little capacity for ketogenesis, ^{14}C-acetoacetate was also substantially diluted, indicating a problem in data interpretation when isotope exchange occurs in cells and tissues.

7.2.4 Isotope Recycling

Most substances (e.g., protein and "nutritionally nonessential" AAs) in the body undergo continuous degradation and re-synthesis, which is collectively referred to as turnover. As a result, the substrate

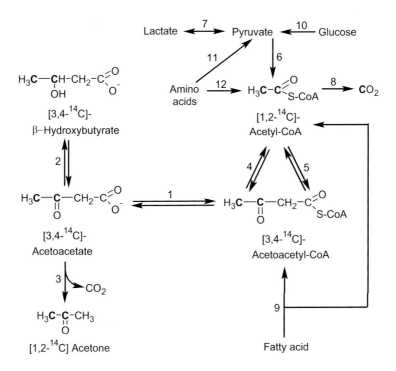

FIGURE 7.9 Isotope exchange. Interconversion of metabolites in cells results in isotope exchange and dilution of labeled precursors. The enzymes catalyzing the indicated reactions are: (1) 3-ketoacid CoA transferase or succinyl-CoA:3-ketoacid CoA transferase; (2) β-hydroxybutyrate dehydrogenase; (3) spontaneous reaction; (4) and (5) acetoacetyl-CoA thiolase; (6) pyruvate dehydrogenase; (7) lactate dehydrogenase; (8) Krebs cycle; (9) β-oxidation; (10) glycolysis; (11) conversion of glucogenic amino acids to pyruvate; and (12) conversion of ketogenic amino acids to pyruvate. The bold letter represents ^{14}C.

and the product of a biochemical reaction can be inter-converted through separate enzymes. When these compounds are labeled, isotope recycling can occur. For example, after L-[U-^{14}C]phenylalanine is incorporated into a protein, this protein will be subsequently degraded to yield L-[U-^{14}C] phenylalanine and other AAs in the cytoplasm where these AAs may be reincorporated into a new molecule of protein. Also, the degradation of L-[2-^{15}N]glutamine by phosphate-activated glutaminase generates free $^{15}NH_3$, some of which can serve as a substrate for L-glutamine synthesis in the same cell and different tissues in the body. Furthermore, L-[U-^{14}C]proline is oxidized to L-[U-^{14}C] pyrroline-5-carboxylate (P5C) by proline oxidase in the mitochondrion, and some of the L-[U-^{14}C]P5C exits to the cytoplasm for conversion into L-[U-^{14}C]proline by P5C reductase. Finally, in the presence of aspartate, [ureido-^{15}N]citrulline is converted into [gunidino-^{15}N]arginine by argininosuccinate synthase and argininosuccinate lyase, and [guanidino-^{15}N]arginine is oxidized to [ureido-^{15}N]citrulline in virtually all animal cells. Thus, recycling of the isotope can be an intracellular (in the same compartment or among organelles) or intercellular process. Note that when [guanidino-^{15}N]arginine is oxidized to produce NO by NO synthase, only 50% of the NO is labeled with because the two nitrogen atoms in ^{15}N because the two nitrogen atoms in the guanidino group of arginine are not distinguished by NO synthase but only one of them is oxidized to NO. When isotope recycling occurs, the SR or IE of the labeled substrate is increased, leading to underestimations of the activities of metabolic pathways, such as protein synthesis, glutaminolysis, and proline oxidation in the above examples (Figure 7.10). One effective means to minimize isotope recycling is to increase the extracellular concentration of the unlabeled substrate (e.g., flooding dose technology *in vivo* and in cell or tissue incubation).

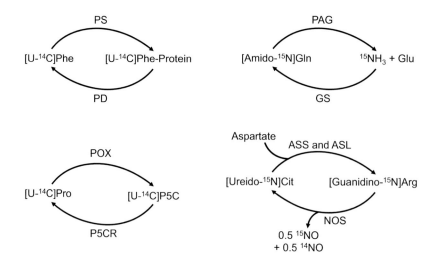

FIGURE 7.10 Isotope recycling. A labeled isotope in a product is reincorporated into its precursor. This can result in an increase in the specific activity or isotope enrichment of the labeled precursor, leading to under-estimations of product formation or metabolic flux. When [guanidino-^{15}N]arginine is oxidized to produce nitric oxide (NO) by NO synthase, only 50% of the NO is labeled with ^{15}N because the two nitrogen atoms in the guanidino group of arginine are not distinguished by NO synthase but only one of them is oxidized to NO. Arg, arginine; ASL, argininosuccinate lyase; ASS, argininosuccinate synthase; Cit, citrulline; Gln, glutamine; Glu, glutamate; GS, glutamine synthetase; NO, nitric oxide; NOS, nitric oxide synthase; PAG, phosphate-activated glutaminase; PD, protein degradation; Phe, phenylalanine; POX, proline oxidase; PS, protein synthesis; P5C, pyrroline-5-carboxylate; P5CR, pyrroline-5-carboxylate reductase.

7.2.5 ISOTOPIC NON-STEADY STATE

When a cell is exposed to a labeled AA at a constant rate (e.g., the incubation or culture of cells or a tissue, or the constant intravenous infusion of a tracer after a priming dose), its intracellular SR or IE increases until it reaches a plateau value, which is referred to as an isotopic steady state (Figure 7.11). The rate at which the SR or IE of an intracellular AA reaches isotopic steady state depends on many factors, including the extracellular concentration of the AA, the activity of AA transporters, size of the metabolic pool of the tracee AA, rates of intracellular protein turnover, as well as the rates of catabolism and/or synthesis of the AA. Ideally, intracellular SR or IE should reach the plateau value as soon as possible and be maintained for a prolonged period of time to minimize confounding issues such as isotope dilution and recycling, as well as under- and over-estimated values of SR or IE, so that the rate of a biochemical reaction can be measured accurately. This is because both the amount of radioactivity or stable isotope in the labeled product and the SR or IE of the labeled precursor are used to calculate product formation or metabolic flux. For example, when skeletal muscle from young chicks is incubated at 37°C in Krebs bicarbonate buffer containing 1 mM L-phenylalanine, L-[2,6-^{3}H]phenylalanine, and physiological concentrations of other AAs found in the plasma, the SR of intracellular L-[2,6-^{3}H]phenylalanine reaches a plateau value within 15 min after initiation of the tissue incubation. Similarly, when piglet enterocytes are incubated at 37°C in Krebs bicarbonate buffer containing 2 mM L-[U-^{13}C]glutamine and physiological concentrations of other AAs found in the plasma, the IE of intracellular L-[U-^{13}C]glutamine reaches a plateau value within 5 min after the initiation of cell incubation. Note that it is the concentration of the tracee (e.g., L-phenylalanine), not the amount of the tracer (e.g., L-[2,6-^{3}H]phenylalanine), that primarily affects the time needed for the SR or IE to reach a plateau value. However, both the concentration of the tracee (e.g., L-phenylalanine) and the amount of the radioactive tracer (e.g., L-[2,6-^{3}H]phenylalanine) or the concentration of the stable isotope tracer (e.g., L-[2,6-^{2}H]phenylalanine) determine the absolute value of SR or IE at isotopic steady state.

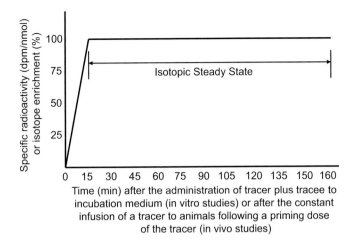

FIGURE 7.11 Isotopic steady state of a tracer in cells (*in vitro* incubation) or the plasma (*in vivo* animal studies) after the constant administration of a radioactive or stable isotope tracer. When a radioactive or stable isotope tracer is administered to cells (*in vitro* incubation) or animals (*in vivo* studies) at a constant rate, the specific radioactivity of the radioisotope or the isotope enrichment of the stable isotope at the site of its metabolism or the plasma can reach a plateau value (e.g., between 15 and 160 min after the addition of a tracer). This is known as an isotopic steady state. *In vitro* studies require the simultaneous presence of both a tracer and its tracee in the incubation medium, whereas only a tracer (but not its tracee) is administered to animals in *in vivo* studies. In animal studies, priming with a large dose of the tracer is generally used to reduce the time for the tracer to reach an isotopic steady state (plateau). Changes in the specific radioactivity of the radioisotope tracer or the isotope enrichment of the stable isotope tracer in the plasma before the start of its constant infusion to the animal are not shown in this figure. In tracer studies, an isotopic steady state in cells should be achieved as soon as possible. The X-axis refers to time after either the addition of a tracer plus its tracee to the incubation medium (*in vitro* studies) or the start of constant intravenous infusion of a tracer to an animal (*in vivo* studies). A plateau value is set at 100 dpm/nmol for a radioisotope or 100% for a stable isotope.

In some experiments, an isotopic steady state may not be obtained over a certain experimental period (Figure 7.12), resulting in an inability to accurately determine product formation from substrates. For example, when skeletal muscle from young chicks is incubated at 37°C in Krebs bicarbonate buffer containing 0.2 mM L-phenylalanine, L-[2,6-³H]phenylalanine, and physiological concentrations of other AAs found in the plasma, the SR of intracellular L-[2,6-³H]phenylalanine does not reach a plateau value within 1 h after the initiation of tissue incubation. Thus, such an incubation condition is not appropriate for determining the rate of protein synthesis in this tissue. Also, in macrophages incubated at 37°C in the Krebs bicarbonate buffer containing [6-¹⁴C]glucose and 5 mM glucose, an isotopic steady state of [6-¹⁴C]glucose is not reached during a 1-h period of incubation, and, therefore, the rate of CO_2 produced from carbon-6 of glucose cannot be accurately determined. A researcher can get around these problems by increasing extracellular concentrations of phenylalanine from 0.2 to 1 mM and by extending the time of macrophage incubation from 1 to 3 h. At the concentration of 1 mM in the incubation medium, phenylalanine does not affect the rates of protein turnover in chick or rat skeletal muscles (as measured with ¹⁴C-tyrosine), compared with 0.2 mM phenylalanine.

7.3 POTENTIAL PITFALLS OF ISOTOPIC STUDIES

The foregoing problems associated with isotopic studies may lead to potential pitfalls if investigators do not have adequate knowledge of both tracer methodologies and metabolism of the molecules under study. These pitfalls may include incorrect data interpretation, misleading conclusions, and unwarranted assumptions, as indicated in the preceding sections. Let's use oxidation of L-[1-¹⁴C]

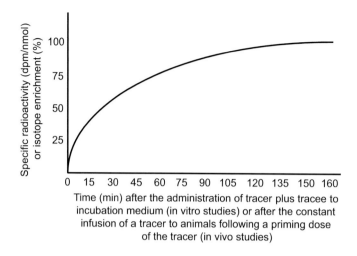

FIGURE 7.12 Isotopic non-steady state of a tracer in cells (*in vitro* incubation) or the plasma (*in vivo* animal studies) after the constant administration of a radioactive or stable isotope tracer. When a radioactive or stable isotope tracer is administered to cells (*in vitro* incubation) or animals (*in vivo* studies) at a constant rate but the extracellular concentration of the tracee is low, the specific radioactivity of the radioisotope or the isotope enrichment of the stable isotope at the site of its metabolism or the plasma does not reach a plateau value within a prolonged period of time (e.g., 160 min in this example). This is known as isotopic non-steady state. In tracer studies, isotopic non-steady state in cells or the plasma should be avoided. The X-axis refers to time after either the addition of a tracer plus its tracee to the incubation medium (*in vitro* studies) or the start of constant intravenous infusion of a tracer to an animal (*in vivo* studies). A plateau value is set at 100 dpm/nmol for a radioisotope or 100% for a stable isotope.

valine and L-[U-^{14}C]valine in rats (Table 7.9) as an example of how to carefully and correctly interpret data from isotopic studies.

In this example, rats were fed either a low-protein diet (2.5% protein) or a high-protein diet (21.5% protein) for 16 days and then, they received a single administration of L-[1-^{14}C]valine or L-[U-^{14}C] valine via enteral feeding. The percentage of the administered L-[U-^{14}C]valine appearing in expired $^{14}CO_2$ during subsequent 1 h was measured. The percentage of L-[U-^{14}C]valine exhaled as $^{14}CO_2$

TABLE 7.9

Production of $^{14}CO_2$ by Rats Fed a Low- or a High-Protein Diet for 1 h after Receiving a Single Enteral Administration of L-[1-^{14}C]Valine or L-[U-^{14}C]Valine[a]

Diet	Labeled AA	% of ^{14}C-Valine Excreted as $^{14}CO_2$
Low Protein	L-[U-^{14}C]Valine	85
High protein	L-[U-^{14}C]Valine	56
Low Protein	L-[1-^{14}C]Valine	46
High Protein	L-[1-^{14}C]Valine	69

Source: Reeds, P.J. 1974. *Br. J. Nutr.* 31:259–270.

[a] Rats were fed a low-protein (2.5% protein) or high-protein (21.5% protein) diet for 16 days. Thereafter, rats were given by tube a single dose of 5 μCi of either L-[U-^{14}C]valine or L-[1-^{14}C] valine per 100 g body-weight. The amino acids were administered in casein hydrolysate supplying a total of 10 μmol valine per 100 g body-weight. $^{14}CO_2$ produced by the individual rats was collected for 1 h immediately after the administration of the isotopes.

within 1 h after the administration of the radioisotope was higher in rats fed the low-protein diet than in rats fed the high-protein diet. These data appear to suggest that feeding rats a high-protein diet reduces valine oxidation in rats. This suggestion would not be consistent with our knowledge of valine metabolism and nutrition in animals. Then, how could these results be explained satisfactorily? To address this question, let's review how $^{14}CO_2$ is produced from the oxidation of L-[1-^{14}C] valine or L-[U-^{14}C]valine. As illustrated in Chapter 4, the oxidative decarboxylation of valine by branched-chain α-ketoacid dehydrogenase releases carbon-1 from valine and the remaining carbons can be oxidized to CO_2 via the Krebs cycle. Concentrations of valine in the plasma are lower in rats fed the low-protein diet compared with rats fed the high-protein diet. Thus, L-[U-^{14}C]valine in the plasma and in cells is diluted to a lesser extent in the rats fed the low-protein diet, as the animals oxidize more L-[U-^{14}C]valine and excrete more $^{14}CO_2$. Note that the dilution of ^{14}C-labeled valine carbons occurs both at the BCKA dehydrogenase step and in the Krebs cycle primarily due to the formation of unlabeled acetyl-CoA from the oxidation of AAs other than valine. Because the complete oxidation of the decarboxylated carbon skeleton of L-[U-^{14}C]valine via the Krebs cycle accounts for 80% of its $^{14}CO_2$ production, isotope dilution in mitochondria is the major reason for the observation that rats fed the low-protein diet produced lesser amounts of $^{14}CO_2$ from L-[U-^{14}C] valine than rats fed the high-protein diet. However, this should not be taken to indicate that feeding a high-protein diet reduces valine oxidation in rats.

In contrast to the experiment involving L-[U-^{14}C]valine, consumption of the low-protein diet reduced the production of $^{14}CO_2$ from L-[1-^{14}C]valine in rats compared with the high-protein diet. Note that $^{14}CO_2$ is generated from L-[1-^{14}C]valine only at the step of oxidative decarboxylation by BCKA dehydrogenase, but not via the Krebs cycle. It is likely that: (1) the dilution of L-[1-^{14}C] valine in the plasma and cells of rats fed the high-protein diet occurs to a relatively lesser extent than the activation of L-[1-^{14}C]valine oxidation for $^{14}CO_2$ production; (2) compared to rats fed the low-protein diet, the high-protein diet stimulates oxidative decarboxylation of L-[1-^{14}C]valine to a much greater extent than that which would be offset by the dilution of L-[1-^{14}C]valine-derived L-[1-^{14}C]α-ketoacid in the cytoplasm and mitochondria. To support these possible explanations, the SR of L-[1-^{14}C]valine in major organs for valine transamination and oxidative decarboxylation should be determined in rats fed the low-protein and high-protein diets.

Because the same amounts of L-[1-^{14}C]valine and L-[U-^{14}C]valine were administered to the rats, the rate of $^{14}CO_2$ production from L-[1-^{14}C]valine should be greater than that from L-[U-^{14}C]valine which has only 20% of its radioactivity in the carboxyl carbon. Thus, in rats fed the high-protein diet, the percentage of L-[1-^{14}C]valine excreted as $^{14}CO_2$ was higher than that of L-[U-^{14}C]valine although the increase was much less than expected. By contrast, in rats fed the low-protein diet, the percentage of L-[1-^{14}C]valine excreted as $^{14}CO_2$ was lower than that of L-[U-^{14}C]valine within 1 h after the administration of the radioisotopes. Such an observation is in striking contrast to expected results and can be explained by additional data on: (1) the SR of L-[1-^{14}C]valine and L-[U-^{14}C] valine, as well as the SR of their α-ketoacids at isotopic steady state; (2) $^{14}CO_2$ production from the radioisotopes at various time times within 1 h of their administration, in major tissues of valine catabolism.

7.4 SUMMARY

Radioisotopes and stable isotopes have been employed in biochemical research for over a half century. Priming with a large dose of the tracer chosen for a study is generally used to reduce the time for the tracer to reach an isotopic steady state (plateau). In these studies, the calculation of product formation is based on the SR of the radioisotope or the IE of the stable isotope in the plasma or at the site of the metabolism of the tracee. Because isotopes occur in nature, the background radioactivity values of a radioactive tracer or the background enrichment values of a stable tracer must be subtracted from the values for biological samples for calculations. The measurements of products should be made at isotopic steady state when the values of SR or IE are constant. The bolus pulse approach is also useful for studying whole-body protein turnover and AA metabolism. Tracer experiments offer the advantages of high specificity and sensitivity over conventional methods. Thus, the use of isotopes can greatly facilitate studies to identify new pathways for AA synthesis and catabolism and to understand the mechanisms responsible for regulating AA metabolism in cells and in the body. Without isotopes, it would not be possible to perform many key biochemical or nutritional experiments (e.g., the oxidation and synthesis of AAs, as well as the synthesis and degradation of protein) at cellular, molecular, and whole-body levels. Common problems encountered in tracer experiments include dilution, randomization, exchange, and recycling of isotopes, as well as isotopic non-steady state in cells or the plasma. As with all biological experiments, adequate knowledge of biology and due caution should be exercised when performing tracer studies. Additionally, all necessary steps must be taken to avoid potential pitfalls leading to incorrect conclusions.

REFERENCES

Allen, D.K. and J.D. Young. 2020. Tracing metabolic flux through time and space with isotope labeling experiments. *Curr. Opin. Biotechnol.* 64:92–100.

Bequette, B.J., N.E. Sunny, S.W. El-Kadi, and S.L. Owens. 2006. Application of stable isotopes and mass isotopomer distribution analysis to the study of intermediary metabolism of nutrients. *J. Anim. Sci.* 84 (Suppl):E50–E59.

Bertolo, R.F.P., J.A. Brunton, P.B. Penzharz, and R.O. Ball. 2003. Arginine, ornithine, and proline interconversion is dependent on small intestinal metabolism in neonatal pigs. *Am. J. Physiol.* 284:E915–E822.

Boelens, P.G., P.A. van Leeuwen, C.H. Dejong, and N.E. Deutz. 2005. Intestinal renal metabolism of L-citrulline and L-arginine following enteral or parenteral infusion of L-alanyl-L-[2,^{15}N]glutamine or L-[2,^{15}N]glutamine in mice. *Am. J. Physiol.* 289:G679–G685.

Brosnan, J.T. 1982. Pathways of carbon flux in gluconeogenesis. *Fed. Proc.* 41:91–95.

Brunengraber, H., J.K. Kelleher, and C. Des Rosiers. 1997. Applications of mass isotopomer analysis to nutrition research. *Annu. Rev. Nutr.* 17:559–596.

Bush, J.A., G. Wu, A. Suryawan, H.V. Nguyen, and T.A. Davis. 2002. Somatotropin-induced amino acid conservation in pigs involves differential regulation of liver and gut urea cycle enzyme activity. *J. Nutr.* 132:59–67.

Castillo, L., T.E. Chapman, M. Sanchez, Y.M. Yu, J.F. Burke, A.M. Ajami et al. 1993. Plasma arginine and citrulline kinetics in adults given adequate and arginine-free diets. *Proc. Natl. Acad. Sci. USA.* 90:7749–7753.

Darmaun, D., D.E. Matthews, and D.M. Bier. 1986. Glutamine and glutamate kinetics in humans. *Am. J. Physiol.* 251:E117–E126.

Deutz, N.E.P., J.J. Thaden, G.A.M. Ten Have, D.K. Walker, and M.P.K.J. Engelen. 2018. Metabolic phenotyping using kinetic measurements in young and older healthy adults. *Metabolism* 78:167–178.

Engelen, M.P.K.J., G.A.M. Ten Have, J.J. Thaden, and N.E.P. Deutz. 2019. New advances in stable tracer methods to assess whole-body protein and amino acid metabolism. *Curr. Opin. Clin. Nutr. Metab. Care* 22:337–346.

Fink, G., S. Desrochers, C. Des Rosiers, M. Garneau, F. David, T. Daloze, B.R. Landau, and H. Brunengraber. 1988. Pseudoketogenesis in the perfused rat heart. *J. Biol. Chem.* 263:18036–18042.

Frank, J.W., J. Escobar, H.V. Hguyen, S.C. Jobgen, W.S. Jobgen, T.A. Davis, and G. Wu. 2007. Oral N-carbamylglutamate supplementation increases protein synthesis in skeletal muscle of piglets. *J. Nutr.* 137:315–319.

Fukagawa, N.K., K.L. Minaker, V.R. Young, D.E. Matthews, D.M. Bier, and J.W. Rowe. 1989. Leucine metabolism in aging humans: effect of insulin and substrate availability. *Am. J. Physiol.* 256:E288–E294.

Garlick, P.J., D.J. Millward, W.P. James, and J.C. Waterlow. 1975. The effect of protein deprivation and starvation on the rate of protein synthesis in tissues of the rat. *Biochim. Biophys. Acta.* 414:71–84.

Gasier, H.G., S.E. Riechman, M.P. Wiggs, S.F. Previs, and J.D. Fluckey. 2009. A comparison of ^{2}H$_2$O and phenylalanine flooding dose to investigate muscle protein synthesis with acute exercise in rats. *Am. J. Physiol.* 297:E252–E259.

Granados, J.Z., G.A.M. Ten Have, A.C. Letsinger, J.J. Thaden, M. Engelen, J.T. Lightfoot, and N.E.P. Deutz. 2020. Activated whole-body arginine pathway in high-active mice. *PLoS One* 15:e0235095.

Hellerstein, M.K. 1991. Relationship between precursor enrichment and ratio of excess M2/excess M1 isotopomer frequencies in a secreted polymer. *J. Biol. Chem.* 266:10920–10924.

Houlihan, D.F., S.J. Hall, C. Gray, and B.S. Noble. 1988. Growth rates and protein turnover in Atlantic cod, *Gadus morhua. Can. J. Fish Aquat. Sci.* 45:951–964.

Kim, I., S. Suh, I. Lee, and R.R Wolfe. 2016. Applications of stable, nonradioactive isotope tracers in *in vivo* human metabolic research. *Exp. Mol. Med.* 48:e203.

Lapierre, H., D.R. Ouellet, R. Berthiaume, R. Martineau, G. Holtrop, and Lobley, G.E. 2008. Distribution of ^{15}N in amino acids during ^{15}N-leucine infusion: impact on the estimation of endogenous flows in dairy cows. *J. Dairy Sci.* 91:2702–2714.

Lobley, G. E. 2003. Protein turnover—what does it mean for animal production? *Can. J. Anim. Sci.* 83:327–340.

Maharjan, P., G. Mullenix, K. Hilton, A. Beitia, J. Weil, N. Suesuttajit et al. 2020. Effects of dietary amino acid levels and ambient temperature on mixed muscle protein turnover in *Pectoralis major* during finisher feeding period in two broiler lines. *J. Anim. Physiol. Anim. Nutr.* 104:1351–1364.

Marliss, E.B., S. Chevalier, R. Gougeon, J.A. Morais, M. Lamarche, O.A.J. Adegoke, and G. Wu. 2006. Elevations of plasma methylarginines in obesity and ageing are related to insulin sensitivity and rates of protein turnover. Diabetologia 49:351–359.

Marshall, C.P. and R.W. Fairbridge. 1999. *Encyclopedia of Geochemistry.* Springer, New York.

Pereira, S., E.B. Marliss, J.A. Morais, S. Chevalier, and R. Gougeon. 2008. Insulin resistance of protein metabolism in type 2 diabetes. *Diabetes* 57:56–63.

Raguso, C.A., P. Pereira, and V.R. Young. 1999. A tracer investigation of obligatory oxidative amino acid losses in healthy, young adults. *Am. J. Clin. Nutr.* 70:474–483.

Reeds, P.J. 1974. The catabolism of valine in malnourished rat. Studies in vivo and in vitro with different labelled forms of valine. *Br. J. Nutr.* 31:259–270.

Schoenheimer, R. and D. Rittenberg. 1938. The application of isotopes to the study of intermediary metabolism. *Science* 87:221–226.

Schoenheimer, R., D. Rittenberg, G.L. Foster, A.S. Keston, and S. Ratner. 1938. The application of the nitrogen isotope N^{15} for the study of protein metabolism. *Science* 88:599–600.

Stoll, B., D.G. Burrin, J. Henry, H. Yu, F. Jahoor, and P.J. Reeds. 1999. Substrate oxidation by the portal drained viscera of fed piglets. *Am. J. Physiol.* 277:E168–E175.

Ten Have, G.A.M., M.P.K.J. Engelen, R.R. Wolfe, and N.E.P. Deutz. 2017. Phenylalanine isotope pulse method to measure effect of sepsis on protein breakdown and membrane transport in the pig. *Am. J. Physiol.* 312:E519–E529.

Ten Have, G.A.M., M. Engelen, R.R. Wolfe, and N.E.P. Deutz. 2019. Inhibition of jejunal protein synthesis and breakdown in pseudomonas aeruginosa-induced sepsis pig model. *Am. J. Physiol.* 316:G755–762.

Watford, M. and G. Wu. 2005. Glutamine metabolism in uricotelic species: variation in skeletal muscle glutamine synthetase, glutaminase, glutamine levels and rates of protein synthesis. *Comp. Biochem. Physiol.* B. 140:607–614.

Wijayasinghe, M.S., L.P. Milligan, and J.R. Thompson. 1983. In vitro degradation of leucine in muscle, adipose tissue, liver, and kidney of fed and starved sheep. Biosci. Rep. 3:1133–1140.

Wilkinson, D.J. 2018. Historical and contemporary stable isotope tracer approaches to studying mammalian protein metabolism. *Mass Spectrom. Rev.* 37:57–80.

Wolfe, R.R. 1993. *Tracers in Metabolic Research.* Alan R. Liss, Inc., New York.

Wu, G. 1997. Synthesis of citrulline and arginine from proline in enterocytes of postnatal pigs. *Am. J. Physiol.* 272:G1382–G1390.

Wu, G. and J.R. Thompson. 1987. Ketone bodies inhibit leucine degradation in chick skeletal muscle. *Int. J. Biochem.* 19:937–943.

Zak, R., A.F. Martin, and R. Blough. 1979. Assessment of protein turnover by use of radioisotopic tracers. *Physiol. Rev.* 59:407–447.

8 Protein Synthesis

Amino acids (AAs) have been known to be components of proteins since the early 1900s. In 1901, A. Kossel (a Nobel laureate) suggested that individual AAs were added to the protein molecule in varying amounts. One year later, E. Fischer (another Nobel laureate) correctly proposed that proteins result from the formation of bonds between the amino group of one AA and the carboxyl group of another AA in a linear structure termed peptides. In the same year, O. Loewi reported that dogs fed a diet consisting of protein-free hydrolysates of pancreatic tissues could maintain positive nitrogen balance, and suggested that animals must synthesize their own body proteins from AAs as the products of the breakdown of dietary protein occurring in the lumen of the small intestine. However, how peptide bonds are formed from AAs in cells puzzled biochemists at that time. A series of isotopic studies by R. Schoenheimer and coworkers in the 1930s showed that ^{15}N-labeled tyrosine and leucine could be incorporated into proteins in animals. Thirty years later, the pathway of protein synthesis was discovered by several groups of scientists using both eukaryotes (organisms with a nucleus enclosed within a nuclear envelope, such as animals, plants, and yeast) and bacteria. Because the K_m values of aminoacyl-tRNA synthases for AAs are lower than those of AA-degrading enzymes (Krebs 1972), protein synthesis takes precedence over AA catabolism in animal cells and microbes (Waterlow 1984). The molecular mechanisms for the nutritional regulation of this biochemical event began to be unfolded in the 1990s when the activation of the mechanistic target of rapamycin (MTOR) signaling pathway by certain AAs (e.g., leucine) in animal cells was discovered (Blommaart et al. 1995). This seminal finding was confirmed *in vivo* (e.g., Anthony et al. 2000; Davis et al. 2008; Suryawan et al. 2011; Yin et al. 2010). In essence, protein synthesis represents a major physiological process for AA utilization in cells. In this chapter, the pathway of intracellular protein synthesis in animals will be described along with its characteristics, significance, and measurement.

8.1 HISTORICAL PERSPECTIVES OF THE PROTEIN SYNTHESIS PATHWAY

The history of studies of the metabolic pathway responsible for protein biosynthesis dates back to the late 1930s when T. Caspersson and J. Brachet found that DNA is localized almost exclusively in the nucleus of the eukaryotic cell, whereas RNA is present primarily in the cytoplasm. J. Brachet also noted that the RNA-containing particles in the cytoplasm are rich in proteins and suggested that these particles are the site of protein synthesis. In 1941, both authors further observed that the amount of cytosolic RNA-protein complexes (later named ribosomes) is positively correlated with the rate of protein synthesis. The 1950s witnessed rapid advances in the field, including (1) K. Porter's discovery in 1952 of the endoplasmic reticulum (an organelle that consists of an interconnected network of tubules, vesicles, and cisternae) in eukaryotes, with the rough endoplasmic reticulum being involved in protein synthesis; (2) G.E. Palade's description of ribosomes consisting of RNA-protein complexes in 1953; (3) G. Gamow's suggestion of a minimum genetic code of three nucleotides in 1954; (4) isolation by M. Grunberg-Manago and S. Ochoa of the enzyme which links RNA nucleotides to form RNA *in vitro* in 1955; (5) the report by A. Kornberg in 1956 that enzymes are necessary for DNA synthesis *in vitro*; and (6) the discoveries by M.B. Hoagland and coworkers that separate enzymes catalyze the activation of different AAs for incorporation into peptides (1956), that cells contain tRNA, which combines with AAs before protein synthesis (1957), and that the DNA polymerase isolated from *E. coli* could catalyze DNA synthesis *in vitro*. In 1958, A.

Tissières and J.D. Watson isolated 70S ribosomes from *E. coli* that contain two subunits (50S and 30S), while F. Crick proposed that DNA determines the sequence of AAs in a polypeptide.

The early 1960s was the beginning of functional studies identifying an essential role for RNA in protein synthesis. Specifically, S. Weiss and J. Hurtwitz independently discovered in 1960 that RNA polymerase (a nucleotidyl transferase) is responsible for the DNA-directed synthesis of RNA. Additionally, five landmark papers published in 1961 showed that: (1) the production of a particular AA sequence by a specific RNA (by M. Nirenberg and H. Mathei); (2) the presence and function of mRNA in protein synthesis (independently reported by F. Jacob and J. Monod, and by S. Brenner, F. Jacob, and M. Meselson); (3) direct evidence that the genetic code is a triplet-deoxynucleotide unit (by F. Crick and J.D. Watson); and (4) the compelling proof that the mRNA molecule is formed on one DNA template strand (by B.D. Hall and S. Spiegelman). Two years later, H.M. Temin reported that, in certain viruses, RNA synthesizes DNA, which in turn codes for proteins. In 1964, the biochemistry of tRNA molecules was uncovered when R.W. Holley identified the nucleotide sequence of the alanine-tRNA molecule in yeast and M. Nirenberg and P. Leder found that the binding of tRNA to the ribosome depends on mRNA as a template. Thus, by the mid-1960s, the pathway for protein synthesis in animal cells had been established, in which DNA is transcribed forming messenger RNA (mRNA), transfer RNA (tRNA), and ribosomal RNA (rRNA, a component of the ribosome), with specific tRNA bringing their corresponding AAs to the mRNA template for the formation of polypeptides.

8.2 BIOCHEMICAL PATHWAYS OF PROTEIN SYNTHESIS IN THE CYTOPLASM OF ANIMAL CELLS

8.2.1 Overall View of Protein Synthesis in the Cytoplasm of Animal Cells

The process of cytosolic protein synthesis in eukaryotes (including humans and other animals) is now well understood and includes five steps: (1) gene transcription; (2) initiation of translation; (3) peptide elongation; (4) termination; and (5) posttranslational modifications (Pain 1996). Steps 2–4 are collectively referred to as mRNA translation (the formation of a polypeptide from AAs on the mRNA template). Note that tRNA is necessary for translation, because mRNA cannot directly recognize AAs but can bind to a tRNA that carries a corresponding AA. In essence, the mRNA synthesized from DNA encodes the polypeptide with each AA designated by a specific codon (three nucleotides). The genetic codes for AAs are summarized in Table 8.1. tRNAs serve as the adaptors to translate genetic information from nucleic acids into proteins with ribosomes as the factories. The overall pathway of cytosolic protein synthesis is illustrated in Figure 8.1.

Cytosolic protein synthesis takes place in all cell types of animals, including those that lack nuclei but retain presynthesized mRNAs, tRNAs, and ribosomes in the cytoplasm, such as reticulocytes (immature red blood cells), erythrocytes (mature red blood cells), and platelets (Kabanova et al. 2009; Mills et al. 2016). This biochemical process is necessary to replace the proteins that are continuously degraded and to maintain their homeostasis in these cells. As indicated in Chapter 4, K_M values (1.5–30 mM) of enzymes for AA degradation are much greater than K_M values (0.2–0.4 mM) of AA-tRNA synthetases for AAs as the building blocks of proteins. Thus, protein synthesis takes precedence over AA degradation in cells under physiological conditions, although all metabolic processes occur simultaneously. After a meal, AAs are used mainly for protein synthesis, and the amount of AAs entering their degradation pathways will depend on their intracellular concentrations, as well as endocrine status and cell signaling. This means that it is very important to maintain a proper balance of AAs for maximum protein synthesis to minimize AA oxidation in animals. Based on the studies of proteolysis (Fagan et al. 1986), the rate of protein synthesis in erythrocytes is likely much lower than that in reticulocytes to maintain particularly high concentrations of hemoglobin in the erythrocytes. Therefore, the rates of protein synthesis vary with cell types and their physiological needs.

TABLE 8.1
The Standard Genetic Codons for Amino Acids in Protein Biosynthesis[a]

First Position (5' End)	Second Position				Third Position (3' End)
	U	**C**	**A**	**G**	
U	Phe	Ser	Tyr	Cys	U
	Phe	Ser	Tyr	Cys	C
	Leu	Ser	Stop	Stop[c]	A
	Leu	Ser	Stop[d]	Trp	G
C	Leu	Pro	His	Arg	U
	Leu	Pro	His	Arg	C
	Leu	Pro	Gln	Arg	A
	Leu	Pro	Gln	Arg	G
A	Ile	Thr	Asn	Ser	U
	Ile	Thr	Asn	Ser	C
	Ile	Thr	Lys	Arg	A
	Met[b]	Thr	Lys	Arg	G
G	Val	Ala	Asp	Gly	U
	Val	Ala	Asp	Gly	C
	Val	Ala	Glu	Gly	A
	Val	Ala	Glu	Gly	G

[a] A codon on the mRNA molecule consists of three nucleotides. One AA in protein can be coded for by more than one codon. For example, Phe is specified by UUU or UUC, and Ser by UCU, UCC, UCA, or UCG.

[b] AUG codes for the initiation signal, as well as internal Met and *N*-formylmethionine residues.

[c] Selenocysteine is incorporated into a selenoprotein during translation elongation and is coded for by an internal UGA stop codon under the guidance of a specific mRNA hairpin structure located further downstream, the SECIS (selenocysteine inserting sequence) element.

A = adenine; C = cytosine; G = guanine; U = uracil

[d] UAG codes for pyrrolysine. Pyrrolysine is incorporated into methylamine methyltransferase in certain archaea and eubacteria.

8.2.2 GENE TRANSCRIPTION IN ANIMAL CELLS

The first step in protein synthesis is the transcription of a DNA gene to form rRNA, mRNA, and tRNA in the nucleus by RNA polymerases I, II, and III, respectively (Palangat and Larson 2012);. The various other types of RNA (e.g., signal recognition particle RNA, small nuclear RNA, and microRNA) are synthesized using the appropriate DNA (Venters and Pugh 2009). Each tRNA contains a trinucleotide sequence (collectively known as an anticodon), which is complementary to a codon in mRNA for a specific AA.

Eukaryotic pre-mRNA requires extensive processing to become mature mRNA before transport through the nuclear pore to the cytoplasm (Hocine et al. 2010). Several steps are required for mRNA processing, which include (1) the exo- and endo-nucleolytic removal of polynucleotide segments; (2) the modification of specific nucleosides; and (3) the addition of nucleotide sequences to the 5' end (five-prime cap, 5' cap) and 3' end [three-prime poly(A) tail]. The 5'-cap (methyl-guanosyl triphosphate) consists of a guanine nucleotide connected to the mRNA via an unusual

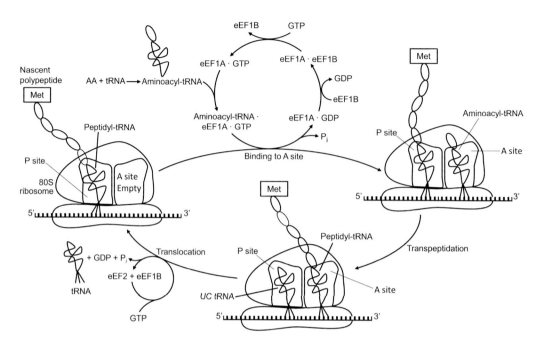

FIGURE 8.1 The biochemical pathway of protein synthesis in animal cells. The 80S ribosome is the functional site for the translation of mRNA into protein. These processes require enzymes (aminoacyl-tRNA synthetase and peptidyltransferase), eukaryotic initiation factors (eIF), elongation factors (eEF), and release factors (eRF). Met-tRNA is the initial aminoacyl-tRNA for protein synthesis in humans and other animals. eEF1A·GTP is required for the binding of an incoming aminoacyl-tRNA to the A site, and eEF1A·GDP is recycled into eEF1A·GTP under the action of eEF1B. Polypeptide elongation is terminated by a terminating codon on the mRNA template. Peptidyltransferase, together with eRF1, hydrolyzes peptidyl-tRNA to release the newly synthesized peptide. The formation of 1 mol protein requires 5 mol ATP.

5′ to 5′ triphosphate linkage and is present on the 5′ end of an mRNA. This guanosine is methylated on the 7 position by guanine-N^7-methyltransferase, with S-adenosylmethionine (SAM) as the donor of a methyl group, to form a 7-methylguanylate cap (m^7G). Further modifications in the mRNA molecule include the possible methylation of the 2′ hydroxy groups of its first two ribose sugars at the 5′ end. The 5′-cap (methyl-guanosyl triphosphate) of mRNA is critical for protection from an RNase (e.g., 5′ exonuclease), recognition of mRNA by the ribosome, and the subsequent binding of mRNA to the 40S ribosomal subunit upon entering the cytoplasm (Lackner and Bähler 2008). In addition, almost all eukaryotic mRNA molecules are polyadenylated at the 3′ end of mRNA via the covalent linkage of a polyadenylyl moiety, and this process occurs during and immediately after the transcription of DNA. Formation of the 3′ poly(A) tail in mRNA involves the cleavage of the 3′ end of the mRNA molecule and the subsequent addition of approximately 200–250 adenine residues from ATP catalyzed by polyadenylate polymerase. This biochemical reaction is enhanced by the nuclear form of poly(A)-binding protein (PABP) through an increase in the activity of poly (A) polymerase. The poly(A) tail and its associated proteins protect mRNA from degradation by exonucleases. The 3′ end polyadenylation is also important for transcription termination in the nucleus.

In eukaryotes, processed RNAs must migrate from the nucleus into the cytoplasm where protein synthesis takes place on the ribosomes of the rough endoplasmic reticulum. Although the movement of mRNA within the nucleus occurs without metabolic energy, ATP is required for the mRNA-protein complex to resume its motion when it becomes stalled within high-density chromatin. The transport of mRNA out of the nucleus is mediated by nuclear pore complexes (consisting of highly conserved protein factors) that are the channels connecting the nucleus and the cytoplasm (Hocine et al. 2010).

8.2.3 INITIATION OF mRNA TRANSLATION INTO PROTEIN IN ANIMAL CELLS

Eukaryotes have circular polyribosomes. Before polypeptide synthesis is initiated, the eukaryotic 80S ribosome (4,200 kDa) is formed from 40S and 60S ribosomal subunits (Budkevich et al. 2008; Kong and Lasko 2012). The steps of this process require initiation factors (Table 8.2). The 40S ribosomal subunit contains an 18S ribosomal RNA and 33 proteins, whereas the 60S ribosomal subunit is comprised of 28S, 5.8S, and 5S ribosomal RNAs, as well as 49 proteins. The 80S ribosomes bind mRNA efficiently in the absence of tRNA. Eukaryotic mRNA generally has only one start site and serves as the template for a single protein.

The initiation of mRNA translation into protein consists of four steps in eukaryotes (Kimball and Jefferson 2010). These processes are as follows: (1) the dissociation of the 80S ribosome into its constituent subunits; (2) the formation of the 43S preinitiation complex from the 40S ribosomal subunit, eIF1A, eIF2·GTP, and Met-tRNA$_i$; (3) the formation of the 48S initiation complex from the 43S complex, mRNA, as well as eIF-4A, 4B, 4E, and 4G; and (4) the formation, from the 48S initiation complex and the 60S ribosomal subunit, of the translationally active 80S ribosome as the site of protein synthesis (Figure 8.2).

TABLE 8.2
Roles of mRNA Translation Factors in Eukaryotic Protein Biosynthesis[a]

Protein Factors	Functions
	(1) Translation Initiation Factors
eIF1	Prevent reassociation of the 40S and 60S subunits; required for the scanning of the ribosome-bound mRNA and initiation-site selection; and promote the assembly of 48S ribosomal complexes
eIF1A[b]	Bind to the 40S subunit of the free 80S ribosome and dissociate the inactive free 80S ribosome to form the 40S and 60S subunits; stabilize the 43S preinitiation complex; and position the initiation Met-tRNA on the start codon of mRNA
eIF1B	Recognize the initiation codon and initiation site; promote the assembly of 48S ribosomal complexes at the initiation codon of a conventional capped mRNA
eIF2 (α, β, γ; GTPase)	Bring the Met-tRNA$_i$ to the 40S ribosome to promote the formation of the 43S; form a ternary complex with GTP and initiator tRNA
eIF2B (GEF)[c]	Catalyzes the exchange of eIF2-bound GDP for GTP to regenerate eIF2
eIF3 (13 subunits)	Bind to the 40S subunit of the free 80S ribosome and dissociate the inactive free 80S ribosome to form the 40S and 60S subunits; promote the assembly of the 40S subunit and the formation of the 48S initiation complex; and the largest scaffolding initiation factor in mammals
eIF4A	An RNA helicase; activate mRNA; and promote the formation of the 48S initiation complex
eIF4E	A cap-binding protein; stimulate the formation of the 48S initiation complex
eIF4B	Activate eIF4A; promote the circularization and activation of the mRNA bound to the active 80S ribosome
eIF4G	eIF4 complex scaffold; bind to the poly(A) tail to stabilize mRNA; and stimulate the formation of the 48S initiation complex
eIF4H[d]	Stimulate eIF4A activity
eIF5A	Promote the formation of translationally active 80S ribosome from the 60S ribosome and the 48S initiation complex
eIF5B	Stimulate the binding of the initiation Met-tRNA to the 40S ribosome; position the initiation Met-tRNA on (GTPase) the start codon of the mRNA; and promote the formation of the translationally active 80S ribosome from the 60S ribosome and the 48S initiation complex
eIF6	Bind to the 60S subunit to inhibit translation initiation; regulate protein synthesis
PABP (nucleus)	Stimulate the formation of a poly (A) tail at the 3′ end of mRNA by increasing the activity of poly (A) polymerase; regulate the length of a newly synthesized poly (A) tail; and stabilize mRNA in the nucleus

(Continued)

TABLE 8.2 (*Continued*)
Roles of mRNA Translation Factors in Eukaryotic Protein Biosynthesis[a]

Protein Factors	Functions
	(2) Translation Elongation Factors
eEF1A	Promote the selection and binding of the incoming amino acid to a polypeptide
eEF1B (2–3 subunits)	Convert eEF1A-GDP to an active state (eEF1A-GTP); modulate the function of release factors and the efficiency of translation termination
eEF2	Catalyze GTP-dependent translocation of peptidyl-tRNA from the A site to the P site of the 80S ribosome
SBP2	Essential for selenoprotein synthesis; bind to the SECIS stem-loop in the 3' UTR of selenoprotein mRNA; and interact with both elongation factors and the ribosomal 28S RNA of the 60S subunit
PABP (cytosolic)	Trigger the binding of (eIF4G) to the poly(A) tail of mRNA in the cytoplasm for the formation of the 48S initiation complex; regulate mRNA decay in the cytoplasm; and interact with a termination factor (eRF3) to regulate the recycling of ribosomes
	(3) Termination Factors
eRF1	Promote the stop-codon-dependent hydrolysis of peptidyl-tRNA
eRF3	Interact with eRF1 and stimulate eRF1 activity in the presence of GTP
	(4) Recycling Factors
eIF3	The principal factor that promotes the splitting of post-termination ribosomes into 60S subunits and tRNA- and mRNA-bound 40S subunits; recruited to 40S subunits during ribosome recycling; and enhance the recycling of post-termination complexes
eIF1	Enhance eIF3 activity; mediate the release of the P-site tRNA from post-termination ribosomes; and promote the recycling of post-termination complexes
eIF1A	Enhance eIF3 activity; promote the recycling of post-termination complexes
eIF3j	A loosely associated subunit of eIF3; enhance eIF3 activity; and ensure the dissociation of mRNA from post-termination ribosomes

eEF, eukaryotic elongation factor; eIF, eukaryotic initiation factor; eRF, eukaryotic release factor; GEF, guanine nucleotide exchange factor; PABP, poly(A)-binding protein; S, Svedberg unit of flotation; SBP2, the SECIS binding protein 2.

[a] Eukaryotes contain more initiation factors than prokaryotes. In prokaryotes, initiation factors are IF1, IF2, and IF3, which correspond to eIF1A, eIF5B, and eIF1 in eukaryotes, respectively; elongation factors are EF-Tu, EF-Ts, and EF-G, which correspond to eEF1A, eEF1B, and eEF2 in eukaryotes, respectively; termination factors are RF1, RF2, and RF3, with RF1 and RF3 corresponding to eRF1 and eRF3 in eukaryotes, respectively; and release factors are RRF and EF-G, which do not homologous factors in eukaryotes.

[b] Formerly designated eIF4c.

[c] Consisting of α, β, γ, δ, and ε subunits.

[d] This gene is deleted in Williams syndrome, a multisystem developmental disorder in humans.

8.2.3.1 Dissociation of Inactive Free 80S Ribosomes into 40s and 60S Subunits

The dissociation of inactive free 80S ribosomes into their constituent 40S and 60S subunits is an essential event in translation and is controlled by initiation factors [e.g., eukaryotic initiation factors (eIF)] and elongation factors [eukaryotic elongation factors (eEF)] (Table 8.2). Under resting or AA-deprivation conditions, nearly all ribosomes in eukaryotes exist in the free 80S form. However, in response to growth stimuli or activators of protein synthesis, the free 80S ribosomes rapidly dissociate into subunits to enter the translation cycle. This process is facilitated by initiation factors and translation factors (Dever 2002). Specifically, when two initiation factors (eIF1A and eIF3) bind to the 40S subunit of the free 80S ribosome, the dissociation of the free 80S ribosome into its 40S and 60S subunits is triggered. In eukaryotes, eEF2 (translocase-2) dissociates the 80S ribosome into its

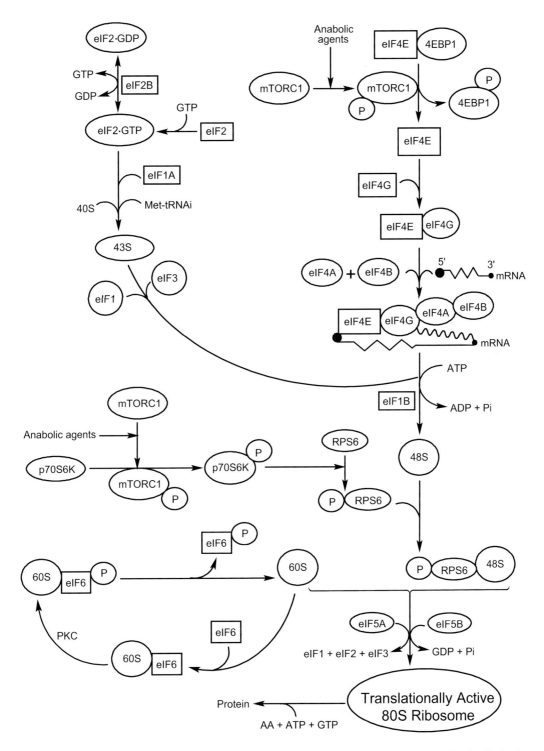

FIGURE 8.2 The biochemical pathway of translation initiation for protein synthesis in animal cells. In the presence of various initiation factors and the mRNA template, 40S and 60S ribosomes combine to form the translationally active 80S ribosome where protein synthesis in the cytoplasm and mitochondria takes place. eIF, eukaryotic initiation factor; 4EBP1, eIF4E-binding protein 1; mTORC1, complex 1 of mammalian or mechanistic target of rapamycin; p70S6K, ribosomal protein S6 kinase 1 (a 70-kDa protein); PKC, protein kinase C; RPS6, ribosomal protein S6; S: Svedberg unit of flotation; UC, uncharged.

subunits in the presence of ATP but not GTP or other nucleoside triphosphates (Demeshkina et al. 2007). After the dissociation of the free 80S ribosome, several eIF (e.g., eIF1, eIF1A, eIF3, and eIF6) may prevent the reassociation of the 40S and 60S subunits.

8.2.3.2 Formation of the 43S Preinitiation Complex

eIF2, a heterotrimer of α, β, and γ subunits, plays an important role in the formation of the 43S preinitiation complex. This elongation factor also catalyzes the translocation of the eukaryotic ribosomes in forward and backward directions (Susorov et al. 2018). In essence, eIF2 in the dephosphorylated state binds GTP to form a binary complex. The latter then binds to Met-tRNA$_i$, generating the eIF2-GTP-Met-tRNA$_i$ complex. tRNA$_i$ is a tRNA that specifically binds the universal initiation codon (AUG) on mRNA to initiate the formation of a protein or polypeptide, and Met-tRNA$_i$ is formed from L-methionine (Met) and tRNAi by aminoacyl-tRNA synthetase.

$$\text{L-Methionine + tRNA}_i \xrightarrow[\text{ATP} \qquad \text{AMP + PPi}]{\text{Methionyl-tRNA}_i \text{ synthetase}} \text{L-Methionyl-tRNA}_i$$

Like other tRNAs, the secondary structure of tRNA$_i$ is a cloverleaf. The eIF2-GTP-Met-tRNA$_i$ complex then binds to the 40S subunit to yield the 43S preinitiation complex, which is stabilized by eIF1A and eIF3. The eIF1A is essential for the transfer of the initiator Met-tRNA$_i$ (as Met-tRNA$_i$·eIF2·GTP ternary complex) to the 40S ribosomal subunit in the absence of mRNA to form the 43S preinitiation complex. This covalent modification occurs after Met-tRNA$_i$ is produced from L-methionine and tRNA$_i$ by methionyl-tRNA synthetase. The Met-tRNAi has an anticodon (i.e., 3′-UAC-5′ for methionine) that binds with the corresponding codon (i.e., the 5′-AUG-3′ start codon for methionine) on the mRNA. The initial AUG codon (encoding for methionine; also the translation initiation codon) on the mRNA signals the interaction of the ribosome with: (1) the mRNA molecule, and (2) the tRNA containing the anticodon.

8.2.3.3 Formation of the 48S Initiation Complex

Several eukaryotic initiation factors (particularly eIF4E and eIF3) are crucial for the formation of the 48S initiation complex. eIF4E (an RNA helicase) recognizes and binds to the 5′ cap structure of mRNA. The phosphorylation of eIF4E-binding protein 1 (4EBP1) by mTOR complex 1 releases eIF4E from the eIF4E·4EBP1 complex (Saxton and Sabatini 2017). This allows eIF4E to bind eIF4G to form the eIF4E·eIF4G binary complex. Because eIF4G is a scaffolding protein that interacts with other transcription factors (eIF3, eIF4A, and eIF4E) and binds to the poly(A) tail, the formation of the eIF4E·eIF4G complex helps recruit eIF4A to mRNA to assemble the eIF4E·eIF4G·eIF4A·mRNA ternary complex. Binding of eIF4G to the poly(A) tail of mRNA is triggered by the cytosolic form of PABP, which also regulates mRNA decay (e.g., via deadenylation) and stability (e.g., changes in secondary and tertiary structures) in the cytoplasm. The complex of eIF4A, eIF4E, and eIF4G is often referred to as eIF4F·eIF4B. The latter contains two RNA-binding domains (one non-specifically interacting with mRNA whereas the second specifically binding the 18S portion of the 40S ribosomal subunit) and acts as an anchor for mRNA, thereby promoting the circularization and activation of the bound mRNA. Note that, in vertebrates, eIF4H is an additional initiation factor with a similar function to eIF4B.

On another arm of initiation that is powered by ATP, eIF1A and eIF3 are recruited to the 43S preinitiation complex, which binds to the capped 5′ end of the mRNA associated with eIF4E, eIF4G, and eIF4A to form the 48S initiation complex. Here, the 5′ cap is used as a recognition signal for ribosomes to bind to the mRNA, and eIF3 functions to promote the assembly of this 48S initiation complex by positioning the mRNA strand near the exit site of the 40S ribosome subunit (Ramanathan et al. 2016). The newly formed 48S complex scans downstream along the 5′-untranslated region (5′-UTR) of the mRNA by moving step-by-step in the 3′ [a poly(A) tail] direction until it encounters the first AUG codon (Ramanathan et al. 2016). IF1B is necessary for the recognition of the initiation codon during the scanning process, which is catalyzed by ATP-dependent helicases. Thus, the 48S initiation complex forms at the initiation codon of a conventional capped mRNA, and this event is promoted by eIF1B. The pairing of the anticodon of Met-tRNA$_i$ with the AUG codon of the mRNA signals that the initial target for polypeptide synthesis has been found.

8.2.3.4 Formation of the Translationally Active 80S Initiation Complex

Ribosomal protein S6 (RPS6) and eIF5 (consisting of eIF5A and eIF5B) are crucial for the formation of the translationally active 80S complex from the 60S ribosome and the 48S initiation complex (which contains the 40S ribosome). After RPS6 is phosphorylated by RPS6 kinase-1 (a 70 kDa protein; p70S6K1), whose activation is catalyzed by MTOR complex-1 (MTORC1), a phosphorylated RPS6 is recruited to the 48S initiation complex (Saxton and Sabatini 2017). Meanwhile, eIF5A, which contains the unusual AA hypusine, acts as a GTPase-activator protein, whereas eIF5B (a GTPase) hydrolyzes the GTP that is bound to eIF2 (the initiation factor that brings the Met-tRNA$_i$ to the 40S ribosome) in the 48S initiation complex. Hydrolysis of the GTP to GDP plus Pi is required for the assembly of the functional 80S ribosome. eIF2B (also known as the guanine nucleotide exchange factor of the GTPase eIF2) promotes the GDP-GTP exchange to regenerate active eIF2, which brings the initiator Met-tRNA$_i$ to the ribosome in the form of the eIF2-GTP·Met-tRNA$_i$ (Bogorad et al. 2018).

The free 60S ribosome joins the 40S ribosome in the 48S initiation complex through a mechanism mediated by eIF6 (also known as p27BBP; the β4 integrin interactor p27). The X-ray structure reveals that when protein synthesis is not activated, the eukaryotic 60S subunit is in complex with eIF6 (Greber 2016). The release of eIF6 from the eIF6-60S complex allows the 60S ribosome to join the 40S ribosome in the 48S initiation complex to form the translationally active 80S initiation complex. The formation of the functional 80S ribosome is associated with the release of eIF1, eIF2, and eIF3. It is now known that eIF6 interacts with RACK1 (a receptor for activated protein kinase C) in the cytoplasm and regulates mRNA translation through its binding to ribosomes (Gallo et al. 2018). Upon stimulation, protein kinase C catalyzes the phosphorylation of eIF6 (an ATP-dependent reaction), leading to its release from the eIF6-60S complex and, consequently, ribosome activation.

The translationally active 80S ribosome contains three RNA-binding sites, designated as A, P, and E (Figure 8.3). The aminoacyl site (also known as acceptor site; A site) binds a new

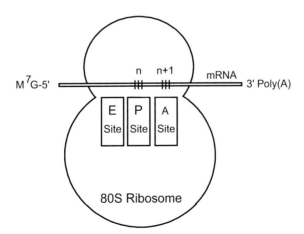

FIGURE 8.3 The 80S ribosome contains three RNA-binding sites designated as A, P, and E. During peptide elongation, the peptidyl moiety from the aminoacyl-tRNA on the P site of the 80S ribosome is transferred to the acceptor end of the existing aminoacyl-tRNA on the A site of the ribosome. The discharged tRNA rapidly dissociates from the P site and is transferred to the E (exit) site before existing the ribosome. M^{7}G, 7-methylguanylate cap; Poly(A), polyadenylyl tail.

aminoacyl-tRNA; the peptidyl site (P site) binds the nascent polypeptide chain linked to the latest aminoacyl-tRNA [namely, binding a peptidyl-tRNA (i.e., a tRNA bound to the peptide being synthesized)]; and the exit site (E site), which allows for the release of deacylated tRNA after peptide bond formation. After translation initiation is completed, the A site of the 80S ribosome is free, whereas the initiator Met-tRNA$_i$ occupies the P site.

8.2.4   Peptide Elongation in Animal Cells

Active translation occurs on the functional 80S ribosome complex where the ribosome reads mRNA in the 5′ to 3′ direction. During this process, each tRNA that carries the corresponding AA moves through the 80S ribosome from the A site to the P site and then exits the ribosome via the E site. Elongation factors are crucial for addition of an AA to a polypeptide and for peptide elongation. Both eEF1A and eEF2 are GTP-binding proteins, and they are remarkably conserved throughout evolution (Greganova et al. 2011). Protein synthesis occurs at a high speed and accuracy, where eukaryotic ribosomes can incorporate 6 AAs into a polypeptide per second and the error rate is $10^{-4}–10^{-3}$ (Ogle and Ramakrishnan 2005). This rapid process of peptide elongation can be divided into the following four steps.

8.2.4.1   Activation of an AA to Form Its Aminoacyl-tRNA

Before an AA is added to a growing peptide, the AA must be bound to a specific tRNA to form aminoacyl-tRNA (AA-tRNA). This AA activation is catalyzed by each of approximately 20 specific aminoacyl-tRNA synthetases besides methionyl-tRNA$_i$ synthetase for L-methionine in eukaryotes. In the reaction of aminoacylation, ATP is hydrolyzed to AMP and PPi. Aminoacyl-tRNA synthesis varies little among contemporary organisms for canonical aminoacyl-tRNA synthesis, i.e., the direct attachment of cognate tRNAs to their corresponding AAs by the 20 canonical aminoacyl-tRNA synthetases. There are mechanisms for AA-tRNA editing to correct mischarged tRNAs as a means of quality control (Ibba and Söll 2001). GTP is required to provide energy for the translocation of AA-tRNA to the A site of the ribosome on the mRNA template. Except for selenocysteine, all AAs that are the building blocks of proteins react directly with their respective tRNA.

$$\text{Amino acid + tRNA} \xrightarrow[\text{ATP} \quad \text{AMP + PPi}]{\text{Aminoacyl-tRNA synthetase}} \text{Aminoacyl-tRNA}$$

8.2.4.2   Addition of an Incoming AA to A tRNA-Bound AA on the 80S Ribosome

Addition of an incoming AA to an existing tRNA-bound AA or peptide on the P site of the 80S ribosome begins as a new aminoacyl-tRNA reads the next codon on the mRNA molecule (Figure 8.4). Overall, this process involves (1) the transfer and binding of an incoming aminoacyl-tRNA to the A site of the ribosome; (2) the covalent linkage of the new tRNA-bound AA to the growing polypeptide chain (peptidyl transfer); and (3) the movement of the newly formed peptidyl-tRNA, together with its bound mRNA, from the A site to the P site of the 80S ribosome (translocation). Elongation factors play an essential role in achieving the accuracy of peptide elongation (Greganova et al. 2011).

8.2.4.3   Transfer and Binding of an Incoming Aminoacyl-tRNA to the A Site

For the cytosolic synthesis of protein, all aminoacyl-tRNAs are formed in the cytoplasm but they are not freely diffusible in this compartment. However, aminoacyl-tRNA synthetases are present in the vicinity of ribosomes and have a capacity to interact with the polyribosomes (assemblies of ribosomes). Additionally, these enzymes are closely associated with elongation factors and the cytoskeletal network. Interestingly, there is evidence that several components of the translation machinery (including aminoacyl-tRNA synthetases, ribosomes, mRNAs, initiation, and elongation factors) are colocalized in animal cells (Rajendran et al. 2018). The supramolecular organization of

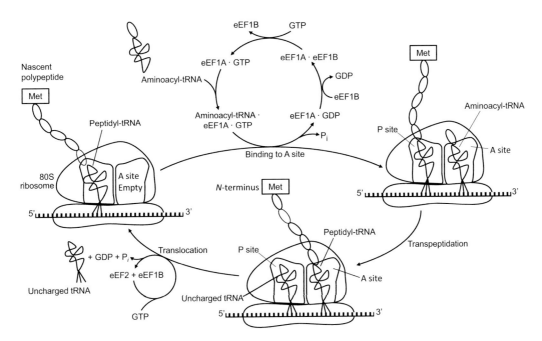

FIGURE 8.4 The pathway of protein synthesis in eukaryotes, including humans and other animals. The 80S ribosome is the functional site for the translation of mRNA into protein. These processes require enzymes (aminoacyl-tRNA synthetase and peptidyltransferase), eukaryotic initiation factors (eIF), elongation factors (eEF), release factors (eRF), and recycling factors. eEF1A·GTP is required for the binding of an incoming aminoacyl-tRNA to the A site, and eEF1A·GDP is recycled into eEF1A·GTP under the action of eEF1B. Polypeptide elongation is terminated by a terminating codon on the mRNA template. Peptidyltransferase, together with eRF1 and eRF3, hydrolyzes peptidyl-tRNA to release the newly synthesized peptide. eRF3 also interacts with the cytosolic PABP to regulate the recycling of ribosomes.

enzymes, proteins, and RNAs may form a metabolon to preferentially channel a newly synthesized aminoacyl-tRNA from the cytoplasm to the ribosomes.

Any aminoacyl-tRNA cannot directly enter the A site. Rather, eEF1A in eukaryotes (or EF-Tu in bacteria) is responsible for the selection and binding of the incoming aminoacyl-tRNA to the A site of the 80S ribosome (Dever 2002). In this process, eEF1A (formerly known as eEF1α; a G-protein) forms a complex with both the new incoming aminoacyl-tRNA and GTP, and the resulting complex then binds to the A site. The interaction of aminoacyl-tRNA with eEF1A stimulates GTP hydrolysis by eEF1A and also causes a conformational change in eEF1A. This causes eEF1A-GDP to detach from the 80S ribosome and leave the aminoacyl-tRNA attached at the A site. Therefore, both the A site and the P site of the 80S ribosome contain their respective aminoacyl-tRNAs (Figure 8.4). After the release of eEF1A-GDP and Pi, eEF1A-GDP can recycle to an active state (eEF1A-GTP) through the action of eEF1B (formerly known as eEF1β).

8.2.4.4   Peptide Bond Formation

Peptidyltransferase in the 60S subunit catalyzes the formation of a peptide bond between the carboxyl group of the existing peptidyl-tRNA occupying the P site and the amino group of the new aminoacyl-tRNA in the A site, with the loss of one molecule of H_2O (Figure 8.5). This enzymatic activity is performed by the 28S ribosomal RNA (a component of the 60S ribosomal subunit) in eukaryotes, and such an RNA is called a ribozyme (Fedor and Williamson 2005). The ribozyme facilitates the formation of the peptide bond through the following mechanisms: (1) lowering the activation entropy of the reaction by strategically positioning the two substrates; (2) placing water in the active site; (3) providing an electrostatic network that stabilizes intermediates of the reaction;

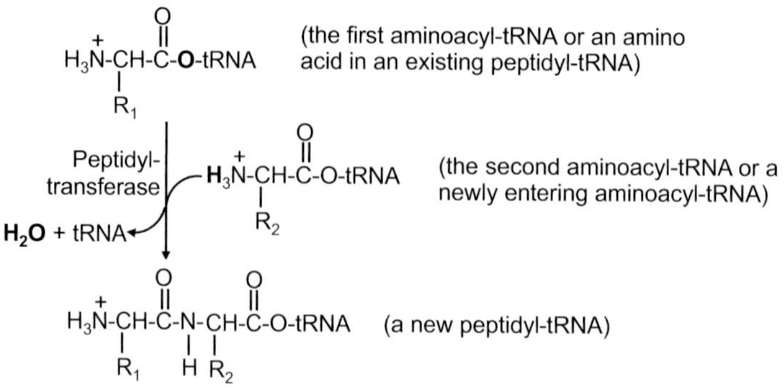

FIGURE 8.5 The formation of a new peptidyl-tRNA on the ribosomes of eukaryotes, including humans and other animals. Peptidyltransferase (a ribozyme, the 28S ribosomal RNA of the 60S ribosomal subunit in eukaryotes) catalyzes the formation of a peptide bond between (1) the carboxyl group of the first aminoacyl-tRNA or an amino acid in an existing peptidyl-tRNA (occupying the P site of the 80 ribosome) and (2) the amino group of the second aminoacyl-tRNA or a newly entering aminoacyl-tRNA (in the A site of the 80 ribosome). This condensation reaction results in the loss of one molecule of H_2O. Note that in prokaryotes, peptidyltransferase is the 23S ribosomal RNA of the 50S ribosomal subunit.

and (4) coordinating proton transfer via a concerted proton shuttle mechanism involving ribose hydroxyl groups on the tRNA substrate. The nucleophilic reaction for the covalent formation of the peptide bond requires no further energy because the AA on the aminoacyl-tRNA is already activated.

8.2.4.5 Translocation of the Newly Formed Peptidyl-tRNA

Upon peptide bond formation, the peptidyl moiety from the AA-tRNA on the P site of the 80S ribosome is transferred to the acceptor end of the existing aminoacyl-tRNA on the A site of the ribosome (Figure 8.4). The discharged tRNA rapidly dissociates from the P site and is transferred to the E site before exiting the ribosome. Simultaneously, eEF2 binds to the ribosome in complex with GTP. This interaction causes a change in the conformation of eEF2 and its activation. The activated eEF2 then hydrolyzes GTP to GDP plus Pi and catalyzes the translocation of the newly formed peptidyl-tRNA, together with its bound mRNA, from the A site to the P site of the 80S ribosome toward the 3′ direction. This frees the A site for another cycle of elongation.

8.2.5 Termination of Peptide Chain Elongation

After multiple cycles of elongation to polymerize AAs into a protein molecule, the completion of polypeptide chain elongation is recognized in the A site by the terminating signal known as the nonsense or terminating codon (e.g., UGA, UAG, or UAA) on the mRNA. Except for the special Sec-tRNA$_{(Sec)}$ (see below), tRNA normally does not have an anticodon that can recognize such a termination codon (Ferré-D'Amaré 2011). Rather, the recognition of a termination codon residing in the A site of the 80S ribosome is performed by eukaryotic protein release factors (eRF) (e.g., eRF1, eRF2, and eRF3), and the stop codon induces the binding of a release factor that prompts the disassembly of the entire ribosome-mRNA complex. Functions of the release factors are modulated by eEF1B. eRF1 recognizes UAA and UAG, whereas eRF2 recognizes UAA and UGA. In complex with GTP, eRF3 (a GTP-binding protein) promotes the binding of eRF1 and eRF2 to the ribosome. In a complex with the peptidyltransferase and GTP, the eRF catalyzes the hydrolysis of the bond between the peptide and the terminal tRNA occupying the P site. Therefore, the newly synthesized peptide and the tRNA are released from the P site. GTP hydrolysis to GDP plus Pi triggers the dissociation of the eRF from the ribosome. eRF3 also interacts with the cytosolic PABP to regulate the recycling of ribosomes. Thereafter, eIF2-GDP is converted into eIF2-GTP by eIF2B (the guanine nucleotide exchange factor), whereas the 80S ribosome dissociates, for recycling, into the 40S and 60S ribosomal subunits, which are utilized for another cycle of protein synthesis (Figure 8.4).

8.2.6 Incorporation of L-Selenocysteine (A Special AA) into Selenoproteins

8.2.6.1 Historical Perspectives of Research on L-Selenocysteine

There is a long history of L-selenocysteine research. Selenium was detected by the Swedish chemist J.J. Berzelius in 1818 as a byproduct of sulfuric acid production and had long been considered to be an industrial hazard for humans and other animals (e.g., causing severely damaged hoofs). However, more than one century later, Jane Pinsent reported in 1953 that selenite (also known as desert rose or gypsum flower; composed of calcium sulfate, $CaSO_4 \cdot 2H_2O$) was required for the optimum activity of formic acid dehydrogenase in *E. coli*. Selenium (Se) was identified by K. Schwarz and C.M. Foltz in the United States in 1957 to be an essential micronutrient for bacteria, mammals, and birds. Subsequently, this element was found to be a cofactor for glutathione peroxidase (Flohé et al. 1973; Rotruck et al. 1973). In support of this notion, Stadtman and colleagues discovered selenocysteine in clostridial glycine reductase (Cone et al. 1976; Turner and Stadtman 1973). Zinoni et al. (1986) reported that UGA (one of the two stop codons in the mRNA) is the genetic codon for selenocysteine that is incorporated into bacterial protein, and this surprise finding was subsequently confirmed in eukaryotes, including humans and other animals. Work in the 1990s has shown that selenocysteine is formed from serine and selenium at the translation step of protein synthesis. In essence, a selenocysteinyl tRNA is first charged with serine, which is then enzymatically modified to form selenocysteine in the presence of selenium. Selenocysteine-containing enzymes include glycine reductase in the clostridia (obligate anaerobes), formate dehydrogenase in bacteria (e.g., *E. coli* and *Salmonella*) and archaea (*Methanococcus vannielii*), hydrogenases in certain anaerobic bacteria, formyl-methanofuran dehydrogenase in archaea (*Methanopyrus kandleri*), glutathione peroxidase in animal tissues (e.g., the liver, kidneys, and blood), and tetraiodothyronine 5'-deiodinase in certain tissues of animals such as thyroid gland, liver, and kidneys (Rother and Krzycki 2010; Stadtman 1996).

8.2.6.2 Formation of Selenocysteine and Its Incorporation into Selenoproteins

Unlike other proteinogenic AAs, free selenocysteine neither exists in cells nor has a cognate aminoacyl-tRNA synthetase. Rather, selenocysteine is incorporated into selenoproteins during translation elongation in animal cells, microbes, and algae via a special synthetic mechanism. In addition, unlike canonical proteinogenic AAs which are coded for directly in the universal genetic code, the incorporation of selenocysteine into selenoproteins in these organisms is encoded by an internal UGA stop codon under the guidance of a specific mRNA hairpin structure located further downstream, the SECIS (selenocysteine inserting sequence) element (Serrão et al. 2018). The SECIS element is defined by characteristic nucleotide sequences and secondary structure base-pairing patterns and differs between eukaryotes and prokaryotes. For example, the SECIS element is typically located in the 3' untranslated region (3' UTR) of the mammalian mRNA but immediately after the UGA codon within the reading frame of the prokaryotic mRNA. The specificity for the stop codon is recognized by tRNASec, whose UCA anticodon is complementary to the UGA stop codon. Note that a specific SECIS-binding protein 2 (SBP2) is essential for selenoprotein synthesis. SBP2 binds to the SECIS stem-loop in the 3' UTR of selenoprotein mRNA, while interacting with both the specialized translation elongation factor and the ribosomal 28S RNA of the 60S subunit (Kossinova et al. 2014).

The Sec-tRNA$_{(Sec)}$ is specifically bound to a specialized translational elongation factor called selenocysteine-tRNA-specific elongation factor (SelB) in a GTP-dependent manner in all known organisms. SelB recognizes only Sec-tRNA$_{(Sec)}$, but not other aminoacyl-tRNAs, and delivers

Sec-tRNA$_{(Sec)}$ to the ribosomal A site. A eukaryotic elongation factor specific for selenocysteine-tRNA (eEF$_{Sec}$) or mammalian SelB (mSelB) has been found in recent years (Dobosz-Bartoszek et al. 2016). The specificity of the Sec-tRNA$_{(Sec)}$ delivery mechanism is conferred by the presence, in Sec-tRNA$_{(Sec)}$, of an extra subunit (SBP2 for mSelB/eEFSec in eukaryotes) or by an extra protein domain (SelB in prokaryotes) which binds to the SECIS elements in a selenoprotein mRNA.

After its binding to SelB (e.g., mSelB in mammals), the selenocysteine tRNA [tRNA$_{(Sec)}$] is initially aminoacylated with serine to form seryl-tRNA$_{(Sec)}$, which is catalyzed by seryl-tRNA ligase (also known as seryl-tRNA synthetase). The selenocysteine tRNAs contain several unique features (including a 10-base (in eukaryotes) or 8-base (in bacteria) pair acceptor stem, a long variable region arm, and substitutions at several well-conserved base positions) and differ substantially from the canonical (conventional and well-established) tRNAs that carry canonical proteinogenic AAs (Serrão et al. 2018). Therefore, the resulting Ser-tRNA$_{(Sec)}$ is not recognized by the normal translation factor (eEF1A in eukaryotes or EF-Tu in bacteria) during translation. Rather, the seryl moiety in Ser-tRNA$_{(Sec)}$ is converted into phosphoserine by O-phosphoseryl-tRNA kinase to form O-phosphoseryl-tRNA$_{(Sec)}$. Subsequently, the O-phosphoseryl residue bound to tRNA$_{(Sec)}$ is converted to a selenocysteine residue by selenocysteine synthase (a pyridoxal phosphate-containing enzyme) in the presence of selenium (in the form of selenophosphate which is generated from selenide and ATP by selenophosphate synthetase). Seryl-tRNA$_{(Sec)}$ is recognized in a special way on the mRNA to insert selenocysteine into a selenoprotein. These biochemical pathways are illustrated in Figure 8.6. In essence, the presence of the specific SECIS prevents the termination of protein biosynthesis and promotes the incorporation of selenocysteine into nascent proteins.

8.2.7   Processing and Export of Newly Synthesized Proteins

8.2.7.1   Posttranslational Modifications of Newly Synthesized Proteins

Most of the newly synthesized proteins have little or no biological activities when released from the ribosome. The polypeptides must undergo appropriate modifications in the cytoplasm and/or on the

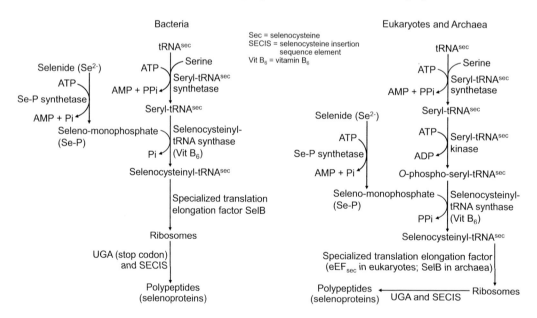

FIGURE 8.6   Formation of selenocysteine from serine and selenium during the mRNA translation process. This biochemical process occurs in bacteria, archaea, and eukaryotes (e.g., humans and other animals). Selenocysteine is incorporated into selenoproteins under the guidance of the UGA code. Free selenocysteine is absent from the cells. Sec, selenocysteine; SECIS, selenocysteine insertion sequence element; Vit B$_6$, vitamin B$_6$.

rough endoplasmic reticulum in eukaryotes (equivalent to becoming mature proteins) (Müller 2018). These posttranslational modifications include (1) proteolytic cleavage [including the removal of the initiating AA (i.e., Met that is located at the N-terminus of the polypeptide in the cytosolic protein synthesis), as well as the C- and N-terminal residues (e.g., signal peptide by signal peptidase); and the limited proteolysis of proproteins or propeptides (inactive proteins or peptides)] and (2) covalent modifications of AA residues in proteins or peptides (Table 8.3). Protein modifications have biological significance and practical implications for research design. For example, while posttranslational modifications of proteins are necessary for their biological activities, the oxidation of proteins may result in their damage. On the other hand, the release of modified AAs (e.g., 3-methylhistidine and 4-hydroxyproline) from proteins can be used to estimate the degradation of myofibrillar proteins in skeletal muscle and connective tissue, respectively.

The multiple forms of lysine residues in the posttranslational modifications of proteins deserve special mentioning. For example, these lysine residues can undergo (1) methylation to form methyl-, dimethyl- and trimethyllysine; (2) acetylation and ubiquitination (important mechanisms for the regulation of protein expression and degradation); (3) hydroxylation to form hydroxylysine in collagen and other types of proteins; and (4) the O-glycosylation of protein-bound hydroxylysine residues in the endoplasmic reticulum and Golgi apparatus to mark certain proteins for secretion from cells (Hellerschmied et al. 2019; Murakami et al. 2012). The extent to which lysine residues are modified may affect the amounts of lysine produced from acid or enzymatic hydrolysis of proteins. Additionally, transglutaminases catalyze the formation of polymerized cross-linking of proteins and, therefore, transglutaminases play an important role in blood coagulation, skin barrier function, and wound healing. For this reason, these enzymes are called nature's biological glues. Thus, since their initial description by D.D. Clarke in 1959, transglutaminases have received increasing interest from life and biomedical scientists (Duarte et al. 2020).

TABLE 8.3
Posttranslational Modifications of Proteins in Cells

Type of Posttranslational Modification	Examples
Proteolytic cleavage	Removal of the initiating AA (e.g., Met or fMet) and the C- and N-terminal residues (e.g., signal peptide by signal peptidase), and limited proteolysis of proproteins (e.g., proinsulin) or propeptides (inactive proteins or peptides)]
Racemization	Interconversion of certain AA residues in proteins (e.g., aspartate in myelin basic protein and β-amyloid protein) from L- to D-isoform
Selenoylation	Co-translational incorporation of selenium into selenoproteins (e.g., GSH peroxidase and thioredoxin reductase)
Covalent modifications of AA residues in proteins or peptides	Formation of chemical bonding by the sharing of one or more electrons (especially pairs of electrons) between atoms
N-Acetylation	Addition of an acetyl group, usually at the N-terminus of proteins (e.g., histone deacetylases and tubulin)
O-Acetylation (Ser/Thr)	Addition of an acetyl group to the hydroxyl group of serine or threonine residues in protein
Adenylylation	Covalent attachment of an AMP molecule to the hydroxyl group of an AA residue in protein
ADP-ribosylation	Addition of one or more ADP-ribose moieties to proteins (e.g., histones and membrane adenylate cyclase)
Biotinylation	Acylation of conserved lysine residues in proteins (e.g., avidin and acyl carrier protein) with biotin
γ-Carboxylation	Addition of a carboxyl group to glutamate residues in proteins (e.g., prothrombin and blood clotting factors)

(Continued)

TABLE 8.3 (*Continued*)
Posttranslational Modifications of Proteins in Cells

Type of Posttranslational Modification	Examples
Disulfide linkage	Coupling of two thiol (–SH) groups in cysteine residues of proteins (e.g., insulin) to form –S–S– linkage
Flavin attachment	Covalent attachment of FAD and FMN to proteins (e.g., NOS and mammalian succinate dehydrogenase)
Glutamylation	Covalent linkage of glutamic acid residues to a γ-carboxyl group of a glutamate residue in proteins (e.g., α-tubulin and β-tubulin)
Glycosylation	Enzyme-catalyzed attachment of carbohydrate to the side chain of proteins (e.g., membrane hormone receptors and lactoferrin) to form glycoproteins
Glycation (non-enzymatic glycosylation)	Covalent bonding of proteins (e.g., hemoglobin and amyloid protein) with a sugar molecule (e.g., glucose and fructose)
Glycylation	Covalent linkage of one or more glycine residues to proteins (e.g., α-tubulin and β-tubulin)
Heme attachment	Attachment of heme to proteins (e.g., cytochromes a and c)
Hydroxylation	Introduction of a hydroxyl group to certain AA (e.g., proline and lysine) residues in proteins (e.g., collagens) to form hydroxylated AA (e.g., 4-hydroxyproline and hydroxylysine)
Methylation	Addition of a methyl group to certain AA (e.g., histidine, lysine, and arginine) residues in proteins (e.g., actin, myosin, and histones) to form methylated AA (e.g., 3-methylhistine and methylated arginines); a type of alkylation
Myristoylation[a]	Covalent attachment of myristate (a 14-carbon saturated fatty acid) to N-terminal glycine residue in proteins (e.g., calcineurin B and the catalytic subunit of AMPK)
S-Nitrosylation	Covalent incorporation of a NO moiety into the thiol group of cysteine in proteins (e.g., NMDA-type glutamate receptor and GSH reductase) to form S-nitrosothiol (SNO)
3-Nitration	Introduction of a nitro (NO_2) group to a tyrosine residue in proteins (e.g., bovine serum albumin and angiotensin II) to form 3-nitrotyrosine
Oxidation[b]	Oxidation of protein by various oxidants
Phosphorylation	Addition of a covalently bound phosphate group into a serine, threonine, or tyrosine reside of proteins (e.g., BCKA dehydrogenase and MTOR) by a protein kinase
Palmitoylation[a]	Covalent attachment of a fatty acid (e.g., palmitic acid) to cysteine and other residues (e.g., serine and threonine) of proteins (e.g., eNOS and CPS-I)
Succinylation	Covalent attachment of a succinyl-CoA molecule to the ε-amino group of a Lys residue in protein residue in protein
Tyrosine sulfation	Addition of a sulfate group to tyrosine residues in proteins (e.g., bovine fibrinopeptide B and G-protein-coupled receptors) to form tyrosine-O-sulfate
Transglutamination	Formation, by transglutaminases, of a covalent bond between a free amine group (e.g., an ε-amino group of a peptide-bound lysine residue) in protein and a γ-carboxamide group (–CO–NH₂) of a peptide-bound glutamine to create an inter- or intramolecular isopeptidyl bond that is highly resistant to proteolysis
Ubiquitination	Formation of the linkage between the protein substrate with ubiquitin

[a] Also known as protein lipidation.

[b] Oxidants include superoxide anion, hydrogen peroxide, hydroxyl radical, NO, peroxynitrite, hypochlorous acid, peroxy radicals, and lipid peroxide. Cysteine and methionine residues are most susceptible to oxidation, but tyrosine, proline, and tryptophan can also be oxidized. Oxidatively modified residues include 3-hydroxytyrosine, 3-chlorotyrosine, 3-nitrated tyrosine (Tyr-NO_2), 5-hydroxyproline, 5-hydroxytryptophan, cysteine sulfenic acid (Cys-SOH), and S-nitrated cysteine. Amino acid residues in proteins can also be modified by reactive oxygen species or carbonate anion radicals to yield protein carbonyls in organisms.

Because collagen accounts for about 1/3 of the total protein in humans and other animals (Chapter 1), it is important to understand how this type of protein undergoes posttranslational modifications and processing. Collagen is formed from AAs (mostly glycine and proline) by fibroblasts through the normal pathway of intracellular protein synthesis described above. The collagen precursor chains that are newly synthesized on ribosomes are called procollagens, which are then processed by the rough endoplasmic reticulum (RER) and Golgi (Myllyharju 2005). Specifically, procollagens are transported into the lumen of the RER to undergo a series of reactions, including (1) the hydroxylation of some proline and lysine residues by RER membrane-bound prolyl hydroxylase (procollagen-proline dioxygenase) and lysyl hydroxylase (procollagen-lysine 5-dioxygenase), respectively; (2) glycosylation (the addition of galactose and glucose residues to certain hydroxylysine residues, as well as the addition of long oligosaccharides to certain asparagine residues in the C-terminal); and (3) the generation of intrachain disulfide bonds between the N- and C-terminal polypeptides to align the three chains and form the triple helix. This procollagen complex moves into the Golgi for further processing (e.g., glycosylation), yielding large electron-dense aggregates. Within the Golgi apparatus, procollagens are packaged into membrane-bound vesicles for secretion into the extracellular space (Lavieu et al. 2014). Specifically, after their processing in the Golgi is completed, the procollagens are secreted by fibroblasts into the extracellular space through exocytosis (Myllyharju 2005). Figure 8.7 summarizes the posttranslational processing of procollagens to

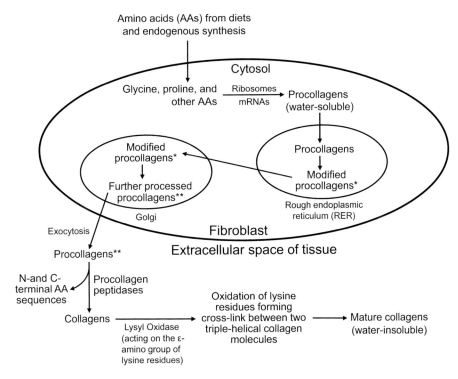

FIGURE 8.7 Processing of procollagens by the rough endoplasmic reticulum (RER) and Golgi apparatus of fibroblasts, as well as the extracellular processing of procollagens to become mature collagens in connective tissue. * Modifications in RER include (1) the hydroxylation of some proline and lysine residues by proline and lysine hydroxylases, respectively; (2) glycosylation (e.g., addition of galactose and glucose residues to certain hydroxylysine residues); and (3) alignment of the three α-chains to form the triple helix. Procollagens are secreted into the extracellular space where they undergo limited N- and C-terminal cleavage, and form cross-links between two triple-helical chains via allysines (intermolecular linkages) to become mature collagens. ** Further modifications in the Golgi apparatus include glycosylation and the packaging of processed procollagens into membrane-bound vesicles for secretion. (Adapted from Li, P. and G. Wu. 2018. *Amino Acids* 50:29–38.)

become mature collagens. The similar mechanisms are also responsible for the export of secretory proteins other than procollagens out of cells.

8.2.7.2 Export of Certain Processed Proteins Synthesized in the Cytosol of Animal Cells into the Extracellular Space

In humans and other animals, proteins that are synthesized in the cytosol of certain cell types and then secreted into the extracellular space include albumin and fibrinogens from hepatocytes, apolipoproteins from hepatocytes and enterocytes, mucins from enterocytes, collagens (as described previously) and other extracellular matrix proteins (e.g., elastins and fibronectins) from fibroblasts, protein/polypeptide hormones from endocrine glands, and β-casein and α-lactalbumin from the mammary epithelial cells of lactating mammals. For example, the liver of the 70-kg healthy human adult synthesizes and releases ~15 g albumin per day (~20% of the daily synthesis of hepatic proteins), which is the most abundant protein in the plasma (70 g/L) and accounts for ~60% of its total proteins (Hou et al. 2020; McIntyre and Rosalki 1994). Albumin plays an important role in the transport of lipids, vitamins, and minerals via the blood circulation and in maintaining the osmolality of the plasma. The hepatic synthesis of 15 g albumin requires ~18 g AAs. Furthermore, in the 70-kg healthy adult human, the rate of the degradation of mature collagens in the extracellular matrix is equal to the rate of their net synthesis (i.e., the rate of procollagens secreted from fibroblasts to the extracellular matrix; 96.5 g/day), with some of the resultant AAs being reused for protein synthesis (Meléndez-Hevia et al. 2009; Wu 2020). In addition, the α- and β-cells of the pancreas synthesize and release glucagon and insulin, respectively. Furthermore, the amounts of deposited protein and exported mucins in the small intestine of the 7.92-kg young pigs are 1.54 and 1.11 g per day, respectively (Hou and Wu 2018). Like animals, the export of proteins from cells occurs in all microorganisms, which is crucial to their survival or pathogenicity (Green and Mecsas 2016).

The liver is the major source of plasma proteins. For example, hepatocytes synthesize and release albumin, immunoglobulins, fibrinogens and other blood clotting factors, apolipoproteins, acute-phase proteins, insulin-like growth factor-I, and AA transaminases into the space of Disse (an extracellular location between a hepatocyte and a sinusoid in the liver), followed by the entry of these proteins into the blood via two pathways (Figure 8.8). Namely, the proteins from the space of Disse enter (1) the hepatic lymphatic system, the thoracic duct, the left subclavian vein, and the right heart, and (2) the sinusoids through the fenestrae (porous sites between endothelial cells of the capillaries) and then move to the hepatic venule (Hou et al. 2020). Plasma proteins (particularly albumin and globulins) are the major determinants of intravascular colloid osmotic pressure, which promotes the absorption of water from the interstitial space into the blood at the capillaries (Morissette 1977). The physiological significance of this process is epitomized by the clinical finding that a reduction in plasma colloid osmotic pressure due to protein malnutrition plays a crucial role in the development of the systemic and pulmonary edema in affected individuals.

Proteins in the plasma equilibrate with those in the interstitial space. For example, in healthy humans and other animals (e.g., pigs), about 40% and 60% of albumin are located in the intravascular plasma and in the extravascular interstitial fluid of tissues (primarily the skin and skeletal muscle), respectively (Dich and Nielsen 1963; Prinsen and de Sain-van der Velden 2004). Thus, the distribution of plasma proteins in the blood and the interstitial space of tissues must be considered when the rates of the syntheses of secreted proteins by hepatocytes and other cell types in the body are determined with the use of tracer or related techniques.

8.3 THE BIOCHEMICAL PATHWAY OF PROTEIN SYNTHESIS IN THE MITOCHONDRIA OF ANIMAL CELLS

Most mitochondrial proteins are synthesized on ribosomes in the cytoplasm. The newly synthesized proteins for subsequent transport into the mitochondrion contain mitochondrion-targeting sequences and are taken up into this organelle by binding to its surface receptor proteins that can

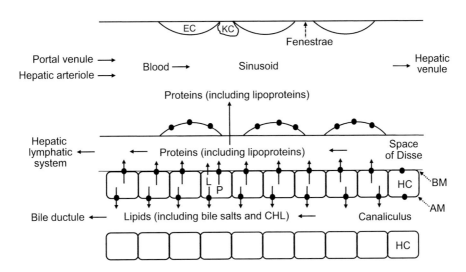

FIGURE 8.8 Export of secreted proteins from the hepatocytes of the liver into the blood. Hepatocytes synthesize many secreted proteins, including albumin, immunoglobulins, fibrinogens and other blood clotting factors, apolipoproteins, acute-phase proteins, insulin-like growth factor-I, and amino acid transaminases. These proteins enter the space of Disse through the basolateral membrane of the hepatocytes, followed by uptake into (1) the hepatic lymphatic system and (2) traversing into the hepatic sinusoid (the capillaries) through the fenestrae (the space between two endothelial cells). Lipids (e.g., glycine- and taurine-conjugated bile acids, phospholipids, unesterified cholesterol, and some conjugated bilirubin) that are synthesized from amino acids and other substrates by hepatocytes are released across the apical (canalicular) membrane of the hepatocytes into the canaliculus (formed from adjacent hepatocytes) and then the bile ductule. The solid circle denotes receptor-mediated endocytosis or a transporter. AM, apical membrane; BM, basolateral membrane; CHL, unesterified cholesterol; HC, hepatocyte; L, lipids; P, proteins.

recognize specific mitochondrion-targeting sequences (Wiedemann and Pfanner 2017). This biochemical process is essential for the integrity and functions of the mitochondria, as well as their adaptations to physiological and environmental alterations. In addition to the cytoplasm, the mitochondria are a source of some proteins.

Research on mitochondrial protein synthesis dates back to the 19th century, when the mitochondrion was discovered. Specifically, the intracellular structures of mitochondria in mammalian cells were observed in the 1840s. The name mitochondrion was coined in 1898 by C. Benda, referring to the Greek "mitos" (thread) and "chondros" (granule) to indicate the appearance of these structures during spermatogenesis. In 1972, protein synthesis within mitochondria was first reported by two independent groups (A. Tzagoloff and P. Meagher in New York, U.S. and H. Weiss in Munchen, Germany). Between 1975 and 1976, physical mapping of mitochondrial DNA was performed for various species. In 1977, mitochondrially translated polypeptides were found to be coded for by mitochondrial DNA. Nucleotide sequences of mitochondrial genes were published in 1979–1980, revealing unique features of the mitochondrial genetic code.

It is now known that the mitochondria in eukaryotes possess their own genome to synthesize a limited number of mitochondrial proteins (e.g., 8 in certain yeasts, 13 in mammals, and approximately 20 in plants) (Kaniak-Golik and Skoneczna 2015). These proteins are subunits of enzyme complexes located on the inner membrane that are involved in respiration and oxidative phosphorylation. The mitochondrial genome encodes all the components required for protein synthesis, as previously described for this biochemical process in the cytoplasm. Mitochondrial translation systems are more similar to those in prokaryotes than in the cytosol of eukaryotes (Ayyub and Varshney 2019). In addition, mitochondrial protein synthesis has some unusual features, including (1) some different codon assignments from the "universal" genetic code; (2) the use of a restricted number of tRNAs to translate all the codons of the genetic code; and (3) unusual structural features of mitochondrial ribosomes (mitoribosomes) such as a higher protein to RNA ratio (Ayyub and Varshney 2019). Itoh et al. (2021) recently reported that mitochondrial ribosomes are confined to the mitochondrial inner membrane to facilitate the membrane insertion of the synthesized proteins.

N-Formylmethionine (fMet), rather than L-methionine, is the initiator AA for mitochondrial protein synthesis on the mRNA. Specifically, L-methionyl-tRNA^{fMet} synthetase catalyzes the formation of L-methionyl-tRNA^{fMet} from L-methionine and tRNA^{fMet}. Then, methionyl-tRNA formyltransferase transfers a formyl group (-HCO-) from N^{10}-formyltetrahydrofolate to L-methionyl-tRNA^{fMet} to generate *N*-fMet-tRNA^{fMet}. fMet is delivered to the 30S ribosome-mRNA complex by the tRNA^{fMet}. The latter has a 3′-UAC-5′ anticodon that binds with the 5′-AUG-3′ start codon on the mRNA. Thus, fMet is coded by the same codon (AUG) as methionine.

$$\text{L-Methionine} + \text{tRNA}^{fMet} \rightarrow \text{L-Methionyl-tRNA}^{fMet} \qquad \left(\text{L-methionyl-tRNA}^{fMet}\text{ synthetase}\right)$$

$$N^{10}\text{-Formyltetrahydrofolate} + \text{L-Methionyl-tRNA}^{fMet} + \text{H}_2\text{O} \rightarrow \text{Tetrahydrofolate}$$

$$+ \ N\text{-Formylmethionyl-tRNA}^{fMet} \qquad \text{(methionyl-tRNA formyltransferase)}$$

Note that erythrocytes in mammals lack mitochondria and, therefore, mitochondrial protein synthesis. By contrast, reticulocytes possess the mitochondria and can synthesize protein in this organelle. It is intriguing that as reticulocytes are maturing, they are gradually losing their mitochondria to develop into erythrocytes. Such a biochemical event is of physiological significance, because the major function of erythrocytes is to transport oxygen in the blood and the presence of mitochondria would consume oxygen and produce reactive oxygen species to potentially damage the cells. A lack of mitochondrial protein synthesis in the erythrocytes can reduce their metabolic rate and demand for energy, thereby ensuring their long life span (~120 days in humans).

8.4 BIOCHEMICAL PATHWAYS OF PROTEIN SYNTHESIS IN THE CYTOSOL OF PROKARYOTES

8.4.1 PROTEIN SYNTHESIS IN THE CYTOSOL OF PROKARYOTES

Prokaryotes (e.g., bacteria) have neither nucleus nor mitochondrion. The pathway of protein synthesis in their cytosol is similar to that in the cytosol of eukaryotes described above. However, there are significant differences in the components and procedures of gene transcription and translation between prokaryotes and eukaryotes (Kapp and Lorsch 2004; Rodnina 2018). These 15 major differences are summarized in Table 8.4 and highlighted in the following paragraphs.

8.4.2 MAJOR DIFFERENCES IN PROTEIN SYNTHESIS BETWEEN PROKARYOTES AND EUKARYOTES

8.4.2.1 Gene Transcription

The processes of gene transcription are similar between eukaryotes and prokaryotes (Gehring et al. 2016; Venters and Pugh 2009). In prokaryotes, as in eukaryotes, most mRNA molecules are polyadenylated at the 3′ end via the covalent linkage of a polyadenylyl moiety. Compared with eukaryotes, the prokaryotic poly(A) tails are generally shorter and less mRNA molecules are polyadenylated. In contrast to eukaryotes, prokaryotic mRNAs have no 5′ caps; both transcription and translation in prokaryotes occur in their cytoplasm and, therefore, do not require transport of RNAs across an organelle after their synthesis. Furthermore, prokaryotic mRNA is essentially mature upon transcription and requires no processing (except in rare cases, such as alternative splicing) or transport (Watson 2013). Thus, gene transcription can be coupled with mRNA translation in prokaryotes.

TABLE 8.4

Differences in Protein Synthesis Between Eukaryotes (e.g., Humans and Other Animals) and Prokaryotes (e.g., Bacteria and Archaea)

Eukaryotes	Prokaryotes
Extensive pre-mRNA processing; transport of processed mRNA from the nucleus to the cytoplasm	Little or no pre-mRNA processing; no mRNA transport; ready to serve as mature mRNA for protein synthesis
Extensive polyadenylation at the 3′ end of mRNA	Shorter poly(A) tails; less mRNAs are polyadenylated
Extensive 5′ caps in mRNA	No 5′ caps in mRNA
Linear polyribosomes	Circular polyribosomes
No coupling between nuclear gene transcription and cytosolic mRNA translation (i.e., spatially and temporally separated)	Coupling between gene transcription and mRNA translation
An mRNA generally has one start site for protein synthesis and serves as a template for the synthesis of one protein	An mRNA can have multiple start sites for protein synthesis and serves as a template for the synthesis of several proteins
80S ribosome (4,200 kDa) consisting of 40S and 60S ribosomes; 18S ribosomal RNA and 33 proteins in the 40S ribosome; 28S, 5.8S, and 5S ribosomal RNAs plus 49 proteins in the 60S ribosome	70S ribosome (2,700 kDa) consisting of 30S and 50S ribosomes; 16S ribosomal RNA and 21 proteins in the 30S ribosome; 23S and 5S ribosomal RNAs plus 31 proteins in the 50S ribosome
15 initiation factors for protein synthesis, including eIF-4A, eIF-4B, eIF-4E, eIF-4G, and eIF-4H	3 initiation factors for protein synthesis: IF1, IF2, and IF3
The 80S ribosome binds mRNA efficiently in the absence tRNA	The 70S ribosome binds mRNA at a greater affinity in the presence than the absence of tRNA
L-Methionine as the amino acid substrate for tRNA$_i$	N-Formylmethionine as the amino acid substrate for tRNA$_i$ in bacteria but L-methionine for tRNA$_i$ in archaea
Elongation factors: eEF1A, eEF1B, eEF2, and SBP2	Elongation factors: EF-Tu, EF-Ts, and EF-G
6 AAs are incorporated into a polypeptide per second	18 AAs are incorporated into a polypeptide per second
Termination factors: RF1, RF2, and RF3	Termination factors: eRF1 and eRF3
Recycling factors: RRF and EF-G	Recycling factors: eIF3, eIF3j, eIF1A, and eIF1
The target of rapamycin cell signaling is the master activator of protein synthesis in the animal kingdom	Lack the target of rapamycin cell signaling

8.4.2.2 Initiation of mRNA Translation into Protein

Prokaryotes have linear polyribosomes. The size and protein quantity of ribosomes in prokaryotes, as well as the number of initiation factors (IFs), are smaller than those in eukaryotes. The prokaryotic active initiation complex (the 70S ribosome, 2700 kDa) consists of 30S and 50S ribosomal subunits. The 30S ribosomal subunit contains a 16S RNA and 21 proteins, whereas the 50S ribosomal subunit is comprised of 23S and 5S ribosomal RNAs, as well as 31 proteins. The 70S ribosomes interact with mRNA at a greater affinity in the presence than in the absence of tRNA. In contrast to eukaryotic mRNA, a prokaryotic mRNA can have multiple start sites and can serve as a template for the synthesis of several proteins. Notably, the target of rapamycin cell signaling is well-conserved in the animal kingdom as the master activator of protein synthesis (Saxton and Sabatini 2017), but is absent from prokaryotes (Roustan et al. 2016).

8.4.2.3 Peptide Elongation and Termination

As in the eukaryotic mitochondria, fMet is the initiator AA for protein synthesis in bacteria (Sherman et al. 1985). Interestingly, like cytosolic protein synthesis, L-methionine is the initiator AA for protein synthesis in archaea (Schmitt et al. 2019). Peptide elongation in prokaryotes requires elongation factors Tu, Ts, and G. Prokaryotic ribosomes can incorporate 18 AAs into a polypeptide per second, 12 more AAs than eukaryotic ribosomes. This helps to explain, in part, why bacteria grow much faster than animal cells. In contrast to eukaryotes, the prokaryotic peptidyltransferase is the 23S ribosomal RNA of the 50S ribosomal subunit.

Some species of bacteria and archaea lack asparaginyl (Asn)- or glutaminyl (Gln)-tRNA synthetases, or both, and, therefore, cannot directly convert asparagine plus ATP into asparaginyl-tRNA or glutamine plus ATP into glutaminyl-tRNA. However, these cells express: (1) a non-discriminating Glu-tRNA synthetase, which can use tRNA^{Glu} or tRNA^{Gln} as a substrate; and (2) a non-discriminating Asp-tRNA synthetase, which can use tRNA^{Asp} or tRNA^{Asn} as a substrate. Therefore, the Glu-tRNA synthetase generates Glu-tRNA^{Gln} from glutamate plus tRNA^{Gln}, and Asp-tRNA synthetase yields Asp-tRNA^{Asn} from aspartate plus tRNA^{Asn}. The resulting mismatched Glu-tRNA^{Gln} from Glu plus tRNA^{Gln} is converted by Glu-tRNA^{Gln} amidotransferase into Gln-tRNA^{Gln} in the presence of glutamine, whereas the resulting mismatched Asp-tRNA^{Asn} from Asp plus tRNA^{Asn} is converted by Asp-tRNA^{Asn} amidotransferase into Asn-tRNA^{Asn} in the presence of asparagine. These unique aminoacylation-transamidation reactions are summarized as follows:

$$Glu + tRNA^{Gln} + ATP \rightarrow Glu\text{-}tRNA^{Gln} + AMP + PPi \quad (Glu\text{-}tRNA \text{ synthetase})$$

$$Glu\text{-}tRNA^{Gln} + Gln + ATP \rightarrow Gln\text{-}tRNA^{Gln} + Glu + ADP + Pi \quad \left(Glu\text{-}tRNA^{Gln} \text{ amidotransferase}\right)$$

$$Asp + tRNA^{Asn} + ATP \rightarrow Asp\text{-}tRNA^{Asn} + AMP + PPi \quad (Asp\text{-}tRNA \text{ synthetase})$$

$$Asp\text{-}tRNA^{Asn} + Asn + ATP \rightarrow Asn\text{-}tRNA^{Asn} + Asp + ADP + Pi \quad \left(Asp\text{-}tRNA^{Asn} \text{ amidotransferase}\right)$$

8.4.3 Incorporation of L-Pyrrolysine (A Special AA) into Proteins of Certain Prokaryotes

L-Pyrrolysine is a building block for the synthesis of specific proteins (e.g., methylamine methyltransferases in a small number of methanogenic archaea, e.g., *Methanosarcina barkeri* and *Methanosarcina* spp.) and bacteria (e.g., Desulfitobacterium hafniense) (Rother and Krzycki 2010). Polycarpo et al. (2004) discovered a specialized aminoacyl-tRNA synthetase (tRNA^{Pyl}) for charging pyrrolysine to tRNA^{Pyl} to form pyrrolysyl-tRNA^{Pyl} in a small number of methanogenic archaea and bacteria. Lysine and tRNA^{Lys} are not substrates of this enzyme. In these prokaryotes, L-pyrrolysine is synthesized from two molecules of L-lysine by three enzymes (PylB, PylC, and PylD) (Tharp et al. 2018). Specifically, one molecule of lysine is first converted into (3R)-3-methyl-D-ornithine, which is then ligated to a second lysine molecule. In this series of biochemical reactions that require ATP and NAD$^+$, an NH$_2$ group is eliminated, followed by cyclization and dehydration steps to yield L-pyrrolysine. L-Pyrrolysine is directly incorporated into the protein during mRNA translation under the direction of a genetic code (UAG on the mRNA template) just like the standard AAs. In most organisms, the UAG codon is the "amber" stop codon.

$$2L\text{-Lysine} + ATP + NAD^+ \rightarrow L\text{-Pyrrolysine} + ADP + Pi + NADH + H^+ \text{ (PylB, PylC, and PylD)}$$

$$L\text{-Pyrrolysine} + tRNA^{Pyl} + ATP \rightarrow L\text{-Pyrrolysine-} tRNA^{Pyl} + AMP + PPi \text{ (pyrrolysyl-tRNA synthetase)}$$

$$L\text{-Pyrrolysine-} tRNA^{Pyl} \rightarrow Protein \text{ (the UAG codonon the mRNA template)}$$

L-Pyrrolysine is the most recent addition to the list of AAs in proteins. It is the 22nd genetically encoded AA in specific proteins of certain prokaryotes, but is not present in humans and other animals. Although special tRNAs are required for the incorporation of L-pyrrolysine and selenocysteine in specialized proteins, the mechanisms for the formation of these two AAs differ in that L-pyrrolysine is synthesized before it is charged to tRNA^{Pyl} but selenocysteine is generated from an AA-tRNA [i.e., seryl-tRNA$_{(Sec)}$] during the mRNA translation.

8.5 BIOCHEMICAL CHARACTERISTICS AND SIGNIFICANCE OF PROTEIN SYNTHESIS

8.5.1 ENERGY REQUIREMENT

Intracellular protein synthesis requires large amounts of energy, primarily in the forms of ATP and GTP. The energy-dependent reactions include (1) AA activation; (2) the entry of tRNA-AA into the A site on the ribosome that requires the cleavage of GTP to GDP; and (3) the translocation of the newly formed peptidyl-tRNA from the A site to the P site on the ribosome. The incorporation of 1 mol AA into protein requires 4 mol ATP and the termination of polypeptide synthesis requires 1 mol GTP, as indicated below.

1. AA activation to AA-tRNA: ATP → AMP + PPi   (2 high-energy phosphate bonds)
2. Entry of tRNA-AA into the A site: GTP → GDP + Pi   (1 high-energy phosphate bond)
3. Translocation of the newly formed peptidyl-tRNA from the A site to the P site: GTP → GDP + Pi   (1 high-energy phosphate bond)
4. Termination of polypeptide synthesis: GTP → GDP + Pi   (1 high-energy phosphate bond)

Thus, 5 mol of high-energy phosphate bonds (equivalent to 5 ATP → 5 ADP + 5 Pi) are required to incorporate 1 mol AAs into 100 g of animal protein. This amounts to 258 kJ for 1 mol AAs, based on 51.6 kJ/mol for one high-energy bond in ATP. To synthesize 100 g protein, whose AA residues are assumed to have an average molecular mass of 100 Daltons, the energy requirement for this event would be 258 kJ. The transport of some AAs by cells also requires ATP (e.g., 0.5 mol ATP/mol AA on average). The energy released during protein biosynthesis helps explain, in part, the phenomenon of "heat increment" after an animal eats a protein meal.

Let's take an adult man in the fed state, for example. Both dietary and endogenous AAs are used to synthesize proteins. To estimate the energy requirement for protein synthesis, we assume that a 70-kg healthy adult man (between 25 and 50 years of age) [ingesting 62 g protein (229 kcal of physiological energy), 421.5 g starch (1,686 kcal of physiological energy), and 65 g fat per day (585 kcal of physiological energy); a total of 2,500 of physiological energy] synthesizes 300 g protein per day, then:

$$300 \text{ g protein} \rightarrow 300/100 = 3 \text{ mol AAs}$$

Let's assume that 0.5 mol ATP is needed by the cell to transport 1 mol of AAs across its plasma membrane.

ATP requirement for protein synthesis: 3 mol AAs × (5 mol ATP/mol AA + 0.5 mol ATP/mol AA) = 16.5 mol ATP

The biological oxidation of 1 mol glucose (180 g), 1 mol AA (on average), 1 mol palmitate, and 1 mol glycerol produces 30, 20, 106, and 18.5 mol ATP, respectively (Chapter 4). If a healthy adult consumes 62 g protein (the molecular weight of the AA residue is 100), 421.5 g starch (the molecular weight of the glucose residue is 162), and 65 g fat (e.g., tripalmitoylglycerol with a molecular weight of 806) per day, with their true digestibilities of 90%, 98%, and 96%, respectively, 14.5% of the dietary energy substrates are oxidized to support whole-body protein synthesis.

ATP produced from dietary intake of 62 g protein = 62 g / 100 g × 0.90 × 20 = 11.2 mol

ATP produced from dietary intake of 421.5 g starch = 421.5 g / 162 g × 0.98 × 30 = 76.5 mol

ATP produced from dietary intake of 65 g fat in diet = 65 g / 806 g × 0.96 × (3 × 106 + 1 × 18.5)

$$= 26.1 \text{ mol}$$

(Note: 1 mol tripalmitoylglycerol contains 3 mol palmitate and 1 mol glycerol.)

The percentage of ATP produced from oxidation of dietary macronutrients that is utilized for protein synthesis is 14.5% [namely, $16.5 \div (11.2 + 76.5 + 26.1) \times 100 = 14.5\%$] in the healthy adult. Note that this calculation does not take, into consideration, the energy required for glucose and glycerol transport, as well as intracellular fatty acid trafficking.

8.5.2   Physiological Significance of Protein Synthesis

Dietary proteins must be converted into tissue proteins to exert their nutritional and physiological roles. This metabolic conversion is accomplished only by the intracellular synthesis of the various types of proteins from AAs. The physiological significance of protein biosynthesis can be readily appreciated because of the vital functions of proteins in animals. Protein synthesis also functions to regulate: (1) intracellular and extracellular concentrations of proteins (including enzymes), (2) replacement of cells, (3) wound healing, and (4) immune responses in organisms.

8.5.2.1   Physiological Functions of Proteins

There are approximately 100,000 different proteins in the animal (Wang et al. 2006). Proteins maintain both cell structure and extracellular structure. In cardiac, skeletal, and smooth muscles, actin and myosin are the major protein constituents of the cellular machinery required for their contraction. Many proteins are enzymes catalyzing biochemical reactions, without which there would be no life. Some proteins regulate gene expression and nutrient metabolism, while protecting the body from oxidative stress and infectious diseases. In addition, as hormones secreted by endocrine glands, proteins mediate cell-to-cell communications in the body. Furthermore, proteins serve to transport and store nutrients (including water and AAs) and oxygen. Finally, proteins are hydrophilic molecules. In general, 1 g of protein is associated with retention of 3 g of water in the body (Wu 2018). Given the various physiological roles of proteins (Table 8.5), a loss of more than 50% of the protein from the body is not compatible with the survival of humans (Leiter and Marliss 1982) and other animals (Wu 2018).

8.5.2.2   Regulation of Protein Concentrations and Animal Growth

Protein synthesis is necessary for replacing the degraded proteins and for maintaining intracellular and extracellular concentrations of proteins in all organisms (Reeds and Lobley 1980). In young

TABLE 8.5
Physiological Functions of Proteins in Animals

Functions	Examples of Proteins Involved
Cell structure	Integral and peripheral membrane proteins
Extracellular structure	Collagen, elastin, and proteoglycans
Enzyme-catalyzed reactions	Dehydrogenase, decarboxylase, and protein kinase
Gene expression	DNA-binding proteins, histones, and repressor proteins
Hormone-mediated effects	Insulin, somatotropin, and placental lactogen
Muscle contraction	Actin, myosin, and tubulin
Osmotic regulation	Proteins (e.g., albumin and fibrinogens) in the plasma
Protection	Blood clotting factors, antibodies, and interferons
Regulation of metabolism	Calmodulin, leptin, and osteopontin
Storage of nutrients and O_2	Ferritin, metallothionein, and myoglobin
Transport of nutrients and O_2	Albumin, hemoglobin, and plasma lipoproteins

animals, protein synthesis plays an important role in determining tissue growth and development, as well as the partitioning of dietary energy into lean tissue gain (Bergen 1974). Rates of protein synthesis in major tissues of young pigs and young rats, as well as adult humans are summarized in Tables 8.6–8.10 (Deng et al. 2009; McNurlan and Garlick 1980; McNurlan et al. 1979). Note that the fractional rate of protein synthesis in the liver of young rats is about 100%/day, meaning that hepatic proteins are almost completely synthesized de novo every 24 h. In adults who do not usually accrete proteins and have lower rates of protein synthesis than the young, protein synthesis remains necessary to maintain protein homeostasis in cells (Waterlow 1984). In all animals, proteins synthesized and exported by cells, such as hepatocytes, enterocytes, and immunocytes, regulate the concentrations of these proteins in the plasma and other extracellular fluids (Bröer and Bröer 2017). For extracellular proteins, the rates of their release from cells are also controlled by exocytosis. The following equation regarding intracellular protein balance applies to all cell types. There could be a positive or negative protein balance in a given tissue or the whole body.

$$\text{Intracellular protein balance} = \text{Rate of protein synthesis} - \text{Rate of protein degradation}$$

Regulation of protein metabolism is the biochemical basis for increasing protein deposition in animal tissues, particularly in skeletal muscle, and for decreasing protein wasting in disease conditions and catabolic states (McAllister et al. 2000; Waterlow 1984). Studies with young pigs by T.A. Davis, P.J. Reeds, and colleagues have shown that an increase in protein accretion in skeletal muscle brought about by protein feeding and AA supplementation results primarily from an increase in protein synthesis rather than a decrease in protein degradation (Davis et al. 1998; 2002, 2008). Changes in the rates of protein synthesis and degradation are also crucial for regulating concentrations of key enzymes in metabolic pathways (see Chapter 10).

8.5.2.3 Production and Replacement of Cells

Protein synthesis is required for the ongoing production of all cells, particularly rapidly proliferating cells such as (1) epithelial cells of the gastrointestinal tract, mammary glands, and skin; (2) reticulocytes; (3) immunologically challenged lymphocytes; and (4) gamete cells of the reproductive system. In addition, reticulocytes are continuously synthesized albeit at a relatively low rate. These cells are vital to the survival and reproduction of organisms. For example, the rapid growth of epithelial cells in the small intestine of neonatal pigs and rats is essential as the cell life span is only 7–20 days depending on age (Klein and McKenzie. 1983; Smith and Jarvis 1978). Some of the intestinal epithelial cells are constantly sloughed off into the gut lumen. New cells are needed to replace the old ones. Also, when an animal is immunologically challenged, T cells and B cells rapidly proliferate so that large amounts of lymphokines and antibodies are generated. An inability for lymphocytes to proliferate in response to activating signals results in impaired immune responses and immunodeficiency.

8.5.2.4 Wound Healing and Recovery from Injury

Successful wound healing is critical to the recovery of patients from injury and to minimize postoperative morbidity and mortality. This process involves (1) the inflammatory phase during which cells of the immune system (e.g., macrophages) produce factors to stimulate the migration and division of cells in a wounded tissue; (2) the proliferative phase characterized by angiogenesis, collagen deposition, granulation tissue formation, epithelialization, and wound contraction by the action of myofibroblasts; and (3) the maturation and remodeling phase during which collagen is synthesized, remodeled, and realigned along tension lines (Rodrigues et al. 2018). Each of these steps requires an enhanced synthesis of multiple proteins from AAs. Increased provision of AAs, particularly arginine, proline, and glycine, improves wound healing in humans and other animals (Li and Wu 2018; Witte and Barbul 2008).

8.5.2.5 Immune Responses and Health

An ability of the host to prevent the invasion of various pathogens depends on both the innate (natural, non-specific) and the acquired (adaptive, specific) immune systems. The innate immune system consists of several integral components: (1) physical barriers (e.g., skin, endothelial cell layer in the respiratory tract, and the gastrointestinal tract); (2) mononuclear phagocytes (e.g., monocytes and macrophages), dendritic cells, polymorphonuclear granulocytes (e.g., neutrophils, eosinophils, and basophils), mast cells, natural killer cells, and platelets; (3) humoral factors, including collectins, complements, lysozymes, C-reactive proteins, and interferons; (4) antimicrobial peptides in the mucosa and lumen of the small intestine; and (5) neutrophil extracellular traps, comprising of DNA and proteins as major structural components (Calder et al. 2002). The acquired immune system consists of T lymphocytes, B lymphocytes, and humoral factors. The bone marrow is primarily responsible for hematopoiesis and lymphopoiesis, while the thymus is required for T-cell development. The spleen, lymph nodes, and the mucosa-associated lymphoid tissues in the gastrointestinal, respiratory, reproductive tracts, and other organs are secondary lymphoid tissues. Antibodies produced by B lymphocytes are highly effective against extracellular pathogens. Both the innate and acquired immune systems require the synthesis of cytokines, antibodies, complements, and other related proteins. Thus, a dietary deficiency of protein or a specific AA (e.g., arginine and glutamine) or other factors that limit protein synthesis will impair immunity and increase the risk for infectious disease (Li et al. 2007). Enhancing the ability of monocytes, macrophages, and other cells of the immune system to synthesize proteins and polypeptides involved in the killing of pathogens has great potential (Chapter 11) to promote the immunological defense of humans and other animals against infections by bacteria, fungi, parasites, and viruses [including coronavirus, such as severe acute respiratory syndrome coronavirus 2 (the virus that causes COVID-19)].

8.6 MEASUREMENTS OF PROTEIN SYNTHESIS

8.6.1 Measurement of Protein Synthesis In Vitro

8.6.1.1 General Considerations

Labeled AA tracers are employed to measure protein synthesis and degradation in isolated tissues, perfused organs, or incubated cells (Adegoke et al. 2003; Baracos et al. 1989; Baracos and Goldberg 1986; Klasing et al. 1987; Tischler et al. 1982, 1984; Wu and Thompson 1990; Zhang et al. 2019). The advantages of *in vitro* methods are numerous. First, the preparation and incubation of tissues or cells are simple, making it possible to study a relatively large number of tissues or cells at one time. Second, the use of contralateral tissues (e.g., skeletal muscle) or cells (e.g., lymphocytes) can decrease experimental errors due to inter-animal differences and increases the power for statistical analysis. Third, experimental conditions can be easily imposed to quickly test a large number of interesting hypotheses. Fourth, *in vitro* methods allow studies of specific cell types, which would be no small undertaking *in vivo*. Fifth, isolated tissues or cells are free of interference from other tissues or interfering factors, thus allowing studies of direct effects of hormones or other substances on protein turnover in a specific tissue or a cell type. Sixth, *in vitro* studies are invaluable for elucidating biochemical mechanisms of protein turnover and for gaining information fundamental to designing *in vivo* studies. Thus, *in vitro* cell or tissue preparations provide a useful tool to study AA biochemistry and nutrition.

  In vitro measurement of protein synthesis has shortcomings. First, the rate of protein synthesis *in vitro* is always lower than that measured *in vivo*. This is due, in part, to the limited diffusion of oxygen into the core of an incubated tissue (e.g., skeletal muscle), thus causing a hypoxic zone. To facilitate oxygen diffusion and substrate transport, it is desirable to use small-size tissues from young rodents, young chickens, and other small animals. The viability of *in vitro* preparations can be assessed by measuring: (1) the linearity of biochemical reactions; (2) intracellular ATP concentration; (3) oxygen consumption; and (4) the integrity of cell structures as indicated by the release of lactate dehydrogenase and the exclusion of trypan blue. Second, incubated tissues (e.g., skeletal muscle) are usually in negative N balance. This, however, may not be true for skeletal muscle isolated from young growing animals (e.g., 9-day-old chicks) or for incubated cells. For incubated muscle, this negative N balance can be improved by mounting the tissue at normal length. Third, *in vitro* data may not necessarily be extrapolated to *in vivo* situations, due to the absence, from the incubated tissue and cells, of mechanisms responsible for maintaining homeostasis in intact animals such as the neuroendocrine and circulatory systems.

8.6.1.2 *In Vitro* **Preparations**

In vitro studies have played, and will continue to play, a major role in advancing our knowledge of protein synthesis. *In vitro* preparations for measuring protein synthesis include (1) perfused organs (e.g., liver, kidneys, heart, lung, intestine, leg muscles, and hemicorpus), (2) incubated tissues or organs (e.g., skeletal muscle (~15–25 mg; quarters of young rat diaphragm), atria, and epididymal fat pads), (3) isolated cells (e.g., myocytes, neutrophils, adipocytes, lymphocytes, hepatocytes, macrophages, enterocytes, tumor cells, skeletal muscle cells, red blood cells, HeLa cells, 3T3 cells, lung cells, L6 myoblasts, and fibroblasts), and (4) cell-free systems. Cells or tissues are usually cultured or incubated for up to 3 h. In isolated cells or tissues, the rate of protein synthesis is usually determined by measuring the rate of incorporation of a labeled AA into newly synthesized protein. This measurement can yield false high values for protein synthesis due to the reincorporation of labeled AAs released during protein degradation into recently synthesized protein. The simplest and most effective strategy to minimize this tracer reincorporation is the use of appropriately high concentrations of the tracee AA (e.g., 1 mM unlabeled phenylalanine) in the incubation (extracellular) medium (Baracos et al. 1989; Wu and Thompson 1990).

Both perfused organs and incubated tissues contain extracellular space. Therefore, the amounts of radioactivity in the extracellular space should be corrected for to determine the intracellular specific radioactivity (SR) of the labeled AA (Chapter 7). This can be done by using a labeled substance (e.g., ^{3}H-inulin) which cannot be taken up by cells of the tissue (Wu and Thompson 1990). Similar considerations are applied to studies involving stable isotopes.

Caution should also be exercised to ensure the viability of a tissue used to measure protein synthesis *in vitro*. In general, an incubated tissue should be small and thin to permit the rapid diffusion of O_2 from the medium into the tissue. Also, the incubation period should be relatively short so that the tissue remains biochemically viable. Some investigators, however, are not aware of these important cautions in their studies and have reported using 500 mg isolated skeletal muscle for incubation, for example. Likewise, some scientists incubated large pieces of skeletal muscle for 96 h. In such studies, the viability of skeletal muscle is questionable.

8.6.1.3 **Choosing A Labeled AA Tracer**

Not all AA tracers can be used to measure protein synthesis. Selection of a tracer AA depends on cell type and tissue. However, the following criteria for choosing an appropriate tracer AA must be considered.

a. The AA tracer or its tracee is neither synthesized nor degraded by the cell or tissue of interest. This facilitates rapid achievement of an intracellular isotopic steady state and the measurement of intracellular SR or isotope enrichment (IE) of the labeled free AAs. Note that labeled AAs that are metabolized in pathways other than through protein turnover can be converted into other labeled intermediates including AAs, or may become diluted, to a large extent, by the synthesis of non-labeled AAs (see Chapter 7).

b. The tracee AA must be transported readily across the plasma membrane and have a small metabolic pool size. This facilitates rapid achievement of intracellular isotopic steady state in the cells or tissue of interest.

c. The tracee AA has no effect on intracellular protein turnover in the cells and tissue of interest. This ensures that the presence of a relatively high concentration of the tracee AA in the incubation or culture medium will not interfere with the effects of tested substances.
d. The isotopically labeled atoms in the tracer cannot be spontaneously exchangeable with non-labeled atoms, and the labeled AA must be of high purity. This helps to prevent the loss and contamination of the tracer AA, while ensuring accurate measurement of protein synthesis.
e. The tracee AA can be analyzed by a reliable method. This ensures accurate measurement of intracellular SR or IE of the free labeled AA in the cells and tissue of interest.
f. The labeled AA should be readily available and relatively economical to help reduce the cost of the studies to allow a number of replicates.

Tracee AAs that meet the above requirements vary with cells and tissue. For example, labeled leucine, valine, or isoleucine can be used to measure protein synthesis in the mammalian and avian liver and hepatocytes (Stoll et al. 1992), but not in skeletal muscle (Baracos et al. 1989; Baracos and Goldberg 1986; Wu and Thompson 1990), because BCAAs are extensively transaminated in skeletal muscle but undergo little catabolism in the liver of mammals and birds (Chapter 4). By contrast, phenylalanine or tyrosine is a good choice for the measurement of protein synthesis in skeletal muscle.

8.6.1.4 Measuring the Rate of Protein Synthesis *In Vitro*

In all studies, extracellular medium must contain physiological levels of AAs found in the plasma or in the lumen of the small intestine, depending on the experimental design. A labeled AA is added into the perfusate or incubation medium. The incorporation of the labeled AA into proteins is measured over a period of time (e.g., 2–3 h) during which the rate of protein synthesis is relatively constant. At the end of the perfusion or incubation, tissue samples or cells are homogenized with an acid (e.g., 5 mL of 10% trichloroacetic acid or 1.5 M $HClO_4$ per 100 mg tissue; or 0.5 mL 10% trichloroacetic acid or 1.5 M $HClO_4$ per 5×10^6 cells) to precipitate proteins and obtain the intracellular free AA pool. The precipitated proteins are solubilized overnight in 0.5 mL Soluene or 1 M NaOH at 60°C. The labeled AA and its tracee in proteins and the intracellular free AA pool are analyzed using various instruments, including high-performance liquid chromatography, liquid scintillation spectrometry, or mass spectrometry. The rate of protein synthesis is generally calculated on the basis of the intracellular SR or IE of the labeled AA in the precursor pool rather than the SR or IE of the aminoacyl-tRNA. This is because the measurement of aminoacyl-tRNA is technically challenging due to its very low concentration in cells and its very high rate of turnover. The rate of protein synthesis measured *in vitro* is expressed often as nmol AA incorporated into protein/mg tissue (Fukls et al. 1975; Wu and Thompson 1991) but sometimes as %/h (Kong et al. 2012; Xi et al. 2012). Let's use a radioactive tracer as an example.

$$\text{Incorporation of AA into protein} = A/F* \div \text{Amount of tissue (mg)} \div \text{Time}$$

A: The amount of radioactivity in the protein (dpm) at the end of the incubation period;
  $F*$: SR of the precursor, namely the labeled free AA in the cell (dpm/nmol);
  t: The duration of protein labeling in tissue;
  K_s: Fractional rate of protein synthesis (%/time);

$$K_s(\%/t) = \left(P*/F*\right) \div \text{Time} \times 100$$

$P*$: SR of the labeled AA in tissue proteins (dpm/nmol).

$$\text{Amount of protein synthesized per unit of time} = K_s \times \text{Protein mass}$$

Example for the calculation of the rate of protein synthesis *in vitro*: Rat soleus muscle (25 mg) is incubated for 2 h at 37°C in the presence of 10 mU/mL insulin, 5 mM D-glucose, 1 mM L- phenylalanine plus L-[U-^{14}C]phenylalanine, and physiological concentrations of other AAs found in the plasma. The SR of ^{14}C-phenylalanine in the incubation medium is 310 dpm/nmol. The intracellular SR of ^{14}C-phenylalanine is 300 dpm/nmol at 15 min of incubation and is maintained constant during the 2-h incubation period. The amounts of ^{14}C-phenylalanine radioactivity and phenylalanine in proteins are 3,500 dpm and 2.8 μmol, respectively. Protein content in skeletal muscle is 20%. What is the rate of protein synthesis in the tissue?

$$\text{Amount of } ^{14}\text{C-Phe radioactivity in protein} = 3,500 \text{ dpm}$$

$$F* = 300 \text{ dpm / nmol Phe}$$

$$\text{Incorporation of AA into protein} = A/F* \div \text{Amount of tissue (mg)} \div \text{Time (h)}$$

$$= 3,500 / 300 \div 25 \text{ mg} \div 2 \text{ h}$$

$$= 0.233 \text{ nmol Phe / mg tissue per h}$$

$$P* = 3,500 \text{ dpm} / 2.8 \text{ μmol Phe} = 1,250 \text{ dpm / μmol Phe} = 1.25 \text{ dpm / nmol Phe}$$

$$K_s = \left(P*/F*\right) \div \text{Time} \times 100\% = 1.25 / 300 \div 2 \text{ h} \times 100\% = 0.208\% / \text{h}$$

$$\text{Amount of protein synthesized per h} = K_s \times \text{Protein mass} = 0.208\% / \text{h} \times 5 \text{ mg} = 0.01 \text{ mg / h}$$

8.6.2   MEASUREMENT OF PROTEIN SYNTHESIS *IN VIVO*

8.6.2.1   General Considerations

Criteria for selection of a tracer AA for *in vivo* studies are the same as for *in vitro* experiments, except that all AAs can be degraded in animals. Many methods have been developed to measure *in vivo* protein synthesis in tissues of humans and other animals, which include (1) the single administration of a tracer AA, (2) flooding dose technique, and (3) constant infusion of a tracer AA (Bergen et al. 1987; Frank et al. 2007; Johnson et al. 2003; Marliss et al. 2006; Reeds and Lobley 1980; Rennie et al. 1994; Zak et al. 1979). Measurement of whole-body protein synthesis based on two or more compartment models has also been validated for use in humans and other animals (Lobley et al. 1980; Waterlow 1984; Wilkinson 2018). The most common methods are the flooding dose technique (Davis and Reeds 2001; Frank et al. 2007; Southorn et al. 1992) and the constant infusion of a tracer (Dillon et al. 2011; Pencharz et al. 1981; Waterlow 1984). However, the experimental approach chosen for measuring tissue protein synthesis *in vivo* should be dictated by the scientific question being addressed.

In vivo methods offer distinct advantages by: (1) allowing studies of protein metabolism under both physiological and pathological conditions, which cannot be absolutely mimicked *in vitro*; (2) providing an invaluable approach to verify *in vitro* findings and their significance in intact animals; and (3) eliminating the need to perform invasive procedures on animals. Disadvantages of *in vivo* studies include the following. First, the number of animals, particularly large animals, used in each experiment is limited by laboratory space and costs. Second, *in vivo* conditions are difficult to control and methodologies are often complicated, thus introducing many variables in data analysis. Third, biological differences between experimental animals can be large, therefore decreasing the sensitivity of the response to treatments. Fourth, it is difficult to study protein turnover in specific cell types *in vivo* due to the presence of and interactions between different cell types within a tissue. Fifth, the interferences of the studied tissue by other tissues exist *in vivo*, making it very difficult to interpret experimental data. Finally, the rates of protein synthesis in tissues are generally under-estimated if they are calculated solely from the isotope abundance of the AA tracer in the plasma without any correction for tracer dilution within the cells (Waterlow 1984).

8.6.2.2 General Terminologies Used in Measuring Protein Turnover *In Vivo*

Radioactive or stable tracers are often used for *in vivo* measurement of protein synthesis in humans and other animals (Davis et al. 1999; Lobley et al. 1980; McNurlan and Garlick 1980; Waterlow 1984; Wray-Cahen et al. 1998). The common terminologies for the kinetics of protein synthesis are described in this section (Figure 8.9). Because a labeled AA in protein can leave the protein pool through protein degradation, terminologies for its kinetics are also introduced herein and are based on those described by Zak et al. (1979). Methods to determine *in vivo* protein degradation in animals will be discussed in more detail in Chapter 9.

A: The amount of radioactivity (dpm for a radioisotope) or mass (nmol for a stable isotope) of the labeled AA in the protein molecule.

P: The amount of a given AA in the total pool of the protein molecule (nmol). Because the AA composition of a protein is constant, P is proportional to the total amount of protein.

P^*: SR (dpm/nmol) of the radioactive tracer AA (e.g., ^{14}C-Phe) or IE (%) of the stable tracer AA in the protein molecule. $P^*=A/P$

F^*: SR (dpm/nmol) of the radioactive tracer AA (e.g., ^{14}C-Phe) or IE (%) of the stable tracer AA in the precursor pool (see Chapter 7 for calculation).

K_s: Fractional rate of the tracer AA entering the protein molecule as a result of protein synthesis.

K_d: Fractional rate of the tracer AA leaving the protein molecule as a result of protein degradation.

K_p: Fractional turnover rate of tracer AA in the protein molecule (i.e., fractional rate of protein synthesis or degradation at steady state when $K_s=K_d$; %/min).

K_F: Rate constant (%/min) for rise of SR or IR of the tracer AA in the free precursor pool to plateau; K_F depends on the tissue and the amount of the labeled AA infused into the body.

$$dP^*/dt = (K_s \times F^*) - (K_d \times P^*)$$

t: The duration of protein labeling in tissue.

In a physiological steady state ($K_s=K_d$), $dP^*/dt = K_p (F^* - P^*)$

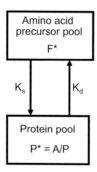

FIGURE 8.9 Common terminologies for the kinetics of *in vivo* protein turnover measured with a tracer amino acid (AA). A labeled AA is incorporated into a protein through protein synthesis, and an AA is released from the protein through protein degradation. A, the amount of radioactivity (dpm for a radioisotope) or mass (nmol for a stable isotope) of the labeled AA in the protein molecule; F^*, specific radioactivity or isotopic enrichment of a tracer AA in the precursor pool; K_d, fractional rate of protein degradation; K_s, fractional rate of protein synthesis; P, the amount of a given AA in the total pool of the protein molecule (nmol); P^*, specific radioactivity or isotopic enrichment of a tracer AA in the protein molecule.

This equation means that the rate of the change of the SR or IE in the protein molecule at any time depends on the difference between the amount of the tracer AA entering the protein molecule from the precursor pool ($K_s \times F^*$) and the amount of the tracer AA leaving the protein molecule through protein degradation ($K_d \times P^*$).

8.6.2.3 Pulse Labeling of Proteins by the Single Administration of a Labeled AA

When a single dose of a labeled AA along with a small amount of the tracee AA is administered into an animal, the precursor-product relationship for SR or IE of the labeled AA is shown in Figure 8.10 with three distinct phases.

Phase 1: $F^* \gg P^*$. This phase is not useful for the measurement of protein turnover.

Phase 2: $F^* = P^*$ (cross-over point). This phase is not useful for the measurement of protein turnover.

Phase 3: $F^* < P^*$. This phase, which may span several hours, can be useful for the measurement of protein turnover. Specifically, the decrease in P^* (SR or IE of the tracer AA in protein) with time is related to the rate of synthesis of new protein. In this phase, F^* is less than P^* because the turnover rate of the labeled AA in the precursor pool is greater than that in the protein pool.

$$dP^*/dt = -K_s \times P^*$$

When K_s is a constant with respect to protein, this equation is integrated to give the following mathematical formula to calculate the fractional rate of protein synthesis.

$$\ln\left(P^*_0/P^*_t\right) = K_s \times t$$

P^*_0 is the SR or IE of the labeled AA in protein at time 0, P^*_t is the SR or IE of the labeled AA in protein at any given time, and t is the duration of measurement of P^* after the administration of a

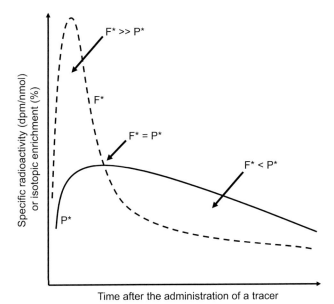

FIGURE 8.10 The precursor-product relationship in the protein pool and the precursor pool in three phases after the single administration of a labeled amino acid (AA) into the animal. F^*, specific radioactivity or isotopic enrichment of a tracer AA in the precursor pool; P^*, specific radioactivity or isotopic enrichment of a tracer AA in the protein molecule. Phase 3 is useful for measuring protein synthesis in tissues. (Adapted from Zak et al. 1979. *Physiol. Rev.* 59:407–447.)

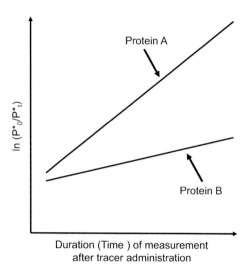

FIGURE 8.11 Measurement of protein synthesis using the pulse labeling method. In Phase 3 of the pulse labeling of proteins (see Figure 8.10), a decline in the specific radioactivity (SR) or isotopic enrichment (IE) of the labeled protein with time can be used to measure the rate of tissue protein synthesis. P^*_0 is the SR or IE of the labeled amino acid (AA) in protein at time 0, P^*_t is the SR or IE of the labeled AA in protein at any given time, and t is a given time during the measurement of P^* after the administration of a tracer. The fractional rate of synthesis of protein A is greater than that of protein B.

tracer. In the plot of ln (P^*_0/P^*_t) as the Y-axis against time (t), the slope is the fractional rate (K_s) of protein synthesis expressed as %/min or %/h (Figure 8.11).

An advantage of the pulse labeling technique is that it can be used to simultaneously determine both rates of synthesis and degradation of a single protein or a group of proteins with similar turn-over rates in a tissue within the same animal. This method, however, is not appropriate for mixed proteins with different synthesis rates because of their complex kinetics in cells. When using the pulse labeling technique, the recycling of a labeled AA into protein can be minimized if [^{14}C] Na_2CO_3 is intravenously administered into a mammal to generate [guanidino-^{14}C]arginine. This is because after [guanidino-^{14}C]arginine is released from protein degradation, the labeled AA is rapidly hydrolyzed to form ^{14}C-urea in the liver.

8.6.2.4 Flooding Dose Technique

The so-called "flooding dose" technique involves the single administration (intravenously, intraperitoneally, or intramuscularly) of large amounts of both tracer [e.g., 150 μCi L-[ring-2,4-^{3}H] phenylalanine per kg body weight (BW)] and tracee AA (e.g., 180 μmol L-phenylalanine/kg BW) into an animal (Fiorotto et al. 2012; Garlick et al. 1994; Tesseraud et al. 2000; Watford and Wu 2005). The goal is to "flood" the entire precursor pool (extracellular and intracellular components) to such an extent that the plasma and intracellular SR are the same. Indeed, a primary assumption of the method that the free AA precursor pool is equilibrated with the true precursor pool (i.e., aminoacyl-tRNA) in tissues (e.g., skeletal muscle, heart, and liver) has been validated for pigs (Davis et al. 1999) and rats (Garlick et al. 1980, 1994). In a short period after the administration of the tracer (e.g., 10 min in rats and chickens after intravenous administration; 30 min in young pigs for intravenous, intraperitoneal, or intramuscular administration), tissues are obtained from the animal for analysis. The fractional rate of protein synthesis (K_s) is calculated as described previously.

There are several practical advantages to the flooding dose technique. Theoretically, it should eliminate uncertainty regarding SR or IE, because the value is the same in all compartments. Second, because the precursor pool is flooded, it should be possible to use only the precursor SR or IE in the plasma to quantify the true value for the intracellular precursor labeled AA, as shown for swine tissues (Table 8.6). Third, it is possible to measure protein synthesis in a short period of time (10–30 min), and this is important for tissues with low rates of protein synthesis (e.g., skeletal muscle and brain), which may otherwise require 4 h or more of constant tracer infusion to achieve a steady-state level of SR or IE. Such an approach also allows for the determination of tissue protein synthesis under metabolic non-steady-state conditions such as feeding, short-term hormone infusion, during exercise, during surgery, and immediately after trauma. Finally, the flooding dose technique is very convenient and useful for measuring synthetic rates of proteins with very short half-lives, as the recycling of the labeled AA into proteins would be minimized. Thus, this method has been extensively used to measure protein synthesis in tissues of rodents, farm animals, and fish,

TABLE 8.6
Specific Radioactivities of L-[4-³H]Phenylalanine in Tissues and Intracellular [4-³H] Phenylalanine-tRNA in the Skeletal Muscle and Liver of Young Pigs Receiving a Flooding Dose of L-Phenylalanine plus L-[4-³H]Phenylalanine[a]

Treatment	Time after ³H-Phe Administration (min)	Blood Free Phenylalanine (Phe)	Skeletal Muscle		Liver	
			Free Phe	Phe-tRNA	Free Phe	Phe-tRNA
Experiment 1 (Fast/Refed)[b]						
Fasted for 24 h	5	1,176±114	---	---	---	---
Refed after 24-h fast	5	1,191±93	---	---	---	---
Fasted for 24 h	15	1,154±109	---	---	---	---
Refed after 24-h fast	15	1,119±70	---	---	---	---
Fasted for 24 h	30	1,107±96	1,074±82	1,053±59	1,039±73	1,069±100
Refed after 24-h fast	30	1,093±62	1,070±77	1,065±55	1,036±81	1,042±140
Experiment 2 (Fed Pigs)[c]						
Saline (intravenous)	5	1,143±91	---	---	---	---
Insulin (intravenous)	5	1,144±92	---	---	---	---
Saline (intravenous)	15	1,100±86	---	---	---	---
Insulin (intravenous)	15	1,108±93	---	---	---	---
Saline (intravenous)	30	1,076±92	1,082±62	1,054±73	1,041±61	1,008±118
Insulin (intravenous)	30	1,068±88	1,046±65	1,062±163	994±74	991±102

Source: Davis, T.A. et al. 1999. *Am. J. Physiol.* 277:E103–E109.

[a] Values for specific radioactivities (dpm of [³H]Phe/nmol Phe) are means±SEM, $n=3$ at 30 min after the administration of L-phenylalanine plus L-[4-³H]phenylalanine. All the measurements were made in 7-day-old pigs. The specific radioactivity of L-[4-³H]phenylalanine in the blood did not differ ($P>0.05$) among the 5-, 10- and 15-min time points after the single administration of a flooding dose of L-phenylalanine [1.5 mmol/kg body weight (BW)] plus 1 mCi of L-[4-³H]phenylalanine.

[b] Two pigs from each of three litters were either fasted for 24 h or refed for 2.75 h after a 24-h fast. Pigs that were refed after the 24-h fast were given three gavage feeds of 30 mL/kg BW of porcine mature milk at 60-min intervals. Pigs received the administration, via the jugular vein catheter, of 10 mL/kg BW of a flooding dose of L-phenylalanine (1.5 mmol/kg BW) plus 1 mCi of L-[4-³H]phenylalanine/kg BW. Samples of the whole blood were taken at 5, 15, and 30 min after the injection of [³H]phenylalanine for measurement of the specific radioactivities of L-[4-³H]Phenylalanine in tissues and [³H]Phe-tRNA in the skeletal muscle (longissimus dorsi muscle) and liver. Refeeding increased ($P<0.05$) the fractional rates of protein synthesis in the skeletal muscle and liver by 65% and 22%, respectively.

[c] Two pigs from each of three litters received intravenous infusion of either saline or insulin (100 ng/kg BW^0.66/min for 4 h; hyperinsulinemic-euglycemic amino acid clamps). The administration of L-phenylalanine plus L-[4-³H]phenylalanine and sample collection were performed as described in Experiment 1. The insulin treatment increased ($P<0.05$) the fractional rate of protein synthesis in the skeletal muscle by 55% and had no effect on that in the liver.

and in human tissues (including skeletal muscle, liver, and intestinal mucosa) and cells (including lymphocytes and tumor cells).

The flooding dose technique has potential limitations. First, the most crucial assumption is that the bolus injection of an AA (e.g., Phe) well in excess of the total body free pool of that AA will not affect the rate of protein synthesis. This technique may not be valid for certain AAs (e.g., leucine, lysine, and arginine) because of their possible effects on the transport of other AAs and on cellular signaling pathways. However, experimental evidence shows that the single administration of a large dose of Phe does not appear to affect tissue protein synthesis during a short time period (e.g., 10 to 30 min) in chickens, rats, and pigs. Second, an additional assumption for the flooding dose technique is that there is no delay in the incorporation of tracer from the free pool to the protein-bound pool. Based on the blood circulation, only a very short period of time (< 15 sec) is required for the transport of a labeled AA from the site of administration to the site of protein synthesis in the tissue of interest. Third, in the flooding dose method, a steady state of the precursor SR or IE is not met because the precursor SR or IE declines with time, which complicates the calculation of the rate of protein synthesis. However, within the short period (e.g., 10–30 min) of protein labeling, the change in the precursor SR or IE is very modest (<5%) and does not significantly alter the rate of tissue protein synthesis. Fourth, the rate of tissue protein synthesis measured by the flooding dose technique may not represent the rate of tissue protein synthesis over a 24-h period, because of diurnal changes in cell metabolism. This concern can be addressed by measuring tissue protein synthesis at various time points of the day, which is a labor- and resource-intensive exercise, or by using the ^2H_2O method (Gasier et al. 2010; Wilkinson et al. 2015).

8.6.2.5 Continuous Infusion of a Tracer AA

The tracer AA can be administered directly into the venous circulation with an initial bolus dosage (priming), followed by a constant infusion of the tracer until the steady-state labeling of the free AA pool is attained (Waterlow 1984; Yang et al. 2012). A priming dose of the isotopically labeled tracer AA is administered before the start of the constant tracer infusion so as to reduce the time needed to achieve the isotopic steady state of the precursor AA. The rate of constant infusion of the tracer must be adequate to ensure the detection of the labeled AA in the free and protein pools of tissues. The solution for the constant infusion of a radioactive or stable isotope tracer does not need to include an addition of its tracee (Garlick et al. 1975; Engelen et al. 2019; Ten Have et al. 2019). The SR or IE of a tracer AA in the blood and in the intracellular compartments increases until an equilibrium is reached during which the precursor SR or IE remains constant (Chapter 7). This kind of metabolic studies usually takes 4–6 h. The mathematical treatment of experimental data is simplified considerably, when the precursor SR or IE is constant. The fractional rate of protein synthesis is calculated from the ratio of protein-bound AA SR to free AA SR (or IE) for tissues (e.g., such as skeletal muscle, heart, and brain) with slow protein turnover (Figure 8.12). A slightly modified equation is used to determine protein synthesis for tissues (e.g., liver and kidney) with high protein turnover rates because the rate constant (K_F) for the rise of SR or IR of the precursor AA in the blood can be readily determined. An example for the calculation of the fractional rate of protein synthesis in the skeletal muscle of adult humans is shown in Table 8.7.

Prolonged constant infusion of the tracer has advantages over the pulse labeling or flooding dose techniques. First, a distinct advantage of the constant infusion method is that whole-body protein synthesis and protein degradation can be measured concurrently with protein synthesis in specific tissues. This makes it possible to estimate the contribution of protein synthesis in different tissues to whole-body protein synthesis in humans and other animals. Second, the rate of protein synthesis can be measured from single samples of tissues, because the kinetics of the free pool labeling can be calculated from the relative amounts of the tracer AA in the protein-bound and precursor AA pools. Third, the SR or IE of the free labeled AA remains constant for a substantial proportion of the infusion period, and therefore, the kinetics of protein labeling are relatively simple. Fourth, the cost of a labeled tracer used in the constant infusion method is lower than that employed in the single

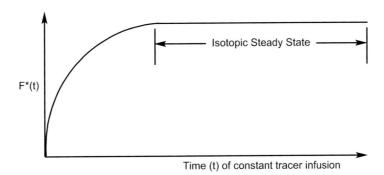

$$\frac{dP^*}{dt} = K_s \, (F^* - P^*) \tag{1}$$

$$F^*(t) = F^*_{max} \times (1 - e^{-K_F t}) \tag{2}$$

$$\frac{P^*}{F^*} = \frac{K_F}{(K_F - K_s)} \times \frac{1 - e^{-K_s t}}{(1 - e^{-K_F t})} - \frac{K_s}{(K_F - K_s)} \tag{3}$$

$$F^*(t) = F^*_{max} \times (1 - e^{-RK_s t}) \tag{4}$$

$$\frac{P^*}{F^*} = \frac{R}{(R - 1)} \times \frac{1 - e^{-K_s t}}{(1 - e^{-RK_s t})} - \frac{1}{(R - 1)} \tag{5}$$

FIGURE 8.12 Measurement of protein synthesis using the constant infusion of a tracer. A tracer amino acid (AA) is infused intravenously into humans or other animals at a constant rate after the short administration of a priming dose of the tracer. The expressions for F^* are substituted in the equation $dP^*/dt = K_s \, (F^* - P^*)$, which is integrated to give mathematical formulae to calculate the fractional rate of protein synthesis depending on tissue type (i.e., tissues with high or slow protein turnover rates). e, the base for natural logarithms; F^*, SR (dpm/nmol) of the radioactive tracer AA or IE (%) of the stable tracer AA in the precursor pool; F^*_{max} is maximum SR (dpm/nmol) of the radioactive tracer AA or maximum IE (%) of the stable tracer AA in the precursor pool; K_F, rate constant (%/min; or %/h) for the rise of SR or IE of the free tracer AA to describe an increase of tracer in the precursor pool; K_s, fractional rate of protein synthesis (%/min or %/h); P^*, SR (dpm/nmol) of the radioactive tracer AA (e.g., ^{14}C-Phe) or IE (%) of the stable tracer AA in the protein molecule; R, ratio of the protein-bound AA to the free AA in tissue; t, the duration of protein labeling in tissue. Equation 1 is applicable to tissues with either a low or a high rate of protein turnover. Equations 2 and 3 are used for tissues with a high rate of protein turnover (e.g., liver and small intestine), whereas Equations 4 and 5 are suitable for tissues with a low rate of protein turnover (e.g., skeletal muscle and heart).

administration of a large dose of a tracer AA used in the flooding dose technique. Thus, the constant infusion technique is preferred in studies with humans (Waterlow 1984) and large farm animals, including cattle, sheep, and pigs (Lobley et al. 1980; Reeds and Lobley 1980). Finally, the constant infusion technique is particularly applicable to tissues (e.g., skeletal muscle) with slow turnover rates, because of the prolonged length of the protein labeling period.

Using the constant infusion method to measure the rate of protein synthesis *in vivo* has shortcomings. First, this method is unsatisfactory in tissues and cells (e.g., the liver and intestinal epithelial cells) with rapid protein turnover rates, because the SR or IE of the free labeled AA rises during the course of the infusion due to the recycling of the labeled AA from the protein pool into the free AA pool. Second, the constant infusion technique is not suitable for use in tissues (the liver and

TABLE 8.7

Calculations of the Fractional Rate of Protein Synthesis in the Skeletal Muscle of Post-Absorptive Adult Humans Receiving Primed Constant Infusion of [²H₅]Phenylalanine[a]

| Time of the Constant Infusion of Tracer | Background-Corrected MPE | | Fractional Rate of Muscle Protein Synthesis (%/day) |
	Muscle Protein (MPE, %)	Intracellular Free ³H-Phe in Muscle (MPEp, %)	
T_1 (120 min)	0.0323	7.6277	---
T_2 (360 min)	0.0586	7.7047	---
ΔMPE in muscle protein over 240 min. (MPE at T_2 − MPE at T_1)	0.0262	---	---
Average MPEp of IC free ³H-Phe in (MPEp at T_1 + MPEp at T_2)/2	---	7.6662	---
Between 120 and 360 min (a 240-min period)	---	---	2.05[b]

Source: Kim et al. 2016. *Exp. Mol. Med.* 48:e203.

Note: IC, intracellular; MPE, background-corrected molar percent enrichment of the tracer; MPEp, background-corrected molar percent enrichment of the tracer at the isotopic steady state (plateau).

[a] Adult humans simultaneously received the primed constant intravenous infusion of L-[ring-²H₅]phenylalanine [prime: 3.07 μmol/kg BW; the rate of constant infusion (F) = 0.084 μmol/kg BW/min]. Blood and skeletal muscle samples were obtained before the isotope administration (for correction of background values) and at the isotopic steady state after the isotope administration. Plasma and muscle samples were analyzed by a mass spectrometer for the tracers and tracees. An isotopic steady state of L-[ring-²H₅]phenylalanine within the skeletal muscle cells was reached by 120 min of the constant infusion of the tracer.

[b] Calculated as [ΔMPE in muscle protein over 240 min/(Average MPEp of IC free ³H-Phe at plateau × Time of tracer infusion (h)] × 24 h × 100% = [0.0262% / (7.6662% × 4 h)] × 24 h × 100% = 2.05%/day.

---

gastrointestinal tract) from which substantial proportions of synthesized proteins are exported, as the rate of protein synthesis is underestimated. Third, in the constant infusion method, the SR or IE of ²H₅-Phe in the venous plasma is similar to, and therefore is generally used as a surrogate of, ²H₅-Phe-tRNA in the skeletal muscle, heart, and liver (Baumann et al. 1994; Ljungqvist et al. 1997). Experimental results have also shown that the IE of [1-¹³C]α-ketoisocaproic acid in the plasma is similar to the IE of [1-¹³C]leucine-tRNA in the skeletal muscle and heart, whereas the intracellular IE of [1-¹³C]leucine in the free pool is close to the IE of [1-¹³C]leucine-tRNA in skeletal muscle (Baumann et al. 1994; Watt et al. 1991). Thus, the IE or SR of the labeled AA in the tissue free AA pool or of its metabolite (e.g., labeled α-ketoisocaproate from infused labeled leucine) is the most reliable measurement of the IE or SR of the aminoacyl-tRNA pool during the constant infusion of a labeled AA (Table 8.8). Fourth, the constant infusion method requires a metabolic steady state, which may not exist under certain nutritional (e.g., feeding), physiological (e.g., during exercise), and diseased (e.g., infection) conditions. Thus, this method is not suitable for measuring acute changes in rates of tissue protein synthesis in humans and other animals. Finally, the constant infusion method is not easily adapted to small animals (e.g., rats, mice, and neonatal pigs) because it is very stressful to physically restrain them for a prolonged period of time.

8.6.2.6 Leucine Oxidation Method

The rate of production of an end product (e.g., ¹⁴C- or ¹³C-labeled CO_2, ¹⁵N-urea, or ³H- or ²H-labeled H_2O) of the oxidation of an appropriately administered AA (e.g., leucine) can be used to calculate the rates of whole-body protein synthesis and protein degradation in humans and other animals (El-Khoury

TABLE 8.8
Isotopic Enrichment of Stable Tracer in Growing Rats and Adult Humans

Metabolite	Isotopic Enrichment (Atom Percent Excess, %) after a Constant Infusion of L-[1-^{13}C,^{15}N]Leucine into Rats[a]		Isotopic Enrichment (Atom Percent Excess, %) after a Constant Infusion of L-[1-^{13}C] Leucine into Adult Humans[b]
	^{13}C	^{15}N	
Arterial plasma leucine	12.3±1.13	6.27±0.65	---
Arterial plasma α-ketoisocaproate	11.48±1.00	---	---
Venous plasma leucine	12.1±1.16	6.09±0.58	6.36±0.56
Venous plasma α-ketoisocaproate	11.22±0.95	---	5.58±0.50
Skeletal muscle free leucine	8.97±0.31	3.37±0.33	4.56±0.40
Skeletal muscle leucyl-tRNA	10.26±0.47	4.72±0.70	4.98±0.43
Liver free leucine	4.12±0.58	3.59±0.6	---
Liver leucyl-tRNA	7.04±0.86	5.49±0.9	---

Source: Watt et al. 1991. *Proc. Natl. Acad. Sci. USA* 88:5892–5896.

[a] Growing rats [250 g of body weight (BW)] received the primed constant intravenous infusion of L-[1-^{13}C,^{15}N]leucine [prime: 0.6 mg/100 g BW; the rate of constant infusion (*F*)=0.6 mg/100 g BW/h] for 1 h. Blood samples and leg muscle were obtained at the end of tracer infusion. Plasma and leg muscle samples were analyzed by a mass spectrometer for the tracers and tracees. Values are means±SEM, for 4 to 6 experiments.

[b] Adult humans received the primed constant intravenous infusion of L-[1-^{13}C]leucine [prime: 0.85 mg/kg BW; the rate of constant infusion (*F*)=1 mg/kg BW/h] for up to 71 h. Blood samples and erector spinae muscle were obtained at the end of tracer infusion. Plasma and muscle samples were analyzed by a mass spectrometer for the tracers and tracees. Values are means±SEM, *n*=8. The fractional rate of protein synthesis in the skeletal muscle was 2.26%/day.

et al. 1995; Marliss et al. 2006; Millward et al. 1996; Waterlow 1984). [1-^{14}C]Leucine or [1-^{13}C]leucine is often used for this purpose because of the following reasons. First, leucine cannot be synthesized in the body. The use of nonessential AAs renders calculation of protein degradation difficult, because both the dietary uptake and synthesis de novo have to be measured. Second, the metabolic fate of leucine is relatively simple and easy to quantify, particularly with carboxyl labeled leucine. For example, the oxidative decarboxylation of [1-^{14}C]leucine or [1-^{13}C]leucine gives labeled CO_2, which can be readily measured. Either [1-^{14}C]leucine or [1-^{13}C]leucine has an additional advantage in that its transamination product, α-ketoisocaproate, can be isolated from the plasma and used to estimate intracellular SR or IE of free labeled leucine. Third, leucine is usually not a limiting AA in the diet for animals. Fourth, leucine is well distributed throughout body proteins and the free pool.

Let us consider the two-compartment model for leucine oxidation in animals (Figure 8.13). This model is based on several assumptions. First, leucine is utilized *in vivo* only via the oxidation pathway and protein synthesis. Second, in physiological and isotopic steady state, the amount of labeled leucine entering the free AA pool equals the amount of the labeled AA leaving this pool. Third, leucine kinetics are representative of whole-body protein kinetics. Fourth, intracellular SR or IE of labeled leucine is the same for leucine oxidation and for protein synthesis. Fifth, CO_2 produced from leucine oxidation is quantitatively recovered in the expired air. Using the leucine oxidation method, labeled leucine is infused intravenously into the animal at a constant rate for 4–6 h as described above. Depending on whether a radioactive or stable isotope is used, the SR or IE of labeled leucine in the plasma at the steady state is measured to calculate the rate of leucine oxidation. The flux (*Q*) of leucine through the free AA pool is determined using intravenous infusion of labeled leucine (Figure 8.14). The relationship between the flux of leucine and the rate of protein synthesis or degradation is described as follows:

$$I + B = E + Z = Q$$

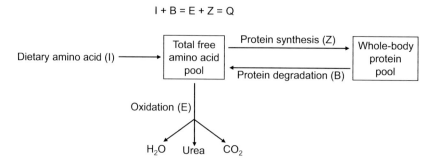

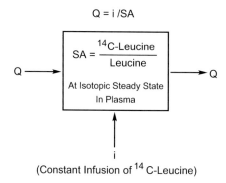

FIGURE 8.13 Measurement of protein synthesis using the leucine oxidation method. [1-^{14}C]Leucine or [1-^{13}C]leucine is infused intravenously into humans or other animals at a constant rate after the short administration of a priming dose of the tracer. E is the rate of leucine oxidation, which can be measured using either [1-^{14}C]leucine ($^{14}CO_2$ production) or [^{15}N]leucine (urinary excretion of ^{15}N-urea); I is the rate of leucine intake from the diet, which can be determined by chemical analysis; B is the rate of whole-body protein degradation; and Z is the rate of protein synthesis.

FIGURE 8.14 Measurement of plasma leucine flux. Plasma leucine flux (Q) is measured using intravenous infusion of labeled leucine at a constant rate. The isotopic steady-state specific radioactivity (SR) or isotopic enrichment (IE) of the labeled free amino acid (AA) in the plasma and the rate of tracer infusion (i) into the study participants are used to calculate the plasma leucine flux, which is also taken to represent whole-body leucine flux.

$$Q = I + B = E + Z$$

where E is the rate of leucine oxidation, which can be measured by [1-^{14}C]leucine ($^{14}CO_2$ production) or [^{15}N]leucine (urinary excretion of ^{15}N-urea); I is the intake of leucine from the diet, which can be determined by chemical analysis; B is the rate of whole-body protein degradation; and Z is the rate of protein synthesis. Based on the estimated content of leucine in the whole-body protein [e.g., 707 µmol leucine/g protein (Waterlow 1995) or 629 µmol leucine/g protein (Pacy et al. 1994) for adult humans], the rate of whole-body protein synthesis is calculated.

$$\text{Protein synthesis } (Z) = Q - E$$

$$\text{Protein degradation } (B) = Q - I$$

A major advantage of the leucine oxidation method is that it can be used to simultaneously determine both the rates of protein synthesis and protein degradation in the whole body. The second advantage is that this method is noninvasive and convenient for determining protein turnover in humans and large animals. Third, the model involves simple and straightforward mathematics. Fourth, the use of SR or IE of labeled α-ketoisocaproate in the plasma is a good indicator of the intracellular SR or IE of labeled leucyl-tRNA in skeletal muscle and heart to determine leucine oxidation and protein synthesis (Baumann et al. 1994; El-Khoury et al. 1995; Watt et al. 1991). This increases the practical usefulness of the leucine oxidation technique in clinical research.

A significant disadvantage of the leucine oxidation method is that it cannot be used to determine the rate of protein synthesis in individual tissues. Additionally, there are potential problems in the accurate and precise determination of the recovery of labeled CO_2 produced from leucine oxidation. When [^{15}N]leucine, [^{15}N]glycine, or [^{15}N]lysine is used to estimate urea production from its oxidation (the end-product method; Duggleby and Waterlow 2005), it usually takes a long time (e.g., 9 h) to completely collect urine samples from study participants before and after tracer administration (Conley et al. 1980; Waterlow 1984). Other disadvantages of the technique include those discussed previously for the AA constant infusion method used to quantify protein synthesis.

8.6.2.7 Use of ^2H_2O to Determine Protein Synthesis in Tissues

An American scientist and Nobel laureate, H. Urey, discovered the isotope deuterium in 1931 and concentrated the stable isotope in water. Three years later, G. de Hevesy and E. Hofer used heavy water (also known as ^2H_2O, D_2O, and deuterium oxide) to determine the rate of water turnover adult humans. Ussing reported in 1937 the incorporation of ^2H_2O into the protein of animal tissues and, using this method, found in 1941 that the proteins of the liver, small intestine, and serum in rats and mice were renewed much more rapidly than those of the kidneys, skeletal muscle, skin, and blood corpuscles, whereas the bodies contained a mixture of rapidly and slowly renewable proteins.

Water participates in all biochemical pathways in humans and other animals. After ^2H_2O is administered into study participants, all AAs in their blood are labeled with ^2H because of the following reactions. First, intracellular and extracellular proteins are degraded in the presence of ^2H_2O to generate ^2H-labeled AAs (with two hydrogen atoms in the amino group of a zwitterionic AA being labeled with ^2H). Second, both the α-amino group and the α-hydrogen atom of the AAs synthesized either de novo or from the existing α-ketoacids in the body can be labeled with ^2H through the transamination of pyruvate with ^2H-labeled AAs (e.g., ^2H-glutamate and ^2H-aspartate). Third, some NADH-, NADPH-, and ammonia-dependent enzymes (e.g., glutamate dehydrogenase and pyrroline-5-carboxylate reductase) that catalyze the reduction of some α-ketoacids in the presence of H^+ can result in the production of ^2H-labeled AAs (e.g., ^2H-glutamate and ^2H-proline). The α-^2H of alanine is derived only from the transamination of pyruvate with an AA (e.g., glutamate and aspartate) in the presence of $^2H^+$. Fourth, the conversion of phosphoenolpyruvate (a product of glucose via glycolysis) into pyruvate by pyruvate kinase results in the incorporation of ^2H into the β-carbon of pyruvate via the protonation of carbanions (Rose and Kuo 1989). The isotopic enrichment of [3-^2H]pyruvate in the body water is increased through the conversion of [3-^2H]pyruvate into [6-^2H]glucose in the presence of $^2H^+$ via NADH-dependent gluconeogenesis and the subsequent metabolism of [6-^2H]glucose via glycolysis to form [3-^2H]phosphoenolpyruvate. In the studies involving the use of ^2H_2O to determine the rate of protein synthesis in humans, rats, mice, and fish, ^2H-alanine was chosen as an AA precursor for the mathematical calculation because ^2H_2O was very rapidly in equilibrium with ^2H-alanine in the plasma (Belloto et al. 2007; Gasier et al. 2010; Wilkinson et al. 2014). Because of rapid hydrogen exchanges between water and alanine, the mass percent excess (MPE) of ^2H-alanine in the plasma of the peripheral blood was 4.09 and 4.12 times that of ^2H_2O in the fed and 8-h fasted rats, respectively (Belloto et al. 2007). When expressed per the α-hydrogen of alanine, the atom percent excess (APE) of ^2H-alanine in the plasma is the same as that of ^2H_2O (Previs et al. 2004). Plateau values for the mass percent excess (MPE) of both ^2H_2O and ^2H-alanine in the plasma of the post-absorptive humans were maintained between 1 and 12 h after their ingestion of ^2H_2O, with the MPE of ^2H-alanine being 3.8 times the MPE of ^2H_2O (Belloto et al. 2007).

After humans and other animals receive the administration of ^2H_2O (99.9% enrichment), it is in such a rapid equilibrium with the body water and free alanine in the blood that the isotopic enrichments of ^2H_2O and ^2H-alanine in the plasma rapidly reached a plateau. In a healthy 70-kg adult human (containing 40 L of water) ingesting 200 mL of ^2H_2O once, a MPE value (0.5%) of the labeled water in the plasma and the whole body could be achieved and maintained for hours (Previs et al. 2004). In both fed and 8-h fasted rats, the plateau values for both ^2H_2O and ^2H-alanine were obtained within 10 min after the intraperitoneal of ^2H_2O (Belloto et al. 2007). Because of the relatively slow turnover of the body water pool with its half-life being about 11 days (Wilkinson et al. 2014), a single bolus dose of ^2H_2O followed by regular oral dosing can effectively maintain the steady-state isotopic enrichments of ^2H_2O and ^2H-alanine in the plasma and of ^2H-alanine in tissues (e.g., the liver, skeletal muscle, and heart) for a prolonged period of time. This can permit the measurement of the synthesis of both total proteins with mixed half-lives and the specific proteins (e.g., myofibrillar proteins) with a long half-life, as well as changes in the rates of their synthesis over days and weeks. For example, the plateau levels of the isotopic enrichments of ^2H_2O and ^2H-alanine in the plasma and of ^2H-alanine in tissues (e.g., the liver, skeletal muscle, and heart) of rats were maintained for at least 80 h after the animals received a single bolus dose of ^2H_2O, followed by regular oral administration through drinking water (Belloto et al. 2007). Similarly, when post-absorptive healthy adult humans consumed a loading dose of ^2H_2O (3 g/L of body water) and thereafter ^2H_2O-enriched water (6 g ^2H_2O/L) at the rate of 150 mL/h for at least 12 h, the isotopic enrichments of ^2H_2O and ^2H-alanine in the plasma were maintained at plateau levels for 12 h (Belloto et al. 2007).

When one molecule of ^2H-alanine is incorporated into protein, two of its three ^2H atoms in the $-NH_3^+$ group are lost due to the formation of a peptide bond (Figure 8.15) and the α-^2H of

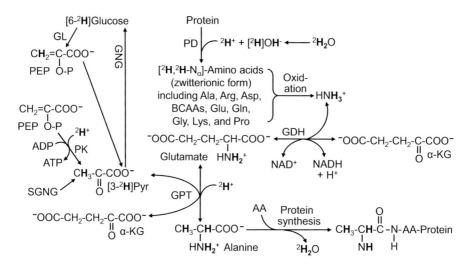

FIGURE 8.15 Use of ^2H_2O for the measurement of protein synthesis in humans and other animals. The ^2H atom from ^2H_2O can be incorporated into alanine via: (1) intracellular and extracellular transamination of pyruvate with an amino acid; (2) degradation of intracellular and extracellular proteins; (3) NADH- and NADPH-dependent reactions in the presence of H^+; and (4) the conversion of phosphoenolpyruvate into pyruvate by pyruvate kinase, which results in the incorporation of ^2H into the β-carbon of pyruvate via the protonation of carbanions. The isotopic enrichment of [3-^2H]pyruvate in the body water is increased through the conversion of [3-^2H]pyruvate into [6-^2H]glucose in the presence of $^2H^+$ via NADH-dependent gluconeogenesis and the subsequent metabolism of [6-^2H]glucose via glycolysis to form [3-^2H]phosphoenolpyruvate. The α-^2H of alanine is derived only from the transamination of pyruvate with an amino acid (e.g., glutamate and aspartate) in the presence of $^2H^+$. ^2H-Alanine is incorporated into protein via protein synthesis, with the loss of two ^2H atoms in the amino group as ^2H_2O. Caution should be exercised in the use of the isotopic enrichments of the precursor and product for the calculation of the fractional rate of the synthesis of intracellular and exported proteins. GL, glycolysis; GNG, gluconeogenesis; PD, protein degradation; PEP, phosphoenolpyruvate; PK, pyruvate kinase; Pyr, pyruvate; SGNG, substrates of gluconeogenesis (e.g., amino acids, lactate, glycerol, and propionate). The bold hydrogen denotes deuterium (^2H).

the alanine residue (alanyl unit) appears in the protein. Thus, the amount of total ^{2}H atoms in the alanine residues of protein does not reflect the amount of total ^{2}H atoms in the free intracellular ^{2}H-alanine that is incorporated into the protein. By contrast, the amounts of the α- and β-^{2}H atoms in the alanine residues of protein can reflect the amounts of the α- and β-^{2}H atoms in the free intracellular ^{2}H-alanine precursor that is incorporated into the protein (Previs et al. 2004). The isotopic enrichments of the α- and β-^{2}H atom in the free intracellular ^{2}H-alanine precursor are greater than those in the alanine residues of protein until all the alanine residues have been incorporated from the labeled precursor into the labeled protein.

The most immediate precursor for protein synthesis is the amino acyl-tRNA. However, as noted previously, this precursor pool is very small and labile in cells, and it is technically difficult to analyze amino acyl-tRNA. Therefore, a surrogate that best approximates the true labeling of the amino acyl-tRNA is often used to calculate the rate of AA incorporation into protein, as noted previously. The following equation, which is based on the MPE of ^{2}H-alanine in protein and the MPE of ^{2}H$_2$O in the plasma, has been used to calculate the fractional rate of tissue protein synthesis (FRS) in human, rat, and mouse studies involving the use of ^{2}H$_2$O (Gasier et al. 2010).

$$\text{FRS} (\% / \text{h}) = \frac{\text{Isotopic enrichment of }^2\text{H-alanine in protein (MPE)}}{\text{Isotopic enrichment of }^2\text{H}_2\text{O in plasma at plateau (MPE)} \times n \times \text{Time (h)}} \times 100$$

where n represents the exchange of ^{2}H between water and alanine detected in the plasma due to the intracellular biochemical reactions that involve ^{2}H$_2$O as indicated previously. Gasier et al. (2010) reported that the value of the n was 3.8 for humans, rats, and mice and was 3.7 for channel catfish. In this equation, $n \times$ the MPE of ^{2}H$_2$O is equivalent to the MPE of free ^{2}H-alanine in the plasma. Similarly, the MPE of ^{2}H-alanine in the plasma of adult humans was 3.8 times the MPE of ^{2}H$_2$O at the isotopic steady state (Belloto et al. 2007).

The ^{2}H$_2$O labeling method is less invasive, less restrictive, less expensive, and more convenient than the traditional AA tracer techniques and can be performed in freely living humans. Study participants can ingest the tracer solution at any time in their routine activities (e.g., during eating, performing a job, and doing exercise). For measurements over days or weeks, a constant isotopic enrichment of ^{2}H$_2$O in the plasma and the body water that is achieved shortly after a single loading dose of ^{2}H$_2$O can be maintained by the replacement of ^{2}H$_2$O and unlabeled water that are lost due to the daily turnover of the body water. Of note, Wilkinson et al. (2015) reported that the rate of myofibrillar protein synthesis in human skeletal muscle measured with ^{2}H$_2$O ingestion was quantitatively comparable to that measured with the traditional phenylalanine tracer (i.e., the primed, continuous intravenous infusion of [^{13}C$_6$]phenylalanine) in both fed and fasted states.

Like other tracer techniques, the ^{2}H$_2$O method has its shortcomings. First, some individuals may experience nausea and vertigo after ingesting an administered dose of ^{2}H$_2$O (Gasier et al. 2010). This potential problem can be alleviated by the more frequent administration of the tracer in the same daily amount. Second, it is unknown whether the MPE of ^{2}H$_2$O in the plasma can represent the true MPE of intracellular alanyl-tRNA. Third, ^{2}H-alanine does not meet the traditional criteria for tracer selection in the studies of protein synthesis, because alanine is extensively synthesized and metabolized in tissues (including the skeletal muscle and liver). The intracellular isotopic enrichment of ^{2}H-alanine is affected by more factors than that of [^{13}C$_6$]phenylalanine in skeletal muscle, and this may also be true for the variations of intracellular MPE values. Thus, on an individual basis, the ^{2}H$_2$O labeling and [^{13}C$_6$]phenylalanine methods did not quantitatively agree in all study participants in their rates of intramuscular myofibrillar protein synthesis (Wilkinson et al. 2015). Likewise, the values of the fractional rates of total proteins or myofibrillar proteins in rat skeletal muscles measured with the ^{2}H$_2$O method differed substantially from those measured with the ^{3}H-phenylalanine flooding technique (Gasier et al. 2009). These discrepancies may result, in part, from the uncertainty of the MPE of the intracellular free ^{2}H-alanine and the fact that protein-bound

^{2}H-alanine may contain a different number of ^{2}H than the free ^{2}H-alanine precursor. For this reason, the MPE values of the α- and β-^{2}H atoms (or simply the α-^{2}H atom) in the intracellular free ^{2}H-alanine at the isotopic steady state and the intracellular protein-bound ^{2}H-alanine should be used to calculate the fractional rate of protein synthesis in cells.

8.6.3 Rates of Whole-Body and Tissue-Specific Protein Synthesis in Humans and Other Animals

The reported rate of whole-body protein synthesis in healthy adult humans (g protein/kg BW/day) ranged from 3.0 to 4.3 as measured with [^{15}N]glycine or [^{15}N]alanine (Pacy et al. 1994; Soares et al. 1991; Waterlow 1984) and was 4.3 (Motil et al. 1981) or 4.37 (Clugston and Garlick 1982) as measured with [1-^{13}C]leucine. Thus, values of whole-body protein synthesis based on the kinetics of [1-^{13}C]leucine are either similar to or higher than those from the kinetics of [^{15}N]glycine or [^{15}N]alanine (Waterlow 1984). This difference is possibly due to a number of variables, such as the age (19–25-year-old young adults, 25–50-year-old adults, or older adults), sex (males or females), dietary protein (e.g., 0.6 or 0.8 g/kg BW/day) and energy intakes (e.g., 30 or 43 kcal/kg BW/day), prior physical activity levels (e.g., minimal or high), and hormonal status of study participants, as well as the use of the leucine-to-protein conversion factor (e.g., ×12.5) to correct for non-collagen protein and leucine content in the body. Note that the content of leucine in the various types of collagen and elastin is much lower than that in non-collagen proteins (Chapter 1). Because the rates of the turnover of collagen and non-collagen proteins differ substantially, an appropriate leucine-to-protein conversion factor should be carefully considered for the calculation whole-body protein synthesis from leucine flux data. A proper AA-to-protein conversion factor is crucial for the accurate calculation of whole-body protein synthesis based on AA kinetics in the whole body. In this regard, it is noteworthy that Pacy et al. (1994) converted leucine kinetic values into protein synthesis by assuming that the leucine content of protein in adult humans is 629 µmol/g. Based on consistent results from some independent studies involving different tracer methods, Waterlow (1995) has estimated that the rate of whole-body protein synthesis in the 70-kg healthy adult human is approximately 300 g/day (or 4.3 g/kg BW/day). In all species of adult mammals, the rates of whole-body protein synthesis (g/kg BW/day) decrease with an increase in their BW (Table 8.9). The rates of whole-body protein synthesis and energy expenditure in adult chickens (27.2 g protein and 300 kJ/kg BW/day) are much greater than those in adult mammals (Muramatsu 1990).

In healthy humans and other animals, there are tissue- and age-specific differences in the rates of protein synthesis (Waterlow 1984; Welle et al. 1995). For example, among all the tissues examined in young rats, the jejunal mucosa has the highest fractional rate of protein synthesis, followed by the liver and the whole small intestine (with a similar rate), bone (soluble fraction), spleen and stomach (with a similar rate), large intestine, skin (with a similar rate), kidney, and lung in descending order (Table 8.10). In young rats, the fractional rate of protein synthesis does not differ among the brain, heart, and skeletal muscle (with mixed fiber types). Similar patterns have been reported for young pigs (Table 8.10). In elderly humans (60–84 years of age), the fractional rate of protein synthesis in skeletal muscle is 20%–30% lower than that in young adults (20–30 years of age) (Breen and Phillips 2011). Thus, the fractional rates of protein synthesis in the whole body and individual tissues of humans and other animals (e.g., rats and pigs) decrease with increased ages (Davis et al. 2008, 2010; Waterlow 1984).

Changes in nutritional and hormonal states, as well as physical activity (Table 8.11) and diseases, affect protein synthesis in humans and other animals. Specifically, the fractional rates of protein synthesis in the whole body and individual tissues of humans and other animals (e.g., rats, pigs, and chicks) decrease in response to food deprivation, protein deficiency, and diseases (e.g., infections, cancer, diabetes, and burn injury) (McNurlan et al. 1980; Tian and Baracos 1989; Waterlow 1984, 1995; Yu et al. 1996), but increase under the conditions of physical activity, lactation, and pregnancy (Baracos et al. 1991; Elango and Ball 2016). This view is supported by the following lines of evidence. First, the fractional rates of protein synthesis in the skeletal muscle, liver, and jejunal mucosa of young rats decrease by 52%, 29%, and 25%, respectively, in response to a 2-day fast (McNurlan

TABLE 8.9
Whole-Body Protein Turnover in Healthy Adult Mammals and in Growing Mammals in the Fed State

Species	Body Weight (BW, kg)	Protein Synthesis (g/kg BW/day)	Protein Degradation (g/kg BW/day)	Metabolic Rate (kJ/kg BW/day)
		Healthy Adult Mammals[a]		
Mouse	0.04	43.5	43.5	760
Rat	0.35	22.0	22.0	364
Rabbit	3.6	9.2	9.2	192
Cat	4.4	8.5	8.5	184
Dog	10.8	10.1	10.1	170
Goat	38	6.6	6.6	177
Sheep	63	5.6	5.6	96
Man	70	4.3[b]	4.3	103[c]
Cattle	500	3.4	3.4	68
Cow	575	3.0	3.0	60
		Growing Mammals		
Rat	0.05 (3 weeks)	34.4	26.1	618
	0.1 (5 weeks)	31.3	25.7	546[d]
	0.211 (8 weeks)	22.0	20.1	450
	0.584 (44 weeks)	18.2	15.5	—
	0.604 (105 weeks)	13.1	13.1	—
Pig	30	13.5	10.4	231
	60	10.1	8.5	148
	90	7.4	6.8	115

Source: Brown, D. and L.E. Mount. 1982. *Livest. Prod. Sci.* 9: 389–398; Kleiber, M. 1947. *Physiol. Rev.* 27:511–541; Motil, K.J. et al. 1981. *Metabolism* 30:783–791; Reeds, P.J. and G.E. Lobley. 1980. *Proc. Nutr. Soc.* 39:43–52; Reeds, P.J. et al. 1980. *Br. J. Nutr.* 43:445–455; Riond et al. 2003. *J. Anim. Physiol. Anim. Nutr.* 87:221–228; Waterlow, J.C. 1984. *Quart. J. Exp. Physiol.* 69:409–438; Waterlow, J.C. 1995. *Annu. Rev. Nutr.* 15:57–92; Wester, T.J. et al. 2006. *FASEB J.* A1045; Williams, C.C. et al. 2001. *J. Anim. Sci.* 79:3128–3136. Goldspink, D.F. and F.J. Kelly. 1984. *Biochem. J.* 217:507–516.

[a] The rate of whole-body protein synthesis equals the rate of whole-body protein degradation in the physiological steady state. This means that adult animals do not gain protein in the whole body.

[b] This value was reported for healthy adult humans by Motil et al. (1981) and is the same as or essentially identical to the values of 4.3, 4.3, 4.24, and 4.37 g/kg BW/day from the studies of Pacy et al. (1994), Soares et al. (1991), Fern et al. (1981), and Clugston and Garlick (1982), respectively. The literature values of whole-body protein synthesis in healthy adult humans vary considerably, ranging from 2.0 to 7.75 g protein/kg BW/day, depending on a number of experimental variables. These factors include the methods used for the assessment of protein turnover, as well as the age, sex, and dietary protein and energy intakes of the study participants.

[c] Calculated on the basis of energy intake of 43 kcal/kg BW/day. This value is similar to that (107 kJ/kg BW/day) reported by Waterlow (1984).

[d] Calculated assuming that whole-body protein turnover contributes to 20% of whole-body energy expenditure.

et al. 1979, 1980). Furthermore, two and four days after the intraperitoneal administration of *E. coli*, the fractional rates of protein synthesis are decreased in skeletal muscle (sartorius muscle) by 42% and 33%, respectively, but are not altered in the liver or heart, compared with the saline-administered (control) group (Tian and Baracos 1989). These findings indicate that reductions of protein synthesis in skeletal muscle are more sensitive to food deprivation or infection than the liver and heart. Second, protein deprivation for 8–9 days reduces the fractional rates of protein synthesis

TABLE 8.10

Fractional Rates of Protein Synthesis in Tissues of Young Mammals in the Fed or Fasted State[a]

Whole Body or Tissue	Young Pigs (35-Day-Old; Fed)[b]	Young Rats (100 g BW)[c,d] Fed	Young Rats (100 g BW)[c,d] 48-h Fasted	Young Rats (130–140 g BW)[e] Fed	Young Rats (130–140 g BW)[e] 48-h Fasted	Lambs (1-Week-Old; Fed)[e,f]
Whole body	---	34	---	---	---	24
Bone (soluble fraction)	---	---	---	90	62	---
Brain	---	17	---	---	---	---
Colon	42	---	---	---	---	38
Heart	31	17	---	20	---	---
Kidney	40	48	---	---	---	---
Liver	84	87–105	62	86	72	111
Lung	58	33	---	33	---	---
Pancreas	76	---	---	---	---	---
Skeletal muscle	12	13	6.2	17	5.8	21
Small intestine	---	103	---	---	---	88
Proximal	60	---	---	---	---	86
Distal	59	---	---	---	---	84
Jejunal mucosa	---	136–140	111	119	---	---
Jejunal serosa	---	60	---	51	---	---
Large intestine	---	62	---	---	---	---
Spleen	57	76	---	68	---	---
Stomach	58	74	---	---	---	56
Skin (soluble fraction)	---	---	---	64	47	24

Note: BW, body weight; "---", data are not available.

[a] Fractional rate of protein synthesis (%/day). The values are the means.

[b] Deng et al. (2009). Longissimus dorsi muscle was used for the measurement of protein synthesis.

[c,d] McNurlan and Garlick (1980), and McNurlan et al. (1979, 1980). The BW of the fed and 48-h fasted rats was approximately 100 and 74 g, respectively.

[e] Garlick et al. (1980) and Preedy et al. (1983). Gastrocnemius muscle was used for the measurement of protein synthesis.

[f] Attaix et al. (1986, 1988); and Attaix and Arnal. (1987). The jejunum and skeletal muscle (tensor fasciae latae) were used for the measurement of protein synthesis. The calculation of tissue protein synthesis was based on the specific radioactivity of the ^{3}H-valine tracer in tissue.

in the skeletal muscle, whole liver, hepatic non-secreted (cellular) protein, hepatic albumin, jejunal mucosa, and jejunal serosa by 73%, 33%, 28%, 54%, 22%, and 36%, respectively (McNurlan et al. 1980). Third, compared with dry (non-lactating) goats, the fractional rates of protein synthesis in the mammary glands, rumen, duodenum, and kidneys of lactating goats are increased by 19-fold, 2-fold, 84%, and 72%, respectively, but those in the skin and skeletal muscle of the hind-limb are decreased by 43% and 19%, respectively, to support milk production (Baracos et al. 1991). Fourth, the absolute rates of whole-body protein synthesis increase by 15% and 25%, respectively, in women during the second and third trimesters of pregnancy (Duggleby and Jackson 2002). Similarly, intermittent mechanical stretching of skeletal muscle stimulates its protein synthesis in a prostaglandin $F_{2\alpha}$-dependent manner (Palmer et al. 1983), whereas resistance exercise enhances MTOR cell signaling in the muscle (Moore et al. 2011). Fifth, the synthesis of hepatic acute-phase proteins increases but the synthesis of skeletal muscle protein decreases in humans and other animals in response to infections (Hallemeesch et al. 2002; Jahoor et al. 1999; Manary et al. 2004; Mansoor

TABLE 8.11

Whole-Body Protein and Myofibrillar Protein Synthesis in Healthy Young and Older Humans before and after 3 Months of Resistance Training[a]

Variable	Young Adults (22- to 31-Year-Old)[b]		Older Adults (62- to 72-Year-Old)[c]	
	Baseline (before Training)	Trained (after Training)[d]	Baseline (before Training)	Trained (after Training)[d]
Body weight of men ($n=5$), kg	77.5±4.3	78.4±4.2	83.1±4.9	83.5±4.2
Body weight of women ($n=4$), kg	58.7±4.9	59.3±4.4	59.8±2.7	61.1±2.9
Lean body mass of men ($n=5$), kg	63.2±3.1	66.5±2.6	64.3±2.7	65.7±3.2
Lean body mass of women ($n=4$), kg	47.9±2.0	48.4±2.1	42.5±2.9	42.4±3.4
Urinary CTN excretion of men ($n=5$), g/day	1.91±0.14	1.78±0.08	1.78±0.15	1.80±0.13
Urinary CTN excretion of women ($n=4$), g/day	1.30±0.04	1.31±0.12	0.95±0.08	0.94±0.08
Leucine appearance, mmol/h	8.2±0.5	8.9±0.6*	7.7±0.7	7.6±0.7[†]
Leucine oxidation, mmol/h	2.0±0.2	1.9±0.2	1.8±0.2	1.7±0.2
Conversion of leucine into protein, mmol Leu/h	6.7±0.4	7.5±0.5*	6.4±0.6	6.4±0.5[†]
Urinary 3-MH excretion, μmol/g creatinine	128±14	153±12	132±7	134±15
FRS of skeletal muscle myofibrillar proteins, %/h	0.061±0.004	0.062±0.005	0.041±0.005[†]	0.045±0.005[†]

Source: Welle, S. et al. 1995. *Am. J. Physiol.* 268:E422–E427.

Note: CTN, creatinine; FRS, fractional rate of synthesis; 3MH, 3-methyl-histidine.

[a] Values are means±SEM, $n=9$ (5 men plus 4 women) for data other than body weight, lean body mass, and urinary creatinine excretion. There were 5 men and 4 women in each age group. The participants consumed a meat-free diet for 3 days, and urine samples collected on Day 3 were analyzed for 3-methyl-histidine and creatinine. On Day 4, after an overnight fast, whole-body leucine kinetics and skeletal muscle myofibrillar protein synthesis were measured using [1-¹³C]leucine and before 24-h urinary excretion and protein synthesis were measured.

[b] The mean body weights of the young men and women were 77.5 and 58.7 kg, respectively.

[c] The mean body weights of the older men and women were 83.1 and 59.8 kg, respectively.

[d] Within 1 month after the baseline measurements were made, study participants performed resistance exercise (weight lifting) every Monday, Wednesday, and Friday for 3 months. After the 3 months of exercise training, all the measurements were made as before training.

* $P<0.05$ vs the corresponding baseline value; † $P<0.05$ vs the corresponding young group.

et al. 1997). Sixth, the fractional rates of protein synthesis in the skeletal muscle and liver of tumor-bearing mice decrease by 70% and 40%, respectively, compared with the control, healthy animals, and this reduction cannot be explained by a 14% decline in food intake per mouse during the last 5 days of the study (Emery et al. 1984). Finally, chemically induced diabetes reduces the fractional rates of protein in the skeletal muscle, whole liver, hepatic non-secreted (cellular) protein, and hepatic albumin by 69%, 49%, 42%, and 43%, respectively, without influencing those in the jejunal mucosa and serosa (McNurlan et al. 1980), suggesting that intestinal protein synthesis may not be sensitive to insulin. The changes in the rates of whole-body and tissue protein synthesis play an important role in the regulation of systemic AA homeostasis.

8.7 SUMMARY

Protein synthesis is essential to life. In both animals and microbes, DNA is transcribed to form rRNA, mRNA, and tRNA in the nucleus by RNA polymerases I, II, and III, respectively, as well as various other types of RNA (e.g., signal recognition particle RNA, small nuclear RNA, and microRNA). Eukaryotic mRNA precursors are processed by 5′ capping, 3′ cleavage and polyadenylation, and

RNA splicing to remove introns before being transported to the cytoplasm, where protein synthesis from AAs on the mRNA template occurs on the ribosomes in the rough endoplasmic reticulum. The mitochondria also contain DNAs and the needed machinery to synthesize a limited number of proteins. The process of cytosolic and mitochondria protein synthesis consists of five stages: activation of amino acids (catalyzed by aminoacyl-tRNA synthase); initiation of polypeptide synthesis (formation of 80S ribosome from 40S and 60S subunits); elongation of polypeptide; termination (recognized by the terminating signal on the mRNA); and posttranslational modifications of peptides (Figure 8.16). The protein synthetic pathway requires a number of eukaryotic initiation factors (e.g., eIF1, eIF2, eIF2B, eIF3, eIF4A, eIF4E, eIF4G, and eIF5), elongation factors (e.g., eEF1A, eEF1B, and eEF2), and release factors. Translation initiation also depends on the phosphorylation of several regulatory proteins, including MTOR, 4EBP1, and p70S6K1. After the newly synthesized proteins are released from the ribosome, they undergo posttranslational modifications (e.g., limited cleavage, acetylation, disulfide linkage formation, methylation, phosphorylation, and/or ubiquitination) to become biologically active. Protein synthesis requires a relatively large amount of energy (~15% of dietary energy intake) but fulfills important physiological functions, including regulating intracellular concentrations of proteins, promoting cell proliferation, and supporting cell replacement. Tracer methodologies have been developed to determine both *in vitro* and *in vivo* rates of protein synthesis in cells, tissues, and the whole body. The most common *in vivo* methods are the flooding dose technique and the constant infusion of a tracer AA. Each of these methods has advantages and disadvantages and should be chosen according to the objectives of studies.

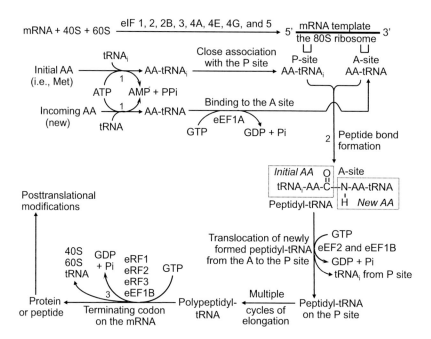

FIGURE 8.16 Protein synthesis from amino acids (AAs) on the cytosolic 80S ribosome in animal cells. The 80S ribosome is formed from 40S and the 60S ribosomes as the site for the translation of mRNA to produce protein. These processes require a variety of eukaryotic initiation factors (eIF), elongation factors (eEF), and release factors (eRF). Polypeptide elongation is terminated by a terminating codon on the mRNA template. The newly synthesized protein or peptide undergoes posttranslational modifications to become biologically active. Enzymes that catalyze the indicated reactions are as follows: (1) aminoacyl-tRNA synthetase, which is specific for each AA; (2) peptidyltransferase (a ribozyme; i.e., 28S rRNA in eukaryotes or 23S rRNA in bacteria), which catalyzes peptide bond formation between two aminoacylated tRNA substrates; and (3) peptidyltransferase, which, together with RF (RF1 in eukaryotes or RF1/RF2 in bacteria), hydrolyzes peptidyl-tRNA to release the newly synthesized peptide.

REFERENCES

Adegoke, O.A., M.I. McBurney, S.E. Samuels, and V.E. Baracos. 2003. Modulation of intestinal protein synthesis and protease mRNA by luminal and systemic nutrients. *Am. J. Physiol.* 284:G1017–G1026.

Anthony, J.C., F. Yoshizawa, T.G. Anthony, T.C. Vary, L.S. Jefferson, and S.R. Kimball. 2000. Leucine stimulates translation initiation in skeletal muscle of postabsorptive rats via a rapamycin-sensitive pathway. *J. Nutr.* 130:2413–2419.

Attaix, D. and M. Arnal. 1987. Protein synthesis and growth in the gastrointestinal tract of the young preruminant lamb. *Br. J. Nutr.* 58:159–169.

Attaix, D., A. Manghebati, J. Grizard, and M. Arnal. 1986. Assessment of *in vivo* protein synthesis in lamb tissues with [³H] valine flooding doses. *Biochim. Biophys. Acta* 882:389–397.

Attaix, D., E. Aurousseau, A. Manghebati, and M. Arnal. 1988. Contribution of liver, skin and skeletal muscle to whole-body protein synthesis in the young lamb. *Br. J. Nutr.* 60:77–84.

Ayyub, S.A. and U. Varshney 2019. Translation initiation in mammalian mitochondria- a prokaryotic perspective. *J. RNA Biol.* 17:165–175.

Baracos, V.E. and A.L. Goldberg. 1986. Maintenance of normal length improves protein balance and energy status in isolated rate skeletal muscles. *Am. J. Physiol.* 251:C588–C596.

Baracos, V.E., M. Langman, and A. Mak. 1989. An *in vitro* preparation of the extensor digitorum longus muscle from the chick (*Gallus domesticus*) for studies of protein turnover. *Comp. Biochem. Physiol. A* 92:555–563.

Baracos, V.E., J. Brun-Bellut, and M. Marie. 1991. Tissue protein synthesis in lactating and dry goats. *Br. J. Nutr.* 66:451–465.

Baumann, P.Q., W.S. Stirewalt, B.D. O'Rourke, D. Howard, and K.S. Nair. 1994. Precursor pools of protein synthesis: a stable isotope study in a swine model. *Am. J. Physiol.* 267: E203–E209.

Belloto, E., F. Diraison, A. Basset, G. Allain, P. Abdallah, and M. Beylot. 2007. Determination of protein replacement rates by deuterated water: validation of underlying assumptions. *Am. J. Physiol.* 292:E1340–E1347.

Bergen, W.G. 1974. Protein synthesis in animal models. *J. Anim. Sci.* 38:1079–1091.

Bergen, W.G., D.R. Mulvaney, D.M. Skjaerlund, S.E. Johnson, and R.A. Merkel. 1987. In vivo and in vitro measurements of protein turnover. *J. Anim. Sci.* 65 (Suppl. 2):88–106.

Blommaart, E.F., J.J. Luiken, P.J. Blommaart, G.M. van Woerkom, and A.J. Meijer. 1995. Phosphorylation of ribosomal protein S6 is inhibitory for autophagy in isolated rat hepatocytes. *J. Biol. Chem.* 270:2320–2326.

Bogorad, A.M., K.Y. Lin, and A. Marintchev. 2018. eIF2B mechanisms of action and regulation: a thermodynamic view. *Biochemistry* 57:1426–1435.

Breen, L. and S.M. Phillips. 2011. Skeletal muscle protein metabolism in the elderly: interventions to counteract the 'anabolic resistance' of ageing. *Nutr. Metab. (Lond)* 8:68.

Bröer, S. and A. Bröer. 2017. Amino acid homeostasis and signalling in mammalian cells and organisms. *Biochem. J.* 474:1935–2963.

Brown, D. and L.E. Mount. 1982. The metabolic body size of the growing pig. *Livest. Prod. Sci.* 9:389–398.

Budkevich, T.V., A.V. El'skaya, and K.H. Nierhaus. 2008. Features of 80S mammalian ribosome and its subunits. *Nucleic Acids Res.* 36:4736–4744.

Calder, P.C., C.J. Field, and H.S. Gill. 2002. *Nutrition and Immune Function.* CAB International, Wallingford, Oxon.

Clugston, G.A. and P.J. Garlick. 1982. The response of protein and energy metabolism to food intake in lean and obese man. *Human Nutrition: Clin. Nutr.* 36C:57–70.

Cone, J.E., R.M. del Rio, J.N. Davis, and T.C. Stadtman. 1976. Chemical characterization of the selenoprotein component of clostridial glycine reductase: identification of selenocysteine as the organoselenium moiety. *Proc. Natl. Acad. Sci. USA* 73:2659–63.

Conley, S.B., G.M. Rose, A.M. Robson, and D.M. Bier. 1980. Effects of dietary intake and hemodialysis on protein turnover in uremic children. *Kidneys Int.* 17:837–846.

Davis, T.A. and P.J. Reeds. 2001. Of flux and flooding: the advantages and problems of different isotopic methods for quantifying protein turnover in vivo: II. Methods based on the incorporation of a tracer. *Curr. Opin. Clin. Nutr. Metab. Care.* 4:51–56.

Davis, T.A., D.G. Burrin, M.L. Fiorotto, P.J. Reeds, and F. Jahoor. 1998. Roles of insulin and amino acids in the regulation of protein synthesis in the neonate. *J. Nutr.* 128 (Suppl. 2):347S–350S.

Davis, T.A., M.L. Fiorotto, H.V. Nguyen, and D.G. Burrin. 1999. Aminoacyl-tRNA and tissue free amino acid pools are equilibrated after a flooding dose of phenylalanine. *Am. J. Physiol.* 277:E103–E109.

Davis, T.A., M.L. Fiorotto, D.G. Burrin, P.J. Reeds, H.V. Nguyen, P.R. Beckett et al. 2002. Stimulation of protein synthesis by both insulin and amino acids is unique to skeletal muscle in neonatal pigs. *Am. J. Physiol.* 282:E880–E890.

Davis, T.A., A. Suryawan, R.A. Orellana, H.V. Nguyen, and M.L. Fiorotto. 2008. Postnatal ontogeny of skeletal muscle protein synthesis in pigs. *J. Anim. Sci.* 86 (Suppl. 14):E13–E18.

Davis, T.A., A. Suryawan, R.A. Orellana, M.L. Fiorotto, and D.G. Burrin. 2010. Amino acids and insulin are regulators of muscle protein synthesis in neonatal pigs. *Animal* 4:1790–1796.

Demeshkina, N., G. Hirokawa, A. Kaji, and H. Kaji. 2007. Novel activity of eukaryotic translocase, eEF2: dissociation of the 80S ribosome into subunits with ATP but not with GTP. *Nucleic Acids Res.* 35:4597–4607.

Deng, D., Y.L. Yin, W.Y. Chu, K. Yao, T.J. Li, R.L. Huang et al. 2009. Impaired translation initiation activation and reduced protein synthesis in weaned piglets fed a low-protein diet. *J. Nutr. Biochem.* 20:544–552.

Dever, T.E. 2002. Gene-specific regulation by general translation factors. *Cell* 108:545–556.

Dich, J. and K. Nielsen. 1963. Metabolism and distribution of ^{131}I-labelled albumin in the pig. *Can. J. Comp. Med. Vet. Sci.* 27:269–273.

Dillon, E.L., S.L. Casperson, W.J. Durham, K.M. Randolph, R.J. Urban, E. Volpi et al. 2011. Muscle protein metabolism responds similarly to exogenous amino acids in healthy younger and older adults during NO-induced hyperemia. *Am. J. Physiol.* 301:R1408–R1417.

Dobosz-Bartoszek, M., M.H. Pinkerton, Z. Otwinowski, S. Chakravarthy, D. Söll, P.R. Copeland, and M. Simonović. 2016. Crystal structures of the human elongation factor eEFSec suggest a non-canonical mechanism for selenocysteine incorporation. *Nat. Commun.* 7:12941.

Duarte, L., C.R. Matte, C.V. Bizarro, and M.A.Z. Ayub. 2020. Transglutaminases: part I - origins, sources, and biotechnological characteristics. *World J. Microbiol. Biotechnol.* 36:15.

Duggleby, S.L. and A.A. Jackson. 2002. Protein, amino acid and nitrogen metabolism during pregnancy: how might the mother meet the needs of her fetus? *Curr. Opin. Clin. Nutr. Metab. Care* 5:503–509.

Duggleby, S.L. and J.C. Waterlow. 2005. The end-product method of measuring whole-body protein turnover. *Br. J. Nutr.* 94:141–153.

El-Khoury, A.E., M. Sanchez, N.K. Fukagawa, and V.R. Young. 1995. Whole body protein synthesis in healthy adult humans;[13]CO_2 technique vs. plasma precursor approach. *Am. J. Physiol.* 268:E174–E184.

Elango, R. and R.O. Ball 2016. Protein and amino acid requirements during pregnancy. *Adv. Nutr.* 7:839S–844S.

Emery, P.W., L. Lovell, and M.J. Rennie. 1984. Protein synthesis measured in vivo in muscle and liver of cachectic tumor-bearing mice. *Cancer Res.* 44:2779–2784.

Engelen, M., G.A.M. Ten Have, J.J. Thaden, and N.E.P. Deutz. 2019. New advances in stable tracer methods to assess whole-body protein and amino acid metabolism. *Curr. Opin. Clin. Nutr. Metab. Care* 22: 337–46.

Fagan, J.M., L. Waxman, A.L. Goldberg. 1986. Red blood cells contain a pathway for the degradation of oxidant-damaged hemoglobin that does not require ATP or ubiquitin. *J. Biol. Chem.* 261:5705–5713.

Fedor, M.J. and J.R. Williamson. 2005. The catalytic diversity of RNAs. *Nat. Rev. Mol. Cell Biol.* 6:399–412.

Fern, E.B., P.J. Garlick, M.A. McNurlan, and J.C. Waterlow. 1981. The excretion of isotope in urea and ammonia for estimating protein turnover in man with (^{15}N) glycine. *Clin. Sci.* 61:217–28

Ferré-D'Amaré, A.R. 2011. Protein synthesis: stop the nonsense. *Nature* 474:289–290.

Fiorotto, M.L., H.A. Sosa Jr, and T.A. Davis. 2012. In vivo measurement of muscle protein synthesis rate using the flooding dose technique. *Methods. Mol. Biol.* 798:245–264.

Flohé, L., E.A. Günzler, and H.H. Schock. 1973. Glutathione peroxidase: a selenoenzyme. *FEBS Lett.* 32:132–134.

Frank, J.W., J. Escobar, H.V. Hguyen, S.C. Jobgen, W.S. Jobgen, T.A. Davis, and G. Wu. 2007. Oral N-carbamylglutamate supplementation increases protein synthesis in skeletal muscle of piglets. *J. Nutr.* 137:315–319.

Fukls, R.M., Li, J.B. and Goldberg, A.L. 1975. Effects of insulin, glucose, and amino acids on protein turnover in rat diaphragm. *J. Biol. Chem.* 250:290–298.

Gallo, S., S. Ricciardi, N. Manfrini, E. Pesce, S. Oliveto, P. Calamita, M. Mancino et al. 2018. 2018. RACK1 specifically regulates translation through its binding to ribosomes. *Mol. Cell. Biol.* 38:e00230–18.

Garlick, P.J., D.J. Millward, W.P.T. James, and J.C. Waterlow. 1975. The effect of protein deprivation and starvation on the rate of protein synthesis in tissues of the rat. *Biochim. Biophys. Acta* 414:71–84.

Garlick, P.J., M.A. McNurlan, and V.R. Preedy. 1980. A rapid and convenient technique for measuring the rate of protein synthesis in tissues by injection of [³H] phenylalanine. *Biochem. J.* 192:719–723.

Garlick, P.J., M.A. McNurlan, P. Essén, and J. Wernerman. 1994. Measurement of tissue protein synthesis rates in vivo: a critical analysis of contrasting methods. *Am. J. Physiol.* 266:E287–E297.

Gasier, H.G., S.E. Riechman, M.P. Wiggs, S.F. Previs, and J.D. Fluckey. 2009. A comparison of ^2H_2O and phenylalanine flooding dose to investigate muscle protein synthesis with acute exercise in rats. *Am. J. Physiol.* 297:E252–E259.

Gasier, H.G., J.D. Fluckey, and S.F. Previs. 2010. The application of ^2H_2O to measure skeletal muscle protein synthesis. *Nutr. Metab. (Lond)* 7:31.

Gehring, A.M., J.E. Walker, and T.J. Santangelo. 2016. Transcription regulation in archaea. *J. Bacteriol.* 198:1906–1917.

Goldspink, D.F. and F.J. Kelly. 1984. Protein turnover and growth in the whole body, liver and kidney of the rat from the foetus to senility. *Biochem. J.* 217:507–516.

Greber, B.J. 2016. Mechanistic insight into eukaryotic 60S ribosomal subunit biogenesis by cryo-electron microscopy. *RNA* 22:1643–1662.

Green, E.R. and J. Mecsas. 2016. Bacterial secretion systems – An overview. *Microbiol. Spectrum* 4:VMBF-0012-2015.

Greganova, E., M. Altmann, and P. Bütikofer. 2011. Unique modifications of translation elongation factors. *FEBS Lett.* 278:2613–2624.

Hallemeesch, M.M., P.B. Soeters, and N.E. Deutz. 2002. Renal arginine and protein synthesis are increased during early endotoxemia in mice. *Am. J. Physiol.* 282:F316–F323.

Hellerschmied, D., Y.V. Serebrenik, L. Shao, G.M. Burslem, and C.M. Crews. 2019. Protein folding state-dependent sorting at the Golgi apparatus. *Mol. Biol. Cell* 30:2097–2347.

Hocine, S., R.H. Singer, and D. Grünwald. 2010. RNA processing and export. *Cold Spring Harb. Perspect Biol.* 2:a000752.

Hou, Y.Q. and G. Wu. 2018. L-Glutamate nutrition and metabolism in swine. *Amino Acids* 50:1497–1510.

Hou, Y.Q., S.D. Hu, X.Y. Li, W.L. He, and G. Wu. 2020. Amino acid metabolism in the liver: nutritional and physiological significance. *Adv. Exp. Med. Biol.* 1265:21–37.

Ibba, M. and D. Söll. 2001. The renaissance of aminoacyl-tRNA synthesis. *EMBO Rep.* 2:382–387.

Itoh, Y., J. Andréll, A. Choi, U. Richter, P. Maiti, R.B. Best et al. 2021. Mechanism of membrane-tethered mitochondrial protein synthesis. *Science* 371:846–849.

Jahoor, F., B. Gazzard, G. Phillips, D. Sharpstone, M. Delrosario, M.E. Fraser et al. 1999. The acute phase protein response to human immunodeficiency virus in human subjects. *Am. J. Physiol.* 276:E1092–E1098.

Johnson, H.A., C.C. Calvert, and K.C. Klasing. 2003. Challenging the assumptions in estimating protein fractional synthesis rate using a model of rodent protein turnover. *Adv. Exp. Med. Biol.* 537:221–237.

Kabanova, S., P. Kleinbongard, J. Volkmer, B. Andrée, M. Kelm, and T.W. Jax. 2009. Gene expression analysis of human red blood cells. *Int. J. Med. Sci.* 6:156–159.

Kaniak-Golik, A. and A. Skoneczna. 2015. Mitochondria–nucleus network for genome stability. *Free Radical Biol. Med.* 82:73–104.

Kapp, L.D. and J.R. Lorsch. 2004. The molecular mechanics of eukaryotic translation. *Annu. Rev. Biochem.* 73:657–704.

Kimball, S.R. and L.S. Jefferson. 2010. Control of translation initiation through integration of signals generated by hormones, nutrients, and exercise. *J. Biol. Chem.* 285:29027–29032.

Klasing, K.C., C.C. Calvert, and V.L. Jarrell. 1987. Growth characteristics, protein synthesis and protein degradation in muscles from fast and slow-growing chickens. *Poultry Sci.* 66:1189–1196.

Klein, R.M. and J.C. McKenzie. 1983. The role of cell renewal in the ontogeny of the intestine. I. Cell proliferation patterns in adult, fetal, and neonatal intestine. *J. Pediatr. Gastroenterol. Nutr.* 2:10–43.

Kong, J. and P. Lasko. 2012. Translational control in cellular and developmental processes. *Nature Rev. Genet.* 13:383–394.

Kong, X.F., B.E. Tan, Y.L. Yin, H.J. Gao, X.L. Li, L.A. Jaeger et al. 2012. L-Arginine stimulates the mTOR signaling pathway and protein synthesis in porcine trophectoderm cells. *J. Nutr. Biochem.* 23:1178–1183.

Kossinova, O., A. Malygin, A. Krol, and G. Karpova. 2014. The SBP2 protein central to selenoprotein synthesis contacts the human ribosome at expansion segment 7L of the 28S rRNA. *RNA* 20:1046–1056.

Krebs, H.A. 1972. Some aspects of the regulation of fuel supply in omnivorous animals. *Adv. Enzyme Regul.* 10:397–420.

Lackner, D.H. and J. Bähler 2008. Translational control of gene expression from transcripts to transcriptomes. *Int. Rev. Cell Mol. Biol.* 271:199–251.

Leiter, L. and E.B. Marliss. 1982. Length of survival during prolonged total fasting may be determined by fat as well as protein stores. *JAMA* 248:2306–2307.

Li, P. and G. Wu. 2018. Roles of dietary glycine, proline and hydroxyproline in collagen synthesis and animal growth. *Amino Acids* 50:29–38.

Li, P., Y.L. Yin, D.F. Li, S.W. Kim, and G. Wu. 2007. Amino acids and immune function. *Br. J. Nutr.* 98:237–252.

Ljungqvist, O.H., M. Persson, G.C. Ford, and K.S. Nair. 1997. Functional heterogeneity of leucine pools in human skeletal muscle. *Am. J. Physiol.* 273:E564–E570.

Lobley, G.E., V. Milne, J.M. Lovie, P.J. Reeds, and K. Rennie. 1980. Whole body and tissues protein synthesis in cattle. *Br. J. Nutr.* 43:491–502.

Manary, M.J., K.E. Yarasheski, R. Berger, E.T. Abrams, C.A. Hart, and R.L. Broadhead. 2004. Whole-body leucine kinetics and the acute phase response during acute infection in marasmic malawian children. *Pediatr. Res.* 55:940–946.

Mansoor, O., M. Cayol, P. Gachon, Y. Boirie, P. Schoeffler, C. Obled, and B. Beaufrère. 1997. Albumin and fibrinogen syntheses increase while muscle protein synthesis decreases in head-injured patients. *Am. J. Physiol.* 273:E898–E902.

Marliss, E.B., S. Chevalier, R. Gougeon, J.A. Morais, M. Lamarche, O.A.J. Adegoke, and G. Wu. 2006. Elevations of plasma methylarginines in obesity and ageing are related to insulin sensitivity and rates of protein turnover. *Diabetologia* 49:351–359.

McAllister, T.A., J.R. Thompson, and S.E. Samuels. 2000. Skeletal and cardiac muscle protein turnover during cold acclimation in young rats. *Am. J. Physiol.* 278:R705–R711.

McIntyre, N. and S. Rosalki. 1994. Tests of the function of the liver. In: *Scientific Foundations of Biochemistry in Clinical Practice* (Williams, D.L. and V. Marks, eds). Elsevier, New York. pp. 383–398.

McNurlan, M.A. and P.J. Garlick. 1980. Contribution of rat liver and gastrointestinal tract to whole-body protein synthesis in the rat. *Biochem. J.* 186:381–383.

McNurlan, M.A., A.M. Tomkins, and P.J. Garlick. 1979. The effect of starvation on the rate of protein synthesis in rat liver and small intestine. *Biochem. J.* 178:373–379.

McNurlan, M.A., V.M. Pain, and P.J. Garlick. 1980. Conditions that alter rates of tissue protein synthesis in vivo. *Biochem. Soc. Trans.* 8:283–285.

Meléndez-Hevia, E., P. De Paz-Lugo, A. Cornish-Bowden, and M.L. Cárdenas. 2009. A weak link in metabolism: the metabolic capacity for glycine biosynthesis does not satisfy the need for collagen synthesis. *J. Biosci.* 34:853–872.

Mills, E.W., J. Wangen, R. Green, and N.T. Ingolia. 2016. Dynamic regulation of a ribosome rescue pathway in erythroid cells and platelets. *Cell Rep.* 17:1–10.

Millward, D.J., A. Fereday, N. Gibson, and P.J. Pacy. 1996. Postprandial protein metabolism. *Bailliere's Clin. Endocrin. Metab.* 10:533–549.

Moore, D.R., P.J. Atherton, M.J. Rennie, M.A. Tarnopolsky, and S.M. Phillips. 2011. Resistance exercise enhances mTOR and MAPK signalling in human muscle over that seen at rest after bolus protein ingestion. *Acta Physiol. (Oxf)* 201:365–372.

Morissette, M.P. 1977. Colloid osmotic pressure: its measurement and clinical value. *Can. Med Assoc. J.* 116:897–900.

Motil, K.J., D.M. Bier, D.E. Matthews, J.F. Burke, and V.R. Young. 1981. Whole body leucine and lysine metabolism studied with $[1-^{13}C]$ leucine and $[\alpha-^{15}N]$ lysine: response in healthy young men given excess energy intake. *Metabolism* 30:783–791.

Müller, M.M. 2018. Post-translational modifications of protein backbones: unique functions, mechanisms, and challenges. *Biochemistry* 57:177–185.

Murakami, H., K. Shimbo, Y. Inoue, Y. Takino, and H. Kobayashi. 2012. Importance of amino acid composition to improve skin collagen protein synthesis rates in UV-irradiated mice. *Amino Acids* 42:2481–2489.

Muramatsu, T. 1990. Nutrition and whole-body protein turnover in the chicken in relation to mammalian species. *Nutr. Res. Rev.* 3:211–228.

Myllyharju, J. 2005. Intracellular post-translational modifications of collagens. *Top. Curr. Chem.* 247:115–247.

Ogle, J.M. and V. Ramakrishnan. 2005. Structural insights into translational fidelity. *Annu. Rev. Biochem.* 74:129–177.

Pacy, P.J., G.M. Price, O. Halliday, and D.J. Millward. 1994. Nitrogen homoestasis in man: the diurnal responses of protein synthesis and degradation and amino acid oxidation for diets with increasing protein intakes. *Clin. Sci.* 86:103–118.

Pain, V.M. 1996. Initiation of protein synthesis in eukaryotic cells. *Eur. J. Biochem.* 236:747–771.

Palangat, M. and D.R. Larson. 2012. Complexity of RNA polymerase II elongation dynamics. *Biochim. Biophys. Acta.* 1819:667–672.

Palmer, R.M., P.J. Reeds, T. Atkinson, and R.H. Smith. 1983. The influence of changes in tension on protein synthesis and prostaglandin release in isolated rabbit muscles. *Biochem. J.* 214:1011–1014.

Pencharz, P.B., M. Masson, F. Desgranges, and A. Papageorgiou. 1981. Total-body protein turnover in human premature neonates: effects of birth weight, intra-uterine nutritional status and diet. *Clin. Sci.* 61:207–215.

Polycarpo, C., A. Ambrogelly, A. Bérubé, S.M. Winbush, J.A. McCloskey, P.F. Crain et al. 2004. An aminoacyl-tRNA synthetase that specifically activates pyrrolysine. *Proc. Natl. Acad. Sci. USA.* 101:12450–12454.

Preedy, V.R., M.A. McNurlan, and P.J. Garlick. 1983. Protein synthesis in skin and bone of the young rat. *Br. J. Nutr.* 49:517–523.

Previs, S., R. Fatica, V. Chandramouli, J. Alexander, H. Brunengraber, and B.R. Landau. 2004. Quantifying rate of protein synthesis in humans by use of ^2H_2O: application to patients with end-stage renal failure. *Am. J. Physiol.* 286:E665–E672.

Prinsen, B.H.C.M.T. and M.G.M. de Sain-van der Velden. 2004. Albumin turnover: experimental approach and its application in health and renal disease. *Clin. Chim. Acta* 347:1–14.

Rajendran, V., P. Kalita, H. Shukla, A. Kumar, and T. Tripathi. 2018. Aminoacyl-tRNA synthetases: structure, function, and drug discovery. *Int. J. Biol. Macromol.* 111:400–414.

Ramanathan, A., G.B. Robb, and S. Chan. 2016. mRNA capping: biological functions and applications. *Nucleic Acids Res.* 44:7511–7526.

Reeds, P.J. and G.E. Lobley. 1980. Protein synthesis: are there real species differences? *Proc. Nutr. Soc.* 39:43–52.

Reeds, P.J., A. Cadenhead, M.F. Fuller, G.E. Lobley, and J.D. McDonald. 1980. Protein turnover in growing pigs. Effects of age and food intake. *Br. J. Nutr.* 43:445–455.

Rennie, M.J., K. Smith, and P.W. Watt. 1994. Measurement of human tissue protein synthesis: an optimal approach. *Am. J. Physiol.* 266:E298–E307.

Riond, J.-L., M. Stiefel, C. Wenk, and M. Wanner. 2003. Nutrition studies on protein and energy in domestic cats. *J. Anim. Physiol. Anim. Nutr.* 87:221–228.

Rodrigues, M., N. Kosaric, C.A. Bonham, and G.C. Gurtner. 2018. Wound healing: a cellular perspective. *Physiol. Rev.* 99:665–706.

Rodnina, M.V. 2018. Translation in prokaryotes. *Cold Spring Harb. Perspect. Biol.* 10:a032664.

Rose, I.A. and D.J. Kuo. 1989. The substrate proton of the pyruvate kinase reaction. *Biochemistry* 28:9579–9585.

Rother, M. and J.A. Krzycki. 2010. Selenocysteine, pyrrolysine, and the unique energy metabolism of methanogenic archaea. *Archaea* 2010:453642.

Rotruck, J.T., A.L. Pope, H.E. Ganther, A.B. Swanson, D.G. Hafeman, and W.G. Hoekstra. 1973. Selenium: biochemical role as a component of glutathione peroxidase. *Science* 179:588–590.

Roustan, V., A. Jain, M. Teige, I. Ebersberger, and W. Weckwerth. 2016. An evolutionary perspective of AMPK-TOR signaling in the three domains of life. *J. Exp. Bot.* 67:3897–3907.

Saxton, R.A and D.M. Sabatini. 2017. mTOR signaling in growth, metabolism, and disease. *Cell* 168:960–976.

Schwarz, K. and C.M. Foltz. 1957. Selenium as an integral part of factor 3 against dietary necrotic liver degeneration. *J. Am. Chem. Soc.* 79:3292–3293.

Serrão, V.H.B., I.R. Silva, M.T.A. da Silva, J.F. Scortecci, A. de Freitas Fernandes, and O.H. Thiemann. 2018. The unique tRNA[Sec] and its role in selenocysteine biosynthesis. *Amino Acids* 50:1145–1167.

Sherman, F., J.W. Stewart, and S. Tsunasawa. 1985. Methionine or not methionine at the beginning of a protein. BioEssays 3:27–31.

Schmitt, E., P. Coureux, A. Monestier, E. Dubiez, and Y. Mechulam. 2019. Start codon recognition in eukaryotic and archaeal translation initiation: a common structural core. *Int. J. Mol. Sci.* 20:939.

Smith, M.W. and L.G. Jarvis. 1978. Growth and cell replacement in the new-born pig intestine. *Proc. R. Soc. Lond.* B. 203:69–89.

Soares, M.J., L.S. Piers, P.S. Shelly, S. Robinson, A.A. Jackson, and J.C. Waterlow. 1991. Basal metabolic rate, body composition and whole-body protein turnover in Indian men with differing nutritional status. *Clin. Sci.* 81:419–425.

Southorn, B.G., J.M. Kelly, and B.W. McBride. 1992. Phenylalanine flooding dose procedure is effective in measuring intestinal and liver protein synthesis in sheep. *J. Nutr.* 122:2398–2407.

Stadtman, T.C. 1996. Selenocysteine. *Annu. Rev. Biochem.* 65:83–100.

Stoll, B., W. Gerok, F. Lang, and D. Häussinger. 1992. Liver cell volume and protein synthesis. *Biochem. J.* 287:217–222.

Suryawan, A., R.A. Orellana, M.L. Fiorotto, and T.A. Davis. 2011. Leucine acts as a nutrient signal to stimulate protein synthesis in neonatal pigs. *J. Anim. Sci.* 89:2004–2016.

Susorov, D., N. Zakharov, E. Shuvalova, A. Ivanov, T. Egorova, A. Shuvalov et al. 2018. Eukaryotic translation elongation factor 2 (eEF2) catalyzes reverse translocation of the eukaryotic ribosome. *J. Biol. Chem.* 293:5220–5229.

Ten Have, G.A.M., M. Engelen, R.R. Wolfe, and N.E.P. Deutz. 2019. Inhibition of jejunal protein synthesis and breakdown in pseudomonas aeruginosa-induced sepsis pig model. *Am. J. Physiol.* 316: G755–G762.

Tesseraud, S., A.M. Chagneau, and J. Grizard. 2000. Muscle protein turnover during early development in chickens divergently selected for growth rate. *Poultry Sci.* 79:1465–1471.

Tharp, J.M., A. Ehnbom, and W.R. Liu. 2018. tRNA^Pyl: structure, function, and applications. *RNA Biol.* 15:441–452.

Tian, S. and V.E. Baracos. 1989. Effect of *Escherichia coli* infection on growth and protein metabolism in broiler chicks (Gallus domesticus). *Comp. Biochem. Physiol. A.* 94:323–331.

Tischler, M., M. Desautels, and A.L. Goldberg. 1982. Does leucine, leucycl tRNA or some metabolite of leucine regulate protein synthesis and degradation in skeletal and cardiac muscle. *J. Biol. Chem.* 257:1613–1621.

Tischler, M.E., A.H. Ost, B. Spina, P.H. Cook, and J. Coffman. 1984. Regulation of protein turnover by glucose, insulin, and amino acids in adipose tissue. *Am. J. Physiol.* 247:C228–C233.

Turner, D.C. and T.C. Stadtman. 1973. Purification of protein components of the clostridial glycine reductase system and characterization of protein A as a selenoprotein. *Arch. Biochem. Biophys.* 154:366–381.

Venters, B.J. and B.F. Pugh. 2009. How eukaryotic genes are transcribed. *Crit. Rev. Biochem. Mol. Biol.* 44:117–141.

Wang, J.J., D.F. Li, L.J. Dangott, and G. Wu. 2006. Proteomics and its role in nutrition research. *J. Nutr.* 136:1759–1762.

Waterlow, J.C. 1984. Protein turnover with special reference to man. *Quart. J. Exp. Physiol.* 69:409–438.

Waterlow, J.C. 1995. Whole-body protein turnover in humans – Past, present, and future. *Annu. Rev. Nutr.* 15:57–92.

Watford, M., and G. Wu. 2005. Glutamine metabolism in uricotelic species: variation in skeletal muscle glutamine synthetase, glutaminase, glutamine levels and rates of protein synthesis. *Comp. Biochem. Physiol. B.* 140:607–614.

Watson, J.D. 2013. *Molecular Biology of the Gene*, 7th edition. Pearson Higher Ed, New York.

Watt, P.W., Y. Lindsay, C.M. Scrimgeour, P.A.F. Chien, J.N.A. Gibson, D.J. Taylor, and M.J. Rennie. 1991. Isolation of aminoacyl-tRNA and its labeling with stable-isotope tracers: use in studies of human tissue protein synthesis. *Proc. Natl. Acad. Sci. USA.* 88:5892–5896.

Welle, S., C. Thornton, and M. Statt. 1995. Myofibrillar protein synthesis in young and old human subjects after three months of resistance training. *Am. J. Physiol.* 268:E422–E427.

Wester, T.J., K. Weidgraaf, and S.F. Forsyth. 2006. Measurement of whole body protein turnover in the adult cat (*Felis catus*). *FASEB J.* 20: A1045.

Wiedemann, N. and N. Pfanner. 2017. Mitochondrial machineries for protein import and assembly. *Annu. Rev. Biochem.* 86:685–714.

Wilkinson, D.J. 2018. Historical and contemporary stable isotope tracer approaches to studying mammalian protein metabolism. *Mass Spectrom. Rev.* 37:57–80.

Wilkinson, D. J., M. V. Franchi, M. S. Brook, M. V. Narici, J. P. Williams, W. K. Mitchell et al. 2014. A validation of the application of D(2)O stable isotope tracer techniques for monitoring day-to-day changes in muscle protein subfraction synthesis in humans. *Am. J. Physiol.* 306:E571–E579.

Wilkinson, D.J., J. Cegielski, B.E. Phillips, C. Boereboom, J.N. Lund, P.J. Atherton, and K. Smith. 2015. Internal comparison between deuterium oxide (D2O) and L-[ring-13C6] phenylalanine for acute measurement of muscle protein synthesis in humans. *Physiol. Rep.* 3:e12433.

Williams, C.C., K.A. Cummins, M.G. Hayek, and G.M. Davenport. 2001. Effects of dietary protein on whole-body protein turnover and endocrine function in young-adult and aging dogs. *J. Anim. Sci.* 79:3128–3136.

Witte, M.B., Barbul, A. 2008. Arginine physiology and its implications for wound healing. *Wound Repair Regeneration* 11:419–423.

Wray-Cahen, D., H.V. Nguyen, D.G. Burrin, P.R. Beckett, M.L. Fiorotto, Reeds, P.J. et al. 1998. Response of skeletal muscle protein synthesis to insulin in suckling pigs decreases with development. *Am. J. Physiol.* 275:E602–609.

Wu, G. 2018. *Principles of Animal Nutrition*. CRC Press, Boca Raton, FL.

Wu, G. 2020. Important roles of dietary taurine, creatine, carnosine, anserine and 4-hydroxyproline in human nutrition and health. *Amino Acids* 52:329–360.

Wu, G. and J.R. Thompson. 1990. The effect of glutamine on protein turnover in chick skeletal muscle. *Biochem. J.* 265:593–598.

Xi, P.B., Z.Y. Jiang, Z.L. Dai, X.L. Li, K. Yao, C.T. Zheng et al. 2012. Regulation of protein turnover by L-glutamine in porcine intestinal epithelial cells. *J. Nutr. Biochem.* 23:1012–1017.

Yang, Y., T.A. Churchward-Venne, N.A. Burd, L. Breen, M.A. Tarnopolsky, and S.M. Phillips. 2012. Myofibrillar protein synthesis following ingestion of soy protein isolate at rest and after resistance exercise in elderly men. *Nutr. Metab.* 9:57.

Yin, Y.L., K. Yao, Z.J. Liu, M. Gong, Z. Ruan, D. Deng et al. 2010. Supplementing L-leucine to a low-protein diet increases tissue protein synthesis in weanling pigs. *Amino Acids* 39:1477–1486.

Yu, Y.M., R.L. Sheridan, J.F. Burke, T.E. Chapman, R.G. Tompkins, and V.R. Young. 1996. Kinetics of plasma arginine and leucine in pediatric burn patients. *Am. J. Clin. Nutr.* 64:60–66.

Zak, R., A.F. Martin, and R. Blough. 1979. Assessment of protein turnover by use of radioisotopic tracers. *Physiol. Rev.* 59:407–447.

Zhang, J.M., W.L. He, D. Yi, D. Zhao, Z. Song, Y.Q. Hou, and G. Wu. 2019. Regulation of protein synthesis in porcine mammary epithelial cells by L-valine. *Amino Acids* 51:717–726.

Zinoni, F., A. Birkmann, T.C. Stadtman, and A. Böck. 1986. Nucleotide sequence and expression of the selenocysteine-containing polypeptide of formate dehydrogenase (formate-hydrogen-lyase-linked) from escherichia coli. *Proc. Natl. Acad. Sci. USA.* 83:4650–4654.

9 Intracellular and Extracellular Degradation of Body Proteins

The seminal work of R. Schoenheimer and coworkers in 1938 and 1939 that involved ^{15}N-labeled tyrosine and leucine in animals revealed, for the first time, dynamic changes of the body's components, including protein and amino acids (AAs). This revolutionary finding directly challenged the long-standing view that structural proteins in the body were in a static state and that dietary protein was only used as a metabolic fuel by humans and other animals (Schoenheimer and Rittenberg 1940). The continuous synthesis and degradation of protein is collectively termed "intracellular protein turnover" (Figure 9.1). This metabolic cycle occurs in nearly all cell types as an essential physiological event. Note that intracellular protein turnover is not a synonym for intracellular protein degradation (also known as proteolysis) because the former is composed of both protein synthesis and protein degradation.

Although the pathway for protein biosynthesis was elucidated in the mid-1960s, many of the pathways for intracellular proteolysis were not well understood until the late 1980s and early 1990s when the ubiquitin-proteasome cascade was discovered (Goldberg and St John 1976; Hershko et al. 1980; Hershko and Ciechanover 1998; Hough et al. 1986). Over the past two decades, there has been growing interest in the intracellular degradation of proteins (including newly synthesized collagen) via not only proteasomes (Coux et al. 2020) but also autophagy (Dikic and Elazar 2018; Noguchi et al. 2020) and the extracellular degradation of body proteins such as mature collagens in the connective tissue (Salsas-Escat et al. 2010; Strzyz 2020). In essence, protein degradation, which is an energy-dependent process, is an endogenous source of AAs for utilization in humans and other animals and also plays a crucial role in the renewal of whole-body proteins necessary for health and well-being (Craik et al. 2011; Goldberg 2003). In this chapter, the biochemical pathways of intracellular and extracellular degradation of body proteins in animals will be described along with the characteristics, significance, measurement, and rates of these processes. They are distinct from the extracellular degradation of food proteins and gastrointestinal secretions by digestive proteases and peptidases in the lumen of the gastrointestinal tract.

9.1 HISTORIC PERSPECTIVES OF INTRACELLULAR PROTEIN DEGRADATION

Research on intracellular protein degradation has spanned over 70 years since R. Schoenheimer published in 1942 his groundbreaking book on the dynamics of whole-body protein turnover in mammals. A decade later, M.V. Simpson reported in 1953 that mammalian cells can degrade

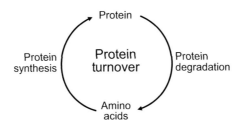

FIGURE 9.1 Intracellular protein turnover in cells. Protein undergoes continuous synthesis and degradation in the cell. These two physiological processes are collectively known as intracellular protein turnover.

461

intracellular proteins and this biochemical event requires metabolic energy. In the same year, C. de Duve discovered that the lysosome is a membrane-bound organelle in cells. In 1955, this organelle was found by C. de Duve to contain cathepsins for degrading cellular proteins. The requirement of metabolic energy for protein breakdown in bacteria (*E. coli*) was reported by J. Mandelstam in 1958, which paved the way for future studies of energy-dependent proteolysis in animal cells. Meanwhile, ongoing work in the area of neurobiology led to the identification of Ca^{2+}-dependent protease (calpain) for degrading intracellular proteins outside the lysosome. Specifically, calpain was extracted for the first time from the rat brain by G. Guroff in 1964, and this work was extended to skeletal muscle and other tissues in the late 1960s (Kohn 1969).

The 1970s witnessed exciting developments in the field of intracellular protein degradation. Specifically, in 1974, G. Goldstein discovered ubiquitin (a 76-AA polypeptide) in eukaryotic cells. In 1977, Etlinger and Goldberg found that protein degradation requires ATP in a reticulocyte preparation without lysosomes and proposed both lysosomal and nonlysosomal systems for intracellular proteolysis. Further studies revealed that the lysosome is not involved in the degradation of most intracellular proteins under basal conditions, indicating a major role for the nonlysosomal pathway for proteolysis in cells. A seemingly unrelated study was published in 1977, which identified the linkage between ubiquitin and histone H2A as an iso-peptide bond (Goldknopf and Busch 1977). However, it is this work that laid a foundation for the future elucidation of how ubiquitin conjugates with a protein targeted for degradation. Thus, in 1978, A. Ciechanover and A. Hershko found that two fractions (I and II) isolated from reticulocytes were required to reconstitute ATP-dependent protein degradation in a cell-free system. The active component in Fraction I turned out to be a small, ~8.5 kDa heat-stable protein, called ATP-dependent proteolysis factor 1 (APF1), which by itself had no activity to degrade protein in the presence or absence of ATP (Ciechanover et al. 1978). Fraction II contained multiple proteins but by itself only had a low ability to degrade protein in the presence or absence of ATP. Both Fractions I and II were required to reconstitute the energy-dependent proteolytic activity that was found in the whole reticulocyte lysates incubated with ATP (Ciechanover et al. 1978).

Much effort in the 1980s and the early 1990s to characterize the two unknown fractions from reticulocytes (Ciechanover et al. 1978) led to the discovery of the ATP- and ubiquitin-dependent proteasome in the 1980s. Specifically, in 1980, A. Hershko and colleagues demonstrated that APF1 is covalently conjugated to protein substrates and proposed that APF1 serves as a signal to stimulate intracellular proteolysis by a downstream protease. In the same year, APF1 was shown to be identical to ubiquitin, linking this polypeptide with intracellular proteolysis, whereas the "multicatalytic protease complex" (later known as the 20S core-particle subcomplex of the 26S proteasome) was identified. Hershko et al. (1983) proposed a three-step ubiquitin-protein ligase cascade that is catalyzed by ubiquitin-activating enzyme (E1), ubiquitin-conjugating enzyme (E2), and ubiquitin-protein ligase (E3). Using the unique cell cycle arrest mutant (ts85) that contains a thermolabile E1 enzyme, Ciechanover et al. (1984) provided compelling evidence for a link between ubiquitination and protein degradation, as the cells failed to degrade normal short-lived proteins in response to heat inactivation. Two years later, Hough et al. (1986) partially purified an ATP-dependent protease that specifically degrades ubiquitin conjugates, and this protease was later called the 26S proteasome. In 1987, A. Hershko correctly proposed that the 20S proteasome is part of the 26S proteasome. Driscoll and Goldberg (1990) identified the proteasome (multicatalytic protease) to be a component of the 1,500-kDa proteolytic complex that degrades ubiquitin-conjugated proteins. Two years later, Hoffman et al. (1992) recognized the multiple forms of the 20S multicatalytic and the 26S ubiquitin- and ATP-dependent proteases (Fraction II) from reticulocyte lysates, thereby completing the answers to the previous questions of the identity and functions of the two unknown fractions that were isolated in 1980 from the same type of cell-free preparations. The discovery of the proteasome was recognized with the 2004 Nobel Prize in Chemistry to Aaron Ciechanover, Avram Hershko, and Irwin Rose.

9.2 PROTEASES AND PEPTIDASES FOR INTRACELLULAR PROTEIN DEGRADATION

Intracellular protein degradation is catalyzed by proteases, with the resulting small peptides being hydrolyzed by peptidases, tripeptidases, and dipeptidases (Rivett 1990). Most proteases are hydrolases (also known as peptidases), but some (e.g., asparagine peptide lyases) are not. Therefore, the terms "proteases" and "peptidases" should not be treated as synonymous. Upon the discovery of intracellular proteolysis in the 1950s, a system of nomenclature for the enzymes was developed. Proteases are classified according to (1) reaction type, (2) the chemical nature of the catalytic site, and (3) their evolutionary relationship to each other, as revealed by AA sequences and enzyme structures (Bond and Butler 1987). The classification and naming of enzymes based on the type of reaction is the primary principle of the enzyme nomenclature of the International Union of Biochemistry and Molecular Biology (IUBMB 1992). Note that the use of impure enzyme preparations in experiments can lead to errors in the classification of proteases.

9.2.1 CLASSIFICATION BY REACTION TYPE

Proteases can be classified as exopeptidases and endopeptidases based on the type of reaction, namely the hydrolysis of a peptide bond formed by AAs in either the terminal region (exopeptidases) or within an internal region (endopeptidases) of a protein (Figure 9.2). Some proteases may have both exopeptidase and endopeptidase properties, and these enzymes include cathepsins B and H (Barrett and Kirschke 1981). Large peptides are degraded by (1) aminopeptidases (that release

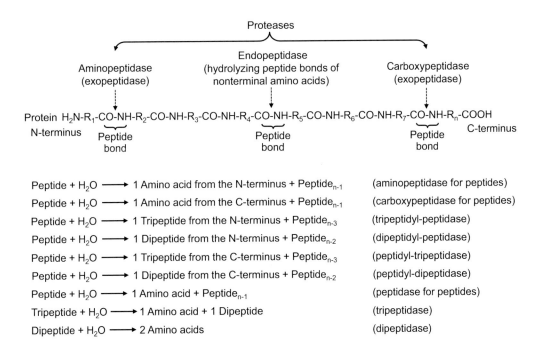

FIGURE 9.2 Roles of proteases, aminopeptidases, carboxypeptidases, tripeptidyl-peptidases, dipeptidyl-peptidases, peptidyl-tripeptidases, peptidyl-dipeptidases, peptidases, tripeptidases, and tripeptidases in animal cells. Note the differences in substrates and/or products between the following pairs of enzymes: (1) aminopeptidases for peptides vs aminopeptidases for proteins, (2) carboxypeptidases for peptides vs carboxypeptidases for proteins, (3) tripeptidyl-peptidases vs peptidyl-tripeptidases, and (4) dipeptidyl-peptidases vs peptidyl-dipeptidases.

a single AA residue from the N-terminus of their substrates), (2) carboxypeptidases (that release a single AA residue from the C-terminus of their substrates), (3) tripeptidyl-peptidase (that release a tripeptide from the N-terminus of their substrates), (4) dipeptidyl-peptidase (that release a dipeptide from the N-terminus of their substrates), (5) peptidyl-tripeptidases (that release a tripeptide from the C-terminus of their substrates), and (6) peptidyl-dipeptidases (that release a dipeptide from the C-terminus of their substrates). Some peptidases remove terminal AA residues that are substituted, cyclized, or linked by isopeptide bonds (namely peptide linkages other than those of α-carboxyl to α-amino groups; e.g., ω-peptidases). When a peptidase exhibits marked preference for a particular AA residue, the name of this AA is used to form a qualifier (e.g., "leucine" aminopeptidase and "proline" endopeptidase). Leucine aminopeptidase preferentially catalyzes the removal of leucine residues at the N-terminus of proteins and peptides, whereas proline endopeptidase hydrolyzes a peptide bond formed from proline within a polypeptide. For enzymes with very complex or broad specificity, alphabetical or numerical serial letters [e.g., peptidyl-dipeptidase A (angiotensin I converting enzyme), peptidyl-dipeptidase B (atrial dipeptidyl carboxyhydrolase), dipeptidyl-peptidase I, and dipeptidyl-peptidase II] are used as the postfix (Rawlings et al. 2012).

9.2.1.1   Exopeptidases (Aminopeptidases and Carboxypeptidases)

Exopeptidases cleave peptide bonds from either the carboxyl (C)- or the amino (N)-terminus of a polypeptide chain and can be further divided into aminopeptidases and carboxypeptidases. Aminopeptidases attack peptide bonds beginning from the N-terminus. Examples of aminopeptidases are leucine aminopeptidase, alanine (alanyl) aminopeptidases, proline (prolyl) aminopeptidase, dipeptidyl-peptidases, and tripeptidyl-peptidases, and pyroglutamyl aminopeptidase. Carboxypeptidases hydrolyze peptide bonds beginning from the C-terminus. Examples of carboxypeptidases are carboxypeptidases A, B, C, D, and E, as well as peptidyl-dipeptidases I (e.g., cathepsin C) and II.

9.2.1.2   Endopeptidases (Proteinases)

Endopeptidases (also known as proteinases) preferentially attack peptide bonds in the inner regions of peptide chains. The presence of free α-amino or α-carboxyl groups in peptides has a negative effect on the activity of these enzymes. Examples of endopeptidases are proteasome, cathepsin D, glutamate (glutamyl) endopeptidase, lysine (lysyl) endopeptidase, proline (prolyl) endopeptidase, serine endopeptidase, cysteine endopeptidase, and oligoendopeptidases. The oligopeptidases act on oligopeptide or polypeptide substrates that are smaller than proteins. Note that the endopeptidases that cleave synthetic substrates consisting of a small number of AAs may not always act on the same sequences present in proteins. This indicates that the sequence and structure of a protein can affect its susceptibility to an endopeptidase. The presence of free α-amino or α-carboxyl groups in peptides or proteins has a negative effect on the activity of these enzymes.

9.2.2   Classification by Catalytic Site

Because of the difficulties in classifying and naming some proteases, an alternative system based on the catalytic site of the enzymes was invented in the 1960s. Thus, carboxypeptidases and endopeptidases are divided into seven subclasses according to catalytic mechanisms: serine, cysteine, aspartate, threonine, glutamate, asparagine, and metallo proteases (Table 9.1), although some endopeptidases (e.g., thermopsin 26 and *Aspergillus* proteinase A) have not yet been assigned to any of these subclasses due to insufficient evidence. Serine- and cysteine-type peptidases have serine and cysteine residues, respectively, at their active sites. Aspartate-type peptidases have two aspartic acid residues at their active sites. Threonine peptidases were first reported in 1995 when the structure of the proteasome was determined and three of its fourteen different subunits were revealed as peptidases possessing an N-terminal threonine. The role of threonine in the active sites of the proteasome helps explain how this large protease acts in cells. Glutamate peptidases (first described

TABLE 9.1
Classification of Proteolytic Enzymes by Catalytic Type

Class	Active Site (AA Residues)	Examples of Inhibitors
Serine	Ser, Asp, His	3,4-DCI, DFP, PMSF, leupeptin, chymostatin, antipain, and aprotinin
Cysteine	Cys, His	Thiol reagents, E-64, leupeptin, chymostatin, antipain, IDA, and cystatin C
Aspartate	Asp, Asp	Pepstatin A
Threonine	Thr	Bortezomib and N-capped dipeptidyl leucine boronic acid
Glutamate	Glu, Gln	PT1 and TA1
Asparagine	Asn	Unknown
Metallo	Zn, Glu, Tyr; or Zn, Glu, His	EDTA, 1,10-phenanthroline, and phosphoramidon

Note: AA, amino acid; 3,4-DCI, 3,4-dichloroisocoumarin; DFP, di-isopropylfluorophosphate; E-64, L-3-carboxy-trans-2,3-epoxypropyl-leucylamido(4-guanidino)butane; IDA, iodoacetate; PMSF, phenylmethylsulphonylfluoride; PT1, 20-residue peptide encoding Glu29 to Thr48 of the *T. emersonii* glutamic peptidase 1 propeptide; TA1, 6-residue transition state analogue: Ac-Phe-Lys-Phe-AHPPA-Leu-Arg-NH2.

---

in 2004; carboxypeptidases) have glutamate and glutamine in the active sites. Asparagine peptide lyases (first described in 2011; also known as asparagine peptide lyases) utilize asparagine as a nucleophile in the active site. Unlike other proteolytic enzymes (which are hydrolases), asparagine peptide lyases are lyases and perform only self-cleavages. Metallopeptidases depend on a metal ion for their catalytic activity.

The use of protease inhibitors has provided an experimental basis for the classification of the proteolytic system (Figure 9.3). The reagent of choice to identify a serine protease is 3,4-dichloroisocoumarin, which reacts rapidly with and irreversibly inhibits a wide range of serine proteases. Aprotinin (a polypeptide) and phenylmethylsulfonyl fluoride are potent inhibitors of serine proteases. E-64 is a rapid, specific, and irreversible inhibitor of many cysteine endopeptidases (e.g., the calpain and papain families) of animal and plant origin and yet does not usually react with low-molecular-mass thiols such as cysteine and dithiothreitol. However, some cysteine proteases from microorganisms (e.g., clostripain and streptopain) are poorly inhibited by E-64 (Katunuma and Kominami 1995). Iodoacetate, iodoacetamide, and *N*-ethylmaleimide (1 mM) can be used as inhibitors of these enzymes, but it should be borne in mind that these reagents react rapidly with low-molecular-mass thiol activators of cysteine peptidases. Chymostatin inhibits both serine cysteine proteases. Pepstatin A is a highly specific and effective inhibitor of all aspartic-type proteases and yet does not usually affect other types of proteases. Importantly, removal of pepstatin A can restore enzyme activity. Inhibitors of threonine proteases, glutamate proteases, and asparagine peptide lyases are under development.

The human and mouse genomes encode about 200 metalloproteinases. A majority of them are secreted from cells or bound to the plasma membrane, and those metalloproteinases that are either secreted or membrane-anchored are designated as astacin. Thus, there are both intracellular (e.g., calpains in skeletal muscle) and extracellular (e.g., matrix collagenases in animals and thermolysin from thermophilic bacteria) metalloproteinases (Bond 2019). Most metalloproteinases are zinc-containing enzymes (called metzincin), and some metalloproteinases require cobalt for their catalytic activities. Zinc can react with a bidentate ligand in coordination chemistry to form a strong complex. One of these ligands is 1,10-phenanthroline, which is widely used to recognize metalloproteinases, many of which are extracellular proteases. Caution should be taken in interpreting data from these kinds of studies. For example, an inhibition of a metalloproteinase by a chelating agent is not necessarily due to the removal of the metal ion from the active site of the enzyme. Additionally, inhibition of proteases by a nonspecific chelating agent (e.g., EDTA) does not indicate that the enzyme is a metalloproteinase, because many proteases of other types are activated by cations (e.g., Ca^{2+} in the calpains).

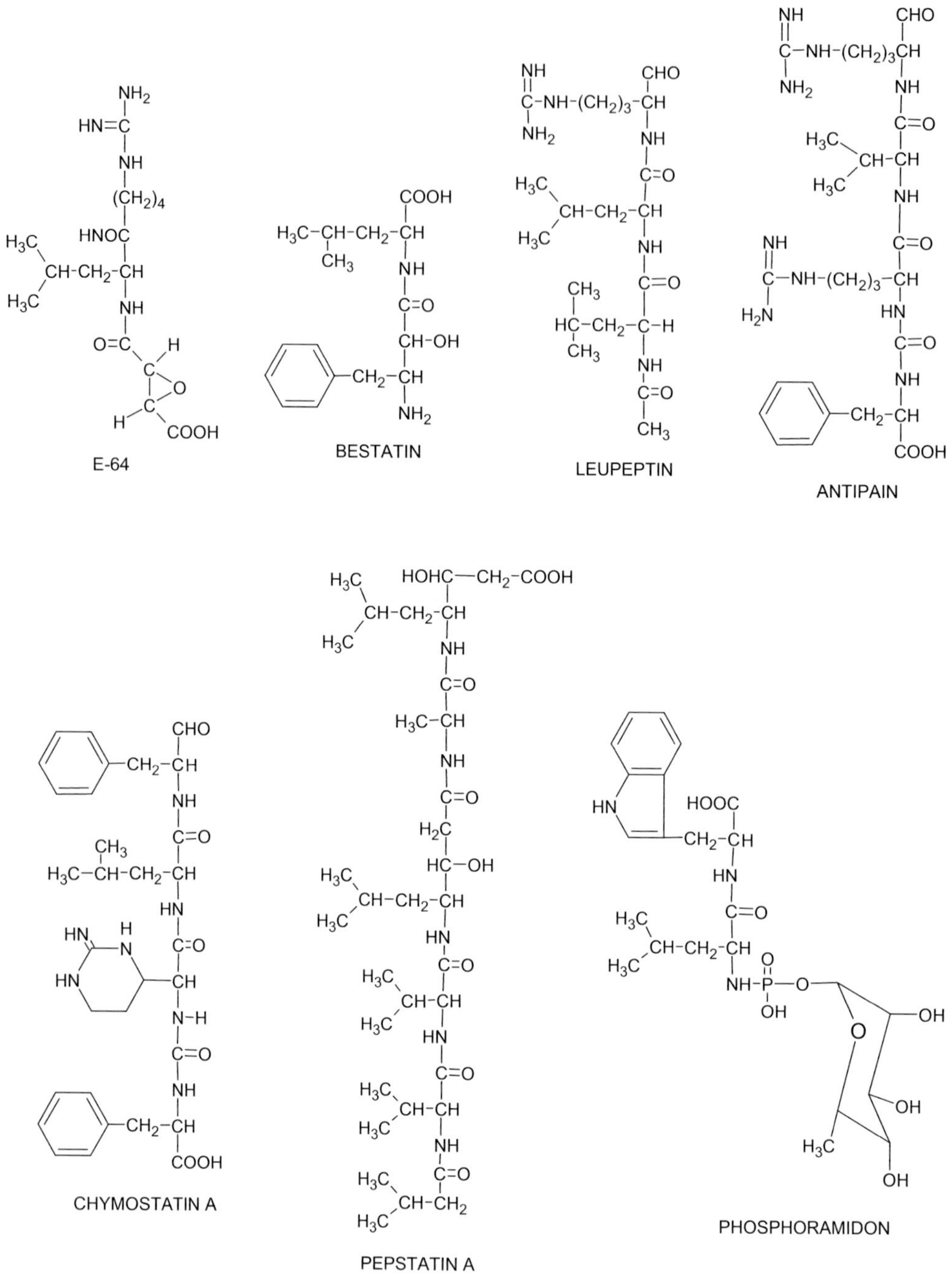

FIGURE 9.3 Structures of some protease inhibitors of microbial origin. These protease inhibitors are small peptides consisting of one or more modified amino acid residues. They inhibit serine, cysteine, aspartate, and metalloproteases in both bacteria and animal cells.

Knowledge of protease inhibitors is essential for the design of biochemical experiments. For example, a mixture of protease inhibitors (final concentrations of 1 mM EDTA, 5 µg/mL phenyl-methylsulfonyl fluoride, 5 µg/mL aprotinin, 5 µg/mL chymostatin, and 5 µg/mL pepstatin A in homogenization medium) is often used to homogenize cells or tissues for inhibiting proteolysis

(Wu 1997). A lack of protease inhibitors in the buffer for the homogenization of cells or tissues (particularly those with high rates of protein turnover, e.g., the small intestine and liver) may result in the complete or partial loss of certain proteins (or enzymes).

9.2.3 CLASSIFICATION BY EVOLUTIONARY RELATIONSHIP

More than 1,000 distinct proteases exist in organisms (Bond 2019). There are 641 and 677 protease genes in the human and the mouse, respectively, constituting ~3% of their genomes. Approximately 450 proteases (endopeptidases and exopeptidases) from over 1,400 organisms (bacteria, archaea, archezoa, protozoa, fungi, plants, animals, and viruses) have been sequenced. The genes encoding many proteases have also been cloned. In addition, X-ray structures have revealed the sites for substrate binding, inhibitor binding, and catalysis on the enzyme molecules. These data provide useful information about the evolutionary and structural relationships among the enzymes, which can be used to provide a third approach to their classification as various families. Such extensive efforts resulted in the development of the MEROPS database (http://www.merops.co.uk), which includes a frequently updated list of all protease sequences. Available evidence shows that enzymes of the same catalytic type can be unrelated in AA sequences (e.g., papain and caspases are unrelated cysteine peptidases; methionyl aminopeptidase and thermolysin are unrelated metalloproteinases). Conversely, proteases of different catalytic types can be evolutionarily related [e.g., the poliovirus picornain 3C is a cysteine peptidase but has a similar structure to trypsin (a serine peptidase)]. Thus, proteases can be classified by structure and sequence similarity. As proposed by N.D. Rawling and A.J. Barrett (1993), proteases with homologous sequences are grouped into families, and families with related structures are grouped into clans. For example, Clan PA includes serine and cysteine peptidases with a structure similar to trypsin. Clan PB includes peptidases with an N-terminal serine nucleophile (e.g., the penicillin G acylase precursor) and an N-terminal cysteine nucleophile (e.g., the penicillin V acylase precursor). Clan PC includes cysteine peptidases [e.g., γ-glutamyl hydrolase and the serine peptidase (dipeptidase E)].

9.3 INTRACELLULAR PROTEOLYTIC PATHWAYS

Intracellular proteins are degraded via highly selective pathways to maintain a dynamic state of protein turnover. Some extracellular proteins (e.g., albumin and insulin) in the interstitial fluid of tissues (e.g., the liver, kidneys, and skeletal muscle) can be taken up by macrophages via pinocytosis (a kind of endocytosis) for intracellular degradation (Swanson and Watts 1995). Proteases are present in the cytoplasm, plasma membrane, and many organelles of the cell (Bond 1987). Besides the cytoplasm and the lysosome, peptidases are present in the plasma membrane, mitochondria, nucleus, and rough endoplasmic reticulum. Thus, since the 1970s, intracellular proteolytic pathways have been classified according to the location of proteases: the lysosomal system and the nonlysosomal system. To date, this nomenclature is still used to include the autophagy-initiated proteolysis in the lysosome and the ATP-dependent proteasomes in the cytoplasm. Both the autophagy and the proteasome are activated in response to oxidative stress and fasting to degrade oxidized proteins and misfolded proteins (Coux et al. 2020; Noguchi et al. 2020).

9.3.1 THE LYSOSOMAL PROTEOLYTIC PATHWAY

9.3.1.1 Entry of Cytosolic Proteins into the Lysosomes via Endocytosis and Autophagy

The lysosome contains many proteases that are tagged with mannose-6-phosphate for targeting into this organelle from the endoplasmic reticulum (Benbrook and Long 2012). Proteins are delivered from the cytoplasm to the lysosome via the endocytic pathway mediated by one or more of the following five mechanisms: (1) endocytosis; (2) crinophagy; (3) macroautophagy; (4) microautophagy; and (5) chaperone-mediated autophagy (Dice 1987; Noguchi et al. 2020). Endocytosis refs to the engulfing of cytosolic proteins into the lysosome through the endosome pathway. Crinophagy (autophagic elimination of granules) involves the direct fusion of the lysosome with secretory granules containing damaged proteins. Macroautophagy is a process whereby a fraction of cytosolic constituents (e.g., proteins, organelles, and membranes) is enclosed and isolated by a double-membrane structure called the phagophore to form an autophagosome, which fuses with the lysosome to become an autolysosome (Figure 9.4). The autophagosome may also fuse with an endosome to form an amphisome (an autophagic vacuole) before fusion with the lysosome. Microphagy refers to the internalization of cytosolic proteins into the lysosome. In chaperone-mediated autophagy, a protein containing a KFERQ sequence is recognized by the cytosolic chaperone protein (heat-shock cognate 70) and cochaperones to form a complex, which is then translocated into the lysosome through its transmembrane protein Lamp-2A.

With the award of the 2016 Nobel Prize in Medicine or Physiology to Yoshinori Ohsumi for his work on autophagy, recent years have witnessed intensive interest in the role of this biochemical pathway under diverse physiological (e.g., growth, development, lactation, reproduction, and fasting) and pathological (e.g., cancer, diabetes, infection, heart disease, and neurological disorders) conditions (Hurley and Young 2017; Noguchi et al. 2020). Macroautophagy is activated by the endoplasmic reticulum stress to degrade oxidized proteins under oxidative stress and misfolded proteins. Although autophagy was originally thought to be a bulk, nonselective "self-eating" degradative process, this event is now known to be also regulated through the selective interaction of a polyubiquitinated protein (e.g., p62) with microtubes-associated protein 1 light chain 3 (Shaid et al. 2013). The selective autophagy occurs constitutively and can be induced by cellular stress signals (Mizushima and Komatsu 2011). Specifically, the lysosome possesses autophagy receptors, which bind both ubiquitinated protein substrates and the autophagy-specific light chain 3 (LC3) modifier on the inner sheath of autophagosomes. The protein substrates and autophagic vacuoles are then selectively transported into the lysosome. Direct translocation of cytosolic proteins means their direct uptake by the lysosome. Figure 9.4 illustrates the formation of autolysosomes during the process of macroautophagy.

9.3.1.2   Proteases in the Lysosomes

Once cytosolic proteins are inside the lysosome, they are denatured due to the low pH and then hydrolyzed by proteases to release AAs (Trivedi et al. 2020). These proteases include (1) cathepsin B (cysteine protease) with both endopeptidase and exopeptidase (C-terminus) activities; (2) cathepsin H (cysteine protease; a glycoprotein) with both endopeptidase and exopeptidase (N-terminus) activities; (3) cathepsin L (a major lysosomal cysteine protease; endopeptidase); (4) cathepsin D (aspartate protease; endopeptidase); (5) cathepsin K (cysteine protease in osteoclasts and bronchial epithelium); and (6) other recently identified proteases, such as cathepsins C (myeloid cells), F (macrophages), O (widespread), V (thymic epithelium), W (CD8+ T cells), and Z (widespread). The optimal pH for lysosomal proteases is 3–5. Thus, some weak bases [e.g., ammonia, methylamine, chloroquine (a drug primarily used to prevent and treat malaria), or monensin (an ionophore)] inhibit lysosomal protein degradation by increasing intralysosomal pH above 5.0. Note that chloroquine also reduces lysosomal proteolysis by decreasing the autophagosome–lysosome fusion in cells (Mauthe et al. 2018).

9.3.1.3   Proteins Degraded by the Lysosomal Proteolytic System

The lysosomal proteolytic system participates in the intracellular degradation of (1) endocytosed proteins, (2) nonmyofibrillar proteins under conditions of nutritional deprivation and stress, (3) oxidized proteins under oxidative stress, (4) misfolded proteins, and (5) organelles and membranes (Ciechanover 2012; Saftig and Puertollano 2021). Studies involving the use of inhibitors of lysosomal enzymes indicate that, in the presence of physiological concentrations of insulin, glucose, and AAs, the lysosomal proteolytic system contributes to the degradation of 30%–35% and 20%–25% of intracellular proteins in mammalian enterocytes (Wu 2018) and skeletal muscle (Furuno et al.

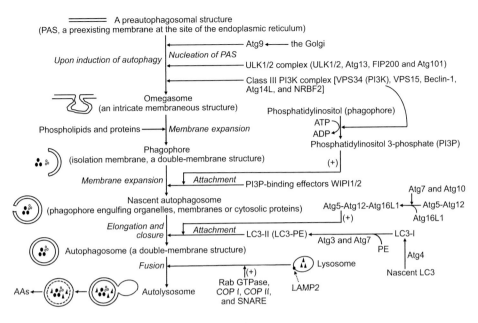

FIGURE 9.4 Formation of an autolysosome and lysosomal proteolysis during the process of autophagy in animal cells. Macroautophagy involves (1) the ULK1/2 complex, which consists of ULK1/2 (kinase), Atg13 (a regulatory subunit), FIP200 (a scaffold for binding and interacting with proteins), and Atg101 (a regulatory subunit); and (2) the class III PI3K complex, which is composed of VPS34 (PI3K activity), VPS15 (a scaffold for binding and interacting with proteins), beclin-1 (a regulatory subunit), Atg14 (endoplasmic reticulum-targeting), and NRBF2 (an activator), and Atg9 (generated by the Golgi). Note that beclin-1 is a mammalian ortholog of the yeast autophagy-related gene 6 (Atg6) and interacts with the class III PI3-kinase signaling complex to promote the formation of autophagic vacuoles. Upon induction of autophagy, ULK1/2 is phosphorylated, and the activated ULK1/2 phosphorylates Atg9 (a transmembrane protein that is generated by the Golgi and localizes to small vesicles) and the class III PI3K. This is followed by the recruitment of the ULK1/2 complex and Atg9 (generated by the Golgi) as a preautophagosomal structure (PAS, a preexisting membrane) at the site of the endoplasmic reticulum to form an omegasome. The latter is an intricate membranous structure that resembles the Greek letter omega in electron microscope pictures. The process of the recruitment of core autophagy factors is called nucleation. The omegasome undergoes expansion through the addition of phospholipids and proteins to generate a phagophore (also known as an isolation membrane), which is a double-membrane structure. At the site of nucleation, the class III PI3K catalyzes the conversion of phosphatidylinositol in the phagophore to phosphatidylinositol 3-phosphate (PI3P). PI3P binds to effectors WIPI1/2 and promotes their attachment to the phagophore and its membrane expansion, yielding a nascent autophagosome that can engulf organelles, membranes, and cytosolic proteins (called a cargo). The nascent autophagosome is elongated and closed after the attachment of LC3-II (LC3-PE) in the presence of the Atg5-Atg12-Atg16L1 complex to make an autophagosome (a double-membrane structure). The LC3-II is formed from PE and LC3-1, with the latter being produced from the nascent (newly synthesized) LC3 under the control of Atg4. The Atg5-Atg12-Atg16L1 complex is generated from Atg5-Atg12 and Atg16L1 in response to the stimulation of Atg7 and Atg10. Under the catalysis of the vesicle- and organelle-identifying Rab GTPase, as well as the facilitation of LAMP2, COP I, COP II, and SNARE, the outer membrane of the autophagosome fuses with the lysosome that is rich in hydrolases (including proteases) to produce an autolysosome. At this stage, its inner membrane is broken down by the lysosomal enzymes, giving rise to the single-membrane autolysosome. The cargo within the autolysosome is degraded by proteases and peptidases to amino acids. Atg, autophagy-related protein; COP, coat-protein complex; FIP200, FAK (focal adhesion kinase) family-interacting protein of 200 kDa; LAMP2, lysosomal membrane-associated protein 2; Rab, Ras-related protein); LC3, microtubule-associated protein light chain 3; NRBF2, nuclear receptor binding factor; PE, phosphatidylethanolamine; PI3K, phosphatidylinositol 3-phosphate kinase; SNARE, soluble NSF (N-ethylmaleimide sensitive factor) attachment protein receptor proteins of vesicle fusion; WIPI, WD (tryptophan-aspartic acid) repeat protein interacting with phosphoinositides; ULK1/2, UNC (uncoordinated)-51-like kinase 1 or 2; and VPS, vacuolar protein sorting.

1990; Lowell et al. 1986; Tiao et al. 1996; Wing et al. 1995), respectively. The lysosomal system is not involved to a significant extent in the degradation of myofibrillar proteins in skeletal, cardiac, or smooth muscle (Lowell et al. 1986).

9.3.2 The Nonlysosomal Proteolytic Pathway

9.3.2.1 Overview of the Nonlysosomal Proteolytic System

A variety of low- and high-molecular-mass proteases are found outside the lysosome. Based on catalytic mechanisms, the nonlysosomal pathway for proteolysis can be divided into (1) the Ca^{2+}-dependent proteolytic system; (2) the caspases; (3) the ATP-dependent, ubiquitin-independent proteolytic system; and (4) the ATP- and ubiquitin-dependent proteolytic system (Goldberg 2003; Etlinger and Goldberg 1977; Varshavsky 2012). All of these protein degradation pathways are present in the cytoplasm and may also be expressed in certain organelles (e.g., peroxisomes, nucleus, and mitochondria). The optimal pH for nonlysosomal proteases is 7–8.

9.3.2.2 The Ca^{2+}-Dependent Proteolytic System (Calpain System)

The calpain system consists of 14 different members of the Ca^{2+}-dependent protease (cysteine proteases) plus calpastatin. Many tissues, including skeletal muscle, contain two well-characterized Ca^{2+}-dependent proteases: μ-calpain and m-calpain (Goll et al. 2008). In skeletal muscle, calpains are concentrated in the I-band and Z-disk areas of the myofibril. The calpains initiate the degradation of myofibrillar protein by disassembling the outer layer of the proteins from the myofibril and releasing them as myofilaments (Goll et al. 2008). Myofilaments undergo further degradation by calpains. No specific AA sequence is recognized by calpains, but these enzymes prefer to hydrolyze peptide bonds consisting of leucine, valine, isoleucine, phenylalanine, and tyrosine residues. Note that the calpains only partially degrade myofibrillar proteins and do not hydrolyze proteins to small peptides or AAs. Available evidence shows that calpains are not responsible for the degradation of the bulk of the sarcoplasmic proteins. However, defects in a muscle-specific calpain (p94) cause the limb-girdle muscular dystrophy type 2A disease (an autosomal recessive disorder) in humans due to an inability to degrade myofibrillar proteins (Richard et al. 1995). These results indicate that either a general, nonspecific increase in proteolysis or a disruption of its normal regulatory mechanisms can result in muscle atrophy.

9.3.2.3 Caspases

Cells express several caspases (cysteine proteases; e.g., caspases 1, 3, and 9), which are responsible for the partial (or limited) degradation of proteins during apoptosis (programmed cell death). The caspases do not require Ca^{2+} for activity but are activated by events (e.g., inflammation and oxidative stress) that initiate apoptosis. These enzymes do not appear to play a major role in the intracellular degradation of proteins (including myofibrillar proteins) in healthy animals, but are crucial for cell signaling in response to necrosis, inflammation, and oxidative stress (Shalini et al. 2015).

9.3.2.4 The ATP-Dependent and Ubiquitin-Independent Proteolytic System

Some proteases (e.g., proteasome) in cells (e.g., skeletal muscle and reticulocytes) hydrolyze proteins in an ATP-dependent and ubiquitin-independent manner (Erales and Coffino 2014). These enzymes are soluble alkaline proteins. Their proteolytic activity is also stimulated by UTP, CTP, and GTP but to a much lesser extent than ATP. ATP is not hydrolyzed by this type of reaction, where ATP targets protein substrates to the proteases (e.g., mitochondrial proteases and 26S proteasome), activates the proteases, and destabilizes the substrate proteins, thereby facilitating the attack of the substrates by the proteases independently of ubiquitin conjugation. This proteolysis system is responsible for the degradation of short-lived proteins, including ornithine decarboxylase. Because these proteins are key regulatory enzymes of metabolic pathways, the ATP-dependent and ubiquitin-independent proteolytic system plays an important role in cell physiology and function.

There is a considerable volume of information on protein degradation in the skeletal muscle and liver, as well as erythrocytes (red blood cells) and reticulocytes in the literature. The focus on skeletal muscle is, in part, historical as early studies employed biochemically viable muscle preparations for mechanistic studies *in vitro*. Muscle is the predominant reservoir of protein in the body, and protein turnover in this tissue is sensitive to regulation by hormones and other factors, including fasting, cytokines, infection, denervation, cancer cachexia, AIDS, cachexia, space flight, bed rest, fatty acids, AAs, and their metabolites (Baracos 1988; Goldberg 2003). Pathological muscle atrophy occurs in both humans and other animals (Bonaldo and Sandri 2013), which necessitates a need to identify mechanism-based therapies. In addition to skeletal muscle, much work on protein degradation has been done with the liver because this organ has a high rate of protein turnover and an active lysosomal proteolytic system and also responds sensitively to various physiological and pathological factors (e.g., glucagon, cAMP, β-agonists, cytokines, fasting, and infection; Mortimore and Pösö 1987). Furthermore, erythrocytes and reticulocytes are very useful for studying the ATP-dependent proteolytic system and the oxidant-induced proteolysis in animal cells for the following reasons. First, erythrocytes lack the ATP-dependent proteolysis, whereas this pathway occurs in reticulocytes (Fagan et al. 1986). Second, oxidized proteins in both erythrocytes and reticulocytes are actively degraded primarily via an ATP-independent process. Third, hemoglobin accounts for >95% of the total soluble protein in erythrocytes, and thus, these cells provide a unique model to measure the rate of the degradation of a homogenous protein. In essence, studies with these different cell types help to elucidate the complex pathways and regulation of intracellular protein degradation, as well as the role of this biochemical process in health and disease.

9.3.2.5 The ATP- and Ubiquitin-Dependent Proteolytic (Proteasome) System

The ATP- and ubiquitin (a 76-AA globular small protein)-dependent proteolytic (proteasome) system is now considered to be the major system responsible for protein degradation within cells (Ciechanover 2012; Goldberg 2003). The proteasome is ubiquitous in eukaryotes and archaea, and is present in bacteria. The proteasome subcomponents are referred to by their Svedberg sedimentation coefficient (S). The most common form of the proteasome is the 26S proteasome, which is approximately 2,000 kDa in molecular mass. This eukaryotic proteasome and its role in proteolysis are described below.

9.3.2.5.1 Structure of the 26S Proteasome

The 26S proteasome contains one 20S proteasome (a hollow proteolytic core particle; 700-kDa) and two 19S regulatory caps with one cap on each end of the core particle (Figure 9.5). The core has openings at its two ends (which allow the target protein to enter) and an enclosed cavity in which proteins are degraded.

In eukaryotic cells, the 20S core particle contains 28 different subunits grouped into 2 classes: α and β subunits, the molecular weights of which range from 20 to 35 kDa. There are seven different gene products for each of the α and β classes. The individual α or β subunits have sequence homology with each other, but they differ markedly from any other proteolytic enzymes. The 20S particle is arranged in four rings of seven subunits each, with the α subunits forming the two outer rings and the β subunits (possessing proteolytic activity, with the β1, β2, and β5 subunits containing functional catalytic sites) forming the two inner rings.

The 19S regulatory particle functions to unfold polypeptides and recognize the substrates for the 20S core particle. This is important because protein molecules cannot enter the catalytic center without first being unfolded. The 19S regulatory complex consists of a lid and a base. The lid consists of eight different polypeptides that are involved in binding polyubiquitin chains and removing them from the polypeptide that is marked to be degraded. The base contains six homologous ATPases and three polypeptides that do not have any ATPase activity. The ATPases use the energy of ATP to (1) unfold the polypeptide entering the proteasome chamber, (2) facilitate substrate binding to the 20S core particle, and (3) attach ubiquitin to the polypeptide.

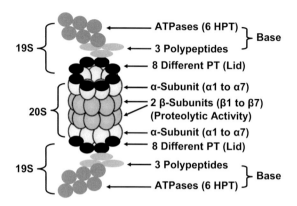

FIGURE 9.5 The 26S proteasome for intracellular protein degradation in animal cells. The 26S proteasome (2,000-kDa) in eukaryotes contains one 20S proteasome and two 19S regulatory caps. The 20S proteasome is a 700-kDa hollow proteolytic core particle that contains multiple peptidase activities. One of the two 19S regulatory caps is located on each end of the core particle. The 19S regulatory complex is composed of multiple ATPases and components for binding protein substrates. HPT, homologous polypeptides; PT, polypeptides.

9.3.2.5.2 Ubiquitin-Dependent Protein Degradation

Ubiquitin-dependent protein degradation in animal cells involves several steps: (1) the activation of ubiquitin by a multienzyme system that involves three conjugation factors and requires the hydrolysis of ATP to AMP plus PPi; (2) the binding of multiple ubiquitin moieties to the protein substrate to form the conjugating enzymes-ubiquitin-protein substrate complex; (3) the ATP-dependent degradation of the protein substrate by the multicatalytic 26S proteasome to yield AAs and small peptides; and (4) the de-ubiquitination of the conjugating enzymes-ubiquitin complex by isopeptidase to regenerate ubiquitin and the conjugating enzymes. This proteolytic pathway is highly specific for substrates and highly conserved among eukaryotic cells (Figure 9.6).

Ubiquitination of proteins (also called ubiquitylation) is necessary before their degradation by the 26S proteasome. This involves the linkage between the protein substrate with ubiquitin (a 76-AA, 8,565-Da protein in all eukaryotic cells) and requires three classes of enzymes: (1) E1 enzyme, which activates the ubiquitin, (2) E2 enzyme, which binds to the ubiquitin molecule, and (3) E3 enzyme, which transfers the ubiquitin molecule to the target protein. Specifically, an ε-amino group of the selected protein is first attached through an isopeptide bond to the C-terminal end ubiquitin. Attachment may also occur through the N-terminal AA of the selected protein, but the N-terminal amino group of many proteins (including most myofibrillar proteins) is blocked by covalent modifications, such as acetylation. This initial step of protein ubiquitination is catalyzed by the ATP-dependent E1 enzyme (ubiquitin-activating enzyme) to produce the E1-substrate-ubiquitin complex and to activate the ubiquitin molecule (Figure 9.6). This reaction is driven by the energy released from the hydrolysis of ATP to AMP and PPi. It is noteworthy that ubiquitin is covalently linked to the protein substrate destined for degradation. In most cases, a chain of at least four ubiquitin molecules must be tagged to the target protein. The ubiquitin-linked protein, commonly called a ubiquitin–protein conjugate, is then recognized and degraded by the ATP-dependent 26S proteasome to form free AAs and peptides ranging from 3 to 23 AA residues (Ciechanover 2012). Most of the oligopeptides contain 6 to 10 AA residues, with an average of 8 AA residues. These resulting small peptides are further broken down to free AAs by di- and tripeptidases in the cell. After proteolysis is completed, ubiquitin, the E2 enzyme, and the E3 enzyme are released from the E2-E3-ubiquitin complex in a reaction catalyzed by ubiquitin isopeptidase (also known as deubiquitinating enzyme) that cleaves the ubiquitin-protein bonds. The resulting ubiquitin, E2 enzyme, and E3 enzyme are reused for the degradation of another protein molecule. Analogous to the role of ornithine in the urea cycle, ubiquitin acts as a catalyst in the pathway of the ubiquitin-dependent

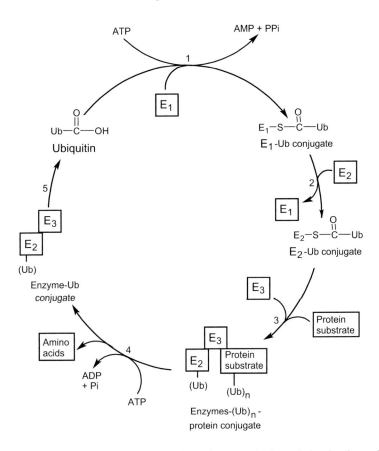

FIGURE 9.6 The ATP-dependent and ubiquitin-dependent protein degradation by the multicatalytic 26S proteasome in animal cells. This initial step of protein ubiquitination is catalyzed by the E1 enzyme to produce the E1-substrate-ubiquitin complex. The activated ubiquitin is transferred to the E2 enzyme, which is also known as the ubiquitin-conjugating enzyme or ubiquitin carrier protein. Subsequently, the E2-ubiquitin complex interacts with the E3 enzyme (also called ubiquitin ligase) to form the E2-E3-ubiquitin complex in which ubiquitin is attached to the E3 enzyme. The E2-E3-ubiquitin complex then conjugates with a targeted protein, and, thereafter, the E2 enzyme catalyzes the transfer of the ubiquitin moiety to the protein substrate yielding the E2-E3-ubiquitin-protein complex. E1, E2, E3: ubiquitin-conjugating enzymes 1, 2, and 3, respectively; Ub, ubiquitin. The enzyme-catalyzed reactions are (1) ATP-dependent activation of ubiquitin by E1 enzyme (ubiquitin-activating enzyme); (2) attachment of activated ubiquitin to E2 enzyme (the ubiquitin-conjugating enzyme or ubiquitin carrier protein); (3) conjugation of the E2-ubiquitin complex with E3 enzyme (ubiquitin ligase); (4) recognition and ATP-dependent degradation of the ubiquitin-linked protein (commonly called a ubiquitin–protein conjugate) by the 26S proteasome to form free amino acids and small peptides; and (5) deubiquitination of the E2-E3-ubiquitin complex catalyzed by ubiquitin isopeptidase (also known as deubiquitinating enzyme). The pathway for the ubiquitin-dependent protein degradation can be regarded as the ubiquitin cycle.

protein degradation. This pathway can be regarded as the intracellular ubiquitin cycle in which ubiquitin brings in the protein substrate for the degradation via a series of coordinated reactions and is regenerated at the end of the proteolysis.

Although the binding of ubiquitinated proteins activates the proteasome's degradative machinery, some ubiquitinated proteins bind to the 26S ribosome but escape proteolysis and are subsequently deubiquitinated and released. Thus, there are complex mechanisms that regulate proteasome activity (VerPlank and Goldberg 2017). Results of recent studies indicate a key regulatory role for the phosphorylation of the proteasome in protein degradation (VerPlank et al. 2019). Specifically, a phosphatase, UBLCP1, binds to the 19S subunit Rpn1. The subunit phosphorylation promotes the association of the 19S regulatory particle with the 20S proteasome to form the 26S complex, thereby stimulating proteolysis. Conversely, dephosphorylation of Rpn1 in the purified proteasome enhances its dissociation into 20S and 19S components, leading to suppressed protein breakdown. Likewise, the phosphorylation of Rpt6 (a component of the proteasome) by protein kinase A increases the proteolytic activity of the 26S proteasome under both *in vitro* and *in vivo* conditions. For example, 26S proteasomes are rapidly activated by diverse hormones (e.g., epinephrine or glucagon) and physiological states (e.g., exercise and fasting) that raise cAMP and cause Rpn6 phosphorylation in skeletal muscle (VerPlank et al. 2019). Because phosphorylation occurs primarily on the α-subunits of the 20S proteasome and the ATPases of the 19S proteasome, it is likely that specific kinases regulate the rate of breakdown of ubiquitinated protein substrates by the 26S proteasome in the different compartments of cells.

9.3.2.5.3 *Functions of the Proteasome*

The ubiquitin-proteasome system functions to (1) selectively degrade short-lived regulatory proteins (e.g., proteins involved in apoptosis or programmed cell death and proteins involved in signaling processes in the cell), abnormal proteins, and most of the long-lived proteins in mammalian cells; (2) regulate cellular processes, such as cell division, cell signaling, and regulation of gene activity; (3) remove misfolded, oxidized, and damaged proteins; (4) in certain immune cells, cleave foreign proteins into smaller pieces called antigenic peptides presented by MHC class I molecules on their cell surface to induce an immune response; and (5) degrade proteins in response to fasting, oxidative stress, heat stress, and infection. The proteasome pathway plays a major role in degrading most of the long-lived myofibrillar proteins (e.g., actin, myosin, troponin, and tropomyosin) and soluble (cytoplasmic) proteins in skeletal muscle. In this tissue, specific interactions between the myofibrillar proteins protect them from ubiquitin-dependent hydrolysis by the 26S proteasome, and the key rate-controlling step of this pathway is their dissociation from the myofibril (contractile filament) that is catalyzed by other proteases (including calpains). Results from studies of skeletal muscles indicate that the activation of the ubiquitin-proteasome pathway is primarily responsible for the rapid loss of proteins from skeletal muscle under various catabolic conditions, such as cancer cachexia, denervation atrophy, fasting, injury, metabolic acidosis, infection, and sepsis (Kitajima et al. 2020). Conversely, impairment of the proteasome activity may play a role in the pathogenesis of tumorigenesis, Huntington's disease, Parkinson's disease, and other neurodegenerative diseases. The past two decades have witnessed tremendous interest in the proteasome in health and disease (Coux et al. 2020).

9.3.2.6 Proteins Degraded by the Nonlysosomal Proteolytic System

Proteases and peptidases outside the lysosomes degrade most intracellular proteins. Acting in concert, the nonlysosomal proteolytic system is responsible for the breakdown of (1) normal short-lived proteins, (2) abnormal, denatured, and aged proteins under basal metabolic conditions, (3) both myofibrillar and nonmyofibrillar proteins under conditions of nutritional deprivation, (4) oxidized proteins under oxidative stress, (5) misfolded proteins; and (6) newly synthesized collagens. Depending on cell type, the nonlysosomal system can contribute to the degradation of 70%–80% of intracellular proteins in the presence of physiological concentrations of insulin, glucose, and AAs (Attaix et al. 2002).

9.4 CHARACTERISTICS AND PHYSIOLOGICAL SIGNIFICANCE OF INTRACELLULAR PROTEIN DEGRADATION

9.4.1 BIOLOGICAL HALF-LIVES OF PROTEINS

Different proteins are degraded at different rates (Goldberg and St John. 1976). Thus, intracellular proteins have remarkably different half-lives that range from several minutes for short-lived proteins to several days for long-lived proteins (Table 9.2). In cells, abnormal proteins are more rapidly

TABLE 9.2

Biological Half-Lives ($T_{1/2}$) of Proteins in Mammalian Tissues

Proteins	Tissue	$T_{1/2}$
a. Short-Lived Proteins ($T_{1/2} < 5\,h$)		
Ornithine decarboxylase	Liver	11 min
δ-Aminolevulinate synthetase		
Soluble (cytosolic)	Liver	0.33 h
Mitochondrial	Liver	1.1 h
RNA polymerase I	Liver	1.3 h
Tyrosine aminotransferase	Liver	2.0 h
Tryptophan oxygenase	Liver	2.5 h
Deoxythymidine kinase	Liver	2.6 h
HMG-CoA reductase	Liver	3.0 h
Serine dehydratase	Liver	4.0 h
Amylase	Liver	4.3 h
b. Proteins with Intermediate Half-Lives ($5\,h \leq T_{1/2} < 50\,h$)		
PEP carboxykinase	Liver	5.0 h
Aniline hydroxylase	Liver	5.0 h
Glucokinase	Liver	12 h
RNA polymerase II	Liver	12 h
Dihydroorotase	Liver	12 h
Glucose-6-P dehydrogenase	Liver	15 h
Glycerol-3-P dehydrogenase	Liver	15 h
Endothelial NO synthase	Vasculature	20 h
c. Long-Lived Proteins ($T_{1/2} > 50\,h$)		
Ornithine aminotransferase	Kidney	4.0 days
	Liver	0.95 days
Arginase	Liver	4.0
Lactate dehydrogenase	Liver	4.3 days
	Kidney	6.1 days
	Heart	8.2 days
	Skeletal muscle	43 days
Aldolase	Skeletal muscle	~20 days
Myosin	Skeletal muscle	~20 days
Actin	Skeletal muscle	~60 days

Source: Dice, J.F. 1987. *FASEB J.* 1:349–357; Goldberg, A.L. and A.C. St John. 1976. *Annu. Rev. Biochem.* 45:747–803; Swick, R.W. and H. Song. 1974. *J. Anim. Sci.* 38:1150–1157.

Note: HMG-CoA, β-Hydroxy-β-methylglutaryl-CoA (also known as 3-hydroxy-3-methylglutaryl-CoA); NO, nitric oxide; 3-P, 3-phosphate; 6-P, 6-phosphate

degraded than normal proteins. Much evidence shows that the rates of degradation of normal proteins vary widely, depending on their functions. For example, enzymes at key metabolic control points may be degraded much faster than those enzymes whose activity is largely constant under physiological conditions. One of the most rapidly degraded proteins is ornithine decarboxylase, which has a half-life of 11 min. By contrast, structural proteins such as actin and myosin in skeletal muscle have a half-life of a month or longer, while hemoglobin essentially lasts for the entire lifetime of the erythrocyte (e.g., ~120 days in humans and 35 days in chickens). To ensure the proper functioning of cells, the half-lives of all proteins must be maintained through proteolysis.

The half-lives of proteins are affected by their physicochemical properties and their structures (Toyama and Hetzer 2013). For example, short-lived proteins tend to be (1) large, acidic, and hydrophobic proteins; (2) proteins with low thermal stability; (3) proteins with attached carbohydrate or phosphate groups; (4) proteins with oxidized cysteine, histidine, and methionine residues; (5) proteins with deaminated glutamine and asparagine residues; or (6) proteins in the absence of stabilizing ligands.

The AA sequence may also partially determine the half-life of a protein. According to the PEST hypothesis, rapidly degrading proteins (e.g., $T_{1/2}<2$h) generally have regions rich in proline (P), glutamate (E), serine (S), and threonine (T) residues (Rogers et al. 1986). Such PEST regions rarely occur in more stable proteins. In addition, the stability of proteins is affected partially by the N-terminal AA residue, which is called the N-end rule. Let's use ß-galactosidase (the enzyme that hydrolyzes lactose to galactose and glucose) as an example (Table 9.3). An obvious difference among these AAs is the size of the side chain. It appears that the stabilizing AAs have small side chains, whereas the side chains of destabilizing AAs tend to be large (Bachmair et al. 1986). It is now known that N-terminal residues of short-lived proteins are recognized by recognition components (called N-recognins), which are essential components of N-degrons (degradation signal or a specific sequence of AAs in the N-terminus of protein) (Tasaki et al. 2012). Known N-recognins in eukaryotes interact with small proteins (including ubiquitin) and mediate protein ubiquitylation and selective proteolysis by the 26S proteasome. Dysregulation of the N-end rule pathway due to mutations in the human *UBR1* gene (encoding ubiquitin-protein ligase E3 component N-recognin 1) causes diseases, such as the Johanson–Blizzard syndrome (an autosomal recessive disorder) characterized by congenital exocrine pancreatic insufficiency, facial dysmorphism, multiple malformations, and often mental retardation (Tasaki et al. 2012).

TABLE 9.3

Effects of the N-Terminal Amino Acid on the Half-Life of β-Galactosidase[a]

N-Terminal Amino Acid	$T_{1/2}$ of β-galactosidase
Met	>20h
Ser	>20h
Ala	>20h
Thr	>20h
Val	>20h
Gly	>20h
Ile	~30min
Glu	~30min
Tyr	~10min
Gln	~10min
Phe	~3min
Leu	~3min
Asp	~3min
Lys	~3min
Arg	~2min

Source: Bachmair, A. et al. 1986. *Science* 234:179–186.
In prokaryotes, once the *N*-formyl-Met is removed, the second residue becomes the N-terminal residue and is subject to the N-end rule.
[a] The N-terminal amino acid of this protein is methionine, which can be excised.

9.4.2 ATP Requirement for Intracellular Protein Turnover

The energy requirement for peptide bond cleavage cannot be explained by thermodynamic considerations, since the hydrolysis of peptide bonds is an exergonic process. However, experimental evidence shows that ATP is required for protein breakdown by (1) ATP-dependent but ubiquitin-independent proteases (2 ATP molecules per peptide bond) and (2) the ATP- and ubiquitin-dependent 26S proteasome (equivalent to 3 ATP molecules per peptide bond) (Figure 9.6). Combining all proteolytic pathways in cells, approximately two ATP molecules are used for the cleavage of one peptide bond in proteins. Based on the example of energy requirement for protein synthesis in healthy adult humans (Chapter 8), it can be estimated that 5.3% [i.e., $(2 \times 3 \, \text{mol ATP}/113.8 \, \text{mol ATP}) \times 100 = 5.3\%$] of dietary energy is utilized for the degradation of 300 g of protein in these individuals.

As indicated previously, body proteins undergo continuous synthesis and breakdown on humans and other animals and both processes consume energy. In adult humans ingesting 56 g of digestible protein and gaining no protein, ~25 g of body protein is irreversibly oxidized to CO_2, ammonia, and urea, whereas 31 g of protein (in the form of AAs) is used for metabolic pathways other than protein synthesis and irreversible AA oxidation (Figure 9.7), and 14.5% of dietary energy is utilized for the synthesis of 300 g of protein/day (Chapter 8). Thus, whole-body protein turnover accounts for about 20% (i.e., 14.5% + 5.3% = 19.8%) of energy metabolism in fed adults. This value perfectly matches the estimation of Waterlow (1995) that whole-body protein turnover contributes 20% of energy expenditure in healthy adult humans.

9.4.3 Physiological Significance of Intracellular Protein Degradation

The intracellular degradation of protein has many functions. First, proteolysis is required to remove aged proteins, abnormal proteins, and denatured proteins due to changes in extracellular and intracellular environments (e.g., pollution, heat stress, as well as oxidative stress induced by free radicals

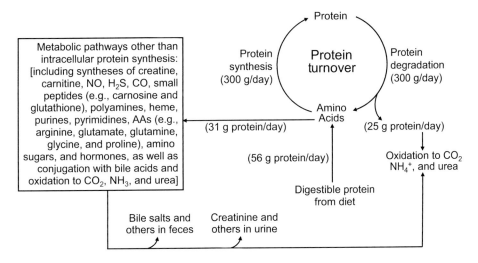

FIGURE 9.7 Whole-body protein turnover and the use of dietary protein for protein synthesis and other metabolic pathways in the 70-kg healthy adult human. A 70-kg healthy adult human ingests 56 g of digestible protein in the diet, synthesizes 300 g of protein, degrades 300 g of protein, and gains no protein. Approximately 25 g of the body protein per day is irreversibly oxidized to CO_2, ammonia, and urea via proteolysis and associated catabolic pathways. Accordingly, ~25 g of digestible dietary protein (in the form of AAs) is used to replace the irreversible loss of the body protein through oxidation to CO_2 and ammonia. Approximately 31 g of digestible dietary protein (in the form of AAs) is used for metabolic pathways other than intracellular protein synthesis. Whole-body protein turnover (protein synthesis plus protein degradation) accounts for about 20% of energy expenditure in the body.

and other oxidants). The presence of abnormal proteins within cells may interfere with normal cellular metabolism, result in changes in cell volume and osmolarity, and cause tissue injury. Second, protein degradation serves to regulate cellular biochemical reactions by removing enzymes and regulatory proteins that are no longer needed. Third, protein degradation plays an important role in adaptation to nutritional deprivation (e.g., such as fasting and lack of dietary protein intake) and pathological conditions (e.g., burn, cancer, infection, inflammation, and injury) by supplying AAs (e.g., alanine, glutamine, and arginine) for gluconeogenesis, ammoniagenesis, ATP production, synthesis of essential proteins, production of neurotransmitters, generation of gaseous signaling molecules, and immune responses. Note that because AA oxidation always occurs in animals even though they have been food-deprived for many days, protein breakdown is necessary to provide AAs under catabolic conditions associated with the irreversible loss of AAs from the body (Table 9.4). In fasted individuals, the urinary loss of nitrogen results from net protein breakdown in the whole body, which should not be taken to indicate dietary protein requirement for the replacement of body protein in a fed state. This is because substantial amounts of the AAs from proteolysis are needed for glucose synthesis in the fasted state to compensate for the lack of carbohydrate intake. Fourth, many newly synthesized proteins must undergo partial degradation (i.e., removal of peptide fragments) to achieve their normal biological activities, to be directed to their appropriate place in the cell, or to be secreted from the cell. Fifth, proteolysis regulates the life span of normal proteins to control their concentrations, cell and whole-body growth, and cell functions that are essential to survival.

Thus, insulin is used in clinical therapy to inhibit muscle proteolysis in type 1 diabetes, and a targeted inhibition of protein degradation in people with muscular atrophy can help to counter skeletal muscle wasting and restore physical activity (Sandri 2013). However, a nonspecific pharmacological inhibition of whole-body proteolysis in healthy individuals or virus-infected patients can cause adverse effects. For example, the use of chloroquine or hydroxychloroquine (which inhibits lysosomal protein degradation in humans and other animals) to treat persons infected with severe acute respiratory syndrome coronavirus 2 [SARS-CoV-2; the virus causing COVID-19)] results in

TABLE 9.4
Urinary Nitrogen Excretion during 6 Days of Fasting in Normal and Obese Adult Humans[a]

Group	Age (yr)	Initial BW (kg)	Final BW (kg)	DPF	1	2	3	4	5	6	0–6	UNE	Loss of BP[c]
												(g/kg BW/day)	
Normal men	23.6	66.3	61.0	13.4	10.7	13.5	14.5[d]	12.2	11.5	11.1	12.2	0.192	1.20
Obese men	24.5	110.5	104.6	14.4	10.7	12.3	14.0[d]	12.6	12.1	10.8	12.1	0.113	0.703
Normal women	22.8	57.4	52.6	8.2	6.6	9.1	9.6[d]	8.9	8.4	7.4	8.3	0.151	0.943
Obese women	23.7	92.0	86.4	11.7	7.8	9.0	9.9[d]	9.5	8.8	8.5	8.9	0.100	0.624

Columns 6–12 are Urinary Nitrogen Excretion (UNE, g/day) by Days of Fasting; last two columns are During a Six-Day Fast[b].

Source: Göschke, H., M. Stahl, and H. Thölen. 1975. *Klin. Wochenschr.* 53:605–610.

Note: BP, body protein; BW, body weight; DPF, the day preceding fast; yr, years; and UNE, urinary nitrogen excretion.

[a] Values are the means for 12 participants per group. The study participants maintained their body weights for 2–3 weeks on a diet with energy of approximately 15%, 35%, and 50% from protein, fat, and carbohydrate, respectively, before the beginning of a six-day fast. During the six-day fast, the study participants were provided with drinking water and weak tea but no vitamin or mineral supplements.

[b] Calculations were based on the average body weight (BW) of the study participants.

[c] Calculated as $N \times 6.25$.

[d] Different from the values on Day 1 and Day 6 ($P \leq 0.01$).

serious heart rhythm problems and other safety issues (including cardiovascular and lymph system disorders, kidney injuries, and liver damage and dysfunction) (FDA 2020).

Because of proteolysis, only a fraction of the synthesized constitutive protein is retained or accreted in tissues or the body (Table 9.5). It is possible that there is no deposition or even a loss of protein in humans and other animals under physiological conditions. For example, protein accretion is zero in weight-stable adults gaining no protein, whereas individuals exhibit a negative protein balance during a short-term fast. However, it should be borne in mind that most of the AAs released from protein degradation are reused for protein synthesis, although the percentage of the intracellular AA recycling varies with tissues, as well as physiological and pathological conditions. Furthermore, as indicated previously, intracellular protein accretion and lean tissue growth [e.g., body weight (BW) gain] depend on not only protein synthesis but also protein degradation. This is clearly illustrated by the finding that the skeletal muscle of fast-growing chickens has a 40% lower fractional rate of protein breakdown and grows more rapidly than the muscle of slow-growing chickens despite no significant difference in the fractional rate of muscle protein synthesis between the two lines of birds (Tesseraud et al. 2000).

Let us use glutamine metabolism in lymphocytes as an example to illustrate the nutritional and physiological importance of intracellular protein degradation. An adult man has 10^{12} lymphocytes, which, in the resting state, utilize 13 mmol glutamine/h/10^{12} cells (Newsholme et al. 1987). Assuming that 10% of glutamine carbons are irreversibly lost as CO_2 and its nitrogen can be efficiently salvaged, net use of glutamine by the lymphocytes of the whole body would be 1.3 mmol/h/10^{12} cells (Wu et al. 2011). Glutamine concentration in the plasma is 0.55 mM or 8.25 mmol in the total extracellular fluid (15 L). This amount of glutamine would be sufficient for utilization by lymphocytes alone for at most 6.4 h, even not considering glutamine utilization by other tissues and cell types, such as the kidneys, small intestine, pancreas, spleen, and macrophages (Chapter 4). Thus, net protein degradation in response to fasting and protein malnutrition is essential to provide glutamine for the immune and other systems of the body.

9.5 MEASUREMENTS OF INTRACELLULAR PROTEIN DEGRADATION

9.5.1 MEASUREMENT OF INTRACELLULAR PROTEIN DEGRADATION IN VITRO

9.5.1.1 General Considerations

Intracellular protein degradation releases free AAs (Figure 9.8). In cells (e.g., enterocytes, mammary epithelial cells, and brown adipocytes) or tissues (e.g., skeletal muscle and small intestine) without an inhibition of protein synthesis, the release of a nonmetabolizable AA depends on the balance between protein degradation and synthesis and is called net protein degradation. The criteria for the selection of an AA to measure intracellular protein degradation are the same as or similar to those used for studies of protein synthesis (Chapter 8). The reincorporation of AAs arising from protein degradation into newly synthesized proteins needs to be taken into account. In a few specific cases, protein degradation may be measured by the release of a nonmetabolizable, modified AA from intracellular proteins (i.e., an AA that has been modified through posttranslational methylation or hydroxylation and cannot be reincorporated into proteins).

$$\text{Net protein degradation} = \text{Protein degradation} - \text{Protein synthesis}$$

$$\text{Protein degradation} = \text{Net protein degradation} + \text{Protein synthesis}$$

In incubated cells or tissues whose pathway of protein synthesis is not inhibited, the release of an AA is an indicator of only net protein degradation, and protein synthesis should be determined simultaneously to calculate the rate of protein degradation. By contrast, when an inhibitor of protein synthesis (e.g., 0.5 mM cycloheximide) is included in the incubation medium, the release of an AA is an indicator of total protein degradation (or simply called protein degradation) in cells or tissues.

TABLE 9.5

Rates of Total Protein Degradation and the Ratios of Protein Accretion to Total Protein Synthesis in the Whole Bodies of Young Mammals, Chickens, and Fish[a]

Species	Ratios of Protein Accretion to Total Protein Synthesis	Total Protein Synthesis Per Day	Total Protein Degradation Per day	Protein Accretion Per Day	BW Gain Per Day	Reference
Preterm human infant (0.85–1.91 kg BW)	0.10	20 g/kg BW	18 kg BW	2.0 g/kg BW	16 g/kg BW	Stack et al. (1989)
Growing rats (100 g BW)	0.18	3.13 g	2.57 g	0.56 g	6.0 g	McNurlan and Garlick (1980)
Rapidly growing pigs (e.g., 10 kg BW)	0.30	167 g	117 g	50 g	350 g	Lobley (2003)
Slow-growing chickens (86 g BW, 2-week-old)	0.40	1.98 g	1.19 g	0.79 g	5.6 g	Tesseraud et al. (2000)
Fast-growing chickens (180 g BW, 2-week-old)	0.53	3.81 g	1.79 g	2.02 g	14.3 g	Tesseraud et al. (2000)
Finishing beef steers[b] (445 kg BW)	0.06	4,133 g	3,885 g	248 g	1,650 g	Lobley (2003)
Atlantic cod (300 g BW)	0.35	1.25 g	0.81 g	0.44 g	3.0 g	Houlihan et al. (1988)

Note: BW, body weight.

[a] Deposition of 1 g of protein in the body is associated with the retention of 3 g of water.

[b] Growing cattle at the final stage of weight gain before slaughter.

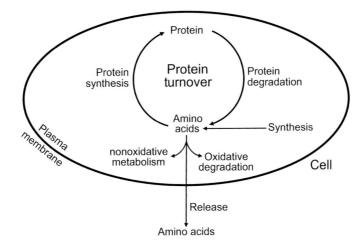

FIGURE 9.8 Release of amino acids (AAs) from intracellular protein degradation in cells or tissues. In cells, the protein undergoes continuous synthesis and degradation, which is collectively referred to as intracellular protein turnover. Protein gain in cells and tissues depends on the balance between the rates of protein synthesis and proteolysis. Most of the AAs released from proteolysis are reincorporated into protein, and some of them may be metabolized via oxidative and nonoxidative pathways. Some AAs may be synthesized de novo in a cell-specific manner. When the rate of protein degradation is greater than the rate of protein synthesis plus AA degradation, cells or tissues release AAs into the extracellular space (e.g., the blood *in vivo* or incubation medium *in vitro*). Those AAs that are neither synthesized nor degraded by the cell or tissue can be used as indicators of protein breakdown. When protein synthesis is inhibited, the release of a nonmetabolizable AA reflects total protein degradation in cells or tissues. When protein synthesis is not inhibited, the release of a nonmetabolizable AA reflects net protein degradation in cells or tissues. Release of nonmetabolizable AA = protein degradation – protein synthesis.

In studies involving the release of a labeled AA from labeled proteins, the inclusion of a high concentration of the unlabeled AA in the incubation medium (e.g., 1 mM Phe in medium for skeletal muscle and intestinal cells) is sufficient to minimize the reincorporation of the labeled tracer AA into the protein pool. A caveat to these methods is that incubated tissues are invariably in net negative N balance, even if they are taken from animals undergoing rapid muscle growth. Finally, as for the measurement of protein synthesis in incubated cells or tissues, in studies to determine protein degradation, the extracellular medium must contain physiological levels of AAs found in the plasma or in the lumen of the small intestine, depending on the experimental design, so that results will have physiological and nutritional relevance.

9.5.1.2 Tracer and Nontracer Methods for Measuring Protein Degradation *In Vitro*

9.5.1.2.1 *The Release of A Labeled AA from Intracellular Labeled Proteins*

Let's use the chick as the sources of skeletal muscle to study protein degradation. A tracer is administered to the animal to generate labeled proteins with both short and long half-lives in skeletal muscle, and the tissue is obtained for incubation after a sufficient period of the *in vivo* isotope labeling. The goal of this method is to generate intracellular labeled proteins for the assessment of *in vitro* proteolysis and is not a pulse labeling technique to estimate the rate of muscle protein degradation *in vivo*. For example, a 9-day-old chick receives a bolus intraperitoneal injection of 0.45 ml of a 0.9% NaCl solution containing 0.4 mM L-phenylalanine (Phe) plus [ring-2,6-^{3}H]Phe (0.83 Ci/mmol) (Tian and Baracos 1989; Wu and Thompson 1990). Twenty-four hours later, extensor digitorum communis muscle is isolated from the chick, respectively. The muscle is washed twice with physiological saline and then preincubated at 37°C for 30 min in 2 mL of oxygenated (95% O_2/5% CO_2) Krebs buffer containing 10 mU/mL insulin, 5 mM D-glucose, 1 mM Phe, and plasma concentrations of other AAs to deplete intracellular free ³H-Phe. Thereafter, the muscle is incubated at 37°C for 2 h in 2 mL of oxygenated Krebs buffer containing 10 mU/mL insulin, 5 mM D-glucose, 1 mM Phe, and plasma concentrations of other AAs to determine the release of ³H-Phe into the medium. The use of high Phe concentration in the medium is to facilitate the release of ³H-Phe from the skeletal muscle and to minimize the reincorporation of intracellular ³H-Phe into proteins. Similar approaches have been applied to studies of protein degradation in the extensor digitorum longus muscle of young rats, the enterocytes of animals, placental cells, mammary epithelial cells, and brown adipocytes (Kong et al. 2012; Tan et al. 2010; Tischler et al. 1982; Zhang et al. 2019). The release of labeled leucine or valine from labeled proteins in hepatocytes is often used as an index of hepatic protein degradation (Vom Dahl et al. 1991).

A major advantage of the tracer technique is that protein degradation can be measured at a high sensitivity in the presence of all AAs and simultaneously with the assessment of intracellular protein synthesis. A disadvantage of this method is that the release of an AA from the cell into extracellular medium may be affected by other AAs if they share a common transport system. This should be verified to ensure that the release of a labeled AA accurately reflects the rate of protein degradation in the studied cells or tissues.

9.5.1.2.2 The Dilution of A Labeled AA

The dilution of a labeled AA is based on the principle that, in a tissue receiving a tracer AA, a decrease in the SR or IE of the labeled AA in the free pool is affected by the extent to which intracellular protein is degraded. For example, a greater dilution of SR or IE of the free labeled AA indicates a higher rate of protein degradation in the cells or tissue. An example is the use of ¹⁵N-Phe to measure protein degradation in rat skeletal muscle perfused with various concentrations of glutamine (MacLennan et al. 1988). Compared with the control (0 mM glutamine), the presence of 2–10 mM glutamine results in less dilution of ¹⁵N-Phe in the collected perfusate, suggesting a role for glutamine to inhibit intramuscular proteolysis. Advantages of this method are high sensitivity, a lack of interference by the processes of protein synthesis, and simplicity. A disadvantage of the technique is that the dilution of a labeled AA may occur due to isotope exchange independent of intracellular protein degradation, as discussed in Chapter 7. For example, the hydrolysis of a small peptide to individual AAs may affect the dilution of SR or IE of the labeled AA precursor.

9.5.1.2.3 The Release of An Indicator AA from Incubated Tissues

Depending on individual tissues (e.g., skeletal muscle, liver, and intestine), the release of an indicator AA is determined to measure intracellular protein degradation in vitro (Figure 9.8). This AA should not be synthesized or degraded by the specific tissue. Examples are given as follows.

a. *The release of Leu or Val from perfused liver*. Leucine, isoleucine, and valine undergo little degradation in the mammalian and avian livers because of the absence or very low activity of hepatic BCAA aminotransferase (Chapter 4). Because transamination with α-ketoglutarate (α-KG) is the first step in BCAA degradation, the absence of BCAA aminotransferase limits the catabolism of BCAA in hepatocytes. Thus, the release of BCAAs from the perfused liver reflects the net rate of proteolysis in this organ when protein synthesis is not inhibited (Vom Dahl et al. 1991).

b. *The release of Tyr or Phe from incubated muscles*. Neither tyrosine (Tyr) nor Phe is degraded in skeletal muscle because of the lack of the necessary enzymes (tyrosine hydroxylase and phenylalanine hydroxylase) (Baracos et al. 1989; Baracos and Goldberg 1986; Klasing and Jarrell 1985; Tischler et al. 1982). Tyr can be measured easily by a sensitive fluorescence method (Baracos et al. 1989), but simple and accurate analysis of all AAs is now made possible by advanced chemical techniques, such as high-performance liquid chromatography (Wu and Meininger 2008). Disadvantages of this method are that (1) Tyr is usually absent from the incubation medium in order to adequately determine the release of a small amount of Tyr; and (2) an inhibitor of protein synthesis is usually present in the medium to block protein synthesis in order to estimate total protein degradation. The absence of Tyr from the incubation medium results in decreased protein synthesis, and cycloheximide itself may inhibit protein degradation in cultured muscle cells.

c. *The release of 3-methylhistidine from actin and myosin.* 3-Methylhistidine is formed from the methylation of protein-bound histidine residues as a posttranslational event and is not a substrate for protein synthesis. Because actin and myosin are present almost exclusively in smooth muscle, cardiac muscle, and skeletal muscle, the release of 3-methylhistidine can be used to estimate protein degradation in these tissues (Goodman 1987). This method is highly specific for measuring actin and myosin degradation, but is beset with analytical problems because it is difficult to analyze 3-methylhistidine in a general laboratory. Additionally, 3-methylhistidine can be released from the hydrolysis of dipeptides (e.g., balenine) independent of intracellular proteolysis.

Although this chapter focuses on intracellular proteolysis, it is worth mentioning in passing that the release of 4-hydroxyproline from an incubated tissue is a useful indicator of the degradation of extracellular collagen in the tissue. 4-Hydroxyproline is a unique proline derivative found exclusively in collagen (extracellular protein) of skeletal muscle, skin, and other connective tissues and is not a substrate for protein synthesis. Thus, the release of 4-hydroxyproline can be directly proportional to collagen breakdown. This method is highly specific for measuring collagen degradation, but is beset with analytical challenges because it is difficult to analyze 4-hydroxyproline in a general laboratory. Also, the release of 4-hydroxyproline may not be used to estimate collagen degradation in tissues (e.g., kidneys, liver, and small intestine) that express 4-hydroxyproline oxidase. This concern can be alleviated through the determination of metabolites (e.g., glycine) of 4-hydroxyproline in those tissues.

9.5.2 Measurement of Intracellular Protein Degradation *In Vivo*

9.5.2.1 General Considerations

Measurements of intracellular protein degradation *in vivo* involve the use of a labeled AA (Claydon et al. 2012; Waterlow 1984). Stable isotope tracers are often used in humans and large farm animals, because they are ethically acceptable and safe for studies (Bier and Matthews 1982). By contrast, radioactive tracers are good choices for studying *in vivo* protein degradation in rodents and small farm animals because of high sensitivity, easy analysis, and low costs. In rapidly growing young animals, the assessment of intracellular protein degradation can be based on fractional rates of protein synthesis and protein accretion (Mulvaney et al. 1985). However, inherent variability in the measurement of these two components may affect the accuracy of the determination of protein breakdown.

AA metabolism and protein turnover exhibit complex kinetics (Reeds and Davis 1999). Thus, except in tissue biopsy where a small amount of tissue (e.g., muscle and skin) can be obtained after the administration of a tracer, *in vivo* kinetic variables such as AA oxidation, protein synthesis, and protein degradation cannot be directly measured *in vivo* because these physiological processes take place in intracellular pools, which are experimentally inaccessible. An alternative to tissue sampling is necessary for the estimation of protein turnover *in vivo*, which is generally based on tracer kinetics data in the plasma, an easily accessible pool for tracer input and sampling. From these plasma data, one has to make quantitative inferences to the inaccessible metabolic pools of AAs. Therefore, it is essential to have "a model of the system", namely a hypothesis, to account for the metabolic fate of AAs and protein *in vivo* (Pacy et al. 1994). If an animal can be euthanized, the appearance of a labeled AA from a prelabeled protein may indicate the rate of proteolysis. For example, the degradation of newly synthesized collagens in rats has been estimated from the amount of free [^{14}C]4-hydroxyproline in tissues at 30 min after the administration of [^{14}C]proline (Mays et al. 1991).

When the rate of protein synthesis and protein growth in cells or a tissue is known, the rate of protein degradation can be calculated using the following equation. This method is useful for rapidly growing animals.

$$K_d = K_s - K_g$$

K_d (%/day) is the fractional rate of protein degradation. K_g (%/day) is the fractional rate of protein growth, which is determined experimentally based on protein accumulation in the tissue within a given period of time (e.g., 2–7 days depending on age and species). K_s (%/day) is the fractional rate of protein synthesis.

$$K_g(\%/\text{day}) = (P_{t2} - P_{t1})/(P_{t1}) \div t \times 100$$

P_{t2}: Amount of protein at the final time point ($t2$).
P_{t1}: Amount of protein at the initial time point ($t1$).
t: Duration (days) of the experimental period.

The calculation of K_g is based on the assumption that protein growth in cells or a tissue is linear during the experimental period. This assumption should be tested under the experimental conditions of a proposed study.

In the physiological steady state, $K_d = K_s$. Thus, the methods described in Chapter 8 for the measurement of *in vivo* protein synthesis also yield data on the rates of intracellular protein degradation in tissues and the whole body of healthy adults who do not usually gain protein. In addition to these methodologies, unique methods for determining *in vivo* protein degradation in healthy adults, in adults exhibiting negative or positive protein, and in growing animals are outlined in the following sections.

9.5.2.2 Pulse Labeling of Proteins by the Single Administration of A Labeled AA

The precursor-product relationship for SR or IE of the labeled AA after the single administration of a tracer AA is illustrated in Chapter 8. In Phase 3 of the pulse labeling when $F^* < P^*$ (Figure 8.7 of Chapter 8), the decrease in the amount (A) of radioactivity or mass of a tracer in protein with time is proportional to the rate of protein degradation.

F^*: The specific radioactivity (dpm/nmol) of a tracer AA (e.g., ^{14}C-Phe) in the precursor pool.
P^*: The specific radioactivity (dpm/nmol) of the tracer AA (e.g., ^{14}C-Phe) in the protein pool.

$$dA/dt = -K_d \times A$$

When K_d is a constant with respect to protein, this equation is integrated to give the following mathematical formula to calculate the fractional rate of protein degradation (%/t).

$$\ln\left(A_0/A_t\right) = K_d \times t$$

A_0 is the amount of the radioactivity or mass of the labeled AA in protein at time 0, A_t is the amount of the radioactivity or mass of the labeled AA in protein at any given time, and t is the duration of measurement after tracer administration. In the plot of $\ln(A_0/A_t)$ as the Y-axis against time (t), the slope is the fractional rate (K_d) of protein degradation expressed as %/min or %/h (Figure 9.9). Protein A has a greater fractional rate of degradation than protein B.

The half-life of a protein is determined from its K_d. When $A_t = 1/2\ A_0$ [i.e., at the half-life ($T_{1/2}$) of protein],

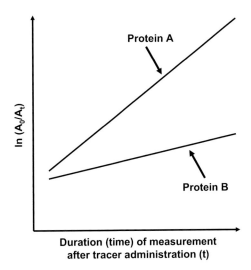

FIGURE 9.9 Measurement of the fractional rate of protein degradation (K_d) using the pulse labeling method. In Phase 3 of the pulse labeling of protein (see Chapter 8), a decline in the amount of the radioactivity or mass of the labeled amino acid (AA) in protein with time can be used to measure the rate of tissue protein degradation. A_0 is the amount of the radioactivity or mass of the labeled AA in protein at time 0, A_t is the amount of the radioactivity or mass of the labeled AA in protein at any given time, and t is the duration of measurement after tracer administration. $T_{1/2} = 0.693/K_d$. K_d is the slope of the regression line. The rate of degradation of protein A is greater than that of protein B.

$$\ln 2 = K_d \times T_{1/2};$$

$$T_{1/2} = (\ln 2)/K_d = 0.693/K_d.$$

This approach also applies to the measurement of the $T_{1/2}$ values of proteins in incubated cells and tissues.

An advantage of the pulse labeling technique is that it is highly sensitive for determining protein degradation in a small amount of a tissue and within a relatively short period of time (likely up to several hours). However, it should be kept in mind that this method is not appropriate for mixed proteins with different rates of degradation or various K_d values.

9.5.2.3 The Leucine Oxidation Method

As discussed in Chapter 8, the production of ^{14}C- or ^{13}C-labeled CO_2 from [1-^{14}C]leucine or [1-^{13}C] leucine constantly infused into humans or other animals can be determined to calculate whole-body protein turnover, including protein degradation (Figure 8.10 of Chapter 8). Excretion of $^{3}H_2O$ or ^{15}N-urea from intravenously infused [6-^{3}H]leucine or [^{15}N]leucine, respectively, can also be used to estimate leucine oxidation. In all these experiments, SR or IE of the precursor pool and products at isotopic steady state should be obtained for the calculation of *in vivo* whole-body protein degradation (Hankard et al. 1998).

9.5.2.4 Urinary Excretion of 3-Methylhistidine

Posttranslational methylation of some histidine residues in actin and myosin proteins generates 3-methylhistidine residues, as indicated previously. After these proteins are hydrolyzed by proteases, 3-methylhistidine is produced by skeletal, smooth, and cardiac muscles and is not reincorporated into proteins (Young et al. 1972). In female adult rats (250 g BW) with a slow rate of protein degradation (1.1%–1.6%/day) in skeletal muscle and a high rate of protein degradation (29%/day) in the intestine, skeletal muscle and intestine contain 86% and 1.9% of the total protein-bound

3-methylhistidine in the body (332 μmol/kg BW), respectively, and account for 38%–52% and 22% of the total 3-methylhistidine excreted in the urine (3.8 μmol/kg BW/day), respectively (Millward and Bates 1983). Much evidence shows that 3-methylhistidine is quantitatively excreted in the urine in some species (including cats, cattle, chickens, deer, frogs, humans, rats, and rabbits) and therefore can be a useful noninvasive technique for measuring whole-body protein degradation in these animals (Marks et al. 1996; Rathmacher and Nissen 1998; Young and Munro 1978). Because skeletal muscle is the major source of urinary 3-methylhistidine, it has been used as an indicator of protein breakdown in this tissue. In some species (e.g., dogs, goats, mice, pigs, and sheep), 3-methylhistidine cannot be quantitatively excreted in the urine and thus is not a useful indicator of muscle protein degradation (Harris and Milne 1980, 1981; Hill et al. 2001; Rathmacher and Nissen 1998). This is because in pigs, sheep, and goats, 3-methylhistidine reacts with β-alanine to form a dipeptide, β-alanyl-L-3-methylhistidine (balenine), which is abundant in skeletal muscle. In dogs, 3-methylhistidine undergoes decarboxylation to form 3-methylhistamine and a large amount of 3-methylhistidine is excreted in the feces. In mice, 3-methylhistidine is also decarboxylated to form 3-methylhistamine, followed by oxidative deamination to yield 1-methylimidazole-4-acetic acid, whereas 3-methylhistidine can be acetylated to N-acetyl-3-methylhistidine (Figure 9.10).

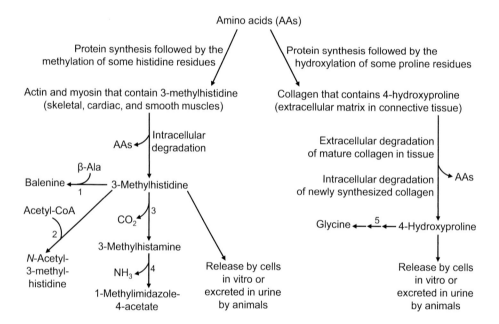

FIGURE 9.10 Use of the release of an indicator amino acid to assess the rates of myofibrillar protein (actin and myosin) and collagen degradation in incubated tissues (or cells) or the whole body. Myofibrillar proteins (actin and myosin) and collagens are synthesized from amino acids (AAs). The posttranslational methylation and hydroxylation of myofibrillar proteins and collagens result in the formation of 3-methylhistidine and 4-hydroxyproline residues, respectively. The degradation of the modified myofibrillar proteins and collagens generates 3-methylhistidine and 4-hydroxyproline, respectively. Both 3-methylhistidine and 4-hydroxyproline are not reincorporated into proteins but may be metabolized in cells. In incubated tissues or cells, the release of 3-methylhistidine and 4-hydroxyproline may be a useful indicator of the breakdown of myofibrillar proteins and collagens, respectively. In species (including humans and rats) that quantitatively excrete 3-methylhistidine in urine, the urinary output of 3-methylhistidine can indicate the breakdown of whole-body or possibly skeletal muscle myofibrillar proteins. Likewise, the urinary excretion of 4-hydroxyproline may reflect the breakdown of whole-body collagens. The enzymes that indicate the catalyzed reactions are (1) balenine synthetase; (2) N-acetyl-3-methylhistidine synthase; (3) 3-methylhistidine decarboxylase; (4) diamine oxidase and aldehyde dehydrogenase; and (5) a series of enzymes for the conversion of 4-hydroxyproline into glycine.

The relative contribution of the skeletal muscle to 3-methylhistidine in the body may depend on many factors such as the metabolic rates of nonskeletal muscle tissues (e.g., the small intestine, cardiac muscle, and skin). In young growing rats, the small intestine contributes significant amounts of 3-methylhistidine due to the rapid turnover rates of intracellular proteins. Additionally, dietary intake of 3-methylhistidine from animal products (e.g., meat and bones) must be considered and corrected for when calculating the production of 3-methylhistidine from the degradation of actin and myosin. Furthermore, concentrations of the dipeptides containing 3-methylhistidine in animal tissues should be constant during a 24-h period of urine collection. Thus, caution should be exercised when using the urinary excretion of 3-methylhistidine as an indicator of skeletal muscle protein breakdown in the body.

9.6 DEGRADATION OF EXTRACELLULAR PROTEINS IN TISSUES

9.6.1 DEGRADATION OF EXTRACELLULAR MATRIX PROTEINS IN TISSUES

9.6.1.1 Extracellular Matrix Proteins

The extracellular matrix consists of various kinds of proteins [including procollagens, mature collagens, elastins, proteoglycans (e.g., aggrecan, perlecan, neurocan, and syndecan), glycoproteins (e.g., fibronectins, osteopontin, and laminins), other proteins (e.g., enzymes), and glycosaminoglycans] (Lu et al. 2011; Wu 2018). These macromolecules are secreted by special cells (e.g., fibroblasts, chondrocytes, macrophages, or neutrophils, depending on the type of protein) within an organ (e.g., the skin, bone, cartilage, intestine, mammary tissue, blood vessels, and placenta) that contains connective tissue. The mature collagens (the major proteins in the extracellular matrix) and elastins form fibrils to contribute to the major tensile strength and viscoelasticity of the connective tissue. Proteoglycans, which are comprised of glycosaminoglycan chains that are long, linearized, and negatively charged due to the presence of sulfate and uronic acid groups, are considered as a special subset of glycoproteins (proteins containing carbohydrate polymers). Proteoglycans provide structural support and mechanical strength to the extracellular matrix and play a role in the modulation of cell growth. Fibronectins bind collagen and cell-surface integrins to modulate cell adhesion, growth, migration, differentiation, and wound healing. Osteopontin (a phosphorylated glycoprotein) binds to transmembrane integrins and extracellular matrix components to regulate cell signal transduction, gene expression, and physiological processes such as implantation and placentation during pregnancy (Denhardt and Guo 1993; Johnson et al. 2003). As part of the basement membrane (an extracellular matrix), laminins interact with other extracellular matrix components to provide support for tissues and mediate the attachment, migration, and organization of cells into tissues. Enzymes in the extracellular matrix include procollagen peptidases, collagenases, and metalloelastase. All extracellular matrix proteins contribute to tissue remodeling during growth, development, and recovery from physical injury. In healthy humans and other animals, the homeostasis of these proteins is properly maintained through their intracellular synthesis (discussed in Chapter 8), intracellular degradation of newly synthesized proteins, export out of cells into the interstitial space, and extracellular degradation of processed/mature proteins.

9.6.1.2 Degradation of Extracellular Matrix Proteins via Proteases and Peptidases

Some of the proteins that have been secreted into the extracellular matrix undergo limited degradation, as well as AA residue-specific modifications. For example, extracellular procollagen peptidases cleave the N-terminal and C-terminal AA sequences (called propeptides) from procollagens to generate collagens. In addition, ADAMTS-2 (a disintegrin and metalloproteinase with thrombospondin motifs-2) also catalyzes the removal of an amino prodomain from procollagen I in the dermis (Apte al. 2009). Furthermore, lysyl oxidase (an extracellular enzyme) acts on the ε-amino group of lysine residues to generate reactive aldehydes (α-aminoadipic-δ-semialdehydes, also called allysines). The latter spontaneously form specific covalent cross-links between two triple-helical chains to stabilize collagen molecules (mature collagen) and contribute to fibril strength (Robins 2007). Note that various matrix metalloproteinases (MMPs) can also release an AA segment from precursor matrix proteins (Lu et al. 2011). This is physiologically important because most MMPs are secreted as inactive enzymes but can be activated when cleaved by extracellular proteinases.

MMPs, ADAMS (a disintegrin and metalloproteinases), and ADAMTS proteinases, as well as elastases are responsible for the degradation of extracellular matrix proteins (Heinz et al. 2010; Lu et al. 2011). These enzymes are released by various cell types, including macrophages, fibroblasts, neutrophils, and tumor cells. Because MMPs, ADAMS, and ADAMTS are zinc-dependent endopeptidases, they are also called metalloproteinases. MMP-1, which is also known as collagenase 1, is activated by MMP-3 (which is also known as stromelysin 1) and MMP-10, as well as plasmin and kallikrein. MMP-3 is activated by plasmin and kallikrein. MMP-8, which is also known as collagenase 2, is activated by MMP-3 and 10, as well as plasmin. MMP-10, which is also known as stromelysin 2, is activated by plasmin and kallikrein. MMP-11, which is also known as stromelysin 3, is activated by plasmin. MMP-12, which is also known as macrophage-derived metalloelastase, degrades not only elastin but also proteoglycans, glycoproteins, and plasminogen in the extracellular matrix. Expression of MMP-12 is enhanced by proinflammatory cytokines, which contribute to the degeneration of connective tissue.

There are over 25 members in the MMP family in animals. In the extracellular matrix, most of the MMPs are not attached to the plasma membranes of the cells, but the membrane-type MMPs (MMP-14, MMP-15, MMP-23, and MMP-24) have a transmembrane domain and a short cytoplasmic tail, and MMP-17 and MMP-25 have glycosylphosphatidylinositol linkages. ADAMS are membrane-anchored metalloproteinases with a functional protease domain outside the plasma membrane and a C-terminal tail in the cytosol. There are over 33 members in the ADAMS family in animals, and some of these enzymes degrade glycoproteins and collagens. ADAMTS proteinases consist of at least 19 members of closely related metalloproteinases. Although MMPs use a wide range of extracellular matrix proteins as substrates, some of the enzymes have more specific targets. For example, certain MMPs for the degradation of selective substrates are MMP-3 and MMP-10 for proteoglycans, fibronectin, and laminin; MMP-1 for collagen III; MMP-8 and MMP-13 for collagen I and collagen II, respectively; both MMP-2 and MMP-9 degrade denatured collagens. Elastases belong to the serine, metallo, or cysteine families of endopeptidases for the degradation of elastins in the extracellular matrix, and these proteins are also substrates for MMP-2, MMP-9, and MMP-12. The degradation of extracellular matrix proteins is illustrated in Figure 9.11.

The concerted actions of MMPs, ADAMS, ADAMTS, and elastases degrade extracellular proteins into AAs. In addition, MMPs, ADAMS, and ADAMTS release glycosaminoglycans and carbohydrate polymers from proteoglycans and glycoproteins, respectively. Extracellular glycosaminoglycans are further metabolized via both the extracellular and intracellular pathways, as described in Chapter 5. The resultant carbohydrate polymers are degraded by specific enzymes to yield their respective oligosaccharides (such as glucose, galactose, mannose, and uronic acid), which are metabolized to pyruvate, lactate, acetyl-CoA, and CO_2 via various pathways in animals (Wu 2018).

Collagen turns over at more rapid rates in normal tissues than intramuscular myofibrillar proteins. For example, the mean rate of collagen degradation is about 3%–5%/day in the skin of adult rats, but is greater than 10%/day in some tissues, such as the lung and periodontal ligament (Laurent 1987). Intracellular degradation of newly synthesized collagen occurs within minutes of its synthesis and occurs at higher rates than the extracellular degradation of mature matrix collagen (Bienkowski 1984). Like noncollagen proteins, the degradation of collagens plays an important role in the regulation of their mass in the extracellular matrix. Of note, collagenases in animals target very specific peptide bonds, whereas collagenases in bacteria have broad substrate specificity. The degradation of extracellular matrix proteins plays an important role in health and disease. For example, osteoarthritis, which is a common debilitating disease in humans associated with collagen degradation, affects over 32.5 million Americans, and most people over the age of 60 will suffer from this disease to some degree of severity (CDC 2020). Another disorder of collagen degradation

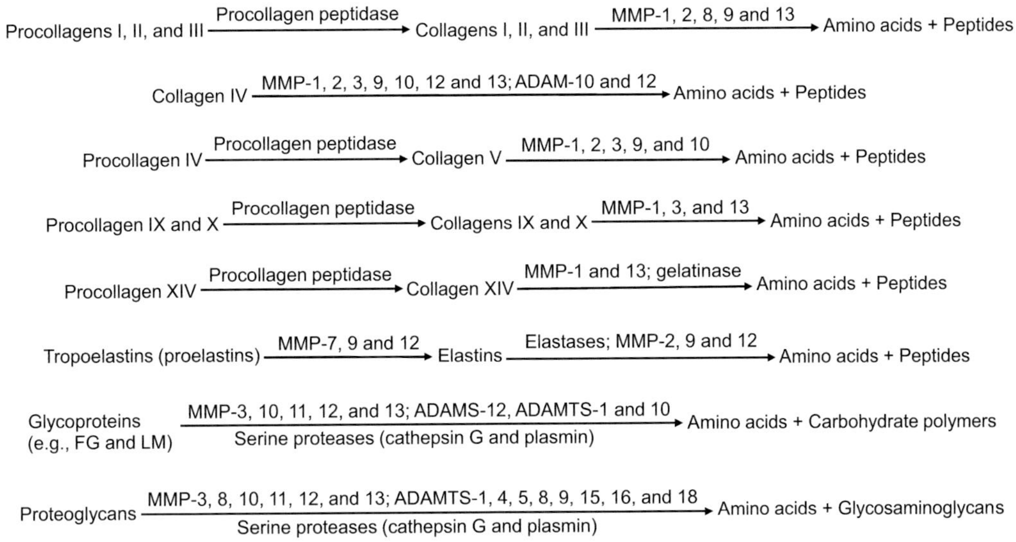

Procollagens I, II, and III $\xrightarrow{\text{Procollagen peptidase}}$ Collagens I, II, and III $\xrightarrow{\text{MMP-1, 2, 8, 9 and 13}}$ Amino acids + Peptides

Collagen IV $\xrightarrow{\text{MMP-1, 2, 3, 9, 10, 12 and 13; ADAM-10 and 12}}$ Amino acids + Peptides

Procollagen IV $\xrightarrow{\text{Procollagen peptidase}}$ Collagen V $\xrightarrow{\text{MMP-1, 2, 3, 9, and 10}}$ Amino acids + Peptides

Procollagen IX and X $\xrightarrow{\text{Procollagen peptidase}}$ Collagens IX and X $\xrightarrow{\text{MMP-1, 3, and 13}}$ Amino acids + Peptides

Procollagen XIV $\xrightarrow{\text{Procollagen peptidase}}$ Collagen XIV $\xrightarrow{\text{MMP-1 and 13; gelatinase}}$ Amino acids + Peptides

Tropoelastins (proelastins) $\xrightarrow{\text{MMP-7, 9 and 12}}$ Elastins $\xrightarrow{\text{Elastases; MMP-2, 9 and 12}}$ Amino acids + Peptides

Glycoproteins (e.g., FG and LM) $\xrightarrow[\text{Serine proteases (cathepsin G and plasmin)}]{\text{MMP-3, 10, 11, 12, and 13; ADAMS-12, ADAMTS-1 and 10}}$ Amino acids + Carbohydrate polymers

Proteoglycans $\xrightarrow[\text{Serine proteases (cathepsin G and plasmin)}]{\text{MMP-3, 8, 10, 11, 12, and 13; ADAMTS-1, 4, 5, 8, 9, 15, 16, and 18}}$ Amino acids + Glycosaminoglycans

FIGURE 9.11 Degradation of extracellular matrix proteins in humans and other animals. Procollagens, tropoelastins, glycoproteins, and proteoglycans are secreted into the extracellular matrix, where procollagens and tropoelastins undergo limited degradation to become mature proteins. Matrix metalloproteinases (MMPs), ADAMS (a disintegrin and metalloproteinases), and ADAMTS (a disintegrin and metalloproteinase with thrombospondin motifs) proteinases, as well as elastases are responsible for the degradation of extracellular matrix proteins. MMPs, ADAMS, and ADAMTS are zinc-dependent endopeptidases and are metalloproteinases. MMP-1 (collagenase 1) is activated by MMP-3 (stromelysin 1) and 10, as well as plasmin and kallikrein. MMP-3, which is also known as stromelysin 1, is activated by plasmin and kallikrein. MMP-8 (collagenase 2) is activated by MMP-3 and MMP-10, as well as plasmin. MMP-10 (stromelysin 2) is activated by plasmin and kallikrein. MMP-11 (stromelysin 3) is activated by plasmin. MMP-12 (macrophage-derived metalloelastase) degrades not only elastin but also proteoglycans, glycoproteins, and plasminogen in the extracellular matrix. Elastases belong to the serine, metallo, or cysteine families of endopeptidases for the degradation of elastins in the extracellular matrix. The degradation of extracellular matrix proteins generates free AAs and bioactive peptides.

is the inherited Ehlers–Danlos syndrome, which is characterized by overly flexible joints that can dislocate, the skin that is translucent and elastic and bruises easily, and the dilation and even rupture of major blood vessels (Malfait et al. 2020). Furthermore, a hallmark of many diseases (including various cancers) is the enhanced degradation of the extracellular matrix proteins in connective tissue (including metastases in bone), leading to high rates of mortality (Phang et al. 2010). Bone metastases lead to a huge amount of morbidity and tremendous pain. Inhibiting excessive collagen degradation under these catabolic conditions may improve the health and well-being of affected patients and extend their lives (Xu et al. 2019).

9.6.2 Degradation of Proteins in the Plasma of Blood

9.6.2.1 Proteins in the Plasma of Blood

The plasma of the blood is rich in proteins, including albumin (the most abundant protein), globulins (including immunoglobulins, Ig), fibrinogens, cytokines, enzymes (e.g., glutamate-pyruvate transaminase, glutamate-oxaloacetate transaminase, and arginase), and hormones (e.g., insulin, growth hormone, and luteinizing hormone). The concentration of total proteins in the plasma of healthy adult humans is 6–8 g/100 mL, with albumin, globulins, and fibrinogens accounting for approximately 59%, 37%, and 4% of the total plasma proteins (Busher 1990; McNeal et al. 2018; Roshal 2013), respectively. Based on the blood volume (~5 L) and the percentage of its plasma (~60%) in a

70-kg healthy adult human, the amounts of albumin, globulins, and fibrinogens in the subject's total plasma (3 L) are approximately 124, 78, and 11 g, respectively. Note that fibrinogens are absent from the serum after the clotting of the blood. Proteins (including albumin) in the plasma can move out of the endothelial cells at various rates into the interstitial fluid of tissues and then return to the blood through the lymphatic circulation. Thus, proteins in the plasma appear in the extravascular space. For example, about 40% and 60% of total albumin in the body (~350 g in a 70-kg adult human) are present in the blood and the interstitial space of tissues, respectively.

9.6.2.2 Extracellular Degradation of Plasma Proteins by Proteases in the Blood and the Interstitial Space of Tissues

Plasma proteins turn over through their extracellular degradation in the blood and their entry into the interstitial space of tissues. Different plasma proteins [such as albumin and immunoglobulins (Ig)] have different half-lives, suggesting that they may be degraded at different rates in the blood. For example, based on the kinetics of proteins in the serum, the half-lives of the following proteins in the whole body of healthy adult humans are as follows: albumin, 19 days; insulin, 5–6 min; IgA (the second most abundant Ig), 6; IgD, 3 days; IgE, 2.5 days; IgG (the most abundant Ig), 23 days; and IgM (the third most abundant Ig), 5 days (Lobo et al. 2004; Prinsen and de Sain-van der Velden 2004). Similarly, based on the kinetics of proteins in the serum, the half-lives of albumin and insulin in the whole body of growing pigs are 8.2 days (Dich and Nielsen 1963) and 24 min (Petersen et al. 2013), respectively, whereas the half-lives of IgA, IgM, and IgG in the whole body of neonatal pigs are 2.6, 2.8, and 9.5 days, respectively (Curtis and Bourne 1973). It appears that the half-lives of proteins in the serum are much shorter than those in the extravascular fluid. For example, the half-lives of intravascular and extravascular albumin in healthy adult humans are 16 h and ~20 days, respectively, and the half-life of albumin in the whole body of young pigs is 8.2 days (Dich and Nielsen 1963). As illustrated in Figure 9.12, the degradation of plasma proteins is carried out by both plasma proteases (an extracellular proteolysis; Altshuler et al. 2012; Aoyagi et al. 1990; Crawley et al. 2011; Romero et al. 1986) and the engulfing macrophages (intracellular proteolysis; Swanson and Watts 1995) in the interstitial space of tissues). Plasma proteases include aminopeptidases, endopeptidases

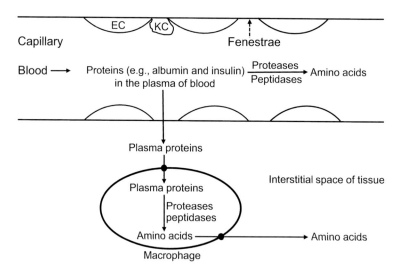

FIGURE 9.12 Degradation of plasma proteins in humans and other animals. The plasma of the blood contains proteases to carry out proteolysis, which include aminopeptidases, plasmin, renin, kinin-kallikreins, ADAMTS13, calcium-dependent proteases, as well as trypsin-, chymotrypsin-, and elastase-like enzymes. Proteins (including albumin) in the plasma can move out of the endothelial cells into the interstitial fluid of tissues, where the proteins are engulfed by macrophages for intracellular proteolysis.

(e.g., plasmin), renin, kinin-kallikreins [serine proteases that release kinins (bradykinin and kallidin; vasodilators) from kininogens], ADAMTS13 (a constitutively active blood metalloprotease that cleaves ultra-large von Willebrand factor (VWF) to produce smaller VWF units, and calcium-dependent proteases, as well as trypsin-, chymotrypsin-, and elastase-like enzymes. Thus, plasma proteins can provide peptides and AAs to tissues and cells in humans and other animals.

9.6.3 Measurement of Extracellular Protein Degradation

[^{14}C]Proline and [^{14}C]4-hydroxyproline have been used to measure the rates of the degradation of collagen in the extracellular space (Bienkowski 1984; Laurent 1987). In addition, the release of labeled [^{14}C]4-hydroxyproline from prelabeled ^{14}C-collagen in an incubated tissue can be employed to assess the degradation of extracellular collagen when intracellular proteasomes and lysosomes are suppressed by specific inhibitors. Furthermore, the intravenous administration of ^{125}I- or ^{131}I-labeled proteins (e.g., albumin) followed by its decay in the plasma is useful to quantify the fractional rate of the proteins in the plasma and the whole body (Prinsen and de Sain-van der Velden 2004). The underlying principles for the tracer methods are the same as described previously for the measurement of intracellular and whole-body protein breakdown.

9.7 RATES OF WHOLE-BODY AND TISSUE-SPECIFIC PROTEIN DEGRADATION IN HUMANS AND OTHER ANIMALS

As discussed in Chapter 8, the reported rates of whole-body and tissue-specific protein turnover in healthy adult humans differ substantially, possibly due to a number of variables, such as age, sex, dietary protein and energy intakes, prior physical activity levels (e.g., minimal or high), and hormonal status of study participants, as well as the use of the leucine-to-protein conversion factor [e.g., ×12.5 (707 µmol leucine/g protein; Waterlow 1995) or ×14.05 (629 µmol leucine/g protein; Lacy et al. 1994) for adult humans]. Thus, comparisons of the published data on the rates of whole-body protein degradation from different studies are complicated because of different experimental conditions. Based on the results of several studies involving different tracer methods, Waterlow (1995) has estimated that the rate of whole-body protein degradation in the 70-kg healthy adult human is approximately 300 g/day (or 4.3 g/kg BW/day). The irreversible oxidation of body protein has been estimated to be ~10% of the total amount of protein breakdown (i.e., 30 g/day) in the 70-kg healthy adult human (Bröer and Bröer. 2017). In all species of adult mammals, the rates of protein degradation in the whole body (expressed as g/kg BW/day) or skeletal muscle decrease with an increase in their BW and age, but rise in response to intermittent mechanical stretching, intensive exercise, infections, injury, stress (e.g., heat, cold, or oxidative stress), metabolic acidosis, intrauterine growth restriction, and diseases (e.g., cancer, diabetes, renal failure, and muscle wasting) (Dodson et al. 2011; Hanna et al. 1989; Palmer et al. 1985; Pencharz et al. 1981; Rattan 2010; Waterlow 1984, 1995).

The physiological and pathological conditions mentioned above may also affect muscle proteolysis in birds. There is evidence that prostaglandin E2 mediates an infection-induced increase in proteolysis in chick skeletal muscle (Tian and Baracos 1989), suggesting a close link between lipid and protein metabolism. Other factors may contribute to the modulation of protein metabolism in avian muscles. In this regard, it is noteworthy that woody muscle myopathy syndrome, which is characterized by myodegeneration, interstitial connective tissue accretion, and fibrosis, has recently been discovered in the breast (pectoralis) muscle of rapidly growing broilers (Sihvo et al. 2014). Whether alterations in intracellular protein turnover due to a deficiency of one or more AAs (e.g., glycine, proline, and glutamine) and a reduction in extracellular proteolysis contributes to the development of this metabolic syndrome in broilers (with a prevalence rate of about 8% in high yielding strains) warrant investigations. Compared with leg muscles, the breast muscle of chickens has 330% higher glutaminase activity, substantially lower concentrations of glutamine and glycine (78% and 53% reductions, respectively), and a 71% lower rate of fractional protein synthesis (Watford and Wu 2005). This may help to explain why the breast muscle (white fibers) rather than leg muscles (primarily red fibers) are susceptible to myopathy in broilers.

The physiological response of humans and other animals to short- and long-term fasting with time-dependent changes in protein metabolism has been a fascinating area of study for over a century. Concentrations of AAs in the plasma and tissues, associated with cycles of fasting-feeding, regulate the process of protein degradation (Fiorotto et al. 2000), with low AA availabilities signaling the need to activate proteolysis through both lysosomal and nonlysosomal pathways (Goldberg 2003). Given adequate intakes of water, vitamins, and minerals, survival is limited by the loss of body protein. Göschke et al. (1975) reported that normal and obese adults (men and women) exhibited a significant increase in urinary nitrogen excretion between Days 1 and 3 of fasting, followed by a steady decline. The response in the early phase results primarily from a decrease in the circulating levels of insulin, leading to increases in both proteolysis and AA catabolism in the whole body (Waterlow 1984). The change in nitrogen loss during the chronic phase of fasting is due to an inhibition of muscle proteolysis by the elevated concentrations of ketone bodies (Thompson and Wu 1991). This is consistent with the contribution of body protein to energy provision in the body, as the biological oxidation of protein provides 15% of the total ATP production in normal men after a 6-day fast but only 5% of the total ATP production in obese women at the end of a 28-day fast. Furthermore, normal men lost more nitrogen than normal women with the same BW, and the same was observed for obese men vs obese women (Göschke et al. 1975). Thus, the sex and duration of fasting, as well as the body fat mass profoundly affect protein metabolism in humans.

9.8 SUMMARY

Intracellular protein degradation, which is a component of intracellular protein turnover, is catalyzed by exopeptidases and endopeptidases. Based on the catalytic sites, proteases are classified as serine, cysteine, aspartate, and metallo proteinases. According to the location of proteases, proteolytic systems are classified as lysosomal (optimal pH 3–5) and nonlysosomal (optimal pH 7–8) systems (Figure 9.13). Lysosomal proteases consist of cathepsins B, H, L, and D and are responsible mainly for the degradation of organelles and membranes, long-lived intracellular proteins, endocytosed proteins, partly myofibrillar proteins, and proteins under conditions of nutrient deprivation and stress, as well as oxidized and misfolded proteins. Autophagy plays a crucial role in this process. Nonlysosomal proteases include calpains, the caspases, ATP-dependent but ubiquitin-independent proteases, and the ATP- and ubiquitin-dependent 26S proteasome and are responsible for the degradation of both short-lived and long-lived proteins, abnormal and denatured proteins, oxidized and misfolded proteins, and newly synthesized collagens. In recent years, much attention has been directed to the structure and functions of the complex 26S proteasome, which contains one 20S core and two 19S regulatory caps. This multiunit protease is highly conserved among eukaryotic cells and is responsible for most of the protein degradation in the cells. Thus, the 26S proteasome functions as a universal degradation machine for a wide variety of protein substrates. Intracellular protein degradation requires a large amount of energy (~2 ATP molecules for hydrolysis of each peptide bond) but is essential for the regulation of many cellular processes, including the cell cycle, gene expression, processing of antigens in the immune system, and responses to oxidative stress. Extracellular matrix proteins (including mature collagens) in tissues are degraded by secreted metalloproteinases (including collagenases) and elastases, whereas plasma proteins (e.g., albumin and insulin) are degraded by extracellular proteases in the plasma and by the engulfing macrophages in the interstitial space of tissues (e.g., the liver, skeletal muscle, skin, and kidneys). To understand the regulatory mechanism of protein homeostasis, both tracer and nontracer methods, including pulse labeling, leucine oxidation, and release of an indicator AA, have been developed to determine the rates of intracellular protein turnover and extracellular proteolysis *in vitro* and *in vivo*. Choice of the methods should be dictated by scientific questions to be asked.

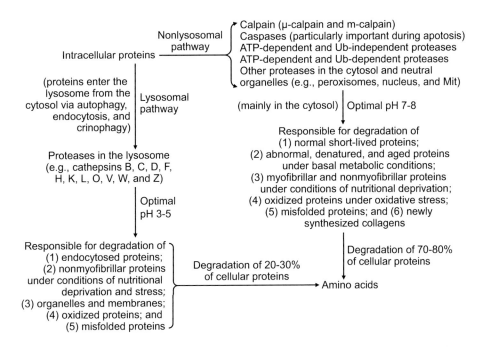

FIGURE 9.13 Degradation of intracellular proteins via the lysosomal and nonlysosomal pathways in animal cells. These two proteolytic systems target different cellular proteins, but also use either the same or different kinds of certain proteins as substrates under certain physiological (e.g., fasting) and proinflammatory (e.g., oxidative stress) conditions. Most of the cellular proteins are degraded by the nonlysosomal pathway. Mit, mitochondria; Ub, ubiquitin.

REFERENCES

Altshuler, A.E., A.H. Penn, J.A. Yang, G.R. Kim, and G.W. Schmid-Schönbein. 2012. Protease activity increases in plasma, peritoneal fluid, and vital organs after hemorrhagic shock in rats. *PLoS One* 7:e32672.

Aoyagi, T., T. Wada, F. Kojima, M. Nagai, S. Harada, T. Takeuchi et al. 1990. Three main components in plasma proteases and their relation to the renin-angiotensin system. *Biotechnol. Appl. Biochem.* 12:258–263.

Apte, S.S. 2009. A disintegrin-like and metalloprotease (reprolysin-type) with thrombospondin type 1 motif (ADAMTS) superfamily---Functions and mechanisms. *J. Biol. Chem.* 284:31493–31497.

Attaix, D., L. Combaret, M.-N. Pouch, and D. Taillandier. 2002. Cellular control of ubiquitin-proteasome-dependent proteolysis. *J. Anim. Sci.* 80 (Suppl. 2):E56–E63.

Bachmair, A., D. Finley, and A. Varshavsky. 1986. In vivo half-life of a protein is a function of its amino-terminal residue. *Science* 234:179–186.

Baracos, V.E. 1988. Role of factors derived from activated macrophages in regulation of muscle protein turnover. *Adv. Exp. Med. Biol.* 240:225–234.

Baracos, V.E. and A.L. Goldberg. 1986. Maintenance of normal length improves protein balance and energy status in isolated rate skeletal muscles. *Am. J. Physiol.* 251:C588–C596.

Baracos, V.E., M. Langman, and A. Mak. 1989. An *in vitro* preparation of the extensor digitorum longus muscle from the chick (*Gallus domesticus*) for studies of protein turnover. *Comp. Biochem. Physiol. A* 92:555–563.

Barrett, A.J. and H. Kirschke. 1981. Cathepsin B, cathepsin H, and cathepsin L. *Methods Enzymol.* 80:535–561.

Benbrook, D.M. and A. Long. 2012. Integration of autophagy, proteasomal degradation, unfolded protein response and apoptosis. *Exp. Oncol.* 34:286–297.

Bienkowski, R.S. 1984. Intracellular degradation of newly synthesized collagen. *Collagen Rel. Res.* 4:399–412.

Bier, D.M. and D.E. Matthews. 1982. Stable isotope tracer methods for in vivo investigations. *Fed. Proc.* 41:2679–2685.

Bonaldo, P. and M. Sandri. 2013. Cellular and molecular mechanisms of muscle atrophy. *Dis. Model Mech.* 6:25–39.

Bond, J.S. 2019. Proteases---History, discovery, and roles in health and disease. *J. Biol. Chem.* 294:1643–1651.

Bond, J.S. and P.E. Butler. 1987. Intracellular proteases. *Annu. Rev. Biochem.* 56:333–364.

Bröer, S. and A. Bröer. 2017. Amino acid homeostasis and signalling in mammalian cells and organisms. *Biochem. J.* 474:1935–2963.

Busher, J.T. 1990. Serum albumin and globulin. In: *Clinical Methods---The History, Physical, and Laboratory Examinations*, 3rd edition (Walker, H.K., Hall, W.D., and Hurst, J.W., eds). Butterworths, Boston, MA. pp. 497–498.

CDC (Centers for Disease Control and Prevention CDC). 2020. *Osteoarthritis (OA).* U.S. Department of Health & Human Services, Washington, DC.

Ciechanover, A. 2012. Intracellular protein degradation---from a vague idea thru the lysosome and the ubiquitin-proteasome system and onto human diseases and drug targeting. *Biochim. Biophys. Acta* 1824:3–13.

Ciechanover, A., Y. Hod, and A. Hershko. 1978. A heat-stable polypeptide component of an ATP-dependent proteolytic system from reticulocytes. *Biochem. Biophys. Res. Commun.* 81:1100–1105.

Ciechanover, A., D. Finley, and A. Varshavsky. 1984. Ubiquitin dependence of selective protein degradation demonstrated in the mammalian cell cycle mutant ts85. *Cell* 37:57–66.

Claydon, A.J., M.D. Thom, J.L. Hurst, and R.J. Beynon. 2012. Protein turnover---measurement of proteome dynamics by whole animal metabolic labelling with stable isotope labelled amino acids. *Proteomics* 12:1194–206.

Coux, O., B.A. Zieba, and S. Meiners. 2020. The proteasome system in health and disease. *Adv. Exp. Med. Biol.* 1233:55–100.

Craik, C.S., M.J. Page, and E.L. Madison. 2011. Proteases as therapeutics. *Biochem. J.* 435:1–16.

Crawley, J.T., R. de Groot, Y. Xiang, B.M. Luken, and D.A. Lane. 2011. Unraveling the scissile bond---how ADAMTS13 recognizes and cleaves von Willebrand factor. *Blood* 118:3212–3221.

Curtis, J. and F.J. Bourne. 1973. Half-lives of immunoglobulins IgG, IgA and IgM in the serum of new-born pigs. *Immunology* 24:147–155.

Denhardt, D.T. and X. Guo 1993. Osteopontin---a protein with diverse functions. *FASEB J.* 7:1475–1482.

Dice, J.F. 1987. Molecular determinants of protein half-lives in eukaryotic cells. *FASEB J.* 1:349–357.

Dich, J. and K. Nielsen. 1963. Metabolism and Distribution of 131 I-labelled Albumin in the Pig. *Can. J. Comp. Med. Vet. Sci.* 27:269–273.

Dikic, I. and Z. Elazar. 2018. Mechanism and medical implications of mammalian autophagy. *Nat. Rev. Mol. Cell Biol.* 19:349–364.

Dodson, S., V.E. Baracos, A. Jatoi, W.J. Evans, D. Cella, J.T. Dalton, and M.S. Steiner. 2011. Muscle wasting in cancer cachexia---Clinical implications, diagnosis, and emerging treatment strategies. *Annu. Rev. Med.* 62:265–279.

Driscoll, J. and A.L. Goldberg. 1990. The proteasome (multicatalytic protease) is a component of the 1500-kDa proteolytic complex which degrades ubiquitin-conjugated proteins. *J. Biol. Chem.* 265:4789–4792.

Erales, J. and P. Coffino. 2014. Ubiquitin-independent proteasomal degradation. *Biochim. Biophys. Acta* 1843:216–221.

Etlinger, J.D. and A.L. Goldberg. 1977. A soluble ATP-dependent proteolytic system responsible for the degradation of abnormal proteins in reticulocytes. *Proc. Natl. Acad. Sci. USA.* 74:54–58.

FDA (Food and Drug Administration). 2020. FDA cautions against use of hydroxychloroquine or chloroquine for COVID-19 outside of the hospital setting or a clinical trial due to risk of heart rhythm problems. https://www.fda.gov/drugs/drug-safety-and-availability/fda-cautions. Accessed April 18, 2021.

Fagan, J.M., L. Waxman, A.L. Goldberg. 1986. Red blood cells contain a pathway for the degradation of oxidant-damaged hemoglobin that does not require ATP or ubiquitin. *J. Biol. Chem.* 261:5705–5713.

Fiorotto, M.L., T.A. Davis, and P.J. Reeds. 2000. Regulation of myofibrillar protein turnover during maturation in normal and undernourished rat pups. *Am. J. Physiol.* 278:R845–R854.

Furuno, K., M.N. Goodman, and A.L. Goldberg. 1990. Role of different proteolytic systems in the degradation of muscle proteins during denervation atrophy, *J. Biol. Chem.* 265:8550–8557.

Goldberg, A.L. 2003. Protein degradation and protection against misfolded or damaged proteins. *Nature* 426:895–899.

Goldberg, A.L. and A.C. St John. 1976. Intracellular protein degradation in mammalian and bacterial cells. *Annu. Rev. Biochem.* 45:747–803.

Goldknopf, I.L. and H. Busch. 1977. Isopeptide linkage between nonhistone and histone 2A polypeptides of chromosomal conjugate-protein A24. *Proc. Natl. Acad. Sci. USA.* 74:864–868.

Goll, D.E., G. Neti, S.W. Mares, and V.F. Thompson. 2008. Myofibrillar protein turnover---the proteasome and the calpains. *J. Anim. Sci.* 86(14 Suppl):E19–E35.

Goodman, M.N. 1987. Differential effects of acute changes in cell Ca^{2+} concentration on myofibrillar and non-myofibrillar protein breakdown in the rat extensor digitorum longus muscle in vitro. Assessment by production of tyrosine and N$^\tau$-methylhistidine. *Biochem. J.* 241:121–127.

Göschke, H., M. Stahl, and H. Thölen. 1975. Nitrogen loss in normal and obese subjects during total fast. *Klin. Wochenschr.* 53:605–610.

Hankard, R.G., D. Hammond, M.W. Haymond, and D. Darmaun. 1998. Oral glutamine slows down whole body protein breakdown in Duchenne muscular dystrophy. *Pediatr. Res.* 43:222–226.

Hanna, J., A. Guerra-Moreno, J. Ang, and Y. Micoogullari. 2019. Protein degradation and the pathologic basis of disease. *Am. J. Pathol.* 189:94–103.

Harris, C.I. and G. Milne. 1980. The urinary excretion of 3-methylhistidine in sheep---an invalid index of muscle protein breakdown. *Br. J. Nutr.* 44:129–140.

Harris, C.I. and G. Milne. 1981. The inadequacy of urinary 3-methylhistidine excretion in the pig as a measure of muscle protein breakdown. *Br. J. Nutr.* 45:423–429.

Heinz, A., M.C. Jung, L. Duca, W. Sippl, S. Taddese, C. Ihling et al. 2010. Degradation of tropoelastin by matrix metalloproteinases – cleavage site specificities and release of matrikines. *FEBS J.* 277:1939–1956.

Hershko, A. and A. Ciechanover. 1998. The ubiquitin system. *Annu. Rev. Biochem.* 67:425–479.

Hershko, A., A. Ciechanover, H. Heller, A.L. Haas, and I.A. Rose. 1980. Proposed role of ATP in protein breakdown---conjugation of protein with multiple chains of the polypeptide of ATP-dependent proteolysis. *Proc. Natl. Acad. Sci. USA.* 77:1783–1786.

Hershko, A., H. Heller, S. Elias, and A. Ciechanover. 1983. Components of ubiquitin-protein ligase system. Resolution, affinity purification, and role in protein breakdown. *J. Biol. Chem.* 258:8206–8214.

Hill, A.S., S.L. Marks, and Q.R. Rogers. 2001. Quantitation of urinary 3-methylhistidine excretion in growing dogs as an index of *in vivo* skeletal muscle catabolism. *J. Nutr. Biochem.* 12:346–350.

Hoffman, L., G. Pratt, and M. Rechsteiner. 1992. Multiple forms of the 20S multicatalytic and the 26S ubiquitin/ATP-dependent proteases from rabbit reticulocyte lysate. *J. Biol. Chem.* 267:22362–22368.

Hough. R., G. Pratt, and M. Rechsteiner. 1986. Ubiquitin-lysozyme conjugates. Identification and characterization of an ATP-dependent protease from rabbit reticulocyte lysates. *J. Biol. Chem.* 261:2400–2408.

Houlihan, D.F., S.J. Hall, C. Gray, and B.S. Noble. 1988. Growth rates and protein turnover in Atlantic cod, *Gadus morhua. Can. J. Fish Aquat. Sci.* 45:951–964.

Hurley, J.H. and L.N. Young. 2017. Mechanisms of autophagy initiation. *Annu. Rev. Biochem.* 86:225–244.

International Union of Biochemistry and Molecular Biology (IUBMB) 1992. *Enzyme Nomenclature.* Academic Press, San Diego, CA.

Johnson, G.A., R.C. Burghardt, F.W. Bazer, and T.E. Spencer. 2003. Osteopontin---roles in implantation and placentation. *Biol. Reprod.* 69:1458–1471.

Katunuma, N. and E. Kominami. 1995. Structure, properties, mechanisms, and assays of cysteine protease inhibitors---cystatins and E-64 derivatives. *Methods Enzymol.* 251:382–397.

Kitajima, Y., K. Yoshioka, and N. Suzuki. 2020. The ubiquitin–proteasome system in regulation of the skeletal muscle homeostasis and atrophy---from basic science to disorders. *J. Physiol. Sci.* 70:40.

Klasing, K.C. and V.L. Jarrell. 1985. Regulation of protein degradation in chick muscle by several hormones and metabolites. *Poultry Sci.* 64:694–699.

Kohn, R.R. 1969. A proteolytic system involving myofibrils and a soluble factor from normal and atrophying muscle. *Lab. Invest.* 20:202–206.

Kong, X.F., B.E. Tan, Y.L. Yin, H.J. Gao, X.L. Li, L.A. Jaeger et al. 2012. L-Arginine stimulates the mTOR signaling pathway and protein synthesis in porcine trophectoderm cells. *J. Nutr. Biochem.* 23:1178–1183.

Laurent, G.J. 1987. Dynamic state of collagen---pathways of collagen degradation in vivo and their possible role in regulation of collagen mass. *Am. J. Physiol.* 252:C1–C9.

Lobley, G.E. 2003. Protein turnover—what does it mean for animal production? *Can. J. Anim. Sci.* 83:327–340.

Lobo, E.D., R.J. Hansen, and J.P. Balthasar. 2004. Antibody pharmacokinetics and pharmacodynamics. *J. Pharma. Sci.* 93:2645–2668.

Lowell, B.B., N.B. Ruderman, and M.N. Goodman. 1986. Evidence that lysosomes are not involved in the degradation of myofibrillar proteins in rat skeletal muscle. *Biochem. J.* 234:237.

Lu, P., K. Takai, V.M. Weaver, and Z. Werb. 2011. Extracellular matrix degradation and remodeling in development and disease. *Cold Spring Harb. Perspect Biol.* 3:a005058.

MacLennan, P.A., K. Smith, B. Weryk, P.W. Watt, and M.J. Rennie. 1988. Inhibition of protein breakdown by glutamine in perfused rat skeletal muscle. *FEBS Lett.* 237:133–136.

Malfait, F., M. Castori, C.A. Francomano, C. Giunta, T. Kosho, and P.H. Byers. 2020. The Ehlers–Danlos syndromes. *Nat. Rev. Dis. Primers* 6:64.

Marks, S.L., Q.R. Rogers, and J.G. Morris. 1996. Quantitative excretion of 3-methylhistidine in urine of cats as a measure of *in vivo* skeletal muscle protein catabolism. *J. Nutr. Biochem.* 7:60–63.

Mauthe, M., I. Orhon, C. Rocchi, X. Zhou, M. Luhr, K.J. Hijlkema et al. 2018. Chloroquine inhibits autophagic flux by decreasing autophagosome-lysosome fusion. *Autophagy* 14:1435–1455.

Mays, P.K., R.J. McAnulty, J.S. Campa, and G.J. Laurent. 1991. Age-related changes in collagen synthesis and degradation in rat tissues. Importance of degradation of newly synthesized collagen in regulating collagen production. *Biochem. J.* 276:307–313.

McNeal, C.J., C.J. Meininger, C.D. Wilborn, C.D. Tekwe, and G. Wu. 2018. Safety of dietary supplementation with arginine in adult humans. *Amino Acids* 50:1215–1229.

McNurlan, M.A. and P.J. Garlick. 1980. Contribution of rat liver and gastrointestinal tract to whole-body protein synthesis in the rat. *Biochem. J.* 186:381–383.

Millward, D.J. and P.C. Bates. 1983. 3-Methylhistidine turnover in the whole body, and the contribution of skeletal muscle and intestine to urinary 3-methylhistidine excretion in the adult rat. *Biochem. J.* 214:607–615.

Mizushima, N. and M. Komatsu. 2011. Autophagy---renovation of cells and tissues. *Cell* 147:728–741.

Mortimore, G.E. and A.R. Pösö. 1987. Intracellular protein catabolism and its control during nutrient deprivation and supply. *Annu. Rev. Nutr.* 7:539–564.

Mulvaney, D.R., R.A. Merkel, and W.G. Bergen. 1985. Skeletal muscle protein turnover in young male pigs. *J. Nutr.* 115:1057.

Newsholme, E.A., P. Newsholme, and R. Curi. 1987. The role of the citric acid cycle in cells of the immune system and its importance in sepsis, trauma and burns. *Biochem. Soc. Symp.* 54:145–162.

Noguchi, M., N. Hirata, T. Tanaka, F. Suizu, H. Nakajima, and J.A. Chiorini. 2020. Autophagy as a modulator of cell death machinery. *Cell Death Dis.* 11:517.

Pacy, P.J., G.M. Price, O. Halliday, and D.J. Millward. 1994. Nitrogen homeostasis in man---the diurnal responses of protein synthesis and degradation and amino acid oxidation for diets with increasing protein intakes. *Clin. Sci.* 86:103–118.

Palmer, R.M., P.A. Bain, and P.J. Reeds. 1985. The effect of insulin and intermittent mechanical stretching on rates of protein synthesis and degradation in isolated rabbit muscle. *Biochem. J.* 230:117–123.

Pencharz, P.B., M. Masson, F. Desgranges, and A. Papageorgiou. 1981. Total-body protein turnover in human premature neonates---Effects of birth weight, intra-uterine nutritional status and diet. *Clin. Sci.* 61:207–15.

Petersen, S.B., F.S. Nielsen, U. Ribel, J. Sturis, and O. Skyggebjerg. 2013. Comparison of the pharmacokinetics of three concentrations of insulin aspart during continuous subcutaneous insulin infusion (CSII) in a pig model. *J. Pharm. Pharmacol.* 65:230–235.

Phang, J.M., W. Liu, and O. Zabirnyk. 2010. Proline metabolism and microenvironment. *Annu. Rev. Nutr.* 30:441–463.

Prinsen, B.H.C.M.T. and M.G.M. de Sain-van der Velden. 2004. Albumin turnover---experimental approach and its application in health and renal disease. *Clin. Chim. Acta* 347:1–14.

Rathmacher, J.A. and S.L. Nissen. 1998. Development and application of a compartmental model of 3-methylhistidine metabolism in humans and domestic animals. *Adv. Exp. Med. Biol.* 445:303–324.

Rattan, S.I. 2010. Synthesis, modification and turnover of proteins during aging. *Adv. Exp. Med. Biol.* 694:1–13.

Rawlings, R.D. and AJ Barrett. 1993. Evolutionary families of metallopeptidases. *Biochem. J.* 290:205–218.

Rawlings, N.D., A.J. Barrett, and A. Bateman. 2012. MEROPS---the database of proteolytic enzymes, their substrates and inhibitors. *Nucleic Acids Res.* 40:D343–D350.

Reeds, P.J. and T.A. Davis. 1999. Off flux and flooding---the advantages and problems of different isotopic methods for quantifying protein turnover in vivo---I. Methods based on the dilution of a tracer. *Curr. Opin. Clin. Nutr. Metab. Care.* 2:23–28.

Richard, I., O. Broux, V. Allamand, F. Fougerousse, N. Chiannilkulchai, N. Bourg et al. 1995. Mutations in the proteolytic enzyme calpain 3 cause limb-girdle muscular dystrophy type 2A. *Cell* 81:27–40.

Rivett, A.J. 1990. Intracellular protein degradation. *Essays Biochem.* 25:39–81.

Robins, S.P. 2007. Biochemistry and functional significance of collagen cross-linking. *Biochem. Soc. Trans.* 35:849–852.

Rogers, S., R. Wells, and M. Rechsteiner. 1986. Amino acid sequences common to rapidly degraded proteins--- the PEST hypothesis. *Science* 234:364–368.

Romero, N., D. Tinker, D. Hyde, and R.B. Rucker. 1986. Role of plasma and serum proteases in the degradation of elastin. *Arch. Biochem. Biophys.* 244:161–168.

Roshal, M. 2013. Thrombin time and fibrinogen determination. In: *Transfusion Medicine and Hemostasis*, 2nd edition (Shaz, B.H., C.D., Hillyer, M., Roshal, and C.S. Abrams, eds). Elsevier, New York, pp. 793–798.

Sandri, M. 2013. Protein breakdown in muscle wasting: Role of autophagy-lysosome and ubiquitin-proteasome. *Int. J. Biochem. Cell Biol.* 45:2121–2129.Saftig, P. and R. Puertollano. 2021. How lysosomes sense, integrate, and cope with stress. *Trends Biochem. Sci.* 46:97–112.

Salsas-Escat, R., P.S. Nerenberg, and C.M. Stultz. 2010. Cleavage site specificity and conformational selection in type I collagen degradation. *Biochemistry* 49:4147–4158.

Schoenheimer, R. and D. Rittenberg. 1940. The study of intermediary metabolism of animals with the aid of isotopes. *Physiol. Rev.* 20:218–248.

Shaid, S., C.H. Brandts, H. Serve, and I. Dikic. 2013. Ubiquitination and selective autophagy. *Cell. Death Differ.* 20:21–30.

Shalini, S., L. Dorstyn, S. Dawar, and S. Kumar. 2015. Old, new and emerging functions of caspases. *Cell Death Differ.* 22:526–539.

Sihvo, H., K. Immonen, and E. Puolanne. 2014. Myodegeneration with fibrosis and regeneration in the pectoralis major muscle of broilers. *Vet. Pathol.* 51:619–623.

Stack, T., P.J. Reeds, T. Preston, S. Hay, D.J. Lloyd, and P.J. Aggett. 1989. ^{15}N tracer studies of protein metabolism in low birth weight preterm infants---A comparison of ^{15}N glycine and ^{15}N yeast protein hydrolysate and of human milk- and formula-fed babies. *Pediatr. Res.* 25:167–172.

Strzyz, P. 2020. Collagen around the clock. *Nat. Rev. Mol. Cell Biol.* 21:120–121.

Swanson, J.A., Watts, C. 1995. Macropinocytosis. *Trends Cell Biol.* 5:424–428.

Swick, R.W. and H. Song. 1974. Turnover rates of various muscle proteins. *J. Anim. Sci.* 38:1150–1157.

Tan, B.E., Y.L. Yin, X.F. Kong, P. Li, X.L. Li, H.J. Gao et al. 2010. L-Arginine stimulates proliferation and prevents endotoxin-induced death of intestinal cells. *Amino Acids* 38:1227–1235.

Tasaki, T., S.M. Sriram, K.S. Park, and Y.T. Kwon. 2012. The N-end rule pathway. *Annu. Rev. Biochem.* 81:261–289.

Tesseraud, S., A.M. Chagneau, and J. Grizard. 2000. Muscle protein turnover during early development in chickens divergently selected for growth rate. *Poultry Sci.* 79:1465–1471.

Tian, S. and V.E. Baracos. 1989. Prostaglandin-dependent muscle wasting during infection in the broiler chick (Gallus domesticus) and the laboratory rat (Rattus norvegicus). *Biochem. J.* 263:485–490.

Thompson, J.R., and G. Wu. 1991. The effect of ketone bodies on nitrogen metabolism in skeletal muscle. *Comp. Biochem. Physiol.* 100B:209–216.

Tiao, G.., J.M. Fagan, V. Roegner, M. Lieberman, J.J. Wang, J.E. Fischer, and P.O. Hasselgren. 1996. Energy-ubiquitin-dependent muscle proteolysis during sepsis is regulated by glucocorticoids, *J. Clin. Invest.* 97:339–348.

Tischler, M., M. Desautels, and A.L. Goldberg. 1982. Does leucine, leucyl tRNA or some metabolite of leucine regulate protein synthesis and degradation in skeletal and cardiac muscle. *J. Biol. Chem.* 257:1613–1621.

Toyama, B.H. and M.W. Hetzer. 2013. Protein homeostasis---Live long, won't prosper. *Nat. Rev Mol. Cell Biol.* 14:55–61.

Trivedi, P.C., J.J. Bartlett, and T. Pulinilkunnil. 2020. Lysosomal biology and function---Modern view of cellular debris bin. *Cells* 9:1131.

Varshavsky, A. 2012. The ubiquitin system, an immense realm. *Annu. Rev. Biochem.* 81:167–176.

VerPlank, J.J.S. and A.L. Goldberg. 2017. Regulating protein breakdown through proteasome phosphorylation. *Biochem. J.* 474:3355–3371.

VerPlank, J.J.S., S. Lokireddy, J. Zhao, and A.L. Goldberg. 2019. 26S Proteasomes are rapidly activated by diverse hormones and physiological states that raise cAMP and cause Rpn6 phosphorylation. *Proc. Natl. Acad. Sci. USA.* 116:4228–4237.

Vom Dahl, S., C. Hallbrucker, F. Lang, W. Gerok, and D. Häussinger. 1991 Regulation of liver cell volume and proteolysis by glucagon and insulin. *Biochem. J.* 278:771–777.

Xu, S., H. Xu, W. Wang, S. Li, H. Li, T. Li et al. 2019. The role of collagen in cancer---from bench to bedside. *J. Transl. Med.* 17:309.

Waterlow, J.C. 1984. Protein turnover with special reference to man. *Q. J. Exp. Physiol.* 69:409–438.

Waterlow, J.C. 1995. Whole-body protein turnover in humans – Past, present, and future. *Annu. Rev. Nutr.* 15:57–92.

Wing, S.S., A.L. Haas, and A.L. Goldberg. 1995. Increase in ubiquitin-protein conjugates concomitant with the increase in proteolysis in rat skeletal muscle during starvation and atrophy denervation, *Biochem. J.* 307:639–645.

Wu, G. 1997. Synthesis of citrulline and arginine from proline in enterocytes of postnatal pigs. *Am. J. Physiol.* 272:G1382–G1390.

Wu, G. 2018. *Principles of Animal Nutrition.* CRC Press, Boca Raton, FL.

Wu, G. and C.J. Meininger. 2008. Analysis of citrulline, arginine, and methylarginines using high-performance liquid chromatography. *Methods Enzymol.* 440:177–189.

Wu, G. and J.R. Thompson. 1990. The effect of glutamine on protein turnover in chick skeletal muscle in vitro. *Biochem. J.* 265:593–598.

Wu, G., F.W. Bazer, G.A. Johnson, D.A. Knabe, R.C. Burghardt, T.E. Spencer et al. 2011. Important roles for L-glutamine in swine nutrition and production. *J. Anim. Sci.* 89:2017–2030.

Young, V.R. and H.N. Munro. 1978. N^τ-Methylhistidine (3-methylhistidine) and muscle protein turnover---an overview. *Fed. Proc.* 37:2291–2300.

Young, V.R., S.D. Alexis, B.S. Baliga, H.N. Munro, and W. Muecke. 1972. Metabolism of administered 3-methylhistidine. Lack of muscle transfer ribonucleic acid charging and quantitative excretion as 3-methylhistidine and its N-acetyl derivative. *J. Biol. Chem.* 247:3592–3600.

Zhang, J.M., W.L. He, D. Yi, D. Zhao, Z. Song, Y.Q. Hou, and G. Wu. 2019. Regulation of protein synthesis in porcine mammary epithelial cells by L-valine. *Amino Acids* 51:717–726.

10 Regulation of Amino Acid Metabolism

A metabolic pool of free amino acids (AAs) in organs (e.g., skeletal muscle, liver, and kidneys), tissues (e.g., the blood, white adipose tissue, and skin), cells (e.g., hepatocytes, macrophages, and lymphocytes), and intracellular organelles (e.g., cytoplasm and mitochondria) is relatively constant in healthy individuals at a given developmental stage (Figure 10.1). This reflects the fine balance between the supply of AAs (exogenous and endogenous) and their utilization. In the postabsorptive state, the concentrations of AAs [including nutritionally essential AAs (EAAs) and so-called nutritionally non-essential AAs (NEAAs)] in the plasma and tissues do not fluctuate substantially so as to maintain desirable concentration gradients between the plasma and tissues or cells (Hou et al. 2020; Jungas et al. 1992; Li et al. 2020; Wester et al. 2015). As illustrated in studies with *rapidly growing pigs, concentrations of most AAs in cells and tissues (except for arginine in the mammalian liver)* are much greater than those in the plasma (Table 10.1). It is noteworthy that concentrations of free AAs in the plasma and tissues vary with species, developmental stage, nutritional state, endocrine status, physical activity, time of the day, and diseased condition (Brosnan 2003; Gilbreath et al. 2021; Gill et al. 1989; Li et al. 2021; Wheatley et al. 2014).

In 1932, W.B. Cannon coined the term "homeostasis", which is defined as a relatively constant state of the body. In other words, homeostasis is the maintenance of the composition of the internal environment that is essential for health, which includes the balances of AAs, ammonia, proteins, carbohydrates (including glucose), lipids, water, acid–base, and electrolytes in the organism (Baker 2005; Burrin and Davis 2004; He and Wu 2020; Wu 2020). Disturbance of homeostasis for either a short or prolonged period of time may result in diseases and even death. Clinical examples in human medicine are hypoargininemia, hyperammonemia, hypercysteinemia, and endothelial dysfunction.

Because of alterations in the rates of AA metabolism brought about by changes in the hormonal and developmental status, circulating levels of many AAs vary greatly during fetal and neonatal periods, as well as under catabolic conditions and in disease. In addition, results of recent studies indicate dynamic changes of free AA concentrations in milk, the skeletal muscle of lactating mammals, and fetal fluids during pregnancy (Agostoni et al. 2000; Wu 2009). For example, concentrations of free glutamine in sow's milk increase from 0.1 to 4 mM between Days 1 and 21 of lactation (Wu and Knabe 1994), and those in ovine allantoic fluid increase from 0.1 to 25 mM between Days 30 and 60 of gestation (Kwon et al. 2003). By contrast, intramuscular concentrations of glutamine decrease by >50% in lactating sows and mares, as well as in humans and other animals with injury and sepsis because of the enhanced release of glutamine from skeletal muscle (Watford 2015). Additionally, arginine, ornithine, and citrulline are unusually abundant in porcine allantoic fluid (e.g., 4–6 mM arginine on Day 40 of pregnancy) and ovine allantoic fluid (e.g., 10 mM citrulline

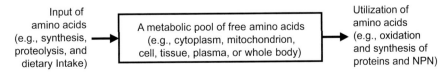

FIGURE 10.1 Regulation of homeostasis of free amino acids by their input and utilization in a metabolic pool, which can be an organ, a tissue, a cell, and an intracellular organelle. The free pool of amino acids is relatively constant in healthy individuals at a given developmental stage. NPN, non-protein nitrogenous substances.

TABLE 10.1

Concentrations of Free Amino Acids in the Plasma, Tissues, and Whole Body of 42-Day-Old Pigs and the Content of Peptide-Bound Amino Acids (PAAs) in Their Skeletal Muscle[a]

Amino acids (AAs)	Free AA in plasma (nmol/mL)	Free AA in tissues or the whole body (nmol/g wet weight of tissue)					PAA in GM muscle or the body (mg/g wet weight of tissue)	
		GM muscle	Brain	Liver	Jejunal mucosa	Whole body	GM muscle	Whole body
Ala	481	1,392	1,021	4,120	2,258	1,046	12.2	9.32
Arg	124	164	121	72	966	126	14.1	9.71
Asp	30	125	2,097	1,506	1,405	139	10.7	5.15
Asn	112	129	134	823	763	102	8.54	6.14
Cys[b]	143	84	203	213	187	65	3.11	1.89
Gln	536	4,581	7,830	3,586	1,149	3,427	10.9	6.75
Glu	103	1,532	8,977	4,017	3,920	1,085	18.6	12.1
Gly	1,072	2,546	1,186	6,854	2,816	1,911	7.50	16.8
His	76	212	105	797	709	158	6.27	2.96
Hyp	62	45	17	30	13	17	0.66	5.42
Ile	131	78	101	304	424	61	10.6	5.07
Leu	162	121	190	616	738	93	16.5	9.81
Lys	108	139	102	497	986	106	15.2	8.64
Met	85	64	79	98	297	50	5.81	2.68
Phe	113	106	128	217	440	82	10.1	4.92
Pro	242	1,836	907	5,033	1,283	1,372	8.02	12.2
Ser	174	254	889	1,159	2,455	191	8.70	6.32
Thr	191	368	1,470	914	831	283	9.74	5.02
Trp	70	53	39	112	203	40	2.73	1.59
Tyr	105	118	124	253	368	88	7.66	3.90
Val	170	126	126	657	1,075	97	12.0	6.04
GABA	0.74	1.8	1,854	69	12	124	–	–
β-Ala	12	749	66	428	16	566	–	–
Cit	76	98	59	60	204	75	–	–
Orn	72	80	32	446	817	129	–	–
Tau	52	9,624	2,816	10,526	10,849	7,338	–	–

[a] Pigs (offspring of Yorkshire × Landrace dams and Duroc × Hampshire sires) were fed a corn- and soybean meal–based diet containing 21% crude protein. At 42 days of age, blood samples were obtained from the jugular vein at 4 h after feeding. Thereafter, pigs were euthanized to obtain tissues for the analyses of free and peptide-bound amino acids (AAs). The content of each AA was calculated on the basis of its intact molecular weight. The content of dry matter was 25% (g/g) in the GM muscle, brain, and liver and was 22% in the jejunal mucosa. The content of true proteins plus peptides in the GM muscle and the whole body was 17.2% and 14.2% of fresh wet tissue weight, respectively.

[b] Total cysteine (cysteine + ½ cystine).

Notes: Cit, citrulline; DM, dry matter; GM, gastrocnemius; GABA, γ-aminobutyrate; Hyp, 4-hydroxyproline; JN, jejunum; Orn, ornithine; PAA, peptide-bound AA (AA in proteins plus peptides); Tau, taurine.

on Day 60 of pregnancy) during early to mid-gestation, compared with their plasma concentrations (e.g., 0.1–0.2 mM arginine and citrulline) (Kwon et al. 2003). Notably, these three AAs plus glutamine represent approximately 70% of total α-AA nitrogen in allantoic and amniotic fluids. A great increase (up to 80-fold) in the concentrations of the arginine family of AAs in allantoic fluid occurs during the most rapid period of placental growth. Also, the concentration of serine in ovine allantoic fluid increases from 0.51 mM on Day 30 of pregnancy to 16.5 mM on Day 140 of pregnancy when serine contributes to 60% of total α-AAs in this fetal fluid (Kwon et al. 2003). Furthermore, the total recoverable amounts of glutamine, leucine, and isoleucine in ovine uterine flushings increase by 20-, 3-, and 14-fold, respectively, between Days 10 and 15 of pregnancy, whereas those of arginine, histidine, ornithine, and lysine increase 8-, 22-, 5-, and 28-fold, respectively, between Days 10 and 16 of gestation (Gao 2020). Such dynamic changes of AA concentrations, along with the homeostasis of AAs, in physiological fluids, occur as a result of the complex and exquisite regulation of AA metabolism (including intracellular protein turnover) in a cell-, tissue-, and species-specific manner. Thus, the quantitative analysis of metabolic control in health and disease is an important area of biochemical research. The major objective of this chapter is to highlight the cellular mechanisms [including the mechanistic target of rapamycin (MTOR) cell signaling] responsible for the regulation of AA metabolism (including protein turnover) in humans and other animals.

10.1 BASIC CONCEPTS IN METABOLISM

10.1.1 Chemical Reactions

The general principles of chemical reactions apply to enzyme-catalyzed reactions in cells and cell-free systems. In a chemical reaction that occurs with no change in the volume of the system, the reaction rate (or velocity) equals the change in concentration of product per unit time. Based on kinetics, there are at least five chemical reaction orders, most of which are relevant to cell metabolism in animals.

Zero-order reaction: The rate of product formation is independent of the substrate concentration but dependent on time.

First-order reaction: The rate of product formation is directly proportional to the substrate (S) concentration $v \propto [S]$.

Second-order reaction: The rate of product formation either depends directly on the concentration of two substrates (S1 and S2) or depends on the square of the concentration of a single substrate (S) $v \propto [S1] \times [S2]$, or $v \propto [S]^2$.

Mixed-order reaction: The rate of product formation depends on the concentration of a reactant raised to a fractional power due to changes in variables (e.g., pH), $v \propto [S]^{1/n}$, $n \geq 2$.

Higher-order reaction: The rate of product formation depends on the concentration of one or more reactants raised to a power greater than 2, $v \propto [S]^n$, $n > 2$; or $v \propto [S_1]^{n1}[S_2]^{n2}$, $n1 + n2 > 2$.

Transmembrane AA transport (e.g., the uptake of aspartate, glutamate, and glycine by enterocytes across their apical membranes) and many reactions of AA metabolism (e.g., intracellular protein turnover, glutamine synthesis, and the urea cycle) require energy and/or reducing equivalents, whereas others produce ATP and/or reducing equivalents (Wu 2018). ATP is the major form of chemical energy that can be converted into all other forms of energy used by living organisms. Therefore, ATP has been described as the "energy currency" of the cell. The ratio of $[ATP]/([ADP]+[AMP])$ is often used to describe the cellular energy status. Some enzymes for AA synthesis and degradation depend on NADH/NAD$^+$ or NADPH/NADP$^+$ as cofactors [e.g., pyrroline-5-carboxylate + NADPH + H$^+$ → proline + NADP$^+$]. An alteration in the redox state is an important mechanism that regulates the synthesis and catabolism of AAs in cells. Additionally, cellular redox signaling affects gene expression and, therefore, the metabolic network (Phang et al. 2010; Wang et al. 2012).

10.1.2 Laws of Thermodynamics as Applied to Amino Acid Metabolism

Thermodynamics was originally applied to physics and engineering, and the laws were formulated to describe the properties of devices such as heat engines (Alberty 2004). The first and second laws of thermodynamics also apply equally well to animals with constant temperature and pressure but the emphasis is somewhat different. For example, there is less emphasis on temperature and pressure in metabolic thermodynamics. The third law of thermodynamics states that the entropy of a pure crystalline substance at absolute zero temperature (0 K) is zero; this law does not apply to animal metabolism and, therefore, is not discussed in this chapter.

10.1.2.1   The First Law of Thermodynamics

The first law of thermodynamics is the law of energy conservation. Any energy that is released by the system (e.g., an animal) must be gained by its surroundings (e.g., the environment). Thus, energy can neither be created nor be destroyed, it can only be converted from one form into another. (Remember that there is no production of energy in humans and other animals!) In other words, the change in chemical energy (internal energy) when one mole of substance A is converted into B is equal to the heat produced plus the work done on the system or the heat consumed plus the work done by the system. The energy absorbed in the forward reaction is equal to the energy released in the reverse reaction. The first law of thermodynamics can be expressed mathematically as:

$$\Delta E = q + w$$

ΔE is the change (Δ) in the internal chemical energy of the system (e.g., chemical reactions, cells, tissues, or animals), q is the heat absorbed by the system, and w is the work done on the system. ΔE is a state function.

When the pressure (P) of the system is constant and its volume (V) may occur (the conditions that likely apply to metabolic reactions in cells, tissues, and animals), the work done on the system can be expressed as follows:

$$w = -P\Delta V$$

The total energy content (enthalpy, H) of the system equals the internal energy of the system plus the product of the system's pressure and volume. The mathematical relationship among enthalpy, internal energy, pressure, and volume of the system can be described as follows:

$$H = E + PV$$

When the pressure of the system is constant and its volume may change, the change in enthalpy of the system (ΔH) can be expressed by the following equation:

$$\Delta H = \Delta E + P\Delta V = q + w + P\Delta V$$

At constant pressure, if there is no change in the volume of the system (i.e., $\Delta V = 0$ and $P\Delta V = 0$),

$$\Delta H = q + w + P\Delta V = q + w$$

Note that $w = 0$ at constant volume for $w = -P\Delta V$, and then $\Delta H = q$.

Similarly, the above equations can also be rearranged into the enthalpy expression at constant pressure, with the same result.

$$\Delta H = \Delta E + P\Delta V = q + w - w = q$$

Like ΔE, ΔH is independent of the chemical pathway by which a process is carried out and depends only on the differences in chemical energy before and after the process has occurred (Newsholme 1984). For example, whether glucose is oxidized either by burning in oxygen in a calorimeter or by a series of biochemical reactions including the glycolysis and Krebs cycle in the brain, ΔH is the same. This is because these processes involve the same substrates and generate the same products, namely, Glucose $+ 6O_2 \rightarrow 6CO_2 + 6H_2O$.

In an insulated system (e.g., a bomb calorimeter) that has no exchange of matter or energy with its surroundings, the whole enthalpy change of the system appears as heat. This is the principle for the use of the bomb calorimeter to measure the total energy content of AAs, proteins, lipids, carbohydrates, metabolites, and foods. Specifically, ΔH values are calculated from the heat produced when a substance or a foodstuff is combusted with excess O_2 in a bomb calorimeter. Thus, all the carbon is oxidized to CO_2, all the hydrogen to H_2O, and all N to nitrogen oxide. In combustion, the oxidation of an AA or a protein is complete with the production of water, CO_2, and nitrogen oxide, whereas AA oxidation is incomplete in animals with nitrogen excreted in the forms of ammonia, urea, uric acid, creatine, and other nitrogenous metabolites. Because of the differences in the end products of combustion and the oxidation of AAs in animals, the biological values of ΔH for AAs are much lower than those obtained from combustion. This is important in calculating the biological energy of AAs and protein in food and in estimating the efficiency of metabolic transformations of AAs in animals (Chapter 4).

10.1.2.2   The Second Law of Thermodynamics

The key to understanding direction and equilibrium in chemical reactions is the second law of thermodynamics, which introduces the concept of change in entropy (ΔS). Spontaneous reactions always proceed with an increase in total entropy (i.e., $\Delta S > 0$). Like enthalpy, entropy's value depends only on the state of a system and not on the route by which it arrives at that state (Newsholme 1984). We can state the second law of thermodynamics as "all processes proceed in a direction that increases the total entropy".

In a formal mathematical term, entropy is the heat (q) absorbed in a thermodynamically reversible reaction (at T K) divided by the absolute temperature (T expressed as Kelvin temperature), namely, $\Delta S = q/T$.

10.1.2.3   The Concept of Free Energy Unifies the First and Second Laws of Thermodynamics

Although the total entropy change is a sufficient criterion upon which to establish which process can and cannot occur, it is not always easy to measure the changes in the entropy of both the reactants and the environment. A change in Gibbs free energy (ΔG), which was originally developed in the 1870s by the American mathematician J.W. Gibbs, defines the equilibrium condition in terms of the enthalpy and entropy of the system at constant temperature and pressure (the conditions that likely apply to the metabolic reactions in cells, tissues, and animals). The *free* energy refers to the available energy that does useful work in a chemical reaction.

$$\Delta G = \Delta H - T\Delta S$$

ΔG: the Gibbs free energy change; ΔH: the enthalpy change; ΔS: the entropy change.
T: Kelvin temperature.

Thus, the Gibbs free energy change provides a unifying principle in thermodynamics. ΔG can be positive, negative, or zero.

If $\Delta G < 0$, the process is spontaneous and is called exergonic.
If $\Delta G > 0$, the process is not spontaneous and is called endergonic.
If $\Delta G = 0$, the system is at equilibrium (no change in free energy and no net flux through a reaction).

$$\Delta G = \Delta G^o + RT \ln X \text{ or } \Delta G = \Delta G^o + 2.3RT \log X$$

ΔG^o: standard free energy change.

$X = [B]/[A]$ (X is a mass action ratio at a given time)

for a reaction involving only one substrate and one product: $A \leftrightarrow B$;

where A is the substrate and B is the product;

for a reaction involving two substrates and two products: $A + 2C \leftrightarrow B + 2D$;

$$X = \left([B] \times [D]^2\right) \big/ \left([A] \times [C]^2\right) \qquad \left(X \text{ is a mass action ratio at a given time}\right),$$

where A and C are substrates, B and D are products, and the number "2" refers to the moles of the given substrate and product.

R: Gas constant (1.987 cal/(K × mol) or 8.314 J/(K × mol). (1 cal = 4.1842 J).

T: Kelvin temperature (K). (37°C = 310 K; 25°C = 298 K; 0°C = 273 K).

At equilibrium, $\Delta G = 0$, and $\Delta G° = -2.3\ RT \log X$.

Note that $\Delta G°'$ (standard free energy change measured at pH 7.0, 25°C, pressure 1 atm, concentrations of all reactants and products at 1 M except for 55.6 M water) is often used to replace $\Delta G°$ in a biological reaction. Values of $\Delta G°$ or $\Delta G°'$ for many reactions involving AAs can be found in the biochemistry literature.

The mass action ratio equals the equilibrium constant when the concentrations of product(s) and reactant(s) are at equilibrium. Based on the second law of thermodynamics, changes in concentrations of substrates and products can affect the net flux through an enzyme-catalyzed reaction. Let us take ornithine aminotransferase (OAT) as an example.

$$\text{Pyrroline-5-carboxylate} \left(\text{P5C}\right) + \text{Glutamate} \leftrightarrow \text{Ornithine} + \alpha\text{-Ketoglutarate}$$

OAT favors either the formation of ornithine from P5C and glutamate or the catabolism of ornithine to generate P5C in the enterocyte depends on the concentrations of reactants of the reaction and the removal of its product via absorption into the portal circulation. An inborn deficiency of OAT causes: (1) hypoornithinemia (a risk factor for ammonia toxicity) in neonates who have low rates of intestinal syntheses of P5C by P5C synthase and of ornithine by arginase and (2) hyperornithinemia (a risk factor for retinal damage) in adults who have a relatively high rate of ornithine production from arginine by arginase in the small intestine and other tissues.

10.1.3 The Concept of Equilibrium in Biochemical Reactions

Biochemical reactions in AA metabolism are basic physiological events in animals (Newsholme 1984). Some reactions are reversible, but others are irreversible. The directionality of the reactions, which is affected by pH, temperature, electrical potential, and ionic strength, as well as the concentrations of reactants and products, plays a significant role in determining the net flux through a given metabolic pathway. Thus, it is important to understand the concept of equilibrium and non-equilibrium reactions. Consider the following hypothetical enzyme-catalyzed reaction in a closed system (no exchange of matter or energy with its surroundings):

$$A \underset{V_r}{\overset{V_f}{\rightleftharpoons}} B$$

Where A and B are reactants; V_f: rate of forward component; V_r: rate of reverse component.

The state, in which the rates of forward and reverse reactions are equal ($V_f = V_r$), is referred to as an equilibrium. An animal is an example of an open thermodynamic system, in which there is a continuous exchange of both matter and energy with its surroundings. In metabolic pathways, some reactions (e.g., most AA transamination reactions) are close to equilibrium ($V_f \approx V_r$), and some (e.g., AA decarboxylation) are far removed from equilibrium ($V_f \gg V_r$, or $V_f \ll V_r$). The equilibrium constant (K_{eq}) is defined as the ratio of concentrations of product and substrate when the reaction is at equilibrium. Under this condition, there is no net work done and no change in ΔG. The equilibrium constant depends on only the stoichiometry of the reaction, not on its mechanism.

$$K_{eq} = \left[B_{eq}\right]/\left[A_{eq}\right] \text{ at equilibrium; for the reaction: } A \leftrightarrow B$$

$$\text{Note: mass action ratio} = [B]/[A]$$

$$K_{eq} = \left(\left[B_{eq}\right] \times \left[D_{eq}\right]^2\right)/\left(\left[A_{eq}\right] \times \left[C_{eq}\right]^2\right) \text{ at equilibrium; for the reaction: } A + 2C \leftrightarrow B + 2D.$$

$$\text{Note: mass action ratio for the above reaction} = \left([B] \times [D]^2\right)/\left([A] \times [C]^2\right)$$

Water and H^+ participate in many biochemical reactions, and they must be considered to balance equations. The concentration of water is 55.6 M [i.e., (1 g × 1000)/(18 × 1 L) = 55.6], whereas the concentrations of H^+ at pH 7.0 and 7.4 are 100 and 40 nM, respectively. If water is the solvent in a chemical reaction, it is not included in K_{eq} calculation. Note that substances whose concentrations are constant during the course of a chemical reaction do not appear in K_{eq} expression. Thus, if water is a reactant or product in an aqueous solution (i.e., water as the solvent), the amount of water as a reactant or product of a chemical reaction is insignificant relative to the amount of water as the solvent, and water concentration rarely changes during the course of the chemical reaction; under these conditions (as occurring in animals and cells), water concentration is considered to be unity or one (1) and is omitted from K_{eq} expression. For example, for the spontaneous dissociation of water ($H_2O \leftrightarrow H^+ + OH^-$), $K_{eq} = ([H^+] \times [OH^-])/[H_2O] = [H^+] \times [OH^-]/1 = [H^+] \times [OH^-]$. In calculating K_{eq} for a reaction, the units of concentrations of substrate(s) and products(s) should be expressed consistently, and the K_{eq} itself does not have any units.

10.1.4 Near-Equilibrium (Reversible) and Non-Equilibrium (Irreversible) Reactions

Reactions in metabolic pathways for AA metabolism can be divided into near-equilibrium (close to equilibrium or reversible reaction in cells) and non-equilibrium (far removed from equilibrium or irreversible reaction in cells). Near-equilibrium reactions are often loosely called equilibrium reactions. A non-equilibrium reaction that is saturated with a pathway substrate may be a flux-generating reaction. Let's consider the following hypothetical reaction in a metabolic pathway.

$$E1 \qquad E2 \qquad E3$$

$$S \underset{0.01}{\overset{10.01}{\rightleftharpoons}} A \underset{90}{\overset{100}{\rightleftharpoons}} B \underset{0.1}{\overset{10.1}{\rightleftharpoons}} P$$

In this enzyme-catalyzed pathway, the initial substrate (S) is converted to its product (A). The intermediate B is formed from A and is continuously converted to P (product). The metabolic significance of near-equilibrium reactions is: (1) allowing an easy reversal of the pathway; (2) conferring relatively high rates of reactions; and (3) providing sensitivity for the regulation of flux through a pathway. Small changes in the concentrations of substrates or products can produce large changes in the metabolic flux. For example, in the $E2$ step, if the forward reaction is increased by 10% due to an increase in [A] or the removal of the intermediate B without a change in the backward reaction, the next flux would double. Thus, the removal of products or substrates determines both the directionality and net flux of the equilibrium reactions. For comparison, the metabolic significance of non-equilibrium reactions is: (1) providing directionality in a metabolic pathway; (2) providing potential sites for the regulation of flux by biological factors (e.g., allosteric factors); and (3) maintaining the concentrations of intermediates while allowing for the rapid transmission of changes in flux through the pathway.

10.1.5 ENZYMES IN BIOCHEMICAL REACTIONS

10.1.5.1 Enzymes as Biological Catalysts

In 1877, the German physiologist Wilhelm Kühne first coined the term "enzyme" as a substance to facilitate the fermentation of sugar to alcohol by yeast. Enzymes are biological catalysts. Most of the enzymes are protein in nature, while certain RNAs have catalytic activity and these RNA molecules are called ribozymes (Johnston et al. 2001). The significance of enzymes in living organisms is not just that of catalysis. The existence of enzymes not only increases the rates of metabolic processes but also enables them to be regulated. As a result of this regulation, individual reactions and metabolic pathways can be integrated into the overall metabolic system which functions so effectively in the whole organism that the homeostasis of AAs, protein, and other nutrients can be precisely maintained in healthy animals. The properties of enzymes include substrate specificity, denaturation, pH dependence, temperature dependence, activation, and inhibition.

Enzyme kinetics are determined extracellularly (e.g., a test tube) using either cell extracts or purified proteins in laboratory studies. The classic Michaelis–Menten equation describes a hyperbolic relationship between initial rate (i.e., catalytic activity) and substrate concentration.

$$V_i = \frac{V_{max}[S]}{K_m+[S]} \qquad \frac{1}{V_i} = \frac{K_m+[S]}{V_{max}[S]} \qquad \frac{1}{V_i} = \frac{K_m}{V_{max}} \times \frac{1}{[S]} + \frac{[S]}{V_{max}[S]}$$

V_{max}: maximum rate of reaction. K_m: Michaelis constant. K_m is defined as the substrate concentration at which the rate of reaction is half-maximal.

A K_m value allows for: (1) estimating the affinity of enzymes toward their substrates with a low or high K_m value indicating a high or low affinity of the enzyme toward the substrate, respectively; (2) assessing whether a particular enzyme plays a role in a metabolic pathway. When a K_m value of an enzyme for its substrate is 100 times the substrate concentration in the cell, it is unlikely that this reaction would have physiological relevance. By contrast, when a K_m value of an enzyme for its substrate is much lower than the intracellular concentration of the substrate (e.g., <1% of the substrate concentration in the cell), it is likely that this reaction is regulated by the availability of a cofactor rather than directly by the substrate. An example is NO synthesis from arginine by NO synthase in endothelial cells, where the K_m value of NO synthase for arginine is only $3\,\mu M$ but the concentrations of arginine are 1–2 mM depending on the concentration of arginine in the extracellular solution. It is now known that the intracellular concentration of tetrahydrobiopterin (an essential cofactor for NO synthase) plays a critical role in regulating NO synthesis by NO synthase in endothelial cells.

10.1.5.2 Reversible Inhibition of Enzymes

An enzyme can be inhibited by both endogenous and exogenous inhibitors. The main classes of reversible enzyme inhibition are known as competitive, non-competitive, and uncompetitive (Segel 1993). Removal of inhibitors can restore enzyme activities. These classes of enzyme inhibition can be distinguished by kinetics and the sites of action of inhibitors, as well as double reciprocal plots (also known as Lineweaver plots) (Figure 10.2).

10.1.5.2.1 Competitive Inhibition

Competitive inhibition occurs at the substrate binding (catalytic site). An inhibitor is usually a substrate analog. In competitive inhibition, K_m value is increased but V_{max} is not altered. Increasing substrate concentration can overcome competitive inhibition. In non-competitive inhibition, inhibitors bear no structural resemblance to the substrate and can bind reversibly either to the free enzyme or to the enzyme-substrate complex. V_{max} is decreased but K_m remains unaltered in non-competitive inhibition, which is usually reversible. An increase in substrate concentration generally does not relieve this type of enzyme inhibition. However, non-competitive inhibition can be alleviated or reversed by reducing the concentration of the inhibitor. In uncompetitive inhibition, an inhibitor

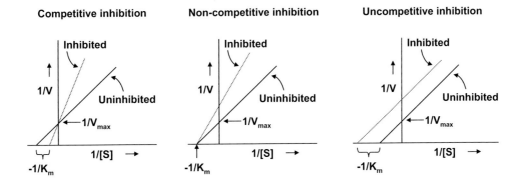

FIGURE 10.2   Double reciprocal plots (also known as Lineweaver–Burk plots) for competitive, non-competitive, and uncompetitive inhibition of enzyme-catalyzed reactions. These three kinds of reversible inhibition are characterized by different enzyme kinetics.

binds with the enzyme-substrate complex. Both K_m and V_{max} are altered in uncompetitive inhibition, which is rare for reactions with single substrates but may occur in multimeric enzymes. Uncompetitive inhibition generally cannot be relieved by increasing substrate concentration but can be reversed by reducing the concentration of the inhibitor.

The competitive inhibition of enzymes is characterized by an increase in K_m (example: inhibition of NOS by N^G-monomethylarginine, inhibition of dihydrofolate reductase by methotrexate, and inhibition of glutamine–fructose-6-phosphate transaminase by glucosamine-6-phosphate).

$$E+S \rightarrow ES$$
$$+$$
$$I$$
$$\downarrow$$
$$EI$$

10.1.5.2.2   Non-competitive Inhibition

Non-competitive inhibition of enzymes is characterized by a decrease in V_{max} (examples: inhibition of phosphofructokinase-I by ATP or citrate, inhibition of intestinal proline oxidase by L-lactate, and inhibition of pyruvate kinase by L-alanine). Some metals, such as arsenic, silver, mercury, and lead are non-competitive inhibitors of enzymes. For example, lead inhibits ferrochelatase, the enzyme that adds iron into protoporphyrin IX to generate heme.

$$E+S \rightarrow ES$$
$$+ \qquad +$$
$$I \qquad I$$
$$\downarrow \qquad \downarrow$$
$$EI \qquad ESI$$

10.1.5.2.3   Uncompetitive Inhibition

Uncompetitive inhibition of enzymes is characterized by decreases in both K_m and V_{max} [examples: inhibition of acylpeptide hydrolase (an enzyme that catalyzes the removal of acetyl-AAs from the N-terminus of peptides and cytoplasmic proteins) by a small peptide inhibitor such as trifluoro-acetylated tetrapeptide, inhibition of δ-aminolevulinate dehydratase by alloxan, and inhibition of acetylcholinesterase by tertiary amines (R_3N)].

10.1.5.3 Irreversible Inhibition of Enzymes

Enzymes can be irreversibly inhibited by substances that usually covalently modify the structures or AA residues of the enzymes. Irreversible inhibitors often contain electrophilic groups such as aldehydes, haloalkanes, alkenes, phenyl sulfonates, or fluorophosphonates. These reactive groups react with the side chains of AAs to form covalent adducts. An example of irreversible enzyme inhibition is the inactivation of acetylcholinesterase (the enzyme hydrolyzes the neurotransmitter acetylcholine) and chymotrypsin (a protease in the lumen of the small intestine) by diisopropylfluorophosphate (a nerve poison). In both enzymes, diisopropylfluorophosphate covalently modifies their active serine sites (e.g., serine-203 of acetylcholinesterase and serine-195 of chymotrypsin) (Pope et al. 2005).

Suicide inhibition is an unusual type of irreversible inhibition in that the enzyme converts the inhibitor into a reactive form in its active site. An example is the inhibition of ornithine decarboxylase (ODC) by α-difluoromethylornithine (DFMO; an analog of ornithine) to reduce the synthesis of polyamines from ornithine and treat African trypanosomiasis (sleeping sickness) (Fairlamb 2003). In this case, ODC catalyzes the decarboxylation of DFMO instead of ornithine followed by the elimination of a fluorine atom from DFMO to convert DFMO into a highly reactive conjugated imine. The latter then reacts with either a cysteine or a lysine residue in the active site of ODC to irreversibly inactivate the enzyme. The concentrations of intracellular polyamines in DFMO-treated cells can be restored through the provision of exogenous putrescine or its metabolites (spermidine and spermine), such as their addition to incubation medium or the oral administration of putrescine (Li et al. 2001; Liu et al. 2019).

10.1.6 Intracellular Compartmentation of Metabolic Pathways

A metabolic pathway can be defined as a series of enzyme-catalyzed reactions in which a molecule is either degraded to simpler products or synthesized from simpler precursors (Newsholme 1984). A pathway can be linear (such as arginine synthesis), cyclic (such as the urea cycle), or spiral (the synthesis of fatty acids from AA-derived acetyl-CoA). In fatty acid synthesis, the same set of enzymes is used repeatedly for chain lengthening. A physiologically useful definition of a metabolic pathway would be a series of enzyme-catalyzed reactions, initiated by flux-generating steps and ending with the formation of products. This latter definition indicates that a metabolic pathway may span more than one organ. For example, the pathway for the synthesis of arginine from glutamine could be considered to be initiated in the small intestine or skeletal muscle depending on the source of glutamine (arterial or enteral diet). An excellent example of intracellular compartmentation of a metabolic pathway is the urea cycle (Watford 2003). It involves both the mitochondrion and the cytosol. Within a compartment, enzymes are closely associated and sequentially pass intermediates along the pathway (Ovadi and Saks 2004). In the hepatic and intestinal urea cycle, the physiological significance of intracellular compartmentation of a metabolic pathway is evident in that ammonia produced in the mitochondrion is locally converted into citrulline, a non-toxic product, for export to the cytosol. Another example is arginine synthesis from glutamine in enterocytes (Wu and Morris 1998).

10.1.7 Metabolic Design Principles

Reading general biochemistry textbooks, students might be led to believe that: (1) all the important principles of metabolic control are well established; (2) metabolic pathways are sequential, isolated events; and (3) the control of a metabolic pathway resides only at a single step. It is worth pointing out that metabolism and its control are not as simplistic as the long-standing dogma of a "rate-limiting step" in a linear reaction sequence implies. John T. Brosnan (2005) states that the metabolic design principles are determined by physical and chemical constraints to minimize: (1) unwanted side reactions by maintaining very low levels of metabolic intermediates; (2) the occurrence of highly reactive chemical groups (e.g., aldehydes); (3) changes in pH, temperature, osmotic pressure, ammonia concentration, and solvent capacity; and (4) excess mass. Fortunately, animals (including humans) have evolved to develop mechanisms ensuring that metabolic chaos does not occur in animals. These mechanisms include: (1) the occurrence of highly active and specific enzymes that catalyze "desired" reactions; (2) compartmentation (e.g., metabolic channeling and reactions within organelles); (3) many rescue and repair reactions (e.g., DNA repair and defense against oxidative stress); and (4) positive and feedback regulation of enzyme-catalyzed reactions.

Two important concepts concerning metabolism have been advanced over the past four decades: distributive metabolic control and metabolon (the supramolecular organization of the enzymes in a single metabolic sequence). The theory of distributive metabolic control states that control can be distributed throughout the metabolic sequence or resides in one or more of the individual steps (Fell 1997). For example, control points for hepatic urea synthesis could be AA or ammonia transport, carbamoyl phosphate synthetase-I (CPS-I), and N-acetylglutamate (NAG) synthase. A metabolon has been defined as a pathway which is organized in a sequential association to convert a substrate into its product (Srere 1985). Isotope-based experimental evidence for this concept has come from the initial study of urea cycle enzymes in hepatocytes and experiments on other pathways, such as branched-chain AA (BCAA) catabolism via BCAA transaminase and branched-chain α-ketoacid (BCKA) dehydrogenase. The interdependence of all metabolic reactions can be demonstrated by the observation that the deletion of a single enzyme of a metabolic pathway results in many changes in a variety of pathways not directly related to the one being studied (Yu et al. 2019). An advantage of a metabolon is to facilitate the transfer of intermediates between enzymes and maintain a high concentration of a substrate in the catalytic site of an enzyme.

10.2   REGULATION OF AMINO ACID METABOLISM

The metabolism of AAs in cells is regulated by their transmembrane transport and the activities of the related enzymes under physiological or pathological conditions (Closs et al. 2006; Li et al. 2008, 2009; Newsholme 1984; Poulin et al. 1992; Strack et al. 1996). Long-term regulation of enzyme activity (i.e., in the order of days) is achieved primarily through changes in gene expression and protein synthesis, as well as protein degradation (Metallo and Vander Heiden 2013; Palii et al. 2009; Suryawan and Davis 2014; Wang et al. 2012). Concentrations of the enzymes with relatively short half-lives (e.g., ODC and tyrosine transaminase) are more sensitive to regulation by protein synthesis and proteolysis than those with relatively long half-lives (e.g., ornithine carbamoyltransferase, glutaminase, and arginase) in the rat liver. An increase in enzyme activity can be achieved by increasing the amount of enzyme protein, which is referred to as enzyme induction. Enzyme induction involves protein synthesis, namely the transcription of DNA to mRNA and the translation of mRNA to protein. Thus, the induction of most enzymes [except for some enzymes (e.g., ODC and the cytosolic δ-aminolevulinate synthetase with short half-lives of 11 min and 0.33 h, respectively)] in cells is generally a slow process. For example, the amount of arginase in the rat liver is increased slowly in response to feeding of high dietary protein (Chapter 6). Conversely, the inhibition of protein synthesis or the activation of protein degradation can result in a decrease in the abundance of enzyme protein.

For the short-term regulation of enzyme activity (i.e., in the order of seconds, minutes, or hours), both *in vitro* and *in vivo* studies of AA metabolism have demonstrated the following regulatory mechanisms in cells: (1) the allosteric regulation of enzymes; (2) the covalent modification of enzymes (e.g., protein phosphorylation, acetylation, methylation, and ubiquitination); (3) the concentrations of activators and inhibitors; (4) phosphorylation potential $[ATP/(ADP \times P_i)]$ or energy status; (5) the concentrations of substrates, cofactors, and products; (6) redox potential; (7) acyl-CoA potential; and (8) cell volume. Alterations in hormones, nutrition (dietary intake of protein, AAs, lipids, carbohydrates, energy, vitamins, and minerals), and cell volume can affect AA metabolism through one or more of these mechanisms (Metallo and Vander Heiden 2013). Because the regulation of gene expression is discussed in Chapter 11, the short-term mechanisms that regulate AA metabolism are detailed in the following sections.

10.2.1 Allosteric Regulation

Allosteric regulation, which was first described for microbial threonine deaminase and aspartate transcarbamylase in 1956, is defined as the regulation of an enzyme by an effector molecule which binds to a regulatory site on the protein other than its active site. Effectors that enhance or decrease enzyme activity are referred to as allosteric activators or inhibitors, respectively. For example, NAG and arginine are allosteric activators of CPS-I and NAG synthase, respectively (Meijer et al. 1990). Additionally, glutamate dehydrogenase is allosterically inhibited by GTP and ATP but activated by ADP and L-Leu (Brosnan and Brosnan 2012). L-Leucine enhances glutamate dehydrogenase activity, thereby stimulating energy metabolism in pancreatic β-cells and their release of insulin (Treberg et al. 2010). In many of the metabolic pathways for microbial AA synthesis, products are allosteric inhibitors of certain key enzymes.

Allosteric effects can be explained by the concerted Monod-Wyman-Changeux (MWC) model proposed by J. Monod, J. Wyman, and J.-P. Changeux in 1965 or by the sequential model described by D.E. Koshland, G. Nemethy, and D. Filmer in 1966. Both models postulate that: (1) the subunits of an enzyme can exist in one of two conformations [tensed (T) or relaxed (R)]; (2) relaxed subunits bind substrate(s) more rapidly than those in the tense state; and (3) conformational changes in the enzyme alter its catalytic activity. However, the two models differ most in their assumptions about subunit interaction and the preexistence of both states. First, the MWC model postulates that the subunits of an enzyme are all connected in such a way that a conformational change in one subunit will be conferred to all other subunits; therefore, all subunits must exist in the same conformation. Therefore, in the MWC model, the binding of an allosteric effector can result in an R or T conformational state. Second, the sequential model states that the subunits of an enzyme are not necessarily connected and may not have the same conformation. According to this model, binding of a substrate to one subunit can increase the affinity of adjacent subunits for the same substrate, thereby enhancing or decreasing enzyme activity.

10.2.2 Reversible Phosphorylation and Dephosphorylation of Protein

In 1906, P.A. Levene at the Rockefeller Institute for Medical Research reported the presence of phosphate in the protein vitellin (known as phosvitin). The same author, working with Fritz Lipmann, identified in 1933 phosphoserine in casein. Twenty years later, E.P. Kennedy at the University of Chicago described in 1954 the enzymatic phosphorylation of animal proteins (casein and mitochondrial proteins). In 1955, Edwin Krebs and Edmond Fischer discovered that radiolabeled ATP donates a phosphate group to the serine residue of muscle glycogen phosphorylase to convert the enzyme from its *b* (inactive) to *a* (active) form. Their subsequent work identified this phosphorylation as part of a protein kinase cascade. This seminal finding resulted in their winning the 1992 Nobel Prize in Physiology or Medicine. It is now known that the activities of some enzymes are regulated by reversible phosphorylation (addition of the phosphoryl group of ATP) and dephosphorylation (removal of a phosphoryl group by hydrolysis) of the enzyme proteins. Protein phosphorylation is catalyzed by a protein kinase (e.g., cAMP-dependent kinase), whereas protein dephosphorylation is performed by a protein phosphatase (Figure 10.3). The AA residues in a protein that are phosphorylated are tyrosine, serine, threonine, and histidine. The protein kinases catalyzing phosphorylation reactions constitute one of the largest protein families known to date, including more than 100 homologous enzymes in yeast and more than 550 in human beings (Manning et al. 2002). This multiplicity of enzymes permits the fine-tuned regulation of metabolic pathways in a tissue-, time-, and substrate-specific manner. Most protein kinases are highly specific for their substrates (proteins), but some have activities toward a broad spectrum of proteins.

Protein phosphorylation and dephosphorylation are not the reverses of one another. The phosphorylation and dephosphorylation mechanism does not involve an alteration in the amount of enzyme protein and therefore allows for the rapid modification of enzyme activity. Phosphorylation of a protein results in its conformational change, leading to the activation or inactivation of enzymatic

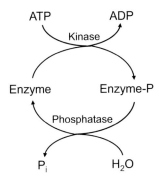

FIGURE 10.3 Regulation of enzyme activity by reversible phosphorylation (addition of the phosphoryl group of ATP) and dephosphorylation (removal of a phosphoryl group by hydrolysis). Protein phosphorylation is catalyzed by a protein kinase, whereas protein dephosphorylation is performed by a protein phosphatase. Protein phosphorylation may increase or decrease enzyme activity depending on individual proteins.

activity. Protein phosphorylation is a highly effective means to regulate the activities of proteins. The major characteristics of this reaction include: (1) modifying the protein structure and its activity from fully active to completely inactive or vice versa; (2) thermodynamically having large free energy to shift the direction of the reaction almost completely in favor of the formation of its products; (3) rapidly occurring in less than a second and lasting for a period of hours; (4) amplifying the action of a single kinase to phosphorylate many target proteins; and (5) linking the energy status of the cell to the regulation of nutrient metabolism.

Some enzymes in AA metabolism are known to undergo phosphorylation and dephosphorylation. Whether phosphorylation of an enzyme results in an increase or a decrease in its catalytic activity varies with individual enzymes. For example, BCKA dehydrogenase is inactivated by phosphorylation and activated by dephosphorylation (Harris et al. 2005). This enzyme is present mainly in the phosphorylated (inactive) form in the heart and skeletal muscle but in the dephosphorylated (active) form in the liver and kidneys. Some hormones (e.g., insulin, growth hormone, cortisol, and glucagon), diets, and other factors influence BCAA metabolism probably via the regulation of phosphorylation and dephosphorylation. For example, feeding animals with high-protein diets increases BCKA dehydrogenase activity in the heart and kidneys by increasing the conversion of the enzyme from the phosphorylated form into the dephosphorylated form. Additionally, insulin and growth hormone stimulate the phosphorylation of BCKA dehydrogenase in bovine mammary epithelial cells, thereby reducing BCAA oxidative decarboxylation, whereas cortisol and glucagon have the opposite effect (Lei et al. 2012a).

In contrast to BCKA dehydrogenase, phenylalanine hydroxylase, tryptophan hydroxylase, tyrosine hydroxylase, and tyrosine aminotransferase are activated by protein phosphorylation and inactivated by protein dephosphorylation (Fitzpatrick 2012). The phosphorylation of phenylalanine hydroxylase, tryptophan hydroxylase, and tyrosine aminotransferase is catalyzed by protein kinase A (a cAMP-dependent kinase), whereas phosphorylation of tyrosine hydroxylase is performed by both protein kinase A and protein kinase C (a Ca^{2+}- dependent kinase) (Dunkley et al. 2004). Through changes in the activities of protein kinase A and protein kinase C, many hormones (including insulin, glucagon, glucocorticoids, and epinephrine) affect the catabolism of aromatic AAs in the liver and possibly other tissues (e.g., the kidneys and brain).

10.2.3 CONCENTRATIONS OF SUBSTRATES AND COFACTORS

Concentrations of substrates and cofactors (e.g., CoA-SH; NADPH, NADH, and tetrahydrobiopterin) play an important role in regulating AA metabolism (Fitzpatrick 1999; Kim et al. 2012; Wu and Thompson 1988). This can be graphically illustrated by BCAA catabolism in skeletal muscle exposed to ketone bodies (Table 10.2). Both acetoacetate and β-hydroxybutyrate inhibit the transamination of

TABLE 10.2

Effects of Ketone Bodies and Pyruvate on Leucine and Valine Transamination in Skeletal Muscle from 24 h Fasted Young Chicks

Addition to incubation medium	Net rate of transamination		Alanine release	Glutamine release
	Leucine	Valine		
		nmol/mg tissue/2 h		
None	1.46 ± 0.08	0.80 ± 0.09	2.05 ± 0.09	1.98 ± 0.11
4 mM AcAc	$0.66 \pm 0.04*$	$0.38 \pm 0.06*$	$1.26 \pm 0.05*$	$2.41 \pm 0.09*$
None	1.40 ± 0.14	0.76 ± 0.07	1.97 ± 0.12	2.01 ± 0.17
4 mM DL-BHB	$0.78 \pm 0.06*$	$0.44 \pm 0.04*$	$1.44 \pm 0.05*$	$2.53 \pm 0.16*$
5 mM Pyruvate	1.34 ± 0.11	0.72 ± 0.04	2.75 ± 0.10	1.78 ± 0.18
5 mM Pyruvate + 4 mM AcAc	1.30 ± 0.08	0.68 ± 0.04	2.89 ± 0.17	1.86 ± 0.14
5 mM Pyruvate	1.42 ± 0.10	0.80 ± 0.08	2.98 ± 0.14	1.87 ± 0.14
5 mM Pyruvate + 4 mM BHB	1.36 ± 0.07	0.82 ± 0.10	2.62 ± 0.20	1.75 ± 0.15

Source: Wu, G. and J.R. Thompson. 1988. *Biochem. J.* 255:139–144.

Note: Values are means $\pm$ SEM, $n = 12$ for BCAA transamination and $n = 10$ for alanine and glutamine release by skeletal muscle. Extensor digitorum communis muscles from 24 h fasted young chicks were incubated at 37°C for 2 h in Krebs bicarbonate buffer, containing 12 mM glucose and 0.3 mM NH₄Cl. Alanine and glutamine release are indicators of their synthesis by the muscle.

AcAc, acetoacetate; BHB, β-hydroxybutyrate.

* $P < 0.01$ vs. the corresponding control.

leucine and valine as well as alanine synthesis while increasing glutamine synthesis, in the skeletal muscle of fasted chicks. The inhibitory effect of ketone bodies on BCAA transamination is prevented by the addition of pyruvate (Figure 10.4). These findings can be explained by the following biochemical mechanisms. First, the inhibition of glycolysis by ketone bodies decreases the production of pyruvate from glucose, resulting in decreased transamination of glutamate with pyruvate to form alanine and α-ketoglutarate (KG). Because of the reduced formation of both pyruvate and oxaloacetate from glucose, α-KG production via citrate and isocitrate is also suppressed. As a result, glutamate is channeled to the production of glutamine, whereas a decrease in α-KG availability ultimately reduces the transamination of BCAAs. In the presence of added pyruvate, α-KG is generated from the transamination of glutamate as well as the metabolism of pyruvate and oxaloacetate and, therefore, is available for BCAA transamination. Consequently, pyruvate promotes alanine synthesis while reducing glutamine synthesis by skeletal muscle (Figure 10.4). The regulation of AA metabolism by ketone bodies plays a crucial role in the adaptation of humans and other animals to food deprivation or low-energy diets, as well as their conservation of body nitrogen and survival under these nutritional conditions (Owen 2005; Thompson and Wu 1991).

Ketone bodies also inhibit the oxidative decarboxylation of BCKAs in extrahepatic tissues (including skeletal muscle, mammary tissue, kidneys, and small intestine) in the absence or presence of pyruvate (Wu and Thompson 1987, 1988). Acetoacetate and β-hydroxybutyrate are readily oxidized to CO_2 and water in these tissues, particularly under food deprivation conditions. The oxidation of ketone bodies consumes large amounts of both CoA-SH and NAD⁺, thereby decreasing the availability of these cofactors for both pyruvate dehydrogenase and BCKA dehydrogenase. Elevation of pyruvate concentrations further reduces the availability of NAD⁺ and CoA-SH for BCKA decarboxylation. The ratios of NADH/NAD⁺ and acyl-CoA/R-COOH can also control the activities of these enzymes and the oxidation of pyruvate and BCKA. Thus, competition for the cofactors of enzymes is a major mechanism responsible for the effect of ketone bodies on inhibiting

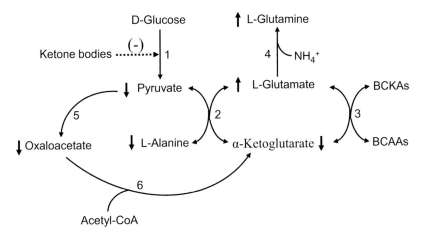

FIGURE 10.4 Mechanisms whereby ketone bodies reduce the transamination of branched-chain amino acids (BCAAs) and alanine synthesis while increasing glutamine synthesis in skeletal muscle. Note that ketone bodies inhibit the production of pyruvate from glucose via glycolysis, thereby suppressing the transamination of glutamate with pyruvate to form alanine and α-ketoglutarate. Glutamate is then channeled to glutamine synthesis. Reduced availability of α- ketoglutarate ultimately impairs BCAA transamination. Provision of exogenous pyruvate prevents the inhibitory effects of ketone bodies on BCAA transamination and alanine synthesis. Enzymes that catalyze the indicated reactions are: (1) enzymes of the glycolysis pathway; (2) glutamate–pyruvate transaminase; (3) BCAA transaminase; (4) glutamine synthetase; (5) pyruvate carboxylase (Mg^{2+}- and ATP-dependent); and (6) some enzymes of the Krebs cycle (citrate synthase, aconitase, and isocitrate dehydrogenase). BCAAs, branched-chain amino acids; BCKAs, branched-chain α-ketoacids.

BCAA catabolism in skeletal muscle (Figure 10.5). This helps mammals and birds to survive a prolonged period of food deprivation and thus is of physiological significance.

10.2.4 CONCENTRATIONS OF ACTIVATORS AND INHIBITORS

The availability of activators and inhibitors can increase and decrease metabolic fluxes, respectively. This concept can be illustrated by the effects of NAG (an allosteric activator of CPS-I; Meijer et al. 1990) and lactate (an inhibitor of proline oxidase; Dillon et al. 1999). Changes in intramitochondrial concentrations of NAG via alterations in the expression of NAG synthase or intramitochondrial levels of glutamate and acetyl-CoA greatly affect the urea cycle in hepatocytes and enterocytes, as well as the intestinal synthesis of citrulline from glutamine, glutamate, and proline in mammals. Several lines of evidence indicate that NAG plays an important role in regulating the intestinal synthesis of citrulline and arginine in postnatal pigs as an animal model (Wu and Morris 1998). First, although OAT and ornithine carbamoyltransferase (OCT) are abundant in pig enterocytes, only ~35% of

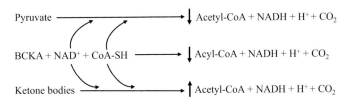

FIGURE 10.5 Mechanisms whereby ketone bodies inhibit the oxidative decarboxylation of pyruvate and branched-chain α-ketoacids (BCKA) in skeletal muscle. Oxidation of ketone bodies consumes both CoA-SH and NAD^+, resulting in the reduced availability of these cofactors for pyruvate dehydrogenase and BCKA dehydrogenase. Thus, competition for the cofactors of enzymes is a major mechanism regulating AA metabolism in cells.

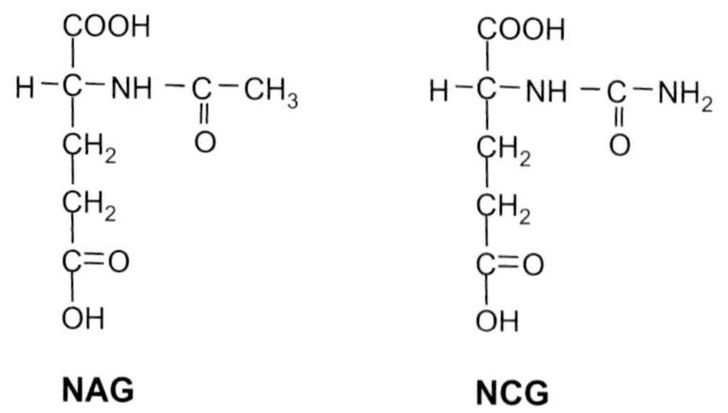

FIGURE 10.6 Chemical structures of *N*-acetylglutamate (NAG) and *N*-carbamoylglutamate (NCG) in the non-ionized form. NCG is a metabolically stable analog of NAG and an effective activator of carbamoyl phosphate synthetase-I in hepatocytes and enterocytes. NAG is hydrolyzed by cytosolic deacetylase in cells, but NCG is not a substrate of this enzyme.

proline-derived P5C is converted into citrulline in enterocytes of 14-day-old pigs. This suggests a low concentration of mitochondrial carbamoyl phosphate in enterocytes of 2- to 3-week-old pigs. Second, mitochondrial NAG concentration was decreased progressively in enterocytes of 7- to 14-day-old pigs, compared with newborn pigs, as was the intestinal synthesis of citrulline and arginine, in association with a marked postnatal decline in enterocyte NAG synthase activity. Third, although the amounts of the intestinal CPS-I protein are similar between 2- and 21-day-old pigs, a low concentration of mitochondrial NAG limits *in vivo* intestinal citrulline and arginine synthesis from both glutamine and proline in suckling piglets. Fourth, *N*-carbamoylglutamate (NCG; a metabolically stable analog of NAG; Figure 10.6) at 2 mM stimulates citrulline production from glutamine and proline in the enterocytes of 14-day-old pigs by 8.7- and 1.6-fold, respectively. Finally, the oral administration of NCG (50 mg/kg BW every 12 h) to young pigs between 4 and 14 days of life enhances concentrations of citrulline and arginine, muscle protein synthesis, and daily weight gains (Wu et al. 2004). Thus, NCG is a novel, effective, and low-cost growth-promoting agent for sow-reared piglets.

Elevated concentrations of lactate in the plasma are associated with severe hypocitrullinemia and hypoargininemia but hyperprolinemia in infants. Additionally, arginine deficiency occurs in adult humans with elevated plasma concentrations of lactate. Because the small intestine is a major organ for initiating proline catabolism via proline oxidase in the body and is the major source of circulating citrulline and arginine in neonates and adults, research was conducted to determine whether lactate is an inhibitor of intestinal synthesis of citrulline and arginine from proline. Kinetics analysis revealed non-competitive inhibition of intestinal proline oxidase by lactate (decreased maximal velocity and unaltered Michaelis constant) (Dillon et al. 1999). Lactate did not affect either activities of other enzymes for arginine synthesis from proline or proline uptake by enterocytes but decreased the synthesis of ornithine, citrulline, and arginine from proline in a concentration-dependent manner. These results demonstrate that lactate inhibits the synthesis of citrulline and arginine from proline via an inhibition of proline oxidase in enterocytes and provide a biochemical basis for explaining hyperprolinemia, hypocitrullinemia, and hypoargininemia in infants with hyperlactacidemia.

10.2.5 Signal Transduction

Signal transduction is defined as a chain of biochemical reactions in cells brought about by their responses to extracellular chemicals (including nutrients, hormones, drugs, toxins, or phytochemicals) (Figure 10.7). For example, hormones (e.g., glucagon) in the blood are chemical signals that control cell metabolism (e.g., stimulation of glycine oxidation in the mitochondria of hepatocytes) (Jois et al. 1989), whereas monosodium glutamate in food confers good taste through its interaction with specialized sensory cells (Wu 2020). Approximately half of the 25 largest protein

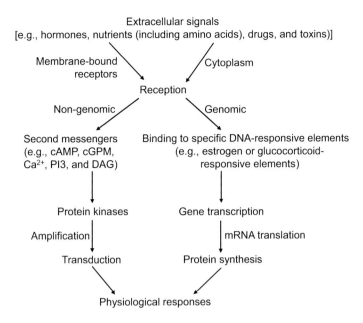

FIGURE 10.7 Signal transduction in cells. The extracellular signal is transduced into the cell via four sequential events. They are interaction of an extracellular chemical (also known as a ligand or the primary messenger) with the plasma membrane, generation of intracellular second messengers, covalent modifications of target proteins, and termination of signaling cascades. The last step, which is not illustrated in this figure, requires the removal of second messengers, reversing protein modification (e.g., switching off protein kinases). DAG, diacylglycerol; PI3, phosphoinositide 3 [also known as inositol-1,4,5-trisphosphate (IP3)].

families encoded by the human genome play important roles in signal transduction, indicating its widespread and diverse information-processing circuits in the body. Signal transduction cascades (also known as a molecular circuit) mediate the sensing and processing of both physiological and non-physiological substances by cells to detect, amplify, and integrate external signals to generate responses in the membrane, cytoplasm, mitochondria, and other intracellular organelles (Gomperts et al. 2002). The biochemical responses include changes in nutrient transport, enzyme activity, gene expression, ion channel activity, or metabolism. Defects in signal transduction can cause: (1) impairments in growth, development, and homeostasis; (2) increased susceptibility to infectious diseases; and (3) obesity, diabetes, cardiovascular disorders, DNA mutation, cancer, and other diseases.

Signal transduction generally includes 4 processes: (1) interaction of an extracellular chemical (also known as a ligand or the primary messenger) with the plasma membrane; (2) generation of intracellular second messengers; (3) covalent modifications of target proteins; and (4) termination of signaling cascades. Note that signal transduction cascades in response to an extracellular ligand may share the common reactions among different species, tissues, and cell types (Gomperts et al. 2002; Meijer and Dubbelhuis 2004). However, the physiological responses to hormones, nutrients, and environmental stimuli may be cell-specific due to the absence of one or more of the above steps and, therefore, do not generally occur in all cell types. For example, cAMP increases the synthesis of tyrosine aminotransferase in the liver and kidneys but not the small intestine or skeletal muscle.

10.2.5.1 Binding of Extracellular Ligands to the Plasma Membrane

Because large molecules (e.g., glucagon and insulin) cannot enter the cytoplasm of the cell, they must bind to specific membrane-associated receptor proteins to initiate signal transduction. Some low-molecular-weight hormones (e.g., epinephrine and norepinephrine) also bind to their target receptors (e.g., the β-adrenergic receptor) on the plasma membrane, which in turn activates G proteins (guanine nucleotide–binding proteins) (Rodbell 1980). The activated G protein stimulates membrane-bound adenylyl cyclase. Receptors for extracellular ligands are intrinsic membrane proteins that have both extracellular and intracellular domains. A binding site on the extracellular domain can specifically recognize its ligand. The interaction between the ligand and the receptor alters the conformational (e.g., tertiary or quaternary) structures of the extracellular and intracellular domains of the receptor. These structural changes of the receptor proteins trigger subsequent generation of intracellular signaling molecules (also known as second messengers).

Many hydrophobic substances (e.g., estrogens, glucocorticoids, and other steroid hormones) can enter the cytoplasm of the cell by diffusing through the plasma membrane to affect gene expression (Rousseau 2013). Once inside the cell, these molecules can bind to proteins (e.g., glucocorticoid receptors) that can interact directly with DNA. The activated receptor is translocated from the cytoplasm to the nucleus through the nucleopore. Inside the nucleus, the receptor complex binds to specific DNA-responsive elements (e.g., glucocorticoid-responsive elements) to activate gene transcription. These effects occur with a time lag of hours or even days. Interestingly, studies over the past three decades have shown that estrogens, glucocorticoids, and other steroid hormones can exert some of their rapid physiological effects through non-genomic mechanisms. The underlying signal transduction involves multiple pathways, including Ca^{2+} influx, phospholipase C activity, cAMP production, as well as mitogen-activated protein kinase, phosphoinositide 3-kinase, and AMP-activated protein kinase signaling cascades that do not directly link with gene transcription (Lösel and Wehling 2003). Thus, steroid hormones exert their physiological effects via both genomic and non-genomic mechanisms.

10.2.5.2 Generation of Intracellular Second Messengers

Intracellular second messengers are usually small molecules that act to relay information from the ligand–receptor (either membrane-bound or cytosolic) complex. These second messengers include cAMP, cGMP, Ca^{2+}, inositol-1,4,5-trisphosphate, diacylglycerol, and nitric oxide (NO), depending on the first messengers (Pollard et al. 2017). These molecules may have the following functions: a) influencing gene expression and other processes; b) amplifying the physiological responses by affecting a number of key protein kinases and the activities of many enzymes, therefore leading to the generation of many second messengers within the cell; c) affecting multiple signaling pathways to create cross talks which can finely tune the regulation of cell metabolism and activity. The second messengers exert their effects via either divergent (e.g., cAMP and cGMP) or common (e.g., cGMP and NO) cell signaling pathways.

10.2.5.3 Covalent Modifications of Target Proteins

The covalent attachment of a molecule to a protein can modify its enzymatic or physiological activity. Most modifications are reversible, but some are not readily reversible. An example is the irreversible attachment of a lipid group to Ras and Src (a protein tyrosine kinase) that are localized to the cytoplasmic face of the plasma membrane. Phosphorylation and dephosphorylation, which are noted in the previous section, are the most common but not the only means of covalent modification in proteins. As noted previously, the activities of many enzymes, membrane channels, and other target proteins are regulated by phosphorylation in virtually every metabolic process. Other types of covalent modifications include acetylation, methylation, and ubiquitination. For example, histones can be rapidly acetylated and deacetylated *in vivo* to affect gene transcription (Wang et al. 2012). However, the acetyltransferase and deacetylase enzymes are themselves regulated by phosphorylation. Also, as will be noted in Chapter 11, methylation of DNA and protein is a well-known mechanism of epigenetic regulation in cells. Finally, the attachment of ubiquitin to a protein targets the degradation of the protein by the proteasome (Chapter 9).

10.2.5.4 Termination of Signaling Cascades

After a signaling process has been initiated and the extracellular information from ligands has been transduced into cells, the signaling cascade must be terminated (Pollard et al. 2017). Mechanisms for the termination of a signaling process include the dephosphorylation, deacetylation, demethylation, deubiquitination of proteins; GTP hydrolysis (in G protein signaling); the internalization, degradation, or recycling of receptors; as well as the degradation of cAMP and cGMP. The corresponding enzymes include protein phosphatases, deacetylases, demethylases, deubiquitinases, GTPase, phosphodiesterases 4, 7, and 8, as well as phosphodiesterases 5, 6, and 9. Switching off protein kinases can prevent the effects of primary ligands on specific cells. If a signaling process is not terminated, cells can lose their responsiveness to new signals. Also, signaling processes that are not terminated properly may lead to organ dysfunction, as well as uncontrolled cell growth and development of cancer.

10.2.6 CHANGES IN CELL VOLUME

All cells express water channels or transporters (aquaporins), and water can rapidly enter most cells through the plasma membrane. Cell volume (primarily determined by intracellular water content) can change in response to alterations in extracellular osmolarity that are affected by nutritional, physiological, and pathological conditions. For example, upon ingestion of a meal and fluids, nutrients (including water) are transported into the cell, leading to cell swelling. Conversely, loss of cellular water in dehydration leads to cell shrinkage. The maintenance of adequate cell volume is a major prerequisite for cell survival, growth, and development. A change in cell volume has recently been proposed as a mediator of cellular metabolism in hepatocytes and other cells (Hoffmann et al. 2009). For example, cell swelling induced by hypo-tonicity or AAs stimulates glycogen synthesis, lipogenesis, glycolysis, and glutaminolysis, but inhibits proteolysis, glycogen breakdown, and urea synthesis, in isolated rat liver preparations. On the other hand, cell shrinkage increases protein degradation and decreases protein synthesis in the perfused rat liver, regardless of whether cell volume is modulated by extracellular osmolarity, AAs, or hormones. Furthermore, cell swelling in hypoosmotic medium decreases, whereas cell shrinkage in hyperosmotic medium increases, the rates of release of glutamine and alanine from incubated rat skeletal muscle (Parry-Billings et al. 1991).

An exciting new development in the metabolism of AAs in cells of the immune system is a role for cell volume in regulating their utilization of both glucose and glutamine. Specifically, decreasing extracellular osmolarity from 336 to 286 mOsmol by decreasing medium NaCl from 119 to 94 mM increases cell volume and the rates of glutamine metabolism and glycolysis in lymphocytes and macrophages (Wu and Flynn 1995). Conversely, increasing extracellular osmolarity from 286 to 386 mOsmol by the addition of 50 and 100 mM D-mannitol progressively decreases cell volume and the rates of glutamine and glucose degradation in both cell types (Wu and Flynn 1995). The findings that glutamine and glucose metabolism in lymphocytes and macrophages are regulated by cell volume changes may have physiological and immunological implications. For example, the cell volume of both lymphocytes and macrophages increases in response to mitogenic stimulation and immunological activation, probably due to alterations in transmembrane transport systems. Although the phosphorylation of protein kinase C has been proposed as a signaling mechanism for the increased cellular metabolism in activated lymphocytes and macrophages (Field et al. 2000), the increased cell volume *per se* may be partially responsible for the increased glutamine and glucose metabolism in these cells in response to mitogenic stimulation. It is also known that the phagocytosis of particles (e.g., starch, latex beads, and microorganisms) by macrophages results in increased glycolysis. However, the underlying mechanisms have not yet been elucidated. Note that both phagocytosis and pinocytosis increase the cell volume of macrophages due to the increased accumulation of particles or solutes inside the cells and the associated increase in the influx of water, possibly through the activation of aquaporins. The increased cell volume induced by phagocytosis may account, in part, for the increased cellular metabolism previously reported for macrophages. As the change in cell volume is an early event in the activation of lymphocytes and macrophages, this may be a mechanism in regulating the function of these cells. Because glutamine and glucose are two major metabolic fuels in lymphocytes and macrophages (Field et al. 2000), a change in cell volume may affect the provision of energy and protein turnover, thereby regulating the function of immunocytes.

10.2.7　Other Mechanisms for the Regulation of Enzyme Activity

Proteolytic activation is the activation of a protein or enzyme (known as a zymogen) by peptide cleavage (Chapter 9). Examples of zymogens are pepsinogen, prothrombin, fibrinogen, proinsulin, and procaspases. Activities of some enzymes (e.g., hormone-sensitive lipase and glucokinase) are also regulated by the intracellular movement to and from the sites of their substrates (e.g., lipid droplets for hormone-sensitive lipase) or between different compartments (e.g., between the nucleus and cytoplasm for glucokinase). Interestingly, palmitoylation inhibits hepatic CPS-I activity (Corvi et al. 2001), whereas both palmitoylation and myristoylation activate eNOS (type-3 NO synthase) in endothelial cells (Aicart-Ramos et al. 2011). In addition, the polymerization of acetyl-CoA carboxylase by allosteric activators (e.g., citrate) increases its catalytic activity and, therefore, the conversion of AAs into fatty acids in the lipogenic tissues, such as white adipose tissue and mammary tissue (Hunkeler et al. 2018). This is another mechanism for the regulation of acetyl-CoA carboxylase activity via protein phosphorylation and dephosphorylation, as well as gene expression at the transcriptional level. Furthermore, the binding of a molecule to the active site of an enzyme can modulate its catalytic activity, leading to either an increase or a decrease in the rate of a biochemical reaction. For example, physiological levels of NO bind to the heme moiety of guanylate cyclase (a heme enzyme), triggering the structural rearrangement of the protein to rapidly activate its enzymatic activity (Kang et al. 2019). By contrast, the activity of aconitase (a non-heme iron enzyme) is inhibited in response to the binding of high concentrations of NO to its iron–sulfur center (Gardner et al. 1997). Thus, multiple mechanisms exist to regulate enzyme activities in animal cells.

10.3　EFFECTS OF NUTRITIONAL AND PHYSIOLOGICAL FACTORS ON AMINO ACID METABOLISM

AA synthesis and catabolism depend on the concentrations of substrates and cell signaling cascades. Therefore, dietary factors and hormones have profound effects on AA metabolism in a cell-, tissue- and species-specific manner. In general, the endogenous synthesis of NEAAs (e.g., arginine, glutamate, and glutamine) is largely independent of their dietary intake or plasma concentrations within physiological ranges. However, AA catabolism is stimulated by dietary AA and protein intakes, as well as by the elevated extracellular concentrations of AAs. Let's use arginine and glutamine as examples because the metabolism of these two AAs in animals has been well characterized and has received much attention over the past three decades. Thus, these examples illustrate some principles of the regulation of AA metabolism.

10.3.1　AA Synthesis

10.3.1.1　Arginine Synthesis

Both enzymological and metabolic data indicate that P5C synthase, proline oxidase, and NAG synthase catalyze key steps in arginine synthesis from glutamine and proline (Wu and Morris 1998). In enterocytes, the synthesis of citrulline and arginine is not subject to feedback inhibition by physiological levels of arginine. For example, the intestinal expression of P5C synthase and proline oxidase is not affected by increasing the dietary intake of arginine within the physiological range (e.g., from 0.5% to 2% arginine in swine and rat diets) (Wu et al. 2016). Similarly, augmenting the concentration of arginine in the arterial plasma of rats from 0.2 to 0.5 mM does not influence the conversion of arterial citrulline into arginine in the kidneys (Dhanakoti et al. 1990). However, the synthesis of citrulline and arginine from glutamine, glutamate, and proline in enterocytes increases with increasing: (1) their extracellular concentrations from 0.5 to 5 mM; (2) the circulating levels of cortisol within the physiological range (e.g., from 21 to 83 μg/L) by stimulating the expression of P5C synthase, proline oxidase, and NAG synthase; and (3) intramitochondrial concentrations of NAG and ammonia (Wu et al. 2009). Likewise, in healthy animals, the renal synthesis of arginine from citrulline increases stoichiometrically with extracellular citrulline, when intracellular aspartate is not a limiting factor (Dhanakoti et al. 1990). By contrast, elevating the extracellular concentrations of lactate from 0.5 to 10 mM dose-dependently inhibits the intestinal synthesis of citrulline from proline by inhibiting proline oxidase activity (Dillon et al. 1999), thereby limiting the availability of citrulline for arginine production by the kidneys. Thus, high circulating levels of lactate during intensive exercise may contribute to lowered concentrations of arginine in the plasma (Hackl et al. 2009; Rose and Richter 2009), which can be ameliorated by the dietary intake of arginine precursors (e.g., citrulline, glutamine, and proline). Collectively, the endogenous synthesis of arginine is exquisitely regulated to maintain concentrations in the plasma and cells at physiological levels.

10.3.1.2 Glutamine Synthesis

BCAA transaminase and glutamine synthetase are two key regulatory enzymes in glutamine synthesis which is subject to feedback inhibition by glutamine. In muscle cells, glutamine synthesis is strongly inhibited by high levels of extracellular glutamine beyond 2 mM primarily because of reduced expression of the glutamine synthetase protein due to destabilization of its mRNA (Wang and Watford 2007). However, animal studies have shown that increasing the extracellular concentrations of BCAAs, glutamate, α-KG, and ammonia within physiological ranges increases glutamine synthesis by skeletal muscle, lactating mammary tissue, white adipose tissue, heart, brain, and lungs (Tekwe et al. 2019; Tischler and Goldberg 1980a, b; Wang et al. 2016a; Wu et al. 1989; Zhang et al. 2019; Yao et al. 2012). In addition, human studies have demonstrated that the dietary intake of BCAAs is effective in promoting glutamine production by skeletal muscle and other tissues both in the fed state and under catabolic conditions as well as during exercise (MacLean and Graham 1993). Similar results have been obtained from experiments involving young pigs and lactating sows (Lei et al. 2012b). This led to the practical use of dietary BCAA supplementation to improve lactation and muscle function in swine (Zhang et al. 2021).

Increasing the concentrations of insulin and glucocorticoids within physiological ranges inhibit and increase glutamine synthesis in skeletal muscle, respectively, by suppressing and stimulating BCAA transamination (Hutson et al. 1980, 2005). Thus, in response to stress factors, such as lactation and elevated environmental temperatures, skeletal muscle mobilizes BCAAs in proteins to synthesize and release glutamine for utilization by other cell types and tissues, including lymphocytes, macrophages, hepatocytes, mammary epithelial cells, small intestine, and kidneys. Likewise, there are marked changes in circulating levels of hormones during lactation. For example, in cows, lactation is associated with elevated concentrations of stress hormones (cortisol and glucagon), but lowered concentrations of anabolic hormones (insulin and growth hormone), in the plasma (Lei et al. 2012b). Increases in extracellular concentrations of the stress hormones and the anabolic hormones promote and inhibit glutamine synthesis in mammary epithelial cells, respectively. These metabolic changes in glutamine synthesis are consistent with the decreased abundance of BCAA transaminase in the presence of anabolic hormones but increased levels of this enzyme in the presence of stress hormones to regulate glutamate and glutamine synthesis. Such coordinated alterations in hormones facilitate milk production by lactating mammals to feed their neonates.

Compartmentation of metabolism is an important regulatory mechanism for glutamine synthesis in tissues, particularly the brain and liver that possess the intercellular glutamine–glutamate cycle and have a limited ability to take up glutamate. Glutamate is a precursor for glutamine synthesis in the brain. However, the blood–brain barrier (BBB), which consists of endothelial cells of the capillary wall, the astrocyte end feet, and pericytes, separates the circulating blood from the brain and is not permeable to glutamate, aspartate, or γ-aminobutyrate (GABA) in the blood (Figure 10.8). Thus, glutamate in the brain must be derived from either AAs (e.g., BCAAs) plus α-KG via BCAA transaminase or ammonia plus α-KG via glutamate dehydrogenase.

There are two isoforms of BCAA transaminase in the central nervous system, with the mitochondrial form (BCATm) in astrocytes but the cytosolic form (BCATc) in neurons (Bixel et al. 2001).

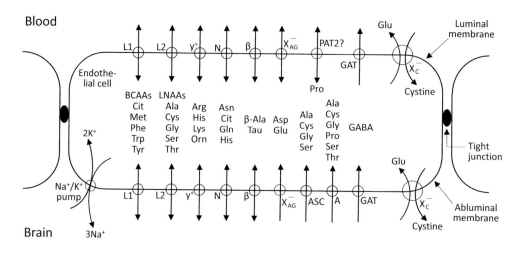

FIGURE 10.8 The blood–brain barrier (BBB) for the selective transport of amino acids. The BBB consists of two polarized membranes: luminal membrane (the blood side) and abluminal membrane (the brain side). Nutrients in the blood must cross both membranes to enter the brain. Three classes of Na^+-independent facilitative AA transporters for large neutral amino acids (L1), cationic AAs (y^+), and acidic AAs (x_G-), as well as one Na^+-dependent AA transport for neutral AAs with a side-chain NH_2 group (N) exist on the luminal membrane. L1 and y^+ are present in both membranes. By contrast, the ASC and imino systems are absent from the luminal membrane of the endothelial cells in the BBB. Thus, large neutral AAs (e.g., branched-chain AAs, phenylalanine, tyrosine, and tryptophan) and basic AAs (e.g., arginine, lysine, histidine, and ornithine) in the blood readily cross the BBB into the brain. Small neutral AAs (e.g., alanine, glycine, serine, and cysteine) in the blood also readily cross the BBB into the brain, but the BBB restricts the entry of physiological concentrations of proline and hydroxyproline from the blood into the brain. The abluminal membrane of the endothelial cells in the BBB contains Na^+-dependent AA transport systems ASC (for small AAs), A (for alanine, serine, glycine, cysteine, threonine, and proline), N (for glutamine, citrulline, asparagine, and histidine), and excitatory AA transporter (EAAT; for acidic AAs and cysteine) for effluxes from the brain into the blood. In healthy humans and other animals, the BBB is impermeable to not only glutamate and aspartate in the blood but also γ-aminobutyrate (GABA) in the blood and the endogenous cerebral GABA. By contrast, GABA readily exists from the brain to the blood to regulate its concentration in the central nervous system. (Reproduced from He, W.L. and G. Wu. 2020. *Adv. Exp. Med. Biol.* 1265:167–185. With permission.)

After the blood-borne BCAAs enter astrocytes, these AAs undergo transamination with α-KG to form BCKAs and glutamate, which is amidated to glutamine by glutamine synthetase. The astrocytes release glutamine and BCKAs, and all these molecules are taken up by neurons, where glutamine is hydrolyzed to glutamate plus ammonia by phosphate-activated glutaminase and BCKAs participate in transamination with glutamate to generate BCAAs and α-KG. Upon stimulation, the neurons release both BCAAs and glutamate, which are taken up by astrocytes for glutamine synthesis. This intercellular glutamine–glutamate cycle between the neurons and astrocytes plays an important role in maintaining the homeostasis of glutamate, which is a precursor of both aspartate and GABA (Figure 10.9).

10.3.2 AA CATABOLISM

10.3.2.1 Arginine Catabolism

Arginine metabolism is regulated by multiple factors that include transport by the cell membrane, nutrients (e.g., lysine, BCAAs, manganese, n-3 fatty acids), hormones (e.g., glucocorticoids, growth hormone, and leptin), cytokines, endotoxins, and endogenously generated substances (e.g., creatine, ornithine, P5C, and methylarginines) (Hobbach and Closs 2020; Wu et al. 2009). Lysine competes with arginine for entry into cells and also inhibits arginase activity. Therefore, an arginine:lysine ratio in the diet is a critical factor influencing arginine utilization in the body. Under normal feeding

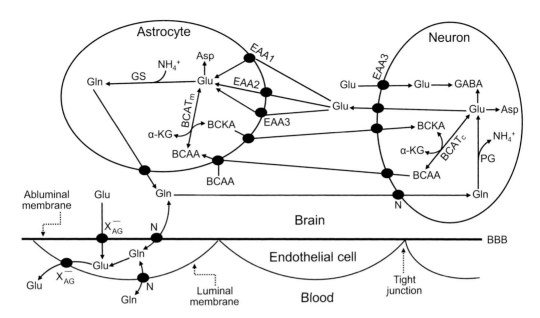

FIGURE 10.9 Compartmentation of glutamine and glutamate metabolism in the astrocytes and neurons of the central nervous system. Astrocytes (a subtype of glial cells) synthesize glutamine from both BCAA- and neuron-derived glutamate. Neurons take up glutamine for glutamate production and upon stimulation release glutamate. The intercellular glutamine–glutamate cycle plays an important role in maintaining the high concentrations of glutamate in the brain, where glutamate is a precursor for the synthesis of γ-aminobutyrate (GABA) and aspartate in a cell-specific manner. BBB, blood–brain barrier; BCATc, branched-chain amino acid transaminase (cytosolic isoform); BCATm, branched-chain amino acid transaminase (mitochondrial isoform); BCKA, branched-chain α-ketoacid; BCKD, branched-chain α-ketoacid dehydrogenase complex; PAG, phosphate-activated glutaminase; GS, glutamine synthetase; α-KG, α-ketoglutarate. (Reproduced from He, W.L. and G. Wu. 2020. *Adv. Exp. Med. Biol.* 1265:167–185. With permission.)

conditions, the total amount of arginine in diets for farm animals and rodents should not be 200% greater than that of lysine (namely, arginine:lysine ratio <3). However, experimental evidence shows that humans can tolerate a greater arginine:lysine ratio in the enteral diet (McNeal et al. 2018).

Glucocorticoids play a major role in upregulating arginine catabolism via the arginase pathway in many cell types, particularly hepatocytes, enterocytes, and macrophages (Morris 2009). By contrast, these hormones inhibit NO generation by suppressing NOS expression and BH4 synthesis (Wu et al. 2009). During weaning, the glucocorticoid surge induces expression of intestinal arginase, resulting in enhanced hydrolysis of arginine for polyamine and proline syntheses (Wu et al. 2018). Interestingly, a high level of circulating cortisol in the fetus during late gestation and in the newborn does not induce arginase expression in their small intestines. Thus, intestinal arginase expression is unresponsive to cortisol during the fetal and early neonatal periods, but the underlying mechanisms are unknown.

Cytokines (e.g., interleukin-4 and interferon-γ), other inflammatory stimuli (e.g., lipopolysaccharide), and cAMP can greatly stimulate the expression of arginase I, arginase II, and ODC in many cell types (Morris 2012). Inflammatory cytokines and endotoxins also strongly induce the expression of NOS2 (type-2 NO synthase) and GTP cyclohydrolase I (which catalyzes the first step in *de novo* BH4 synthesis) in almost all cell types (Shi et al. 2004). Therefore, these substances upregulate arginine degradation for the synthesis of urea, ornithine, proline, polyamines, and NO in a cell-specific manner, and the concentrations of arginine in the plasma are reduced markedly in response to infection or inflammation.

N^G-monomethyl-L-arginine (NMMA) and asymmetric dimethylarginine (ADMA) are competitive inhibitors of all NOS isoforms ($K_i = 1.0$–$1.6\,\mu M$) (Wu and Morris 1998). However, concentrations of NMMA and ADMA are relatively low in the plasma of healthy individuals (0.5–1 μM) compared with those of arginine (100–250 μM), depending on the nutritional state and developmental stage. There are reports that 1 μM NMMA or ADMA does not affect NO synthesis in endothelial cells cultured in the presence of 0.2 mM L-arginine (Kohli et al. 2004). Although much higher concentrations of NMMA and ADMA (e.g., 5–10 μM) can occur in patients with obesity, diabetes, cardiovascular disease, and renal dysfunction and can inhibit NO synthesis by cells, the physiological significance of endogenous methylarginines in the regulation of NO production by endothelial cells and other cell types remains to be defined (Tsikas and Wu 2015).

10.3.2.2 Glutamine Catabolism

Two distinct isoforms of phosphate-activated glutaminase (the liver and kidney types) catalyze the first and key regulatory step of glutamine catabolism in humans and other animals (Chapter 4). In all cell types studied, increasing the extracellular concentrations of glutamine from 0.5 to 5 mM increases the hydrolysis of glutamine to glutamate and ammonia in a dose-dependent manner, ensuring that glutamine (an inhibitor of NO synthesis in endothelial cells; Meininger and Wu 1997) will not inhibit NO-dependent blood circulation under physiological conditions. In the kidneys, further degradation of glutamate relieves its potential inhibitory effect on the mitochondrial glutaminase, thereby allowing the complete catabolism of glutamine to form 2 molecules of ammonia and 5 molecules of CO_2. In the small intestine and liver of many species, including dogs, humans, pigs, and rats, glutamine degradation is stimulated by elevated levels of glucocorticoids and glucagon within physiological ranges to enhance the intestinal synthesis of citrulline and hepatic production of glucose (Wu 1998). Thus, glutamine catabolism is augmented in diabetic animals due to the enhanced expression of phosphate-activated glutaminase (Curthoys and Watford 1995), resulting in increased requirements for dietary AAs (including glutamine and BCAAs). Furthermore, compartmentation exists for the regulation of glutamine catabolism within cells and organs, as discussed previously.

Acid–base balance strongly affects glutamine utilization in a cell-specific manner to maximize its supply to the kidneys (Welbourne 1987). In response to metabolic acidosis, the following coordinated changes in interorgan glutamine metabolism occur. First, uptake of arterial glutamine by the small intestine and lymphocytes (which amount to approximately 1.5 kg in the adult human) is markedly inhibited by elevated extracellular levels of H^+ to spare glutamine for use by the kidneys. Second, oxidation of glutamine in the liver is reduced by a low pH and this organ releases glutamine into the circulation. Third, the renal activity of phosphate-activated glutaminase, as well as the uptake and catabolism of glutamine by the kidneys of acidotic animals is greatly enhanced to generate NH_3 for removing excess H^+ as NH_4^+. Interestingly, a similar pattern of glutamine catabolism occurs in pregnant mothers with fetal alcohol syndrome, resulting in a reduced transfer of glutamine from mother to fetus and, therefore, reduced concentration of glutamine in the fetal circulation (Ramadoss et al. 2008; Sawant et al. 2014). Importantly, this new knowledge led to the development of glutamine supplementation as a novel strategy to ameliorate acid–base imbalance and intrauterine growth retardation in alcoholic gestating mothers (Sawant et al. 2014, 2015; Washburn et al. 2013).

10.3.3 INTRACELLULAR PROTEIN TURNOVER

10.3.3.1 Mechanistic Target of Rapamycin Cell Signaling (Mechanistic Target of Rapamycin Cell Signaling Complexes 1 and 2)

Mechanistic target of rapamycin (MTOR) is a major component of a cell signaling pathway that provides a mechanism for the regulation of protein synthesis and cytoskeleton remodeling, as well as intracellular protein degradation via autophagy (Figure 10.10). MTOR is a highly conserved serine/threonine protein kinase and is also known as FK506-binding protein 12-rapamycin-associated protein 1 (FRAP-1). The MTOR system consists of MTOR complex 1 (MTORC1) and MTOR complex 2 (MTORC2), which are structurally and functionally distinct in cells. Nutrients signal to MTORC1 through the lysosome-associated Rag GTPases (Sabatini 2017).

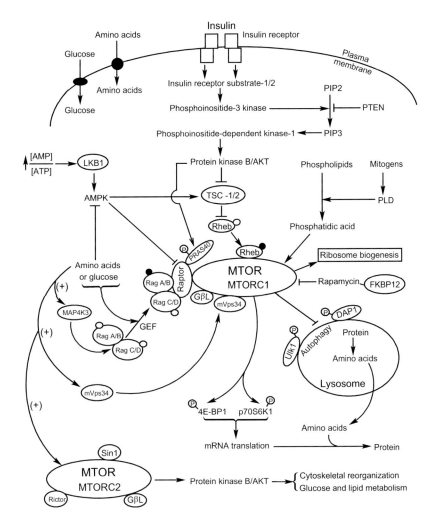

FIGURE 10.10 The MTOR1 signaling in the regulation of intracellular protein turnover. The mechanistic target of rapamycin (MTOR) integrates nutrient and other cellular signals to increase protein synthesis and inhibit protein degradation via autophagy. MTOR complex-1 (MTORC1) is composed of four components: MTOR (a highly conserved serine/threonine protein kinase), raptor (regulatory-associated protein of TOR), mLST8 (MTOR-associated protein, LST8 homolog), and PRAS40 (a raptor-interacting protein that binds to MTORC1). MTORC1 can be activated by certain AA through protein phosphorylation. Specifically, AA may bind to the Rag complex (Rag A/B and Rag C/D), triggering an exchange between GDP with GTP in the Rag A/B protein and MTOR phosphorylation. Activated MTOR phosphorylates eIF4E-binding protein-1 (4E-BP1) and ribosomal protein S6 kinase-1 (p70S6K1), thereby stimulating mRNA translation for protein synthesis. MTOR is inhibited by TSC-1/2 (tuberous sclerosis complex-1/2) whose activity is enhanced by AMPK (AMP-activated protein kinase) but suppressed by protein kinase B (also known as AKT). Phosphorylation of AKT in response to insulin and other growth factors relieves an inhibitory effect of TSC-1/2 on MTOR. Additionally, certain nutrients (e.g., glutamine, arginine, leucine, and glucose) and phosphatidic acid stimulate MTOR phosphorylation and thus increase its activity. Oxidation of AA, glucose, and fatty acids reduces the cellular ratio of AMP:ATP, therefore suppressing AMPK activity via liver kinase B1 (LKB1; also known as serine/threonine kinase 11). Activated MTOR also inhibits lysosomal proteolysis via autophagy by phosphorylating death-associated protein 1 (DAP1) and Ulk1; GEF, guanine nucleotide exchange factor; MAP4K3, a conserved Ser/Thr kinase; mVps34, mammalian vacuolar protein–sorting mutant 34; PIP2, phosphatidylinositol-4-5,-bisphosphate; PIP3, phosphatidylinositol-3,4-5,-triphosphate; PLD, phospholipase D; PRAS40, proline-rich Akt substrate of 40 kDa; PTEN, phosphatase and tensin homolog; RHEB, Ras homolog enriched in brain (a Ras family GTPase); RICTOR, rapamycin-insensitive companion of TOR; SIN1, stress-activated MAP kinase–interacting protein 1; Ulk1, Unc-51-like kinase 1. Open circle = GDP; solid circle = GTP. The sign (+) denotes activation by amino acids.

10.3.3.1.1 Mechanistic Target of Rapamycin Complex 1

MTORC1 is composed of the following: MTOR, raptor (regulatory-associated protein of TOR), mLST8 [MTOR-associated protein, LST8 homolog; also known as G protein beta subunit-like (GβL)], and PRAS40 (the proline-rich Akt substrate of 40 kDa; a raptor-interacting protein that binds MTOR). PRAS40 is dissociated from MTOR under conditions (e.g., sufficient AAs) that activate MTOR signaling. Conversely, PRAS40 binds the MTOR kinase domain under conditions (e.g., nutrient deprivation) that inhibit MTOR signaling. MTORC1 has long been known to be inhibited by rapamycin, a microbial product that was discovered in the bacterium *Streptomyces hygroscopicus* of soil samples from the island of Rapa Nui in 1972 (Sehgal et al. 1975).

In response to certain AAs (e.g., arginine, glutamine, glycine, leucine, proline, tryptophan, and valine), MTOR1 is activated when its Ser^{2448} residue is phosphorylated by an upstream kinase (Kim and Guan 2011). The underlying mechanisms are complex and remain largely unknown. Some lines of evidence suggest that AAs exert their effects by stimulating: (1) GTPases (Rag A/B and Rag C/D), which then bind raptor; (2) MAP4K3 (a conserved Ser/Thr kinase), which binds Rag A/B and Rag C/D; and (3) mVps34 (mammalian vacuolar protein–sorting mutant 34), which activates RHEB (Ras homolog) enriched in brain (a Ras family GTPase). Activated MTOR phosphorylates two downstream target proteins: ribosomal protein S6 kinase-1 (S6K1) and 4E-BP1 (eIF4E-binding protein-1, a translational repressor protein). An increase in S6K1 phosphorylation results in hyperphosphorylation of ribosomal protein S6 and thus facilitates the translation of mRNAs for protein synthesis (see Chapter 8). In a non-phosphorylated state, 4E-BP1 binds eIF4E (an initiation factor) with high affinity and, thus, eIF4E cannot bind eIF4G (an initiation factor) to form the translationally active eIF4F–eIF4G complex. Conversely, phosphorylation of 4E-BP1 reduces its binding affinity for eIF4E, relieving the translational repression of 4E-BP1 on the binding of eIF4E to eIF4G and generating the translationally active eIF4F–eIF4G complex. Activation of MTORC1 by certain AAs (e.g., arginine, leucine, glutamine, and glycine) also inhibits autophagy and, therefore, the lysosome protein degradation in cells [e.g., hepatocytes (Blommaart et al. 1995) and enterocytes (Xi et al. 2012)]. Insulin, insulin-like growth factor, some AAs, and α-KG are known to stimulate the phosphorylation of MTORC1 in a cell-specific manner, thereby regulating the intracellular turnover and concentrations of protein (Dennis et al. 2011).

10.3.3.1.2 Mechanistic Target of Rapamycin Complex 2

MTORC2 contains MTOR, RICTOR (rapamycin-insensitive companion of TOR), mLST8, and SIN1 (stress-activated MAP kinase–interacting protein 1). Although MTORC2 was previously thought to be insensitive to rapamycin, emerging findings from both *in vitro* and *in vivo* studies indicate that chronic exposure of cells to rapamycin also inhibits MTORC2 (Guertin et al. 2009; Lamming et al. 2012). Like MTORC1, MTORC2 is activated when it is phosphorylated by a protein kinase, but MTORC2 is relatively poorly understood and few MTORC2 effectors/substrates have been identified (Fu and Hall 2020). AMP-activated protein kinase, GTPases, Wnt3A, and Wnt7A have been reported to activate MTORC2 in in eukaryotes (Knudsen et al. 2020). The MTORC2 signaling pathway involves the production of PI3, and some of its events include the promotion of MTORC2-ribosome association. To date, MTORC2 is known to phosphorylate mainly AGC (protein kinase A, G and C families) kinases in cells, including Akt (also known as protein kinase B), protein kinase C, and serum- and glucocorticoid-induced kinases 1 at their hydrophobic motif and turn motif (Oh and Jacinto 2011). For example, Ser473 in the hydrophobic motif of Akt and Thr450 in the turn motif of Akt are phosphorylated in response to activation signals (e.g., insulin, growth factors, serum, glucose, and certain AAs such as glutamine and leucine). In addition, MTORC2 can also phosphorylate Ser477 and Thr479 at the C terminus of Akt in proliferating cells (Liu et al. 2014).

Results of recent studies indicate that MTORC2 phosphorylates protein kinase B/Akt and may function to regulate cell proliferation, differentiation, migration, and cytoskeletal reorganization (Wang et al. 2016b). There is growing interest in MTORC2 in the regulation of nutrient metabolism. Specifically, studies involving liver-specific RICTOR knockout mice revealed a critical role for hepatic MTORC2 in glucose and lipid metabolism via insulin-induced Akt signaling (Hagiwara et al. 2012). These mice lacked Akt Ser473 phosphorylation and exhibited reductions in hepatic glucokinase and sterol regulatory element–binding protein 1c (SREBP1c) activities, resulting in enhanced gluconeogenesis, hyperglycemia, and hyperinsulinemia but impaired glycolysis, reduced lipogenesis, and hypolipidemia. Expression of constitutively active Akt2 in MTORC2-deficient hepatocytes restored both glycolysis and lipogenesis, whereas overexpression of glucokinase normalized glycolysis but not lipogenesis (Hagiwara et al. 2012). Thus, hepatic MTORC2 activates glycolysis and lipogenesis through Akt, glucokinase, and SREBP1c signaling. In support of this view, emerging evidence shows that MTORC2 is required for insulin-mediated suppression of hepatic gluconeogenesis. Therefore, chronic administration of rapamycin impairs glucose tolerance and insulin action in the whole body. In some mammalian cells (e.g., Hela, HEK293, and MCF7), a mixed group of AAs (EAAs + NEAAs) can activate MTORC2 through the phosphoinositide-3 kinase and Akt pathway (Manning and Toker 2017; Tato et al. 2011).

10.3.3.2 Factors That Affect Intracellular Protein Turnover

A better understanding of the factors affecting intracellular protein turnover is essential to increase protein deposition in animals and to reduce negative N balance in organisms under catabolic conditions (Chapter 9). Much of our current knowledge about the regulation of AA metabolism, including intracellular protein turnover, has been generated from studies involving various cytokines released by cells of the immune system (Figure 10.11). The following general conclusions can be made regarding the effects of diverse factors on protein synthesis and degradation in animal tissues and the whole body. First, increasing dietary intake of AAs or extracellular concentrations of

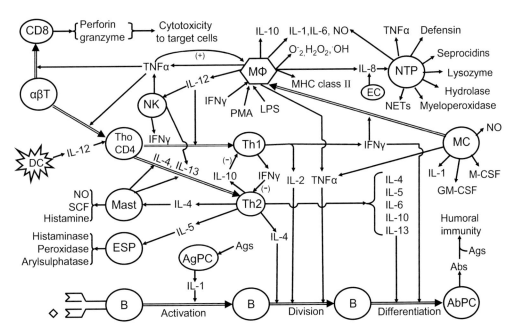

FIGURE 10.11 Cytokines and other regulatory molecules released by cells of the immune system that regulate AA metabolism, including intracellular protein turnover in animals. Abbreviations: αβ T, αβ T cell; Abs, antibodies; Ags, antigens; AbPC, antibody-producing cells; AgPC, antigen-presenting cells; B, B lymphocytes; CD8, cytotoxic T cells carrying CD8 marker; DC, dendritic cell; EC, endothelial cells; ESP, eosinophil; GM-CSF, granulocyte/macrophage colony-stimulating factor; IFNγ, interferon γ; IL, interleukin; LPS, lipopolysaccharide; MΦ, macrophage; M-CSF, macrophage colony-stimulating factor; Mast, mast cells; MC, monocyte, NETs, neutrophil extracellular traps; NK, natural killer cells; NO, nitric oxide; NTP, neutrophil; PMA, phorbol myristate acetate; SCF, stem cell factor; Th0 CD4, T cells carrying CD4 marker; Th1, T helper cell 1; Th2, T helper cell 2; TNFα, tumor necrosis factor α. Note that macrophages are classified as inflammatory (M1) and anti-inflammatory (M2) and that the balance between M1 and M2 cells affects the immune response. (Reproduced from Li, P. et al. 2007. *Br. J. Nutr.* 98:237–252. With permission.)

AAs stimulates protein synthesis and inhibits intracellular protein degradation in tissues (including the small intestine, liver, heart, kidneys, and skeletal muscle) (Bertrand et al. 2013; Wu 2009). Second, energy substrates (e.g., glucose, saturated fatty acids, and ketone bodies) have a little direct effect on protein synthesis while inhibiting protein degradation in diverse tissues (including skeletal muscle, heart, and liver) of healthy animals (Sugden and Fuller 1991; Wu and Thompson 1990). There were reports that chronic exposure to saturated fatty acids (e.g., palmitate) impaired insulin sensitivity and reduced protein synthesis while upregulating proteolytic systems in C2C12 muscle cells (Perry et al. 2018), suggesting a role for elevated saturated fatty acids in metabolic syndrome in persons with type 2 diabetes mellitus. Third, anabolic hormones (e.g., insulin, growth hormone, and insulin-like growth factor-1) primarily promote protein synthesis, whereas catabolic hormones (glucocorticoids), metabolic acidosis, and inflammatory cytokines activate proteolysis (Costamagna et al. 2015; Flynn et al. 2020; Sugden and Fuller 1991). Insulin is the most potent hormone to stimulate protein synthesis and suppress proteolysis in skeletal muscle (Suryawan and Davis 2014). Fourth, by stimulating protein synthesis and inhibiting protein degradation, feeding adequate amounts of high-quality protein is the most attractive way to promote protein deposition in the whole body (Reeds 1989). Fifth, like bed rest and space flight, a lack of muscle contraction reduces protein synthesis and possibly has no effect on proteolysis in skeletal muscle cells (Stein and Schluter 1997; Vandenburgh et al. 1999), leading to muscle atrophy (e.g., loss of muscle mass and strength). However, the effects of radiation during space flight may result in protein oxidation (Fang et al. 2002), thereby possibly stimulating protein breakdown in skeletal muscle and other tissues. Finally, both the fractional rate of protein synthesis and the fractional rate of protein degradation decrease with age (Chapters 8 and 9). In elderly persons who exhibit a gradual loss of body protein, the fractional rate of protein synthesis is slower than the fractional rate of protein degradation in various tissues, resulting in a gradual loss of body proteins. This may be due to remarkable reductions in: (1) the sensitivity of skeletal muscle and other tissues to anabolic hormones and nutrients (e.g., AAs) (Wilkinson et al. 2018); (2) the circulating levels of anabolic AAs (e.g., arginine) (Wu et al. 2020); and (3) NO synthesis in microvascular endothelial cells due to a deficiency of tetrahydrobiopterin (Delp et al. 2008) in aging persons than in growing individuals or young adults. Thus, enhancing protein balance through improvements in AA nutrition is fundamental to increase resistance to cellular stress, improve muscle strength, and extend the life span of individuals.

Our current knowledge about the regulation of protein metabolism has been built, to a great extent, on studies involving skeletal muscle (Frost and Lang 2008; Goldberg and St John 1976), mainly because of two reasons. First, the skeletal muscle represents 40% and 45% of the body weight in healthy young and adult animals (including fish), respectively, and is the largest reservoir of both free and peptide-bound AAs in animals (Sandoval et al. 2020; Li et al. 2021). Second, a dramatic loss of intramuscular proteins occurs in response to numerous catabolic conditions, such as starvation, low intake of dietary protein, infection, diabetes, denervation, hyperthyroidism, and heat stress (Chapters 8 and 9); therefore, effective means to reverse the negative protein balance are highly desirable. Collective evidence from extensive studies worldwide has shown that many factors can affect protein turnover in skeletal muscle. These factors include: (1) dietary intakes of energy, protein, AAs, and other nutrients (Table 10.3); (2) hormones, hormone-like factors, and other physiological factors (Table 10.4); and (3) stress (including oxidative stress and space flight) and pathological factors (Table 10.5). Note that most of these published studies involved a mixed group of proteins in skeletal muscle, which contains three types of proteins: (1) sarcoplasmic (cytosolic); (2) myofibrillar; and (3) stromal. Sarcoplasmic proteins represent 30–35% of total protein in the muscle by weight. Myofibrillar proteins, which constitute the myofibrillar (contractile) structure in skeletal muscle, account for 55–60% of total protein in the muscle by weight (Sandoval et al. 2020; Southorn et al. 1990). The major myofibrillar proteins are actin and myosin, but more than 15 other proteins are associated with the myofibrillar structure. Therefore, care should be taken to interpret the effects of nutritional, physiological, pathological, and environmental factors on the synthesis and degradation of specific proteins in skeletal muscle.

TABLE 10.3
Nutritional Factors That Affect Protein Turnover in Skeletal Muscle

Factors	Protein synthesis	Protein degradation	Net effect
Frequency of Feeding			
Intermittent feeding	Increase	No effect	Anabolic
Dietary Protein and Energy Intake			
High energy intake	Increase	Decrease	Anabolic
Low energy intake	Decrease	Increase	Catabolic
High-protein intake			
High quality	Increase	Decrease	Anabolic
Low quality	Increase	Increase	Catabolic
Low-protein intake	Decrease	No effect	Catabolic
Fasting			
Short term	Decrease	Increase	Catabolic
Long term	Decrease	Decrease	Preserve nitrogen
Amino Acids and Their Metabolites			
Arginine	Increase	Decrease	Anabolic
Citrulline	Increase	Decrease	Anabolic
Glutamine	Increase	Decrease	Anabolic
Glycine	Increase	Decrease	Anabolic
β-Hydroxy-β-methylbutyrate	Increase	No effect	Anabolic
Leucine	Increase	Decrease	Anabolic
Proline	Increase	No effect	Anabolic
Mixture of EAAs	Increase	Decrease	Anabolic
α-Ketoglutarate	Increase	Decrease	Anabolic
α-Ketoisocaproate	No effect	Decrease	Anabolic
Other Nutritional Factors			
Calcium	No effect	Increase	Catabolic
Glucose	No effect	Decrease	Anabolic
Saturated fatty acids	No effect	Decrease	Anabolic
n-3 Fatty acids	Increase	No effect	Anabolic
n-6 Fatty acids	No effect	Increase	Catabolic
Ketone bodies			
Fed state	Decrease	No effect	Catabolic
Fasted state	Decrease	Decrease	Preserve nitrogen
Magnesium	Required	Decrease	Anabolic
Zinc	Increase	No effect	Anabolic

Note: EAAs, nutritionally essential amino acids.

10.3.4 BLOOD FLOW AS A REGULATOR OF AMINO ACID METABOLISM *IN VIVO*

In intact animals, AA metabolism is controlled at both cellular and systematic levels, including inter-organ cooperation (Chapters 3, 4, and 5). For example, the intestinal absorption of AAs and their transport among tissues, as well as placental-fetal nutrient and O_2 transfer in gestating dams, are dependent on adequate rates of blood flow (Reynolds et al. 2006; Satterfield et al. 2010). Furthermore, metabolic products (e.g., ammonia and CO_2) are carried through blood circulation from peripheral tissues to specific target organs (e.g., liver and lungs) for disposal. Thus, the regulation of blood flow

TABLE 10.4

Hormones, Hormone-Like Factors, and Other Physiological Factors That Affect Protein Turnover in Skeletal Muscle

Factors	Protein synthesis	Protein degradation	Net effect
Hormones			
Estradiol	Increase	Decrease	Anabolic
Glucocorticoids			
Fed state, low dose	Decrease	No effect	Catabolic
Fed state, high dose	Decrease	Increase	Catabolic
Fasted state	Decrease	Increase	Catabolic
Growth hormone	Increase	No effect	Anabolic
Insulin	Increase	Decrease	Anabolic
Progesterone	Increase	No effect	Anabolic
Testosterone	Increase	Decrease	Anabolic
Triiodothyronine			
Physiological dose	*Increase*	*Increase*	*No change*
High dose	Increase	Increase	Catabolic
Hormone-Like Factors			
Insulin-like growth factors I and II	Increase	Decrease	Anabolic
β-Agonists[a]	Increase	No effect	Anabolic
Synthetic steroids[b]	Increase	No effect	Anabolic
Prostaglandin E_2	No effect	Increase	Catabolic
Prostaglandin $F_{2\alpha}$	Increase	No effect	Anabolic
Other Physiological Factors			
Aging[c]	Decrease	Decrease	Catabolic
Cell volume expansion	Increase	Decrease	Anabolic
During exercise	Decrease	Increase	Catabolic
Post-exercise[d]	Increase	Increase	Anabolic
Muscle contraction	Increase	Increase	Anabolic
Pregnancy	Increase	No effect	Anabolic
Space flight	Decrease	Either no effect or increase	Catabolic

[a] Including cimaterol, clenbuterol, isoproterenol, and ractopamine.

[b] Including zeranol, trenbolone acetate, and estradiol-17β.

[c] Compared with neonates. Elderly persons exhibit a lower rate of fractional protein synthesis and a higher rate of fractional protein degradation in skeletal muscle, compared with young adults.

[d] When individuals receive adequate intakes of protein or amino acids and energy after exercise.

is not only vital to life but is also an important mechanism for the modulation of the metabolism of AAs and other nutrients. For example, uteroplacental blood flow is a major determinant of AA transfer from mother to fetus and, therefore, fetal survival and growth in mammals (Figure 10.12).

Compelling evidence shows that physiological levels of NO stimulate blood flow, thereby increasing the supply of AAs, fatty acids, glucose, and oxygen to tissues for protein synthesis and mitochondrial oxidation of energy substrates *in vivo* (Jobgen et al. 2006). Additionally, increased uptakes of dietary AAs [e.g., arginine (the nitrogenous precursor of NO) and ornithine] by insulin-sensitive tissues can promote blood flow into skeletal muscle, as well as the synthesis of polyamines (putrescine, spermidine, and spermine) (Wu et al. 2009). This, in turn, can enhance DNA synthesis, angiogenesis, mitochondrial biogenesis, and oxidative capacity in cells (Bazer et al. 2015).

TABLE 10.5
Stress and Pathological Factors That Affect Protein Turnover in Skeletal Muscle

Factors	Protein synthesis	Protein degradation	Net effect
Stress Factors			
Acidosis	Decrease	Increase	Catabolic
Cold stress	Decrease	Increase	Catabolic
Free radicals/oxidants	Decrease	Increase	Catabolic
Heat stress	Decrease	Increase	Catabolic
Lymphokines			
Interleukin-1	No effect	Increase	Catabolic
Interleukin-6	No effect	Increase	Catabolic
Tumor necrosis factor-α	No effect	Increase	Catabolic
Pathological Factors			
Burn	Decrease	Increase	Catabolic
Cancer	Decrease	Increase	Catabolic
Denervation	No effect	Increase	Catabolic
Diabetes	Decrease	Increase	Catabolic
Fever	Decrease	Increase	Catabolic
Inflammation and sepsis	Decrease	Increase	Catabolic
Injury	Decrease	Increase	Catabolic
High concentrations of nitric oxide	Decrease	Increase	Catabolic
Obesity	Decrease	Increase	Catabolic

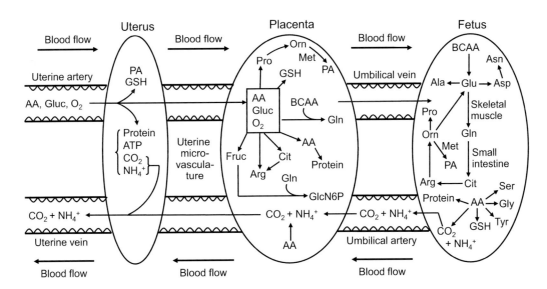

FIGURE 10.12 Provision of AA from mother to fetus via NO-dependent uteroplacental blood flow in the gestating mammal. The uterine artery in the mother delivers oxygen, AA, and other nutrients from the maternal arterial blood to the uterus and, through the uterine microvasculature, to the placenta. Subsequently, the umbilical vein supplies these substances from the placenta to the fetus. Uptake of a nutrient by the uterus or the fetus is determined on the basis of the Fick principle: uptake = blood flow rate × $(A - V)$, where $(A - V)$ represents the difference in arteriovenous concentration of the nutrient across the uterus or the fetus. Fruc, fructose; Gluc, glucose; GlcN6P, glucosamine-6-phosphate; GSH, glutathione; Orn, ornithine; PA, polyamines.

Thus, although either nanomolar or micromolar concentrations of NO inhibit oxygen consumption by isolated mitochondria *in vitro*, physiological levels of NO enhance whole-body energy expenditure in obese persons, brown adipose tissue mass (and its blood flow), and the loss of excessive white adipose tissue from the body (McKnight et al. 2010).

10.4 SUMMARY

Metabolism of AAs involves both near-equilibrium and non-equilibrium reactions, which are under the control of the first and second laws of thermodynamics (namely energy conservation and the notion that an inherent direction occurs in a chemical reaction). Either type of reaction offers distinct biochemical advantages. Precise regulation of metabolic pathways is essential to the survival, growth, development, and health of organisms. Of particular interest, knowledge about the complex mechanisms responsible for metabolic control helps us gain a more complete understanding of AA synthesis, catabolism, and utilization under both physiological and pathological conditions. The intracellular concentrations and localization of enzymes, their covalent and non-covalent modifications, as well as the intracellular concentrations of cofactors, activators, and inhibitors affect the activities of enzymes in cells. Changes in these variables may take seconds, minutes, hours, or days, depending on individual proteins, cell type, developmental stages, and animal species. Although much useful knowledge about enzyme kinetics is based on *in vitro* experiments, what is demonstrated in test tubes does not always take place in intact cells and, even if occurring, may not affect metabolic flux *in vivo* that is also regulated by rates of blood flow to affect the uptake of AAs and other nutrients, as well as the removal of their metabolites. Additionally, it should be borne in mind that *in vivo* concentrations of macromolecules in cells are exceedingly high and there are protein-protein interactions, but such characteristics may be absent from cell lysates or purified enzymes. Therefore, caution should be exercised in extrapolating studies involving *in vitro* preparations to the whole animal. Finally, the regulation of AA metabolism via intracellular protein synthesis and degradation is also controlled by the MTOR cell signaling. AAs are important nutrient signals to activate MTORC1 and MTORC2, thereby increasing protein synthesis, inhibiting proteolysis, preventing or alleviating oxidative stress, and enhancing cytoskeletal reorganization. Thus, MTOR is an attractive target for the regulation of AA metabolism (including intracellular protein turnover) in animal cells. A better understanding of the complex mechanisms responsible for the regulation of AA metabolism will not only greatly advance the field but will also have important implications for the development of new means to improve the immunity, growth, health, and reproduction of humans and other animals.

REFERENCES

Agostoni, C., B. Carratu, C. Boniglia, A.M. Lammardo, E. Riva, and E. Sanzini. 2000. Free glutamine and glutamic acid increase in human milk through a three-month lactation period. *J. Pediatr. Gasteroenterol. Nutr.* 31:508–512.

Aicart-Ramos, C., R. Ana, V. Rodriguez-Crespo. 2011. Protein palmitoylation and subcellular trafficking. *Biochim. Biophys. Acta* 1808:2981–2994.

Alberty, R. 2004. A short history of the thermodynamics of enzyme-catalyzed reactions. *J. Biol. Chem.* 279:27831–27836.

Baker, D.H. 2005. Comparative nutrition and metabolism: explication of open questions with emphasis on protein and amino acids. *Proc. Natl. Acad. Sci. USA* 102:17897–17902.

Bazer, F.W., G.A. Johnson, and G. Wu. 2015. Amino acids and conceptus development during the peri-implantation period of pregnancy. *Adv. Exp. Med. Biol.* 843:23–52.

Bertrand, J., A. Goichon, P. Déchelotte, and M. Coëffier. 2013. Regulation of intestinal protein metabolism by amino acids. *Amino Acids* 45:443–450.

Bixel, M., Y. Shimomura, S. Hutson, and B. Hamprecht. 2001. Distribution of key enzymes of branched-chain amino acid metabolism in glial and neuronal cells in culture. *J. Histochem. Cytochem.* 49:407–418.

Blommaart, E.F., J.J. Luiken, P.J. Blommaart, G.M. van Woerkom, and A.J. Meijer. 1995. Phosphorylation of ribosomal protein S6 is inhibitory for autophagy in isolated rat hepatocytes. *J. Biol. Chem.* 270:2320–2326.

Brosnan, J.T. 2003. Interorgan amino acid transport and its regulation. *J. Nutr.* 133:2068S–2072S.

Brosnan, J.T. 2005. Metabolic design principles: chemical and physical determinants of cell chemistry. *Adv. Enzyme Regul.* 45:27–36.

Brosnan J.T. and M.E. Brosnan. 2012. Glutamate: a truly functional amino acid. *Amino Acids* 45:413–418.

Burrin, D.G. and T.A. Davis. 2004. Proteins and amino acids in enteral nutrition. *Curr. Opin. Clin. Nutr. Metab. Care* 7:79–87.

Closs, E.I., J.-P. Boissel, A. Habermeier, and A. Rotmann. 2006. Structure and function of cationic amino acid transporters (CATs). *J. Membr. Biol.* 213:67–77.

Corvi, M.M., C.L. Soltys, and L.G. Berthiaume. 2001. Regulation of mitochondrial carbamoyl-phosphate synthetase 1 activity by active site fatty acylation. *J. Biol. Chem.* 276:45704–45712.

Costamagna, D., P. Costelli, M. Sampaolesi, and F. Penna. 2015. Role of inflammation in muscle homeostasis and myogenesis. *Mediators Inflamm.* 2015:805172.

Curthoys, N.P. and M. Watford. 1995. Regulation of glutaminase activity and glutamine metabolism. *Annu. Rev. Nutr.* 15:133–159.

Dhanakoti, S.N., J.T. Brosnan, G.R. Herzberg, and M.E. Brosnan. 1990. Renal arginine synthesis: studies *in vitro* and *in vivo*. *Am. J. Physiol.* 259:E437–442.

Delp, M.D., B.J. Behnke, S.A. Spier, G. Wu, and J.M. Muller-Delp. 2008. Aging diminishes endothelium-dependent vasodilation and tetrahydrobiopterin content in rat skeletal muscle arterioles. *J. Physiol.* 586:1161–1168.

Dennis, M.D., J.I. Baum, S.R. Kimball, and L.S. Jefferson. 2011. Mechanisms involved in the coordinate regulation of mTORC1 by insulin and amino acids. *J. Biol. Chem.* 286:8287–8296.

Dillon, E.L., D.A. Knabe, and G. Wu. 1999. Lactate inhibits citrulline and arginine synthesis from proline in pig enterocytes. *Am. J. Physiol.* 276:G1079–G1086.

Dunkley, P.R., L. Bobrovskaya, M.E. Graham, E.I. Von Nagy-Felsobuki, and P.W. Dickson. 2004. Tyrosine hydroxylase phosphorylation: regulation and consequences. *J. Neurochem.* 91:1025–1043.

Fairlamb, A.H. 2003. Chemotherapy of human African trypanosomiasis: current and future prospects. *Trends Parasitol.* 19:488–494.

Fang, Y.Z., S. Yang, and G. Wu. 2002. Free radicals, antioxidants, and nutrition. *Nutrition* 18:872–879.

Fell, D. 1997. *Understanding the Control of Metabolism*. Portland Press, London.

Field, C.J., I. Johnson, and V.C. Pratt. 2000. Glutamine and arginine: immunonutrients for improved health. *Med. Sci. Sports Exerc.* 32:S377–388.

Fitzpatrick, P.F. 1999. Tetrahydropterin-dependent amino acid hydroxylases. *Annu. Rev. Biochem.* 68:355–381.

Fitzpatrick, P.F. 2012. Allosteric regulation of phenylalanine hydroxylase. *Arch. Biochem. Biophys.* 519:194–201.

Flynn, N.E., M.H. Shaw, and J.T. Becker. 2020. Amino acids in health and endocrine function. *Adv. Exp. Med. Biol.* 1265:97–109.

Frost, R.A. and C.H. Lang. 2008. Regulation of muscle growth by pathogen-associated molecules. *J. Anim. Sci.* 86(Suppl. 14):E84–E93.

Fu, W. and M.N. Hall. 2020. Regulation of mTORC2 signaling. *Genes (Basel)* 11(9):1045.

Gao, H. 2020. Amino acids in reproductive nutrition and health. *Adv. Exp. Med. Biol.* 1265:111–131.

Gardner, P.R., G. Costantino, C. Szabó, and A.L. Salzman. 1997. Nitric oxide sensitivity of the aconitases. *J. Biol. Chem.* 272:25071–25076.

Gilbreath, K.R., F.W. Bazer, M.C. Satterfield, and G. Wu. 2021. Amino acid nutrition and reproductive performance in ruminants. *Adv. Exp. Med. Biol.* 1285:43–61.

Gill, M, France, J, Summers, B.W. McBride, and L.P. Milligan. 1989. Mathematical integration of protein metabolism in growing lambs. *J. Nutr.* 119:1269–1286.

Goldberg, A.L., and A.C. St John. 1976. Intracellular protein degradation in mammalian and bacterial cells: Part 2. *Annu. Rev. Biochem.* 45:747–803.

Gomperts, B.D., I.M. Kramer, and P.E. Tatham. 2002. *Signal Transduction*. Academic Press, San Diego, CA.

Guertin, D.A., D.M. Stevens, M. Saitoh, S. Kinkel, K. Crosby, and J.H. Sheen et al. 2009. mTOR complex 2 is required for the development of prostate cancer induced by Pten loss in mice. *Cancer Cell.* 15:148–59.

Hackl, S., R. van den Hoven, M. Zickl, J. Spona, and J. Zentek. 2009. The effects of short intensive exercise on plasma free amino acids in standardbred trotters. *J. Anim. Physiol. Anim. Nutr.* 93:165–173.

Hagiwara, A., M. Cornu, N. Cybulski, P. Polak, C. Betz, F. Trapani et al. 2012. Hepatic mTORC2 activates glycolysis and lipogenesis through Akt, glucokinase, and SREBP1c. *Cell Metab.* 15:725–738.

Harris, R.A., M. Joshi, N.H. Jeoung, and M. Obayashi. 2005. Overview of the molecular and biochemical basis of branched-chain amino acid catabolism. *J. Nutr.* 135:1527S–1530S.

He, W.L. and G. Wu. 2020. Metabolism of amino acids in the brain and their roles in regulating food intake. *Adv. Exp. Med. Biol.* 1265:167–185.

Hobbach, A.J. and E.I. Closs. 2020. Human cationic amino acid transporters are not affected by direct nitros(yl)ation. *Amino Acids* 52:499–503.

Hoffmann, E.K., I.H. Lambert, and S.F. Pedersen. 2009. Physiology of cell volume regulation in vertebrates. *Physiol. Rev.* 89:193–277.

Hou, Y.Q., S.D. Hu, X.Y. Li, W.L. He, and G. Wu. 2020. Amino acid metabolism in the liver: nutritional and physiological significance. *Adv. Exp. Med. Biol.* 1265:21–37.

Hunkeler, M., A. Hagmann, E. Stuttfeld, M. Chami, Y. Guri, H. Stahlberg, and T. Maier. 2018. Structural basis for regulation of human acetyl-CoA carboxylase. *Nature* 558:470–474.

Hutson, S.M., C. Zapalowski, T.C. Cree, and A.E. Harper. 1980. Regulation of leucine and alpha-ketoisocaproic acid metabolism in skeletal muscle. Effects of starvation and insulin. *J. Biol. Chem.* 255:2418–2426.

Hutson, S.M., A.J. Sweatt, and K.F. LaNoue. 2005. Branched-chain amino acid metabolism: implications for establishing safe intakes. *J. Nutr.* 135:1557S–1564S.

Jobgen, W.S., S.K. Fried, W.J. Fu, C.J. Meininger, and G. Wu. 2006. Regulatory role for the arginine-nitric oxide pathway in metabolism of energy substrates. *J. Nutr. Biochem.* 17:571–588.

Johnston, W.K., P.J. Unrau, M.S. Lawrence, M.E. Glasner, and D.P. Bartel. 2001. RNA-catalyzed RNA polymerization: accurate and general RNA-templated primer extension. *Science* 292:1319–1325.

Jois, M., B. Hall, K. Fewer, and J.T. Brosnan. 1989. Regulation of hepatic glycine catabolism by glucagon. *J. Biol. Chem.* 264:3347–3351.

Jungas, R.L., M.L. Halperin, and J.T. Brosnan. 1992. Quantitative analysis of amino acid oxidation and related gluconeogenesis in humans. *Physiol. Rev.* 72:419–448.

Kang, Y., R. Liu, J. Wu, and L. Chen. 2019. Structural insights into the mechanism of human soluble guanylate cyclase. *Nature* 574:206–210.

Kim, J. and K.L. Guan. 2011. Amino acid signaling in TOR activation. *Annu. Rev. Biochem.* 80:1001–1032.

Kim, J.Y., G.W. Song, G. Wu, and F.W. Bazer. 2012. Functional roles of fructose. *Proc. Natl. Acad. Sci. USA* 109:E1619–E1628.

Knudsen, J.R., A.M. Fritzen, D.E. James, T.E. Jensen, M. Kleinert, and E.A.Richter. 2020. Growth factor-dependent and -independent activation of mTORC2. *Trends Endocrinol. Metab.* 31:13–24.

Kohli, R., C.J. Meininger, T.E. Haynes, W. Yan, J.T. Self, and G. Wu. 2004. Dietary L-arginine supplementation enhances endothelial nitric oxide synthesis in streptozotocin-induced diabetic rats. *J. Nutr.* 134:600–608.

Kwon, H., T.E. Spencer, F.W. Bazer, and G. Wu. 2003. Developmental changes of amino acids in ovine fetal fluids. *Biol. Reprod.* 68:1813–1820.

Lamming, D.W., L. Ye, P. Katajisto, M.D. Goncalves, M. Saitoh, D.M. Stevens et al. 2012. Rapamycin-induced insulin resistance is mediated by mTORC2 loss and uncoupled from longevity. *Science* 335:1638–1643.

Lei, J., D.Y. Feng, Y.L. Zhang, S. Dahanayaka, X.L. Li, K. Yao et al. 2012a. Hormonal regulation of leucine catabolism in mammary epithelial cells. *Amino Acids* 45:531–41.

Lei, J., D.Y. Feng, Y.L. Zhang, F.Q. Zhao, Z.L. Wu, A. San Gabriel et al. 2012b. Nutritional and regulatory role of branched-chain amino acids in lactation. *Front. Biosci.* 17:2725–2739.

Li, H., C.J. Meininger, J.R. Hawker Jr., T.E. Haynes, D. Kepka-Lenhart, S.K. Mistry et al. 2001. Regulatory role of arginase I and II in nitric oxide, polyamine, and proline syntheses in endothelial cells. *Am. J. Physiol.* 280:E75–E82.

Li, P., Y.L. Yin, D.F. Li, S.W. Kim, and G. Wu. 2007. Amino acids and immune function. *Br. J. Nutr.* 98:237–252.

Li, P., S.W. Kim, X.L. Li, S. Datta, W.G. Pond, and G. Wu. 2008. Dietary supplementation with cholesterol and docosahexaenoic acid increases the activity of the arginine-nitric oxide pathway in tissues of young pigs. *Nitric Oxide* 19:259–265.

Li, P., S.W. Kim, X.L. Li, S. Datta, W.G. Pond, and G. Wu. 2009. Dietary supplementation with cholesterol and docosahexaenoic acid affects concentrations of amino acids in tissues of young pigs. *Amino Acids* 37:709–716.

Li, X.Y., S.X. Zheng, and G. Wu. 2020. Amino acid metabolism in the kidneys: nutritional and physiological significance. *Adv. Exp. Med. Biol.* 1265:71–95.

Li, X.Y., S.X. Zheng, and G. Wu. 2021. Nutrition and functions of amino acids in fish. *Adv. Exp. Med. Biol.* 1285:133–168.

Liu, P., Z. Wang, and W. Wei. 2014. Phosphorylation of Akt at the C-terminal tail triggers Akt activation. *Cell Cycle* 13:2162–2164.

Liu, B.M., X.R. Jiang, L. Cai, X.M. Zhao, Z.L. Dai, G. Wu, and X.L. Li. 2019. Putrescine mitigates intestinal atrophy through suppressing inflammatory response in weanling piglets. *J. Anim. Sci. Biotechnol.* 10:69.

Lösel, R. and M. Wehling. 2003. Nongenomic actions of steroid hormones. *Nat. Rev. Mol. Cell Biol.* 4:46–56.

MacLean, D.A. and T.E. Graham. 1993. Branched-chain amino acid supplementation augments plasma ammonia responses during exercise in humans. *J. Appl. Physiol.* 74:2711–2717.

Manning, B.D. and A. Toker. 2017. AKT/PKB signaling: navigating the network. *Cell* 169:381–405.

Manning, G., G.D. Plowman, T. Hunter, and S. Sudarsanam. 2002. Evolution of protein kinase signaling from yeast to man. *Trends Biochem. Sci.* 27:514–520.

McKnight, J.R., M.C. Satterfield, W.S. Jobgen, S.B. Smith, T.E. Spencer, C.J. Meininger et al. 2010. Beneficial effects of L-arginine on reducing obesity: potential mechanisms and important implications for human health. *Amino Acids* 39:349–357.

McNeal, C.J., C.J. Meininger, C.D. Wilborn, C.D. Tekwe, and G. Wu. 2018. Safety of dietary supplementation with arginine in adult humans. *Amino Acids* 50:1215–1229.

Meijer, A.J., and P.F. Dubbelhuis. 2004. Amino acid signalling and the integration of metabolism. *Biochem. Biophys. Res. Commun.* 313:397–403.

Meijer, A.J., W.H. Lamers, and R.A. Chamuleau. 1990. Nitrogen metabolism and ornithine cycle function. *Physiol. Rev.* 70:701–748.

Meininger, C.J. and G. Wu. 1997. L-Glutamine inhibits nitric oxide synthesis in bovine venular endothelial cells. *J. Pharmacol. Exp. Ther.* 281:448–453.

Metallo, C.M. and M.G. Vander Heiden. 2013. Understanding metabolic regulation and its influence on cell physiology. *Mol. Cell* 49:388–398.

Morris, S.M. Jr. 2009. Recent advances in arginine metabolism: roles and regulation of the arginases. *Br. J. Pharmacol.* 157:922–930.

Morris, S.M. Jr. 2012. Arginases and arginine deficiency syndromes. *Curr. Opin. Clin. Nutr. Metab. Care* 15:64–70.

Newsholme, E.A. 1984. *Biochemistry for the Medical Sciences.* Wiley, New York.

Oh, W.J. and E. Jacinto. 2011. mTOR complex 2 signaling and functions. *Cell Cycle* 10:2305–2316.

Ovadi, J., and V. Saks. 2004. On the origin of intracellular compartmentation and organized metabolic systems. *Mol. Cell. Biochem.* 256:5–12.

Owen, O.E. 2005. Ketone bodies as a fuel for the brain during starvation. *Biochem. Mol. Biol. Educ.* 33:246–251.

Palii, S.S., C.E. Kays, C. Deval, A. Bruhat, P. Fafournoux, and M.S. Kilberg. 2009. Specificity of amino acid regulated gene expression: analysis of gene subjected to either complete or single amino acid deprivation. *Amino Acids* 37:79–88.

Parry-Billings, M., S.J. Bevan, E. Opara, and E.A. Newsholme. 1991. Effects of changes in cell volume on the rates of glutamine and alanine release from rat skeletal muscle *in vitro. Biochem. J.* 276:559–561.

Perry, B.D., J.A. Rahnert, Y. Xie, B. Zheng, M.E. Woodworth-Hobbs, and S.R. Price. 2018. Palmitate-induced ER stress and inhibition of protein synthesis in cultured myotubes does not require Toll-like receptor 4. *PLoS One* 13:e0191313.

Phang, J.M., W. Liu, and O. Zabirnyk. 2010. Proline metabolism and microenvironmental stress. *Annu. Rev. Nutr.* 30:441–463.

Pollard, T.D., W.C. Earnshaw, J. Lippincott-Schwartz, and G. Johnson. 2017. *Second Messengers. Cell Biology,* 3rd edition. Elsevier, New York. pp. 443–462.

Pope, C., S. Karanth, and J. Liu. 2005. Pharmacology and toxicology of cholinesterase inhibitors: uses and misuses of a common mechanism of action. *Environ. Toxicol. Pharmacol.* 19:433–446.

Poulin, R., L. Lu, B. Ackermann, P. Bey, and A.E. Pegg. 1992. Mechanism of the irreversible inactivation of mouse ornithine decarboxylase by α-difluoromethylornithine. Characterization of sequences at the inhibitor and coenzyme binding sites. *J. Biol. Chem.* 267:150–158.

Ramadoss, J., G. Wu, and T.A. Cudd. 2008. Chronic binge ethanol mediated acidemia reduces availability of glutamine and related amino acids in maternal plasma of pregnant sheep. *Alcohol* 42:657–666.

Reeds, P.J. 1989. Regulation of protein turnover. In: *Animal Growth Regulation* (Campion, D.R., G.J. Hausman, and R.J. Martin, ed). Plenum Press, New York. pp. 183–210.

Reynolds, L.P., J.S. Caton, D.A. Redmer, A.T. Grazul-Bilska, K.A. Vonnahme, P.B. Borowicz et al. 2006. Evidence for altered placental blood flow and vascularity in compromised pregnancies. *J. Physiol.* 572:51–58.

Rodbell, M. 1980. The role of hormone receptors and GTP-regulatory proteins in membrane transduction. *Nature* 284:17–22.

Rose, A.J. and E.A. Richter. 2009. Regulatory mechanisms of skeletal muscle protein turnover during exercise. *J. Appl. Physiol.* 106:1702–1711.

Rousseau, G. 2013. Fifty years ago: the quest for steroid hormone receptors. *Mol. Cell. Endocrinol.* 375:10–13.

Sabatini, D.M. 2017. Twenty-five years of mTOR: uncovering the link from nutrients to growth. *Proc. Natl. Acad. Sci. USA* 114:11818–11825.

Sandoval, C., G. Wu, S.B. Smith, K.A. Dunlap, and M.C. Satterfield. 2020. Maternal nutrient restriction and skeletal muscle development: consequences for postnatal health. *Adv. Exp. Med. Biol.* 1265:153–165.

Satterfield, M.C., F.W. Bazer, T.E. Spencer, and G. Wu. 2010. Sildenafil citrate treatment enhances amino acid availability in the conceptus and fetal growth in an ovine model of intrauterine growth restriction. *J. Nutr.* 140:251–258.

Sawant, O.B., J. Ramadoss, G.D. Hankins, G. Wu, and S.E. Washburn. 2014. Effects of L-glutamine supplementation on maternal and fetal hemodynamics in gestating ewes exposed to alcohol. *Amino Acids* 46:1981–1996.

Sawant, O.B., G. Wu, and S.E. Washburn. 2015. Maternal L-glutamine supplementation prevents prenatal alcohol exposure-induced fetal growth restriction in ewes. *Amino Acids* 47:1183–1192.

Segel, I.H. 1993. *Enzyme Kinetics*. Wiley, New York.

Sehgal, S.N., H. Baker, and C. Vézina. 1975. Rapamycin (AY-22,989), a new antifungal antibiotic. II. Fermentation, isolation and characterization. *J. Antibiot. (Tokyo)* 28:727–732.

Shi, W., C.J. Meininger, T.E. Haynes, K. Hatakeyama, and G. Wu. 2004. Regulation of tetrahydrobiopterin synthesis and bioavailability in endothelial cells. *Cell Biochem. Biophys.* 41:415–433.

Southorn, B.G., R.M. Palmer, and P.J. Garlick. 1990. Acute effects of corticosterone on tissue protein synthesis and insulin-sensitivity in rats *in vivo*. *Biochem. J.* 272:187–191.

Srere, P.A. 1985. The metabolon. *Trends Biochem. Sci.* 10:109–110.

Stein, T.P. and M.D. Schluter. 1997. Human skeletal muscle protein breakdown during spaceflight. *Am. J. Physiol.* 272:E688–E695.

Strack, P.R., L. Waxman, and J.M. Fagan. 1996. Activation of the multicatalytic endopeptidase by oxidants. Effects on enzyme structure. *Biochemistry* 35:7142–7249.

Sugden, P.H. and S.J. Fuller. 1991. Regulation of protein turnover in skeletal and cardiac muscle. *Biochem. J.* 273:21–37.

Suryawan, A. and T.A. Davis. 2014. Regulation of protein degradation pathways by amino acids and insulin in skeletal muscle of neonatal pigs. *J. Anim. Sci. Biotechnol.* 5:8.

Tato, I., R. Bartrons, F. Ventura, and J.L. Rosa. 2011. Amino acids activate mammalian target of rapamycin complex 2 (mTORC2) via PI3K/Akt signaling. *J. Biol. Chem.* 286:6128–6142.

Tekwe, C.D., K. Yao, J. Lei, X.L. Li, A. Gupta, Y.Y. Luan et al. 2019. Oral administration of α-ketoglutarate enhances nitric oxide synthesis by endothelial cells and whole-body insulin sensitivity in diet-induced obese rats. *Exp. Biol. Med.* 244:1081–1088.

Thompson, J.R. and G. Wu. 1991. The effect of ketone bodies on nitrogen metabolism in skeletal muscle. *Comp. Biochem. Physiol. B* 100:209–216.

Tischler, M.E. and A.L. Goldberg. 1980a. Production of alanine and glutamine by atrial muscle from fed and fasted rats. *Am. J. Physiol.* 238:E487–E493.

Tischler, M.E. and A.L. Goldberg. 1980b. Leucine degradation and release of glutamine and alanine by adipose tissue. *J. Biol. Chem.* 255:8074–8081.

Treberg, J.R., M.E. Brosnan, M. Watford, and J.T. Brosnan. 2010. On the reversibility of glutamate dehydrogenase and the source of hyperammonemia in the hyperinsulinism/hyperammonemia syndrome. *Adv. Enzyme Regul.* 50:34–43.

Tsikas, D. and G. Wu. 2015. Homoarginine, arginine, and relatives: analysis, metabolism, transport, physiology, and pathology. *Amino Acids* 47:1697–1702.

Vandenburgh, H., J. Chromiak, J. Shansky, M. Del Tatto, and J. Lemaire. 1999. Space travel directly induces skeletal muscle atrophy. *FASEB J.* 13:1031–1038.

Wang, X. and M. Watford. 2007. Glutamine, insulin and glucocorticoids regulate glutamine synthetase expression in C2C12 myotubes, Hep G2 hepatoma cells and 3T3 L1 adipocytes. *Biochim. Biophys. Acta* 1770:594–600.

Wang, J.J., Z.L. Wu, D.F. Li, N. Li, S.V. Dindot, M.C. Satterfield et al. 2012. Nutrition, epigenetics, and metabolic syndrome. *Antioxid. Redox Signal.* 17:282–301.

Wang, L., D. Yi, Y.Q. Hou, B.Y. Ding, K. Li, B.C. Li et al. 2016a. Dietary supplementation with α-ketoglutarate activates mTOR signaling and enhances energy status in skeletal muscle of lipopolysaccharide-challenged piglets. *J. Nutr.* 146:1514–1520.

Wang, X.Q., G. Wu, and F.W. Bazer. 2016b. mTOR: the master regulator of conceptus development in response to uterine histotroph during pregnancy in ungulates. In: *Molecules to Medicine with mTOR* (Maiese, K., ed). Elsevier, New York. pp. 23–35.

Washburn, S.E., O.B. Sawant, E.R. Lunde, G. Wu, and T.A. Cudd. 2013. Acute alcohol exposure, acidemia or glutamine administration impacts amino acid homeostasis in ovine maternal and fetal plasma. *Amino Acids* 45:543–554.

Watford, M. 2003. The urea cycle. *Biochem. Mol. Biol. Educ.* 31:289–297.

Watford, M. 2015. Glutamine and glutamate: nonessential or essential amino acids? *Anim. Nutr.* 1:119–122.

Welbourne, T.C. 1987. Interorgan glutamine flow in metabolic acidosis. *Am. J. Physiol.* 253:F1069–F1076.

Wester, T.J., G. Kraft, D. Dardevet, S. Polakof, I. Ortigues-Marty, D. Rémond, and I. Savary-Auzeloux. 2015. Nutritional regulation of the anabolic fate of amino acids within the liver in mammals: concepts arising from *in vivo* studies. *Nutr. Res. Rev.* 28:22–41.

Wheatley, S.M., S.W. El-Kadi, A. Suryawan, C. Boutry, R.A. Orellana, H.V. Nguyen et al. 2014. Protein synthesis in skeletal muscle of neonatal pigs is enhanced by administration of β-hydroxy-β-methylbutyrate. *Am. J. Physiol.* 306:E91–E99.

Wilkinson, D.J., M. Piasecki, and P.J. Atherton. 2018. The age-related loss of skeletal muscle mass and function: measurement and physiology of muscle fibre atrophy and muscle fibre loss in humans. *Ageing Res. Rev.* 47:123–132.

Wu, G. 1998. Amino acid metabolism in the small intestine. *Trends Comp. Biochem. Physiol.* 4:39–74.

Wu, G. 2009. Amino acids: metabolism, functions, and nutrition. *Amino Acids* 37:1–17.

Wu, G. 2018. *Principles of Animal Nutrition.* CRC Press, Boca Raton, FL.

Wu, G. 2020. Metabolism and functions of amino acids in sense organs. *Adv. Exp. Med. Biol.* 1265:201–217.

Wu, G., and J.R. Thompson. 1987. Ketone bodies inhibit leucine degradation in chick skeletal muscle. *Int. J. Biochem.* 19:937–943.

Wu, G., and J.R. Thompson. 1988. The effect of ketone bodies on alanine and glutamine metabolism in isolated skeletal muscle from the fasted chick. *Biochem. J.* 255:139–144.

Wu, G., and J.R. Thompson. 1990. The effect of ketone bodies on protein turnover in isolated skeletal muscle from the fed and fasted chick. *Int. J. Biochem.* 22:263–268.

Wu, G., and D.A. Knabe. 1994. Free and protein-bound amino acids in sow's colostrum and milk. *J. Nutr.* 124:415–424.

Wu, G., and N.E. Flynn. 1995. Regulation of glutamine and glucose metabolism by cell volume in lymphocytes and macrophages. *Biochim. Biophys. Acta* 1243:343–350.

Wu, G., and S.M. Morris Jr. 1998. Arginine metabolism: nitric oxide and beyond. *Biochem. J.* 336:1–17.

Wu, G., J.R. Thompson, G. Sedgwick, and M. Drury. 1989. Formation of alanine and glutamine in chick (*Gallus domesticus*) skeletal muscle. *Comp. Biochem. Physiol. B* 93:609–613.

Wu, G., D.A. Knabe, and S.W. Kim. 2004. Arginine nutrition in neonatal pigs. *J. Nutr.* 134:2783S–2390S.

Wu, G., F.W. Bazer, T.A. Davis, S.W. Kim, P. Li, J.M. Rhoads et al. 2009. Arginine metabolism and nutrition in growth, health and disease. *Amino Acids* 37:153–168.

Wu, Z.L., Y.Q. Hou, S.D. Hu, F.W. Bazer, C.J. Meininger, C.J. McNeal, and G. Wu. 2016. Catabolism and safety of supplemental L-arginine in animals. *Amino Acids* 48:1541–1552.

Wu, G., F.W. Bazer, G.A. Johnson, and Y.Q. Hou. 2018. Arginine nutrition and metabolism in growing, gestating and lactating swine. *J. Anim. Sci.* 96:5035–5051.

Wu, C.S., Q. Wei, H. Wang, D.M. Kim, M. Balderas, G. Wu et al. 2020. Protective effects of ghrelin on fasting-induced muscle atrophy in aging mice. *J. Gerontol. Ser. A* 75:621–630.

Xi, P.B., Z.Y. Jiang, Z.L. Dai, X.L. Li, K. Yao, C.T. Zheng et al. 2012. Regulation of protein turnover by L-glutamine in porcine intestinal epithelial cells. *J. Nutr. Biochem.* 23:1012–1017.

Yao, K., Y.L. Yin, X.L. Li, P.B. Xi, J.J. Wang, J. Lei et al. 2012. Alpha-ketoglutarate inhibits glutamine degradation and enhances protein synthesis in intestinal porcine epithelial cells. *Amino Acids* 42:2491–2500.

Yu, T., Y. Dabirian, Q. Liu, V. Siewers, and J. Nielsen. 2019. Strategies and challenges for metabolic rewiring. *Curr. Opin. Syst. Biol.* 15:30–38.

Zhang, J.M., W.L. He, D. Yi, D. Zhao, Z. Song, Y.Q. Hou, and G. Wu. 2019. Regulation of protein synthesis in porcine mammary epithelial cells by L-valine. *Amino Acids* 51:717–726.

Zhang, Q., Y.Q. Hou, F.W. Bazer, W.L. He, E.H. Posey, and G. Wu. 2021. Amino acids in swine nutrition and production. *Adv. Exp. Med. Biol.* 1285:81–107.

11 Physiological Functions and Nutritional Supplementation of Amino Acids

Amino acids (AAs) serve not only as the building blocks of proteins but also as signaling molecules in cell physiology (Bazer et al. 2015; Beaumont and Blachier 2020; Closs et al. 2000; Ruth and Field 2013; Suryawan et al. 2020). Furthermore, AAs are regulators of food intake, gene expression, the protein phosphorylation cascade, and cell-to-cell communication (Wu 2009). Additionally, AAs are key precursors for the syntheses of hormones and low-molecular-weight nitrogenous substances, with each having enormous biological importance (Table 11.1). Physiological concentrations of AA metabolites [e.g., carbon monoxide (CO), creatine, catecholamines (e.g., dopamine, epinephrine, and norepinephrine), glutathione (GSH), nitric oxide (NO), hydrogen sulfide (H_2S), polyamines (putrescine, spermidine, and spermine), homoarginine, serotonin, taurine, D-AAs, and thyroid hormones] are required for cellular functions, including antioxidative, anti-inflammatory, and immune responses (Agostinelli et al. 2010; Bazer et al. 2015; Blachier et al. 2015; Field et al. 2000; Le Floc'h et al. 2011; Rodionov et al. 2019; Tsikas et al. 2018). However, elevated levels of other products [e.g., ammonia, γ-aminobutyrate (GABA), homocysteine, and dimethylarginines] are pathogenic factors for neurological disorders, oxidative stress, and cardiovascular disease (He and Wu 2020; Jakubowski 2019; Li et al. 2020a). Thus, an optimal balance among AAs in the diet and circulation is crucial for whole-body homeostasis. There is growing recognition that AAs regulate key metabolic pathways that are necessary for maintenance, growth, development, reproduction, lactation, productivity, immunity, and health. These AAs, which are called functional AAs in nutrition, include arginine, cysteine, glutamate, glutamine, glycine, leucine, methionine, proline, and tryptophan. Dietary supplementation with one or a mixture of these AAs is beneficial for (1) improving the embryonic, fetal, and postnatal survival of offspring; (2) enhancing antioxidative capacity and immunity; (3) preventing and ameliorating health problems at various stages of the life cycle, including fetal growth restriction [indicated by low body weight (BW) at birth], neonatal morbidity and mortality, weaning-associated intestinal dysfunction and wasting syndrome, metabolic syndrome (e.g., hyperglycemia, dyslipidemia, obesity, diabetes, and cardiovascular disease), and infertility; and (4) optimizing the efficiency of metabolic transformations to enhance muscle growth, milk production, and athletic performance, while preventing excess white fat deposition and reducing adiposity (Durante 2020; Flynn et al. 2020; Ren et al. 2020; Wang et al. 2010; Wu 2010). The physiological functions of AAs along with their use for dietary supplementation and therapy are highlighted in this chapter and are further discussed in Chapter 12 on inborn errors of metabolism.

11.1 ROLES OF AAs IN PROTEIN AND SMALL-PEPTIDE SYNTHESES

11.1.1 PROTEIN SYNTHESIS

The primary purpose of AAs in humans and other animals is to serve as building blocks for proteins, which are essential components of the body and are required for cell growth, development, and function. The protein synthetic pathway in cells is illustrated in Chapter 8. This biochemical process requires a large amount of energy. Note that not all proteins contain each of the 20 canonical proteinogenic AAs in animal cells. For example, mature bovine, human and porcine insulin lack

TABLE 11.1
Physiological Functions of Amino Acids and Their Metabolites in Humans and Other Animals[a]

Amino Acid	Metabolites or Direct Action	Major Functions
Amino acids	Proteins	Structural components of the body; cell growth, development, and function; colloidal properties
	Peptides	Hormones, antibiotics, metabolic regulation, and antioxidants
	Ammonia	Substrate for carbamoyl phosphate synthetase II and glutamate dehydrogenase; bridging amino acid and glucose metabolism; regulation of acid-base balance
Alanine	Directly	Inhibition of pyruvate kinase and hepatic autophagy; gluconeogenesis; transamination; glucose-alanine cycle; interorgan metabolism and transport of both carbon and nitrogen
β-Alanine	Directly	A component of coenzyme A and pantothenic acid
	Dipeptides	Carnosine (β-alanyl-L-histidine), carcinine (β-alanyl-histamine), anserine (β-alanyl-1-methyl-L-histidine), and balenine (β-alanyl-3-methyl-histidine) with antioxidative effects; improvements of skeletal muscle function and exercise performance; osmolytes
Arginine	Directly	Activation of MTOR and AMPK signaling pathways; antioxidant; regulation of hormone secretion; allosteric activation of N-acetylglutamate synthase; ammonia detoxification; regulation of gene expression; immune function; activation of tetrahydrobiopterin synthesis; nitrogen reservoir; methylation of proteins; deimination (formation of citrulline) of arginine residues in proteins[b]
	Nitric oxide	Signaling molecule; regulator of food intake, nutrient metabolism, vascular tone, hemodynamics, angiogenesis, spermatogenesis, embryogenesis, fertility, immune function, hormone secretion, wound healing, neurotransmission, tumor growth, mitochondrial biogenesis, energy metabolism, and cell function
	Agmatine	Inhibition of NOS, ornithine decarboxylase, and monoamine oxidase; ligand for α_2-adrenergic and imidazoline receptors; precursor for the synthesis of putrescine
	Ornithine	Ammonia detoxification; syntheses of proline, glutamate, and polyamines; mitochondrial integrity; wound healing; precursor for the synthesis of putrescine
	Methylarginines	Competitive inhibition of NOS
Asparagine	Directly	Cell metabolism and physiology; regulation of gene expression and immune function; ammonia detoxification; function of the nervous system
	Acrylamide[c]	Oxidant; cytotoxicity; gene mutation; low food quality
Aspartate	Directly	Purine, pyrimidine, asparagine, and arginine synthesis; transamination; urea cycle; activation of NMDA receptors; synthesis of inositol and β-alanine
	D-Aspartate	Activation of NMDA receptors in the brain
Citrulline	Directly	Antioxidant; arginine synthesis; osmoregulation; ammonia detoxification; N reservoir in the conceptus
Cysteine	Directly	Disulfide linkage in protein; transport of sulfur
	Taurine	Antioxidant; regulation of cellular redox state; an osmolyte
	H_2S	A signaling molecule; regulation of cell metabolism; killing of pathogens; vasodilation; neurological function

(Continued)

TABLE 11.1 (*Continued*)
Physiological Functions of Amino Acids and Their Metabolites in Humans and Other Animals[a]

Amino Acid	Metabolites or Direct Action	Major Functions
Glutamate	Directly	Glutamine, citrulline, and arginine synthesis; bridging the urea cycle with the Krebs cycle; transamination; ammonia assimilation; flavor enhancer; activation of NMDA receptors; *N*-acetylglutamate synthesis; a metabolic fuel in animal cells, particularly enterocytes
	γ-Aminobutyrate	Inhibitory or excitatory neurotransmitter, depending on age, type of receptor, and the region of the brain; regulation of neuronal excitability throughout the nervous system; modulation of muscle tone; inhibition of T-cell response and inflammation
Glutamine	Directly	Regulation of protein turnover through cellular MTOR signaling; regulation of cell volume; gene expression; and immune function; a major fuel for rapidly proliferating cells; inhibition of apoptosis; syntheses of purine, pyrimidine, ornithine, citrulline, arginine, proline, and asparagine; nitrogen reservoir; synthesis of NAD(P)
	Glu and Asp	Excitatory neurotransmitters; components of the malate shuttle; cell metabolism; ammonia detoxification; major fuels for enterocytes; alanine synthesis
	Glucosamine-6-P	Synthesis of amino sugars and glycoproteins; inhibition of NO synthesis; anti-inflammation; angiogenesis; cell growth and development; inhibition of the pentose cycle
	Ammonia	Renal regulation of acid-base balance; synthesis of glutamate and carbamoyl phosphate
Glycine	Directly	Inhibiting calcium influx through activation of a glycine-gated channel in the cell membrane; purine and serine synthesis; synthesis of porphyrins and heme; inhibitory neurotransmitter in the central nervous system; co-agonist with glutamate for NMDA receptors; antioxidant; anti-inflammation; one-carbon metabolism; conjugation with bile acids
	Heme	Hemoproteins (e.g., hemoglobin, myoglobin, catalase, and cytochrome c); production of carbon monoxide (a signaling molecule); storage of iron in the body
	Bilirubin	Natural ligand of aryl hydrocarbon receptor in the cytoplasm
Histidine	Directly	Protein methylation; hemoglobin structure and function; antioxidative dipeptides; one-carbon metabolism
	Histamine	Allergic reaction; vasodilator; activation of central acetylcholine secretion; stimulation of secretions by the gastrointestinal tract
	Imidazoleacetate	Analgesic and narcotic actions
	Urocanate	Modulation of the immune response in the skin; protecting the skin against ultraviolet radiation
Isoleucine	Directly	Synthesis of glutamine and alanine; balance among BCAAs
Leucine	Directly	Regulation of protein turnover through cellular MTOR signaling and gene expression; activator of glutamate dehydrogenase; BCAA balance; flavor enhancer
	Gln and Ala	Many metabolic functions
	HMB	Regulation of immune response and skeletal muscle protein synthesis
Lysine	Directly	Regulation of nitric oxide synthesis; antiviral activity (treatment of herpes simplex); protein methylation (e.g., trimethyllysine in calmodulin), acetylation, ubiquitination, and *O*-linked glycosylation

(*Continued*)

TABLE 11.1 (*Continued*)

Physiological Functions of Amino Acids and Their Metabolites in Humans and Other Animals[a]

Amino Acid	Metabolites or Direct Action	Major Functions
	5-Hydroxylysine	Structure and function of collagen
Methionine	Homocysteine	Oxidant; independent risk factor for cardiovascular disease; inhibition of nitric oxide synthesis
	Betaine	Methylation of homocysteine to methionine; one-carbon unit metabolism; precursor for glycine synthesis
	Cysteine	Cellular metabolism and nutrition
	SAM	Methylation of proteins and DNA; creatine, epinephrine, and polyamine synthesis; regulation of gene expression; one-carbon metabolism
	Taurine	Antioxidant; osmoregulation; organ development; vascular, muscular, cardiac, and retinal functions; anti-inflammation; conjugation with bile acids
	Phospholipids	Synthesis of lecithin and phosphatidylcholine cell signaling
Phenylalanine	Directly	Activation of tetrahydrobiopterin (a cofactor for NOS) synthesis; synthesis of tyrosine and phenylacetylglutamate; neurological development and function
Proline	Directly	Collagen structure and function; neurological function; osmoprotectant; activation of MTOR; a sensor of cellular energy status; an antioxidant; a regulator of the differentiation of cells (including embryonic stem cells)
	H_2O_2	Killing pathogens; intestinal integrity; a signaling molecule; an oxidant required for innate immunity
	P5C	Cellular redox state; DNA synthesis; lymphocyte proliferation; ornithine, citrulline, arginine, and polyamine synthesis; gene expression; stress response
	4-Hydroxyproline	Structure and function of collagen; glycine synthesis
	3-Hydroxyproline	Structure and function of collagen
Serine	Directly	Required for the conversion of homocysteine into cystathionine in methionine catabolism; one-carbon metabolism; syntheses of cysteine, purine, pyrimidine, ceramide, choline, and phosphatidylserine; synthesis of tryptophan in bacteria; gluconeogenesis (particularly in ruminants); protein phosphorylation
	Glycine	Many metabolic and regulatory functions
	D-Serine[d]	Activation of NMDA receptors in the brain
Theanine	Directly	An amino acid (glutamine analogue) in tea leaves; antioxidant; increasing concentrations of γ-aminobutyrate, dopamine, and serotonin in the brain; neuroprotective effect
Threonine	Directly	Synthesis of the mucin protein that is required for maintaining intestinal integrity and function; immune function; protein phosphorylation and O-linked glycosylation; glycine synthesis
Tryptophan	Serotonin	Neurotransmitter; inhibiting the production of inflammatory cytokines and superoxide; regulation of food intake; improvements in mood, cognition, behavior, and nocturnal sleep in humans; reduction in aggressive behavior
	N-Acetylserotonin	Inhibitor of tetrahydrobiopterin synthesis; antioxidant; inhibition of the production of inflammatory cytokines and superoxide
	Melatonin	Antioxidant; inhibition of the production of inflammatory cytokines and superoxide; circadian rhythms (through the synthesis in the retina and the pineal gland)

(Continued)

TABLE 11.1 (*Continued*)
Physiological Functions of Amino Acids and Their Metabolites in Humans and Other Animals[a]

Amino Acid	Metabolites or Direct Action	Major Functions
	Anthranilic acid	Inhibiting the production of proinflammatory T helper 1 cytokines; preventing autoimmune neuroinflammation; enhancing immune function
	Niacin	A component of NAD and NADP, coenzymes for many oxidoreductases; posttranslational modifications of proteins, including poly(ADP-ribose) polymerases
	Indoles[e]	Natural ligands of aryl hydrocarbon receptor in the cytoplasm; regulation of immune responses
	Kynurenate	Neuromodulatory activity; antiexcitotoxic and anticonvulsant effects
Tyrosine	Directly	Protein phosphorylation, nitrosation, and sulfation
	Dopamine	Neurotransmitter; regulation of immune response
	EPN and NEPN	Neurotransmitters; cell metabolism
	Melanin	Antioxidant; inhibition of the production of inflammatory cytokines and superoxide; immunity; energy homeostasis; sexual activity; stress response; pigmentation of the skin and hair
	T3 and T4	Regulation of energy and protein metabolism, as well as growth and development
Valine	Directly	Synthesis of glutamine and alanine; balance among BCAAs
Arg and Met	Polyamines	Gene expression; DNA and protein synthesis; ion channel function; apoptosis; signal transduction; antioxidants; cell function; cell proliferation and differentiation
Arg, Met, and Gly	Creatine	Antioxidant; antiviral; antitumor; energy metabolism in the heart, skeletal muscle, brain, reproductive tract, and other tissues; neurological and muscular development and function
Cys, Glu, and Gly	Glutathione	Free radical scavenger; antioxidant; cell metabolism (e.g., the formation of leukotrienes, mercapturate, glutathionylspermidine, glutathione-nitric oxide adduct, and glutathionyl proteins); signal transduction; gene expression; apoptosis; cellular redox; immune response
Gln, Asp, and Gly	Nucleic acids	Coding for genetic information; gene expression; cell cycle and function; protein and uric acid synthesis; lymphocyte proliferation; facilitation of wound healing
	Uric acid	Antioxidant; the major end product of amino acid oxidation in avian species
Lys, Met, and Ser	Carnitine	Transport of long-chain fatty acids into mitochondria for oxidation; storage of energy as acetylcarnitine; an antioxidant
Ser and Met	Choline	A component of acetylcholine (a neurotransmitter); and phosphatidylcholine (a structural lipid in the membrane); precursor for the synthesis of betaine (a methyl donor in the one-carbon metabolism), sarcosine, and glycine

[a] Unless indicated, amino acids (except for glycine, taurine, β-alanine, and γ-aminobutyrate) mentioned herein are L-amino acids.

[b] Including myelin basic protein, filaggrin, and histone proteins.

[c] Formed when asparagine reacts with reducing sugars or reactive carbonyls at high temperature.

[d] Synthesized from L-serine by serine racemase.

[e] Including indole acetic acid, kynurenine, and tryptamine.

Note: BCAAs, branched-chain amino acids; SAM, *S*-adenosylmethionine; EPN, epinephrine; HMB, β-hydroxy-β-methylbutyrate; MTOR, mechanistic target of rapamycin; NEPN, norepinephrine; NOS, nitric oxide synthase; T$_3$, triiodothyronine; and T$_4$, thyroxine.

both tryptophan and methionine. In addition, animal proteins do not contain pyrrolysine, but it is a rare proteinogenic AA in certain bacteria (Chapter 1).

11.1.2 SMALL-PEPTIDE SYNTHESIS

As noted in Chapter 5, many small peptides with enormous physiological importance are synthesized from AAs. These peptides include (1) antibiotics produced by bacteria and the intestinal mucosa, (2) GSH (a tripeptide), (3) dipeptides (carnosine, carcinine, anserine, and balenine in a species-specific manner), and (4) physiologically important small peptides consisting of 9 or 10 AA residues, including opioid peptides. Note that anserine is not synthesized in humans but it is abundant in cattle and many other animals (e.g., pigs and poultry). In some but not all of these peptides, two cysteine residues form a disulfide linkage (–S–S–). A synthetic dipeptide widely used in the food industry is aspartame (Asp-Phe-O-CH$_3$), which is approximately 200 times sweeter than sucrose (Magnuson et al. 2007). Examples of the physiologically important small peptides synthesized by animals are listed here.

Angiotensin II (10 AAs):	Asp-Arg-Val-Tyr-Ile-His-Pro-Phe-His-Leu (NH$_2$)
Bradykinin (9 AAs):	Arg-Pro-Pro-Gly-Phe-Ser-Pro-Phe-Arg (NH$_2$)
Oxytocin (9 AAs):	Cys-Tyr-Ile-Gln-Asn-Cys-Pro-Leu-Gly (NH$_2$)
Arginine vasopressin (9 AAs):	Cys-Tyr-Phe-Gln-Asn-Cys-Pro-Arg-Gly (NH$_2$)
Kallidin (10 AAs):	Lys-Arg-Pro-Pro-Gly-Phe-Ser-Pro-Phe-Arg (NH$_2$)
Lysine vasopressin (9 AAs):	Cys-Tyr-Phe-Gln-Asn-Cys-Pro-Lys-Gly (NH$_2$)

11.2 ROLES OF AAs IN THE SYNTHESIS OF NONPEPTIDE MOLECULES AND OTHER METABOLITES

11.2.1 SYNTHESIS OF NONPEPTIDE MOLECULES

AAs are substrates for the synthesis of nonpeptide hormones (e.g., epinephrine, norepinephrine, and thyroxine), low-molecular-weight nitrogenous substances (e.g., ammonia, carnitine, creatine, dopamine, NO, GABA, nucleotides, polyamines, homoarginine, and thyroxine), and other molecules [e.g., CO and H$_2$S]. Some of these synthetic pathways require S-adenosylmethionine (SAM) as the methyl group donor (Bieber 1988; Mudd et al. 2007). Each of these AA metabolites has enormous biological importance. For example, AAs play a major role in gaseous signaling (see Section 11.2.2.1). Physiological concentrations of AA metabolites are essential to whole-body homeostasis, reproduction, lactation, growth, development, immunity, and health. However, excessive amounts of some metabolites (e.g., ammonia, homocysteine, and asymmetric dimethylarginine) are pathogenic factors for neurological disorders, oxidative stress, and cardiovascular disease (Durante 2020; Hou et al. 2020; Wu 2020a). There is growing recognition that metabolites of AAs at physiological concentrations are cell signaling molecules that affect gene expression, the protein phosphorylation cascade, neurotransmission, nutrition, and metabolic pathways in humans and other animals (Table 11.2).

An important physiological role of AAs is to regulate neurotransmission in the central nervous system (He and Wu 2020). Thus, normal AA metabolism is essential for maintaining good mental health (including behavior) in humans and other animals. Conversely, abnormal AA metabolism possibly due to a combination of genetic defects and environmental factors may contribute to mental disorders. The latter include depression, attention deficit-hyperactivity disorder, substance use disorders (drug addiction), autism spectrum disorder, bipolar disorder, and schizophrenia. In the United States, nearly one in five U.S. adults (51.5 million in 2019) live with a mental illness, ranging

TABLE 11.2

Important Roles for Amino Acids and Their Metabolites in the Nutrition and Metabolism of Humans and Other Animals

1. Food intake, as well as nutrient absorption and metabolism (e.g., nutrient transport, protein turnover, fat synthesis and oxidation, glucose synthesis and oxidation, amino acid synthesis and oxidation, urea and uric synthesis for ammonia detoxification, and efficiency of food utilization)
2. Cellular signaling via MTOR, cAMP, and cGMP pathways, as well as the generation of NO, CO, and H_2S
3. Hormone synthesis and secretion (e.g., insulin, glucagon, growth hormone, prolactin, placental lactogen, and epinephrine)
4. Regulation of endothelial cell function, blood flow, and lymph circulation
5. Immune function and health (e.g., T-cell proliferation and B-cell maturation, antibody production by B cells, killing of pathogens, as well as the prevention and mitigation of obesity, diabetes, and metabolic syndrome)
6. Reproduction and lactation (e.g., spermatogenesis, male fertility, female fertility, ovulation, ovarian steroidogenesis, embryonic implantation and survival, placental angiogenesis and growth, fetal growth and development, and lactogenesis)
7. Acid-base balance, neurotransmission, extracellular and intracellular osmolarity[a], antioxidative defense, and whole-body homeostasis
8. Postnatal survival, growth, and development, as well as tissue regeneration and remodeling

[a] Osmolarity is defined as osmoles of solute/L of solution (e.g., the serum, plasma, blood, or fetal fluid), and osmolality as osmoles of solute/kg of solvent (e.g., water). In physiology and medicine, scientists and clinicians tend to use the term "osmolarity" for convenience.

from a mild to a moderate and to a severe degree of severity (NIMH 2021). Knowledge of AA metabolism and its regulation in tissues, particularly the brain, can help to develop effective means to prevent and treat neurological abnormalities.

11.2.2 Gaseous Signaling via Nitric Oxide, Carbon Monoxide, and Hydrogen Sulfide

11.2.2.1 Chemical Properties of AA-Derived Gases

NO, CO, and H_2S are lipophilic, colorless molecules that easily penetrate biological membranes and exert their effects independent of membrane receptors (Kharitonov et al. 1995; Kots et al. 2011; Li et al. 2009). NO and CO are odorless, but H_2S and SO_2 each have a characteristic strong, pungent odor (e.g., the smell of rotten eggs for H_2S). NO is a highly reactive free radical, whereas CO, H_2S, and SO_2 are strong reducing agents. None of these gases are stable in physiological solutions. Particularly, NO is rapidly oxidized to nitrite (NO_2^-) and nitrate (NO_3^-) as stable products in the body. Because of its rapid oxidation by oxygen, hemoglobin, and other oxidants, NO has an exceedingly short half-life (<5 s) in cells and tissues (Durante 2020). CO is oxidized to CO_2, in the biological system. CO_2 reacts with H_2O via carbonic anhydrase to form H_2CO_3, which is in chemical equilibrium with H^+ plus HCO_3^-. The half-lives of CO in the blood circulation are 22–120 and 40–75 min, respectively, for humans (Shimazu et al. 2000) and pigs (Aberg et al. 2004). In physiological solutions, H_2S exists in equilibrium with HS^-, whereas SO_2 spontaneously reacts with water to yield sulfurous acid (H_2SO_3) and then sulfite (SO_3^{2-}) (Moore and Whiteman 2015). In addition, H_2S is enzymatically oxidized to thiosulfate ($S_2O_3^{2-}$) and sulfate (SO_4^{2-}) in the mitochondria by specific enzymes, sulfide:quinone oxidoreductase, persulfide dioxygenase, rhodanese, and sulfite oxidase (Bouillaud and Blachier 2011; Beltowski 2015). The half-lives of H_2S in the blood of rats, pigs and cows are 2.5, 1.3 and 0.86 min, respectively (Whitfield et al. 2008).

As gases, NO, CO, H_2S, and SO_2 are exhaled by the lungs (Durante 2020; Moore and Whiteman 2015). The remaining amounts are oxidized in the body, as noted previously. The end products of their oxidation in cells and tissues, which include nitrite, nitrate, HCO_3^-, sulfite, and sulfate, are excreted from the body primarily by the kidneys (via urine) and, to a lesser extent, by the large intestine (via feces).

11.2.2.2 Functions of Nitric Oxide

NO is a signaling molecule in animals (Figure 11.1). Physiological concentrations of NO enhance (1) angiogenesis; (2) cell signal transduction; (3) embryogenesis; (4) expression of genes related to tissue growth and development, oxidation of energy substrates, and antioxidative responses; (5) mitochondrial biogenesis and respiration; (6) secretion of hormones (e.g., insulin, growth hormone, prolactin, and placental lactogen); (7) immune responses and the killing of pathogens; (8) intestinal motility and mucosal integrity; (9) neurotransmission; (10) transport and metabolism of nutrients; (11) ovulation in females; (12) spermatogenesis in males; (13) thermogenesis and control of body temperature; (14) vasodilation and cardiovascular function; and (15) wound healing.

Among the first identified functions of NO were its roles as the major endothelium-derived relaxing factor, a mediator of the immune response, a neurotransmitter, a cytotoxic free radical, and a

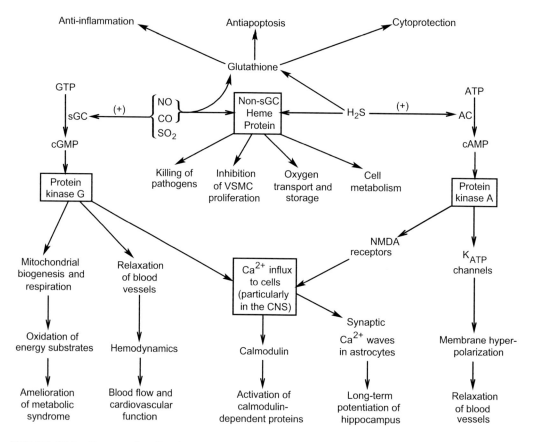

FIGURE 11.1 Gaseous signaling in cells via cGMP-dependent and cAMP-dependent, as well as cGMP-independent and cAMP-independent pathways in animal cells. Physiological levels of both NO and CO activate guanylate (guanylyl) cyclase to generate cGMP, which stimulates cGMP-dependent protein kinase. H_2S activates adenylate cyclase activity to yield cAMP, which stimulates cAMP-dependent protein kinase. NO, CO, and H_2S enhance glutathione synthesis to protect cells from oxidative stress. These gases also play important roles in innate and cell-mediated immunities, including cytoprotection for immunocytes, the modulation of inflammatory responses, reductions in the production of proinflammatory cytokines, and increases in the production of anti-inflammatory cytokines. AC, adenylate cyclase; CNS, central nervous system; and sGC, soluble guanylate cyclase. The sign (+) denotes activation.

widespread signaling molecule (Boger et al. 2007; Closs et al. 2000; Ignarro et al. 2001; Ricciardolo et al. 2004). Thus, NO participates in virtually every cellular and organ function in the body. In blood vessels, NO released by endothelial cells activates guanylyl cyclase in adjacent smooth muscle cells, thereby elevating the concentrations of cellular cGMP and causing smooth muscle relaxation (Moncada and Higgs 1993). As such, physiological concentrations of NO produced by the endothelial isoform of eNOS [type 3 NO synthase (NOS)] are essential for regulating vascular tone and hemodynamics (Moncada and Higgs 1993). In addition, NO stimulates angiogenesis (the formation of new blood vessels from preexisting ones), which plays an important role in physiological events (e.g., wound healing, vascular remodeling, ovulation, and placental growth) and in pathological conditions (e.g., tumor growth, myocardial infarction, and diabetic retinopathy). Furthermore, NO inhibits leukocyte adhesion, platelet aggregation, superoxide generation, the expression of vascular cell adhesion molecules and monocyte chemotactic peptides, proliferation of smooth muscle cells, and the release of endothelin 1 (a vasoconstrictor). Thus, NO is a vasodilator, antiatherogenic, antiproliferative, and antithrombotic factor in the cardiovascular system (Durante 2020; Wu and Meininger 2000).

Physiological concentrations of NO also regulate the transport and metabolism of nutrients, including glucose, fatty acids, and AAs in animals (Jobgen et al. 2006). As a signaling molecule, increasing the availability of NO in the physiological range stimulates glucose and fatty-acid uptake, as well as glucose and fatty-acid oxidation in skeletal muscle, heart, liver, and adipose tissue, while inhibiting the syntheses of glucose, glycogen, and fat in target tissues (e.g., liver and adipose), and enhancing lipolysis in white adipocytes. Thus, a chronic inhibition of NO synthesis causes hyperlipidemia and fat accretion in rats (Khedara et al. 1999), whereas dietary arginine supplementation (e.g., 1.25% arginine-HCl in drinking water for 10 weeks) reduces fat mass in obese diabetic fatty rats (Fu et al. 2005). The underlying mechanisms responsible for the beneficial health effects of physiological concentrations of NO may involve multiple cGMP-dependent pathways (McKnight et al. 2010). First, NO stimulates the phosphorylation of AMP-activated protein kinase (AMPK), resulting in (1) decreased levels of malonyl-CoA via the inhibition of acetyl-CoA carboxylase and activation of malonyl-CoA decarboxylase and (2) decreased expression of genes related to lipogenesis and gluconeogenesis (glycerol-3-phosphate acyltransferase, sterol regulatory element-binding protein 1c, and phosphoenolpyruvate carboxykinase). Second, NO increases the phosphorylation of hormone-sensitive lipase and perilipins, leading to the translocation of the lipase to the surface of neutral lipid droplets and hence the stimulation of lipolysis. Third, NO activates the expression of peroxisome proliferator-activated receptor γ (PPARγ) coactivator-1α, thereby enhancing mitochondrial biogenesis, oxidative phosphorylation, and development of brown adipose tissue. Fourth, NO increases blood flow to insulin-sensitive tissues, promoting the uptake of energy substrates and the removal of their oxidation products via the circulation. Modulation of the arginine-NO pathway through dietary supplementation with L-arginine or L-citrulline may aid in the prevention and treatment of metabolic syndrome in obese humans and companion animals and in reducing unfavorable fat mass in animals of agricultural importance (Li et al. 2021b; Wu 2020c; Zhang et al. 2021).

As a free radical species, NO has two facets in its biology. As an oxidant, high or pathological concentrations of NO inhibit nearly all enzyme-catalyzed reactions through protein oxidation (Dai et al. 2013a; Jobgen et al. 2006). Proteins inactivated by NO include (1) heme-containing proteins, including cytochromes (e.g., cytochromes b, c, c_1, and aa_3) in the mitochondrial respiratory chain; (2) enzymes containing nonheme iron (also known as iron-sulfur proteins), including aconitase of the Krebs cycle, as well as NADH dehydrogenase, succinate dehydrogenase, and coenzyme Q reductase of the mitochondrial electron transport system; and (3) proteins that undergo S-nitrosothiol modification, including creatine kinase, insulin-receptor substrate 1, and protein kinase B. NO also reacts with H_2O_2 to form $ONOO^-$, another potent oxidant. Elevated levels of NO and peroxynitrite readily oxidize biomolecules (e.g., proteins, AAs, lipids, and DNA), which lead to cell injury and death. This cytotoxic effect of NO is responsible for the killing of pathogens by activated macrophages and other phagocytes in the immune system. The pathogens include bacteria, parasites, fungi, and viruses, including coronaviruses such as severe acute respiratory syndrome coronavirus (SARS-CoV; Åkerström et al. 2005) and SARS-CoV-2 [the virus causing the coronavirus disease-2019 (Covid-19); Akaberi et al. 2020]. Of note, excessive NO is deleterious to mammalian cells and mediates the pathogenesis of many diseases, including the autoimmune destruction of pancreatic β cells in type 1 diabetes mellitus, arthritis, glomerulonephritis, and neurological disorders. In addition, when excess NO is produced by all NOS isoforms under septic and inflammatory conditions, life-threatening hypotension occurs in animals.

11.2.2.3 Functions of Carbon Monoxide

Unlike NO, CO is not an oxidant and, therefore, does not directly cause oxidative damage to AAs or macromolecules (Li et al. 2009). However, like NO, CO reversibly binds heme-containing proteins, including oxyhemoglobin, myoglobin and cytochrome c oxidase, and soluble guanylyl cyclase. CO, a product of heme oxygenase (HO), binds the enzyme's physiological substrate (heme), and this reaction may be a mechanism for regulating CO bioavailability (Wu and Wang 2005). Because physiological concentrations of CO activate the conversion of GTP to cGMP, which triggers cGMP-dependent kinases and the phosphorylation of target proteins, this gas can elicit a series of physiological responses (e.g., relaxation of vascular smooth muscle cells, vasodilation, and mitochondrial biogenesis) (Figure 11.1).

CO is a neural messenger that differs markedly from classical neurotransmitters (e.g., glutamate, acetylcholine, and noradrenaline) in biosynthesis, chemical nature, cellular localization, and mechanisms of action (Queiroga et al. 2015). In neurons, CO, either alone or in combination with NO, enhances the synthesis of cGMP from GTP. CO acts downstream from the N-methyl-D-aspartate (NMDA) receptor as a retrograde messenger at synapses and stimulates long-term potentiation (a type of synaptic plasticity used as a mechanism of learning) in the hippocampus. Endogenous CO may also play an important role in memory processing.

Physiological concentrations of CO have potent cytoprotective effects, particularly on neurons (Wu and Wang 2005). Overexpression of the heme oxygenase 1 (HO1) gene protects dopaminergic neurons against the neurotoxicity induced by 1-methyl-4-phenylpyridinium. By contrast, *HO1* knockout mice exhibit a profound lesion in the brain following the administration of NMDA into the striatum. Moreover, overexpression of HO2 protects olfactory receptor neurons from glutathione depletion-induced apoptosis. The neuroprotective action of CO is a new addition to the long list of the functions of glycine and heme in humans and other animals (Goebel and Wollborn 2020).

CO can also modulate the functions of the immune system (Nakahira et al. 2006; Otterbein et al. 2000). For example, high concentrations of CO above physiological ranges inhibit microbial growth and kill pathogenic organisms, but also induce apoptosis and tissue injury via the NF-κB cell signaling pathway (Li et al. 2009). This notion is further substantiated by the following lines of evidence. First, CO is a key modulator of NO-mediated antiapoptotic and anti-inflammatory functions in hepatocytes and macrophages, as these effects are absent in mice lacking HO1 or receiving HO1 inhibitors. Similar results were obtained for human enterocytes treated with enterohemorrhagic *Escherichia coli*. Second, CO derived from HO1 prevents reactive oxygen species-induced translocation of toll-like receptors (TLR) 2, 4, 5, and 9 into lipid rafts in macrophages, thereby inhibiting TLR signaling and conferring potent anti-inflammatory effects. Third, CO reduces NO synthesis by iNOS (inducible NOS) in hepatocytes and intestinal cells, decreases the circulating levels of proinflammatory cytokines [e.g., interleukins 1β and 6, and tumor necrosis factor-α (TNF-α)], and increases the production of anti-inflammatory cytokines (e.g., interleukin 10) via the p38 mitogen-activated protein kinase pathway. Also, inhaled CO at physiological doses confers anti-inflammatory effects against ventilator-induced lung injury.

Like NO, CO can regulate the metabolism of energy substrates in mitochondria (Ryter et al. 2006). At high doses above physiological ranges, CO inhibits cytochrome c oxidase, thereby reducing substrate oxidation and ATP production. Addition of a CO donor (5–30 μM) to the incubation medium results in a dose-dependent increase in the oxidation of glucose and oleic acid in both the adipose tissue and the skeletal muscle of rats (McKnight et al. 2010). Thus, upregulation of CO synthesis, within physiological ranges, may reduce adiposity. In support of this notion, oral administration of arginine via drinking water increases NOS1 and HO3 expression in the adipose tissue of both Zucker diabetic fatty rats (Fu et al. 2005) and diet-induced obese rats (Jobgen et al. 2009a, b), while reducing fat gain and improving whole-body insulin sensitivity in both animal models. Similarly, partly through the regulation of nutrient metabolism via cGMP signaling, dietary supplementation with arginine reduces fat mass and enhances antioxidative capacity primarily through changes in the expression of genes in growing-finishing pigs (Tan et al. 2009). Furthermore, arginine supplementation [e.g., adding 0.8% arginine to the basal diet between Days 14 and 28 (Li et al. 2014) or between Days 30 and 114 of gestation (Mateo et al. 2007)] increases embryonic/fetal survival and growth in gilts. Weekly intraperitoneal administration of an HO1 inducer (cobalt protoporphyrin, 3 mg/kg BW) to obese diabetic mice for 6 weeks reduces visceral and subcutaneous fat, concentrations of proinflammatory cytokines (e.g., interleukins 6 and 1β, and TNFα), and glucose in the plasma (Li et al. 2008). In addition, arginine supplementation improves whole-body insulin sensitivity, as well as the metabolic profiles of fatty acids and glucose in the plasma of rats with chemically induced diabetes (Kohli et al. 2004), obese rats with type 2 diabetes mellitus (Fu et al. 2005), and diet-induced obese rats (Jobgen et al. 2009a,b). These findings indicate that CO may ameliorate the adverse effects of obesity and metabolic syndrome in humans and other animals.

11.2.2.4 Functions of Hydrogen Sulfide

H_2S is another gas recently recognized to play an important role in the cardiovascular system through a number of mechanisms (Figure 11.1). First, there may be cross-talk between various gaseous signaling pathways. Particularly, physiological levels of H_2S modulate the arginine-NO pathway in the endothelial cells of the aorta and induce vascular dilation (Li et al. 2009). For example, H_2S improves survival after cardiac arrest and cardiopulmonary resuscitation via an eNOS-dependent mechanism in mice. Second, increasing physiological concentrations of H_2S can increase cGMP availability in the vasculature, which in turn triggers cGMP-dependent kinases and the phosphorylation of target proteins that elicit a series of physiological responses (e.g., relaxation of vascular smooth muscle cells, vasodilation, and mitochondrial biogenesis). Third, H_2S has a Ca^{2+}-dependent effect on vasodilation via cGMP-independent mechanisms that may involve (1) direct stimulation of ATP-sensitive K^+ channels and membrane hyperpolarization; (2) a decrease in the production of oxidants; and (3) Ca^{2+}/calmodulin signaling in vascular smooth muscle cells. Fourth, physiological levels of H_2S inhibit myocardial injury induced by oxidants (e.g., homocysteine), thereby maintaining the circulatory system in the normal state.

H_2S is a novel mediator of neurological functions (Moore and Whiteman 2015). The H_2S released from astrocytes or glia surrounding the synapses facilitates induction of hippocampal long-term potentiation via activation of NMDA receptors. This gas also increases Ca^{2+} concentrations in glial cells and induces Ca^{2+} waves in astrocytes to mediate glial signal transduction. Furthermore, H_2S has an anti-inflammatory effect by augmenting GSH availability in neurons. This conclusion is based on evidence that (1) H_2S increases γ-glutamylcysteine synthase activity either by direct activation of the enzyme or through a posttranscriptional mechanism (e.g., enhancement of mRNA translation and/or inhibition of protein degradation); (2) H_2S enhances concentrations of cAMP that activate protein kinase A, leading to NMDA phosphorylation and the opening of Ca^{2+} channels; and (3) H_2S stimulates ATP-sensitive K^+ channels in neuronal cells, causing the efflux of K^+ and membrane hyperpolarization.

Finally, H_2S can regulate cell metabolism (Li et al. 2009). For example, H_2S is an inhibitor of cytochrome C in the mitochondrial electron transport system. Thus, nontoxic levels of H_2S decrease cellular oxidative metabolism, attenuate the production of reactive oxygen species, and possibly increase the longevity of animals. H_2S may be an oxygen sensor, thereby modulating the response of cells to hypoxia. In the lumen of the large intestine where concentrations of total and free H_2S are in millimolar and micromolar ranges, physiological concentrations of H_2S regulate the metabolism of short-chain fatty acids (including butyrate), glucose, and glutamine, while modulating the proliferation of colonocytes and possibly tumorigenesis and the progression of colon cancer (Beaumont and Blachier 2020). Therapeutic applications of H_2S in clinical medicine are being actively investigated.

11.2.3 Roles of Select AAs

11.2.3.1 Arginine

Arginine has crucial roles in nutrition and metabolism (Wu et al. 2009). First, as a major building block for protein synthesis, arginine represents 14% of total nitrogen in body protein. In addition, there are multiple pathways for arginine catabolism to generate ornithine, polyamines, proline, glutamate, agmatine, creatine, homoarginine, and NO (Chapters 4 and 5). Each of these substances has enormous biological importance (see other sections of this chapter). Thus, arginine requirements by the fetus, young animals, and adults are particularly high. Second, arginine is required for maintaining hepatic urea synthesis in an active state. Third, arginine stimulates the secretion of growth hormone and insulin and activates the mechanistic target of rapamycin (MTOR) cell signaling in humans and other animals, thereby playing an important role in regulating protein synthesis and degradation (Chapter 10). Fourth, arginine increases the proliferation and migration of enterocytes by activating MTOR and focal adhesion kinase, respectively. Fifth, arginine inhibits the expression of pro-oxidative and lipogenic genes, while increasing the expression of genes (e.g., PPARγ coactivator-1α and AMPK kinase, and glutathione synthase) related to mitochondrial biogenesis, development of brown adipose tissue, antioxidative responses, and oxidation of energy substrates (e.g., fatty acids and glucose) in a cell-specific manner.

Compelling evidence shows that dietary supplementation with arginine is beneficial for improving cardiovascular health, immunity, neurological function, muscular activity, wound healing, fertility in both males and females, nutrient absorption, mitochondrial biogenesis, and insulin sensitivity, while reducing hyperglycemia, dyslipidemia, obesity, high blood pressure, atherosclerosis, infections, embryonic and fetal deaths, and diarrhea (Table 11.3). For example, through the activation of the MTOR cell signaling pathway to stimulate protein synthesis and inhibit proteolysis in skeletal muscle, dietary supplementation with 1% arginine promotes lean tissue gain in animals (Jobgen et al. 2009; Kim et al. 2013; Tan et al. 2009). Similarly, administration of arginine is effective in enhancing exercise endurance and muscle force generation in humans (Fricke et al. 2008), and also in reducing inflammation and maintaining muscle integrity in a mouse model of Duchenne muscular dystrophy (Hnia et al. 2008), the most common muscle wasting disease. This beneficial effect of arginine results, in part, from increases in blood flow across skeletal muscle as well as the associated uptake of nutrients and oxygen by this organ. Because muscle wasting occurs in astronauts or bed-rest patients, it is important to determine whether this disorder can be prevented by dietary arginine supplementation. The actions of arginine on the vasculature and other tissues are mediated by both NO-dependent and NO-independent mechanisms (Table 11.4). The favorable effect of L-arginine in treating many common health problems is unique among AAs and offers great promise for improved health and well-being in humans and other animals.

TABLE 11.3
Roles of Arginine in the Growth, Health, and Diseases of Humans and Other Animals

Roles of Arginine	Effect	Mediators
Cardiovascular disorders		
Coronary and peripheral arterial diseases	↓	NO and possibly homoarginine
Heart failure, stroke, and ischemia–reperfusion injury	↓	NO and possibly homoarginine
Sickle cell anemia and vasculopathy	↓	NO

(Continued)

TABLE 11.3 (*Continued*)

Roles of Arginine in the Growth, Health, and Diseases of Humans and Other Animals

Roles of Arginine	Effect	Mediators
Endothelial dysfunction in patients with CVRF		
Aging and hyperhomocysteinemia	↓	NO
Diabetes, hypertension, and smoking	↓	NO and possibly homoarginine
Hypercholesterolemia and high-fat feeding	↓	NO
Hormone secretion		
Growth hormone, glucagon, insulin, and prolactin	↑	NO and ornithine
Placental lactogen and progesterone	↑	NO and ornithine
Immune function		
B-cell maturation and antibody production	↑	NO, PA, and PS
Killing pathogens (bacteria, fungi, parasites, and virus)	↑	NO
T-cell proliferation and cytokine production	↑	NO, PA, and PS
Metabolism		
BAT growth and energy-substrate oxidation	↑	cGMP, PA, cAMP, and NO
Cell signaling (AMPK, MTOR, and cGMP)	↑	NO and Arg
Lactogenesis and neonatal growth and development	↑	Arg, NO, MTOR, PA, and proline
Mitochondrial biogenesis and function	↑	cGMP, PA, and NO
Protein synthesis and muscle growth	↑	MTOR and PA
Ammonia detoxification via the urea cycle	↓	Arg, NAG, and ornithine
Obesity, insulin resistance, and dyslipidemia	↓	AMPK, Arg, and NO
Orotic aciduria and gout	↓	NAG and ornithine
Production of ROS and oxidative stress	↓	Arg, creatine, PA, and NO
Protein degradation and apoptosis	↓	MTOR, NO, and autophagy
Reproduction		
Embryo implantation, survival, and growth	↑	NO, PA, PS, and MTOR
Fetal survival, growth, and health	↑	NO, PA, PS, and MTOR
Ovulation, ovarian steroidogenesis, and oocyte quality	↑	NO and PA
Placental angiogenesis, growth, and function	↑	NO, PA, PS, and MTOR
Spermatogenesis, sperm quality, and male fertility	↑	NO, PA, and PS
Uterine contractility and preterm labor	↓	NO
Erectile dysfunction	↓	NO
Preeclampsia in human pregnancy and animal models	↓	NO
Skeletal muscle and brain function	↑	Creatine, NO, and PS
Tissue injury and repair		
Cystic fibrosis and lung injury	↓	NO, PA, and proline
Gastrointestinal, liver, and vessel injury	↓	NO, PA, and proline
Necrotizing enterocolitis in infants	↓	NO, PS, PD, and PA
Renal disease with systemic hypertension	↓	NO
Severe malaria, ulcers, and mitochondrial myopathy	↓	NO
Tissue integrity, wound healing, and angiogenesis	↑	NO, PA, proline, and PS
Tumor growth		
Tumorigenesis at early stages	↓	NO
Tumorigenesis at late stages	↑	PA, proline, ornithine, and PS

Note: The symbols "↑" and "↓" denote enhancement and inhibition (or prevention), respectively. AMPK, AMP-activated protein kinase; BAT, brown adipose tissue; CVRF, cardiovascular risk factors; MTOR, mechanistic target of rapamycin (protein kinase); NAG, *N*-acetylglutamate; NO, nitric oxide; PA, polyamines; PS, protein synthesis; ROS, reactive oxygen species.

TABLE 11.4
Nitric Oxide (NO)-Dependent and NO-Independent Actions of L-Arginine on the Vasculature of Humans and Other Animals

NO-Dependent Vascular and other metabolic Actions	NO-Independent Vascular Actions
↑ GC and smooth muscle cell relaxation	↑ EC membrane polarization and transport activity
↑ Vasodilation and the flow of blood to tissues	↑ Expression of GTP-CH1 for BH4 synthesis
↑ Transport of water across the cell membrane	↑ Expression of GSH-synthetic genes in cells
↑ Glucose transport and oxidation by tissues	↑ MTOR cell signaling and protein synthesis
↑ Brown adipose tissue development	↑ Brown adipose tissue development
↑ Oxidation of fatty acids in tissues	↑ Production of agmatine and homoarginine
↑ Anti-inflammatory responses	↑ CO production and signaling
↑ Killing pathogens (e.g., bacteria and viruses)	↑ Beneficial bacteria in the intestine
↑ EC proliferation and angiogenesis	↑ Extracellular and intracellular pH
↓ Endothelin 1 release by EC	↑ Release of insulin, GH, glucagon, and prolactin
↓ Leukocyte adhesion to blood vessel wall	↑ Synthesis of ornithine, creatine, Pro, and PA
↓ Platelet aggregation within blood vessel	↑ Plasmin generation and fibrinogenolysis
↓ Superoxide production by EC	↓ Leukocyte adhesion to non-EC matrix
↓ Expression of cell adhesion molecules	↓ FA profile, oxygenation, and viscosity of blood
↓ Expression of monocyte chemotactic peptides	↓ Angiotensin-converting enzyme activity
↓ Obesity and dyslipidemia	↓ Homocysteine in blood
↓ Cardiovascular disease (including hypertension)	↓ Lactate, ammonia, and ketone bodies in blood
↓ Proliferation of vascular smooth muscle cells	↓ Release of O_2^- and H_2O_2 and lipid peroxidation
↓ EC mitochondrial injury and apoptosis	↓ Formation of TXB_2, fibrin, and platelet-fibrin

Note: CO, carbon monoxide; EC, endothelial cell; FA, fatty acid; GC, guanylyl cyclase; GH, growth hormone; GSH, glutathione; GTP-CH1, GTP-cyclohydrolase-1; MTOR, mechanistic target of rapamycin; PA, polyamines; Pro, proline; TXB_2, thromboxane B_2. The symbols ↑ and ↓ denote increase and decrease, respectively.

Over the past decade, there has been growing interest in the role of homoarginine (a physiological metabolite of arginine) in the health and disease of humans and other animals (Ajinkya et al. 2016; Jensen et al. 2020). Less than 0.025% and 0.045% of ingested arginine are metabolized to homoarginine in pigs and rats, respectively (Hou et al. 2016). Concentrations of homoarginine in the plasma are relatively low (approximately $2\,\mu M$) in healthy humans (Marescau et al. 1985) and rats (Hou et al. 2015), but increase up to $20\,\mu M$ in hyperargininemic patients (Marescau et al. 1985), and decrease in diabetic mice (Wetzel et al. 2019). Emerging evidence shows that homoarginine can regulate the metabolism of arginine and other nutrients by inhibiting arginine transport across the cell membranes, arginase, as well as liver and bone alkaline phosphohydrolases, while serving as a substrate for NOS (Atzler et al. 2015; Tsikas et al. 2018). Whether homoarginine has a beneficial or an adverse effect on NO production likely depends on cell type, extracellular and intracellular concentrations of arginine, and activities of competing pathways for homoarginine and arginine metabolism. Of note, low concentrations of homoarginine in the plasma are associated with a high risk of cardiovascular (Atzler et al. 2015) and renal (Wieczorek-Surdacka et al. 2019) diseases in humans and animals. Accordingly, dietary supplementation with homoarginine [via either drinking water (50 mg/L) or a miniosmotic pump (0.72 mg/kg BW/day)] for 12 weeks prevents kidney damage in diabetic mice (Wetzel et al. 2019).

11.2.3.2 Glutamine

Physiological functions of glutamine include its roles in (1) modulating the secretion of hormones (e.g., increasing the release of insulin and growth hormone, but reducing the production of glucocorticoids), (2) participating in multiple metabolic pathways (e.g., nucleotide and arginine syntheses), and (3) regulating gene expression and signal transduction in cells (Wu et al. 2011a). Through its oxidation pathway, glutamine is a major energy substrate for rapidly dividing cells, including enterocytes and immunologically challenged lymphocytes, and other cell types (e.g., kidneys during food deprivation, reticulocytes, and activated macrophages), providing ATP for intracellular protein turnover, nutrient transport through the plasma membrane, cell growth and migration, as well as the maintenance of the integrity of cells (Blachier et al. 2015; Dominique 2016). The formation of ammonia from glutamine is vital for renal regulation of the acid-base balance in animals, particularly under acidotic conditions. Glutamine is also a precursor for the synthesis of purine and pyrimidine nucleotides (Chapter 5) that are essential for the proliferation of cells, including embryonic cells, trophoblasts, intraepithelial lymphocytes, and mucosal cells. Importantly, glutamine is a major AA for the endogenous synthesis of citrulline and arginine in most mammals, including pigs, cattle, and sheep, via the intestinal-renal axis, with the circulating level of citrulline serving as a useful noninvasive biomarker of intestinal mass and function. This synthetic pathway compensates for (1) a deficiency of arginine [a nutritionally essential AA (EAA) for young mammals] in milk during the suckling period and (2) the extensive catabolism of dietary arginine by the small intestine of postweaning animals. In addition, glutamine [an AA that is synthesizable *de novo* in animal cells (AASA)] is converted into alanine in enterocytes through the glutaminolysis pathway, which compensates for a relatively low concentration of alanine in milk for suckling neonates, including calves, human infants, lambs, and piglets. Furthermore, glutamine is required for the formation of *N*-acetylglucosamine-6-phosphate, a common substrate for the synthesis of glycoproteins and glycosaminoglycans (e.g., hyaluronic acid) that are particularly abundant in mucosal cells, plasma membranes, placentae, and conceptuses (Curi et al. 2005; Kim et al. 2012). As a precursor of glutamate, glutamine plays a role in the synthesis of glutathione, the most abundant small-molecular-weight antioxidant in animal cells.

Besides its roles as a major substrate for multiple metabolic pathways, glutamine has a plethora of key regulatory functions in animals (Wu 2009). For example, glutamine modulates the expression of genes that beneficially regulate nutrient metabolism and cell survival, including ODC, heat-shock proteins, and NOS in multiple cell types. Heat-shock proteins are crucial for protecting cells from death, whereas NOS catalyzes arginine oxygenation to form NO, a signaling molecule that regulates many cellular functions. In activated macrophages, expression of inducible NOS is critical for the killing of pathogens (e.g., bacteria, fungi, virus, and parasites) by macrophages and this depends on the availability of glutamine (Wu and Meininger 2002). Notably, ODC is a key enzyme for converting ornithine into polyamines, which stimulate DNA and protein synthesis. In addition, glutamine increases the intestinal expression of genes that are necessary for cell growth and removal of oxidants, while reducing the intestinal expression of genes that promote oxidative stress and immune activation (Wang et al. 2008). The transcription of a gene to mRNA may be regulated by glutamine through one or more of the following mechanisms: (1) the alteration of the specificity of RNA polymerase for promoters; (2) the binding of repressors to noncoding DNA sequences that are near or overlap the promoter region; and (3) changes in the availability of transcription factors (e.g., upregulation and downregulation of coactivators and corepressors). Likewise, dietary supplementation with 1% glutamine repressed the unfolded protein response and oxidative stress in the small intestine of weanling piglets (He et al. 2019). Furthermore, glutamine regulates the metabolism of the arginine and serine families of AAs and reduces the catabolism of most AA (including nutritionally essential and nonessential AA such as BCAAs, lysine, and glutamate) in jejunal and ileal bacteria (Dai et al. 2013b). This may help to explain, in part, the finding that dietary supplementation with 1% glutamine to mice shifts the colonic microbiota toward a more healthy profile by increasing Bacteroidetes and decreasing Firmicutes (Ren et al. 2014b).

Cell signaling pathways are also regulated by glutamine (Blachier et al. 2015; Rhoads and Wu 2009; Xi et al. 2012). For example, in the presence of physiological concentrations of glucose, glutamine activates MTOR in many cell types, including skeletal muscle, the small intestine, and placental cells through the phosphorylation of this well-conserved protein kinase, thereby stimulating protein synthesis as well as inhibiting intracellular autophagy proteolysis (Chapter 10). There is also evidence

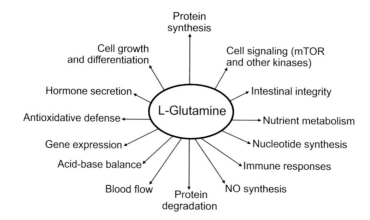

FIGURE 11.2 Physiological functions of glutamine in humans and other animals. Glutamine can regulate multiple physiological processes in diverse cell types, including gene expression, cell signaling, antioxidative responses, intracellular protein turnover, immune function, nitric oxide synthesis, and acid–base balance. These effects of glutamine are cell and tissue-specific, and interorgan cooperation is necessary for glutamine to exert some of its beneficial actions in the whole body.

that glutamine affects the activities of AMPK, extracellular signal-related kinase, Jun kinase, and mitogen-activated protein kinase (MAPK), thereby initiating a cascade of protein phosphorylation and a series of physiological responses. At present, it is not known whether glutamine directly or indirectly phosphorylates MTOR and other protein kinases. Furthermore, glutamine modulates the production of NO and CO in diverse cell types (e.g., macrophages and endothelial cells), which are important gaseous signaling molecules in the body (Li et al. 2009; Wu and Meininger 2002). Exquisite integration of these glutamine-dependent regulatory networks affects cell proliferation, migration, differentiation, metabolism, homeostasis, survival, and function (Figure 11.2).

11.2.3.3 Glutamate

Glutamate is one of the most abundant free and protein-bound AAs in animal cells (Brosnan and Brosnan 2013). It is an immediate precursor for the synthesis of glutamine, which is essential for many synthetic pathways, and also has regulatory functions in cell metabolism and physiology, as noted previously. Notably, through its extensive oxidation to CO_2, glutamate is a major metabolic fuel for enterocytes of the small intestine in mammals, birds, fish, and crustaceans (Beaumont and Blachier 2020; Hou and Wu 2018a; Li et al. 2020b, 2021a). Via transamination reactions, glutamate also donates the amino group for the intracellular synthesis of many AAs (e.g., alanine, aspartate, glycine, serine, and proline) that either compensate for their relative deficiencies in diets or contribute to interorgan nitrogen metabolism. In addition, the formation of glutamate from ammonia plus α-KG by glutamate dehydrogenase (GDH) not only scavenges ammonia (a substance that is highly toxic to the central nervous system *in vivo*), but also bridges nitrogen and carbohydrate metabolism in cells. Furthermore, glutamate and its decarboxylation product (GABA) are the major excitatory neurotransmitter and the major inhibitory neurotransmitter, respectively, within the central nervous system (Table 11.5). As a result, glutamate is key to controlling the behavior, function, and homeostasis of humans and other animals (He and Wu 2020). Likewise, glutamate is required for the synthesis of GSH (the most potent low-molecular-weight antioxidant in cells; Wu et al. 2004) and the formation of polyglutamated folate cofactors (that participate in one-carbon metabolism; Stover and Field 2011). Thus, physiological concentrations of glutamate (0.5 to 2 mM; present in the jejunal lumen) enhance barrier and antioxidative functions in porcine intestinal epithelial cells, as indicated by increases in cell viability, transepithelial electrical resistance, and membrane integrity, as well as the abundances of the tight junction proteins occludin, claudin 3, zonula occludens (ZO)-2, and ZO-3 (Jiao et al. 2015). These metabolic functions of glutamate provide the

TABLE 11.5

Neurotransmitters or Neuromodulators in the Central Nervous System of Animals

Neurotransmitter	Precursor(s)	Function
Acetylcholine	Choline and acetyl-CoA	Neurotransmitters and neuromodulators in the brain; modulation of arousal, attention, memory, and motivation
γ-Aminobutyrate	Glutamate (ultimately BCAAs)	The principal inhibitory neurotransmitter in the brain; a major inhibitory neurotransmitter in the spinal cord (50% sharing with glycine); regulation of food intake
Aspartate	Glutamine, glutamate, and BCAAs	A major excitatory neurotransmitter in the brain
Carbon monoxide (CO)	Heme (ultimately glycine)	A neurotransmitter and a neuromodulator in the brain; modulation of synaptic plasticity and neuronal activity; modulation of LTP
Dopamine	Tyrosine	A neurotransmitter in the brain; modulation of learning, motor control, reward, emotion, and executive function; inhibition of food intake
Epinephrine	Tyrosine	A neurotransmitter in the brain; enhancer of memory formation processes
Glutamate	Glutamine, BCAAs, and possibly ammonia plus α-KG	The primary excitatory neurotransmitter in the brain; primary mediator of neuron system plasticity
Glycine	Serine, 4-hydroxyproline	A major inhibitory neurotransmitter in the spinal cord and lower brain stem; a co-agonist with glutamate at NMDA receptors in the brain
Hydrogen sulfide (H_2S)	Cysteine	A neurotransmitter and a neuromodulator in the brain; modulation of synaptic plasticity and neuronal activity; facilitating the induction of hippocampal LTP; potentiating the activity of NMDA receptors
Histamine	Histidine	A neurotransmitter in the brain and spinal cord; inhibition of food intake; promotion of wakefulness; control of motivational behavior
Nitric oxide (NO)	Arginine	A neurotransmitter and a neuromodulator in the brain; modulation of synaptic plasticity and neuronal activity; inhibiting the activity of NMDA receptors at physiological levels
Nonopioid NPs[a]	Amino acids	Neurotransmitters and neuromodulators in the brain; modulation of analgesia, hypothermia, and locomotion; involved in the regulation of dopamine pathways
Norepinephrine	Tyrosine	A neurotransmitter in the brain; modulation of emotion, sleep, attention, focus, and learning in the brain; modulation of response to the ANS
Opioid peptides[b]	Amino acids	Neurotransmitters and neuromodulators in the brain and spinal cord; modulation of pain perception, analgesia, and euphoria; modulation of the actions of other neurotransmitters
Serotonin	Tryptophan	A neurotransmitter in the brain and gastrointestine; modulation of neuropsychological processes and neural activity; in the brain, inhibition of food intake; in the small intestine, endocrine cells synthesize and release serotonin to stimulate gastrointestinal motility and food intake

Source: He, W.L. and G. Wu. 2020. *Adv. Exp. Med. Biol.* 1265:167–185.

[a] Including (1) neurotensin (a 13-amino acid neuropeptide that plays a role in regulating the release of luteinizing hormone and prolactin from the anterior pituitary gland and has a significant interaction with the dopaminergic system in the brain; and (2) cholecystokinin (CCK) that is produced by endocrine cells of the small intestine and acts as a neurotransmitter and a neuro-modulator in the gut and brain. CCK is composed of different numbers of amino acid residues (e.g., CCK58, CCK33, CCK22, and CCK8), depending on the posttranslational modification of its 150-amino acid precursor, preprocholecystokinin.

[b] Methionine-enkephalin (a pentapeptide), leucine-enkephalin (a pentapeptide), and related neuropeptides (e.g., endorphins) are generated from the degradation of proteins and serve as endogenous opioid neurotransmitters. Opiates (e.g., morphine; naturally present) and opioids (e.g., heroin; synthetic substances) mimic the effects of the neuropeptides.

Note: ANS, autonomic nervous system; CCK, cholecystokinin; α-KG, α-ketoglutarate; LTP, long-term potentiation; NMDA receptor, *N*-methyl-D-aspartate receptor (a glutamate receptor and an ion channel protein present in nerve cells); NPs, neurotransmitter peptides biochemical basis for the finding that dietary supplementation with 1%–4% monosodium gluta-mate (MSG) to piglets increased jejunal villus height, DNA content, and antioxidative capacity, as well as whole-body growth, while dose-dependently reducing the incidence of diarrhea during the first week after weaning (Rezaei et al. 2013). Moreover, glutamate interacts with specific umami taste receptors in the tongue and the gastrointestinal tract to elicit Ca^{2+}- and NO-dependent cell signaling and nutrient sensing, thereby stimulating food intake and gut motility (San Gabriel and Uneyama 2013; Wu 2020a; Zhang et al. 2013). Finally, glutamate is uniquely present in proteins (e.g., blood clotting factors) for posttranslational carboxylation to form dicarboxyl glutamyl resi-dues that bind calcium, thereby activating the biological functions of the proteins. Thus, glutamate plays critical roles in nutrition, metabolism, and cell signaling to maintain tissue- and whole-body homeostasis in humans and other animals.

11.2.3.4 Glycine

Glycine has crucial roles in both nutrition and metabolism (Li and Wu 2018). First, glycine represents 11.5% of total AAs (14.5% of AA nitrogen) in body proteins. Protein synthesis accounts for 80% of whole-body glycine needs by neonates, such as calves, human infants, lambs, and piglets. Of note,

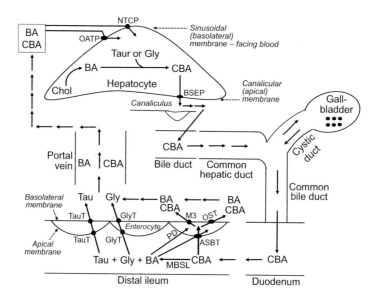

FIGURE 11.3 Physiological roles of taurine and glycine in the hepatic conjugation of bile acids and the enterohepatic circulation of bile salts in humans and other animals. The transport of bile salts from the liver to the duodenum and the return of bile salt from the distal ileum to the liver via the enterohepatic cir-culation in humans. Conjugated bile acids are exported by the ATP-dependent bile salt export pump out of the hepatocyte through its canalicular (apical) membrane into the canaliculus. The bile salts subsequently enter bile ducts, the common hepatic duct, and the gallbladder. During digestion, the bile salts are secreted from the gallbladder to the common bile duct and then the duodenum. In the distal ileum, a fraction of bile salts is hydrolyzed by microbial bile salt hydrolases to form bile acids and taurine or glycine. Taurine, glycine, and bile salts are efficiently taken up by the enterocytes of the distal ileum via specific transport-ers. The substances are transported in the blood for uptake by the hepatocyte via its sinusoidal basolateral membrane. During each enteral-hepatic cycle, about 95% of the liver-derived bile salts are reabsorbed to the liver. ASBT, apical sodium-dependent bile salt/acid transporter (in ileal enterocytes); BA, bile acids (unconjugated), BSEP, bile salt export pump; CBA, conjugated bile acids; Gly, glycine; GlyT, glycine trans-porters; M3, multidrug resistance protein 3; MBSL, microbial bile salt hydrolases; NTCP, Na^+-taurocholate-cotransporting polypeptide; OATP family, organic anion-transporting polypeptide family; OSTα/β, organic solute transporter subunit α/β; PD, passive diffusion; Tau, taurine; and TauT, taurine transporters. (Reprinted from Wu, G. 2020b. *Amino Acids* 52:329–360.)

there are multiple pathways for glycine utilization to generate glutathione, creatine, purines (RNA and DNA), heme (hemoglobins), and serine, all of which have crucial physiological functions (see other sections of this chapter) (Wang et al. 2013). For example, heme-containing proteins are crucial for oxygen transport and mitochondrial biogenesis. Second, glycine, like taurine, is a major AA for the conjugation of bile acids in animals, which play a key role in the digestion and absorption of lipids and lipid-soluble vitamins (Figure 11.3). Third, through glycine-gated chloride channels in leukocytes and macrophages, glycine modulates intracellular Ca^{2+} levels, thereby regulating the production of cytokines and superoxide, as well as immune function. Fourth, glycine is a neurotransmitter in the central nervous system, thereby regulating locomotion, food intake, and whole-body homeostasis. Specifically, glycine is a major inhibitory neurotransmitter in the spinal cord and lower brain stem and is a co-agonist with glutamate at NMDA receptors (glutamate and ion channel protein receptors that are activated after binding with both glycine and glutamate) in the brain to exert an excitatory effect on the neuron. Fifth, glycine suppresses endoplasmic reticulum (ER) stress, inhibits the action of CHOP [C/EBP homologous protein; also known as growth arrest and DNA damage-inducible gene 153 (GADD153), an apoptotic protein], and prevents oxidative stress and apoptosis of animal cells [e.g., the epithelial cells of the small intestine (Fan et al. 2019; Wang et al. 2014a)]. Likewise, dietary supplementation with glycine to mice attenuates the lipopolysaccharide (LPS)-induced apoptosis of hepatocytes and the infiltration of inflammatory cells into the liver (Zhang et al. 2020). Sixth, glycine, like serine, participates in one-carbon unit metabolism to promote DNA synthesis and cell proliferation (Bazer et al. 2021). Finally, glycine activates the MTOR cell signaling pathway and attenuates the expression of genes related to protein breakdown [muscle-specific ring finger 1 (MuRF1) and muscle atrophy F-box (MAFbx)/atrogin 1] in skeletal muscle cells (Sun et al. 2016). Both MuRF1 and atrogin 1 are muscle-specific E3 ubiquitin ligases implicated in intracellular protein degradation. Similarly, glycine stimulates protein synthesis and inhibits proteolysis in the enterocytes of the small intestine (Wang et al. 2014a). Thus, dietary supplementation with glycine can alleviate oxidative stress and reduce obesity in Zucker diabetic fatty rats (Simmons et al. 2020).

11.2.3.5 Proline

Proline is a unique AA both chemically and biochemically (Phang et al. 2008). On a per gram basis, the requirement of proline for whole-body protein synthesis is the highest among all AAs (Li and Wu 2018). Growing evidence shows that proline is a key regulator of multiple biochemical and physiological processes in cells, including enterocytes, placenta, tumors, bacteria, and parasites (Bringaud et al. 2012; Li and Wu 2018; Phang et al. 2010). For example, proline is a major nitrogenous substrate for the synthesis of polyamines in the neonatal small intestine (Wu et al. 2000) and in the placentae (Wu et al. 2005) of mammals. This discovery is significant because both tissues are characterized by high rates of protein synthesis and cell proliferation. Pathways exist for the synthesis of polyamines from proline via proline oxidase and ornithine decarboxylase. Additionally, proline and its metabolite (P5C) regulate the expression of genes (e.g., those for antioxidative responses) and cellular signaling pathways that are crucial to health and disease (Phang et al. 2010). Interestingly, proline can scavenge free radicals and this antioxidant property of proline may explain why its concentrations increase markedly in response to cellular oxidative stress. Furthermore, proline plays a role in regulating the MTOR activation pathway (Liu et al. 2019; Pistollato et al. 2010), which integrates signals from nutrients (glucose and AAs), cellular energy status, growth factors, and various stress factors to affect cell growth and function. Therefore, proline acts in concert with other AAs (including arginine, glutamine, glycine, and leucine) to enhance protein synthesis in animal cells.

Proline is an EAA for poultry because P5C is not synthesized *de novo* and the conversion of arginine into proline in birds is inadequate relative to physiological requirements (He et al. 2021; Wu 2009). Proline is a conditionally essential AA for young mammals (including piglets) and patients with burns due to inadequate endogenous synthesis via the arginase and P5C synthase pathways relative to needs (Chapter 3). Additionally, endogenous synthesis of proline from glutamate cannot meet the requirements for proline by many species of fish (Li et al. 2020b). Therefore, proline is now considered to be an EAA or conditionally essential AA for fish in both early life and adult stages. The essential requirement for proline as a nutrient for poultry, young mammals, and wounded individuals is supported by several lines of experimental evidence. First, supplementing 0.0%, 0.2%, 0.4%, and 0.8% proline to a chemically purified diet containing 1% arginine and 10% glutamate dose-dependently increased daily weight gains (from 11.88 to 13.38 g/day) of young chickens without affecting their feed intake (an average of 114 g/chick) (Graber et al. 1970). Second, supplementing 0%, 0.35%, 0.7%, 1.05%, 1.4%, or 2.1% proline to a proline-free chemically defined diet containing 0.48% arginine and 2% glutamate dose-dependently improved daily weight gains (from 342 to 411 g/day) and feed efficiency (g feed/g gain; from 1.66 to 1.35) of young pigs, while reducing concentrations of urea in the plasma by one-half (Kirchgessner et al. 1995). Notably, increasing the dietary content of proline from 0.0 and 2.1% enhanced daily N retention from 1.27 to 1.53 g/(kg BW)$^{0.75}$ (Kirchgessner et al. 1995). Similarly, supplementing 1% proline to a corn- and soybean meal-based diet enhanced jejunal villus height (+16.4%), small-intestinal weight (+9.2%), and body-weight gain (+13.8%) without affecting feed intake in weanling pigs (Wu et al. 2011b). Third, dietary proline is necessary for promoting tissue repair and N balance in humans and other animals with wounds and burns (Barbul 2008). Fourth, dietary supplementation with 0.07%, 0.14%, and 0.28% hydroxyproline (a metabolite of proline) to a plant protein-based diet for 88 days enhanced the weight gain of Atlantic salmon by 8.1%, 14%, and 11%, respectively (Aksnes et al. 2006). Fifth, dietary supplementation with 0.50% proline to mice from embryonic day 0.5 (E0.5) to E12.5 or term enhanced placental nutrient transport and development, as well as embryonic and fetal survival (Liu et al. 2019, 2020). Collectively, these findings have important implications for proline as an essential nutrient in birds, mammals, and fish.

11.2.3.6 Tryptophan

The metabolism of tryptophan in the body occurs via the 5-hydroxyindole and the kynurenine pathways (Fernstrom 2013). Major metabolic products from the 5-hydroxyindole pathway are serotonin (5-hydroxytryptamine) and melatonin (N-acetyl-5-methoxytryptamine), whereas important products from the kynurenine pathway are kynurenine and kynurenic acid (Chapter 4). Besides animal cells, the gut microbiota can metabolize tryptophan and produce indole, indole-3-acetic acid, indole-3-propionic acid, 3-methylindole (skatole), and tryptamine through either deamination or decarboxylation. The 5-hydroxyindole pathway mainly exists in the gastrointestinal tract and the nervous system, and the kynurenine pathway occurs in many tissues (mainly the liver, brain, and intestine). As a result of microbial catabolism, a large amount of tryptophan metabolites is present in the hindgut (Dai et al. 2019). Through direct actions and its versatile metabolites, tryptophan plays crucial roles in regulating endocrine, immunological, neurological (e.g., behavior), cardiovascular, intestinal (e.g., gut motility), and reproductive functions, as well as signaling through the gut–brain axis (Dai et al. 2015). For example, physiological concentrations of tryptophan (0.4 and 0.8 mM present in the jejunal lumen) activate the MTOR cell signaling to stimulate protein synthesis and inhibit protein degradation in porcine intestinal epithelial cells, while enhancing the expression of tryptophan transporters and tight junction proteins in these cells (Wang et al. 2015a). Also, increasing the total dietary content of tryptophan from approximately 0.2% to 1% for 15 days augmented daily weight gain (+20.4%) and serotonin concentration in the hypothalamus (+186%), while reducing cortisol concentration in the saliva (−48.6%), whole-body lipid peroxidation (indicated by a 30% decrease in plasma malondialdehyde concentration), aggressive behavior, and the frequencies of sitting and lying down (Shen et al. 2012). Likewise, adequate provision of tryptophan enhances the resistance of animals to infections (Bessede et al. 2014), while improving mood, cognition, behavior, and nocturnal sleep in humans (Fernstrom 2013; Strasser et al. 2016). Furthermore, dietary supplementation with tryptophan via drinking water (0.1 mg/g BW/day) enhanced colonic immune responses and alleviated colitis in dextran sodium sulfate-challenged mice partly by modulating the interactions of serotonin with the 5-hydroxytryptamine receptors 1A and 4 that are present in neutrophils and macrophages (Wang et al. 2020). Similarly, dietary supplementation with

0.2% or 0.4% tryptophan to a corn- and soybean meal-based diet (containing 0.2% tryptophan) improved the intestinal mucosal barrier function in weaned piglets partly by altering the population and metabolism of tryptophan-metabolizing microbiota (Liang et al. 2018, 2019). Thus, there is growing interest in the physiological functions of tryptophan.

11.2.4 ROLES OF SELECT NITROGENOUS PRODUCTS OF AAS

Physiological functions of nitrogenous AA metabolites are summarized in Table 11.1. The physiological roles of NO have been highlighted previously. In the following sections, functions of the nitrogenous metabolites are summarized. These substances include polyamines, creatine, GSH, nucleotides, taurine, histamine, melanin, melatonin, carnosine, and glucosamine.

11.2.4.1 Functions of Polyamines

Much is known about the biochemical properties of polyamines and their roles in health and disease (Agostinelli 2020). At physiological pH, putrescine, spermidine, and spermine have 2, 3, and 4 positive charges, respectively. These alkaline molecules can greatly affect the intracellular milieu. As polycationic substances, polyamines participate in many cellular processes through binding to RNA, DNA, nucleotide triphosphate, proteins, and other negatively charged molecules. In animals, physiological concentrations of polyamines enhance (1) angiogenesis; (2) DNA and protein synthesis; (3) embryogenesis; (4) expression of genes related to metabolism and growth of cells and tissues (e.g., brain, liver, skeletal muscle, brown adipose tissue, and lymphoid organs); (5) the production of antibodies and immune responses; (6) intestinal maturation; (7) ion channel function; (8) proliferation and differentiation of cells; (9) apoptosis, NMDA receptor activity, and cell signal transduction; (10) spermatogenesis; (11) wound healing; and (12) secretions of hormones. However, excessive amounts of polyamines are toxic to cells, partly due to the production, by spermine oxidase, of acrolein (CH_2=CH–CHO) from spermidine and spermine (Pegg 2013), which is more toxic than reactive oxygen species (O_2^-, H_2O_2 and $\cdot OH$) (Igarashi et al. 2020).

Polyamines participate in the posttranslational modifications of some proteins in cells. Of particular interest, J.E. Folk and colleagues discovered in 1980 that spermidine is required for the modification of eIF5A by deoxyhypusine synthase [also known as spermidine:eIF5A-lysine 4-aminobutyltransferase (propane-1,3-diamine-forming) or [eIF5A-precursor]-lysine:spermidine 4-aminobutyltransferase (propane-1,3-diamine-forming)] to form the hypusine residue that is critical for eukaryotic translation (Park and Wolff 2018). Specifically, this enzyme catalyzes the transfer of a moiety (a 4-aminobutyl group) of spermidine to the active site (lysine residue) of eIF5A to yield (eIF5A-precursor)-deoxyhypusine, which is converted into a hypusine residue by deoxyhypusine hydroxylase (a Fe^{2+}-dependent monooxygenase; DOHH). The long and basic side chain of the hypusine residue promotes eIF5A-mediated translation elongation by stimulating eIF5A activity, facilitating peptide bond formation, and enhancing translation termination through the release of polypeptides. The overall reaction is as follows:

$$[eIF5A\text{-precursor}]\text{-lysine} + \text{Spermidine} \rightarrow [eIF5A\text{-precursor}]\text{-deoxyhypusine} + \text{Propane-1,}$$
$$3\text{-diamine (deoxyhypusine synthase)}$$

$$[eIF5A\text{-precursor}]\text{-deoxyhypusine} + AH_2 (\text{electron acceptor}) + O_2 \rightarrow [eIF5A\text{-precursor}]\text{-hypusine}$$
$$+ A + H_2O \text{ (DOHH)}$$

Hypusine [N^ε-(4-amino-2-hydroxybutyl) lysine; an unusual basic amino acid]

When [eIF5A-precursor]-hypusine is degraded by protease, hypusine ([N^ε-(4-amino-2-hydroxybutyl) lysine]; an unusual basic amino acid) is released. This AA was originally isolated from a trichloroacetic acid-soluble extract of the bovine brain in 1971. Among animal tissues, the brain and testes have the highest concentrations of free and protein-bound hypusine, respectively (Abbruzzese et al. 1988). The free hypusine is also present in a form that is bound to GABA in the central nervous system. The concentration of hypusine in the brain is developmentally regulated, as its concentration in brain protein is the highest in the first 2 weeks of postnatal life and then steadily decreases until adulthood. This underscores the role of adequate lysine nutrition in neurological growth and development.

Polyamines are also physiological substrates for some transglutaminases that catalyze the formation of an isopeptide bond (an amide bond) between a primary amine or the γ-NH_2 group of a glutamine residue in a polypeptide chain and the ε-NH_2 of a lysine residue of another polypeptide chain, with the subsequent release of ammonia (Agostinelli et al. 2010). Depending on the donor of the amine group, there are two types of transglutaminase (also known as nature's biological glues), with isoforms 1 and 2 incorporating amines into proteins or cross-linked proteins, respectively. Mammalian transglutaminases require Ca^{2+} as a cofactor, but bacterial transglutaminases do not have such a requirement (Griffin et al. 2002). Bonds formed by transglutaminases exhibit high resistance to proteolytic degradation. Transglutaminases also catalyze the removal of the $-NH_2$ group in the side chain of glutamine residues in proteins (deamidation). Thus, transglutaminase-catalyzed reactions can result in the incorporation of small-molecular-weight amines into the γ-glutamine sites of proteins to form stable inter- or intramolecular cross-linking, which confers the biological activity of proteins. For example, the polyaminated phospholipase A2 has a specific activity approximately three-fold higher than that of phospholipase A2 without polyamination (Cordella-Miele et al. 1993). In addition, polyamines regulate the activities of transglutaminases in the gastrointestinal mucosa and in other cell types (e.g., colonocytes, lymphocytes, placental cells, and tumors). Furthermore, glutamine residues in certain proteins (e.g., blood coagulation protein factor XIII, as well as skin and hair proteins) undergo modifications by transglutaminases to yield biologically active proteins (Griffin et al. 2002).

$$\text{Protein-Gln-}NH_2 + \text{Primary amine}\left(H_2\text{N-R}\right) = \text{Protein-Gln-NH-R} + NH_3 \quad \left(\text{Transglutaminases 1}\right)$$

$$\text{Protein-Gln-}NH_2 + H_2\text{N-}CH_2\text{-Lys-Protein} = \text{Protein-Gln-NH-}CH_2\text{-Lys-Protein} + NH_3$$
$$\left(\text{Transglutaminases 2}\right)$$

$$\text{Protein-Gln-}NH_2 + H_2O = \text{Protein-Glu} + NH_3 \quad \left(\text{Deamidation by transglutaminases}\right)$$

When cells are stimulated with growth factors, one of the first crucial events is the induction of polyamine synthesis, which precedes increases in DNA replication and protein synthesis (Pegg 2016). An increase in the expression of genes involved in polyamine synthesis (e.g., arginase I or II and ODC) promotes the proliferation of cells (e.g., endothelial cells, enterocytes, and vascular smooth muscle cells), but depletion of cellular polyamines by inhibition of these genes arrests cell division (Ignarro et al. 2001; Li et al. 2001; Wei et al. 2001). These functions of polyamines are epitomized by clinical findings from studies with humans and other animals. For example, in humans, mutations in the spermine synthase gene increase spermidine concentrations and decrease spermine concentrations, resulting in Snyder–Robinson syndrome, an X-linked recessive condition characterized by mental retardation, skeletal defects, hypotonia, and movement disorders (Becerra-Solano et al. 2009). In addition, in Gyro mice, an X-chromosomal deletion of the spermine synthase gene leads to the depletion of spermine, which, in turn, causes growth restriction, sterility, deafness, neurological abnormalities, and a tendency to sudden death (Meyer et al. 1998). In mice, knockout of the ODC gene is embryonic lethal, and the impaired growth of the embryonic disk can be prevented through oral administration of putrescine via drinking water to the dam up to the early stages of implantation (Pendeville et al. 2001). In sheep, the rate of polyamine synthesis is greatest in placentomes and endometria between Days 30 and 60 of gestation when their growth and morphological changes are most rapid (Kwon et al. 2003), but an inhibition of the translation of ODC1 mRNA through the intrauterine delivery of morpholino antisense oligonucleotides results in a failure of 50% conceptuses to develop morphologically and functionally (Wang et al. 2014b, Lenis et al. 2018). Interestingly, the normal conceptuses in those ewes with ODC1 knockout exhibit compensatory increases in the expression of arginine decarboxylase and agmatinase to produce putrescine, spermidine, and spermine, indicating that sheep have an alternative pathway to synthesize polyamines for embryonic survival and development (Wang et al. 2014b).

11.2.4.2 Functions of Creatine

Creatine is taken up into cells by Na^+/Cl^--coupled (i.e., sodium- and chloride-dependent) creatine transporter 1 (Figure 11.4). Creatine kinase (also known as creatine phosphokinase) converts creatine and ATP into phosphocreatine (a high-energy compound; also known as creatine phosphate) and ADP. This enzyme is expressed at high levels in most of the cells and tissues that have high energy requirements, including the brain, kidneys, retinal photoreceptor cells, spermatozoa, testis, uterus, placenta, skin, enterocytes, and the sensory hair cells of the inner ear, as well as skeletal, cardiac and smooth muscles (Wyss and Kaddurah-Daou 2000). The phosphocreatine/creatine kinase system is characterized by cell- and tissue-specific isoforms of creatine kinase, which are differentially localized in the cytoplasm and mitochondria to fulfill the need for metabolic channeling and efficient provision of energy. For example, skeletal muscle and the brain express both cytosolic and mitochondrial creatine kinases to utilize ATP generated via glycolysis and the mitochondrial electron transport system, respectively. Therefore, distinct isoforms of creatine kinase are associated with sites of ATP production in vertebrates. Creatine kinase may "buffer" the cellular phosphorylation potential and regulate the activity of intracellular ATPases. Interestingly, the liver does not contain creatine kinase or phosphocreatine (Wyss and Kaddurah-Daou 2000). Low levels of hepatic creatine kinase activity that were previously reported by some researchers might have resulted from the presence of adenylate kinase in the enzyme assay.

The ability of cells to generate phosphocreatine from excessive ATP at the resting state and the utilization of phosphocreatine for rapid regeneration of ATP in response to high demands for energy provide a mechanism for maintaining ATP homeostasis (Wallimann et al. 2011; Wu 2020b). Creatine enters target cells via its transporter. In the cytosol, phosphocreainte/creatine is in equilibrium with ATP/ADP via the action of soluble creatine kinase, which is coupled to glycolytic enzymes for accepting ATP from glycolysis and to ATP utilization via ATP-dependent processes. The latter include the syntheses of protein, nucleic acids, AAs, and glutathione; proteolysis via the ubiquitin-dependent proteasomes; cell remodeling; and the transport of nutrients across the plasma membrane. Similarly, the mitochondrial isoform of creatine kinase located in the outer mitochondrial membrane is coupled to adenine nucleotide translocator for accepting the ATP generated from the electron transport system. The mitochondrial phosphocreatine is transported into the cytosol via the voltage-dependent anion channel. The cytosolic and mitochondrial isoforms of creatine kinase are encoded by two different genes. In the subcellular compartments, the phosphocreainte/creatine shuttle is tightly and functionally connected to ATP production and utilization. Thus, creatine plays an important role in cellular energy metabolism in a temporal and spatial manner, particularly in the nervous, muscular, and reproductive systems. Therefore, defects in creatine synthesis result in neurological and muscular dysfunction and possibly reproductive failure (Philip et al. 2020). Additionally, there is increasing evidence that creatine scavenges free radicals, has antioxidative and antiapoptotic functions, reduces inflammatory responses, and improves glucose tolerance in humans. Finally, creatine may regulate the expression of transcription factors and other proteins in diverse cell types, such as the upregulation of creatine transporter 1 expression in skeletal muscle (Brault et al. 2003) and the downregulation of arginine:glycine amidinotransferase in the kidneys and pancreas (Deminice et al. 2011). Furthermore, phosphocreatine plays an important role in the provision of energy to animal tissues and cells under hypoxic conditions and during intensive

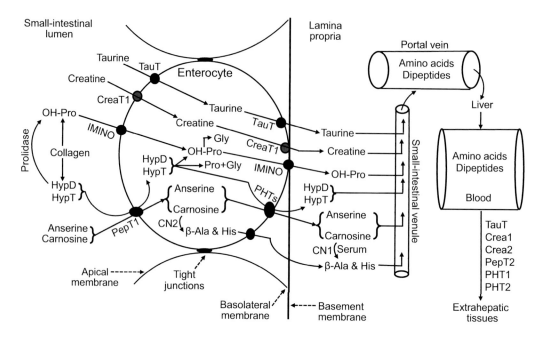

FIGURE 11.4 Intestinal absorption of creatine, taurine, carnosine, anserine, and 4-hydroxyproline and their transport via the blood circulation in humans and other animals. Dietary collagen is hydrolyzed by proteases, peptidases, and prolidase to free amino acids as well as 4-hydroxyproline and its peptides. Dietary taurine, creatine, carnosine, anserine, and 4-hydroxyproline are taken up by the enterocyte across its apical membrane via specific transports. Inside the cell, taurine, creatine, and anserine are not degraded, some of the 4-hydroxyproline-containing peptides are hydrolyzed to 4-hydroxyproline and its peptides, some 4-hydroxyproline is oxidized to glycine, and carnosine undergoes limited catabolism. Taurine, creatine, carnosine, anserine, and 4-hydroxyproline, as well as the products of carnosine hydrolysis (β-alanine and histidine) exit the enterocyte across its basolateral membrane into the lamina propria of the intestinal mucosa via specific transporters. The absorbed nutrients are transported in the blood in the free forms for uptake by extraintestinal tissues via specific transporters. Note that the distribution of PHT1/2 in tissues is species-specific in that human skeletal muscle expresses PHT1, but not PHT2, whereas mouse skeletal muscle expresses both PHT1 and PHT2. β-Ala, β-alanine; CAT, cationic amino acid transporter; CN1, carnosinase 1 (serum carnosinase); CN2, carnosinase 2 (tissue carnosinase); CreaT1, creatine transporter 1; CreaT2, creatine transporter 2; GAT, γ-aminobutyrate transporter; HypD, 4-hydroxyproline-containing dipeptides; HypT, 4-hydroxyproline-containing tripeptides; OH-Pro, 4-hydroxyproline; PAT1, proton-(H+-coupled) and pH-dependent but Na+- and Cl⁻-independent transporter for taurine (low-affinity, high-capacity transporter); PepT1, peptide transporter 1; PepT2, peptide transporter 2; PHT1/2, peptide/histidine transporters 1 and 2; and TauT, taurine transporters. (Reprinted from Wu, G. 2020b. *Amino Acids* 52:329–360.)

physical activity, thereby reducing risks for injury or death in individuals who are susceptible to global oxygen deprivation and asphyxic episodes (LaRosa et al. 2017).

The beneficial effects of oral administration of creatine on improving the health and exercise performance of humans and other animals, including the prevention of fat accumulation in the livers of rats fed a high-fat diet (Deminice et al. 2011), are summarized in Table 11.7. Note that absorbed dietary creatine undergoes limited phosphorylation (only 1% of ingested creatine) in the intestinal mucosa, and nearly 99% of orally ingested creatine enters the portal circulation for utilization by extraintestinal tissues (Jäger et al. 2011). Due to the very low rate of creatine loss (1.7%/day) in the whole-body pool (creatine plus creatine phosphate), continuous supplementation with creatine is not necessary to achieve the saturation of creatine in skeletal muscle (Wu 2020b). Nonetheless, dietary supplementation with a low dose of creatine (e.g., 3 g of creatine monohydrate per day for 28 days in a 76-kg man) results in a steady accumulation of creatine in skeletal muscle, and the saturation of creatine in the muscle (142 mmol/kg dry matter) occurs by Day 28 (Hickner et al. 2010). Furthermore, dietary supplementation with 5% creatine for 18 days to gestating mice before birth asphyxia increased the survival of neonatal females and males by 12% and 19%, respectively (Ellery et al. 2016). Finally, supplementing the diet of gilts with 20 g creatine/day between Day 110 of pregnancy and farrowing (~ Day 140) reduced the number of piglets dying due to overlay by the sows and increased myelination in the brain stem on postnatal Day 2 (Vallet et al. 2013). Thus, creatine can help to improve the health and well-being of both humans and other animals.

11.2.4.3 Functions of Glutathione

GSH participates in many cellular reactions (Meister and Anderson 1983; Sies 1999). First, GSH directly and effectively scavenges free radicals and other reactive oxygen species (e.g., hydroxyl radical, lipid peroxyl radical, peroxynitrite, and H_2O_2) and also acts indirectly through enzymatic reactions. In such reactions, GSH is oxidized to form GSSG, which is then reduced to GSH by the NADPH-dependent glutathione reductase. In addition, glutathione peroxidase (a selenium-containing enzyme) catalyzes the GSH-dependent reduction of H_2O_2 and other peroxides. Second, GSH reacts with various electrophiles, physiological metabolites (e.g., estrogen, melanins, prostaglandins, and leukotrienes), and xenobiotics (e.g., bromobenzene and acetaminophen) to form mercapturates (Figure 11.5). These reactions are initiated by glutathione-S-transferase (a family of Phase II detoxification enzymes). Third, GSH conjugates with NO to form an *S*-nitroso-glutathione adduct, which is cleaved by the thioredoxin system to release GSH and NO. Recent evidence suggests that the targeting of endogenous NO is mediated by intracellular GSH. Additionally, both NO and GSH are necessary for the hepatic action of insulin-sensitizing agents, indicating their critical role in regulating lipid, glucose, and AA utilization. Fourth, GSH serves as a substrate for formaldehyde dehydrogenase, which converts formaldehyde and GSH to *S*-formyl-glutathione. *S*-Formyl-glutathione is hydrolyzed by *S*-formyl-glutathione hydrolase to formate, and this reaction regenerates GSH (Figure 11.6). The removal of formaldehyde (a carcinogen) is of physiological

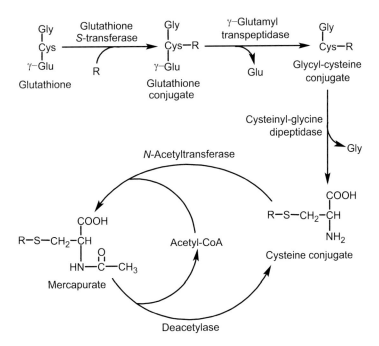

FIGURE 11.5   Role of glutathione in mercapturate formation in humans and other animals. R, various electrophiles, physiological metabolites (e.g., estrogen, prostaglandins, leukotrienes, and melanins), and foreign compounds or xenobiotics (e.g., bromobenzene and acetaminophen) that can conjugate with glutathione.

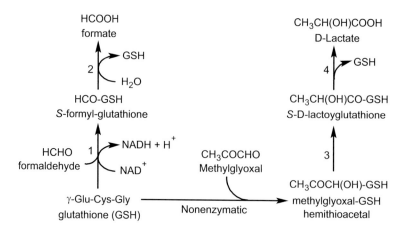

FIGURE 11.6 Role of glutathione in formaldehyde removal and D-lactate synthesis in humans and other animals. Formaldehyde is a potential carcinogen, and D-lactate is a microbial metabolite in the gastrointestinal tract. Thus, glutathione plays important roles in reducing risk for cancers and maintaining the ecosystem of the gastrointestinal microbiota. The enzymes that catalyze the indicated reactions are (1) formaldehyde dehydrogenase; (2) S-formyl-glutathione hydrolase; (3) glyoxalase I; and (4) glyoxalase II.

importance, because it is produced from the metabolism of methionine, choline, methanol, sarcosine, and xenobiotics (via the cytochrome P450-dependent monooxygenase system of the endoplasmic reticulum). Fifth, GSH is required for the conversion of prostaglandin H_2 into prostaglandins D_2 and E_2 by endoperoxide isomerase. Sixth, GSH is involved in the glyoxalase system that converts methylglyoxal to D-lactate, a pathway active in microorganisms including those in the lumen of the small and large intestines (Figure 11.7). Finally, the glutathionylation of proteins, including thioredoxin, ubiquitin-conjugating enzyme, and cytochrome c oxidase, plays an important role in antioxidative defense, proteolysis, and cell respiration.

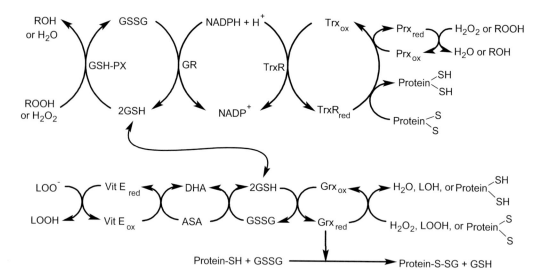

FIGURE 11.7 Role of glutathione in thiol and free radical homeostasis. AsA, ascorbic acid; DHA, dehydroascorbic acid; Grx, glutaredoxin; GR, glutathione reductase; GSH, reduced glutathione; GSH-Px, glutathione peroxidase; GSSG, glutathione disulfide (oxidized glutathione); LH, lipid; LOO, lipid peroxyl radical; LOOH, lipid hydroperoxide; ox, oxidized form; Prx, peroxiredoxin; red, reduced form; ROH, alkyl alcohol; ROOH, alkyl hydroperoxide; Trx, thioredoxin; and TrxR, thioredoxin reductase.

GSH serves vital functions in animals (Table 11.6). Adequate concentrations of GSH are necessary for the proliferation of cells, including hepatocytes, trophoblasts, lymphocytes, and intestinal epithelial cells. GSH also plays an important role in spermatogenesis, sperm maturation, and oocyte development in male and female reproductive systems. In addition, GSH is essential for the activation of T lymphocytes and polymorphonuclear leukocytes, as well as cytokine production, and therefore for mounting successful immune responses when the host is immunologically challenged. Shifting the GSH/GSSG redox toward the oxidizing state activates several cell signaling pathways (including protein kinase B, protein phosphatases 1 and 2A, calcineurin, nuclear factor κB, c-Jun N-terminal kinase, apoptosis signal-regulated kinase 1, and mitogen-activated protein kinase), thereby reducing cell proliferation and increasing apoptosis. Thus, oxidative stress (a deleterious imbalance between the production and removal of reactive oxygen/nitrogen species) plays a key role in the pathogenesis of many diseases, including cancer, inflammation, kwashiorkor (predominantly due to protein deficiency), seizure, Alzheimer's disease, Parkinson's disease, sickle cell anemia, human immunodeficiency virus (HIV)/acquired immune deficiency syndrome (AIDS) and other viruses, heart attack, stroke, obesity, and diabetes (Wu et al. 2004). In humans and other animals (including fish), hepatic dysfunction reduces the ability of the liver to synthesize glutathione for

---

TABLE 11.6
Roles of Glutathione in Animal Metabolism and Physiology

Antioxidant Defense

Scavenging of free radicals and other reactive species

Removal of hydrogen peroxide, lipid peroxides, and related metabolites

Prevention of the oxidation of biomolecules (e.g., proteins and DNA)

Maintenance of thiol homeostasis

Immune Responses

Improvements in the functions of the cells of the immune system

Increases in lymphocyte proliferation and antibody production

Increases in both innate and adaptive immunities

Reductions in inflammation and in risks for infectious diseases

Reductions in the infiltrations of leukocytes into tissues

Killing of pathogens (including bacteria and viruses) by activated macrophages

Metabolism

Synthesis of leukotrienes and prostaglandins

Synthesis of isovalthine and isobuteine in some Felidae species

Conversion of formaldehyde to formate

Production of D-lactate from methylglyoxal

Formation of mercapturates from electrophiles

Formation of glutathione-NO adduct

Storage and transport of cysteine

Regulation

Intracellular redox status

Signal transduction and gaseous signaling

Gene expression

DNA and protein synthesis and proteolysis

Cell proliferation and apoptosis

Cytokine production and immune response

Protein glutathionylation

Function and integrity of membranes and mitochondria

local antioxidative functions and its release into the blood, thereby contributing to systemic oxidative stress and the darkening of tissues such as the heart and skin due to the presence of oxidized molecules (e.g., protein and lipids) (Hou et al. 2020). The overall antioxidative reactions involving GSH are discussed in Chapter 5. An improvement in cellular and plasma glutathione concentrations may play an important role in reducing the susceptibility of humans and other animals to severe acute respiratory syndrome (SARS-CoV; Wu et al. 2004) and COVID-19 (Polonikov 2020; Silvagno et al. 2020) caused by a coronavirus.

11.2.4.4 Functions of Purine and Pyrimidine Nucleotides

Purines and pyrimidines have versatile functions in cells (Fumagalli et al. 2017). First, DNA stores genetic information as the gene and its structure represent the chemical basis of heredity in organisms, including animals, plants, bacteria, and yeasts. This discovery by James Watson and Francis Crick in 1953 was one of the major scientific achievements in the 20th century. DNA directs the synthesis of RNA (including mRNA, tRNA, rRNA, sRNA, miRNA, and siRNA) and, therefore, protein synthesis in cells (Chapter 8). Second, ATP and other nucleoside triphosphates (i.e., GTP and CTP) drive endergonic reactions in synthetic and catabolic pathways. These reactions also generate the phosphorylated metabolites (e.g., glucose-6-phosphate and fructose-6-phosphate) that normally cannot escape the cell because of negative charges in their phosphate group. As high-energy intermediates, UDP-glucose and UDP-galactose participate in the synthesis of complex carbohydrates, and CDP-acylglycerol in the formation of lipid derivatives. In addition, GTP participates in protein synthesis and G protein signaling and serves as the substrate for the generation of tetrahydrobiopterin in cells (Chapter 10). Third, nucleotides are components of FAD, FMN, NAD, NADP, CoA, and SAM, which participate in many reactions, including oxidation, dehydrogenation, and methylation. Fourth, nucleotides have regulatory roles in physiology and metabolism. For example, cGMP and cAMP are second messengers in hormone-mediated or gaseous (e.g., NO, CO, and H_2S) signaling. In addition, ATP and ADP can regulate the activities of enzymes (e.g., α-ketoacid dehydrogenase complex) and mitochondrial oxidative phosphorylation. Furthermore, since Robert Berne and Eckehard Gerlach independently reported in 1963 that adenosine (a product of ATP degradation) causes hypoxic coronary vasodilation, much has been learned about the metabolism and physiology (e.g., anti-inflammatory and neuroprotection) of this purine nucleoside and its transmembrane receptors (e.g., A1, A2A, A2B, and A3) in cells. There is much interest in the role of milk-borne nucleotides in the healthy immune development of mammalian neonates (Field 2005).

11.2.4.5 Functions of Taurine

Taurine is transported into cells by Na^+- and Cl^--dependent transporters, TauT, GAT2, and GAT3, as well as PAT1 (a H^+-coupled, pH-dependent but Na^+- and Cl^--independent transporter), with TauT being the major transporter under physiological conditions (Figure 11.4). Taurine is a highly abundant free β-AA in bile, vertebrate retina (e.g., 50 mM in the rat), milk, skeletal muscle, heart, brain, and many other tissues. Concentrations of taurine in mammalian and avian cells range from 5 to 60 mM, depending on species and cell type (Wright et al. 1986). A 70-kg person has ~70 g taurine, with the human skeletal muscle, heart, retina, and placenta containing 15–20, 28–40, 20–35, and 20–35 mM taurine, respectively. Much evidence shows that taurine is present at high concentrations in the animal kingdom (including insects and arthropods). This is also true for certain marine algae (e.g., Rhodophyceae), but taurine is generally absent from other algae (e.g., Chlorophyceae), which live mainly in fresh water, as well as from the bacterial and plant kingdoms (Hou et al. 2019). Until the early 1970s, taurine was thought to be a biochemically inert molecule. However, a critical role for taurine in nutrition was suggested in 1975 with the discovery that retinal degeneration occurs in taurine-deficient cats. In the same year, it was found that the feeding of infant formulas without taurine could result in cardiac and retinal dysfunction in preterm neonates. Importantly, these problems can be reversed by adding taurine to the infant formulas (Geggel et al. 1985).

Taurine plays major roles in the physiology and nutrition of humans and other animals, including serving as (1) a nutrient to conjugate bile acids to form bile salts in the liver that facilitate intestinal absorption of dietary lipids (including lipid-soluble vitamins) and eliminate cholesterol in bile via the fecal route (Figure 11.3); (2) a major antioxidant, anti-inflammatory, and antiapoptotic factor in the body; (3) a physiological stabilizer of cell membranes; (4) a regulator of Ca^{2+} signaling, fluid homeostasis in cells, and retinal photoreceptor activity; (5) a contributor to osmoregulation; (6) a key component of nerve and muscle conduction networks; (7) a stimulator of neurological development; (8) an inhibitory neurotransmitter in the central nervous system; and (9) *N*-halogenation with hypochlorous acid (HOCl) and hypobromous acid (HOBr) to kill pathogens (Wu 2020b).

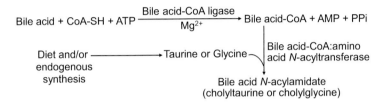

Much evidence shows that taurine exerts beneficial effects on cardiovascular (including protection against ischemia–reperfusion injury, maintaining cell membrane structure, and reducing blood pressure), digestive, endocrine, immune, muscular, neurological, reproductive, and visual systems (Table 11.7). For example, in activated granulocytes and neutrophils, taurine undergoes *N*-halogenation with HOCl and HOBr by the halide-dependent myeloperoxidase system to generate taurine chloramine (*N*-chlorotaurine) and taurine bromamine (*N*-bromotaurine), which can kill bacteria, fungi, parasites, and viruses; potentiate the phagocytic activity of macrophages; and confer anti-inflammatory effects (Marcinkiewicz and Kontny 2014). Interestingly, dietary supplementation with taurine (2% taurine in drinking water) for 28 weeks reduced the expression of adipogenic genes (PPAR-α, PPAR-γ, C/EBP-α, C/EBP-β, and AP2) in white adipose tissue and inhibited the development of obesity in a high-fat diet-induced obese mouse model (Kim et al. 2019). Note that absorbed dietary taurine is not degraded by the intestinal mucosa and all of it enters the portal circulation.

$$H_2O_2 + H^+ + Cl^- \rightarrow H_2O + HOCl \ \left(pK_a = 7.54\right) \quad \left[\text{myeloperoxidase (a heme enzyme)}\right]$$

$$H_2O_2 + H^+ + Br \rightarrow H_2O + HOBr \ \left(pK_a = 8.65\right) \quad \left[\text{myeloperoxidase (a heme enzyme)}\right]$$

$$Taurine + HOCl \rightarrow N\text{-Chlorotaurine} + H_2O \quad \left[\text{halide-dependent myeloperoxidase system}\right]$$

$$Taurine + HOBr \rightarrow N\text{-Bromotaurine} + H_2O \quad \left[\text{halide-dependent myeloperoxidase system}\right]$$

11.2.4.6 Functions of Histamine

There is a rich history of studies of histamine functions in animals. Specifically, the original work on the physiological function of histamine dates back to 1910 when two British physiologists, G. Barger and H.H. Dale, reported that histamine produces tonic contraction of the uterus. Such an effect of histamine was independently confirmed by F. Kutscher in the same year. Many actions of histamine (including vasodilation and induction of hypotension) on multiple organs were revealed by H.H. Dale and P.P. Laidlaw in 1910. By 1932, it had been established that histamine induces allergic reactions. D. Bovet was credited for chemically synthesizing the first antihistamine drug in 1937. A large amount of histamine produced by mast cells (bone marrow-derived tissue-dwelling cells) causes the allergic reaction by serving as the endogenous ligand of histamine receptors H1R-H4R (a class of G protein-coupled receptors) (Thangam et al. 2018). The expression of these

TABLE 11.7

Beneficial Effects of Dietary Taurine, Creatine, Carnosine, Anserine, and 4-Hydroxyproline on Human Health[a]

Dosage	Persons	Benefits	System
		Taurine	
1.5–2.25 g/day for 12 weeks	Children maintained on long-term PNWT	Prevention of electroretinographic abnormality	Retinal health
0.4 or 1.6 g/day for 2 weeks	Healthy adults	Decreases in platelet aggregation and thromboxane release from platelets	Cardiovascular health
1.5 g/day for 90 days	Patients with IDDM	Increase in platelet taurine and a decrease in platelet aggregation	Cardiovascular health
3 g/day for 7 weeks	Overweight or obese adults	Decreases in body weight, plasma TAGs, and atherogenic index	Cardiovascular and metabolic health
3 g/day for 60 days	Adults with mild or borderline HPT	Decrease in blood pressure	Cardiovascular health
3 g/day for 30–45 days	Patients with CHF	Decrease in left ventricular end-diastolic volume and increase in serum creatinine	Cardiovascular and metabolic health
3 g/day for 6 weeks	Patients with CHF	Improvement in cardiac function	Cardiovascular health
6 g/day for 3 weeks	Healthy adults fed a high-fat diet (40% energy from fats)	Decreases in total cholesterol, LDL, and LDL-cholesterol concentrations in serum	Cardiovascular and metabolic health
6 g/day for 1 week	Patients with hypertension	Decrease in blood pressure	Cardiovascular health
2 g/day for 4 weeks	Patients with chronic liver disease	Amelioration of muscle cramps	Skeletal muscle and metabolic health
9–12 g/day for 52 weeks	Patients with MELAS	Reduce the recurrence of stroke-like episodes	Cardiovascular and metabolic health
1–6 g/day for up to 2 weeks	Healthy adults	Improve endurance exercise performance	Skeletal muscle and metabolic health
	Creatine (Cr) in the Form of Cr Monohydrate (CrM) as Cr Phosphate (CrP)		
20 g CrM/day for 6 days; 2 g CrM/day for 22 days	Healthy adult men	Improve muscular strength and reduce intensive exercise-associated muscle damage	Skeletal muscle health
4 g CrM/day for 6 weeks	Healthy adult men and women	Enhance anaerobic power and strength	Skeletal muscle health
4 g CrM/day for 6 weeks	Healthy adult men	Enhance sprint cycling performance	Skeletal muscle health
10–20 g CrM or CrP/day for 6 weeks[b]	Healthy adult men	Enhance muscular strength and lean tissue mass in the body	Skeletal muscle and metabolic health
3 g CrM/day for weeks or months	Healthy adult men and women	Improve antioxidative capacity, exercise performance, and recovery	Skeletal muscle and metabolic health
3 g CrM/day for weeks or months	Patients with neurodegenerative diseases	Improve neurological and muscular function	Neurological and muscle health
		Carnosine	
116 mg/day for 8 weeks	Patients with gastric ulcers	Enhance gastric healing	Gastric health
1.5 g/day for 30 days	Patients with Parkinson's disease	Improve neurological function	Neurological health
2 g/day for 3 months	Patients with Schizophrenia	Improve neurological function	Neurological health

(Continued)

TABLE 11.7 (Continued)
Beneficial Effects of Dietary Taurine, Creatine, Carnosine, Anserine, and 4-Hydroxyproline on Human Health[a]

Dosage	Persons	Benefits	System
0.8 g/day for 8 weeks	Patients with autistic spectrum disorder	Improve behavior as well as social and communication skills	Neurological health
1 g/day for 12 weeks	Patients with type 2 diabetes	Improve metabolic profiles; decrease protein glycosylation and body fat	Cardiovascular and metabolic health
2 g/day for 12 weeks	Overweight or obese persons	Improve metabolic profiles; increase lean tissue mass in the body	Cardiovascular and metabolic health
0.5–2 g/day for up to 6 months	Patients with heart failure	Enhance cardiac output and improve the quality of life	Cardiovascular and metabolic health
		Anserine	
10 or 100 mg/45 kg body weight	Adults undergoing OGTT	Reduce glucose concentration in blood	Metabolic health
Anserine and carnosine mix[c]	Elderly persons	Maintain adequate blood flow to the brain, preserve verbal episodic memory, and improve resting-state network connectivity	Neurological health
Anserine and carnosine mix[c]	Elderly persons	Attenuate cognitive impairment	Neurological health
Anserine and carnosine mix[c]	Elderly persons	Inhibit the production of inflammatory cytokines	Metabolic health and immunity
Anserine and carnosine mix[c]	Elderly persons	Enhance muscular strength and exercise performance	Skeletal muscle health
0.01–0.6 g/day for weeks or months	Adults	Ameliorate stress; enhance physical strength; improve metabolic profiles, immunity, neurological function, and wound healing; promote lactation	Endocrine, metabolic, immune, skeletal muscle, and neurological health
		4-Hydroxyproline in the Form of Collagen Hydrolysate (CH)	
2.5 or 5 g CH/day for 8 weeks	Adult women	Improve skin elasticity	Skin health
5 g CH/day for 6 weeks	Adult women	Enhance moisture content in the epidermis	Skin health
10 g CH/day for 8 weeks	Adult women	Improve collagen density in the dermis and the structure of collagen network	Skin health
5 g CH/day for 8 weeks	Adult women	Improve facial skin conditions	Skin health
5 g CH/day for 1 year	Postmenopausal women	Improve mineral density in bones	Bone health
10 g CH/day for 24 weeks	Postmenopausal women	Mitigate osteoporosis	Bone health
10 g CH/day for 60 days	Persons with knee osteoarthritis	Ameliorate joint pain	Bone health

Source: Wu, G. 2020b. *Amino Acids* 52:329–360.

[a] There were no side effects for the ingestion of taurine, creatine, carnosine, anserine, and hydroxyproline at the indicated dosages on all the studies.

[b] 20 g CrM or CrP/day for 3 days, followed by 10 g CrM or CrP/day for 39 days.

[c] 1 g of anserine and carnosine mix/day, 3:1 (g/g), for 3 months.

Note: CHF, congestive heart failure; HPT, hypertension; IDDM, insulin-dependent diabetes mellitus; LDL, low-density lipoproteins; MELAS, mitochondrial myopathy, encephalopathy, lactic acidosis, and stroke-like episodes; OGTT, oral glucose tolerance test; PNWT, parenteral nutrition (supply of nutrients through intravenous infusion) without taurine; TAGs, triacylglycerols.

receptors is cell- and tissue-specific: H1R in many cells (including mast cells) that are involved in type 1 hypersensitivity reactions, H2R in Th1 lymphocytes for cytokine production, H3R in the blood–brain barrier, and H4R in mast cells. In addition, histamine plays a role in regulating acetylcholine secretion by the central nervous system and in the functions of the gastrointestinal tract (e.g., stimulation of gastric acid secretion).

11.2.4.7 Functions of Melanin

In the skin of humans and other animals, a color pigment is localized in the membrane-bound organelles (melanosomes) of specialized cells (melanocytes) in the basal layer of the epidermis. Pigmentation by melanin (a metabolite of tyrosine) has important biological, cosmetic, and social significance (Lambert et al. 2019). Eumelanin and pheomelanin are two known forms of melanin in the body. There are two types of eumelanin based on their colors: black or brown. Eumelanin occurs in tissues (e.g., skin and feathers) and hair. Another common biological melanin is pheomelanin, which is a polymer of benzothiazine units. There are two types of pheomelanin based on their colors: red or yellow. Pheomelanin is largely responsible for red hair. Dark-skinned animals and people have more melanin than light-skinned individuals. By acting as a sunscreen, melanin protects the skin from ultraviolet light. Increased production of melanin can result in freckles in the skin. Results of recent studies indicate that melanin can influence physiological and behavioral functions, including stress response, energy homeostasis, anti-inflammation, immunity, sexual activity, aggressiveness, and resistance to oxidative injury (Lambert et al. 2019).

11.2.4.8 Functions of Melatonin

The pineal gland and retina receive information about the state of the diurnal light–dark cycle to produce and secrete melatonin (a metabolite of tryptophan) (Cipolla-Neto and Amaral 2018). Melatonin is a hormone and its circulating levels vary in a daily cycle, thereby regulating the circadian rhythms and sleep–wake pattern of animals, including birds, humans, and sheep. At physiological levels, melatonin serves as an antioxidant, protecting nuclear and mitochondrial DNA as well as cell membranes, proteins, and lipids from oxidative injury. Melatonin regulates neurological function (e.g., memory and mood), aging, and immunity in animals (including humans). This hormone also affects mating behavior and reproductive function in seasonal breeders. Melatonin exerts its beneficial effects on animals through (1) antioxidative reactions; (2) changes in nutrient metabolism (e.g., an increase in fatty acid and glucose oxidation in skeletal muscle but a decrease in hepatic lipogenesis); and (3) activation of melatonin receptors (G protein-coupled receptors) on the plasma membrane to trigger the transmission of cell signaling. At present, oral administration of melatonin is a therapy for the sleep disorders that result from circadian rhythm abnormalities and for the alleviation of jet lag due to travel (Cipolla-Neto and Amaral 2018).

11.2.4.9 Functions of Carnosine and Related Dipeptides

Dietary carnosine is absorbed by the enterocytes of the small intestine across their apical membrane via peptide transporter 1 (Figure 11.4). Within the enterocytes, a limited amount of carnosine is hydrolyzed by carnosinase 2 into β-alanine and histidine, and the intracellular carnosine is exported by peptide/histidine transporters 1 and 2 out of the enterocyte across its basolateral membrane into the lamina propria of the small-intestinal mucosa. Nearly all of the ingested carnosine enters the portal circulation (Wu 2020b). In the blood, carnosine is rapidly hydrolyzed by serum carnosinase into β-alanine and histidine, which are subsequently reused for carnosine synthesis by skeletal muscle, heart, and the olfactory bulb of the brain.

Within cells, dipeptides containing histidine or its derivatives are potent quenchers of reactive oxygen, nitrogen, and carbonyl species (Boldyrev et al. 2013). Much work has been done on carnosine. Emerging evidence also shows that carnosine acts on histamine H1 or H3 receptors and on the hypothalamic suprachiasmatic nucleus, a master regulator of the circadian clock in animals. Additionally, through activating the signaling cascades involving mitogen-activated protein kinase and cGMP-dependent protein kinase while inhibiting proapoptotic signaling, carnosine affects the activities of both sympathetic and parasympathetic nerves innervating the adrenal glands, brown adipose tissue, kidneys, liver, pancreas, stomach, and white adipose tissue. This results in beneficial changes in appetite, digestion, absorption, blood pressure, glucose metabolism, lipolysis, and thermogenesis. Containing a histidine moiety, carnosine and carnosine-like dipeptides also play a role in pH buffering, which is of physiological importance in contracting skeletal muscle. In addition, as a positively charged molecule, carnosine can neutralize ATP (~5 mM, a negatively charged molecule). Thus, based on the report of J. Bergstrom in 1974 that human skeletal muscle contains relatively high concentrations of carnosine, studies in the 1980s demonstrated a positive relationship between intramuscular β-alanine concentration and exercise performance in adults. An increase in intramuscular concentrations of these dipeptides brought about by either *in vivo* synthesis or dietary supplementation may help remove hydrogen ions that are generated from enhanced glycolysis during intensive exercise. Furthermore, carnosine plays a role in scavenging oxidants, preventing protein glycation, chelating copper, and ameliorating telomere shortening. Finally, concentrations of carnosine, carnosine-like dipeptides, and their acetylated metabolites in skeletal muscle may not only influence the flavor and taste of meat, but also help identify its species of origin. The beneficial effects of dietary supplementation with carnosine on human health and exercise performance are summarized in Table 11.7.

Although anserine is not synthesized by primates, including humans (Mannion et al. 1992), it is abundant in the skeletal muscles of nonprimate mammals (e.g., cattle, sheep, and pigs), birds, and certain fish (e.g., salmon, tuna, and trout) (Everaert et al. 2019; Wu 2020b). Of note, anserine is the major histidine-containing dipeptide in the skeletal muscles of dog, cat, lion, rabbit, agouti, mouse, kangaroo, wallaby, opossum, cod, smelt, marlin, whiting, croaker, tuna, Japanese char, salmon, and trout (Boldyrev et al. 2013). Anserine has physiological functions similar to those of carnosine, including H+ buffering, antioxidation, modulation of muscle contractility (e.g., excitation and contraction through transmembrane potential maintenance and electromechanical coupling), and regulation of metabolism (Boldyrev et al. 2013). However, as a methylated metabolite of carnosine, anserine has some biochemical properties that are different from those of carnosine. For example, in contrast to carnosine, anserine does not chelate copper and may not regulate nitric oxide availability in cells (Boldyrev et al. 2013). Also, although anserine and carnosine exhibit equivalent antioxidative activities, anserine (1 mM), but not carnosine (1 mM), increased the protein and mRNA levels of heat-shock protein 70 in renal tubular cells treated with 25 mM glucose or 20–100 μM hydrogen peroxide (Peters et al. 2018). Furthermore, anserine, but not carnosine, inhibits carnosinase activity (Derave et al. 2019). Thus, besides its independent effects, anserine may potentiate the action of carnosine in the body.

In humans and other animals, dietary anserine is absorbed by the small intestine, transported in the blood, and taken up by extraintestinal tissues as described previously for dietary carnosine (Figure 11.4), except that the rates of catabolism of anserine to β-alanine and 1-methyl-histidine by serum carnosinase (carnosinase 1) in the plasma and by carnosinase 2 in nonblood tissues are lower than those for carnosine. However, the circulating anserine is cleared rapidly as is carnosine. As summarized in Table 11.7, dietary supplementation with anserine or anserine-rich chicken meat extracts (also containing carnosine) has beneficial effects on the metabolic, neurological, immunological, cardiovascular, and renal functions of humans and other animals (Wu 2020b).

11.2.4.10 Functions of 4-Hydroxyproline

4-Hydroxyproline is taken up into cells primarily by the Na+-dependent system IMINO transporter (all cell types) and the system NBB transporter (present on the brush border of the enterocytes of the small intestine), as well as the Na+-independent system L transporter (all cell types) (Figure 11.4). Most of the diet-derived 4-hydroxyproline-containing di- and tripeptides are not hydrolyzed by the small intestine during the first pass and, therefore, enter the portal circulation (Brandsch 2006). Inside the enterocyte, some of the 4-hydroxyproline-containing tri- and dipeptides undergo hydrolysis by peptidases and/or cytosolic prolidase to form free AAs, including 4-hydroxyproline. Dietary supplementation with 4-hydroxyproline increases its concentration in the plasma (Wu et al. 2011b).

4-Hydroxyproline has structural, physiological, and nutritional significance in humans and other animals (Wu et al. 2019). As a key component of collagen, proline and 4-hydroxyproline permit the sharp twisting of the collagen helix. This allows for establishing and maintaining the rigid structure of the collagen molecule in connective tissues, particularly skin, tendon, cartilage, bone, blood vessels, and the basement membrane (e.g., the intestinal lamina propria; a thin, fibrous, extracellular matrix of tissue that separates an epithelium from its underlying stromal tissue), as well as protecting other tissues in the body (Phang et al. 2010). In addition, the presence of 4-hydroxyproline in the Gly–X–Y collagen peptides reduces chemotaxis and blocks apoptosis in neutrophils, while the hydroxylation of two proline residues in hypoxia-inducible factor-α to form 4-hydroxyproline under normoxic oxygen conditions triggers the proteasomal degradation of the protein to regulate its abundance. Furthermore, as an activator of the apoptotic cascade, oxidation of 4-hydroxyproline by 4-hydroxyproline oxidase to reactive oxygen species can inhibit the growth of cancer cells and promote their death (Phang and Liu 2012). Moreover, 4-hydroxyproline can scavenge oxidants, suppress NF-κB activation, regulate the intracellular redox state, and stimulate the expression of antioxidative enzymes in cells, while inhibiting the production of hydroxyl radical via the Fenton reaction. Finally, multiple tissues in humans and other animals synthesize glycine from 4-hydroxyproline. This metabolic pathway is not dependent on folate (whose provision in diets is quantitatively low relative to glycine requirements) and, therefore, allows for the provision of glycine from the inter-organ metabolism of AAs (e.g., arginine, glutamine, glutamate, ornithine, and proline) other than the tetrahydrofolate-dependent hydroxymethyl transferation of serine. The synthesis of glycine from 4-hydroxyproline plays an important role in maintaining the homeostasis of glycine, as typical diets can meet, at most, 20% and 14% of daily glycine needs in milk-fed neonates and adult humans (Wu 2020b). The benefits of dietary supplementation with 4-hydroxyproline in humans are summarized in Table 11.7.

11.2.4.11 Functions of Glucosamine

Elevated levels of glucosamine inhibit (1) constitutive NO synthesis in endothelial cells by reducing pentose cycle activity and, therefore, the intracellular levels of NADPH and (2) inducible NO synthesis in immunologically activated macrophages and other cell types by suppressing the expression of the iNOS protein (Wu and Meininger 2002). Thus, glucosamine may exhibit either beneficial or detrimental effects on animals, depending on physiological or pathophysiological conditions. For example, as an inhibitor of endothelial cell synthesis of NO, superoxide anion, and peroxynitrite (ONOO⁻), glutamine exerts cardioprotective, neuroprotective, and anti-inflammatory effects during ischemia–reperfusion injury. Accordingly, glucosamine can alleviate or prevent endothelial cell activation and endothelial cell oxidative damage brought about by endotoxin and inflammatory factors (e.g., TNF-α and NF-κB). Furthermore, oral administration of glucosamine can ameliorate (1) cartilage degeneration in osteoarthritis; (2) collagen degeneration in chondrocytes; and (3) atherosclerosis aggravated by chronic arthritis. Thus, glucosamine is widely used as a dietary supplement to treat osteoarthritis in humans and other animals (Salazar et al. 2014).

On the other hand, glucosamine mediates insulin resistance in diabetes and may also have important implications in diabetes-associated cardiovascular complications and the metabolic syndrome (Marshall et al. 1991). The activity of GFAT is enhanced in both the endothelial cells and the skeletal muscle of diabetic animals. In addition, plasma concentrations of glucose and glutamine, as well as tissue concentrations of fructose 6-phosphate, are elevated in diabetic persons with poor metabolic control. Thus, increases in both GFAT activity and concentrations of its substrates enhance the synthesis of glucosamine in endothelial cells and skeletal muscle under hyperglycemic conditions. These findings may explain, in part, decreased endothelial NO synthesis and impaired endothelium-dependent relaxation in diabetes. For this reason, dietary supplementation with glucosamine may not be recommended for (1) diabetic patients, (2) individuals with impaired NO synthesis by endothelial cells, or (3) individuals with physiological activation of NO-dependent angiogenesis in tissues (e.g., gestating mammals with rapidly growing placentae, females with ovulating ovaries; and pregnant or lactating mothers with high rates of cell proliferation in the mammary gland). Inhibition of GFAT may improve cardiovascular function in people with obesity and diabetes. At present, it remains unknown whether a beneficial outcome of glucosamine on alleviating osteoarthritis in obese and diabetic patients outweighs its potential adverse effect on exacerbating insulin resistance. However, a comprehensive review of published clinical studies concluded that oral administration of glucosamine at a daily dose of 21 or 45 mg/kg BW for periods of up to 3 years did not affect fasting blood glucose concentrations or insulin sensitivity in healthy persons, individuals with diabetes, or those with impaired glucose tolerance (Simon et al. 2011).

11.2.4.12 AAs and Their metabolites as Natural Ligands and Activators of Aryl Hydrocarbon Receptors

Tryptophan and its metabolites (e.g., indole acetic acid, kynurenine, and tryptamine), as well as bilirubin (a metabolite of heme), are natural ligands and activators of the aryl hydrocarbon receptor (AhR; also known as dioxin receptor) (Rothhammer and Quintana 2019). AhR is a cytosolic ligand-activated transcription factor in many cell types and tissues (e.g., enterocytes, hepatocytes, lymphoid cells, lungs, and brain), and AhR is normally present in a dormant state in association with a complex consisting of HSP90, XAP2 (hepatitis B virus X-associated protein), and p23. Upon ligand binding, AhR undergoes a conformational change, leading to the exposure of a nuclear localization signal. Thereafter, the ligand-activated AhR translocates into the nucleus, dissociates from the complex, and forms a heterodimer with the closely related Arnt protein in the nucleus. This, in turn, enhances the expression of target genes including cytochrome P450s, which are a superfamily of hemoproteins that catalyze the monooxygenation of various endogenous and exogenous substrates before their excretion in urine and feces. In addition, AhR plays a role in regulating anti-inflammatory pathways and numerous other physiological processes, such as cell metabolism and differentiation. For example, activation of AhR is beneficially associated with the downregulation of NF-κB expression and anti-inflammatory responses in the small-intestinal mucosa, lungs, and brain. This may be an important mechanism for tryptophan and other AAs to modulate intestinal function and gut-associated chronic diseases. Thus, AhR serves as an intracellular sensor for integrating nutrients and related substances with adaptation and survival responses in health and disease.

11.2.5 FUNCTIONS OF AAs IN SENSING

AAs play an important role in the growth, development, and functions of sense organs (Wu 2020a). These specialized organs are the eyes, ears, nose, tongue, and skin, which provide senses of sight, hearing, smell, taste, and touch, respectively, to aid the survival, development, learning, and adaptation of humans and other animals (including fish). The chemosensory transduction involves AAs or their metabolites. The physiological sensing responses help humans and other animals to avoid foods with strong bitter tastes, sour tastes, or unusual (e.g., bad or strong) smell, and to protect the organisms against consuming toxic substances or toxic foods.

To date, there is a large database on AA metabolism and function in the eye and skin under normal (e.g., developmental changes and physiological responses) and pathological (e.g., nutritional and metabolic diseases, nutrient deficiency, infections, and cancer) conditions (Wu 2020d). Important metabolites of AAs for chemosensing include (1) NO and polyamines (from arginine), melanin and dopamine (from phenylalanine and tyrosine), and serotonin and melatonin (from tryptophan) in both the eye and the skin; (2) γ-aminobutyrate (from glutamate) in the retina; (3) urocanic acid and histamine (from histidine) in the skin; (4) certain AAs for the nose [e.g., acidic AAs (aspartate and glutamate); basic AAs (arginine and lysine); glutamine and small neutral AAs (glycine, alanine, serine, and possibly cysteine); and large neutral AAs (methionine, BCAAs, and phenylalanine) and possibly cysteine]; (5) some AA metabolites for the nose [e.g., hydrogen sulfide (H_2S) and methyl mercaptan (methanethiol, CH_3-SH) produced in the tongue and oral cavity as the sources of bad breath in humans]; and (6) glutamate in the digestive tract.

As indicated in Chapter 1, AAs confer five basic taste qualities (sweet, sour, bitter, umami, and salty tastes) through sense signaling in the tongue and the gastrointestinal tract (San Gabriel and Uneyama 2013; Wu 2020d). Taste cells express different taste receptors (transmembrane proteins) for different tastants. The gene *Tas2R* encodes for bitter receptor proteins, whereas the gene *Tas1R* encodes for sweet and umami receptor proteins. Taste receptors for bitter, sweet, and umami tastants are all transmembrane G protein-coupled receptors composed of a GTP-binding α subunit and βγ subunit. Sour and salty taste receptors are H^+ and Na^+ channels, respectively. Specifically, sour taste is initiated by protons (H^+ ions) acting on specific receptors [e.g., hyperpolarization-activated and cyclic-nucleotide-gated (HCN) channels, HCN1 and HCN4] in a subset of taste cells on the tongue and palate epithelium. The sodium (salt) taste receptor or the epithelial Na^+ channel (ENaC), which is also known as the sodium (salt) taste receptor, mediates the passive influx of Na^+ ions through the ion channel via a Na^+ concentration gradient to depolarize taste receptor cells, leading to changes in their membrane potential and excitement. The detailed mechanisms for AA sensing in the digestive tract are discussed in Section E.3 of this chapter. A synergism exists between glutamate and 5′-nucleotides to enhance the response of taste cell receptors to glutamate (San Gabriel et al. 2005, 2009). In mammals (including humans and rats), the response of the taste cell receptors to a mixture of L-glutamate plus 5′-inosinate is approximately 8 and 1.7 times, respectively, greater than that to glutamate alone. Mammalian milk contains not only abundant L-glutamate but also 5′-inosinate, and these nutrients are also present in the lumen of the small intestine as shown for AAs (Wu 2020a). This contributes to explaining why human infants and neonatal livestock enjoy consuming their mothers' milk.

11.2.6 FUNCTIONS OF D-AAs

Animals and microbes can synthesize, from L-AAs, D-AAs, including D-aspartate, D-serine, D-alanine, and D-glutamate. High concentrations of D-aspartate, D-serine, and D-alanine occur in the endocrine glands, with amounts varying with the type of gland. For example, D-aspartate is present at relatively high concentrations in the pituitary, pineal, thyroid, and adrenal glands, as well as testes; D-serine in the hypothalamus; and D-alanine in both the pituitary gland and the pancreas (Baccari et al. 2020). By contrast, the concentrations of D-leucine, D-proline, and D-glutamate are generally low in mammalian and avian tissues. Over the past decades, there has been growing interest in the physiological functions of D-amino acids in humans and other animals (Billard 2012; Flynn et al. 2020).

11.2.6.1 Functions of D-Alanine

The physiological functions of D-alanine in animals are largely unknown. Experimental evidence from rodent studies suggests that D-alanine is an agonist of the glycine site on the NMDA subtype glutamate receptor, thereby possibly affecting memory function and synaptic plasticity (Baccari et al. 2020). In support of this suggestion, there are reports that (1) inadequate activity of this receptor is associated with schizophrenia (a neurological disorder) in humans; (2) oral administration of D-alanine can improve the cognitive ability of patients with this disease; and (3) the reduced production of D-alanine by microflora is linked to antibiotic-induced psychosis (Abe et al. 2005; Lee et al. 2020). In addition, the concentration of D-alanine in the brain and pancreas of rats is related to diurnal and nocturnal (circadian) behaviors, but the underlying mechanisms remain elusive (Flynn et al. 2020). Besides its neurological effects, D-alanine may affect cell metabolism. For example, through the production of H_2O_2, D-alanine may regulate cellular redox signaling at low concentrations but induce cytotoxic oxidative stress at high concentrations in tumors. Interestingly, in aquatic crustaceans and some bivalve mollusks, a large amount of free D-alanine usually accumulates under high salinity stress to possibly serve as a major regulator of intracellular osmolality (Chapter 3).

11.2.6.2 Functions of D-Aspartate

D-Aspartate is the precursor for the important neurotransmitter agonist, NMDA (Baccari et al. 2020; D'Aniello 2007). D-Aspartate binds and activates NMDA receptors to affect long-term potentiation and spatial memory. Moreover, administration of D-aspartate to old mice is able to rescue the physiological age-related decay of hippocampal long-term potentiation (Errico et al. 2012). In mice, an increase in concentrations of D-aspartate completely suppresses long-term depression at corticostriatal synapses and attenuates the prepulse inhibition deficits produced by the psychotomimetic drugs (amphetamine and MK-801). Thus, depletion of D-aspartate racemase in newborn neurons causes severe defects in the dendritic development in the hippocampus of adult mice. Similarly, a reduction in D-aspartate results in a phenotype resembling a deficiency of D-aspartate racemase, which indicates an important role for this enzyme in adult neurogenesis. In addition to its action on the neurological system, D-aspartate is associated with the functional maturation of endocrine glands during the postnatal period, as well as with the synthesis and release of different hormones in rodents (Baccari et al. 2020). These hormones include gonadotropin-releasing hormone, growth hormone, prolactin, progesterone, oxytocin, luteinizing hormone, and testosterone. Thus, administration of D-aspartate to adult men and women can increase the circulating levels of reproductive hormones in animals (Errico et al. 2012).

11.2.6.3 Functions of D-Serine

D-Serine is an endogenous ligand for the glycine site of the NMDA receptor and functions as a novel neurotransmitter (MacKay et al. 2019). Selective degradation of D-serine by D-AA oxidase attenuates NMDA receptor-mediated neurotransmission. Conversely, the inhibitory effects of this enzyme are fully reversed by exogenous D-serine. Thus, in the nervous system, D-serine appears to be a more selective agonist of the NMDA receptor than glycine, the AA which exhibits biphasic effects by acting both as an inhibitory transmitter at strychnine-sensitive glycine receptors and as a co-excitatory transmitter with glutamate at the NMDA receptor (He and Wu 2020). There is evidence that a reduction in the activity of brain D-serine racemase is associated with the development of schizophrenia, Alzheimer's disease, and age-related memory loss (Guercio and Panizzutti 2018). Based on these findings, D-serine has been proposed to be a novel pharmacologic agent to treat these diseases.

11.3 REGULATORY ROLES OF AAs IN FOOD INTAKE, NUTRIENT METABOLISM, AND GENE EXPRESSION

11.3.1 REGULATORY ROLES OF AAs IN FOOD INTAKE

Food intake by animals is affected by the taste, quantity, and quality of dietary protein, and by dietary AAs (He and Wu 2020). Specifically, food consumption by animals is depressed in response to (1) a severe deficiency of dietary protein or an individual AA (particularly an EAA or conditionally essential AA); (2) a distortion of the dietary pattern of AAs when protein intake is either high or low; and (3) a substantial increase in dietary protein or AA content. Under all of these conditions, changes in feeding behavior are associated with substantial alterations in concentrations of many AAs (especially those that are the precursors for the synthesis of neurotransmitters) in the lumen of the stomach and small intestine, as well as the plasma and brain. Interestingly, high dietary protein contributes to satiety to a greater extent than an isocaloric amount of fat or carbohydrate, further supporting a crucial role for AAs in the control of food consumption. Thus, the amount and balance of supplemental AAs can either stimulate or suppress food intake, depending on individual AAs, composition of AAs and other nutrients in the basal diet, as well as endocrine status and developmental stage. For example, supplemental arginine and glycine (1% and 2% in the diet, respectively) moderately stimulate, but supplemental glutamine and leucine (2% and 4% in the diet, respectively) substantially depress, food intake by young pigs fed a typical corn- and soybean meal-based diet (Wu 2018). The underlying mechanisms are complex and involve hormonal, neuronal, and metabolic signals generated from the digestive system [including the stomach, small intestine, pancreas (insulin, amylin, and glucagon), liver, and large intestine], central nervous system, and other organs [e.g., white adipose tissue (leptin)]. In support of this view, there is much evidence that ingested protein can evoke satiation by inducing both gastrointestinal distention and the release of peptides from enteroendocrine cells (Westerterp-Plantenga et al. 2009).

At the stomach level, a variety of neurotransmitters, neuromodulators (e.g., glutamate, acetylcholine, NO, calcitonin-gene-related peptide, and substance P), and other peptides [including ghrelin and bombesin-related peptides (e.g., gastrin-releasing peptide and neuromedin B produced by gastric myenteric neurons)] are utilized to control gastric emptying (He and Wu 2020). These substances also act to relay signals from the mechanoreceptors on the gastric wall to the brain by vagal and spinal sensory nerves. In the small intestine, cholecystokinin (produced by I cells in duodenal and jejunal mucosae) and products of its endoproteolytic cleavage, as well as glucagon-like peptide 1, oxyntomodulin, and peptide YY (produced by L cells in the distal small intestine and colon), serve as primary satiation signals to inhibit food intake. By contrast, ghrelin stimulates food intake by animals, and physiological levels of glutamate increase gastric emptying and intestinal motility.

At the brain level, both the direct blood pathway and the indirect neuromediated (mainly vagus-mediated) pathway contribute to the effects of dietary AAs on food intake (Tomé 2004). Dietary intake of protein and AAs affects the concentrations of AAs, peptides, hormones, glucose, and fatty acids that act on different sites in the brain (the area postrema and the anterior piriform cortex for AAs, and the arcuate nucleus for hormones such as insulin and leptin) (Wu 2018). Interestingly, the area postrema localized near the nucleus of the solitary tract receives information directly from the blood, whereas an AA chemosensor system occurs in the anterior piriform cortex of the brain (Jordi et al. 2013). AA imbalances result in (1) altered concentrations of EAAs or limiting AAs in specific sites of the brain, such as the anterior prepyriform cortex, anterior cingulated cortex, locus coeruleus, and nucleus of solitary tract; and (2) impaired synthesis and reduced concentrations of neurotransmitters (e.g., NO, glutamate, glycine, serotonin, and norepinephrine) in the prepyriform region; and (3) activation of the general AA control nonderepressing 2 (GCN2) enzyme system in the highly excitable anterior piriform cortex of the brain, which increases phosphorylation of eukaryotic initiation factor (eIF2α) to block general protein synthesis (Gietzen and Aja 2012; Hao et al. 2005). However, results of recent studies indicate that the regulation of food intake by dietary EAA content in mice is independent of the proposed GCN2 pathway and other undescribed mechanisms exist for their rapid sensing of dietary EAAs (Leib and Knight 2016).

The neuron-mediated pathway of AA sensing transfers preabsorptive and visceral information to the forebrain through the vagal nerve that innervates the stomach, the duodenum, and the liver (components of the oro-sensory zone) to control neural circuits (Jordi et al. 2013). For example, the lateral hypothalamus secretes peptides (orexin, melanin-concentrating hormone, and neuropeptide Y) to increase food intake, as reported for the effect of ghrelin. By contrast, satiation factors (e.g., leptin) desensitize the brain to hunger signals and inhibit the release of neuropeptide Y, thereby suppressing food intake (Westerterp-Plantenga et al. 2009). These mechanisms aid in our understanding of how dietary protein or AA affects the food intake, food preference, and nutritional adaptation of animals.

11.3.2 Regulatory Roles of AAs in Nutrient Metabolism

There are species differences in the synthesis and catabolism of nutrients as well as the excretion of their metabolites among animal species (Buentello and Gatlin III 2000, 2001; Campbell et al. 1983; Chadwick and Wright 1999; Chiu et al. 1986; Wu 2018). Many lines of evidence identify AAs as regulators of nutrient metabolism in mammals, birds, and aquatic animals (Anderson 1981; He et al. 2021; Li et al. 2021a,b; Wu 2009). First, arginine is an allosteric activator of NAG synthase, a mitochondrial enzyme that converts glutamate and acetyl-CoA into NAG (an allosteric activator of CPS-I). Thus, arginine and glutamate maintain the hepatic urea cycle in an active state for ammonia detoxification. Second, alanine inhibits pyruvate kinase, thereby regulating gluconeogenesis and glycolysis to ensure net glucose production by hepatocytes during periods of food deprivation. Third, glutamate and aspartate mediate the transfer of reducing equivalents across the mitochondrial membrane and thus regulate glycolysis and cellular redox state. Fourth, arginine and phenylalanine increase GTP cyclohydrolase I expression and activity, thereby increasing the availability of tetrahydrobiopterin for NO synthesis and the hydroxylation of aromatic AAs. The arginine-NO pathway can also be modulated by a number of other AAs, including taurine, lysine, glutamate, homocysteine, and asymmetric dimethylarginine, to exert their physiological and pathological effects. For example, NO synthesis by endothelial cells is stimulated by physiological levels of arginine, citrulline, and taurine, but inhibited by elevated levels of lysine, glutamine, homocysteine, and asymmetric dimethylarginine (Wu and Meininger 2002).

Fifth, arginine increases the expression of key proteins and enzymes (e.g., AMPK and PGC-1α) responsible for mitochondrial biogenesis in brown adipose tissue and substrate oxidation in insulin-sensitive tissues (e.g., skeletal muscle, liver, and white adipose tissue), thereby reducing excess fat mass in obese animals (Figure 11.8). Likewise, glutamine regulates ion and nutrient transport as well as oxidative defense, signal transduction, and protein turnover (e.g., stimulation of protein synthesis and inhibition of protein degradation in enterocytes), therefore preventing intestinal atrophy

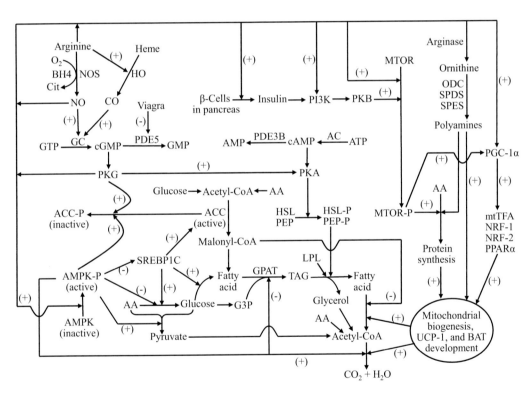

FIGURE 11.8 A proposed mechanism for L-arginine to enhance substrate oxidation and reduce adiposity via the cGMP and AMPK signaling pathways in obese animals. Abbreviations: AA, amino acids; AC, adenylyl cyclase; ACC, acetyl-CoA carboxylase; AMPK, AMP-activated protein kinase; BH4, tetrahydrobiopterin; Cit, citrulline; GC, guanylyl cyclase; G3P, glycerol-3-phosphate; GPAT, glycerol-3-phosphate acyltransferase; HO, heme oxygenase; HSL, hormone-sensitive lipase; LPL, lipoprotein lipase; MTOR, mammalian target of rapamycin; mtTFA, mitochondrial transcription factor A; NO, nitric oxide; NOS, nitric oxide synthase; NRF, nuclear respiration factor; ODC, ornithine decarboxylase; PDE5, phosphodiesterase 5; PDE3B, phosphodiesterase 3B; PEP, perilipins; PGC-1α, peroxisome proliferator-activated receptor γ (PPAR-γ) coactivator 1α; PKA, cAMP-dependent protein kinase A; PKG, cGMP-dependent protein kinase G; PPARα, peroxisome proliferator-activated receptor α; SPDS, spermidine synthase; SPES, spermine synthase; SREBP-1c, sterol regulatory element-binding protein 1c; and TAG, triacylglycerols.

and enhancing growth in animals (e.g., weanling pigs) with intestinal damage and dysfunction. In addition, as noted above, H_2S and CO, which are products of cysteine and heme degradation, respectively, may also play signaling roles in nutrient metabolism (e.g., stimulation of glucose and fatty acid oxidation).

Sixth, metabolism of AAs (glycine, histidine, methionine, and serine), along with vitamins (B_6, B_{12}, and folate), actively participates in one-carbon metabolism and plays a key role in the provision of methyl donors for DNA and protein methylation (Figure 11.9), thereby regulating gene

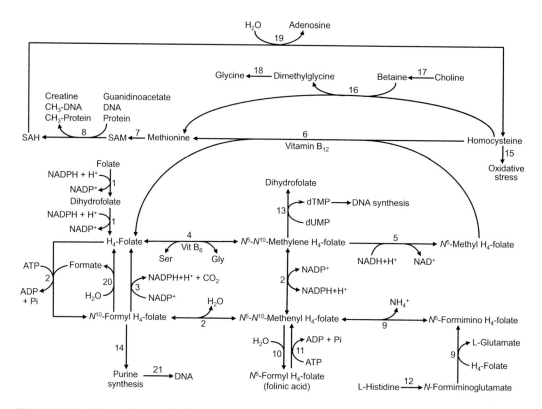

FIGURE 11.9 One-carbon metabolism for the provision of methyl donors in cells. Folate, histidine, methionine, and serine participate in the transfer of one-carbon units for the synthesis of purines and DNA, as well as methylation reactions in animals. The enzymes that catalyze the indicated reactions are (1) folate reductase; (2) N^5-N^{10}-methylene H_4-folate dehydrogenase (a trifunctional enzyme possessing N^{10}-formyl H_4-folate synthetase, N^5-N^{10}-methylene H_4-folate dehydrogenase, and N^5-N^{10}-methenyl H_4-folate cyclohydrolase activities in the cytosol of mammalian cells; a bifunctional enzyme possessing N^5-N^{10}-methylene H_4-folate dehydrogenase and N^5-N^{10}-methenyl H_4-folate cyclohydrolase activities in the mitochondria of mammalian cells); (3) N^{10}-formyl H_4-folate dehydrogenase; (4) serine hydroxymethyl transferase; (5) N^5-N^{10}-methylene H_4-folate reductase; (6) methionine synthase; (7) S-adenosylmethionine synthase; (8) S-adenosylmethionine as a major methyl group donor in methyltransferase reactions; (9) formiminotransferase cyclodeaminase (a bifunctional enzyme possessing glutamate formiminotransferase and formimidoyl H_4-folate cyclodeaminase activities); (10) serine hydroxymethyl transferase, N^5-N^{10}-methenyl H_4-folate cyclohydrolase, and spontaneous reaction at pH 4–7.0; (11) N^5-N^{10}-methenyl H_4-folate synthetase; (12) a sequential series of enzymes: histidase, urocanase, and imidazolone propionate hydrolase; (13) thymidylate synthase; (14) formyltransferase; (15) an oxidant for cells; (16) betaine:homocysteine methyltransferase; (17) choline dehydrogenase; (18) enzymes for glycine synthesis (dimethylglycine oxidase and sarcosine oxidase); (19) S-adenosylhomocysteine hydrolase; (20) N^{10}-formyl H_4-folate synthetase; (21) enzymes for DNA synthesis. dTMP, deoxythymidine 5′-monophosphate; dUMP, deoxyuridine 5′-monophosphate; Gly, glycine; H_4-folate, tetrahydrofolate; SAH, S-adenosylhomocysteine; SAM, S-adenosylmethionine; Ser, serine; and Vit, vitamin.

expression and the biological activities of proteins (Bazer et al. 2021; Field et al. 2018). Seventh, leucine allosterically activates GDH. In the pancreas, this effect of leucine results in enhanced secretion of insulin from β cells via a series of biological responses. Specifically, a leucine-induced increase in GDH activity stimulates glutamate oxidation, leading to an elevated ratio of intracellular [ATP]/[ADP]. This, in turn, inhibits the plasma membrane-bound ATP-gated K^+ channel, resulting in membrane depolarization, an influx of extracellular Ca^{2+}, and the exocytosis of insulin granules from pancreatic β cells. Finally, the complex interorgan metabolism of AAs among the liver, skeletal muscle, intestine, and immune cells maximizes glutamine availability for renal ammoniagenesis under acidotic conditions, while producing arginine, proline, and glutathione to meet physiological and nutritional needs (Figure 11.10).

11.3.3 REGULATORY ROLES OF AAs IN GENE EXPRESSION AND CELL SIGNALING

11.3.3.1 Regulatory Roles of AAs in Gene Expression

Regulation of gene expression by AAs can occur at any step in the highly specific processes that involve the transfer of information encoded in a gene into its product (RNA and/or protein) (Figure 11.11). These biochemical events are transcription, translation, and posttranslational modifications. In both eukaryotic and noneukaryotic cells, transcription is controlled by transcription factors, which are proteins that bind to specific DNA sequences. Transcription factors act either alone or in combination with other proteins, by promoting (as activators) or inhibiting (as repressors) the recruitment of RNA polymerases to specific genes (Brasse-Lagnel et al. 2010). Actinomycin D, an anticancer agent produced by *Streptomyces antibioticus*, blocks gene transcription by inhibiting both DNA and RNA polymerases. In bacteria, gene expression is often suppressed by the accumulation of products. For example, an increase in glucose concentration can suppress the expression of genes that encode for enzymes hydrolyzing lactose and galactose in *E. coli*. Such a regulatory mechanism also exists in mammalian cells for some enzymes (e.g., the inhibition of argininosuccinate lyase expression by arginine in hepatocytes).

Translation (both mRNA stability and efficiency of polypeptide formation) is also a step for the control of protein synthesis (Brasse-Lagnel et al. 2010). Results from cell culture studies indicate that a deficiency of an AA will result in the increased availability of uncharged tRNA that binds and activates the general control nonderepressible protein 2 (GCN2), which is an eIF-2α kinase. GCN2 phosphorylates eIF-2α, leading to a decrease in global protein synthesis (Castilho et al. 2014). However, under conditions of nutrient deprivation, some mRNAs may undergo enhanced translation via mechanisms involving activating transcription factor 4 (ATF4, the mammalian counterpart of the yeast GCN4; Hinnebusch 2005). In addition, an excessive amount of an AA may downregulate or upregulate the expression of genes, depending on its side chains and target proteins. For example, glutamine stimulates ASS gene expression in Caco-2 cells at the transcriptional level (Brasse-Lagnel et al. 2003), but reduces GS protein levels in mouse C2C12 skeletal muscle cells probably at the posttranslational level (Wang and Watford 2007). Moreover, either an excess or a deficiency of arginine modulates global gene expression in mammalian cells (Leong et al. 2006), whereas methionine deficiency stimulates osteopontin expression in hepatocytes through the hypomethylation of DNA and protein (Sahai et al. 2006). Consistent with results from these *in vitro* studies, microarray analyses indicate that dietary supplementation with glutamine or arginine increases the expression of antioxidative genes and reduces the expression of proinflammatory genes in the small intestine and adipose tissue (Fu et al. 2005; Jobgen et al. 2009b; Wang et al. 2008). Additionally, dietary intake of methionine (Rees et al. 2006), glutamine (Zhu et al. 2018), or arginine (Wu et al. 2018) may affect the expression of the fetal genome, fetal growth and survival, and pregnancy outcomes in mammals.

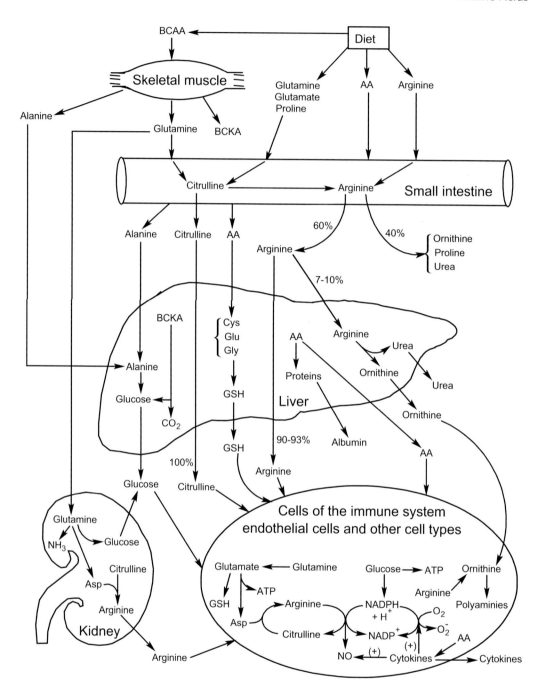

FIGURE 11.10 Interorgan metabolism of branched-chain amino acids (BCAA), glutamine, and arginine and its role in immune function. Skeletal muscle takes up BCAA from the arterial blood, synthesizes both alanine and glutamine from BCAA and α-ketoglutarate, and releases these two amino acids into the circulation. The small intestine utilizes glutamine to synthesize citrulline, which is converted into arginine in the kidneys, cells of the immune system, and other cell types. The liver is the primary organ for the synthesis of glutathione from glutamate, glycine, and cysteine and of glucose from alanine for use by extrahepatic cells (including immunocytes) and tissues. Abbreviations: AA, amino acids; Asp, aspartate; BCAA, branched-chain amino acids; BCKA, branched-chain α-ketoacids; GSH, glutathione; and NO, nitric oxide.

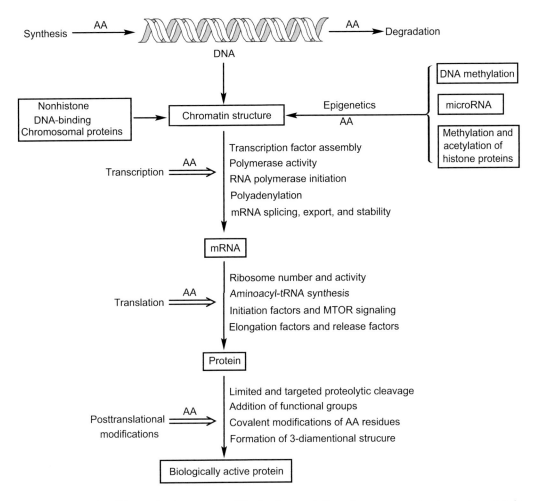

FIGURE 11.11 Possible mechanisms responsible for the regulation of gene expression by amino acids in cells. Amino acids may regulate gene expression in animal cells at transcriptional, translational, and post-translational levels, as well as via microRNA expression and epigenetic modifications of DNA molecules. These effects of amino acids (AA) may be cell- and tissue-specific.

11.3.3.2 Regulatory Roles of AAs in Epigenetics

Effects of AAs on gene expression may be mediated, in part, by epigenetics through the action of SAM, a metabolite of methionine (Phang et al. 2013). Epigenetics is defined as stable and heritable alterations in gene expression through covalent modifications of DNA and core histones without changes in the DNA sequence. Four mechanisms responsible for mediating epigenetic effects are (1) chromatin modifications, (2) DNA methylation (occurring at the 5′-position of cytosine residues within CpG dinucleotides throughout the mammalian genome), (3) histone modifications (acetylation, methylation, phosphorylation, ubiquitination, and sumoylation), and (4) RNA-based mechanisms such as small noncoding RNAs or inhibitory RNAs. The enzymes involved in these reactions include (1) specific DNA methyltransferases (*DNMT1*, *DNMT3a*, and *DNMT3b*) (Figure 11.12); (2) protein methyltransferases (e.g., histone methyltransferases) for regulation of gene expression (Figure 11.13); (3) DNA demethylases; (4) histone acetylase (lysine acetyltransferase); (5) GCN5-related N-acetyltransferase (a superfamily of acetyltransferase), and (6) histone deacetyltransferase.

1. DNA methylation

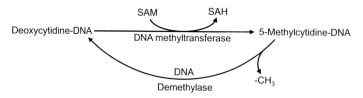

2. Histone acetylation

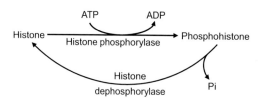

3. Histone methylation

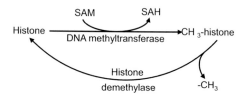

4. Histone phosphorylation

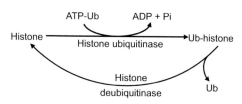

5. Histone ubiquitination

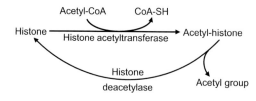

FIGURE 11.12 Biochemical reactions involving DNA methylation and histone modifications. The latter include acetylation, methylation, phosphorylation, and ubiquitination. These reactions are localized in the specific compartments of the cell. *S*-adenosylmethionine is required for the methylation of both DNA and histone protein. SAH, *S*-adenosylhomocysteine; SAM, *S*-adenosylmethionine; and Ub, ubiquitin.

Epigenetic regulation of gene expression is also mediated by small-interfering RNAs or small noncoding RNAs that act through their respective pathways to induce SAM-dependent DNA methylation or histone modifications to silence or enhance gene expression (Mittal 2004; Nikam and Gore 2018). In mammals, the small noncoding RNAs include Piwi RNA and microRNA (miRNA). The biogenesis of mature (functional) miRNA containing ~22 nucleotides from its miRNA gene involves both the nucleus and the cytoplasm in mammalian cells (Figure 11.14). Piwi RNA is restricted to the germ line (e.g., testes in males and oocytes in females) and regulates gene expression possibly through the sequence-specific targeting of heterochromatin formation factors to mobile elements in the genome and the degradation of mobile element transcripts. By contrast, miRNAs are widespread in cells and tissues to regulate gene expression at the posttranscriptional level. Since the discovery of *lin-4* as the first miRNA in 1993, ~1,000 miRNAs have been identified, annotated, and catalogued for humans. Emerging evidence shows a key role for AAs in regulating miRNA expression in animal cells. For example, supplementing arginine to the diet of pregnant swine increases the expression of miRNA-15b/16 and miRNA-221/222 and endothelial NO synthesis in the porcine umbilical vein (Liu et al. 2012). Additionally, dietary supplementation with an EAA enhances the abundances of miRNA-499, miRNA-208b, and miRNA-23a, as well as protein synthesis in human skeletal muscle (Drummond et al. 2009). AA-induced changes in epigenetics contribute to the fetal programming of postnatal growth, metabolism, and health in humans and other animals (Wang et al. 2012; Ji et al. 2016).

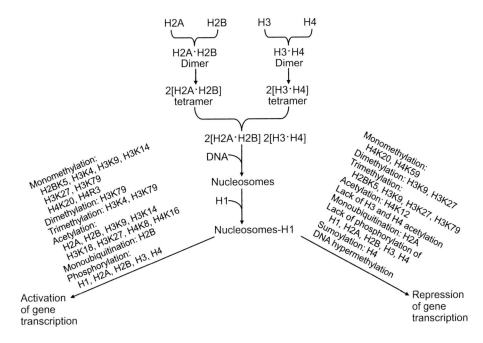

FIGURE 11.13 Roles of histone modifications in the regulation of gene transcription. Methylation of histones, acetylation, or ubiquitination can either activate or repress gene expression, depending on specific histone proteins and the sites of modifications. In a variety of cell types, histone methylation is generally associated with transcriptional repression, but methylation of some lysine (e.g., lysine 4 of histone 3) and arginine residues (e.g., those on H3 and H4) of histones can result in transcriptional activation. In general, phosphorylation of histones promotes transcription, DNA repair, and apoptosis. Abbreviations: H, histone; K, lysine residue; and R, arginine residue.

11.3.3.3 Regulatory Roles for AAs in Cell Signaling

Some AAs (e.g., arginine, glutamate, glutamine, glycine, leucine, proline, and tryptophan) are activators of many cell signaling pathways (Chapter 10). These pathways involve MTOR, cAMP-dependent kinases, cGMP-dependent kinases, G protein-coupled receptors, AMPK, and MAPK (Dar and Shokat 2011; Gui et al. 2012; Suryawan and Davis 2011). These are complex networks of metabolic regulation, but all of them are regulated by protein phosphorylation and protein dephosphorylation mechanisms. These pathways also involve the activation of various proteins in the cytoplasm and the nucleus (Chapter 10).

AMPK is a heterotrimeric enzyme consisting of three subunits: a catalytic α subunit as well as regulatory β and γ units. AMPK acts as a sensor for cellular energy and is activated by an increase in the [AMP]/[ATP] ratio (Jobgen et al. 2006). Activation of AMPK occurs via protein phosphorylation by an established upstream AMPK kinase, LKB1. The overall effect of AMPK activation is to inhibit the ATP-consuming pathways (e.g., lipogenesis, gluconeogenesis, glycogenesis, and protein synthesis), while stimulating the ATP-producing pathways (e.g., glycolysis, as well as fatty acid and glucose oxidation).

Members of the MAPK family include extracellular signal-regulated kinases (ERK1 and ERK2), c-Jun NH(2)-terminal kinase (JNK), p38 MAPK, and ERK5 (Figure 11.15). ERK activates a number of transcription factors and protein kinases. This results in transmission of signals from many extracellular agents (including glutamine) to intracellular organelles, thereby regulating cellular processes, including (1) gene expression; (2) cell proliferation, differentiation, and migration; (3) mitosis and cell survival; and (4) cell cycle progression (Rhoads and Wu 2009). Jun was originally identified in 1994 as a kinase that binds and phosphorylates c-Jun on Ser-63 and Ser-73

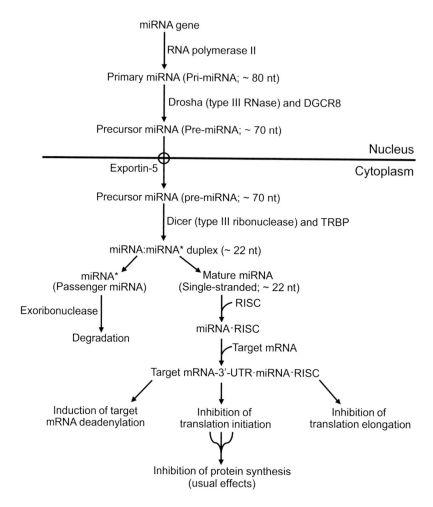

FIGURE 11.14 Biogenesis of microRNA and its role in the regulation of gene expression. The biogenesis of mature (functional) miRNA from its miRNA gene involves both the nucleus and cytoplasm in mammalian cells. A single-stranded mature (functional) miRNA with approximately 22 nucleotides (nt) binds the 3'-untranslated region of the target mRNA. This usually results in decreased protein synthesis through the induction of mRNA deadenylation, reduction of translation initiation, and inhibition of translation elongation. Note that Argonaute proteins bind small RNAs and play an important role in RNA silencing processes. DGCR8, associated protein DGCR8 of Drosha (also known as Pasha); TRBP, transacting RNA-binding protein; miRNA*, passenger strand miRNA for degradation; RISC, RNA-induced silencing complex (RISC) containing several components, including Argonaute proteins, the PW182 protein, and the fragile X mental retardation protein.

within its transcriptional activation domain, whereas p38 MAPK was first isolated in 1993 as a 38-kDa protein that underwent rapid tyrosine phosphorylation in response to endotoxin stimulation. Both JNK and p38 MAPK are responsive to stress stimuli, such as cancers, cytokines, inflammatory signals, protein synthesis inhibitors, heat shock, and osmotic shock to contribute to apoptosis and inflammation (Wagner and Nebreda 2009). In response to extracellular signals (e.g., growth factors), ERK5 translocates to the nucleus, where this kinase regulates gene expression by phosphorylating and activating a number of transcription factors. Activation of the ERK5 signaling pathway has been implicated in physiological functions (e.g., cell survival, proliferation, and differentiation) and in pathological processes (e.g., carcinogenesis, cardiac hypertrophy, and atherosclerosis). Although both ERK1/2 and ERK5 respond to extracellular growth factors, ERK5 has a key

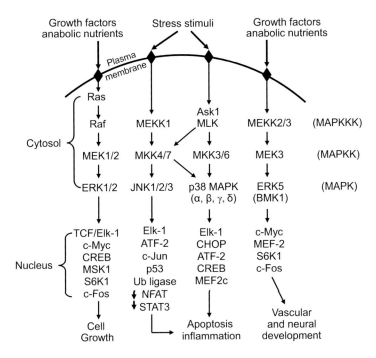

FIGURE 11.15 Cell signaling pathways induced by mitogen-activated protein kinases (MAPK). Four members of the MAPK family are extracellular signal-regulated kinases (ERK1 and ERK2), c-Jun NH(2)-terminal kinase (JNK), p38 MAPK, and ERK5. AP-1, activating protein 1; ASK1, apoptosis signal-regulating kinase 1; ATF, activating transcription factor; CHOP, CCAAT/enhancer-binding protein-homologous protein; CREB, cAMP response element-binding protein; Elk-1, E 26-like transcription factor; ERK5 (also known as BMK1, ERK/big MAP kinase 1); MEF2C, myocyte-specific enhancer factor 2C; MEK, MAPK/ERK kinase; MEKK, MEK kinase; MLK, mixed lineage kinase; MSK1, stress-activated protein kinase 1; NFAT, nuclear factor of activated T cells; Raf, rapidly accelerated fibrosarcoma protein (a protein kinase); Ras, rat sarcoma protein (a small GTPase); S6K1, ribosomal S6 kinase 1; STAT3, signal transducer and activator of transcription 3 (an acute response factor); TCF, ternary complex factor; and Ub, ubiquitin.

role in cardiovascular development, vascular integrity, neural differentiation, and myocyte fusion (Nithianandarajah-Jones et al. 2012).

G protein (also known as guanine nucleotide-binding protein)-coupled receptors (GPCRs) are seven-transmembrane domain receptors that can sense extracellular AAs (e.g., glutamate) and other molecules (e.g., pheromones, hormones, and neurotransmitters) and activate cAMP and phosphatidylinositol cell signaling pathways (Venkatakrishnan et al. 2013). Specifically, binding of the GPCR to a ligand changes the conformational structure of the GPCR, allowing for its catalytic role as a guanine nucleotide exchange factor. The GPCR then activates an associated G protein by exchanging its bound GDP for GTP. The G protein's α subunit, together with the bound GTP, then dissociates from the β and γ subunits to either activate signaling proteins (e.g., adenylyl cyclase, phospholipases C and A2, as well as calcium and potassium channels), or directly act on the target proteins. Experimental evidence shows that the GPCR participates in (1) the sense of smell, taste, visual signals, and cell density; (2) neurotransmission and neurological function; (3) immunity; and (4) mood and behavior (Venkatakrishnan et al. 2013).

11.4 ROLES FOR AAs IN THE IMMUNE RESPONSE

Leukocytes are an important component of the immune system in all animals and require AAs for growth, development, and functions (Calder et al. 2002). Adequate AA nutrition is essential for the development of immunocytes (cells of the immune system) and successful defense against invading pathogens (Calder et al. 2002; Ren et al. 2020; Ruth and Field 2013). Thus, Wu (2018, 2020b) has recently suggested that AAs and their derivatives (e.g., arginine, glutamine, glycine, proline, and tryptophan, as well as taurine, creatine, carnosine, and 4-hydroxyproline) may enhance the immunological defense of humans and other animals against infections by bacteria, fungi, parasites, and viruses (including coronaviruses, such as SARS-CoV and SARS-CoV-2) through improving the metabolism and functions of lymphocytes, monocytes, macrophages, and other cells of the immune system. Furthermore, by improving the function of the immune system, AAs (e.g., glutamine) can inhibit tumorigenesis and cancer growth (Shewchuk et al. 1997). This section provides a brief review of the pertinent literature related to the defense against infectious diseases in humans and other animals, including fish and crustaceans (e.g., shrimp and lobsters).

11.4.1 Immune Systems in Animals

11.4.1.1 Immune Systems in Mammals and Birds

Mammals and birds are protected from various pathogens by both innate (natural, nonspecific) and acquired (adaptive, specific) immune systems (Figure 11.16). These two systems are highly interrelated through various kinds of T lymphocytes and B lymphocytes (also called T cells and B cells), as well as cytokines and signaling molecules (Field et al. 2000; Li et al. 2007). In both mammals and birds, T lymphocytes are produced in the bone marrow and migrate via the blood to the thymus (a specialized primary lymphoid organ of the immune system), where they (called thymocytes)

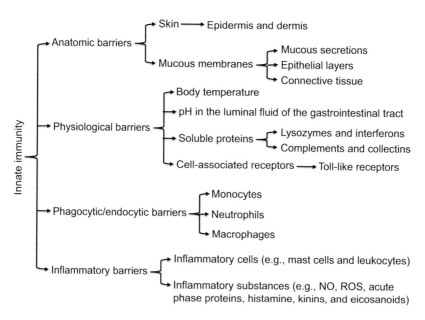

FIGURE 11.16 Innate immunity in humans and other animals. Innate immunity includes physical/anatomical, physiological, phagocytic/endocytic, and inflammatory barriers. The skin and the surface of mucous membranes contribute to physical/anatomical barriers. The physiological barriers of innate immunity consist of body temperature, pH (i.e., gastric acidity), and various soluble factors (e.g., lysozymes, interferons, and complements) and cell-associated molecules (e.g., toll-like receptors). Phagocytosis and endocytosis are also components of the innate immune system that includes specialized cells, such as blood monocytes, neutrophils, and tissue macrophages. In response to tissue damage by invading pathogens, a complex set of inflammatory reactions is triggered, including interactions among various inflammatory cells and proinflammatory molecules (i.e., acute phase proteins and histamine).

develop into mature cells. By contrast, B lymphocytes are produced and mature in (1) the bone marrow in mammals and (2) the bursa of Fabricius (located just dorsal to the cloaca) in birds. These physiological processes require the sufficient synthesis of proteins from AAs.

The innate immune system can rapidly respond to invading microbes, but its major disadvantages include nonspecificity and a lack of memory effect. When the evading pathogens are not fully cleared by the innate immune system over a short period of time, the adaptive immune system is activated within days to destroy the infectious agents. In the acquired immune system, each lymphocyte carries surface receptors for a single antigen, thereby conferring a highly specific immune response. This immune system becomes effective over a few days after initial stimulation and possesses immunological memory (Field et al. 2002). B lymphocytes are unique in their ability to produce and release specific antibodies in humoral immunity. The antibodies can neutralize pathogenic microorganisms (including viruses) or toxins by (1) binding to them, (2) activating complement proteins in the plasma for the destruction of bacteria by phagocytes, (3) immobilizing bacteria, and (4) opsonizing various pathogens. When pathogens escape humoral immunity, they are targeted by the cell-mediated immunity through the production of cytokines (e.g., interferon-γ) and other cytotoxic proteins by T lymphocytes such as cytotoxic T cells after the peptide fragments of pathogens are presented by the major histocompatibility complex on the host cell's surface and recognized by T cells (Childs et al. 2019). Because each lymphocyte carries surface receptors for a single antigen, the acquired immune response is highly specific.

The innate and acquired immune systems are regulated by a highly interactive network of chemical communications, which includes the synthesis of the antigen-presenting molecules, immunoglobulins, and cytokines (Field et al. 2002). Both immune systems are highly dependent upon the availability of AAs for the synthesis of these proteins and polypeptides, as well as other molecules of enormous biological importance. These substances include NO, superoxide, hydrogen peroxide, histamine, GSH, and anthranilic acid (Table 11.1). Individual AAs affect immune responses either directly or indirectly through their metabolites. While the immune system is vital to health, it can be dysfunctional under certain conditions, resulting in the development of autoimmune and hypersensitivity diseases, such as insulin-dependent diabetes mellitus, rheumatoid arthritis, and asthma (Calder et al. 2002).

11.4.1.2 Immune Systems in Fish and Crustaceans

Fish have both innate and acquired immune systems as do mammals. In contrast to mammals, fish lack bone marrow, lymph nodes, and adrenal glands, but possess the head kidney that serves as a hematopoietic, lymphoid, and endocrine organ for the production of erythrocytes (red blood cells), cytokines, antibodies, and some hormones (Li et al. 2020a). Thus, the head kidney plays an important role in both innate and adaptive immunities in fish. Furthermore, the skin [coated by the mucus (consisting of glycoproteins) secreted by goblet cells], lateral line, and gills of fish are the first line of defense against pathogens.

Crustaceans, like other invertebrates, lack adaptive immune systems and depend solely on the innate immune system to defend against infectious pathogens (Vazquez et al. 2009). The prophenoloxidase activating system (the proPO-system) and associated factors are important mediators of immunity in crustaceans. The proPO is activated by substances of microbial origins (e.g., β-1,3-glucans, LPS, and peptidoglycans) that stimulate the circulating hemocytes (large granular hemocytes, small granular hemocytes, and hyaline cells). These cells act through the direct sequestration and killing of infectious agents and via the synthesis and exocytosis of a battery of bioactive molecules such as antimicrobial peptides, reactive oxygen species, and NO (Closs et al. 2000; Rodríguez-Ramos et al. 2010; Söderhäll and Cerenius 1992). Along with hemocytes, crustaceans have plasma proteins or humoral factors, such as lectin, α-2 macroglobulin responsible for clotting, LPS-binding protein, β-glucan-binding protein, antimicrobial peptides, and lysosomes (Trichet 2010; Vazquez et al. 2009). Thus, adequate AA nutrition is particularly important for protecting crustacean (including shrimp and crabs) from infectious diseases.

11.4.1.3   Intestinal Immunity and Health in Animals

In all animals, the gut interacts with dietary AAs (including arginine, glutamine, proline, tryptophan) and other stimuli (e.g., a diversity and number of microorganisms) to influence local and whole-body immune responses (Ren et al. 2020). Intestinal health requires the maintenance of mucosal homeostasis via finely orchestrated communications among epithelial, endothelial, mesenchymal, and immune cells (Ruth and Field 2013; Salinas 2015). Aquatic species (including fish, shrimp, and crabs) are continuously challenged in an environment rich in potential pollutants and pathogens (e.g., bacteria, parasites, fungi, and viruses) that enter their bodies through mucosal epithelial barriers (Parra et al. 2015; Salinas 2015). In addition, under conditions of aquaculture, fish are commonly raised in high densities in cages, ponds, or tanks and, therefore, are often exposed to poor water quality (e.g., elevated concentrations of ammonia and low concentrations of dissolved oxygen), undernutrition, and other stress factors (e.g., overcrowding and heat stress). Thus, compared to terrestrial animals, aquatic animals (particularly farmed fish) have greater risks for infectious diseases that cause high rates of morbidity and mortality. There is evidence that adequate intake of dietary protein plays an important role in improving health and reducing risk for infectious diseases in fish (Li et al. 2009; Shoemaker et al. 2015).

11.4.1.4   Assessments of Immune Function in Animals

There are multiple, complex methods for assessing immune function in individuals, depending on experimental conditions, the availability of analytical facilities, and the investigator's interest. The classic functional measurements *in vivo* include (1) the delayed-type hypersensitivity response measured by skin testing; (2) serum antibody titers or humoral immunity in response to primary or secondary (booster) immunization; (3) blood levels of different lymphocyte subsets as well as serum concentrations of cytokines and other immune mediators; (4) weights of lymphoid organs; and (5) morbidity and recovery from infectious disease (Li et al. 2007). The *in vitro* assays of immune function examine (1) the metabolism of immunocytes; (2) lymphocyte blastogenesis (cell proliferation) in response to mitogens; (3) cell morphology and apoptosis; (4) the phagocytosis of particles by monocytes and macrophages; and (5) the production of antibodies, cytokines, and low-molecular-weight cytotoxic substances (Figure 11.17).

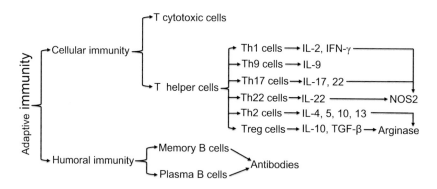

FIGURE 11.17   The adaptive immune system in humans and other animals. Two major populations of lymphocytes, B cells and T cells, participate in the adaptive immunity. Humoral immunity requires B cells (plasma or memory B cells) and specific antibodies, whereas cellular immunity depends on T cells [T helper (Th) or T cytotoxic cells)] and cytokines. Th cells are further divided into six Th subsets (Th1, Th2, Th9, Th17, Th22, and Treg) based on the cytokines they secrete. In macrophages, arginine is metabolized by inducible nitric oxide synthase (NOS2) to generate NO and citrulline (Cit), or by arginase to form ornithine (Orn) and polyamines. Proinflammatory cytokines released by Th1, Th17, and Th22 cells enhance NOS2 activity, while anti-inflammatory cytokines from Th2 and Treg cells activate arginase. Arginine and NOS2 compete for arginine to regulate NO and polyamine syntheses by macrophages.

11.4.2　Protein Malnutrition and Compromised Immunity

Malnutrition (particularly dietary deficiency of protein) and infection are major obstacles to the survival, health, growth, and reproduction of animals and humans worldwide (Childs et al. 2019). This global concern has led to the development of nutritional immunology as a new scientific discipline that integrates nutrition and immunology research methodologies to define a role for nutrients in the metabolism and function of the cells of the immune system at molecular, cellular, tissue, and whole-body levels. There is much evidence that a deficiency of dietary protein compromises both the innate and adaptive immune systems in humans and other animals (Li et al. 2007). This remains a significant nutritional problem in developing countries and in the subpopulations (e.g., the elderly or the hospitalized patients) of people in developed nations. Although dietary supplementation with high-quality protein may be effective in improving protein nutritional status in malnourished individuals, this is not feasible for patients who cannot tolerate enteral feeding. Consequently, defining the roles of individual AAs in immune responses can aid in developing effective strategies to improve health and prevent infectious diseases.

As substrates for the synthesis of proteins (including cytokines) and peptides in the immune system, all the canonical proteinogenic AAs are required for optimal immune responses in humans and other animals (Wu et al. 2009). Certain AAs, such as arginine, glutamine, glycine, and tryptophan, are particularly important for defenses against infectious pathogens and immune-mediated tissue injury. These AAs are highlighted in the following paragraphs.

11.4.2.1　Arginine

Besides metabolic disorders, arginine also plays an important role in immune responses, thereby decreasing risks for infectious diseases and other immune-mediated chronic disorders (Popovic et al. 2007). Notably, arginine regulates the production of antibodies by B cells, as well as T-cell receptor expression and B-cell development (Bansal et al. 2004; De Jonge et al. 2002), thereby positively contributing to both innate and acquired immunities. In support of this notion, dietary supplementation with 1% or 2% arginine (approximately 1 or 2 times the arginine content of the regular diet) to tumor-bearing or septic rats increases thymic weight, the number of thymic lymphocytes, T-lymphocyte proliferation, the cytotoxicity of specific cells (T lymphocyte, macrophages, and natural killer cells), interleukin-2 production, interleukin-2 receptor expression on T lymphocytes, and the delayed-type hypersensitivity response (Li et al. 2007). Further, dietary supplementation with 1% arginine-HCl enhanced the immune status of pregnant sows and neonatal pigs, thereby reducing morbidity and mortality in response to infectious pathogens (Wu et al. 2009). Conversely, inadequate intake of dietary arginine impairs NO synthesis by both constitutive and inducible NOS in mammals (Wu and Meininger 2002), indicating a role for adequate arginine nutrition in immune function. Furthermore, dietary supplementation with 0.93% arginine to adult mice increases the abundance of *Bacteroidetes* but decreases the abundance of *Firmicutes* in the jejunum and ileum, thus positively altering the microbial population in the gut (Ren et al. 2014a). Moreover, arginine is required for defense against viruses, bacteria, fungi, malignant cells, intracellular protozoa, and parasites in mammals, birds, terrestrial animals, lower vertebrates, and invertebrates (Li et al. 2007; Ruth and Field 2013; Wu et al. 2009).

The effect of arginine on tumorigenesis appears to depend on its stage. For example, low-dose oral supplementation of arginine (50 mg/kg BW/day) for 1 year decreased the total number of tumors and increased survival in mice via NO-mediated cytotoxicity against tumor cells and blocking the formation of lipid peroxidation products (Lubec et al. 1996). Likewise, arginine supplementation (1% arginine in drinking water) during the initiation stage of carcinogenesis decreased colorectal tumor production and crypt cell hyperproliferation, but arginine supplementation during the promotion stage stimulated colorectal tumor growth due to the excessive production of polyamines (Ma et al. 1999). Therefore, as part of the immune system, optimal arginine nutrition can improve the health and immunity of humans and other animals to protect individuals from infectious diseases and cancers due to immune imbalances.

Arginine beneficially regulates immune responses through both innate and adaptive immune systems (Popovic et al. 2007; Ren et al. 2018; Wu 2013). In the innate immunity, arginine influences the expression of toll-like receptors and antimicrobials, the phagocytic activity of immunologically activated macrophages, antioxidative enzymes, tight junction proteins, and intestinal mucosal barrier through the production of polypeptides, NO, and polyamines. In adaptive immunity, arginine affects the responses of T helper cells, the activity of cytotoxic T cells, as well the production of cytokines and antibodies against specific pathogens through MTOR and other cell signaling pathways (Figure 11.17). Thus, it is imperative to determine whether dietary supplementation with arginine or citrulline may enhance the immunity of humans against the current global COVID-19 pandemic. New knowledge about the regulation of arginine on host immunity can aid in designing sound therapeutic means to effectively prevent and treat bacterial, parasitic, and viral infections.

11.4.2.2 Glutamine

Glutamine, a major energy substrate for cells of the immune system (including lymphocytes and macrophages), plays an important role in their function and homeostasis (Cruzat and Newsholme 2017; Ren et al. 2014b). In addition, as a major source of glutamate, glutamine regulates the synthesis of glutathione for protecting cells from oxidative stress (Wu et al. 2004). As an essential precursor for the synthesis of purine and pyrimidine nucleotides, glutamine is required for the proliferation of lymphocytes. Thus, increasing extracellular concentrations of glutamine from 0.01 to 0.5 mM (a physiological level in the plasma) dose-dependently increases lymphocyte proliferation (Wu et al. 1992). The immunological functions of glutamine have been discussed in detail by Calder and Yaqoob (1999), Cruzat and Newsholme (2017), Field et al. (2002), Li et al. (2007), Marino and Calder (2017), Melis et al. (2004), Newsholme et al. (1999), Ren et al. (2014b), and Ruth and Field (2013). The major findings are summarized in the following paragraphs.

First, glutamine is necessary for the proliferation of lymphocytes in response to stimulation by T-cell mitogens and activation of protein kinase C. Second, the addition of 2 mM glutamine to culture medium prevented apoptosis, stimulated cell growth, and promoted antibody production in lymphocytes. Third, maximal NO production by activated macrophages occurs in the presence of an extracellular concentration of 1 mM glutamine. Fourth, at or near physiological levels in the plasma, glutamine (0.5–2 mM) modulates the production of cytokines by monocytes and macrophages. Indeed, a sufficient supply of extracellular glutamine (e.g., 2 mM) is required for the maximal production of interleukin (IL)-1 and TNF-α by murine macrophages and of IL-6 and IL-8 by human monocytes. Fifth, the maximum phagocytic activity of murine macrophages depends on adequate provision of extracellular glutamine (0.6 mM). Similarly, glutamine (0.5–2 mM) influences the expression of various genes related to (1) intercellular interactions; (2) the production of cytokines by T lymphocytes; (3) the phagocytosis of immunoglobulin G or complement-opsonized particles by macrophages; (4) antigen presentation; and (5) the opsonization of human monocytes. Sixth, glutamine (0.1–30 mM) in the culture medium enhances the bactericidal function of neutrophils isolated from burn patients in a dose-dependent manner. Finally, glutamine (2 mM) affects the lytic potential of cultured lymphokine-activated killer cells and is required for the activation of natural killer cells that are capable of spontaneous cytolytic activity against a variety of tumor cells through the production of cytokines.

In vivo animal studies show that enteral or parenteral provision of glutamine enhances the immunity of the host. For example, dietary supplementation with 4% glutamine maintains intramuscular glutamine concentrations and normalizes lymphocyte function in early-weaned pigs challenged with endotoxin. Additionally, supplementation with 3.5% glutamine to a casein-based diet (containing 1.9% glutamine) increases the ability of macrophages to produce TNF-α, IL-1b, and IL-6 and the responsiveness of lymphocytes to mitogens. Further, dietary provision of 2% glutamine is essential for the maintenance of gut-associated lymphoid tissues and for the synthesis of secretary immunoglobulin A by the small intestine, thereby preventing TNF-α-induced bacterial transloca-tion from the lumen of the gut into the circulation. Moreover, dietary supplementation with 2% or 4% glutamine increases the survival of mice after bacterial challenges, improves tumor-directed cytotoxic activity of natural killer cells in rats, and reduces the growth of implanted tumors in rats. Likewise, parenteral provision of glutamine (2 g/100 mL) attenuates the adverse effects of total par-enteral nutrition (TPN) on the gut and respiratory tract immunities in rats and enhances the survival of rats after endotoxin and bacterial challenges.

Findings from a majority of human clinical trials indicate that glutamine supplementation in the form of free glutamine or alanyl-glutamine dipeptide (8–30 g of oral glutamine per day or 0.3 g of alanyl-glutamine/kg BW/day in TPN) is beneficial for the immune system in patients with burn injury and gastrointestinal surgical operations, as well as in critically ill patients. These effects are indicated by increases in lymphocyte number and function, as well as reductions in infectious complications, hospital stay, morbidity, and mortality. Notably, a randomized, double-blind study with 28 patients undergoing major abdominal surgery demonstrated that preoperative glutamine supplementation via TPN improved nitrogen balance, increased lymphocyte function, augmented leukotriene production by neutrophils, reduced the incidence of infection, and shortened hospital stays (Morlion et al. 1998). Similar results have been reported for patients receiving bone marrow transplants (McBurney et al. 1994). Consistent with the favorable clinical outcomes, patients receiv-ing glutamine in TPN (5 g/100 mL) exhibited higher total concentrations of blood lymphocytes (including CD4 and CD8 T lymphocytes) when compared with patients receiving glutamine-free TPN (Ziegler et al. 1998). In addition, oral administration of glutamine (27 mg/kg BW) increased concentrations of growth hormone in the plasma of humans (Welbourne, 1995), which in turn bene-ficially modulated the immune system (Newsholme et al. 1999). Thus, a reduced availability of glu-tamine may impair immune function, thereby increasing the susceptibility of humans to infectious diseases. Because these published clinical studies involved a relatively small number of people, the efficacy of glutamine should be verified in a larger, multicenter study.

11.4.2.3 Glutamate

Glutamate plays versatile roles in the metabolism and function of cells, including leukocytes (Brosnan and Brosnan. 2013). In addition, glutamate is the major precursor of aspartate (which is required for the synthesis of purine and pyrimidine nucleotides in lymphocytes, as well as the recy-cling of iNOS-derived citrulline into arginine in activated macrophages) and glutathione (an anti-inflammatory and antiviral peptide; Wu et al. 2004). Intracellular glutamate is also crucial for the proliferation of lymphocytes, as well as the maintenance of NO production by macrophages via the formation of aspartate (Wu and Meininger 2002). Furthermore, glutamate regulates iNOS expres-sion in certain tissues (e.g., brain), thereby indirectly modulating the immunocompetence of ani-mals (Wu and Meininger, 2002). There are reports that GSH stimulates the activation (Hamilos and Wedner 1985) and proliferation (Hamilos et al. 1989) of human peripheral lymphocytes, while fine-tuning the innate immune response through interferon signaling (Diotallevi et al. 2017) through the activation of macrophages to produce NO (Buchmüller-Rouiller et al. 1995). Moreover, glutamate is a substrate for the synthesis of GABA, which is present in both lymphocytes and macrophages (Stuckey et al. 2005). Interestingly, T cells express GABA receptors, which mediate an inhibitory effect of GABA on their proliferation. Importantly, dietary glutamate, glutamine, and aspartate, which are the major metabolic fuels for enterocytes (Wu 2009), help maintain intestinal barrier integrity and prevent the translocation of intestinal microorganisms to the systemic circulation. Besides its role in leukocyte metabolism, glutamate is an excitatory neurotransmitter in central and peripheral nervous systems, acting on ionotropic and metabotropic receptors, which play a role in modulating the immune systems (Li et al. 2007). In support of this view, Lin et al. (1999) reported that supplementation with 4% and 8% glutamate to a glutamine- and glutamate-free diet enhanced delayed-type hypersensitivity and lymphocyte proliferation responses in rats recovering from methotrexate treatment. This beneficial effect of dietary glutamate was dose-dependent and more pronounced after a longer period of supplementation (Lin et al. 1999). These results suggest that dietary glutamate is necessary for maintaining an optimal immune status under conditions of immunosuppression. Due to the important functions of glutamate in the nutrition and physiology of humans and other animals, this AA must not be used as an isonitrogenous control in nutrition experiments. The validity of conclusions from previous studies involving the use of glutamate for such a purpose should be critically reevaluated (Hou and Wu 2018a; Li et al. 2020a).

11.4.2.4 Glycine

As an essential precursor of purine nucleotides, glutathione, and heme, and as a potent antioxidant and a scavenger of free radicals, glycine is essential for the proliferation and antioxidative defense of leukocytes (Li et al. 2007). There is also molecular and pharmacological evidence for a glycine-gated chloride channel in leukocytes (Froh et al. 2002). The activation of this channel suppresses the agonist-induced opening of L-type voltage-dependent calcium channels and, thus, attenuates intracellular concentrations of Ca^{2+}. As a result, glycine plays a role in regulating the production of cytokines by leukocytes and immune function (Zhong et al. 2003). This view is supported by findings from *in vitro* studies showing that an increase in extracellular glycine concentration (0.1–1 mM) within the physiological range activated a glycine-gated chloride channel and hyperpolarized the plasma membrane in a variety of cells types, including macrophages, monocytes, lymphocytes, and neutrophils (Froh et al. 2002). In macrophages stimulated by LPS, glycine (0.1–1 mM) reduced the influx of Ca^{2+} and an increase in its intracellular concentration, thereby blunting the production of superoxide, IL-1, and TNF-α (Wheeler and Thurman, 1999). Glycine did not affect IL-2 production in T cells in response to stimulation by immobilized anti-CD3 antibody, but inhibited cell proliferation in a dose-dependent manner (0.1–1 mM) by attenuating an increase in intracellular concentration of Ca^{2+} (Stachlewitz et al. 2000). Further, the addition of 2 mM glycine to the culture medium prevented apoptosis and enhanced antibody production by B lymphocytes (Duval et al. 1991).

There is also *in vivo* evidence that glycine reduces inflammatory reactions and morbidity in pathogen-infected animals (Chen et al. 2020; Wang et al. 2013; Zhang et al. 2020; Zhong et al. 2013). First, a deficiency of dietary glycine impaired immune responses in chickens treated with LPS, which was alleviated by its dietary supplementation. Likewise, dietary supplementation with 5% glycine to rats infected with a lethal dose of LPS reduced the concentrations of TNF-α in the plasma and improved their survival rate. Similarly, supplementation with 1% glycine to a liquid milk diet for calves alleviated inflammation and attenuated the increase in body temperature following infection with a low dose of endotoxin. Second, glycine protected animals against peptidoglycan polysaccharide-induced arthritis, chemically and stress-induced gastrointestinal mucosal injury, the ischemia and reperfusion injury of a variety of organs, and shock caused by hemorrhage, endotoxin, and sepsis. In particular, dietary supplementation with 5% glycine ameliorated experimental colitis in rat models induced by the intracolonic administration of 2,4,6-trinitrobenzene sulfonic acid or the oral administration of dextran sulfate sodium. In both models of gut inflammation, dietary supplementation with 5% glycine abolished increases in the colonic expression of IL-1b and TNF-α, cytokine-induced neutrophil chemoattractants, and macrophage-derived inflammatory proteins, thereby ameliorating diarrhea and BW loss. Third, dietary supplementation with glycine (5 g/kg BW/day for 6 days) attenuated the LPS-induced apoptosis of hepatocytes and infiltration of inflammatory cells into the liver and lungs of mice, as well as intestinal-weight loss. Collectively, these findings indicate that glycine is a novel anti-inflammatory, immunomodulatory, and cytoprotective nutrient. Clinical trials are warranted to determine the efficacy of dietary glycine supplementation to improve immune functions in humans and other animals.

11.4.2.5 Tryptophan

The products of tryptophan catabolism include serotonin, *N*-acetylserotonin, melatonin, and anthranilic acid (Chapter 4). The immunological functions of tryptophan and its metabolites have been discussed in detail by Amobi et al. (2017), Biefer et al. (2017), Le Floc'h et al. (2011, 2018), Li et al. (2007), Moffett (2003), and Platten et al. (2005). First, tryptophan catabolism increases to generate anthranilic acid through the indoleamine 2,3-dioxygenase (IDO) pathway during inflammation or in response to stimulation by LPS or certain cytokines. Second, serotonin, melatonin, and N-acetylserotonin enhance host immunity by inhibiting the production of superoxide, scavenging free radicals, and attenuating the production of TNF-α. In addition, N-acetylserotonin is an inhibitor of sepiapterin reductase, an enzyme for the synthesis of tetrahydrobiopterin. By modulating inducible NO synthesis, this tryptophan metabolite affects both innate and acquired immune systems. Third, anthranilic acid inhibits the production of proinflammatory Th1 cytokines and prevents autoimmune neuroinflammation. Because there is a progressive decline in tryptophan concentrations in the plasma of animals with inflammation, its catabolism plays a critical role in the functions of both macrophages and lymphocytes. Fourth, a deficiency of tryptophan resulting from IFN-γ treatment is associated with the antiproliferative effect of this cytokine on intracellular parasites and tumors. An increase in the production of IFN-γ is required for its inhibitory effect on the growth of parasites and tumors in the presence of elevated concentrations of tryptophan. Fifth, a pharmacological inhibition of IDO suppresses T-cell activity and induces fetal allograft rejection in mice. Sixth, N-(3,4,-dimethoxycinnamoyl) anthranilic acid, an orally active synthetic derivative of the tryptophan metabolite anthranilic acid, protects paralyzed mice from experimental autoimmune encephalomyelitis. Furthermore, tryptophan catabolism plays a role in immune responses and cancer immunity by producing a local immunosuppressive environment that is able to control T-cell homeostasis and self-tolerance during inflammation.

Adequate provision of dietary tryptophan is crucial for the health of animals (Li et al. 2007, 2021b). For example, a deficiency of dietary tryptophan impairs the immune response in chickens, which is reversed by its supplementation. Conversely, oral administration of 300 mg of tryptophan to rats enhances both phagocytosis by activated macrophages and the innate immune response. Likewise, dietary supplementation with 0.22% tryptophan increases resistance to bacterial and parasitic infections in protein-deficient rats fed a 20% zein (a class of prolamin protein in corn) diet. In addition, there are reports that dietary supplementation with 0.36% or 0.5% tryptophan [corresponding to 8 or 11 times the tryptophan content (0·044%, on a dry matter basis) of commercial feed] reduces cannibalism in fish and cortisol-mediated immune suppression in the rainbow trout. Based on scientific evidence, crystalline tryptophan is now used for managing the health of animals.

11.4.3 Unifying Mechanisms Responsible for the Roles of AAs in Immunity

Protein malnutrition, starvation, and many pathological conditions associated with compromised immunity (e.g., sepsis, cancer, and AIDS) result in reduced concentrations of most AAs in the plasma (Li et al. 2007, 2009, 2020a). There is growing interest in the role of AAs in the immune functions of mammals, birds, fish, and other species. Findings from recent studies support an important role for AAs in immune responses as they regulate (1) the activation of T lymphocytes, B lymphocytes, natural killer cells, and macrophages; (2) cellular redox state, gene expression, and lymphocyte proliferation; and (3) the production of antibodies, cytokines, and other cytotoxic substances (including NO and superoxide). In addition, NO, CO, and H_2S, metabolites of arginine, glycine, and cysteine, respectively, play an important role in both innate and cell-mediated immunities via gaseous signaling pathways (Figure 11.1). Increasing evidence shows that dietary supplementation of specific AAs to animals with malnutrition and infectious disease enhances the immune status, thereby reducing morbidity and mortality. Arginine, BCAAs, glutamine, glutamate, glycine, histidine, methionine, tryptophan, and cysteine precursors are the best prototypes. However, because of a negative impact of imbalance and antagonism among AAs on nutrient intake and utilization, care should be exercised in developing effective strategies for enteral or parenteral provision to maximize health benefits. Such measures must be based on knowledge about the biochemistry, nutrition, and physiology of AAs, their roles in immune responses, nutritional and pathological states of individuals, and expected treatment outcomes. Recent advances in leukocyte AA metabolism are critical for the development of effective means to prevent and treat immunodeficiency diseases, as well as immune-related cancers, neurological disorders, obesity, and cardiovascular dysfunction. AAs and related metabolites hold great promise for improving health and preventing infectious diseases in animals and humans (Wu 2020b).

11.5   USE OF AAs IN HUMAN NUTRITION AND HEALTH, AND IN CELL CULTURE

Because of their important physiological functions, AAs are utilized for many purposes worldwide, including (1) medical and pharmaceutical therapies; (2) dietary supplements; (3) food additives and flavors; (4) manufacturing of cosmetic and toiletry products; and (5) cell culture. These applications, with emphasis on humans and farm animals, are highlighted in the following sections.

11.5.1   USE OF AAs IN MEDICAL AND PHARMACEUTICAL THERAPY

Based on his observation that dogs fed for 6 days a synthetic AA diet containing glucose, fructose, glycerol, and fatty acids maintained a positive N balance, O. Abderhalden first predicted in 1912 the possibility of parenteral nutrition consisting of a mixture of AA and other essential nutrients for humans and other animals. This prediction came true in 1956 when crystalline AAs were first included as components of a TPN solution for intravenous administration to patients. Since then, both EAAs and AASAs have been used increasingly in the nutritional support of the patients who cannot eat, tolerate enteral feeding, or adequately synthesize AAs (Smriga 2020). These patients may have gastrointestinal diseases, coma, surgical operations, feeding difficulties, underdeveloped organs, and/or inborn errors of metabolism (e.g., defects of urea cycle enzymes). For example, arginine has been used to treat hypoargininemia-induced hyperammonemia in preterm infants since the early 1970s. Glutamine is often included in TPN solution to manage patients with small-intestinal atrophy and damage. In addition, intravenous administration of BCAAs, BCKAs, arginine, or glutamine is effective in improving the nitrogen balance in catabolic patients. Furthermore, intravenous infusion of arginine can ameliorate fetal growth retardation and pulmonary hypertension in humans and other animals. Thus, when oral ingestion is not possible or viable, TPN is now used widely in human clinical medicine and has received much attention from practicing veterinarians. Finally, TPN solutions or enteral diets supplemented with arginine, BCAAs, glutamine, and N-acetylcysteine can be beneficial for (1) enhancing T-cell function, antibody production, and immune cell-mediated wound healing; (2) reducing susceptibility to infectious diseases and inflammation; and (3) shortening ventilator days, the time for intensive care unit, and hospital stay.

BCAAs have been proposed to treat patients with liver cirrhosis (the scarring of the liver) or hepatic encephalopathy (brain dysfunction as a result of severe liver disease) because the concentrations of BCAAs in the plasma decrease but those of aromatic AAs increase in these patients (Campollo et al. 1992; Holeček 2018). Under those conditions, the hepatic urea cycle is impaired, resulting in (1) hyperglycemia that stimulates BCAA transamination and oxidation in red and white skeletal muscles and (2) a decrease in the catabolism of aromatic AAs by the liver (Holeček et al. 2011). These metabolic changes result from adaptations of the individuals to the liver diseases because the transamination of BCAAs with α-KG generates glutamate and the amination of glutamate with ammonia forms glutamine in extrahepatic tissues (e.g., skeletal muscle and brain) as a mechanism to remove ammonia from the blood. Thus, dietary supplementation with BCAAs may promote anabolic pathways and remove ammonia, therefore alleviating the syndromes of liver cirrhosis (the scarring of the liver) or hepatic encephalopathy (Tajiri and Shimizu 2013). However, there is no consensus regarding the efficacy of such a nutritional treatment for liver disorders (Holeček 2018). At present, hyperammonemia is managed by restricting dietary protein intake and administering benzoate or phenylbutyrate to remove ammonia (Chapter 6).

Elemental diets containing crystalline AAs were first developed in the 1960s as space foods for the American NASA Apollo Project. Over the past 60 years, enteral feeding of an AA mixture has become part of nutritional therapy for patients with food allergies, inflammatory diseases, Crohn's disease, and metabolic syndrome (Hoffer 2016). Examples for medical and pharmaceutical therapy involving AAs and their derivatives include the oral administration of N-acetylcysteine, arginine, BCAAs, glutamine, and tryptophan to ameliorate drug-induced liver damage, necrotizing enterocolitis in infants, hepatic encephalopathy, short bowel syndrome, and sleeping disorders, respectively. BCAAs are also beneficial for ameliorating hypoalbuminemia and emaciation in patients with uncomplicated hepatic cirrhosis. Moreover, alanine, glycine, lysine, tryptophan, and DOPA are used to treat muscular degeneration, eczema, herpes simplex, depression, and Parkinson's disease, respectively.

In the pharmaceutical industry, AAs are used to synthesize water-soluble regulators of biochemical pathways. For example, cysteine, glutamate, glutamine, and ornithine are the precursors of N-acetylcysteine, N-carbamoylglutamate, N-acetylglutamine, and α-KG-ornithine, respectively. Additionally, AAs are the raw materials for the chemical synthesis of peptides or peptide-like substances. Examples are L-alanyl-L-glutamine, glycyl-L-glutamine, D-glutamyl-D-glutamate, L-ornithine-L-aspartate, angiotensin-converting-enzyme inhibitors, angiotensin II receptor antagonists, HIV protease inhibitors, antiviral agents (e.g., Valaciclovir), antidiabetic agents (e.g., Nateglinide), antibiotics (e.g., ampicillin), polyarginines, and vitamins (e.g., folic acid and pantothenic acid from glutamate and β-alanine, respectively).

Topical use of AAs can be effective to increase their provision to the skin for health management. For example, lysine can be used to treat cold sores (red, fluid-filled blisters that are usually near the mouth or other areas of the face), which are caused by the herpes simplex virus, in humans (Figure 11.18). Specifically, a lysine cream can be applied to human skin areas affected by the herpes simplex virus (Gaby 2006). The therapeutic dose of topical lysine is at least 100 times greater than the amount of arginine in the skin. Alternatively, the oral administration of 3 g lysine-HCl (3 × 1 g)/day to adult humans for 6 months is effective to prevent and treat the frequently recurrent herpes simplex virus, without any adverse effect (Griffith et al. 1987). The underlying mechanism involves the competitive transport of basic AAs by virus-infected cells (Figure 11.18). A high concentration of lysine inhibits not only the uptake of arginine and ornithine by the host cells but also

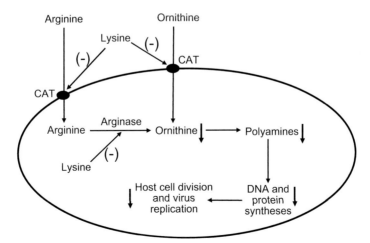

FIGURE 11.18 The role of lysine in the prevention and treatment of the herpes simplex virus in humans and other animals. Elevated concentrations of lysine inhibit the uptake of arginine and ornithine by the cells containing the herpes simplex virus, as well as arginase activity, resulting in the reduced synthesis of polyamines required for nucleotide synthesis and the replication of the virus. This leads to the killing of the virus.

arginase activity, thereby reducing the intracellular concentrations of both arginine and ornithine for the generation of polyamines. Because polyamines are essential for the synthesis of nucleotides and protein, their deficiency inhibits host cell division and virus replication.

11.5.2 Use of AAs as Dietary Supplements

11.5.2.1 Definition

A dietary supplement is a substance taken by mouth to provide a nutrient that humans and other animals may not obtain adequately from their regular diets relative to their optimal growth, development, and health. In the United States and some other countries, many AAs and related substances are available in food stores for human consumption (Roberts 2016). They include β-alanine, arginine, carnosine, citrulline, creatine, glucosamine, glutamate, glutamine, glycine, leucine, lysine, and tryptophan. In the United States, these AAs are classified as GRAS (generally recognized as safe). Alanine, which is used to treat human muscular atrophy by inhibiting pyruvate kinase (a key enzyme of glycolysis), is not sold in general stores of the United States because this AA is considered by the FDA to be a therapeutic drug.

11.5.2.2 Use of AAs in Human Nutrition

Individuals use AA supplements for different purposes, including the maintenance of skeletal muscle, lean tissue gain, white-fat loss, overall well-being, the optimization of fetal and postnatal growth, good taste, the control of mood and behavior, sleep quality, muscle strength, exercise endurance, sports performance, and the improvement of immunity. For example, individuals with an inherited inability to synthesize AAs, such as arginine, asparagine, glutamine, serine, and glycine, are supplemented with these AAs in enteral or parenteral diets. In some developing countries, where the consumption of high-quality proteins is limited, dietary supplementation with limiting AAs (e.g., lysine, methionine, tryptophan, and arginine) may be effective in (1) increasing the growth of children and preventing short stature; (2) delaying the onset and process of aging; and (3) reducing infectious and chronic diseases, while improving the general health in both the young and the elderly. This can also apply to a subset of the population with limited resources in developed nations. Globally, deficiencies of AAs frequently occur in individuals of specific age-groups and can be prevented by dietary supplementation. For example, results of recent studies indicate that 70% of the homebound elderly in the United States are deficient in at least one EAA (Dasgupta et al. 2005). There is evidence that dietary supplementation with a mixture of AAs (arginine, histidine, isoleucine, leucine, lysine, methionine, phenylalanine, threonine, and valine) enhances lean body mass, muscle strength, and physical function in the elderly, compared with the placebo group (Patterson et al. 2019). In addition, arginine is taken orally to augment the synthesis of NO (the major vasodilator and an inhibitor of platelet adhesion to blood vessel walls), enhance fertility, and improve metabolic profiles (Wu et al. 2009). Moreover, tryptophan is used to prevent insomnia by increasing the synthesis of serotonin and melatonin (neurotransmitters) in the brain (Fernstrom 2013). Likewise, glutamine and glycine are used to prevent and treat diarrhea in humans and other mammals (Rhoads and Wu 2009; Wang et al. 2013), whereas MSG is added as a flavor to the food to stimulate appetite in the elderly humans (San Gabriel and Uneyama 2013). Furthermore, human infants fed taurine-free- or taurine-deficient formulas will greatly benefit from taurine supplementation. Likewise, because cow's milk is severely deficient in arginine, infant formulas based on dried milk preparations can be enriched with this AA to improve the balance of all AAs in the food. Finally, oral cysteine can alleviate cobalt, selenium, and inorganic arsenic toxicities through chelation with those minerals in the small intestine (Baker and Czarnecki-Maulden 1987). However, cysteine exacerbates organic pentavalent arsenic toxicity by acting as a reducing agent to facilitate the conversion of organic pentavalent arsenicals (e.g., roxarsone and arsanilic acid) into the more toxic trivalent state (Baker and Czarnecki-Maulden 1987). This also underscores the various effects of AAs in animals, depending on the types of biochemical reactions.

11.5.2.3 Use of AAs in Animal Nutrition and Production

Over the past 70 years, animal production has greatly benefited from dietary supplementation with some AAs. Farm animals (e.g., chickens, pigs, cows, sheep, fish, and shrimp) are usually fed plant-based diets that generally contain low levels of lysine, methionine, threonine, and tryptophan (Apper-Bossard et al. 2013; Ballantyne 2001; Bucking et al. 2013; Hou et al. 2019; Li and Wu 2020a). These four AAs are also generally low in plant protein-based fishmeal replacement diets (Chu et al. 2014; Conceição et al. 2002; Li et al. 2020a). Deficiencies of those AAs limit the maximum growth and production performance of livestock, poultry, fish, and crustaceans, while impairing their immunity and increasing their susceptibility to infectious diseases. To partially correct this problem, DL-methionine was first used in the late 1950s as a feed supplement for broiler chickens. In the 1960s, L-lysine-HCl became commercially available for piglet diets. The 1980s witnessed the beginning of the use of L-threonine and L-tryptophan as supplements for swine and poultry feeds to enhance growth, improve immune function, and reduce glucocorticoid-induced stress. In the 1990s and 2000s, there was interest in the use of isoleucine and valine to improve milk production by lactating sows, but reported results were inconsistent likely due to different experimental conditions. The ratios of leucine, isoleucine, and valine are critical for the efficacy of their supplementation to animals (Sun et al. 2015; Wu 2018). In the past decade, rumen-protected lysine came into use for ruminants (e.g., cows and beef cattle) to increase the milk production of lactating cows and the growth performance of postweaning calves (Schwab and Broderick. 2017). Furthermore, the α-ketoacids of methionine are now available as substitutes for crystalline DL-methionine in the formulations of ruminant and nonruminant diets (Zhang et al. 2015).

Although traditional research logically focused on dietary supplementation with EAAs, recent advances in the physiological roles of AASAs and functional AAs have resulted in their use in swine, poultry, and fish production systems (Andersen et al. 2016; Coutinho 2017; Wu 2018; Zhang et al. 2021). For example, in 2005, a mixture of glutamate and glutamine was first produced for feeding postweaning pigs and chickens in some countries (including Brazil and Mexico) to prevent intestinal atrophy and improve feed efficiency. Dietary supplementation with glutamine (Wu et al. 2011a), glutamate (Rezaei et al. 2013), or glycine (Wang et al. 2014c) improves intestinal growth and development, as well as lean tissue gain in young pigs. However, the US Food and Drug Administration (FDA) does not currently allow the use of glutamine or glutamate as a supplement to animal feeds without approval by each intended state due to historic reasons, although the FDA approves the use of glutamine and glutamate as food supplements for humans. These reasons include (1) the absence of data on glutamine content in feedstuffs due to previous analytical problems, (2) the lack of sufficient glutamine research in livestock nutrition and production prior to the 1990s, and (3) the failure to describe glutamine as a component of proteins in classic animal nutrition textbooks before the 1990s. Nonetheless, based on compelling scientific evidence, both glutamate and glutamine have been approved by many states (including Texas, Minnesota, and North Carolina) of the United States as dietary supplements for farm animals (including livestock and poultry). In many regions of the world, feed-grade glutamate and glutamine are widely used to enhance the efficiency of animal production (including aquaculture) (Hou and Wu 2018a; Li et al. 2020b). Furthermore, based on discoveries driven by basic research, arginine (Progenos™) was first marketed in 2006 to enhance embryonic survival and litter size in gilts and sows. Of particular note, feed-grade arginine is now commercially available to feed livestock, poultry, fish, crustaceans, and companion animals worldwide (EFSA 2018). Arginine can also be used to promote lean tissue growth, reduce whole-body white fat, and enhance immunity in livestock, avian species, and fish (He et al. 2021; Li et al. 2020c; Wu et al. 2018).

Advantages of dietary supplementation with AAs in animal production include (1) balancing AA composition in the diet; (2) reducing total protein content in the diet without compromising maximal growth or production performance; (3) minimizing the impact of animal production on environmental pollution; (4) improving health status and reducing infectious diseases and the associated costs of treatment; (5) enhancing feed efficiency and economic returns; and (6) mitigating the global shortage of animal-protein resources. Alternative sources of crystalline AAs are animal by-products (including ruminant meat and bone meal and hydrolyzed feather meal), which contain abundant amounts of all the canonical proteinogenic AAs (including arginine, BCAAs, glycine, and proline) plus 4-hydroxyproline and taurine (Li and Wu 2020; Li et al. 2020d).

11.5.3   USE OF AAs OR THEIR DERIVATIVES AS FOOD ADDITIVES

11.5.3.1   AAs as Food Additives

Food or feed additives are substances added to food or feed to preserve or create flavor, enhance its taste and appearance, and/or improve its nutritional value (Roberts 2016). As noted in Chapter 1, individual AAs alone, or in combination, have different chemical properties and, therefore, are used as food additives to generate different flavors. Thus, seasonings can be made of one or more AAs, hydrolyzed vegetable protein, hydrolyzed animal protein, or small peptides. Examples are (1) the addition of AAs (e.g., glutamate) to processed foods (e.g., frozen meals, hamburger, instant noodles, sausage, snack cakes, and soup base); (2) heat-induced browning of products containing added AAs and carbohydrate; (3) the use of sulfur-containing AAs (e.g., cysteine, cystine, and methionine) to produce good flavors in foods and increase the extensibility of bread dough; (4) a mixture of AAs and other ingredients used to create the flavor of crab, shrimp, and fish-cake products; (5) the use of L-alanine and L-aspartic acid to improve the flavor of soft drinks; and (6) the use of L-phenylalanine and L-aspartic acid for the synthesis of aspartame (a methyl ester of L-aspartic acid and L-phenylalanine dipeptide; a widely used artificial sweetener) by researchers at the G.D. Searle & Company of the United States in 1965.

A popular food additive made from an AA is MSG (San Gabriel and Uneyama 2013). It has been used for over 100 years as a seasoning to impart the savory taste quality generally described as "*umami*", which is one of the five basic tastes. Guanosine monophosphate and inosine monophosphate amplify the taste intensity of glutamate. A combination of these two nucleotides plus glutamate and other components in some foods (e.g., mushroom extracts) are responsible for the good taste of their soups.

11.5.3.2   Mechanisms for AA-Induced Sensing in the Gastrointestinal Tract

11.5.3.2.1   Taste Cells on the Tongue and the Gastrointestinal Tract

Humans receive tastes through sensory organs (called taste buds) on the tongue, other regions of the mouth, and the gastrointestinal tract. According to their morphology, taste cells are classified into four types: type I (dark), type II (light), type III (intermediate), and type IV (Roper 2006). Type I cells have voltage-gated outward currents, but lack voltage-gated inward currents. These cells are glial like (e.g., transmitter clearance and functional isolation of other taste cell types) and express the glutamate–aspartate transporter and the ecto-ATPase, nucleoside triphosphate diphosphohydrolase-2, and oxytocin receptors. Thus, type I taste cells are generally thought to have a support function in the taste bud, similar to astrocytes in the nervous system. In addition, these cells may function in salt taste transduction.

Type II cells, also known as "receptor" cells, have voltage-gated Na^+ and K^+ currents, as well as receptors and transduction machineries for bitter, sweet, and umami taste stimuli. The specification of these cells appears to be controlled by a homeodomain protein known as Skn-1a. Type 2 taste cells express the taste-specific G protein (gustducin) on the plasma membrane and the selective cation channel known as transient receptor potential melastatin 5 (TRPM5). These cells contain taste receptor type 1, member 1 (Tas1R1); taste receptor type 1, member 2 (Tas1R2); taste receptor type 1, member 3 (Tas1R3); taste receptor type 2 (Tas2R); and metabotropic glutamate receptors (mGluRs), including taste-mGluR4, truncated-mGluR1, and mGluR2/3. The mGluR4, Tas1R1, and Tas1R3 sense umami taste, Tas1R2 and Tas1R3 sense sweet taste, and Tas2R senses bitter taste.

These taste receptors are all cell-specific G protein-coupled receptors, which activate the gustducin upon its binding to a ligand (tastant).

Type III cells form conventional synapses with the gustatory neurons innervating the taste buds and, therefore, are also known as "synaptic cells". These cells have voltage-gated Na^+, K^+, and Ca^{2+} currents and express specific channels to sense acids. The nonselective cation channel PKD2L1 is expressed exclusively in type III cells as the sour taste receptor. Type III taste cells may use serotonin and norepinephrine as neurotransmitters. Thus, these cells make prominent synapses with afferent nerve fibers and sense the sour taste.

Type IV taste cells have a rounded shape and their plasma membrane is located at the basal portion of the taste buds. These cells (also known as basal cells) are rapidly dividing progenitor cells (stem cells) that differentiate into the other types of taste cells. Thus, type IV taste cells replace aged and damaged taste cells (type I to III) during the rapid cell turnover in taste buds. Full physiological functions of type IV taste cells remain to be elucidated.

Sodium salt transduction is mediated by amiloride-sensitive epithelial sodium channels (ENaC). Specifically, Na^+ salt transduction involves the passage of Na^+ into the receptor cell through passive, amiloride-blockable ion channels on the apical membrane of the receptor cell. The ENaC present in taste cells comprises three homologous subunits (a, b, and g) and is functionally similar to that in other $Na+$-transporting epithelia. Additionally, Na^+ and probably other cations (e.g., K^+) can pass through the tight junctions between cells in the taste bud to interact with basolateral ion channels. The apical ion channel is gated by acids, which allows the entry of cations. Changes in intracellular concentrations of these ions result in the depolarization of the taste receptor cell and the release of neurotransmitters at the synapses with the sensory nerve fibers.

In addition to the four types of taste cells and ENaC, the gastrointestinal tract possesses multiple cell types that can sense luminal nutrients, including the enteroendocrine L and K cells as well as brush cells (also called tuft cells or caveolated cells) and enterocytes (San Gabriel and Uneyama 2013). The enteroendocrine L and K cells can sense sweeteners and secrete hormones (e.g., glucagon-like peptide 1 by L cells and glucose-dependent insulinotropic polypeptide). Brush cells express gustducin and TRPM5, and, therefore, may likely be chemosensory cells in the gastrointestinal tract. These cells express phospholipase C-γ2 rather than the C-β2 isoform and may also sense bitter taste.

11.5.3.2.2 AA Sensing in the Tongue

The taste sensations of foods, dietary supplements, and other orally administered substances originate at the tongue epithelium (Wu 2020a). Different AAs have different taste qualities: bitter, sour, sweet, and umami (see Chapter 1). The most studied AA in chemical sensing by the tongue is glutamate (San Gabriel and Uneyama. 2013). While species differences exist in the expression of taste receptors, the results of recent studies indicate that the human tongue has specific receptors for L-glutamate and can detect the umami taste independent of their location on the tongue. These glutamate receptors are (1) Tas1R1 and Tas1R3; and (2) mGluRs, including taste-mGluR4, truncated-mGluR1, and mGluR2/3. To date, three known umami (meaty, broth-like, or savory taste) substances are glutamate, 5′-inosine monophosphate, and 5′-guanosine monophosphate.

As noted above, Tas1R1, Tas1R3, and mGluRs are G protein-coupled receptors acting on similar signaling molecules, including G proteins βγ, phospholipase C-β2, phosphoinositide 3 (PI3)-kinase, and calcium (Figure 11.19). Specifically, in type II taste cells, receptor binding initiates a transduction cascade leading to (1) activation of phospholipase C-β2; (2) an inositol trisphosphate (IP_3)-mediated increase in intracellular Ca^{2+} concentrations due to the release of Ca^{2+} from intracellular stores and the activation of voltage-gated basolateral calcium channels; (3) Ca^{2+}-dependent activation of the monovalent-selective cation channel TRPM5; (4) Na^+-induced depolarization of the plasma membrane; (5) the release of ATP as a synaptic transmitter; and (6) activation of sensory neurons on the tongue. These neurons then send electrical impulses to the cerebellum to interpret

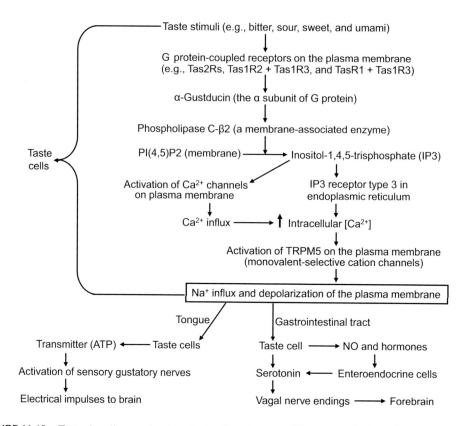

FIGURE 11.19 Taste signaling mechanisms in the digestive tract of humans and other animals. Extracellular taste stimuli induce a series of chemosensing cascade reactions that are common in both the tongue and the gastrointestinal tract. NO, nitric oxide; TRPM5, transient receptor potential melastatin 5 (selective cation channel); Tas1R1, taste receptor type 1, member 1; Tas1R2, taste receptor type 1, member 2; Tas1R3, taste receptor type 1, member 3; and Tas2R, taste receptor type 2 (Tas2R).

and identify taste quality. Thus, taste nerves play an afferent role in AA sensing (namely receiving information and then sending it to the brain for processing and interpretation).

In addition to Tas1R1, Tas1R3, and mGluRs, taste cells of the tongue also express NMDA receptors and non-NMDA ionotropic glutamate receptors (iGluRs). These NMDA and non-NMDA iGluRs on the basal membrane (but not the taste pore) can directly detect glutamate released by the nerve endings as a neurotransmitter, leading to the activation of the two types of glutamate receptors and subsequent cell signaling. Thus, NMDA receptors and non-NMDA iGluR in taste cells may be indirectly involved in the perception of umami taste.

11.5.3.2.3 AA Sensing in the Gastrointestinal Tract

AA sensing in the gastrointestinal tract and the tongue shares common steps in signal transduction between ligand binding and the depolarization of the plasma membrane of taste cells (Figure 11.19). However, chemosensing in the gastrointestinal tract (e.g., the gastric mucosa, duodenum, and ileum) involves an enhanced release of NO and possibly gut hormones from taste cells (Uneyama et al. 2006). Subsequently, these molecules stimulate enteroendocrine cells to synthesize and release serotonin. Taste cells may also directly generate and release serotonin to amplify taste signal transduction. Serotonin acts on the vagal nerves that transmit electrical impulses to the forebrain, including the cortex, hypothalamus, and limbic areas.

Evidence from a limited number of studies shows that nutrient sensing in the gastrointestinal tract may also involve chemosensing mechanisms other than the taste receptor pathways

(Hundal and Taylor 2009; San Gabriel and Uneyama 2013). This alternative route of nutrient sensing is known as the postingestion effect, which can modulate flavor preference, food intake, and mood. For example, the absence of Tas1R3, TRPM5, or PI3 receptor type 3 does not completely abolish the detection of sweet or umami substances by the mouse intestine. Furthermore, transgenic mice lacking taste receptor-mediated signaling components (e.g., gut Tas1R3) still exhibit the postingestion effect. Results from intraduodenal infusion studies indicate that nutrient sensing independent of the taste receptor-mediated taste signal transduction originates in the upper part of the small intestine. The possible underlying mechanisms include the composition of food (e.g., the content of protein, AAs, carbohydrates, fatty acids), production of metabolites in the intestinal lumen and mucosa (Table 11.1), the stimulation of vagal nerve activity, changes in intestinal secretion of hormones and other factors, as well as NMDA- and iGluRs-dependent cell signaling.

11.5.4 Use of AAs in Cosmetic and Toiletry Products

AAs have a high water-holding capacity and, thus, are used as moisturizing factors in cosmetics (particularly creams and emulsions) to retain water in the skin (Burnett et al. 2013). Typical cosmetics contain ~40% AAs and ~12% pyrrolidone carboxylic acid (formed from the cyclodehydration of glutamic acid). Generally speaking, serine is the most abundant AA in the mixture of moisturizing factors, followed by the descending order: (1) citrulline; (2) alanine, glycine, aspartic acid, and threonine; (3) leucine, ornithine, and tyrosine; (4) lysine; (5) valine, arginine, and histidine; (6) phenylalanine; (7) glutamic acid; and (8) proline. Some cosmetic products may contain 10% or more arginine as a surfactant neutralizer. Furthermore, current cleansing products contain glutamic acid, glycine, alanine, or β-alanine that condense with fatty acids via acylation. Additionally, the condensation of lysine with fatty acids is widely used to prepare lubricating cosmetic powders. Finally, some hair conditioner products contain glutamic acid, glycine, or arginine to obtain different pH values in solutions. Notably, these AA-based "environmentally friendly" materials that can be readily metabolized by microbes have low irritation to the skin and are biodegradable surfactants.

11.5.5 Use of AAs in Cell Culture

The availability of AAs has made it possible for the culture of animal cells in nutrition and biomedical research. Although AA-enriched culture media are sold by many companies, the concentrations of AAs are usually 4 to 10 times the concentrations in the plasma of humans and other animals. For example, commercial cell culture medium typically contains 2 to 4 mM glutamine, 0.4 mM arginine, and 1.2 mM lysine. Those high concentrations will mask any effects of physiological concentrations of AAs in cell cultures. For example, when the basal culture medium contains 0.4 mM arginine, which maximally stimulates the MTOR cell signaling and protein synthesis in ovine and porcine trophectoderm cells, the supplementation of 0.2 mM arginine (physiological concentration found in the plasma) to this basal medium does not have a detectable effect on the MTOR pathway in these cells when compared with the control (without arginine supplementation) (Kim et al. 2013; Kong et al. 2012; Wang et al. 2015b). Without caution, such findings would have been interpreted to indicate an inability of the physiological concentrations of arginine to activate the MTOR cell signaling or enhance protein synthesis in these placental cells. However, a physiological concentration of arginine (e.g., 0.2 mM) does activate the MTOR cell signaling to enhance protein synthesis and inhibit proteolysis in trophectoderm cells (Kim et al. 2013; Kong et al. 2012) and other cell types, including enterocytes, brown adipocytes, and mammary epithelial cells. Thus, physiological concentrations of AAs (e.g., those found in the plasma, the intestinal luminal fluid, or uterine luminal fluid, depending on research objectives) must be used for cell culture, so that experimental results are relevant to the physiology and nutrition of humans and other animals. This should be borne in mind when conducting cell culture studies.

11.6 EFFICACY AND SAFETY OF DIETARY AA SUPPLEMENTATION

11.6.1 Efficacy of AA Supplementation

Crystalline AAs in the diet are directly available for absorption by the small intestine. Therefore, they are absorbed into the enterocytes of the small intestine and appear in the portal vein more rapidly than peptide-bound AAs released from protein digestion (Wu 2018). This may result in a transient imbalance among AAs in the systemic circulation, the extent of which likely depends on both the quality and quantity of dietary protein, as well as the supplemental amount of AAs. Such a phenomenon raises some questions about the bioequivalence of supplemental AAs relative to AAs in dietary proteins and peptides. However, experimental evidence from studies with humans, pigs, chickens, and rats consistently indicates that crystalline AAs have high nutritional values when added to a diet deficient in those AAs (Baker 2009; Blachier et al. 2015; Fernstrom 2013; Hou and Wu 2018a; Smriga and Torii 2003; Wu et al. 2018). Examples are provided in the preceding sections. This may also be true for some AAs supplemented to the diets of certain species of fish and crustaceans (Li et al. 2021a,b). For ruminants (e.g., cattle, sheep, and goats), most AAs (e.g., arginine, glutamine, lysine, and methionine) must be protected from degradation in the rumen, with the exceptions of citrulline and glutamate, and possibly aspartate (Gilbreath et al. 2021).

11.6.2 Safety of AA Supplementation

Because it is unethical to feed toxic doses or severe imbalances of AAs to humans, the true upper limits for the levels of supplemental AAs for infants, children, and adults are largely unknown. Thus, the Institute of Medicine (2006) does not provide data on the tolerable upper levels of dietary AA intakes by infants, children, or adults. Table 11.8 summarizes values on safety levels for dietary supplementation with AAs to young, adult (nonpregnant), and gestating swine. When intakes are equally divided daily in three meals, healthy adult humans can well tolerate the amounts of AAs provided from the ingestion of 2 g beef protein/kg BW/day. This is equivalent to the dietary intake (mg/kg of BW/day) of Ala, 105; Arg, 140; Asn, 85; Asp, 105; Cys, 28; Glu, 190; Gln, 115; Gly, 75; His, 65; Ile, 105; Leu, 170; Lys, 185; Met, 65; Phe, 86; Pro, 76; Ser, 85; Thr, 90; Trp, 26; Tyr, 78; and Val, 120 (Hou and Wu 2018b). There is evidence that healthy adult humans can tolerate 3.5 g protein/kg BW/day (Bilsborough and Mann 2006). Thus, the estimated tolerable upper levels of dietary AA intakes for healthy adults are likely 1.75 times those listed above. Expressed per kg BW, human infants and children tolerate greater amounts of dietary AAs than adults due to greater metabolic rates in the former. Extensive research has also shown that supplementing appropriate amounts of an AA (usually 0.2%–2.5% of the diet on a dry matter basis, depending on the individual AAs, age, and species) is generally safe for animals, including swine (Table 11.8). Examples of the safety of the supplementation with arginine, glutamine, and glutamate in humans and other animals will be highlighted in the following sections.

11.6.2.1 Imbalances and Antagonisms among AAs

Results of recent studies indicate the absence of a systematic pattern of adverse effects of the oral AA administration in adult humans, which precludes the selection of "No Observed Adverse Effect Level" or "Lowest Observed Adverse Effect Level" as the usual approach to identify a tolerable upper level of intake for AAs (Shao and Hathcock 2008). Thus, investigators have developed a newer method for risk assessment. Such a method is to determine the Observed Safe Level or the Highest Observed Intake, which is defined by FAO/WHO as the highest intake level with the sufficient evidence of safety.

Excessive amounts of one or more AAs relative to other AAs in a TPN solution or enteral feeding can result in severe adverse effects, including reduced food intake, abnormal behavior, and impaired growth, owing to AA imbalances (disproportionate amounts of AAs; a term first used by S.W. Hier in 1944) or antagonism (mutually adverse and opposing actions of AA; a term first used by W.L.

TABLE 11.8

The No Observed Adverse Effect Levels (NOAELs) for Supplementation with Amino Acids to Typical Diets for Swine[a]

Amino Acid	Young Swine[b]		Adult Swine (Nonpregnant)[c]		Gestating Swine[d]	
	% of Supplemental AA in Diet	Content of AA in the Basal Diet (%)	% of Supplemental AA in Diet	Content of AA in the Basal Diet (%)	% of Supplemental AA in Diet	Content of AA in the Basal Diet (%)
Ala	2.5	1.3	2.7	0.94	2.2	0.78
Arg	2.0	1.3	2.2	1.1	1.0	0.70
Asn	2.0	0.94	2.2	0.77	1.0	0.58
Asp	4.0	1.3	4.2	1.1	2.0	0.76
Cys	0.38	0.37	0.38	0.30	0.25	0.23
Gln	1.0	1.8	1.0	1.6	1.0	1.2
Glu	≥4.0	1.7	≥4.0	1.5	2.0	1.1
MSG	2.0	1.7 (Glu)	2.0	1.5 (Glu)	2.0	1.1 (Glu)
Gly	2.0	0.88	2.0	0.85	2.0	0.55
His	0.50	0.57	0.63	0.44	0.50	0.33
Ile	1.1	0.89	1.3	0.74	1.0	0.51
Leu	2.2	1.8	2.4	1.6	2.0	1.2
Lys	1.4	1.4	1.4	0.90	0.80	0.58
Met	0.40	0.36	0.4	0.28	0.25	0.18
Phe	1.0	0.99	1.1	0.86	0.80	0.60
Pro	2.0	1.6	2.2	1.4	2.0	1.0
Ser	2.0	0.79	2.0	0.83	1.5	0.45
Thr	0.80	0.85	0.80	0.65	0.50	0.49
Trp	0.40	0.25	0.40	0.21	0.30	0.17
Tyr	1.2	0.76	1.3	0.70	0.80	0.45
Val	2.0	1.0	2.2	0.82	1.5	0.65
Cit	2.0	0.0	2.0	0.0	1.0	0.0

Source: Zhang, Q. et al. 2021. *Adv. Exp. Med. Biol.* 1285:81–107.

[a] alues are expressed on the as-fed basis, with the dietary content of dry matter being 90%.

[b] Neonatal or weanling pigs. The dietary content of crude protein is 20%.

[c] Grower-finisher pigs, lactating sows, and adult boars. The dietary content of crude protein is 14%–18%.

[d] Early period of gestation. If 0.8% of arginine is supplemented to the diet, the supplementation should not start before Day 14 of gestation. The dietary content of crude protein is 12%, and dietary intake is 2 kg/day. During late gestation, dietary intake can be increased to 2.2–2.5 kg per day, depending on the maternal nutritional status. The total supplemental amount of nitrogen should not exceed 12.5% of the nitrogen content in the basal diet.

Note: Cit, L-citrulline; MSG, monosodium glutamate; the α-carboxyl group of glutamic acid forms a salt with sodium.

Brickson in 1948). AA imbalances may occur among AAs regardless of their chemical structure and can be prevented by the addition of one or more of the limiting AA to the diet. By contrast, AA antagonism commonly occurs among chemically or structurally related AAs (e.g., lysine-arginine-ornithine, leucine-isoleucine-valine, and threonine-tryptophan) and can be overcome by the addition of chemically or structurally similar AAs. AA imbalance or antagonism may result from (1) impairments of the intestinal absorption of AAs and the transport of AAs by extraintestinal cells; (2) disturbances in AA metabolism and homeostasis; (3) reductions in the generation of signaling molecules (e.g., GABA, NO, CO, and H_2S); and (4) the excess production of toxic substances (e.g., ammonia and homocysteine). Thus, as for all other nutrients (e.g., glucose, fatty acids, minerals, and vitamins), excessive amounts of supplemental AAs or their metabolites (via intravenous or enteral administration) can be toxic to organisms and this must be avoided in dietary formulations and clinical therapies. Safety levels for AA supplementation must be established by well-controlled studies with humans and other animals. There may be species differences in AA imbalance or antagonism such that mammals, birds, fish, crustaceans, and other animals tolerate different ratios of dietary AAs. Likewise, within the same species, nutritional, physiological, and environmental factors [for example, dietary intakes of nutrients (e.g., total amounts of protein, energy, and vitamins), developmental stage, endocrine status, and air pollution] may affect AA imbalances and antagonisms.

11.6.2.2 Arginine as an Example for the Safety of AA Supplementation

Let's use L-arginine as an example for the safety of AA supplementation. L-arginine is stable under sterilization conditions (e.g., high temperature and high pressure) and is not toxic to cells (Wu et al. 2009). However, arginine shares the same transmembrane transporters with other basic AAs (e.g., lysine and ornithine) in cells, improper ratios of these AAs may affect their plasma and intracellular concentrations, possibly leading to metabolic disorders (Chapter 4). Extensive studies have shown that the administration of arginine at an appropriate dose, chemical form, and means is safe for humans and other animals. For example, neonatal pigs, growing-finishing pigs, and pregnant pigs tolerate large amounts of chronic supplemental L-arginine-HCl (at least 0.62, 0.32, 0.21, and 2.14 g arginine/kg BW/day, respectively) administered via enteral diets without any adverse effects (Wu et al. 2016). Likewise, based on food intake, growth, general appearance, and physiological parameters (e.g., hormones, enzymes, and metabolites in the plasma), rats fed a casein-based semi-purified diet (containing 0.61% L-arginine) between 6 and 19 weeks of age well tolerated dietary supplementation with arginine (as arginine-HCl) via drinking water (0, 1.8, or 3.6 g arginine/kg BW/day) (Yang et al. 2015). These supplemental doses of L-arginine were equivalent to 0, 286, and 573 mg arginine/kg BW/day, respectively, in humans. Similarly, growth, metabolic, and histological analyses indicated that dietary supplementation with up to 5% arginine was safe in both male and female rats for at least 13 weeks (Tsubuku et al. 2004a). This level of supplementation was equivalent to 3.3 and 3.9 g arginine/kg BW/day in male and female rats, respectively, based on their food intake per kg BW. Additionally, long-term intravenous infusion of L-arginine-HCl to ewes at 81 mg/kg BW/day between Days 60 and 147 (term) of gestation is safe for both mother and fetus. On the basis of the finding that the intake of dry matter by adult humans is ~10% of that for adult rats, an adult human can likely tolerate an enteral supplemental dose of L-arginine of at least 0.21–0.57 g/kg BW/day (or 15–40 g/day for a 70 kg subject).

In support of the data from animal studies, the intravenous infusion of L-arginine (up to 0.5 g L-arginine-HCl/kg BW for infants or 30 g L-arginine-HCl for an adult over 30–60 min) or the oral administration of L-arginine (9 g L-arginine-HCl/day for an adult) generally has no adverse effects on humans (McNeal et al. 2016). In a double-blind, placebo-controlled trial with 16 healthy adult males, the oral administration of 20 g L-arginine/day for 4 weeks did not result in any adverse effect as determined using standard clinical chemistry indices. Likewise, healthy adults could tolerate the oral administration of 40 g L-arginine/day for 1 week (duration of the study). Similarly, results from other trials indicated no side effects of the oral administration of 21 and 42 g arginine/day to patients with hypercholesterolemia and cystic fibrosis for 4 and 6 weeks, respectively. Healthy adult humans can tolerate dietary supplementation with 30 g arginine (as arginine-HCl) per day for 90 days (McNeal et al. 2018). It is important that arginine be taken in divided doses on each day of administration to (1) prevent gastrointestinal tract disorders due to abrupt production of large amounts of NO; (2) increase the availability of circulating arginine over a longer period of time; and (3) avoid a potential imbalance among AAs.

However, higher oral doses of L-arginine-HCl (>9 g/day) are occasionally associated with nausea, gastrointestinal discomfort, and diarrhea for some people, which may result from a rapid and excess production of NO by the gastrointestinal tract and from impaired intestinal absorption of other dietary basic AAs (lysine and histidine) (McNeal et al. 2016). Also, supplementing 4% or more arginine to diets for animals can cause skin lesions, reduce food intake, and inhibit growth

(Wu et al. 2009). A solution to this potential problem may be the alternative use of L-citrulline, a precursor for arginine synthesis (Faure et al. 2012; Wu and Meininger 2000). As a neutral AA, L-citrulline does not compete with basic AAs for transport by cells, its conversion to arginine consumes one mole of ammonia in the form of aspartate, and its administration does not require equimolar HCl. Thus, enteral or parenteral L-citrulline may be particularly useful for patients with elevated ammonia concentrations, impaired L-arginine transport, enhanced intestinal L-arginine catabolism, abnormal muscle function, or a high activity of constitutively expressed arginase. Finally, because excessive production of NO is destructive to cells, it would not be advisable to administer L-arginine to animals or patients with severe infections, active inflammatory or autoimmune disorders, active malignancy (e.g., late stages of tumorigenesis), or pathological angiogenesis.

11.6.2.3 Glutamine as an Example for the Safety of AA Supplementation

Glutamine itself is not toxic to cells, as large amounts of glutamine (e.g., 4 mM or approximately 8–15 times physiological concentration in the plasma of mammals) are usually included in the culture medium for all human and animal cell lines (Curi et al. 2005). However, the central nervous system is highly sensitive to ammonia generated from glutamine degradation in the body (Chapter 6). Based on a comprehensive review of published studies, Shao and Hathcock (2008) have indicated that *healthy adult humans can tolerate the oral administration of up to 14 g glutamine/day without any adverse effects.* Adult athletes showed no adverse response to dietary supplementation with 28 g glutamine/day for 14 days (Gleeson 2008). Adult patients undergoing bone marrow transplantation reported improvements in mood and well-being after receiving a TPN solution containing >20 g glutamine/day (Young et al. 1993). Likewise, the addition of glutamine (0.35 g/kg BW/day; as 0.5 g alanyl-glutamine/kg BW/day) to a TPN solution did not have any negative effect on critically ill patients (Dechelotte et al. 2006). Similarly, postsurgery patients had no adverse response to the administration of glutamine (0.5 g/kg BW; as alanyl-glutamine) via TPN feeding (Jiang et al. 1993). However, concerns over the safety of glutamine supplementation have arisen from two clinical studies with TPN-fed or enterally fed patients in the intensive care unit. First, an intravenous provision of glutamine (0.35 g/kg BW/day; as 0.5 g alanyl-glutamine) could increase mortality in critically ill patients with multiorgan failure and maintained on mechanical ventilation (Heyland et al. 2013). Second, 28-day enteral feeding of high-protein diets supplemented with immune-modulating nutrients (including glutamine) to critical patients managed with mechanical ventilation increased mortality (van Zanten et al. 2014). It is unknown whether (1) the alanine released from the intravenously administered alanyl-glutamine or other factors may contribute to the adverse effect of the nutritional intervention, (2) glutamine may interact with a high-protein enteral diet to cause hyperammonemia or other metabolic/physiological abnormalities (e.g., reduced blood flow to tissues) in the intensive care unit patients, and (3) the nonglutamine immune-modulating nutrients (e.g., vitamins and ω-3 polyunsaturated fatty acids) supplemented to the enteral diets may contribute to increased mortality in those patients. Nonetheless, the American Society for Parenteral and Enteral Nutrition (McClave et al. 2016), Society for Clinical Care Medicine (McClave et al. 2016), and the European Society for Parenteral and Enteral Nutrition (Singer et al. 2019) now recommend that glutamine supplementation may be used for patients with burn injury or intestinal dysfunction and possibly for some elective surgery patients, but not for patients with multiorgan failures. Clearly, the use of glutamine in clinical nutrition requires the careful design of diets and the careful monitoring of vital physiological variables.

Extensive feeding studies have shown the safety of appropriate doses of supplemental glutamine in swine and rodents (Watford 2008; Wong et al. 2011; Wu et al. 2011a; Zhu et al. 2018). For example, short- and long-term supplementation with glutamine at an appropriate dose (e.g., up to 1% in diet on an as-fed basis; 90% dry matter content in the diet) is safe for neonatal, gestating, and lactating swine. Based on feed intake, the supplemental doses of glutamine per kg BW for neonatal, gestating, and lactating swine are 1.0, 0.20, and 0.32 g/kg BW/day, respectively, in addition to the glutamine in the basal diets (1.2, 0.24, and 0.55 g glutamine/kg BW/day, respectively), without any adverse effects (Wu et al. 2011). In all of these experiments, dietary supplementation with up to 1% glutamine (on an as-fed basis) for 3 weeks did not result in feed-intake reduction, sickness, or death in any pigs. In addition, no side effects of glutamine supplementation of up to 1% in the diet (on an as-fed basis) were observed in postweaning pigs within at least 3 months after termination of a 2-week, 1-month, or 3-month period of supplementation. However, a high supplemental dose of glutamine (e.g., 2% glutamine in a corn- and soybean meal-based diet for weanling piglets) may have an undesirable effect (e.g., reduced feed intake) due to an AA imbalance plus increased amounts of ammonia in the plasma and this must be avoided in dietary supplementation and clinical therapy. Furthermore, growth, metabolic, and histological analyses indicated that dietary supplementation with 1.25% glutamine was safe for both male and female rats for at least 13 weeks (Tsubuku et al. 2004b). This level of supplementation was equivalent to 0.83 and 0.96 g glutamine/kg BW/day in male and female rats, respectively, based on their food intake per kg BW (Tsubuku et al. 2004b).

Broiler chickens (from birth to market weight) well tolerated 1% supplemental glutamine in diets between 7 and 42 days or between 2 and 42 days of age without any adverse effects on feed intake, growth, or health (Abdulkarimi et al. 2019; Ayazi 2014). Similarly, 21- to 42-day-old turkey poults did not exhibit any adverse response to dietary supplementation with 0.7% glutamine (Salmanzadeh and Shahryar 2013). Moreover, dietary supplementation with 0.8 or 1% glutamine for 40–42 days had no negative effects on laying hens (Dong et al. 2010) or laying guinea fowl (Gholipour et al. 2017). Based on reduced feed intake, reduced weight gain, and abnormal intestinal morphology, broilers did not tolerate dietary supplementation with ≥2% glutamine (Bartell and Batal 2007; Khempaka et al. 2011; Soltan 2009). However, in view of intestinal health, growth performance, and feed efficiency, ducklings well tolerated dietary supplementation with 2% glutamine (Zhang et al. 2017a). Thus, there is a species difference in the sensitivity of poultry to dietary glutamine intake.

Like terrestrial animals, the small intestine of fish also extensively oxidizes glutamine to CO_2 (Wu et al. 2020a). Results of extensive research have shown that (1) dietary supplementation with glutamine (up to 3%) does not have adverse or undesirable effects on fish; (2) diets containing a total of up to 5% glutamine (dry matter basis) are not toxic to hybrid striped bass and largemouth bass; (3) dietary glutamine supplementation has beneficial effects on the growth, health, and feed efficiency of fish without adverse effects on health (Li et al. 2020b). For example, channel catfish could well tolerate dietary supplementation with 3% glutamine for 70 days (Pohlenz et al. 2012a, b), and turbots grew well when their typical diets were supplemented with 2% glutamine for 84 days (Zhang et al. 2017b). Also, grass carp did not exhibit any adverse response to dietary supplementation with at least 2% glutamine for 80 days (Yan and Zhou 2006). Similar results were obtained for red drum (Cheng et al. 2011), hybrid striped bass (Cheng et al. 2012), half-smooth tongue sole (*Cynoglossus semilaevis* Günther) postlarvae (Liu et al. 2015), and gilthead seabream (Coutinho et al. 2016). Considering glutamine content (1.5%–2%) in the basal diets, various species of fish can tolerate 4%–5% of glutamine in enteral diets (Li et al. 2020b).

11.6.2.4   Glutamate as an Example for the Safety of AA Supplementation

Different cells use glutamate for different purposes. For example, the enterocytes of the small intestine actively take up and oxidize a large amount of glutamate from its lumen (e.g., 1–10 mM) as a major energy substrate (Chapter 4), glutamate activates the taste cells of the tongue and the gastrointestinal tract via signal transduction (San Gabriel and Uneyama 2013), and glutamate is the major excitatory neurotransmitter in the central nervous system with its extracellular concentrations being <50 μM (He and Wu 2020). The intake of glutamate by adult humans from most habitual diets is about 10–20 g/day (Tomé 2018). There has been a long-standing debate about the safety of the ingestion of glutamate or its salt (MSG) by humans, possibly due to (1) a lack of understanding of glutamate catabolism in the small intestine and (2) the associated intake of sodium from MSG. In the gastrointestinal tract, MSG is ionized to form glutamate and Na^+. Humans and other animals need sodium to maintain the normal physiological functions of all tissues, including the small intestine, large intestine, liver, spleen, heart, brain, skeletal muscle, and kidneys, as well as cells of the immune system (Wu 2018). Nearly all dietary glutamate is metabolized by the small intestine to produce CO_2, water, AAs, glutathione (an antioxidant), and lactate, and only about 3%–5% of dietary glutamate enters the portal circulation (Chapter 4). Thus, dietary intake of glutamate or MSG within physiological levels has little effect on the concentrations of glutamate in blood and other tissues of humans and other animal models (e.g., pigs and rats; Hou and Wu 2918). People generally like the taste of MSG and healthy adults can well tolerate the consumption of up to 10 g of supplemental MSG per day, depending on the amount of glutamate intake from diets. For example, healthy adult humans had no adverse clinical responses to a single oral dose of MSG up to 150 mg/kg BW (Fernstrom et al. 1996; Graham et al. 2000), or the chronic daily consumption of MSG at up to 147 g/day (about 2 g MSG/kg BW/day for a 70 kg person) for at least 34 days (Bazzano et al. 1970). Likewise, patients with psychiatric disorders well tolerated 45 g MSG/day (about 0.6 g/kg BW/day; three divided doses of 15 g or about 0.2 g/kg at each dosing) for at least 12 weeks (Himwich et al. 1955). Only minor side effects, typically nausea, occasionally occurred at such high doses (Himwich et al. 1955). The long-standing claim that the intake of MSG in foods causes the "Chinese Restaurant Syndrome" in humans (an illness characterized by weakness, numbness, palpitations, and headaches after the overconsumption of MSG as a seasoning) is unfounded (Beyreuther et al. 2007; Fernstrom 2018). Note that neurological damage can occur in animals (e.g., rodents, nonprimates, and fish) receiving the subcutaneous, intraperitoneal, intravenous, or intrahippocampal administration of MSG or glutamate, because the MSG or glutamate administered via these means does not undergo the first-pass catabolism in the small intestine. This is completely different than the oral ingestion of MSG or glutamate by humans and other animals.

Extensive feeding studies have shown the safety of appropriate doses of supplemental glutamate in swine (Hou and Wu 2918). For example, 7- to 21-day-old low-birth-weight and normal-birth-weight piglets reared by sows did not show any adverse response to the oral administration of 2 g of glutamate/kg BW/day for at least 2 days. Also, based on general observations (e.g., behavior, skin health, and hair), feed intake, growth, body composition, as well as hematological and blood chemistry tests, dietary supplementation with 0.5%, 1%, 2%, and 4% MSG (equivalent to 0.432%, 0.864%, 1.73%, and 3.46% glutamate, respectively) to pigs between 21 and 42 days of age for 21 days had no adverse effects on the animals (Rezaei et al. 2013). These supplemental doses of 0%, 0.5%, 1%, 2%, and 4% MSG provided pigs with 0, 175, 332, 659, and 1263 mg glutamate/kg BW/day, respectively, beyond the amount of glutamate intake from the basal diet (710–789 mg/kg BW/day) at the feed intake of 36.5–41.3 g/kg BW/day. Likewise, long-term supplementation of diets with 1%–4% glutamate for growing-finishing pigs (30–90 kg BW) was safe for at least ~120 days (Kirchgessner et al. 1993). In addition, the inclusion of 10% crystalline glutamic acid in the purified diets of 10–20 kg (Chung and Baker 1992) and 20- to 50-kg pigs (Wang and Fuller 1989) did not affect their growth or health. Likewise, no adverse effects were observed in lactating sows fed diets supplemented with up to 2% MSG (Hou and Wu 2018). Based on these results, pigs at all production stages can well tolerate dietary supplementation with at least 2% glutamate or MSG without any adverse effects.

Studies with other mammalian species have also shown a lack of adverse effects of short- and long-term dietary supplementation with large doses of glutamate or MSG. For example, the oral administration of MSG to male and female weanling mice via the enteral diet or drinking water at the doses of 46 and 21 g/kg BW/day, respectively, did not result in adverse effects, including no hypothalamic lesions (Heywood et al. 1977). Furthermore, a two-generation study demonstrated that the oral administration of MSG (0.064% MSG in drinking water) to adult female mice throughout mating, gestation, and lactation, and to their offspring until they reached 32 weeks of age did not affect growth, girth size, abdominal fat weight, body composition, or reproductive performance (Nakamura et al. 2013). These results indicate that the oral administration of MSG does not trigger insulin resistance, dyslipidemia, or hepatic steatosis (Nakamura et al. 2013). Likewise, dietary supplementation with 1%, 2%, or 4% MSG to male and female rats for 2 years had no adverse effects on BW gain, food intake, food conversion ratio, hematology, blood chemistry, organ weights, or mortality in comparison with control rats receiving the basal diet (Owen et al. 1978).

Young chicks well tolerated 10% glutamate in diets for at least 2 weeks without any adverse effects on feed intake, growth, or health (Maruyama et al. 1976). Similarly, 8- to 14-day-old chicks fed purified diets containing 10% or 12% glutamate exhibited normal rates of feed intake, daily weight gains, and feed efficiency, as compared with age-matched chicks fed a conventional corn- and soybean meal-based diet containing 24.5% crude protein (Sasse and Baker 1973). Supplementing 1% glutamate to a typical corn- and soybean meal-based diet for 42 days (Olubodun et al. 2015) or 1.1% MSG to similar basal diets for 21 days (Ma et al. 2011) was safe for broilers. This was also observed for 1- to 21-day-old chickens exposed to heat stress (Porto et al. 2015). Finally, dietary supplementation with 2.4% glutamate to laying hens fed a 16.3% crude-protein diet for 140 days did not adversely influence their feed intake or egg production, compared with the control group fed a 17% crude-protein diet (Bezerra et al. 2015). Thus, a safe level of total dietary glutamate is at least 12% (dry matter basis) for chickens.

There is considerable evidence that dietary supplementation with glutamate (at least 10%) or MSG (at least 7%) does not result in adverse or undesirable effects on fish fed diets containing 35%–60% crude protein (Li et al. 2020b). For example, Atlantic salmon well tolerated a dietary supplementation with 1.5% glutamate for 1 year (Larsson et al. 2014), and gilthead seabream juveniles grew well when their typical diets were supplemented with 4% glutamate for 52 days (Caballero-Solares et al. 2015). Also, grass carp did not exhibit any adverse response to dietary supplementation with 0.8% and 1.6% glutamate for 56 days (Zhao et al. 2015). Similar results were obtained for rainbow trout receiving dietary supplementation with 1% and 2% glutamate for 8 weeks (Yoshida et al. 2016).

It must be recognized that there are differences in the metabolism of nutrients among individuals (Carlson et al. 1989; Walker and Lupien 2000) and intestinal glutamate utilization may be influenced by the dietary intakes of other nutrients (Hou and Wu 2018). It is possible that a very small percentage of people, particularly those with gut dysfunction, may not have the ability to catabolize a large amount of dietary MSG or glutamate and, therefore, are sensitive to MSG or glutamate intake. To date, those possible metabolic alterations have not been demonstrated in humans or other animals.

11.7 SUMMARY

By serving as substrates for the synthesis of both polypeptides and other nitrogenous substances that have enormous physiological significance, AAs have both nutritional and regulatory roles in humans and other animals (Figure 11.20). Cell signaling, protein modifications, antioxidative defense, chemical sensing, and epigenetic regulation of transcription are five emerging roles for AAs and their metabolites in organisms. These nutrients are essential to the functions of all cell types and, therefore, whole-body homeostasis, survival, growth, and development. AAs play important roles in preventing metabolic and infectious diseases and in treating certain disorders in digestive, neurological, muscular, reproductive, and cardiovascular systems. Increasing evidence suggests important roles for D-alanine, D-aspartate, and D-serine in neuroendocrine function as well as for D-alanine in intracellular osmotic regulation in certain aquatic animals. Along with L-glutamate and glycine, the D-AAs modulate the activity of the NMDA receptor, which plays critical roles in synaptic plasticity, memory storage, excitotoxicity, neuronal development, and behavior. When diets cannot provide adequate amounts of certain AAs (e.g., arginine, glutamine, glutamate, glycine, proline, and tryptophan), their supplementation can beneficially prevent their deficiency, enhance food intake, protect cells from oxidative stress, optimize immune responses, improve health, modulate physical behavior, and alter body composition (e.g., an increase in skeletal muscle and a decrease in white adipose tissue). When using AAs in dietary supplementation

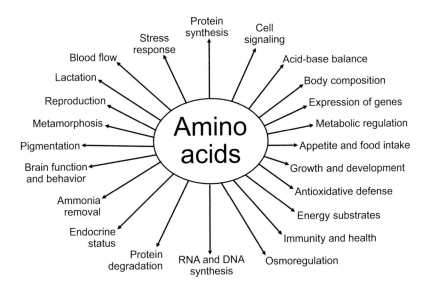

FIGURE 11.20 Roles of amino acids in nutrition and metabolism of humans and other animals. Besides serving as building blocks for proteins, amino acids have multiple regulatory functions in cell signaling and metabolism. Some nonproteinogenic amino acids (e.g., taurine) are vital for the homeostasis of tissues and organs, such as the eyes, heart, brain, and skeletal muscle. These nutrients are crucial for the optimum growth, development, and health of humans and other animals (including swine, ruminants, poultry, fish, and shrimp).

and medical therapy, their chemical properties, balances, antagonisms, and safety must be taken into consideration to maximize the desired nutritional and physiological effects and prevent any undesirable outcomes.

REFERENCES

Abbruzzese, A., V. Liguori, and M.H. Park. 1988. Deoxyhypusine hydroxylase. *Adv. Exp. Med. Biol.* 250:459–466.

Abdulkarimi R., M.H. Shahir, and M. Daneshyar. 2019. Effects of dietary glutamine and arginine supplementation on performance, intestinal morphology and ascites mortality in broiler chickens reared under cold environment. *Asian-Australas. J. Anim. Sci.* 32:110–117.

Abe, H., N. Yoshikawa, M.G. Sarower, and S. Okada. 2005. Physiological function and metabolism of free D-alanine in aquatic animals. *Biol. Pharm. Bull.* 28:1571–1577.

Aberg, A.M., M. Hultin, P. Abrahamsson, and J.E. Larsson. 2004. Circulatory effects and kinetics following acute administration of carbon monoxide in a porcine model. *Life Sci.* 75:1029–1039.

Agostinelli, E. 2020. Biochemical and pathophysiological properties of polyamines. *Amino Acids* 52:111–117.

Agostinelli, E., M.P Marques, R. Calheiros, F.P. Gil, G. Tempera, N. Viceconte et al. 2010. Polyamines: fundamental characters in chemistry and biology. *Amino Acids* 38:393–403.

Ajinkya, S., G. Nawaratna, S.D. Hu, G. Wu, and G. Lubec. 2016. Decreased hippocampal homoarginine and increased nitric oxide and nitric oxide synthase levels in rats parallel training in a radial arm maze. *Amino Acids* 48:2197–2204.

Akaberi, D., J. Krambrich, J. Ling, C. Luni, G. Hedenstierna, J.D. Jarhult et al. 2020. Mitigation of the replication of SARS-CoV-2 by nitric oxide in vitro. *Redox Biol.* 37:101734.

Åkerström, S., M. Mousavi-Jazi, J. Klingström, M. Leijon, Å. Lundkvist, and A. Mirazimi. 2005. Nitric oxide inhibits the replication cycle of severe acute respiratory syndrome coronavirus. *J. Virol.* 79:1966–1969.

Aksnes, A., H. Mundheim, and J. Toppe. 2006. The effect of dietary hydroxyproline supplementation on salmon (*Salmo salar* L.) fed high plant protein diets. *Aquaculture* 275:242–249.

Amobi, A., F. Qian, A.A. Lugade, and K. Odunsi. 2017. Tryptophan catabolism and cancer immunotherapy targeting IDO mediated immune suppression. *Adv. Exp. Med. Biol.* 1036:129–144.

Andersen, S.M., R. Waagbo, and M. Espe. 2016. Functional amino acids in fish nutrition, health and welfare. *Front Biosci* 8:143–169.

Anderson, P.M. 1981. Purification and properties of the glutamine- and *N*-acetyl-L-glutamate-dependent car-bamoyl phosphate synthetase from liver of *Squalus acanthias*. *J. Biol. Chem.* 256:12228–12238.

Apper-Bossard, E., A. Feneuil, A. Wagner, and F. Respondek. 2013. Use of vital wheat gluten in aquaculture feeds. *Aquatic Biosyst.* 9:21.

Atzler, D., E. Schwedhelm, and C.U. Choe. 2015. L-Homoarginine and cardiovascular disease. *Curr. Opin. Clin. Nutr. Metab. Care* 18:83–88.

Ayazi, M. 2014. The effect of dietary glutamine supplementation on performance and blood antioxidant status of broiler chickens under continuous heat stress condition. *Int J Farming Allied Sci* 3:1213–1219.

Baccari, G.C., S. Falvo, A. Santillo, F.D.G. Russo, and M.M. Di Fiore. 2020. D-Amino acids in mammalian endocrine tissues. *Amino Acids* 52:263–1273.

Baker, D.H. 2009. Advances in protein-amino acid nutrition of poultry. *Amino Acids* 37:29–41.

Baker, D.H. and G.L. Czarnecki-Maulden. 1987. Pharmacologic role of cysteine in ameliorating or exacerbat-ing mineral toxicities. *J. Nutr.* 117:1003–1010.

Ballantyne, J.S. 2001. Amino acid metabolism. *Fish Physiol.* 20:77–107.

Bansal, V., P. Rodriguez, G. Wu, D.C. Eichler, J. Zabaleta, F. Taheri, and J.B. Ochoa. 2004. Citrulline can preserve proliferation and prevent the loss of CD3 ζ chain under conditions of low arginine. *JPEN* 28:423–430.

Barbul, A. 2008. Proline precursors to sustain mammalian collagen synthesis. *J. Nutr.* 138:2021S–2024S.

Bartell, S.M. and A.B. Batal. 2007. The effect of supplemental glutamine on growth performance, devel-opment of the gastrointestinal tract, and humoral immune response of broilers. *Poult. Sci.* 86:1940–1947.

Bazer, F.W., G.A. Johnson, and G. Wu. 2015. Amino acids and conceptus development during the peri-implantation period of pregnancy. *Adv. Exp. Med. Biol.* 843:23–52.

Bazer, F.W., H. Seo, G.A. Johnson, and G. Wu. 2021. One-carbon metabolism and development of the concep-tus during pregnancy: lessons from studies with sheep and pigs. *Adv. Exp. Med. Biol.* 1285:1–15.

Bazzano, G., J.A. D'Elia, and R.E. Olson. 1970. Monosodium glutamate: feeding of large amounts in man and gerbils. *Science* 169:1208–1209.

Beaumont, M. and F. Blachier. 2020. Amino acids in intestinal physiology and health. *Adv. Exp. Med. Biol.* 1265:1–20.

Becerra-Solano, L.E., J. Butler, G. Castañeda-Cisneros, D.E. McCloskey, X. Wang, A.E. Pegg et al. 2009. A missense mutation, p.V132G, in the X-linked spermine synthase gene (SMS) causes Snyder-Robinson syndrome. *Am. J. Med. Genet. A* 149:328–335.

Beltowski, J. 2015. Hydrogen sulfide in pharmacology and medicine – an update. *Pharmacol. Rep.* 67:647–658.

Bessede, A., M. Gargaro, M.T. Pallotta, D. Matino, G. Servillo, C. Brunacci et al. 2014. Aryl hydrocarbon receptor control of a disease tolerance defence pathway. *Nature* 511:184–190.

Bezerra, R.M., F.G.P. Costa, P.E.N. Givisiez, C. de Castro Goulart, R.A. dos Santos, and M.R. de Lima. 2015. Glutamic acid supplementation on low protein diets for laying hens. *Acta Sci. Anim. Sci.* 37:129–134.

Beyreuther, K., H.K. Biesalski, J.D. Fernstrom, P. Grimm, W.P. Hammes, U. Heinemann et al. 2007. Consensus meeting: monosodium glutamate – an update. *Eur. J. Clin. Nutr.* 61:304–313.

Bicudo, Á.J., R. Y. Sado, and J.E. Cyrino. 2009. Dietary lysine requirement of juvenile pacu *Piaractus meso-potamicus* (Holmberg, 1887). *Aquaculture* 297:151–156.

Bieber, L.L. 1988. Carnitine. *Annu. Rev. Biochem.* 57:261–283.

Biefer, H.R.C., A. Vasudevan, and A. Elkhal. 2017. Aspects of tryptophan and nicotinamide adenine dinucleo-tide in immunity: a new twist in an old tale. *Int. J. Tryptophan Res.* 10:1–8.

Billard, J.-M. 2012. D-Amino acids in brain neurotransmission and synaptic plasticity. *Amino Acids* 43:1851–1860.

Bilsborough, S. and N. Mann. 2006. A review of issues of dietary protein intake in humans. *Int. J. Sport Nutr. Exerc. Metab.* 16:129–152.

Blachier, F., X.F. Kong, G. Wu, D. Tomé, A. Lancha Jr, M. Andriamihaja, and Y.L. Yin. 2015. Endotoxemia and glutamine. In: *Glutamine in Clinical Nutrition and Health* (Rajendram, R., V.R. Preedy, and V.B. Patel, eds). Springer, New York. pp. 125–139.

Boger, R.H., S.M. Bode-Boger, R.P. Brandes, L. Phivthong-ngam, M. Bohme, R. Nafe et al. 2007. Dietary L-arginine reduces the progression of atherosclerosis in cholesterol-fed rabbits: comparison with lovas-tatin. *Circulation* 96:1282–1290.

Boldyrev, A.A., G. Aldini, and W. Derave. 2013. Physiology and pathophysiology of carnosine. *Physiol. Rev.* 93:1803–1845.

Bouillaud, F. and F. Blachier. 2011. Mitochondria and sulfide: a very old story of poisoning, feeding, and signaling? *Antioxid. Redox. Signal* 15:379–391.

Brandsch, M. 2006. Transport of L-proline, L-proline-containing peptides and related drugs at mammalian epithelial cell membranes. *Amino Acids* 31:119–136.

Brasse-Lagnel, C., A. Fairand, A. Lavoinne, and A. Husson. 2003. Glutamine stimulates argininosuccinate synthetase gene expression through O-glycosylation of Sp1 in Caco-2 cells. *J. Biol. Chem.* 278:52504–52510.

Brasse-Lagnel, C.G., A.M. Lavoinne, and A.S. Husson. 2010. Amino acid regulation of mammalian gene expression in the intestine. *Biochimie* 92:729–735.

Brault, J.J., K.A. Abraham, and R.L. Terjung. 2003. Muscle creatine uptake and creatine transporter expression in response to creatine supplementation and depletion. *J. Appl. Physiol.* 94:2173–2180.

Bringaud, F., M.P. Barrett, and D. Zilberstein. 2012. Multiple roles of proline transport and metabolism in trypanosomatids. *Front. Biosci.* 17:349–374.

Brosnan, J.T. and M.E. Brosnan. 2007. Creatine: endogenous metabolite, dietary, and therapeutic supplement. *Annu. Rev. Nutr.* 27:241–261.

Brosnan, J.T. and M.E. Brosnan. 2013. Glutamate: a truly functional amino acid. *Amino Acids* 45:413–418.

Buchmüller-Rouiller, Y., S.B. Corrandin, J. Smith, P. Schneider, A. Ransijn, C.V. Jongeneel, and J. Mauël. 1995. Role of glutathione in macrophage activation: effect of cellular glutathione depletion on nitrite production and leishmanicidal activity. *Cell. Immunol.* 164:73–80.

Bucking, C., C.M. LeMoine, P.M. Craig, and P.J. Walsh. 2013. Nitrogen metabolism of the intestine during digestion in a teleost fish, the plainfin midshipman (*Porichthys notatus*). *J. Exp. Biol.* 216:2821–2832.

Buentello, J.A. and D.M. Gatlin III. 2000. The dietary arginine requirement of channel catfish (Ictalurus punctatus) is influenced by endogenous synthesis of arginine from glutamic acid. *Aquaculture* 188:311–321.

Buentello, J.A. and D.M. Gatlin III. 2001. Plasma citrulline and arginine kinetics in juvenile channel catfish, *Ictalurus punctatus*, given oral gabaculine. *Fish. Physiol. Biochem.* 24:105–112.

Burnett, C.L., B. Heldreth, W.F. Bergfeld, D.V. Belsito, R.A. Hill, C.D. Klaassen et al. 2013. Safety assessment of α-amino acids as used in cosmetics. *Int. J. Toxicol.* 32:41S–62S.

Caballero-Solares, A., I. Viegas, M.C. Salgado, A.M. Siles, A. Sáez, I. Metón et al. 2015. Diets supplemented with glutamate or glutamine improve protein retention and modulate gene expression of key enzymes of hepatic metabolism in gilthead seabream (*Sparus aurata*) juveniles. *Aquaculture* 444:79–87.

Calder, P.C. and P. Yaqoob. 1999. Glutamine and the immune system. *Amino Acids* 17:227–241.

Calder, P.C., C.J. Field, and H.S. Gill. 2002. *Nutrition and Immune Function.* CABI, Wallingford.

Campbell, J.W., P.L. Aster, and J.E. Vorhaben. 1983. Mitochondrial ammoniagenesis in liver of the channel catfish Ictalurus punctatus. *Am. J. Physiol.* 244:R709–R717.

Campollo, O., D. Sprengers, and N. McIntyre. 1992. The BCAA/AAA ratio of plasma amino acids in three different groups of cirrhotics. *Rev. Invest. Clin.* 44:513–518.

Carlson, H.E., J.T. Miglietta, M.S. Roginsky, and L.D. Steglink. 1989. Stimulation of pituitary hormone secretion by neurotransmitter amino acids in humans. *Metabolism* 38:1179–1182.

Castilho, B.A., R. Shanmugam, R.C. Silva, R. Ramesh, B.M. Himme, and E. Sattlegger. 2014. Keeping the eIF2 alpha kinase Gcn2 in check. *Biochim. Biophys. Acta* 1843:1948–1968.

Chadwick, T.D. and P.A. Wright. 1999. Nitrogen excretion and expression of urea cycle enzymes in the atlantic cod (*Gadus morhua* L.): a comparison of early life stages with adults. *J. Exp. Biol.* 202:2653–2662.

Chamberlin, M.E., H.C. Glemet, and J.S. Ballantyne. 1991. Glutamine metabolism in a holostean (*Amia calva*) and teleost fish (*Salvelinus namaycush*). *Am. J. Physiol.* 260:R159–R166.

Chen, J.Q., Y.H. Jin, Y. Yang, Z.L. Wu, and G. Wu. 2020. Epithelial dysfunction in lung diseases: effects of amino acids and potential mechanisms. *Adv. Exp. Med. Biol.* 1265:57–70.

Cheng, Z., A. Buentello, and D.M. Gatlin III. 2011. Effects of dietary arginine and glutamine on growth performance, immune responses and intestinal structure of red drum, *Sciaenops ocellatus*. *Aquaculture* 319:247–252.

Cheng, Z., D.M. Gatlin III, and A. Buentello. 2012. Dietary supplementation of arginine and/or glutamine influences growth performance, immune responses and intestinal morphology of hybrid striped bass (*Morone chrysops × Morone saxatilis*). *Aquaculture* 362:39–43.

Childs, C.E., P.C. Calder, and E.A. Miles. 2019. Diet and immune function. *Nutrients* 11:1933.

Chiu, Y.N., R.E. Austic, and G.L. Rumsey. 1986. Urea cycle activity and arginine formation in rainbow trout (*Salmo gairdneri*). *J. Nutr.* 116:1640–1650.

Chu, Z.J., Y. Gong, Y.C. Lin, Y.C Yuan, W.J. Cai, S.Y. Gong, and Z. Luo. 2014. Optimal dietary methionine requirement of juvenile Chinese sucker, *Myxocyprinus asiaticus*. *Aquac. Nutr.* 20:253–264.

Chung, T.K. and D.H. Baker. 1992. Ideal amino acid pattern for ten kilogram pigs. *J. Anim. Sci.* 70:3102–3111.

Cipolla-Neto, J. and F.G.D. Amaral. 2018. Melatonin as a hormone: new physiological and clinical insights. *Endocr. Rev.* 39:990–1028.

Closs, E.I., J.S. Scheld, M. Sharafi, and U. Förstermann. 2000. Substrate supply for nitric-oxide synthase in macrophages and endothelial cells: role of cationic amino acid transporters. *Mol. Pharmacol.* 57:68–74.

Conceição, L.E.C., I. Rønnestad, and S.K. Tonheim. 2002. Metabolic budgets for lysine and glutamate in unfed herring (*Clupea harengus*) larvae. *Aquaculture* 206:305–312.Cordella-Miele, E., L. Miele, S. Beninati, and A.B. Mukherjee. 1993. Transglutaminase-catalyzed incorporation of polyamines into phospholipase A2. *J. Biochem.* 113:164–173.

Coutinho, F.F. 2017. Potential benefits of functional amino acids in fish nutrition. Ph.D. Dissertation. Universidade do Porto, Porto, Portugal.

Coutinho, F., C. Castro, E. Rufino-Palomares, B. Ordóñez-Grande, M.A. Gallardo, A. Oliva-Teles, and H. Peres. 2016. Dietary glutamine supplementation effects on amino acid metabolism, intestinal nutrient absorption capacity and antioxidant response of gilthead sea bream (*Sparus aurata*) juveniles. *Comp. Biochem. Physiol. A* 191:9–17.

Cruzat, V.F. and P. Newsholme. 2017. An introduction to glutamine metabolism. In: *Glutamine: Biochemistry, Physiology, and Clinical Applications* (Meynial-Denis, D., ed). CRC Press: Boca Raton, FL. pp. 1–18.

Curi, R., C.J. Lagranha, S.Q. Doi, D.F. Sellitti, J. Procopio, T.C. Pithon-Curi et al. 2005. Molecular mechanisms of glutamine action. *J. Cell. Physiol.* 204:392–401.

Dai, Z.L., Z.L. Wu, Y. Yang, J.J. Wang, M.C. Satterfield, C.J. Meininger et al. 2013a. Nitric oxide and energy metabolism in mammals. *BioFactors* 39:383–391.

Dai, Z.L., X.L. Li, P.B. Xi, J. Zhang, G. Wu, and W.Y. Zhu. 2013b. L-Glutamine regulates amino acid utilization by intestinal bacteria. *Amino Acids* 45:501–512.

Dai, Z.L., Z.L. Wu, S.Q. Hang, W.Y. Zhu, and G. Wu. 2015. Amino acid metabolism in intestinal bacteria and its potential implications for mammalian reproduction. *Mol. Hum. Reprod.* 21:389–409.

Dai, Z.L., S.Q. Sun, H. Chen, M.Y. Liu, L.H. Zhang, Z.L. Wu et al. 2019. Analysis of tryptophan and its metabolites by high-performance liquid chromatography. *Methods Mol. Biol.* 2030:131–142.

D'Aniello, A. 2007. D-Aspartic acid: an endogenous amino acid with an important neuroendocrine role. *Brain Res. Rev.* 53:215–234.

Dar, A.C. and K.M. Shokat. 2011. The evolution of protein kinase inhibitors from antagonists to agonists of cellular signaling. *Annu. Rev. Biochem.* 80:769–795.

Dasgupta, M., J.R. Sharkey, and G. Wu. 2005. Inadequate intakes of indispensable amino acids among homebound older adults. *J. Nutr. Elder.* 24:85–99.

De Jonge, W.J., K.L. Kwikkers, A.A. Te Velde, S.J.H. van Deventer, M.A. Nolte, R.E. Mebius et al. 2002. Arginine deficiency affects early B cell maturation and lymphoid organ development in transgenic mice. *J. Clin. Invest.* 110:1539–1548.

Dechelotte, P., M. Hasselmann, L. Cynober, B. Allaouchiche, M. Coeffier, B. Hecketsweiler et al. 2006. L-alanyl-L-glutamine dipeptide-supplemented total parenteral nutrition reduces infectious complications and glucose tolerance in critically ill patients: the French controlled, randomized, double-blind, multicenter study. *Crit. Care Med.* 34:598–604.

Deminice, D., R.P. da Silva, S.G. Lamarre, C. Brown, G.N. Furey, S.A. McCarter et al. 2011. Creatine supplementation prevents the accumulation of fat in the livers of rats fed a high-fat diet. *J. Nutr.* 141:1799–1804.

Derave, W., B. De Courten, and S.P. Baba. 2019. An update on carnosine and anserine research. *Amino Acids* 51:1–4.

Diotallevi, M., P. Checconi, A.T. Palamara, I. Celestino, L. Coppo, A. Holmgren et al. 2017. Glutathione finetunes the innate immune response toward antiviral pathways in a macrophage cell line independently of its antioxidant properties. *Front. Immunol.* 8:1239.

Dominique, M.-D. 2016. Glutamine metabolism in advanced age. *Nutr. Rev.* 74:225–236.

Dong, X., C. Yang, S. Tang, Q. Jiang, and X. Zou. 2010. Effect and mechanism of glutamine on productive performance and egg quality of laying hens. *Asian-Aust. J. Anim. Sci.* 23:1049–1056.

Drummond, M.J., E.L. Glynn, C.S. Fry, S. Dhanani, E. Volpi, and B.B. Rasmussen. 2009. Essential amino acids increase microRNA-499, -208b, and -23a and downregulate myostatin and myocyte enhancer factor 2C mRNA expression in human skeletal muscle. *J. Nutr.* 139:2279–2284.

Durante, W. 2020. Amino acids in circulatory function and health. *Adv. Exp. Med. Biol.* 1265:39–56.

Duval, D., C. Demangel, K. Munierjolain, S. Miossec, and I. Geahel. 1991. Factors controlling cell proliferation and antibody production in mouse hybridoma cells 1. Influence of the amino acid supply. *Biotechnol. Bioeng.* 38:561–570.

EFSA. 2018. Safety and efficacy of L-arginine produced by fermentation with *Escherichia coli* NITE BP-02186 for all animal species. *EFSA J.* 16:5276.Ellery, S.J., D.A. Larosa, M.M. Kett, P.A. Della Gatta, R.J. Snow, D.W. Walker, and H. Dickinson. 2016. Dietary creatine supplementation during pregnancy: a study on the effects of creatine supplementation on creatine homeostasis and renal excretory function in spiny mice. *Amino Acids* 48:1819-1830.

Ellery, S.J., D.A. Larosa, M.M. Kett, P.A. Della Gatta, R.J. Snow, D.W. Walker, and H. Dickinson. 2016. Dietary creatine supplementation during pregnancy: a study on the effects of creatine supplementation on creatine homeostasis and renal excretory function in spiny mice. *Amino Acids* 48:1819–1830.

Errico, F., F. Napolitano, R. Nisticò, and A. Usiello. 2012. New insights on the role of free D-aspartate in the mammalian brain. *Amino Acids* 43:1861–1871.

Everaert, I., G. Baron, S. Barbaresi, E. Gilardoni, C. Coppa, M. Carini et al. 2019. Development and validation of a sensitive LC–MS/MS assay for the quantification of anserine in human plasma and urine and its application to pharmacokinetic study. *Amino Acids* 51:103–114.

Fan, X.X., S. Li, Z.L. Wu, Z.L. Dai, J. Li, X.L. Wang, and G. Wu. 2019. Glycine supplementation to breast-fed piglets attenuates postweaning jejunal epithelial apoptosis: a functional role of CHOP signaling. *Amino Acids* 51:463–473.

Faure, C., A. Raynaud-Simon, A. Ferry, V. Daugé, L. Cynober, C. Aussel, and C. Moinard. 2012. Leucine and citrulline modulate muscle function in malnourished aged rats. *Amino Acids* 42:1425–1433.

Fernstrom, J.D. 2013. Large neutral amino acids: dietary effects on brain neurochemistry and function. *Amino Acids* 45:419–430.

Fernstrom, J.D. 2018. Monosodium glutamate in the diet does not raise brain glutamate concentrations or disrupt brain functions. *Ann. Nutr. Metab.* 73(Suppl. 5):43–52.

Fernstrom, J.D., J.L. Cameron, M.H. Fernstrom, C. McConaha, T.E. Weltzin, and W.H. Kaye. 1996. Short-term neuroendocrine effects of a large oral dose of monosodium glutamate in fasting male subjects. *J. Clin. Endocrinol. Metab.* 81:184–191.

Field, C.J. 2005. The immunological components of human milk and their effect on immune development in infants. *J. Nutr.* 135:1–4.

Field, C.J., I. Johnson, and V.C. Pratt. 2000. Glutamine and arginine: immunonutrients for improved health. *Med. Sci. Sports Exerc.* 32:S377–S388.

Field, C.J., I.R. Johnson, and P.D. Schley. 2002. Nutrients and their role in host resistance to infection. *J. Leuk. Biol.* 71:16–32.

Field, M.S., E. Kamynina, J. Chon, and P.J. Stover. 2018. Nuclear folate metabolism. *Annu. Rev. Nutr.* 38:219-243.

Flynn, N.E., M.H. Shaw, and J.T. Becker. 2020. Amino acids in health and endocrine function. *Adv. Exp. Med. Biol.* 1265:97–109.

Folk, J.E., M.H. Park, S.I. Chung, J. Schrode, E.P. Lester, and H.L. Cooper. 1980. Polyamines as physiological substrates for transglutaminases. *J. Biol. Chem.* 255:3695–3700.

Fricke, O., N. Baecker, M. Heer, B. Tutlewski, and E. Schoenau. 2008. The effect of L-arginine administration on muscle force and power in postmenopausal women. *Clin. Physiol. Funct. Imaging* 28:307–311.

Friedman, M. and C.E. Levin. 2012. Nutritional and medicinal aspects of D-amino acids. *Amino Acids* 42:1553–1582.

Froh, M., R.G. Thurman, and M.D. Wheeler. 2002. Molecular evidence for a glycine-gated chloride channel in macrophages and leukocytes. *Am. J. Physiol.* 283:G856–G863.

Fu, W.J., T.E. Haynes, R. Kohli, J. Hu, W. Shi, T.E. Spencer et al. 2005. Dietary L-arginine supplementation reduces fat mass in Zucker diabetic fatty rats. *J. Nutr.* 135:714–721.

Fumagalli, M., D. Lecca, M.P. Abbracchio, and S. Ceruti. 2017. Pathophysiological role of purines and pyrimidines in neurodevelopment: unveiling new pharmacological approaches to congenital brain diseases. *Front. Pharmacol.* 8:941.

Gaby, A.R. 2006. Natural remedies for herpes simplex. *Altern. Med. Rev.* 11:93–101.

Geggel, H., M. Ament, and J. Heckenlively. 1985. Nutritional requirement for taurine in patients receiving long-term, parenteral nutrition. *N. Engl. J. Med.* 312:142–146.

Gholipour, V., M. Chamani, H.A. Shahryar, A. Sadeghi, and M.A. Afshar. 2017. Effects of dietary L-glutamine supplement on performance, egg quality, fertility and some blood biochemical parameters in Guinea fowls (*Numida meleagris*). *Kafkas Univ. Vet. Fak. Derg.* 23:903–910.

Gietzen, D.W. and S.M. Aja. 2012. The brain's response to an essential amino acid-deficient diet and the circuitous route to a better meal. *Mol. Neurobiol.* 46:332–348.

Gilbreath, K.R., F.W. Bazer, M.C. Satterfield, and G. Wu. 2021. Amino acid nutrition and reproductive performance in ruminants. *Adv. Exp. Med. Biol.* 1285:43–61.

Gleeson, M. 2008. Dosing and efficacy of glutamine supplementation in human exercise and sport training. *J. Nutr.* 138:2045S–2049S.

Goebel, U. and J. Wollborn. 2020. Carbon monoxide in intensive care medicine-time to start the therapeutic application?! *Intensive Care Med. Exp.* 8:2.

Graber, G., N.K. Allen, and H.M. Scott. 1970. Proline essentiality and weight gain. *Poult. Sci.* 49:692–697.

Graham, T.E., V. Sgro, D. Friars, and M.J. Gibala. 2000. Glutamate ingestion: the plasma and muscle free amino acid pools of resting humans. *Am. J. Physiol.* 278:E83–E89.

Griffin, M., R. Casadio, and C.M. Bergamini. 2002. *Transglutaminases: nature's biological glues. Biochem. J.* 368:377–396.

Griffith, R.S., D.E. Walsh, K.H. Myrmel, R.W. Thompson, and A. Behforooz. 1987. Success of L-lysine therapy in frequently recurrent herpes simplex infection. Treatment and prophylaxis. *Dermatologica* 175:183–190.

Guercio, G.D. and R. Panizzutti. 2018. Potential and challenges for the clinical use of D-serine as a cognitive enhancer. *Front. Psychiatry.* 9:14.

Gui, T., Y. Sun, A. Shimokado, and Y. Muragaki. 2012. The roles of mitogen-activated protein kinase pathways in TGF-β-induced epithelial mesenchymal transition. *J. Signal Transduct.* 2012:289243.

Hamilos, D.L. and H.J. Wedner. 1985. The role of glutathione in lymphocyte activation. I. Comparison of inhibitory effects of buthionine sulfoximine and 2-cyclohexene-1-one by nuclear size transformation. *J. Immunol.* 135:2740–2747.

Hamilos, D.L., P. Zelarney, and J.J. Mascali. 1989. Lymphocyte proliferation in glutathione-depleted lymphocytes: direct relationship between glutathione availability and the proliferative response. *Immunopharmacology* 18:223–235.

Hao, S., J.W. Sharp, C.M. Ross-Inta, B.J. McDaniel, T.G. Anthony, R.C. Wek et al. 2005. Uncharged tRNA and sensing of amino acid deficiency in mammalian piriform cortex. *Science* 307:1776–1778.

He, W.L. and G. Wu. 2020. Metabolism of amino acids in the brain and their roles in regulating food intake. *Adv. Exp. Med. Biol.* 1265:167–185.

He, Y., X.X. Fan, N. Liu, Q.Q. Song, J. Kou, Y.H. Shi et al. 2019. L-Glutamine represses the unfolded protein response in the small intestine of weanling piglets. *J. Nutr.* 149:1904–1910.

He, W.L., P. Li, and G. Wu. 2021. Amino acid nutrition and metabolism in chickens. *Adv. Exp. Med. Biol.* 1285: 109–131.

Heyland, D., J. Muscedere, P.E. Wischmeyer, D. Cook, G. Jones, M. Albert et al. 2013. A randomized trial of glutamine and antioxidants in critically ill patients. *New Eng. J. Med.* 368:1489–1497.

Heywood, R., R.W. James, and A.N. Worden. 1977. The ad libitum feeding of monosodium glutamate to weanling mice. *Toxicol. Lett.* 1:151–155.

Hickner, R.C., D.J. Dyck, J. Sklar, H. Hatley, and P. Byrd. 2010. Effect of 28 days of creatine ingestion on muscle metabolism and performance of a simulated cycling road race. *J. Int. Soc. Sports Nutr.* 7:26.

Himwich, H.E., K. Wolff, A.L. Hunsicker, and W.A. Himwich. 1955. Some behavioral effects associated with feeding sodium glutamate to patients with psychiatric disorders. *J. Nerv. Ment. Dis.* 121:40–49.

Hinnebusch, A.G. 2005. Translational regulation of GCN4 and the general amino acid control of yeast. *Annu. Rev. Microbiol.* 59:407–450.

Hnia, K., J. Gayraud, G. Hugon, M. Ramonatxo, S. De La Porte, S. Matecki, and D. Mornet. 2008. L-arginine decreases inflammation and modulates the nuclear factor-kappaB/matrix metalloproteinase cascade in mdx muscle fibers. Am. J. Pathol. 172:1509–1519.

Hoffer, L.J. 2016. Human protein and amino acid requirements. *JPEN* 40:460–474.

Holeček, M. 2018. Branched-chain amino acids in health and disease: metabolism, alterations in blood plasma, and as supplements. *Nutr. Metab.* 15:33.

Holeček, M., R. Kandar, L. Sispera, and M. Kovarik. 2011. Acute hyperammonemia activates branched-chain amino acid catabolism and decreases their extracellular concentrations: different sensitivity of red and white muscle. *Amino Acids* 40:575–584.

Hou, Y.Q. and G. Wu. 2018a. L-Glutamate nutrition and metabolism in swine. *Amino Acids* 50:1497–1510.

Hou, Y.Q. and G. Wu. 2018b. Nutritionally essential amino acids. *Adv. Nutr.* 9:849–851.

Hou, Y.Q., S.C. Jia, G. Nawaratna, S.D. Hu, S. Dahanayaka, F.B. Bazer, and G. Wu. 2015. Analysis of L-homoarginine in biological samples by HPLC involving pre-column derivatization with *o*-phthalaldehyde and *N*-acetyl-L-cysteine. *Amino Acids* 47:2005–2014.

Hou, Y.Q., S.D. Hu, S.C. Jia, G. Nawaratna, D.S. Che, F.L. Wang et al. 2016. Whole-body synthesis of L-homoarginine in pigs and rats supplemented with L-arginine. *Amino Acids* 2016;48:993–1001.

Hou, Y.Q., W.L. He, S.D. Hu, and G. Wu. 2019. Composition of polyamines and amino acids in plant-source foods for human consumption. *Amino Acids* 51:1153–1165.

Hou, Y.Q., S.D. Hu, X.Y. Li, W.L. He, and G. Wu. 2020. Amino acid metabolism in the liver: nutritional and physiological significance. *Adv. Exp. Med. Biol.* 1265:21–37.

Hundal, H.S. and P.M. Taylor. 2009. Amino acid transceptors: gate keeper of nutrient exchange and regulators of nutrient signaling. *Am. J. Physiol.* 296:E603–E613.

Igarashi, K., T. Uemura, and K. Kashiwagi. 2020. Assessing acrolein for determination of the severity of brain stroke, dementia, renal failure and Sjögren's syndrome. *Amino Acids* 52:119–127.

Ignarro, L.J., G.M. Buga, L.H. Wei, P.M. Bauer, G. Wu, and P. del Soldato. 2001. Role of the arginine-nitric oxide pathway in the regulation of vascular smooth muscle cell proliferation. *Proc. Natl. Acad. Sci. USA* 98:4202–4208.

Institute of Medicine. 2006. *Protein and Amino Acids. Dietary Reference Intakes: The Essential Guide to Nutrient Requirements*. National Academies Press, Washington, DC.

Jäger, R., M. Purpura, A. Shao, T. Inoue, and R.B. Kreider. 2011. Analysis of the efficacy, safety, and regulatory status of novel forms of creatine. *Amino Acids* 40:1369–1383.

Jakubowski, H. 2019. Homocysteine modification in protein structure/function and human disease. *Physiol. Rev.* 99:555–604.

Jensen, M., C. Müller, E. Schwedhelm, P. Arunachalam, M. Gelderblom, T. Magnus et al. 2020. Homoarginine- and creatine-dependent gene regulation in murine brains with L-arginine:glycine amidinotransferase deficiency. *Int. J. Mol. Sci.* 21:1865.

Ji, Y., Z.L. Wu, Z.L. Dai, K.J. Sun, J.J. Wang, and G. Wu. 2016. Nutritional epigenetics with a focus on amino acids: Implications for the development and treatment of metabolic syndrome. *J. Nutr. Biochem.* 27:1–8.

Jiang, Z.M., L.J. Wang, Y. Qi, T.H. Liu, M.R. Qiu, N.F. Yang, and D.W. Wilmore. 1993. Comparison of parenteral nutrition supplemented with L-glutamine or glutamine dipeptides. *J. Parenter. Enteral Nutr.* 17:134–141.

Jiao, N., Z.L. Wu, Y. Ji, B. Wang, Z.L. Dai, and G. Wu. 2015. L-Glutamate enhances barrier and anti-oxidative functions in intestinal porcine epithelial cells. *J. Nutr.* 145:2258–2264.

Jobgen, W.S., S.K. Fried, W.J. Fu, C.J. Meininger, and G. Wu. 2006. Regulatory role for the arginine-nitric oxide pathway in metabolism of energy substrates. *J. Nutr. Biochem.* 17:571–588.

Jobgen, W.J., C.J. Meininger, S.C. Jobgen, P. Li, M.-J. Lee, S.B. Smith et al. 2009a. Dietary L-arginine supplementation reduces white-fat gain and enhances skeletal muscle and brown fat masses in diet-induced obese rats. *J. Nutr.* 139:230–237.

Jobgen, W., W.J. Fu, H. Gao, P. Li, C.J. Meininger, S.B. Smith et al. 2009b. High fat feeding and dietary L-arginine supplementation differentially regulate gene expression in rat white adipose tissue. *Amino Acids* 37:187–198.

Jordi, J., B. Herzog, S.M. Camargo, C.N. Boyle, T.A. Lutz, and F. Verrey. 2013. Specific amino acids inhibit food intake via the area postrema or vagal afferents. *J. Physiol.* 591:5611–5621.

Kharitonov, S.A., G. Lubec, B. Lubec, M. Hjelm, and P.J. Barnes. 1995. L-arginine increases exhaled nitric oxide in normal human subjects. *Clin. Sci.* 88:135–139.

Khedara, A., T. Goto, M. Morishima, J. Kayashita, and N. Kato. 1999. Elevated body fat in rats by the dietary nitric oxide synthase inhibitor, L-N$^\omega$-nitroarginine. *Biosci. Biotech. Biochem.* 63:698–702.

Khempaka, S., S. Okrathok, L. Hokking, B. Thukhanon, and W. Molee. 2011. Influence of supplemental glutamine on nutrient digestibility and utilization, small intestinal morphology and gastrointestinal tract and immune organ developments of broiler chickens. *Int. J. Anim. Vet. Sci.* 5:497–499.

Kim, J.Y., G.H. Song, G. Wu, H.J. Gao, G.A. Johnson, and F.W. Bazer. 2013. Arginine, leucine, and glutamine stimulate proliferation of porcine trophectoderm cells through the MTOR-RPS6K-RPS6-EIF4EBP1 signal transduction pathway. *Biol. Reprod.* 88:113.

Kim, K.S., M.J. Jang, S. Fang, S.G. Yoon, I.Y. Kim, J.K. Seong et al. 2019. Anti-obesity effect of taurine through inhibition of adipogenesis in white fat tissue but not in brown fat tissue in a high-fat diet-induced obese mouse model. *Amino Acids* 51:245–254.

Kirchgessner, M., F.X. Roth, and B.R. Paulicks. 1993. Effects of adding glutamic acid to low protein diets for fattening pigs on criteria of growth and carcass composition. *Agribiol. Res.* 46:346–358.

Kirchgessner, M., J. Fickler, and F.X. Roth. 1995. Effect of dietary proline supply on N-balance of piglets. 3. Communication on the importance of nonessential amino acids for protein retention. *J. Anim. Physiol. Anim. Nutr.* 73:57–65.

Kim, J.Y., G.W. Song, G. Wu, and F.W. Bazer. 2012. Functional roles of fructose. *Proc. Natl. Acad. Sci. USA* 109:E1619–E1628.

Kim, J.Y., G.H. Song, G. Wu, H.J. Gao, G.A. Johnson, and F.W. Bazer. 2013. Arginine, leucine, and glutamine stimulate proliferation of porcine trophectoderm cells through the MTOR-RPS6K-RPS6-EIF4EBP1 signal transduction pathway. *Biol. Reprod.* 88:113.

Kohli, R., C.J. Meininger, T.E. Haynes, W. Yan, J.T. Self, and G. Wu. 2004. Dietary L-arginine supplementation enhances endothelial nitric oxide synthesis in streptozotocin-induced diabetic rats. *J. Nutr.* 134:600–608.

Kong, X.F., B.E. Tan, Y.L. Yin, H.J. Gao, X.L. Li, L.A. Jaeger et al. 2012. L-Arginine stimulates the mTOR signaling pathway and protein synthesis in porcine trophectoderm cells. *J. Nutr. Biochem.* 23:1178–1183.

Kots, A.Y., K. Bian, and F. Murad. 2011. Nitric oxide and cyclic GMP signaling pathway as a focus for drug development. *Curr. Med. Chem.* 18:3299–3305.

Kwon, H., G. Wu, F.W. Bazer, and T.E. Spencer. 2003. Developmental changes in polyamine levels and synthesis in the ovine conceptus. *Biol. Reprod.* 69:1626–1634.

Lambert, M.W., S. Maddukuri, K.M. Karanfilian, M.L. Elias, and W.C. Lambert. 2019. The physiology of melanin deposition in health and disease. *Clin. Dermatol.* 37:402–417.

LaRosa, D.A., S.J. Ellery, D.W. Walker, and H. Dickinson. 2017. Understanding the full spectrum of organ injury following intrapartum asphyxia. *Front. Pediatr.* 5:16.

Larsson, T., E.O. Koppang, M. Espe, B.F. Terjesen, A. Krasnov, H.M. Moreno et al. 2014. Fillet quality and health of Atlantic salmon (*Salmo salar* L.) fed a diet supplemented with glutamate. *Aquaculture* 426:288–295.

Lee, C.L., T.A. Qiu, and J.V. Sweedler. 2020. D-Alanine: distribution, origin, physiological relevance, and implications in disease. *Biochim. Biophys. Acta* 1868:140482.

Le Floc'h, N., W. Otten, and E. Merlot. 2011. Tryptophan metabolism, from nutrition to potential therapeutic applications. *Amino Acids* 41:1195–1205.

Le Floc'h, N., A. Wessels, E. Corrent, G. Wu, and P. Bosi. 2018. The relevance of functional amino acids to support the health of growing pigs. *Anim. Feed Sci. Technol.* 245:104–116.

Lei, J., D.Y. Feng, Y.L. Zhang, F.Q. Zhao, Z.L. Wu, A. San Gabriel et al. 2012. Nutritional and regulatory role of branched-chain amino acids in lactation. *Front. Biosci.* 17:2725–2739.

Leib, D.E. and Z.A. Knight. 2016. Re-examination of dietary amino acid sensing reveals a GCN2-independent mechanism. *Cell Rep.* 13:1081–1089.

Lenis, Y.Y., G.A. Johnson, X.Q. Wang, W.W. Tang, K.A. Dunlap, M.C. Satterfield et al. 2018. Functional roles of ornithine decarboxylase and arginine decarboxylase during the peri-implantation period of pregnancy in sheep. *J. Anim. Sci. Biotechnol.* 9:10.

Leong, H.X., C. Simkevich, A. Lesieur-Brooks, B.W. Lau, C. Fugere, E. Sabo, and N.L. Thompson. 2006. Short-term arginine deprivation results in large-scale modulation of hepatic gene expression in both normal and tumor cells: microarray bioinformatics analysis. *Nutr. Metab.* 3:37.

Li, P. and G. Wu. 2018. Roles of dietary glycine, proline and hydroxyproline in collagen synthesis and animal growth. *Amino Acids* 50:29–38.

Li, P. and G. Wu. 2020. Composition of amino acids and related nitrogenous nutrients in feedstuffs for animal diets. *Amino Acids* 52:523–542.

Li, H., C.J. Meininger, J.R. Hawker Jr., T.E. Haynes, D. Kepka-Lenhart, S.K. Mistry et al. 2001. Regulatory role of arginase I and II in nitric oxide, polyamine, and proline syntheses in endothelial cells. *Am. J. Physiol.* 280:E75–E82.

Li, P., Y.L. Yin, D.F. Li, S.W. Kim, and G. Wu. 2007. Amino acids and immune function. *Br. J. Nutr.* 98:237–252.

Li, M., D.H. Kim, P.L. Tsenovoy, S.J. Peterson, R. Rezzani, L.F. Rodella et al. 2008. Treatment of obese diabetic mice with a heme oxygenase inducer reduces visceral and subcutaneous adiposity, increases adiponectin levels, and improves insulin sensitivity and glucose tolerance. *Diabetes* 57:1526–1535.

Li, X.L., F.W. Bazer, H. Gao, W. Jobgen, G.A. Johnson, P. Li et al. 2009. Amino acids and gaseous signaling. *Amino Acids* 37:65–78.

Li, X.L., F.W. Bazer, G.A. Johnson, R.C. Burghardt, J.W. Frank, Z.L. Dai et al. 2014. Dietary supplementation with L-arginine between days 14 and 25 of gestation enhances embryonic development and survival in gilts. *Amino Acids* 46:375–384.

Li, X.Y., S.X. Zheng, and G. Wu. 2020a. Amino acid metabolism in the kidneys: nutritional and physiological significance. *Adv. Exp. Med. Biol.* 1265:71–95.

Li, X.L., S.X. Zheng, and G. Wu. 2020b. Nutrition and metabolism of glutamate and glutamine in fish. *Amino Acids* 52:671–691.

Li, S.L., Y.C. Zhang, N. Liu, J.Q. Chen, L.N. Guo, Z.L. Dai et al. 2020c. Dietary L-arginine supplementation reduces lipid accretion by regulating fatty acid metabolism in Nile tilapia (*Oreochromis niloticus*). *J. Anim. Sci. Biotechnol.* 11:82.

Li, X.Y., T. Han, S.X. Zheng, and G. Wu. 2021a. Nutrition and functions of amino acids in aquatic crustaceans. *Adv. Exp. Med. Biol.* 1285:169–197.

Li, X.Y., S.X. Zheng, and G. Wu. 2021b. Nutrition and functions of amino acids in fish. *Adv. Exp. Med. Biol.* 1285:133–168.

Liang, H.W., Z.L. Dai, X.S. Ma, N. Liu, Y. Ji, J.Q. Chen et al. 2018. Dietary L-tryptophan modulates the structural and functional composition of the intestinal microbiome in weaned piglets. *Front. Microbiol.* 9:1736.

Liang, H.W., Z.L. Dai, J. Kou, K.J. Sun, J.Q. Chen, Y. Yang et al. 2019. Dietary L-tryptophan supplementation enhances the intestinal mucosal barrier function in weaned piglets: Implication of tryptophan-metabolizing microbiota. *Int. J. Mol. Sci.* 20:20.

Lin, C.M., S.F. Abcouwer, and W.W. Souba. 1999. Effect of dietary glutamate on chemotherapy-induced immunosuppression. *Nutrition* 15:687–696.

Liu, X.D., X. Wu, Y.L. Yin, Y.Q. Liu, M.M. Geng, H.S. Yang et al. 2012. Effects of dietary L-arginine or *N*-carbamylglutamate supplementation during late gestation of sows on the miR-15b/16, miR-221/222, VEGFA and eNOS expression in umbilical vein. *Amino Acids* 42:2111–2119.

Liu, J.W., K.S. Mai, W. Xu, and Q.H. Ai. 2015. Effects of dietary glutamine on survival, growth performance, activities of digestive enzyme, antioxidant status and hypoxia stress resistance of half-smooth tongue sole (*Cynoglossus semilaevis* Günther) post larvae. *Aquaculture* 446:48–56.

Liu, N., Z.L. Dai, Y.C. Zhang, J.Q. Chen, Y. Yang, G. Wu et al. 2019. Maternal L-proline supplementation enhances fetal survival and placental nutrient transport in mice. *Biol. Reprod.* 100:1073–1081.

Liu, N., J.Q. Chen, Y. He, H. Jia, D. Jiang, S. Li et al. 2020. Effects of maternal L-proline supplementation on inflammatory cytokines at the placenta and fetus interface of mice. *Amino Acids* 52:587–596.

Lubec, B., H. Hoeger, K. Kremser, G. Amann, D.Y. Koller, and J. Gialamas. 1996. Decreased tumor incidence and increased survival by one year oral low dose arginine supplementation in the mouse. *Life Sci.* 58:2317–2325.

Ma, Q., K.E. Williamson, D. O'Rourke, and B.J. Rowlands. 1999. The effects of L-arginine on crypt cell hyperproliferation in colorectal cancer. *J. Surg. Res.* 81:181–188.

Ma, X.Y., G.L. Zhou, Y.C. Lin, Z.Y. Jiang, C.T. Zheng, and F. Chen. 2011. Effects of sodium glutamate supplementation on growth performance and meat flavor of yellow-feathered broilers. *Chinese J. Anim. Nutr.* 23:410–416.

MacKay, M., M. Kravtsenyuk, R. Thomas, N.D. Mitchell, S.M. Dursun, and G.B. Baker. 2019. D-Serine: potential therapeutic agent and/or biomarker in schizophrenia and depression? *Front. Psychiatry* z10:25.

Magnuson, B.A., G.A. Burdock, J. Doull, R.M. Kroes, G.M. Marsh, M.W. Pariza et al. 2007. Aspartame: a safety evaluation based on current use levels, regulations, and toxicological and epidemiological studies. *Crit. Rev. Toxicol.* 37:629–727.

Mannion, A.F., P.M. Jakeman, M. Dunnett, R.C. Harris, and P.L. Willan. 1992. Carnosine and anserine concentrations in the quadriceps femoris muscle of healthy humans. *Eur. J. Appl. Physiol. Occup. Physiol.* 64:47–50.

Marcinkiewicz, J. and E. Kontny. 2014. Taurine and inflammatory diseases. *Amino Acids* 46:7–20.

Marescau, B., I.A. Qureshi, P. De Deyn, J. Letarte, R. Ryba, and A. Lowenthal. 1985. Guanidino compounds in plasma, urine and cerebrospinal fluid of hyperargininemic patients during therapy. *Clin. Chim. Acta* 146:21–27.

Marino, L.V. and P.C. Calder. 2017. Glutamine and the immune system. In: *Glutamine: Biochemistry, Physiology, and Clinical Applications* (Meynial-Denis, D., ed). CRC Press, Boca Raton, FL. pp. 293–314.

Marshall, S., V. Bacote, and R. Traxinger. 1991. Discovery of a metabolic pathway mediating glucose-induced desensitization of the glucose transport system. Role of hexosamine biosynthesis in the induction of insulin resistance. *J. Biol. Chem.* 266:4706–4712.

Maruyama, K., M.L. Sunde, and A.E. Harper. 1976. Is L-glutamic acid nutritionally a dispensable amino acid for the young chick? *Poult. Sci.* 55:45–60.

Mateo, R.D., G. Wu, F.W. Bazer, J.C. Park, I. Shinzato, and S.W. Kim. 2007. Dietary L-arginine supplementation enhances the reproductive performance of gilts. *J. Nutr.* 137:652–656.

McBurney, M., L.S. Young, T.R. Ziegler, and D.W. Wilmore. 1994. A cost-evaluation of glutamine-supplemented parenteral nutrition in adult bone marrow transplant patients. *J. Am. Diet. Assoc.* 94:1263–12666.

McClave, S.A., B.E. Taylor, R.G. Martindale, M.M. Warren, D.R. Johnson, C. Braunschweig et al. 2016. Guidelines for the provision and assessment of nutrition support therapy in the adult critically ill patient: Society of Critical Care Medicine (SCCM) and American Society for Parenteral and Enteral Nutrition (A.S.P.E.N.). *JPEN* 40:159–211.

McKnight, J.R., M.C. Satterfield, W.S. Jobgen, S.B. Smith, T.E. Spencer, C.J. Meininger et al. 2010. Beneficial effects of L-arginine on reducing obesity: Potential mechanisms and important implications for human health. *Amino Acids* 39:349–357.

McNeal, C.J., C.J. Meininger, D. Reddy, C.D. Wilborn, and G. Wu. 2016. Safety and effectiveness of arginine in adults. *J. Nutr.* 146:2587S–2593S.

McNeal, C.J., C.J. Meininger, C.D. Wilborn, C.D. Tekwe, and G. Wu. 2018. Safety of dietary supplementation with arginine in adult humans. *Amino Acids* 50:1215–1229.

Meister, A. and M.E. Anderson. 1983. Glutathione. *Annu. Rev. Biochem.* 52:711–760.

Melis, G.C., N. ter Wengel, P.G. Boelens, and P.A.M. van Leeuwen. 2004. Glutamine: recent developments in research on the clinical significance of glutamine. *Curr. Opin. Clin. Nutr. Metab. Care* 7:59–70.

Meyer, R.A. Jr., C.M. Henley, M.H. Meyer, P.L. Morgan, A.G. McDonald, C. Mills and D.K. Price. 1998. Partial deletion of both the spermine synthase gene and the *Pex* gene in the X-linked hypophosphatemic, Gyro (Gy) mouse. *Genomics* 48:289–295.

Mittal, V. 2004. Improving the efficiency of RNA interference in mammals. *Nat. Rev. Genet.* 5:355–365.

Moffett, J.R. 2003. Tryptophan and the immune system. *Immunol. Cell Biol.* 81:247–265.

Moncada, S. and A. Higgs. 1993. The L-arginine-nitric oxide pathway. *New Engl. J. Med.* 329:2002–2012.

Moore, P.K. and M. Whiteman. 2015. *Chemistry, Biochemistry and Pharmacology of Hydrogen Sulfide.* Springer, New York.

Morlion, B.J., P. Stehle, P. Wachtler, H. Siedhoff, M. Koller, W. Konig et al. 1998. Total parenteral nutrition with glutamine dipeptide after major abdominal surgery: a randomized, double-blind, controlled study. *Ann. Surg.* 227:302–308.

Mudd, S.H., J.T. Brosnan, M.E. Brosnan, R.L. Jacobs, S.P. Stabler, R.H. Allen et al. 2007. Methyl balance and transmethylation fluxes in humans. *Am. J. Clin. Nutr.* 85:19–25.

Nakahira, K., H.P. Kim, X.H. Geng, A. Nakao, X. Wang, N. Murase et al. 2006. Carbon monoxide differentially inhibits TLR signaling pathways by regulating ROS-induced trafficking of TLRs to lipid rafts. *J. Exp. Med.* 203:2377–2389.

Nakamura, H., Y. Kawamata, T. Kuwahara, M. Smriga, and R. Sakai. 2013. Long-term ingestion of monosodium L-glutamate did not induced obesity, dyslipidemia or insulin resistance: a two-generation study in mice. *J. Nutr. Sci. Vitaminol.* 59:129–135.

National Institute of Mental Health (NIMH 2021) Mental illness. U.S. National Institutes of Health. https://www.nimh.nih.gov/health/statistics/mental-illness.shtml. Accessed April 18, 2021.

Newsholme, P., R. Curi, T.C.P. Curi, C.J. Murphy, C. Garcia, and M.P. de Melo. 1999. Glutamine metabolism by lymphocytes, macrophages, and neutrophils: its importance in health and disease. *J. Nutr. Biochem.* 10:316–324.

Nikam, R.R. and K.R. Gore. 2018. Journey of siRNA: Clinical developments and targeted delivery. *Nucleic Acid Ther.* 28:209–224.

Nithianandarajah-Jones, G.N., B. Wilm, C.E.P. Goldring, J. Müller, and M.J. Cross. 2012. ERK5: structure, regulation and function. *Cell. Signal.* 24:2187–2196.

Olubodun, J.O., I. Zulkifli, A.S. Farjam, M. Hair-Bejo, and A. Kasim. 2015. Glutamine and glutamic acid supplementation enhances performance of broiler chickens under the hot and humid tropical condition. *Italian J. Anim. Sci.* 14:3263.

Otterbein, L.E., F.H. Bach, J. Alam, M. Soares, H.T. Lu, M. Wysk et al. 2000. Carbon monoxide has anti-inflammatory effects involving the mitogen-activated protein kinase pathway. *Nat. Med.* 6:422–428, 2000.

Owen, G., C.P. Cherry, D.E. Prentice, and A.N. Worden. 1978. The feeding of diets containing up to 4% monosodium glutamate to rats for 2 years. *Toxicol. Lett.* 1:221–226.

Park, M.H. and E.C. Wolff. 2018. Hypusine, a polyamine-derived amino acid critical for eukaryotic translation. *J. Biol. Chem.* 293:18710–18718.

Patterson, S.D., M. Waldron, and O. Jeffries. 2019. Proteins and amino acids and physical exercise. In: *Nutrition and Skeletal Muscle* (Walrand, S., ed). Academic Press, San Diego, CA. pp. 183–196.

Pendeville, H., N. Carpino, J.-C. Marine, Y. Takahasi, M. Muller, J.A. Martial, and J.L. Cleveland. 2001. The ornithine decarboxylase gene is essential for cell survival during early murine development. *Mol. Cell. Biol.* 21:6549–6558.

Pegg, A.E. 2013. Toxicity of polyamines and their metabolic products. *Chem. Res. Toxicol.* 26:1782–1800.

Pegg, A.E. 2016. Functions of polyamines in mammals. *J. Biol. Chem.* 291:4904–14912.

Peters, V., V. Calabrese, E. Forsberg, N. Volk, T. Fleming, H. Baelde et al. 2018. Protective actions of anserine under diabetic conditions. *Int. J. Mol. Sci.* 19:2751.

Phang, J.M. and W. Liu. 2012. Proline metabolism and cancer. *Front. Biosci.* 17:1835–1845.

Phang, J.M., S.P. Donald, Pandhare J, and Y. Liu. 2008. The metabolism of proline, as a stress substrate, modulates carcinogenic pathways. *Amino Acids* 35:681–690.

Phang, J.M., W. Liu, and O. Zabirnyk. 2010. Proline metabolism and microenvironmental stress. *Annu. Rev. Nutr.* 30:441–463.

Phang, J.M., W. Liu, and C. Hancock. 2013. Bridging epigenetics and metabolism: role of non-essential amino acids. *Epigenetics* 8:231–236.

Philip, M., R.J. Snow, P.A. Della Gatta, N. Bellofiore, and S.J. Ellery. 2020. Creatine metabolism in the uterus: potential implications for reproductive biology. *Amino Acids* 52:1275–1283.

Pistollato, F., L. Persano, E. Rampazzo, and G. Basso. 2010. L-Proline as a modulator of ectodermal differentiation in ES cells. *Am. J. Physiol.* 298:C979–C981.

Platten, M., P.P. Ho, S. Youssef, P. Fontoura, H. Garren, E.M. Hur et al. 2005. Treatment of autoimmune neuroinflammation with a synthetic tryptophan metabolite. *Science* 310:850–855.

Pohlenz, C. and D.M. Gatlin III. 2014. Interrelationships between fish nutrition and health. *Aquaculture* 431:111–117.

Pohlenz, C., A. Buentello, A.M. Bakke, and D.M. Gatlin III. 2012a. Free dietary glutamine improves intestinal morphology and increases enterocyte migration rates, but has limited effects on plasma amino acid profile and growth performance of channel catfish *Ictalurus punctatus*. *Aquaculture* 370–371:32–39.

Pohlenz, C., A. Buentello, W. Mwangi, and D.M. Gatlin DM III. 2012b. Arginine and glutamine supplementation to culture media improves the performance of various channel catfish immune cells. *Fish Shellfish Immunol.* 32:762–768.

Polonikov, A. 2020. Endogenous deficiency of glutathione as the most likely cause of serious manifestations and death in COVID-19 patients. *ACS Infect. Dis.* 6:1558–1562.

Popovic, P.J., H.J. Zeh, and J.B. Ochoa. 2007. Arginine and immunity. *J. Nutr.* 137:1681S–1686S.

Porto, M.L., P.E.N. Givisiez, E.P. Saraiva, F.G.P. Costa, A.L.B. Moreira Filho, M.F.S. Andrade et al. 2015. Glutamic acid improves body weight gain and intestinal morphology of broiler chickens submitted to heat stress. *Rev. Bras. Cienc. Avic.* 17:355–362.

Queiroga, C.S.F., A. Vercelli, and H.L.A. Vieira. 2015. Carbon monoxide and the CNS: challenges and achievements. *Br. J. Pharmacol.* 172:1533–1545.

Rees, W.D., F.A. Wilson, and C.A. Maloney. 2006. Sulfur amino acid metabolism in pregnancy: the impact of methionine in the maternal diet. *J. Nutr.* 136:1701S–1705S.

Ren, W.K., S. Chen, J. Yin, J.L. Duan, T.J. Li, G. Liu et al. 2014a. Dietary arginine supplementation of mice alters the microbial population and activates intestinal innate immunity. *J. Nutr.* 144:988–995.

Ren, W.K., J.L. Duan, J. Yin, G. Liu, Z. Cao, X. Xion et al. 2014b. Dietary L-glutamine supplementation modulates microbial community and activates innate immunity in the mouse intestine. *Amino Acids* 46:2403–2413.

Ren, W.K., Y.L. Yin, B.Y. Zhou, F.W. Bazer, and G. Wu. 2018. Roles of arginine in cell-mediated and humoral immunity. In: *Nutrition, Immunity, and Infection* (Calder, P. and A.D. Kulkarni, eds). CRC Press, Boca Raton, FL. pp. 333–348.

Ren, W.K., P. Bin, Y.L. Yin, and G. Wu. 2020. Impacts of amino acids on the intestinal defensive system. *Adv. Exp. Med. Biol.* 1265:133–151.

Rezaei, R., D.A. Knabe, C.D. Tekwe, S. Dahanayaka, M.D. Ficken, S.E. Fielder et al. 2013. Dietary supplementation with monosodium glutamate is safe and improves growth performance in postweaning pigs. *Amino Acids* 44:911–923.

Rhoads, J.M. and G. Wu. 2009. Glutamine, arginine, and leucine signaling in the intestine. *Amino Acids* 37:111–122.

Ricciardolo, F.L.M., P.J. Sterk, B. Gaston, and G. Folkerts. 2004. Nitric oxide in health and disease of the respiratory system. *Physiol. Rev.* 84:731–765.

Roberts, A. 2016. The safety and regulatory process for amino acids in Europe and the United States. *J. Nutr.* 146:2635S–2642S.

Rodionov, R.N., H. Begmatov, N. Jarzebska, K. Patel, M.T. Mills, Z. Ghani et al. 2019. Homoarginine supplementation prevents left ventricular dilatation and preserves systolic function in a model of coronary artery disease. *J. Am. Heart Assoc.* 8:e012486.

Rodríguez-Ramos, T., Y. Carpio, J. Bolívar, G. Espinosa, J. Hernández-López, T. Gollas-Galván et al. 2010. An inducible nitric oxide synthase (NOS) is expressed in hemocytes of the spiny lobster *Panulirus argus*: cloning, characterization and expression analysis. *Fish Shellfish Immunol.* 29:469–479.

Roper, S.D. 2006. Cell communication in taste buds. *Cell. Mol. Life Sci.* 63:1494–1500.

Rothhammer, V. and F.J. Quintana. 2019. The aryl hydrocarbon receptor: an environmental sensor integrating immune responses in health and disease. *Nat. Rev. Immunol.* 19:184–197.

Ruth, M.R. and C.J. Field. 2013. The immune modifying effects of amino acids on gut-associated lymphoid tissue. *J. Anim. Sci. Biotechnol.* 4:27.

Ryter, S.W., J. Alam, and A.M.K. Choi. 2006. Heme oxygenase-1/carbon monoxide: from basic science to therapeutic applications. *Physiol. Rev.* 86:583–650.

Sahai, A., X.M. Pan, R. Paul, P. Malladi, R. Kohli, and P.F. Whitington. 2006. Roles of phosphatidylinositol 3kinase and osteopontin in steatosis and aminotransferase release by hepatocytes treated with methionine-choline-deficient medium. *Am. J. Physiol.* 291:G55–G62.

Salazar, J., L. Bello, M. Chávez, R. Añez, J. Rojas, and V. Bermúdez. 2014. Glucosamine for osteoarthritis: biological effects, clinical efficacy, and safety on glucose metabolism. *Arthritis* 2014:432463.

Salinas, I. 2015. The mucosal immune system of teleost fish. *Biology* 4:525–539.

Salmanzadeh, M. and H.A. Shahryar. 2013. Effects of dietary supplementation with glutamine on growth performance, small intestinal morphology and carcass traits in turkey poults under heat stress. *Revue Med. Vet.* 164:476–480.

San Gabriel, A. and H. Uneyama. 2013. Amino acid sensing in the gastrointestinal tract. *Amino Acids* 45:451–461.

San Gabriel, A., H. Uneyama, S. Yoshie, and K. Torii. 2005. Cloning and characterization of a novel mGluR1 variant from vallate papillae that functions as a receptor for L-glutamate stimuli. *Chem. Senses* 30 (Suppl 1):i25–26.

San Gabriel, A., T. Maekawa, H. Uneyama, and K. Torii. 2009. Metabotropic glutamate receptor type 1 in taste tissue. *Am. J. Clin. Nutr.* 90:743S–746S.

Sasse, C.E. and D.H. Baker. 1973. Modification of the Illinois reference standard amino acid mixture. *Poult. Sci.* 52:1970–1972.

Schwab, C.G. and G.A. Broderick. 2017. A 100-year review: protein and amino acid nutrition in dairy cows. *J. Dairy Sci.* 100:10094–10112.

Shao, A. and J.N. Hathcock. 2008. Risk assessment for the amino acids taurine, L-glutamine and L-arginine. *Reg. Toxicol. Pharmacol.* 50:376–399.

Shen, Y.B., G. Voilqué, J.D. Kim, J. Odle, and S.W. Kim. 2012. Effects of increasing tryptophan intake on growth and physiological changes in nursery pigs. *J. Anim. Sci.* 90:2264–2275.

Shewchuk, L.D., V.E. Baracos, and C.J. Field. 1997. Dietary L-glutamine supplementation reduces the growth of the Morris Hepatoma 7777 in exercise-trained and sedentary rats. *J. Nutr.* 127:158–166.

Shimazu, T., H. Ikeuchi, H. Sugimoto, C.W. Goodwin, A.D. Mason Jr., and B.A. Pruitt Jr. 2000. Half-life of blood carboxyhemoglobin after short-term and long-term exposure to carbon monoxide. *J. Trauma.* 49:126–131.

Shoemaker, C., D.H. Xu, B. LaFrentz, and S. LaPatra. 2015. Overview of fish immune system and infectious diseases. In: *Dietary Nutrients, Additives and Fish Health* (Lee, C.S., C. Lim, D.M. Gatlin III, and C.D. Webster, eds). Wiley, Hoboken, NJ. pp. 1–24.

Sies, H. 1999. Glutathione and its role in cellular functions. *Free Radic. Biol. Med.* 27:916–921.

Silvagno, F., A. Vernone, and G.P. Pescarmona. 2020. The role of glutathione in protecting against the severe inflammatory response triggered by COVID-19. *Antioxidants* 9:624.

Simmons, R.M., S.M. McKnight, A.K. Edwards, G. Wu, and M.C. Satterfield. 2020. Obesity increases hepatic glycine dehydrogenase and aminomethyltransferase expression while dietary glycine supplementation reduces white adipose tissue in Zucker diabetic fatty rats. *Amino Acids* 52:1413–1423.

Simon, R.R., V. Marks, A.R. Leeds, and J.W. Anderson. 2011. A comprehensive review of oral glucosamine use and effects on glucose metabolism in normal and diabetic individuals. *Diabetes Metab. Res. Rev.* 27: 14–27.

Singer, P., A.R. Blaser, M.M. Berger, W. Alhazzani, P.C. Calder, M.P. Casaer et al. 2019. ESPEN guideline on clinical nutrition in the intensive care unit. *Clin. Nutr.* 38:48–79.

Smriga, M. 2020. International regulations on amino acid use in foods and supplements and recommendations to control their safety based on purity and quality. *J. Nutr.* 150:2602S–2605S.

Smriga, M. and K. Torii. 2003. L-Lysine acts like a partial serotonin receptor 4 antagonist and inhibits serotonin-mediated intestinal pathologies and anxiety in rats. *Proc. Natl. Acad. Sci. USA* 100:15370–15375.

Söderhäll, K. and L. Cerenius. 1992. Crustacean immunity. *Annu. Rev. Fish Dis.* 2:3–23.

Soltan, M.A. 2009. Influence of dietary glutamine supplementation on growth performance, small intestinal morphology, immune response and some blood parameters of broiler chickens. *Int. J. Poult. Sci.* 8:60–68.

Stachlewitz, R.F., X. Li, S. Smith, H. Bunzendahl, L.M. Graves, and R.G. Thurman. 2000. Glycine inhibits growth of T lymphocytes by an IL-2-independent mechanism. *J. Immunol.* 164:176–182.Stover, P.J. and M.S. Field. 2011. Trafficking of intracellular folates. *Adv. Nutr.* 2:325–331.

Strasser, B., J.M. Gostner, and D. Fuchs. 2016. Mood, food, and cognition: role of tryptophan and serotonin. *Curr. Opin. Clin. Nutr. Metab. Care* 19:55–61.

Stuckey, D.J., D.C. Anthony, J.P. Lowe, J. Miller, W.M. Palm, P. Styles et al. 2005. Detection of the inhibitory neurotransmitter GABA in macrophages by magnetic resonance spectroscopy. *J. Leukoc Biol.* 78:393–400.

Sun, Y.L., Z.L. Wu, W. Li, C. Zhang, K.J. Sun, Y. Ji, B. Wang et al. 2015. Dietary L-leucine supplementation enhances intestinal development in suckling piglets. *Amino Acids* 47:1517–1525.

Sun, K.J., Z.L. Wu, Y. Ji, and G. Wu. 2016. Glycine regulates protein turnover by activating Akt/mTOR and inhibiting expression of genes involved in protein degradation in C2C12 myoblasts. *J. Nutr.* 146:2461–2467.

Suryawan, A. and T.A. Davis. 2011. Regulation of protein synthesis by amino acids in muscle of neonates. *Front. Biosci.* 16:1445–1460.

Suryawan, A., M. Rudar, M.L. Fiorotto, and T.A. Davis. 2020. Differential regulation of mTORC1 activation by leucine and β-hydroxy-β-methylbutyrate in skeletal muscle of neonatal pigs. *J. Appl. Physiol.* 128:286–295.

Tajiri, K. and Y. Shimizu. 2013. Branched-chain amino acids in liver diseases. *World J. Gastroenterol.* 19:7620–7629.

Tan, B.E., Y.L. Yin, Z.Q. Liu, X.G. Li, H.J. Xu, X.F. Kong et al. 2009. Dietary L-arginine supplementation increases muscle gain and reduces body fat mass in growing-finishing pigs. *Amino Acids* 37:169–175.

Thangam, E.B., E.A. Jemima, H. Singh, M.S. Baig, M. Khan, C.B. Mathias et al. 2018. The role of histamine and histamine receptors in mast cell-mediated allergy and inflammation: The hunt for new therapeutic targets. *Front. Immunol.* 9:1873.

Tomé, D. 2004. Protein, amino acids and the control of food intake. *Br. J. Nutr.* 92(Suppl. 1):S27–S30.

Tomé, D. 2018. The roles of dietary glutamate in the intestine. *Ann. Nutr. Metab.* 73(Suppl.) 5:15–20.

Trichet, V.V. 2010. Nutrition and immunity: an update. *Aquac. Res.* 41:356–372.

Tsikas, D., A. Bollenbach, E. Hanff, and A.A. Kayacelebi. 2018. Asymmetric dimethylarginine (ADMA), symmetric dimethylarginine (SDMA) and homoarginine (hArg): the ADMA, SDMA and hArg paradoxes. *Cardiovasc. Diabetol.* 17:1.

Tsubuku, S., K. Hatayama, K. Mawatari, M. Smriga, and T. Kimura. 2004a. Thirteen-week oral toxicity study of L-arginine in rats. *Int. J. Toxicol.* 23:101–105.

Tsubuku, S., K. Hatayam, K. Mawatari, M. Smriga, and T. Kimura. 2004b. Thirteen week oral toxicity study of L-glutamine in rats. *Int. J. Toxicol.* 23:107–112.

Uneyama, H., A. Nijjima, A. San Gabriel, and K. Torii. 2006. Luminal amino acid sensing in the rat gastric mucosa. *Am. J. Physiol.* 291:G1163–G1170.

Vallet, J.L., J.R. Miles, and L.A. Rempe. 2013. Effect of creatine supplementation during the last week of gestation on birth intervals, stillbirth, and preweaning mortality in pigs. *J. Anim. Sci.* 91:2122–2132.

Van Zanten, A.R.H., F. Sztark, U.X. Kaisers, S. Zielmann, T.W. Felbinger, A.R. Sablotzki et al. 2014. High-protein enteral nutrition enriched with immune-modulating nutrients vs standard high protein enteral nutrition and nosocomial infections in the ICU. *JAMA* 312:514–524.

Vazquez, L., J. Alpuche, G. Maldonado, C. Agundis, A. Pereyra-Morales, and E. Zenteno. 2009. Immunity mechanisms in crustaceans. *Innate Immunity* 15:179–188.

Venkatakrishnan, A.J., X. Deupi, G. Lebon, C.G. Tate, G.F. Schertler, and M.M. Babu. 2013. Molecular signatures of G-protein-coupled receptors. *Nature* 494:185–194.

Wagner, E.F. and A.R. Nebreda. 2009. Signal integration by JNK and p38 MAPK pathways in cancer development. *Nat. Rev. Cancer* 9:537–549.

Walker, R. and J.R. Lupien. 2000. The safety evaluation of monosodium glutamate. *J. Nutr.* 130:1049S–1052S.

Wallimann, T., M. Tokarska-Schlattner, and U. Schlattner. 2011. The creatine kinase system and pleiotropic effects of creatine. *Amino Acids* 40:1271–1296.

Wang, T.C. and M.F. Fuller. 1989. The optimum dietary amino acid patterns for growing pigs. 1. Experiments by amino acid deletion. *Br. J. Nutr.* 62:77–89.

Wang. X. and M. Watford. 2007. Glutamine, insulin and glucocorticoids regulate glutamine synthetase expression in C2C12 myotubes, Hep G2 hepatoma cells and 3T3 L1 adipocytes. *Biochim. Biophys. Acta* 1770:594–600.

Wang, J.J., L.X. Chen, P. Li, X.L. Li, H.J. Zhou, F.L. Wang et al. 2008. Gene expression is altered in piglet small intestine by weaning and dietary glutamine supplementation. *J. Nutr.* 138:1025–1032.

Wang, W.W., X.F. Zeng, X.B. Mao, G. Wu, and S.Y. Qiao. 2010. Optimal dietary true ileal digestible threonine for supporting mucosal barrier in the small intestine of weanling pigs. *J. Nutr.* 140:981–986.

Wang, J.J., Z.L. Wu, D.F. Li, N. Li, S.V. Dindot, M.C. Satterfield et al. 2012. Nutrition, epigenetics, and metabolic syndrome. *Antioxid. Redox Signal.* 17:282–301.

Wang, W.W., Z.L. Wu, Z.L. Dai, Y. Yang, J.J. Wang, and G. Wu. 2013. Glycine metabolism in animals and humans: implications for nutrition and health. *Amino Acids* 45:463–477.

Wang, W.W., Z.L. Wu, G. Lin, S.D. Hu, B. Wang, Z.L. Dai, and G. Wu. 2014a. Glycine stimulates protein synthesis and inhibits oxidative stress in pig small-intestinal epithelial cells. *J. Nutr.* 144:1540–1548.

Wang, X.Q., W. Ying, K.A. Dunlap, G. Lin, M.C. Satterfield, R.C. Burghardt et al. 2014b. Arginine decarboxylase and agmatinase: an alternative pathway for de novo biosynthesis of polyamines for development of mammalian conceptuses. *Biol. Reprod.* 90:84.

Wang, W.W., Z.L. Dai, Z.L. Wu, G. Lin, S.C. Jia, S.D. Hu et al. 2014c. Glycine is a nutritionally essential amino acid for maximal growth of milk-fed young pigs. *Amino Acids* 46:2037–2045.

Wang, H., Y. Ji, G. Wu, K.J. Sun, Y.L. Sun, W. Li et al. 2015a. L-Tryptophan activates mammalian target of rapamycin and enhances expression of tight junction proteins in intestinal porcine epithelial cells. *J. Nutr.* 145:1156–1162.

Wang, X.Q., R.C. Burghardt, J.J. Romero, T.R. Hansen, G. Wu, and F.W. Bazer. 2015b. Functional roles of arginine during the peri-implantation period of pregnancy. III. Arginine stimulates proliferation and interferon tau production by ovine trophectoderm cells via nitric oxide and polyamine-TSC2-MTOR signaling pathways. *Biol. Reprod.* 92(3):75.

Wang, B., S.Q. Sun, M.Y. Liu, H. Chen, N. Liu, Z.L. Wu et al. 2020. Dietary L-tryptophan supplementation regulates colonic serotonin homeostasis and inhibits gut inflammation in mice with dextran sodium sulfate-induced colitis. *J. Nutr.* 150:1966–1976.

Watford, M. 2008. Glutamine metabolism and function in relation to proline synthesis and the safety of glutamine and proline supplementation. *J. Nutr.* 138:2003S–2007S.

Wei, L.H., G. Wu, S.M. Morris Jr., and L.J. Ignarro. 2001. Elevated arginase I expression in rat aortic smooth muscle cells increases cell proliferation. *Proc. Natl. Acad. Sci. USA* 98:9260–9264.

Welbourne, T.C. 1995. Increased plasma bicarbonate and growth hormone after an oral glutamine load. *Am. J. Clin. Nutr.* 61:1058–1061.

Westerterp-Plantenga, M.S., A. Nieuwenhuizen, D. Tomé, S. Soenen, and K.R. Westerterp. 2009. Dietary protein, weight loss, and weight maintenance. *Annu. Rev. Nutr.* 29:21–41.

Wetzel, M.D., T. Gao, M. Venkatachalam, S.M. Morris Jr., and A.S. Awad. 2019. L-Homoarginine supplementation prevents diabetic kidney damage. *Physiol. Rep.* 7:e14235.

Wheeler, M.D. and R.G. Thurman. 1999. Production of superoxide and TNF-α from alveolar macrophages is blunted by glycine. *Am. J. Physiol.* 277:L952–L959.

Whitfield, N.L., E.L. Kreimier, F.C. Verdial, N. Skovgaard, and K.R. Olson. 2008. Reappraisal of H_2S/sulfide concentration in vertebrate blood and its potential significance in ischemic preconditioning and vascular signaling. *Am. J. Physiol.* 294:R1930–1937.

Wieczorek-Surdacka, E., E. Hanff, B. Chyrchel, M. Kuźniewski, A. Surdacki, and D. Tsikas. 2019. Distinct associations between plasma osteoprotegerin, homoarginine and asymmetric dimethylarginine in chronic kidney disease male patients with coronary artery disease. *Amino Acids* 51:977–982.

Wong, A.W., B.A. Magnuson, K. Nakagawa, and R.G. Bursey. 2011. Oral subchronic and genotoxicity studies conducted with the amino acid, L-glutamine. *Food Chem. Toxicol.* 49:2096–2102.

Wright, C.E., H.H. Tallan, Y.Y. Lin, and G.E. Gaull. 1986. Taurine: biological update. *Annu. Rev. Biochem.* 55:427–453.

Wu, G. 2009. Amino acids: metabolism, functions, and nutrition. *Amino Acids* 37:1–17.

Wu, G. 2010. Functional amino acids in growth, reproduction and health. *Adv. Nutr.* 1:31–37.

Wu, G. 2013. Arginine and immune function. In: *Diet, Immunity, and Inflammation* (Calder, P.C. and P. Yaqoob, eds). Woodhead Publishing, Cambridge, UK. pp. 523–543.

Wu, G. 2018. *Principles of animal nutrition.* CRC Press, Boca Raton, FL.

Wu, G. 2020a. Metabolism and functions of amino acids in sense organs. *Adv. Exp. Med. Biol.* 1265:201–217.

Wu, G. 2020b. Important roles of dietary taurine, creatine, carnosine, anserine and hydroxyproline in human nutrition and health. *Amino Acids* 52:329–360.

Wu, G. 2020c. Management of metabolic disorders (including metabolic diseases) in ruminant and nonruminant animals. In: *Animal Agriculture: Challenges, Innovations, and Sustainability* (Bazer, F.W., G.C. Lamb, and G. Wu, eds). Elsevier, New York. pp. 471–492.

Wu, G. 2020d. Metabolism and functions of amino acids in sense organs. *Adv. Exp. Med. Biol.* 1265:201–217.

Wu, G., and C.J. Meininger. 2000. Arginine nutrition and cardiovascular function. *J. Nutr.* 130:2626–2629.

Wu, G., and C.J. Meininger. 2002. Regulation of nitric oxide synthesis by dietary factors. *Annu. Rev. Nutr.* 22:61–86.

Wu, L. and R. Wang. 2005. Carbon monoxide: endogenous production, physiological functions, and pharmacological applications. *Pharmacol. Rev* 57:585–630.

Wu, G., C.J. Field, and E.B. Marliss. 1992. Enhanced glutamine and glucose metabolism in cultured rat splenocytes stimulated by phorbol myristate acetate plus ionomycin. *Metabolism* 41:982–988.

Wu, G., N.E. Flynn, and D.A. Knabe. 2000. Enhanced intestinal synthesis of polyamines from proline in cortisol-treated piglets. *Am. J. Physiol.* 279:E395–E402.

Wu, G., Y.Z. Fang, S. Yang, J.R. Lupton, and N.D. Turner. 2004. Glutathione metabolism and its implications for health. *J. Nutr.* 134:489–492.

Wu, G., F.W. Bazer, J. Hu, G.A. Johnson, and T.E. Spencer. 2005. Polyamine synthesis from proline in the developing porcine placenta. *Biol. Reprod.* 72:842–850.

Wu, G., F.W. Bazer, T.A. Davis, S.W. Kim, P. Li, J.M. Rhoads et al. 2009. Arginine metabolism and nutrition in growth, health and disease. *Amino Acids* 37:153–168.

Wu, G., F.W. Bazer, G.A. Johnson, D.A. Knabe, R.C. Burghardt, T.E. Spencer et al. 2011a. Important roles for L-glutamine in swine nutrition and production. *J. Anim. Sci.* 89:2017–2030.

Wu, G., F.W. Bazer, R.C. Burghardt, G.A. Johnson, S.W. Kim, D.A. Knabe et al. 2011b. Proline and hydroxy-proline metabolism: implications for animal and human nutrition. *Amino Acids* 40:1053–1063.

Wu, Z.L., Y.Q. Hou, S.D. Hu, F.W. Bazer, C.J. Meininger, C.J. McNeal, and G. Wu. 2016. Catabolism and safety of supplemental L-arginine in animals. *Amino Acids* 48:1541–1552.

Wu, G., F.W. Bazer, G.A. Johnson, and Y.Q. Hou. 2018. Arginine nutrition and metabolism in growing, gestat-ing and lactating swine. *J. Anim. Sci.* 96:5035–5051.

Wu, Z.L., Y.Q. Hou, Z.L. Dai, C.A. Hu, and G. Wu. 2019. Metabolism, nutrition and redox signaling of hydroxyproline. *Antioxid. Redox Signal.* 30:674–682.

Wyss, M. and R. Kaddurah-Daouk. 2000. Creatine and creatinine metabolism. *Physiol. Rev.* 80:1107–1213.

Xi, P.B., Z.Y. Jiang, Z.L. Dai, X.L. Li, K. Yao, C.T. Zheng et al. 2012. Regulation of protein turnover by L-glutamine in porcine intestinal epithelial cells. *J. Nutr. Biochem.* 23:1012–1017.

Yan, L. and X.Q. Zhou. 2006. Dietary glutamine supplementation improves structure and function of intestine of juvenile Jian carp (*Cyprinus carpio* var. Jian). *Aquaculture* 256:389–394.

Yang, Y., Z.L. Wu, S.C. Jia, S. Dahanayaka, S. Feng, C.J. Meininger et al. 2015. Safety of long-term dietary supplementation with L-arginine in rats. *Amino Acids* 47:1907–1920.

Yoshida, C., M. Maekawa, M. Bannai, and T. Yamamoto. 2016. Glutamate promotes nucleotide synthesis in the gut and improves availability of soybean meal feed in rainbow trout. *SpringerPlus* 5:1021.

Young, L.S., R. Bye, M. Scheltinga, T.R. Ziegler, D.O. Jacobs, and D.W. Wilmore. 1993. Patients receiving glutamine supplemented intravenous feedings report an improvement in mood. *JPEN* 17:422–427.

Zhang, J., Y.L. Yin, X.G. Shu, T.J. Li, F.N. Li, B.E. Tan et al. 2013. Oral administration of MSG increases expression of glutamate receptors and transporters in the gastrointestinal tract of young piglets. *Amino Acids* 45:1169–1177.

Zhang, S., E.A. Wong, and E.R. Gilbert. 2015. Bioavailability of different dietary supplemental methionine sources in animals. *Front. Biosci. E* 7:478–490.

Zhang, Y., L. Zhao, Y. Zhou, C. Diao, L. Han, N. Yinjie et al. 2017a. Glutamine ameliorates mucosal damage caused by immune responses to duck plague virus. *Dose-Response* 2017:1–11.

Zhang, K., K. Mai, W. Xu, Z. Liufu, Y. Zhang, M. Peng et al. 2017b. Effects of dietary arginine and glutamine on growth performance, nonspecific immunity, and disease resistance in relation to arginine catabolism in juvenile turbot (*Scophthalmus maximus* L.) *Aquaculture* 468:246–254.

Zhang, Y.C., H. Jia, Y.H. Jin, N. Liu, J.Q. Chen, Y. Yang et al. 2020. Glycine attenuates LPS-induced apoptosis and inflammatory cell infiltration in mouse liver. *J. Nutr.* 150:1116–1125.

Zhang, Q., Y.Q. Hou, F.W. Bazer, W.L. He, E.A. Posey, and G. Wu. 2021. Amino acids in swine nutrition and production. *Adv. Exp. Med. Biol.* 1285:81–107.

Zhao, Y., Y. Hu, X.Q. Zhou, X.Y. Zeng, L. Feng, Y. Liu et al. 2015. Effects of dietary glutamate supplementa-tion on growth performance, digestive enzyme activities and antioxidant capacity in intestine of grass carp (*Ctenopharyngodon idella*). *Aquac. Nutr.* 21:935–941.

Zhong, Z, Wheeler MD, Li X, M. Froh, P. Schemmer, M. Yin et al. 2003. L-Glycine: a novel antiinflammatory, immunomodulatory, and cytoprotective agent. *Curr. Opin. Clin. Nutr. Metab. Care* 6:229–240.

Zhu, Y.H., T.T. Li, S.M. Huang, W. Wang, Z.L. Dai, C.P. Feng et al. 2018. Maternal L-glutamine supplemen-tation during late-gestation improves intrauterine growth restriction-induced intestinal dysfunction in piglets. *Amino Acids* 50:1289–1299.

Ziegler, T.R., R.L. Bye, R.L. Persinger, L. Young, J. Antin, and D.W. Wilmore. 1998. Effects of glutamine supplementation on circulating lymphocytes after bone marrow transplantation: a pilot study. *Am. J. Med. Sci.* 315:4–10.

12 Inborn Errors of Amino Acid Metabolism

The term "inborn errors of metabolism" was coined in 1908 by the British physician Archibald Garrod who reported the first case of inherited disorders of cystine metabolism in humans. Since then, over 80 disorders of inborn metabolism of amino acids (AAs) have been reported for humans (Aliu et al. 2018; Endo et al. 2004; Kožich and Stabler 2020; Rumping et al. 2020). Many of these diseases are autosomal recessive disorders, as two copies of the recessive, defective gene (one from each parent) occur on autosomal chromosomes (see the section below). The mutations of genes cause a partial or complete absence of proteins (including enzymes) and cofactors for: (1) the transport (including intestinal absorption and renal reabsorption) or the synthesis or catabolism of AAs; (2) the impaired detoxification of ammonia via the urea cycle and glutamine synthesis; and (3) the impaired syntheses of bioactive molecules, such as glutathione, creatine, carnitine, polyamines, and nitric oxide (NO) (Figure 12.1). The clinical diagnosis often includes analyses of metabolites in the plasma, urine, and cerebrospinal fluid. Concentrations of AA metabolites in these fluids depend on a plethora of factors, including: (1) the digestion of dietary protein; (2) the intestinal absorption of AAs into the portal circulation; (3) the uptake of AAs from the plasma by extraintestinal tissues; (4) the cell-specific synthesis and catabolism of AAs; (5) the rate of intracellular protein turnover (synthesis and degradation); (6) the reabsorption of luminal AAs by the renal proximal tubules into the blood; and (7) the excretion of AAs by the kidneys. Thus, changes in the concentrations of AAs and their metabolites in physiological fluids reflect complex biochemical processes and should be interpreted carefully.

Because of their physicochemical properties, excessive AAs in circulation are removed from the body via excretion in the urine. All diseases are associated with alterations in the metabolism of one or more AAs. However, a severe deficiency of an enzyme (an actual deficit or abnormal form of the protein) in pathways for AA degradation or synthesis has long been recognized to result in characteristic elevations or reductions in AAs and their metabolites in the plasma

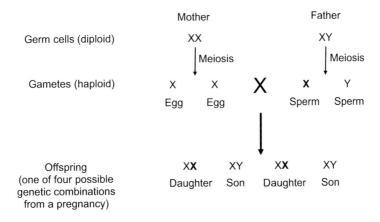

FIGURE 12.1 Contribution of gene mutations to the inborn errors of amino acid (AA) metabolism in humans and other animals. Defects in intestinal AA transporters impair AA absorption by the intestine. Defects in enzymes, their cofactors, or transmembrane AA transport can reduce the synthesis or degradation of AAs in animal cells, leading to either deficiencies or excesses of AAs and their metabolites, depending on the causes. Disruption of AA homeostasis results in metabolic diseases or disorders. X and Y, sex chromosomes.

and urine. It is noteworthy that changes in either a group of related AAs or all AAs in physiological fluids can be brought about by renal dysfunction. In the kidneys, each nephron filters the arterial blood entering this organ. The filtrate flows along the length of the nephron, where its epithelial cells normally reabsorb AAs into the blood through the actions of multiple transporters (Camargo et al. 2013). For example, three transporters encoded by three different genes are responsible for the reabsorption of imino acids and glycine in the kidney proximal tubule: a common transporter for both imino acids and glycine and a specific transporter each for glycine and imino acids (Bröer and Palacín 2011). Excessive accumulation of AAs and their metabolites in the kidneys can cause injury, electrolyte imbalance, acid–base imbalance, hypertension, ammonia toxicity, and even death.

Knowledge about inborn errors of AA metabolism has led to the rapid development of "molecular medicine" over the past half-century. Furthermore, the fact that inherited defects in AA-synthetic enzymes result in metabolic defects and deaths in humans (Spodenkiewicz et al. 2016) exemplifies the nutritional and physiological importance of endogenous AA syntheses and also indicates that dietary intake alone is insufficient for maintaining the homeostasis of biosynthesizable AAs in the body (Hou et al. 2015, 2016). The major inborn errors of AA metabolism are highlighted in this chapter.

12.1 ROLES OF CHROMOSOMES IN GENETIC INHERITANCE AND GENE MUTATIONS

Offspring inherit genetic materials (DNAs) from their parents to express phenotypes (traits or characteristics; e.g., physical appearance, skin and hair color, body weight and height, and behavior) (Figure 12.2). Humans normally have 46 chromosomes arranged in 23 pairs (two chromosomes per pair, with one chromosome from each parent), including one pair of chromosomes called sex chromosomes (XX for females and XY for males). A male receives X and Y chromosomes from his mother and father, respectively, whereas a female obtains an X chromosome

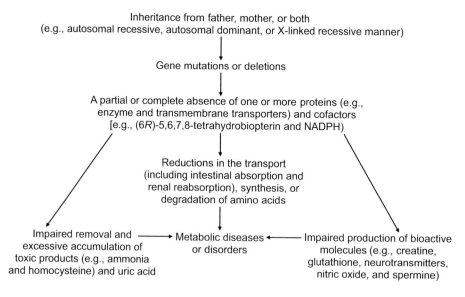

FIGURE 12.2 Inheritance of offspring's genetic materials from parents. Germ cells (diploid) divide and undergo meiosis to produce gametes (haploid; e.g., eggs and sperms) that contain half of the chromosomes present in the germ cells. Female gametes have equal chances to be fertilized by male gametes, generating one of four possible genetic combinations in a pregnancy. X, sex chromosome.

from her mother and another X chromosome from her father. In animal cells, each chromosome contains different segments (genes) of DNA. A phenotype is controlled by two variant (allele) forms of a gene located at the same position in the pair of chromosomes, with one allele inherited from each parent.

12.1.1 AUTOSOMAL DOMINANT OR AUTOSOMAL RECESSIVE INHERITANCE

Dominant and recessive genes are determinants for phenotypes. In one pair of chromosomes (except for the pair of X and Y chromosomes in males), a dominant gene on a chromosome overrides a different variant of the same gene (called a recessive gene) on the other paired chromosome to express a phenotype. Carrying a dominant gene on any chromosome will result in a disease or a disorder. By contrast, the presence of two copies of the same recessive gene in non-sex chromosomes (also called autosomes) is required for the occurrence of a disease or a disorder (being affected) in an individual. In other words, a recessive gene in autosomes is expressed with a characteristic phenotype (i.e., a disease or disorder) *only* when the offspring has two recessive copies for that gene. The terms "autosomal dominant or autosomal recessive inheritance" are used to describe the expression of gene variants on non-sex chromosomes. Examples of autosomal dominant disorders are Huntington's disease, familial hypercholesterolemia, and protoporphyria, whereas examples for autosomal recessive disorders include Tay–Sachs disease, sickle cell anemia, cystic fibrosis, and phenylketonuria (PKU) (Scriver et al. 2001). Note that many inborn errors of AA metabolism are inherited in an autosomal recessive manner (Aliu et al. 2018; Kožich and Stabler 2020; Rumping et al. 2020), meaning that the defective gene responsible for a disorder is located on an autosome and the two alleles of the defective gene (one from each parent) are required for the expression of an inborn error of metabolism.

12.1.2 X-LINKED DOMINANT OR RECESSIVE INHERITANCE

The expression of gene variants on sex chromosomes is termed X-linked dominant, X-linked recessive, or Y-linked. Examples for X-linked dominant disorders are hypophosphatemic rickets (vitamin D–resistant rickets) and ornithine carbamoyltransferase (OCT) deficiency, whereas examples for X-linked recessive disorders include autism spectrum disorders, gout, hemophilia A, and Duchenne muscular dystrophy (Scriver et al. 2001). The X-linked dominant or recessive inheritance results from mutations in genes on the X chromosome, and the occurrence of phenotypes (diseases or disorders) depends on the sex (male or female) of offspring and the parental source of the mutated gene (father, mother, or both) (Table 12.1). In X-linked dominant inheritance, a mutation in one variant of an X-linked gene will result in disease in both male and female offspring. Likewise, in the X-linked dominant inheritance, a male (who has only one X chromosome) will be affected with a disease or disorder if any mutated gene is present on his X chromosome (that is from his mother). By contrast, because a female has two X chromosomes, she will not be affected with a disease when possessing only a single copy of a mutated recessive gene on an X chromosome despite carrying the mutated gene. Thus, in X-linked disorders, a father passes mutated X chromosome genes only to his daughters but not to his sons, whereas a mother passes mutated X chromosome genes to both her daughters and sons. Some common inborn errors of AA metabolism are inherited in the X-linked recessive manner, and these disorders affect more males than females.

12.2 INHERITED DISEASES RESULTING FROM ABNORMAL AMINO ACID METABOLISM

Diseases resulting from inborn errors of AA metabolism in humans are summarized in Table 12.2 and discussed in the following sections. Some of these disorders also occur in animals but are less studied. Characteristic phenotypes in affected individuals are manifested in response to alterations

TABLE 12.1

Occurrence of Diseases or Disorders in Offspring in X-Linked Dominant and X-Linked Recessive Inheritance[a]

Type of inheritance	Sex	Offspring		Carriers of a mutated gene on the X chromosome		
		Inheritance of the mutated gene	Occurrence of disease	Both parents	Father	Mother
X-linked dominant	Male	Yes (50%)	Yes[b]	Yes[c]	–	–
	Female	Yes (100%)	Yes[b]	Yes[c]	–	–
	Male	No	No	–	Yes[c]	–
	Female	Yes (100%)	Yes[b]	–	Yes[c]	–
	Male	Yes (50%)	Yes[b]	–	–	Yes[c]
	Female	Yes (50%)	Yes[b]	–	–	Yes[c]
X-linked recessive	Male	Yes (100%)	Yes[b]	Yes[c]	–	–
	Female	Yes (100%)	Yes[b]	Yes[c]	–	–
	Male	Yes (50%)	Yes[b]	–	Yes[c]	Carrier but not affected
	Female	Yes (100%)	Yes (50%)	–	Yes[c]	Carrier but not affected
	Male	No	No	–	Yes[c]	–
	Female	Yes (100%)	No	–	Yes[c]	–
	Male	Yes (100%)	Yes[b]	–	–	Carrier and affected[d]
	Female	Yes (100%)	No	–	–	Carrier and affected[d]
	Male	Yes (50%)	Yes[b]	–	–	Carrier but not affected
	Female	Yes (50%)	No	–	–	Carrier but not affected

[a] Male gets an X chromosome from his mother and a Y chromosome from his father, whereas a female gets an X chromosome from her mother and another X chromosome from her father. In the X-linked dominant inheritance, carrying a mutated gene on an X chromosome will result in a disease or disorder (being affected). In the X-linked recessive inheritance, carrying a mutated gene on an X chromosome may or may not result in a disease or disorder, depending on the sex of offspring and the parental source of the mutated X chromosome; a male carrying a mutated gene on his X chromosome will be affected with a disease, but a female will be affected only when carrying the same mutated gene on both of her X chromosomes.

[b] Those offspring will develop a characteristic disease if they inherit a mutated X chromosome gene.

[c] Affected with a disease as well.

[d] The mother carries the same mutated gene on both of her X chromosomes.

Note: The number in the parentheses indicates the chances for offspring to inherit the mutated gene. The sign "–" denotes the absence of a mutated gene from an X chromosome.

in the metabolism of either all or certain AAs. Because some AAs and certain AA metabolites are neurotransmitters (Chapter 11), the symptoms of most inborn errors of AA metabolism include mental disorders. Methods for treating inborn errors of AA metabolism, except for specific organ transplantation or gene therapy and the management of specific symptoms, are highlighted along with their causes and consequences. Note that therapies for certain inborn errors of AA metabolism have been approved by the U.S. Food and Drug Administration (FDA).

12.2.1 All or Most Amino Acids

12.2.1.1 Fanconi Syndrome

This disorder results from a general defect in the reabsorption of all AAs, bicarbonate, glucose, phosphate, and uric acid from the lumen of the proximal renal tubules into the blood, leading to their elevated excretion in the urine (Foreman 2019). Fanconi syndrome may be secondary to a kidney injury in at least ten inherited diseases [including cystinosis (the most common example

TABLE 12.2
Inborn Errors of Amino Acid Metabolism

AA or related substance	Name of disease or disorder	Cause
1. All Amino Acids		
All AAs	Fanconi syndrome	Defect in renal reabsorption of all AAs
All AAs	Galactosemia	Deficiency of G1PUT
All AAs	Wilson's disease	Defect in hepatic copper-binding P-type ATPase
2. Asparagine and Dicarboxylic (DCB) Amino Acids		
Asparagine	Asparagine deficiency	Deficiency of asparagine synthetase
DCB AA	DCB aminoaciduria	Mutations of X_{AG}^- (SLC1A1)
3. Basic Amino Acids		
Arginine, lysine, and ornithine	Lysinuric protein intolerance	Defect in the transport of basic AAs
Ornithine	Hyperornithinemia in adults	Deficiency of ornithine aminotransferase
Ornithine	Gyrate in adults	Deficiency of ornithine aminotransferase
4. Branched-Chain Amino Acids		
Isoleucine, leucine, and valine	Maple syrup urine	Deficiency of BCKA dehydrogenase
Leucine	Isovaleric acidemia	Deficiency of isovaleryl-CoA dehydrogenase
Isoleucine	Methylbutyric acidemia	Deficiency of 2-methylbutyryl-CoA dehydrogenase
5. Carnitine		
Carnitine	Primary carnitine deficiency	Defect in carnitine transport
Trimethyllysine	Carnitine deficiency	Deficiency of trimethyllysine dioxygenase
6. Creatine		
Arginine and glycine	Creatine deficiency	Deficiency of arginine:glycine amidinotransferase
Guanidinoacetate	Creatine deficiency	Deficiency of guanidinoacetate methyltransferase
Creatine	Creatine deficiency	Defect in creatine transporter
7. Glutamate		
γ-Aminobutyrate	Neurological dysfunction	Deficiency of γ-aminobutyrate transaminase
Glutamate	Hypoargininemia	Deficiency of P5C synthase
Glutamate	HI/HA syndrome	Superactivity of glutamate dehydrogenase
8. Glutamine		
Glutamine	Glutamine deficiency	Deficiency of glutamine synthetase
Glutamine	Hyperglutaminemia	Deficiency of phosphate-activated glutaminase
9. Glutathione		
Glutathione	Glutathione deficiency	Deficiency of γ-glutamyl-cysteine synthetase
Glutathione	Glutathione deficiency	Deficiency of glutathione synthetase
5-Oxoproline	5-Oxoprolinuria	Deficiency of 5-oxoprolinase
10. Glycine		
Dimethylglycine	Glycine synthesis defect	Deficiency of dimethylglycine dehydrogenase
Glycine	Glycinuria	Defect in renal reabsorption of glycine
Glycine	Ketotic hyperglycinemia	Possibly due to organic acidurias
Glycine	Non-ketotic hyperglycinemia	Deficiency of the glycine cleavage system
Glycine	Sarcosinemia	Deficiency of sarcosine dehydrogenase

(Continued)

TABLE 12.2 (*Continued*)
Inborn Errors of Amino Acid Metabolism

AA or related substance	Name of disease or disorder	Cause
	11. Heme	
Bilirubin	Dubin–Johnson syndrome	Deficiency of MRP2 in the liver
Bilirubin	Jaundice	Deficiency of UGT1A1 or G6PDH
Heme	Protoporphyria	Defect in heme synthesis
	12. Histidine	
Histidine	Cerebromacular degeneration	Defect in renal reabsorption of imidazoles
Histidine	Histidinemia	Deficiency of histidinase
Histidine	Mastocytosis	Deficiency of histidine decarboxylase
Histidine	Urocanic aciduria	Deficiency of urocanase
	13. Phenylalanine (Phe) and Tyrosine (Tyr)	
Phenylalanine	Phenylketonuria, type-I	Deficiency of phenylalanine hydroxylase
Phenylalanine	Phenylketonuria, type-II	Deficiency of tetrahydrobiopterin
Tyrosine	Albinism	Deficiency of tyrosinase
Tyrosine	Alkaptonuria (black urine disease)	Deficiency of homogentisate oxidase
Tyrosine	Hypertyrosinemia, type I	Deficiency of fumarylacetoacetase
Tyrosine	Hypertyrosinemia, type II	Deficiency of tyrosine transaminase
Tyrosine	Hypertyrosinemia, Type III	Deficiency of 4-hydroxyphenylpyruvate dioxygenase (HPD)
Tyrosine	Pheochromocytoma	Excessive catabolism of tyrosine to form catecholamines
Phe, Tyr, and Trp	AADC deficiency	Decrease of AADC activity in brain
	14. Proline and 4-Hydroxyproline (OH-Pro)	
OH-Pro	Hyperhydroxyprolinemia	Deficiency of hydroxyproline oxidase
Proline, OH-Pro, and glycine	Iminoglycinuria	Defect in the proton-coupled AA transporter gene
Proline	Disorder of POHP dipeptides	Deficiency of prolidase
Proline	Hyperprolinemia, type-I	Deficiency of proline dehydrogenase
Proline	Hyperprolinemia, type-II	Deficiency of P5C dehydrogenase
	15. Purines	
Purine	Gout	Superactivity of PRPS and deficiency of HGPRT
Purine	Immunodeficiency	Deficiency of adenosine deaminase
Purine	Immunodeficiency	Deficiency of purine nucleoside phosphorylase
Purine	Kidney stone and failure	Deficiency of APRT
Purine	Lesch–Nyhan syndrome	Almost complete deficiency of HGPRT
Purine	Muscle weakness	Myoadenylate deaminase deficiency
Purine	Xanthinuria	Deficiency of xanthine oxidase
Purine	ADSL deficiency	Deficiency of ADSL
	16. Pyrimidines	
Pyrimidine	β-Aminoisobutyric aciduria	Deficiency of AIB:glutamate transaminase
Pyrimidine	Familial pyrimidinemia	Deficiency of dihydropyrimidine dehydrogenase
Pyrimidine	Hyper-β-alaninemia	Deficiency of β-alanine:α-ketoglutarate transaminase
Pyrimidine	Orotic aciduria	Deficiency of UMP synthase or the urea cycle

(Continued)

TABLE 12.2 (*Continued*)
Inborn Errors of Amino Acid Metabolism

AA or related substance	Name of disease or disorder	Cause
17. Serine		
Serine	Hypophosphatasia	Deficiency of alkaline phosphatase
Serine	Hyposerinemia	Deficiency of phosphoglycerate dehydrogenase
18. Sulfur-Containing Amino Acids		
Cystine	Cystinuria	Defect in renal transport of cystine
Cystine	Cystinosis	Defect in cystine transport across the lysosomal membrane
Methionine	Homocyst(e)inuria	Deficiency of cystathionine synthetase
Methionine	Cystathioninuria	Deficiency of cystathionase
Methionine	Hypermethioninemia	Deficiency of methionine adenosyltransferase
19. Tryptophan		
Tryptophan	Carcinoid	Excessive tryptophan catabolism
Tryptophan	Hartnup	Defect in the transport of Trp and other neutral amino acids
20. The Urea Cycle		
Ammonia	Hyperammonemia	Deficiency of carbamoyl phosphate synthase-I
Arginine	Hyperargininemia	Deficiency of type-1 arginase
Argininosuccinate	Argininosuccinic aciduria	Deficiency of argininosuccinate lyase
Citrulline	Hypercitrullinemia, type-I[a]	Deficiency of argininosuccinate synthase
Citrulline	Hypercitrullinemia, type-II[b]	Deficiency of citrin (mitochondrial Asp/Glu exchanger)
Glutamate	Hyperammonemia	Deficiency of NAG synthase
Ornithine	Hyperornithinemia	Deficiency of ornithine carbamoyltransferase
Ornithine	HHH syndrome	Mutations in mitochondrial ornithine transporter 1
21. Other Organic Acidurias		
Glycine and OH-Pro	Hyperoxaluria	Defect in oxidation of glycine and hydroxyproline
Isoleucine, methionine, threonine, and valine	Propionic academia	Deficiency of propionyl-CoA carboxylase
Isoleucine, methionine, threonine, and valine	Methylmalonic acidemia	Deficiency of methylmalonyl-CoA mutase
Lysine and tryptophan	Ketoadipic academia	Deficiency of 2-ketoadipate dehydrogenase
Lysine and tryptophan	Glutaric academia	Deficiency of glutaryl-CoA dehydrogenase
22. Polyamines		
Spermidine	Snyder–Robinson syndrome	Deficiency of spermine synthase
Spermine	Mucopolysaccharidoses	Possibly reduced ability to degrade spermine

[a] This disorder usually occurs in newborn infants.

[b] This disorder is characterized by neonatal intrahepatic cholestasis. In adults, the disease is often triggered by certain medications, infections, and alcohol consumption.

Note: AADC, aromatic L-amino acid decarboxylase; ADSL, adenylosuccinate lyase; AIB, β-aminoisobutyrate; APRT, adenine phosphoribosyltransferase; BCAAs, branched-chain amino acids; BCKA, branched-chain α-ketoacid; G1PUT, galactose-1-phosphate uridyltransferase; G6PDH, glucose-6-phosphate dehydrogenase; HHH, hyperornithinemia–hyperammonemia–homocitrullinuria; HI/HA syndrome, hyperinsulinism and hyperammonemia; MRP2, multidrug-resistance–associated protein 2; NAG, *N*-acetylglutamate; P5C, pyrroline-5-carboxylate; UGT1A1, uridine diphosphoglucuronate glucuronosyltransferase 1A1; UMP, uridine monophosphate.

in children), tyrosinemia, glycogenosis, mitochondrial disorders, Wilson's disease, galactosemia, hereditary fructose intolerance, Lowe syndrome, and Dent disease] and also may be an isolated condition. Inhibition of the endocytic process mediated by the megalin membrane glycoprotein may be primarily responsible for Fanconi syndrome. Defects in ATP production may also contribute to a low ability of the renal tubules to reabsorb AAs and related molecules into the blood. Persons with this disease exhibit acidosis, aminoaciduria, cystinosis, dehydration, glycosuria, growth failure, hyperchloremia, hyperuricosuria, hypokalemia, liver enlargement, osteomalacia, and proteinuria. Treatment of Fanconi syndrome depends on its cause.

12.2.1.2 Galactosemia

Galactosemia results from a deficiency of galactose-1-phosphate uridyltransferase, an enzyme that converts galactose-1-phosphate and uridine triphosphate to uridine diphosphate galactose (Coman et al. 2010). In this autosomal recessive disorder, the direct conversion of galactose (formed from lactose in milk) into glycogen is limited or absent, thereby allowing the metabolism of galactose into monosaccharides (including xylulose-5-phosphate and glucose-6-phosphate) that provide carbon skeletons for the synthesis of alanine, glutamate, and related AAs in the liver of mammals, including humans (Wu 2018). Thus, affected patients have elevations in the concentrations of galactose and galactitol (a product of galactose degradation by aldose reductase) in the plasma and urine and of AAs in the urine (generalized aminoaciduria), but a reduced concentration of glucose in the plasma. The majority of infants with galactosemia are identified by newborn screening in the United States. Infants with galactosemia exhibit lethargy, vomiting, diarrhea, failure of growth, and jaundice. The progression of this disease leads to ataxia, cataracts (due to galactitol accumulation in the optic lens), enlargement and cirrhosis of the liver, convulsions (rapid and uncontrollable shaking), premature ovarian failure, and mental retardation. A galactose-restricted diet is very effective to treat life-threatening manifestations in affected infants.

12.2.1.3 Wilson's Disease

Wilson's disease (also known as hepatolenticular degeneration; an autosomal recessive disorder) results from a defect of a hepatic type of copper-binding P-type ATPase, which is responsible for directing the efflux of copper from the liver (Bandmann et al. 2015). Thus, copper is not excreted from the liver into the bile or blood circulation, resulting in: 1) the accumulation of copper in the liver, brain, kidneys, red blood cells, and urine and 2) a decrease in serum Cu^{2+} and serum ceruloplasmin. Interestingly, affected individuals exhibit an increase in the urinary excretion of all AAs (generalized aminoaciduria) due to the impaired reabsorption of AAs from the lumen of the proximal renal tubules into the blood without elevations of AA concentrations in the plasma. This is thought to be secondary to metalloprotein complexes in the proximal renal tubular brush border. Relatively large amounts of peptides are also excreted in the urine of individuals with Wilson's disease likely because of their impaired renal transport. These patients suffer from liver damage, neurological dysfunction, skeletal musculature abnormality, and personality change. They also have a green or golden pigment ring around the corner of their eyes due to the deposition of copper in the cell membrane. Treatment of Wilson's disease includes low dietary copper and lifelong administration of D-penicillamine to chelate copper.

12.2.2 ASPARAGINE AND ASPARTATE

12.2.2.1 Asparagine Synthetase Deficiency

This autosomal recessive disorder was originally discovered in 2013. It results from a deficiency of asparagine synthetase (Ruzzo et al. 2013). In humans, the glutamine-dependent asparagine synthetase catalyzes the transfer of an amide group from glutamine to aspartic acid via a β-aspartyl-AMP intermediate to form asparagine (Chapter 3). Patients have a reduction in the plasma concentration of asparagine but an increase in the plasma concentration of glutamine and aspartate. The individuals exhibit congenital microcephaly, intellectual disability, progressive cerebral atrophy, and intractable seizures. Dietary supplementation with asparagine (at an initial dose of 50 mg/kg BW/day to a gradual increase to 100 mg/kg BW/day) for 24 months is well tolerated by affected children (from the age of 3 years and 9 months to 5 years and 9 months; or from the age of 21 months to 3 years and 9 months) and can inhibit their disease progression (Sprute et al. 2019). These findings indicate that asparagine synthesis is essential for neurological development and function.

12.2.2.2 Dicarboxylic Aminoaciduria

This autosomal recessive disorder is caused by loss-of-function mutations in an anionic AA transporter X_{AG}^- (SLC1A1, also known as EAAT3 and EAAC1; Bailey et al. 2011). X_{AG}^- is the major epithelial transporter of: (a) aspartate and glutamate in the kidneys and the intestinal apical membrane and (b) glutamate within the interneuronal synaptic cleft. As a result, these two acidic AAs are not absorbed from the lumen of the small intestine or by the renal tubules into the blood. Affected individuals excrete about 100–250 times more aspartate and glutamate than healthy individuals, depending upon the duration of the preceding fasting period (Teijema et al. 1974). When the patient is not hypoglycemic, plasma AA concentrations are normal, except for moderate hyperprolinemia. However, during recurrent hypoglycemia, the patient has a decrease in glycogenic AAs and an increase in branched-chain AAs (BCAAs). Furthermore, they exhibit an impairment in the growth and development of the thyroid gland and the whole body, as well as a tendency toward hypoglycemia upon fasting. There is no cure for dicarboxylic aminoaciduria. Its treatment is to alleviate the symptoms (e.g., oral sodium bicarbonate to correct acidosis) and complications.

12.2.3 BASIC AMINO ACIDS

12.2.3.1 Lysinuric Protein Intolerance

This extremely rare autosomal recessive disorder, most common in Finland, results from defects in the absorption of basic AAs (arginine, lysine, and ornithine) from the lumen of the small intestine and in the reabsorption of these AAs from the lumen of the renal proximal tubules into the blood (Noguchi and Takahashi 2019). Thus, concentrations of arginine, lysine, and ornithine are reduced in the plasma but are elevated in the urine (due to increased excretion from the kidneys). The transport defects in the endothelial cells and non-polarized cells (e.g., lymphocytes and macrophages) also contribute to impairments in NO synthesis from arginine, resulting in abnormal blood flow and impaired immunity. Affected individuals also have elevated levels of glutamine, glycine, and orotic acid in the plasma and urine primarily due to their increased syntheses (Chapter 3). Patients experience hypoargininemia, growth retardation, hyperammonemia, vomiting, convulsions, and coma, as well as skeletal, immunological, pulmonary, renal, and cardiovascular abnormalities. A deficiency of arginine and ornithine also impairs the function of the urea cycle and leads to hyperammonemia after the consumption of a protein-rich meal. Treatment includes: (1) a protein-restricted diet supplemented with lysine, ornithine, and citrulline (e.g., 5 g/day for a 70-kg adult) and (2) medications to remove excess AAs and ammonia in the blood.

12.2.3.2 Hyperornithinemia

Hyperornithinemia is caused by a deficiency of ornithine aminotransferase (OAT) in adult humans (Valle and Simell 2001). This is an autosomal recessive disorder. Affected individuals have elevated levels of ornithine in the plasma (up to 1.4 mM) and urine (up to 10 mM). Concentrations of glutamate, glutamine, lysine, creatine, and creatinine in the plasma are moderately reduced. Patients with hyperornithinemia experience two distinct disorders: (1) hyperornithinemia–hyperammonemia–homocitrullinemia (HHH) syndrome in infants due to a deficiency of arginine synthesis in the small intestine and (2) gyrate atrophy of the choroid and retina (progressive chorioretinal degeneration as an autosomal recessive trait) in adults due to ornithine-induced cell damage. Mental retardation also occurs in these individuals. Treatment includes: (1) a protein-restricted diet supplemented with citrulline (e.g., 5 g/day for a 70-kg adult) and (2) the use of sodium benzoate and/or sodium or glycerol phenylbutyrate to remove excess ammonia in the blood.

12.2.4 Branched-Chain Amino Acids

12.2.4.1 Maple Syrup Urine Disease

This disease (also known as branched-chain ketoaciduria) occurs in persons with a severe deficiency of BCKA dehydrogenase, the enzyme that decarboxylates BCAA-derived BCKAs to acyl-CoA (Chuang and Shih 2001). This is an autosomal recessive metabolic disorder. The estimated prevalence of Maple syrup urine disease is around 1/150,000 live births worldwide but is seen in up to 1:200 live births in certain Mennonite populations. This disease is characterized by: (1) the excretion of urine that possesses an unpleasant but sweet odor similar to that of maple syrup; (2) elevated levels of all three branched-chain AAs (leucine, isoleucine, and valine) in the plasma, urine, and spinal fluid; and (3) relatively large amounts of BCKAs. Patients with Maple syrup urine disease suffer from pathological changes in the central nervous system, convulsions, mental retardation, respiratory distress, and feeding difficulties. Fortunately, the vast majority are detected by neonatal screening in the United States, Canada, and many other countries and treated with protein- and leucine-restricted diets.

12.2.4.2 Isovaleric Acidemia

This autosomal recessive disorder (also known as isovaleric aciduria) results from a deficiency of isovaleric acid CoA dehydrogenase (Cohn et al. 1978). This enzyme catalyzes the conversion of isovaleric acid CoA to β-methylcrotonyl-CoA in the metabolic pathway of leucine catabolism (Chapter 4). Affected individuals have severe catabolic attacks with metabolic acidosis and are accompanied by elevated levels of: (1) isovalerate in the plasma and urine; (2) isovalerylcarnitine in the plasma; and (3) isovalerylglycine in the urine. Isovalerylcarnitine and isovalerylglycine are formed from the conjugation of isovalerate with carnitine and glycine, respectively. A unique feature of isovaleric acidemia is a distinctive odor of sweaty feet due to the accumulation of isovalerate in physiological fluids and tissues. Infants with the acute neonatal form exhibit poor feeding, severe episodes of vomiting, and profound ketoacidosis, progressing to coma and death. These patients may experience dehydration, hyperammonemia, hypocalcemia, hepatomegaly, hyper/hypoglycemia, depressed bone marrow function, thrombocytopenia, and pancreatitis. Treatment includes: (1) a protein-restricted diet and (2) medications to remove isovaleric acid in the blood. Affected individuals should avoid triggers (e.g., fasting and infections) that can cause a metabolic crisis.

12.2.4.3 Methylbutyric Acidemia

This disorder is an autosomal recessive disorder specific to isoleucine catabolism because of a deficiency of 2-methylbutyryl-CoA dehydrogenase (Korman 2006). This enzyme catalyzes the conversion of 2-methylbutyryl-CoA to tiglyl-CoA (also known as α-methylcrotonoyl-CoA or 2-methylcrotonoyl-CoA; Chapter 4). The affected individuals have elevations in the concentrations of isoleucine, 2-methylbutyrate, 2-methylbutyrylglycine, and 2-methylbutyrylcarnitine in their physiologic fluids (including the plasma and urine). The symptoms include poor feeding, lethargy, hypoglycemia, hypothermia, dehydration, and apnea. Treatment involves a protein-restricted and carbohydrate-sufficient diet.

12.2.5 Carnitine

12.2.5.1 Primary Carnitine Deficiency

This autosomal recessive disorder results from a deficiency of a carnitine transporter due to a mutation of the *SLC22A5* gene (El-Hattab and Scaglia 2015). The metabolic problems can be triggered by periods of fasting or by illnesses, such as viral infections. In this disorder, cells cannot take up carnitine from the circulation, resulting in a severe deficiency in the transfer of long-chain fatty acids from the cytoplasm to mitochondria for β-oxidation. Clinical symptoms of this disorder may include severe brain dysfunction (encephalopathy), a weakened and enlarged heart (cardiomyopathy), confusion, vomiting, muscle weakness, and hypoglycemia (due to impaired gluconeogenesis). Some individuals may be asymptomatic. However, all affected individuals are at risk for heart failure, liver abnormality, skeletal muscle dysfunction, and possibly sudden death. Treatment involves life-long dietary supplementation with L-carnitine.

12.2.5.2 Trimethyllysine Dioxygenase Deficiency

This disorder, which has low penetrance (2%–4%), is a common X-linked recessive disorder in humans, affecting only male offspring (Ziats et al. 2015). Trimethyllysine (TML) dioxygenase is a mitochondrial enzyme encoded by the *TMLHE* gene, which catalyzes the conversion of TML to hydroxy-TML in the first step of carnitine biosynthesis. The affected subject has increased concentrations of TML and decreased concentrations of hydroxy-TML and γ-butyrobetaine in the plasma, urine, and brain. Interestingly, *TMLHE* deficiency is a risk factor for autism, and its symptoms can be alleviated by lifelong dietary supplementation with L-carnitine.

12.2.6 CREATINE

12.2.6.1 Arginine: Glycine Amidinotransferase Deficiency

The deficiency of arginine:glycine amidinotransferase (AGAT) is the third inborn error of creatine metabolism to be reported in humans as an autosomal recessive disorder (Item et al 2001). AGAT catalyzes the first step of creatine synthesis, resulting in the formation of guanidinoacetate and ornithine from arginine and glycine (Chapter 5). Affected individuals have reduced concentrations of guanidinoacetate and creatine in tissues, as well as reduced excretion of guanidinoacetate. Patients develop mental retardation and muscular abnormalities (including weakness and structural myopathy). Oral administration of creatine can reverse the adverse effects of AGAT deficiency (Braissant et al. 2011).

12.2.6.2 Guanidinoacetate Methyltransferase Deficiency

This disorder was the first inborn error of creatine metabolism to be discovered. It is an autosomal recessive disorder (Schulze 2003). This enzyme catalyzes the formation of creatine from guanidinoacetate and *S*-adenosylmethionine (SAM) (Chapter 5). Guanidinoacetate is a product of arginine catabolism catalyzed by arginine:glycine amidinotransferase. Affected individuals have excessive amounts of guanidinoacetate in their body fluids but low concentrations of creatine in their tissues (including the brain as indicated by proton magnetic resonance). These individuals exhibit impairments in muscular and neurological developments, as well as neurological symptoms, including muscular hypotonia and weakness, epilepsy, and autistic behavior. Treatment involves lifelong dietary supplementation with creatine.

12.2.6.3 The X-Linked Creatine Transporter Deficiency

This disorder results from a mutation in the *SLC6A8* gene and was the second inborn error of creatine metabolism to be discovered in humans (Salomons et al. 2003). In this X-linked recessive disorder, cells cannot take up creatine from the circulation, resulting in a severe deficiency of creatine and abnormal energy metabolism in the central nervous system and muscles (Chapter 11). Affected patients exhibit X-linked mental retardation, expressive speech and language delay, epilepsy, developmental delay, and autistic behavior. Dietary supplementation with creatine cannot reverse the adverse effects of creatine transporter deficiency. Treatment includes dietary supplementation with L-arginine, glycine, and methionine.

12.2.7 GLUTAMATE

12.2.7.1 Gamma Aminobutyric Acid Transaminase Deficiency

A deficiency of gamma aminobutyric acid (GABA) transaminase impairs the catabolism of GABA (a product of glutamate decarboxylation) to form succinic semialdehyde (Jaeken et al. 1984; Koenig et al. 2017). This autosomal recessive disorder is characterized by the elevated concentrations of

GABA (up to 5 μM), homocarnosine (up to 25 μM; a dipeptide of GABA and histidine), β-alanine (up to 0.5 μM) in cerebrospinal fluid (CSF); growth hormone (up to 40 ng/mL) in the serum; as well as the urinary excretion of GABA. Affected patients experience severe psychomotor retardation, leukodystrophy, hypotonia, hyperreflexia, and growth acceleration. Treatment involves the intravenous administration of flumazenil (a GABA-A benzodiazepine receptor antagonist, 1.7 mg/kg BW/ day; Koenig et al. 2017).

12.2.7.2 Hyperinsulinism and Hyperammonemia Syndrome

This autosomal dominant disorder results from the dominantly expressed, gain-of-function mutations of glutamate dehydrogenase (GDH), which catalyzes the interconversion of glutamate to α-ketoglutarate and ammonia in the mitochondrion (Pinney et al. 2008). This enzyme occurs widely in the brain, kidneys, liver, and pancreatic β-cells. Patients with hyperinsulinism and hyperammonemia (HI/HA) syndrome have elevated levels of insulin (due to its enhanced secretion from pancreatic β-cells) and ammonia (due to GDH activation), hypoglycemia (due to hyperinsulinemia), an increased frequency of generalized seizures even in the absence of hypoglycemia, and spinocerebellar degeneration. The HI/HA syndrome can be treated with diazoxide, a K_{ATP} channel agonist to normalize concentrations of glucose and insulin in the plasma. Treatment includes: (1) a protein-restricted diet and (2) the use of diazoxide to reduce insulin secretion by pancreatic β-cells.

12.2.7.3 Pyrroline-5-Carboxylate Synthase Deficiency

The deficiency of pyrroline-5-carboxylate (P5C) synthase occurs in humans as an autosomal recessive disorder (Baumgartner et al. 2005). This condition results in impaired conversion of glutamate to P5C, which is the carbon backbone and a nitrogen source for the intestinal synthesis of ornithine, citrulline, and arginine (Chapter 3). Infants with this disease have low concentrations of ornithine, citrulline, and arginine in the face of elevated concentrations of ammonia and glutamine in their plasma. The clinical features in the first weeks after birth include hypotonia, dysmorphic signs, pes planus (flat feet), and clonic seizures. The progression of the disease leads to neurodegeneration, peripheral neuropathy, joint laxity, skin hyperelasticity, bilateral subcapsular cataracts, convulsions, mental retardation, and poor growth. Treatment involves dietary supplementation with L-citrulline (e.g., 5 g/day for a 70-kg adult).

12.2.8 GLUTAMINE

12.2.8.1 Glutamine Synthetase Deficiency

This autosomal recessive disorder results from mutations of the *GS* gene that encodes for glutamine synthetase, the enzyme catalyzing the conversion of ammonia and glutamate into glutamine (Häberle et al. 2006; Spodenkiewicz et al. 2016). Fetuses with severe glutamine synthetase (GS) deficiency have intrauterine growth retardation. Despite enteral nutrition or total parenteral nutrition, affected newborn infants have a near absence of free glutamine in the serum (only 2 μM) compared with a normal value of 500–600 μM in the serum, non-detectable glutamine in the urine, and low glutamine concentration in the cerebrospinal fluid (only 11 μM). They exhibit hyperammonemia, cerebral abnormalities, and severe neurological problems (no spontaneous movements, no responsiveness, no primitive reflexes, marked axial hypotonia, and convulsions). These infants die from multiple organ failure in the first month after birth. In a less severe variant of GS deficiency, affected individuals have a low concentration of glutamine in the serum [126 μM on day 16 after birth and <100 μM at 3 years of age (approximately <20% of the normal value)]; these patients have hyperammonemia, frequent seizures and convulsions, chronic encephalopathy, severe neurological disease, and severe retardation of growth and development, but can survive up to at least 3 years of age. Thus, depending on the severity of hypoglutaminemia, GS deficiency is not always a lethal disorder early in life. Treatment includes enteral or parenteral supplementation with glutamine. Findings from this inborn error of metabolism indicate that: (1) endogenous synthesis of glutamine by the fetus and the neonate plays an essential role in maintaining their glutamine homeostasis and (2) the intake of dietary glutamine by gestating mothers or by neonates is insufficient for their optimal growth, development, health, and survival.

12.2.8.2 Phosphate-Activated Glutaminase Deficiency

This disorder occurs in patients with hereditary protein intolerance (Malmquist and Hetter 1970). Phosphate-activated glutaminase plays a major role in hydrolyzing glutamine to glutamate and ammonia (Chapter 4). Affected individuals have reduced numbers of leucocytes and granulocytes and also exhibit brain atrophy, intellectual impairment, progressive cortical atrophy, and marked skeletal fragility. The infants have poor tolerance to foods containing a high level of protein, likely due to a low rate of glutamine utilization. Recently, van Kuilenburg et al. (2019) reported a glutaminase mutation in humans due to short tandem repeat expansion in the *GLS* gene. Affected individuals exhibited an early-onset delay in overall development, progressive ataxia, and elevated concentrations of glutamine in plasma (1,800–2,209 µM), and cerebellar atrophy. Furthermore, Rumping et al. (2019) identified a loss-of-function mutation in the glutaminase gene in humans as an autosomal recessive disorder. Affected infants had an elevated concentration of glutamine in the plasma. They experienced respiratory difficulty, marked muscular hypotonia, and seizures, and they died within 40 days after birth. This indicates either a toxic level of glutamine, an insufficient intracellular provision of glutamate, or both. At present, there is no established therapy for glutaminase deficiency. Dietary supplementation with glutamate, aspartate, and alanine to affected individuals may be beneficial at least for the function and integrity of their small intestine.

12.2.9 GLUTATHIONE

12.2.9.1 γ-Glutamyl-Cysteine Synthetase Deficiency

The deficiency of γ-glutamyl-cysteine synthetase is a defect in glutathione (GSH) biosynthesis (Ristoff et al. 2000). This is an autosomal recessive disorder. Because γ-glutamyl-cysteine synthetase catalyzes the formation of γ-glutamyl-cysteine from glutamate and cysteine (Chapter 5), a mutation of this enzyme results in a severe deficiency of GSH. Affected individuals may have only 5% of reduced glutathione in cells, including erythrocytes, leading to a reduced capacity for antioxidative defense and a short lifespan for red blood cells. Thus, patients suffer from spinocerebellar degeneration and hereditary hemolytic anemia while having an increased risk for infectious disease. Treatment should include the avoidance of: (1) drugs (phenobarbital, acetylsalicylic acid, and sulfonamides) that can inhibit glucose-6-phosphate dehydrogenase deficiency, e.g., phenobarbital, acetylsalicylic acid, and sulfonamides) and (2) factors that can cause oxidative stress. In addition, a methionine- and cysteine-restricted diet supplemented with antioxidants (including vitamin C and vitamin E) may help to alleviate oxidative injury in cells.

12.2.9.2 Glutathione Synthetase Deficiency

This autosomal recessive disorder is also characterized by reduced concentrations of GSH in cells (Njålsson et al. 2005). This enzyme catalyzes the condensation of γ-glutamylcysteine and glycine to form glutathione (Chapter 5). Persons with GSH synthetase deficiency have unexplained jaundice at birth and markedly elevated excretion of 5-oxoproline in their urine. Affected individuals exhibit oxidative stress, progressive neurologic disorders, hemolytic anemia, and metabolic acidosis. Treatment includes: (1) a methionine- and cysteine-restricted diet; (2) correction of metabolic acidosis with oral sodium bicarbonate; and (3) dietary supplementation with vitamin C and vitamin E.

12.2.9.3 5-Oxoprolinuria

This disorder (possibly an autosomal recessive disorder) results from a deficiency of 5-oxoprolinase (Almaghlouth et al. 2011; Ristoff and Larsson 2007). This enzyme converts 5-oxoproline to glutamate in the pathway of GSH synthesis (Chapter 5). Children experience recurrent episodes of vomiting, enterocolitis, diarrhea, urolithiasis, abdominal pain, and psychomotor developmental delay. Despite normal glomerular and tubular function tests, affected individuals have elevated levels of 5-oxoproline in plasma and massive excretion in urine. Treatment includes: (1) correction of metabolic acidosis with oral sodium bicarbonate and (2) a protein-restricted diet to reduce nitrogen loads.

12.2.10 GLYCINE

12.2.10.1 Dimethylglycine Dehydrogenase Deficiency

This autosomal recessive disorder due to a mutation of the dimethylglycine dehydrogenase gene has been reported for one patient (McAndrew et al. 2008). This mitochondrial enzyme catalyzes the demethylation of dimethylglycine to form sarcosine in the pathway of glycine synthesis from choline (Chapter 3). Affected individuals (diagnosed at 38 years of age) have elevated levels of dimethylglycine in their urine and serum, which are 20- and 100-fold higher than normal values, respectively. The patient has chronic muscle weakness and fatigue and a fish-like body odor but otherwise has no central nervous system symptoms. The intensity of the odor increases with physiological stress (e.g., illness). Treatment may include: (1) a dimethylglycine-restricted diet and (2) dietary supplementation with sarcosine, glycine, or their combination.

12.2.10.2 Glycine Encephalopathy

This is an autosomal recessive disorder also known as non-ketotic hyperglycinemia or NKHG (Tada and Kure 1993). It is relatively prevalent with an incidence of as high as 1:55,000 in the Northern European populations. Second, to PKU, glycine encephalopathy is the next most common disorder of AA metabolism. This disease results primarily from a deficiency of the glycine cleavage system, which converts glycine to ammonia and CO_2 in the mitochondria (Chapter 4). Thus, affected individuals have elevated levels of glycine in their plasma (up to 1.8 mM), cerebral spinal fluid (up to 0.28 mM), tissues (particularly the brain), and urine. There are several forms of glycine encephalopathy, with varying severity of neurological dysfunction and seizures. NKHG is coined to distinguish it from "ketotic hyperglycinemia", propionic acidemia, and other inherited metabolic disorders. Treatment includes: (1) a protein-restricted diet; (2) the intravenous or oral administration of sodium benzoate (which reacts with glycine to form hippurate) to reduce glycine concentration in the blood; and (3) the use of dextromethorphan (an NMDA receptor antagonist) to block some of the harmful effects of excessive glycine.

12.2.10.3 Glycinemia

This autosomal recessive disorder is characterized by ketotic hyperglycinemia (Soriano et al. 1967). The possible cause of this disorder is the enzymatic inhibition of the catabolism of glycine and related AAs by toxic metabolites generated in organic acidurias. Clinical symptoms include ketosis, dehydration, lethargy, vomiting, neutropenia, leukopenia, hypo-γ-globulinemia, and mental retardation. Also, these children suffer from prolonged bouts of hiccups. Affected infants have elevated levels of ketone bodies, glycine (up to 1.5 mM), other AAs (e.g., serine, alanine, isoleucine, and valine) in the plasma, as well as increased urinary excretion of ketone bodies and glycine. The treatment for glycine encephalopathy can be applied to the management of individuals with glycinemia.

12.2.10.4 Glycinuria

This is a sex-linked recessive disorder that has been reported for females (Oberiter 1978). This disease results from a defect in the renal reabsorption of glycine into the blood, leading to an excessive excretion of glycine in the urine. Most of the patients experience nephrolithiasis. Persons with glycinuria have a normal concentration of glycine in their plasma but excrete 0.5–1 g glycine in their urine daily. Treatment involves oral rehydration and a protein-restricted diet that provides a reduced amount of AAs, particularly of glycine, serine, and threonine.

12.2.10.5 Sarcosinemia

This autosomal recessive disorder (also known as hypersarcosinemia) results from a deficiency of sarcosine dehydrogenase (Scott 2001), a mitochondrial enzyme that catalyzes thedemethylation of sarcosine to form glycine (Chapter 3). Affected individuals have elevated levels of sarcosine in their plasma (up to 0.76 mM) and increased urinary excretion (up to 8 mmol/day). Patients may experience low appetite, vomiting, growth retardation, hypertension, hypoactivity, cardiomyopathy, irritability, muscle tremors, and mental retardation. Treatment may involve a dimethylglycine- and sarcosine-restricted diet.

12.2.10.6 Sideroblastic Anemia

Sideroblastic anemia is a form of anemia in which the bone marrow produces ringed sideroblasts (erythroid precursors) containing pathologic iron deposits within mitochondria, rather than healthy red blood cells. This is an autosomal recessive nonsyndromic congenital disorder caused by mutations in the gene *SLC25A38* encoding the erythroid specific mitochondrial carrier family protein for glycine transport (Guernsey et al. 2009). It is now known that the gene *SLC25A38* is crucial for the biosynthesis of heme in eukaryotes.

12.2.11 Heme Synthesis and Catabolism Disorders

Heme (iron protoporphyrin), a metalloporphyrin with iron as the central atom, is a building block for many hemoproteins. This porphyrin is synthesized from glycine and succinate mainly in the bone marrow (to yield hemoglobin) and in the liver (to produce cytochrome P450 enzymes). The metabolic pathways for the synthesis and catabolism of heme are described in Chapter 5.

12.2.11.1 Dubin–Johnson Syndrome (Conjugated Hyperbilirubinemia)

This is an autosomal recessive disorder caused by the accumulation of glucuronide-conjugated bilirubin in the liver due to a mutation in the canalicular multiple drug-resistance protein 2 (MRP2) that secretes the conjugated bilirubin into the bile (Strassburg 2010). Excess conjugated bilirubin enters the blood and is deposited as a yellowish substance (bile pigment) in the eyes and skin to cause jaundice. Approximately 80%–99% of affected individuals have intermittent jaundice caused by excess bilirubin (bile pigment). In addition, they have a black liver (Figure 12.3) because polymerized epinephrine metabolites are accumulated in the lysosomes due to impaired excretion (Morii and Yamamoto 2016). In contrast to unaffected individuals who have a ratio of coproporphyrin III to coproporphyrin I as about 3.5:1 (g/g) in the urine, this ratio is inverted in patients with Dubin–Johnson syndrome. The disorder affects all races, but there is a high incidence (1:1,300) in Persian Jews (Zlotogora 2015). A protein- and iron-restricted diet may be beneficial for affected individuals.

12.2.11.2 Gilbert's Syndrome or Crigler–Najjar Syndrome

This is an autosomal recessive disorder caused by the abnormal metabolism of bilirubin, resulting in an inherited form of non-hemolytic jaundice (Fretzayas et al. 2012). In this condition which affects up to 5% of individuals in the United States, jaundice results from hyperbilirubinemia due to a deficiency of uridine diphosphoglucuronate glucuronosyl transferase 1A1 (UGT1A1) or glucose-6-phosphate dehydrogenase (G6PDH). UGT1A1 catalyzes the degradation of bilirubin derived from heme, which is released from the breakdown of hemoglobin due to the lysis of red blood cells (Chapter 5). Therefore, a partial deficiency of this enzyme results in the accumulation of bilirubin in the plasma (>18 mg/L). There are two UGT1A1 deficiency syndromes depending on either a partial or a complete absence of the enzyme: Gilbert's syndrome (mild phenotype; type-2), Crigler–Najjar syndrome (intermediate phenotype, type-2, and severe phenotype, type-1). G6PDH catalyzes the conversion of NADP$^+$ to NADPH in the pentose phosphate pathway of glucose metabolism. Limited production of NADPH reduces the antioxidative capacity of the body and increases the vulnerability of red blood cells to oxidative stress. This may shorten the life span of these cells, causing them

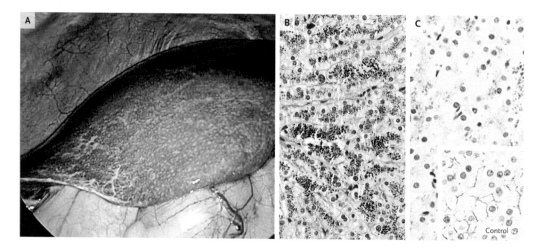

FIGURE 12.3 The appearance and morphology of the liver of a 48-year-old woman with Dubin–Johnson syndrome. The concentration of total bilirubin in the serum was 4.6 mg/dL [79 μM; compared with the reference range for healthy control, 0.2–1.2 mg/dL (3–21 μM)]. A laparoscopic examination revealed a grossly black appearance (Panel a). A biopsy specimen showed coarse, deep brown, pigmented granules on periodic acid–Schiff staining (Panel b), primarily at the canalicular pole of the hepatocytes and especially in the pericentral zones. There was no expression of multidrug-resistance–associated protein 2 (MRP2) in the patient (Panel c; compared with the healthy control specimen [inset]). (Reproduced from Morii, K. and T. Yamamoto. 2016. *N. Engl. J. Med.* 375:e1. With permission.)

to release more hemoglobin for the production of heme and bilirubin. Patients with hyperbilirubinemia exhibit a yellowish color in the skin, eyes, and mucous membranes.

Individuals with Gilbert's syndrome and type-2 Crigler–Najjar syndrome have no disease-related symptoms other than occasional non-symptomatic jaundice. However, those with Crigler–Najjar type 1 have no active *UGT1A1* gene product and, as a result, have severe indirect hyperbilirubinemia, leading to bilirubin deposition in the brain called kernicterus and, therefore, severe developmental delay. They are treated initially with phototherapy, exchange transfusion, and plasmapheresis, but the only cure is liver transplantation.

12.2.11.3 Protoporphyria

The chelation of porphyrin with Fe^{2+} by ferrochelatase (also known as heme synthase) to form heme (Chapter 5) is the first step in the synthesis of hemoglobin, the major oxygen carrier in blood. Protoporphyria is a rare autosomal dominant disorder (also known as erythropoietic protoporphyria) due to a deficiency of ferrochelatase (Lecha et al. 2009). Affected individuals have elevated levels of protoporphyrin in their plasma, tissues, and urine. Patients may experience very painful acute photosensitivity, skin lesions (Figure 12.4), hepatobiliary disease, and liver failure. Prolonged

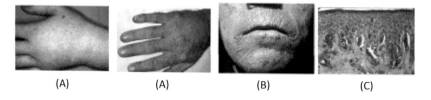

(A)   (A)   (B)   (C)

FIGURE 12.4 Symptoms of protoporphyria in humans. Acute photosensitivity reaction of the skin (a), chronic skin lesions of the skin (b), and the deposition of periodic acid–Schiff-positive substances around papillary blood vessels and dermoepidermal junction (c) in patients with protoporphyria. (Reproduced from a photo freely available in the public domain from Lecha, M. et al. 2009. *Orphanet J. Rare Dis.* 4:19. http://www.ojrd.com/content/4/1/19.)

exposure to the sun can lead to edema and blistering in the skin. Treatment of protoporphyria includes: the avoidance of sunlight and ultraviolet (UV) light, dietary supplementation with vitamin D (compensating for the lack of subcutaneous synthesis of vitamin D_3 from 7-dehydrocholesterol), and the use of creams for tanning and protective clothing.

12.2.12 HISTIDINE

12.2.12.1 Histidinemia

Histidinemia is an autosomal recessive disorder (Taylor et al. 1991). It results from a deficiency of histidase (the enzyme which converts histidine to urocanate and NH_4^+), leading to elevated levels of histidine in the plasma (as much as 15 times the normal value), as well as an increase in the urinary excretion of histidine, imidazolepyruvate, imidazolelactate, and imidazoleacetate. Persons with histidinemia have little urocanic acid in their skin or sweat. This disease is associated with developmental delay, mental retardation, speech defects, and learning difficulties. Treatment involves a histidine-restricted diet.

12.2.12.2 Mastocytosis

Rarely, babies and children are found to have chronic urticarial, or hives, and other allergic symptoms. Mastocytosis is an autosomal recessive disorder caused by the excessive production of histamine by histidine decarboxylate in mast cells due to KIT (a receptor tyrosine kinase) mutations (Orfao et al. 2007). Affected individuals have an excessive number of apparently normal mast cells in the skin and, occasionally, in other tissues and organs (including the bone marrow, gastrointestinal tract, liver and spleen, central nervous system, heart, or blood). Patients with this disorder have elevated urinary excretion of histamine and its metabolite (1-methylimidazole-4-acetate). Symptoms of mastocytosis include a severe urticarial skin rash, edema, enlargement of the liver and spleen, erythema, diarrhea, and tachycardia. Drug therapy (histamine H_1 and H_2 blockers and the avoidance of triggering factors) focuses on stabilizing mast cell membranes, reducing the severity of the attacks, and blocking the action of inflammatory mediators. A histidine- and histamine-restricted diet (e.g., non-fish and non-shrimp foods) may be beneficial for affected individuals.

12.2.12.3 Tay–Sachs Disease

This is an autosomal recessive disease of cerebromacular degeneration. It is most prevalent in individuals of Ashkenazi Jewish ancestry (Filho and Shapiro 2004). The disorder results from a defect in sphingolipid metabolism due to a deficiency of hexosaminidase A. It is a lysosomal enzyme that catalyzes the hydrolysis of terminal N-acetyl-D-hexosamine residues in N-acetyl-β-D-hexosaminides to release N-acetylglucosamine and N-acetylgalactosamine. Thus, the deficiency of this enzyme causes an accumulation of GM2 (the second monosialic ganglioside discovered) gangliosides (glycosphingolipids) in neurons and possibly some other cell types, resulting in a progressive loss of neurological function and an impairment of the renal reabsorption of imidazole compounds into the blood. Affected individuals have increased urinary excretion of anserine, carnosine, histidine, and methylhistidines. A diagnostic clue in patients with cerebromacular degeneration is the presence of a cherry-red spot in the macula upon eye examination. These individuals suffer from blindness, deafness, paralysis, and disorders of the central nervous system. The affected patients may benefit from a diet consisting of meat that contains large amounts of anserine, carnosine, and histidine.

12.2.12.4 Urocanic Aciduria

This is an autosomal recessive disorder that results from a deficiency of urocanase, which is also known as urocanate hydratase (Espinós et al. 2009). In the liver, urocanase converts urocanic acid (a product of histidine catabolism by histidinase) to 4-imidazolone-5-propionic acid and subsequently to glutamate. This disorder is characterized by elevated levels of urocanic acid in both the plasma and the urine. Clinical symptoms, which are generally benign and various, include intermittent ataxia, psychomotor dysfunction, aggressive behavior, and mental retardation. A histidine-restricted diet (e.g., non-fish and non-shrimp foods) may be beneficial for affected individuals.

12.2.13 Phenylalanine and Tyrosine

12.2.13.1 Albinism

Oculocutaneous albinism (OCA) is an autosomal recessive disorder caused by a deficiency of tyrosinase (tyrosine hydroxylase) in melanocytes (Opitz et al. 2004; Sreelatha et al. 2009). This enzyme oxidizes tyrosine to dihydroxyphenylalanine (DOPA) (an intermediate in melanin biosynthesis) by a BH4-dependent mechanism (Chapter 5). The defect in melanin production results in reduced or no pigment in the eyes, skin, and hair (Figure 12.5). Albinism is associated with a number of vision defects, such as poor development of retinal pigment epithelium, photophobia, nystagmus (irregular rapid movement of the eyes back and forth or in a circular motion), optic nerve hypoplasia (the underdevelopment of the optic nerve), and astigmatism (blurred vision due to the inability of the optics of the eye to focus a point object into a sharp, focused image on the retina). A lack of skin pigmentation also increases risks for sunburn and skin cancers.

Treatment of OCA involves the use of sunglasses to protect the eyes from the sun's UV rays, as well as suitable clothing and sunscreen creams to protect the skin. Affected individuals may also benefit from: (1) a tyrosine-restricted diet and (2) oral administration of L-DOPA or melanin. Of note, results of recent studies indicated that oral administration of nitisinone (2 mg/day for an adult) increased hair and skin pigmentation in patients with OCA (Adams et al. 2019). Nitisinone is an FDA-approved medication for the treatment of type-I tyrosinemia. This drug inhibits 4-hydroxyphenylpyruvate dioxygenase (HPD) [the enzyme catalyzing the conversion of 4-hydroxyphenylpyruvate (a product of tyrosine hydroxylation) into homogentisate], thereby reducing the accumulation of toxic byproducts (e.g., succinylacetone) of tyrosine catabolism via the transamination pathway.

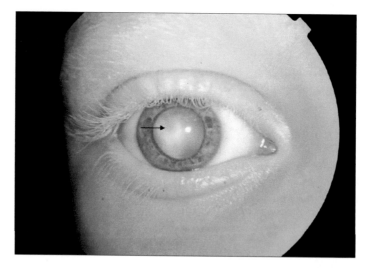

FIGURE 12.5 Abnormal colorization in the eyes of persons with oculocutaneous albinism. The red pupil (arrow) occurs due to inadequate absorption of light from a hypopigmented retina. The patient also exhibits hypopigmented eyelashes, eyebrows, and light iris. (Reproduced from a photo freely available in the public domain from Sreelatha, O.K. et al. 2008. *Oman J Ophthalmol.* 2:43–45. https://europepmc.org/article/med/21234225.)

Nitisinone (also known as NTBC, [2-nitro-4-trifluoromethylbenzoyl]-1,3-cyclohexanedione)

12.2.13.2 Ocular Albinism, Type 1

This is an X-linked recessive disorder caused by mutations in the G protein-coupled receptor 143 (GPR143) gene that plays an important role in the pigmentation (coloring) of the eyes and skin from tyrosine-derived melanin (Oetting 2002). The gene is expressed in the retinal pigment epithelium of the eyes and melanocytes. The incidence of ocular albinism, type 1, is about 1:50,000. It is the most common form of ocular albinism. Affected males lack pigmentation of the retina, experience vision deficits (which are present at birth), and develop photophobia while exhibiting normal skin and hair pigmentation. Treatment involves the use of sunglasses to protect the eyes from the sun's UV rays, as well as suitable clothing and sunscreen creams to protect the skin. Affected individuals may also benefit from the oral administration of melanin.

12.2.13.3 Alkaptonuria (Black Urine Disease)

This autosomal recessive disorder is caused by a deficiency of homogentisate oxidase, which oxidizes homogentisate to maleylacetoacetate in the metabolic pathway of phenylalanine and tyrosine catabolism (Zatkova 2011). This disease is characterized by increased urinary excretion of homogentisate (up to 0.5 g/day). The urine from patients becomes black on standing due to the oxidation of homogentisate by atmospheric oxygen. Persons with alkaptonuria suffer from ochronosis, which is named after the characteristic pigmentation (ochre color) of the connective tissue in the eyes seen upon microscopic examination. They also have abnormal dark spots on the whites of their eyes. Although alkaptonurics generally do not exhibit clinically adverse symptoms early in life, they subsequently develop darkening of the tendons and cartilages due to pigment deposition. After the age of 30, a blue–black color of the skin can be evident (e.g., around the mouth, eyes, and ears; Phornphutkul et al. 2002), and the pigmentation increases in intensity with age (Figure 12.6). Treatment includes: (1) a protein-restricted diet; (2) dietary supplementation with vitamin C to stimulate the oxidation homogentisate to maleylacetoacetate (Chapter 4); and (3) oral administration of nitisinone (2 mg/day for an adult).

12.2.13.4 Aromatic L-Amino Acid Decarboxylase Deficiency

This autosomal recessive disorder results from a deficiency of aromatic L-amino acid decarboxylases in the brain (Montioli et al. 2014). These enzymes convert: (a) DOPA (a metabolite of phenylalanine and tyrosine) into dopamine and (b) 5-hydroxytryptophan (a metabolite of tryptophan hydroxylation) into serotonin. Thus, the neurotransmitters, dopamine, norepinephrine, epinephrine, and serotonin, are deficient in the central nervous system and the peripheral tissues, while the concentrations of DOPA and 5-hydroxytryptophan in neurons are markedly increased. Symptoms usually appear during the first year of life. Affected individuals exhibit developmental delay, intellectual disability, abnormal behavior, gastrointestinal dysmotility, and autonomic dysfunction. Treatment includes: (1) a protein-restricted diet and (2) oral administration of dopamine and serotonin.

12.2.13.5 Hypertyrosinemia

Hypertyrosinemia occurs due to either a deficiency of cytosolic tyrosine transaminase (oculocutaneous tyrosinemia), 4-HPD, or fumarylacetoacetate hydrolase (Chapter 4), and thus consists of three types. This disease is characterized by elevated levels of tyrosine in the plasma (up to 3 mM) and elevated excretion in the urine (up to 2 g/day). Affected patients experience painful corneal erosions with photophobia, liver failure, cirrhosis, skin lesions, kidney disturbances, peripheral neuropathy, and mental retardation. Treatment varies with the type of hypertyrosinemia and, in all cases,

A

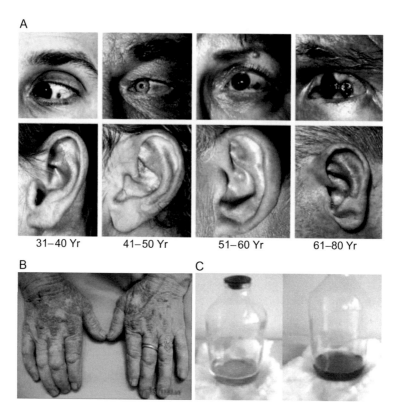

31–40 Yr   41–50 Yr   51–60 Yr   61–80 Yr

B   C

FIGURE 12.6 Ochronotic pigmentation of sclerae and ear cartilage, as well as dark urine from humans with alkaptonuria. This disorder results from a defect of homogentisate oxidase (an enzyme in tyrosine catabolism via the transamination pathway), leading to accumulation of homogentisate in tissues and urine. Affected individuals exhibit: (1) ochronosis (dark pigment deposits on connective tissue in the eyes) and abnormal pigmentation in the eyes and skin, with the symptoms becoming worse with age (Panel a, Reproduced from Phornphutkul C. et al. 2002. *N. Engl. J. Med.* 347:211–221. With permission.); (2) abnormal skin due to degenerative collagenous palmar plaques in a 60-year-old affected woman (Panel b, Reproduced from a photo freely available in the public domain from Vasudevan, B. et al. 2009. *Indian J. Dermatol.* 54:299–301. https:// www.e-ijd.org/text.asp?2009/54/3/299/55650.); and (3) fresh urine from a 38-year-old affected man that later turned dark after long standing (Panel c, Reproduced from a photo freely available in the public domain from Kanniyan K. et al. 2014. *J. Orthop. Case Reports.* 4:29–32. http://europepmc.org/article/PMC/4719265.)

patients can benefit from a protein-restricted diet that provides a reduced amount of AAs, particularly phenylalanine (which is converted into tyrosine by BH4-dependent phenylalanine hydroxylase in the liver and kidneys) and tyrosine.

Type-I tyrosinemia (an autosomal recessive disorder) is a life-threatening, early-onset disorder of tyrosine metabolism caused by a defect of the gene for fumarylacetoacetase (Mitchell et al. 2001), which catalyzes the last step in the tyrosine degradation pathway (Chapter 4). This disorder is characterized by the accumulation of maleylacetoacetate and fumarylacetoacetate, and their by-products [succinylacetone (a potent inhibitor of 5-aminolevulinic acid dehydratase), resulting in the accumulation of 5-aminolevulinic acid (a neurotoxic substance) in the blood and succinylacetoacetate] that are toxic to cells, particularly the liver and kidneys. Succinylacetone is the most useful metabolite to make the diagnosis in a neonate or young infant with liver disease. Tyrosinemia type I is most common among individuals with French–Canadian ancestry and is particularly prevalent in the Saguenay–Lac Saint-Jean region of Quebec with the incidence of 1 in 1,850 births. Symptoms include hepatic abnormalities, liver failure in the early stage, abnormal kidney structure, renal tubular acidosis, growth failure, hypophosphatemic rickets, neurological disorders, yellowing of the

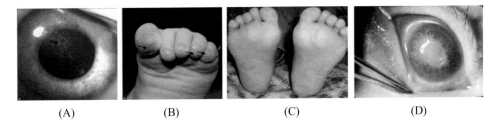

(A)   (B)   (C)   (D)

FIGURE 12.7   Abnormal skin color and lesions in patients with type-II tyrosinemia. Affected infants exhibit grossly symmetrical pseudodendritic subepithelial corneal opacities (a), punctate hyperkeratotic patches on feet (b), lesions, and abnormal color on feet (c), and abnormal eyes (e.g., keratitis and corneal opacity in tyrosinemia). (Panels a and b: Reproduced from a photo freely available in the public domain from Mohite, A.A. and J. Abbott. 2018. *Indian J. Ophthalmol.* 66:449. https://europepmc.org/article/pmc/pmc5859607; Panel c: Reproduced from a photo freely available in the public domain from Altamimi, E. and Alnsour, R. 2014. *Int. J. Clin Med. Imaging* 1(7):1–2. doi:10.4172/ijcmi.1000237; and Panel d: Reproduced from a photo freely available in the public domain at the University of Arizona (Tucson, Arizona, USA); https://disorders.eyes.arizona.edu/disorders/tyrosinemia-type-ii.)

skin, and porphyria-like symptoms. Affected individuals are at increased risk for hepatocellular carcinoma. The condition previously was lethal without liver transplantation but is now treatable with nitisinone (Chinsky et al. 2017). Type-II tyrosinemia (also known as Richner–Hanhart syndrome; an autosomal recessive disorder) results from a deficiency of tyrosine aminotransferase, a major enzyme initiating tyrosine degradation in the liver and kidneys (Mitchell et al. 2001). This causes the elevations of the concentrations of tyrosine and its metabolites (4-hydroxyphenylpyruvate, 4-hydroxyphenyllactate, and 4-hydroxyphenylacetate) in the plasma, cerebrospinal fluid, and urine. In untreated patients, the concentration of tyrosine in the plasma can be as high as 1.2 mM (about ten times the normal value). Symptoms of type-II tyrosinemia include tyrosine crystal deposition in the corneal epithelial cells, leading to photophobia, excessive lacrimation, and burning sensation. Affected patients exhibit skin abnormalities (mainly in the palm of the hand and the sole of the foot; Figure 12.7), normal development to intellectual disability (mild to severe), and in some cases seizures, tremor, and ataxia. The incidence of type-II tyrosinemia is less than 1/250,000. Dietary restriction of tyrosine and phenylalanine is recommended to maintain tyrosine concentrations in the plasma at 200–500 µM while maintaining adequate phenylalanine intake.

Type-III tyrosinemia (formerly known as tyrosinosis) is an autosomal recessive disorder caused by a defect of the 4-HPD gene (Kogut et al. 1967; Mitchell et al. 2001). This enzyme oxidizes *p*-hydroxyphenylpyruvate to homogentisate and depends on ascorbate and Cu^{2+} for its catalytic activity. In affected individuals, the concentrations of tyrosine and its metabolites (4-hydroxyphenylpyruvate, 4-hydroxyphenyllactate, and 4-hydroxyphenylacetate) are substantially increased in their blood (e.g., up to a 5-fold increase in plasma tyrosine) and urine. The most common syndrome is intellectual disability, which can vary from mild to severe. Other findings include psychomotor delay, intermittent ataxia, drowsiness, cirrhosis, severe hypophosphatemic rickets, and renal tubular defects. A milder form of HPD deficiency is Hawkinsin (the accumulation of 4-dihydroxy-cyclohexyl acetic acid), and affected patients show slow growth and metabolic acidosis in the first years after birth, but appear to be asymptomatic later in life. Treatment involves the dietary restriction of both phenylalanine and tyrosine to maintain its plasma concentrations close to physiological ranges.

12.2.13.6   Hypothyroidism

Although most individuals with hypothyroidism are afflicted by the autoimmune inflammation of the thyroid, thyroid dysfunction can be caused by a deficiency of dehalogenase activity or a defect in the utilization of iodide in the thyroid gland as an autosomal recessive disorder (Afink et al. 2008). The individuals lacking dehalogenase have elevated levels of monoiodotyrosine and diiodotyrosine in the plasma and urine after the administration of iodine. By contrast, the individuals who cannot utilize inorganic iodide fail to iodinate tyrosyl compounds in the metabolic pathway of thyroid hormone synthesis. In any case, patients have low concentrations of triiodothyronine and thyroxine in their plasma, leading to compensatory thyroid hyperplasia followed by the degeneration of the thyroid gland and replacement with fibrous tissue. Some of the affected individuals may experience congenital nerve deafness. As mentioned, in most cases, hypothyroidism is secondary, for example, to surgery, radiation therapy, iodine deficiency, or an autoimmune disease called Hashimoto's thyroiditis, rather than to a primary mutation, although a congenital form has been recognized. Treatment involves oral administration of thyroid hormone, such as synthetic levothyroxine [3,5,3′, 5′-tetraiodo-L-thyronine; a synthetic form of thyroxine (T4)]. Levothyroxine is converted into triiodothyronine (T3) in the body.

12.2.13.7 Phenylketonuria

Phenylketonuria (PKU) was the first inborn error of metabolism shown to affect the neurological function of humans (Figure 12.8). It was first identified in 1934 by the Norwegian physician, Ivar Asbjørn Følling, who observed an elevation of phenylketones in the urine of two siblings with both unusual odor and intellectual disability (Centerwall and Centerwall 2000). This disease results from an impaired conversion of phenylalanine into tyrosine due to a deficiency of either phenylalanine hydroxylase (type-I PKU) or its essential cofactor, BH4 (type-II PKU) (Williams et al. 2008). BH4 deficiency is caused by mutations of one of the genes which encode enzymes for the biosynthesis (GTP cyclohydrolase I or 6-pyruvoyl-tetrahydropterin synthase) or regeneration (pterin-4a-carbinolamine dehydratase or dihydropteridine reductase). Individuals with PKU are unable to break down the phenylalanine present in dietary proteins and artificial sweeteners (aspartame).

Affecting one in 10,000–15,000 newborn babies in the United States, both type-I and type-II PKU are autosomal recessive disorders (Williams et al. 2008). Patients with type-I or type-II PKU have an increased concentration of phenylalanine. In addition, persons with type-II PKU also have increases in the plasma concentrations of tyrosine and phenylalanine due to defects in the catabolism of these two AAs but decreases in the plasma concentrations of serotonin, dopamine, and melanin due to reductions in their synthesis via BH4-dependent pathways. All PKU patients exhibit an increased

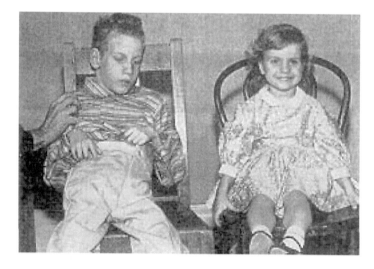

FIGURE 12.8 Two siblings carrying a mutated phenylalanine hydroxylase gene. The untreated 11-year-old boy (on the left) has phenylketonuria and is severely retarded. However, his 2-year-old sister (on the right), who was diagnosed with phenylketonuria in early infancy and promptly treated with dietary therapy, has normal development. (Reproduced from a photo freely available in the public domain at https://drustapbio.fandom.com/wiki/Phenylketonuria.)

urinary excretion of phenylalanine, phenylpyruvate (due to phenylalanine degradation via an alternative transamination pathway), phenyllactate, phenylacetylglutamine, α-hydroxyphenylpyruvate, and related compounds, but a decreased urinary excretion of serotonin and 5-hydroxyindoleacetate. These patients also have abnormal muscle tone, dysfunctional tendon reflexes, eczema, convulsions, mental retardation, seizures, and brain damage. The standards of treatment continue to be either a low-phenylalanine diet for both type-I and type-II PKU or the oral administration of BH4 for type-II PKU, depending on the molecular basis of the disease. After 2018, two novel therapies have also been approved for PKU treatment. First, a novel enzyme therapy with a PEGylated recombinant phenylalanine ammonia lyase that breaks down phenylalanine (called Palynziq) has become the only enzyme therapy for the disease. Second, the FDA has approved the drug sapropterin dihydrochloride (Kuvan®), which is a form of BH4, to assist with the breakdown of phenylalanine for type-II PKU. Current research for PKU treatment includes: (1) gene therapy to correct for a deficiency of phenylalanine hydroxylase or GTP cyclohydrolase-I and (2) an oral "designer probiotic", which is a genetically engineered microbe to degrade some dietary phenylalanine before its absorption by the small intestine (Isabella et al. 2018).

12.2.13.8 Pheochromocytoma

Pheochromocytoma is a unique tumor of the adrenal medulla (Figure 12.9) or the ganglia of the sympathetic nervous system that produces excessive amounts of epinephrine and norepinephrine from tyrosine (Crona et al. 2017). It is an autosomal dominant disorder and is characterized by the growth of noncancerous (benign) tumors in structures called paraganglia (groups of cells near the nerve cell bunches called ganglia). One or more enzymes of the pathway for catecholamine synthesis are highly expressed or activated in the affected cells. This disease is characterized by the increased excretion of epinephrine, norepinephrine, metanephrine, normetanephrine, and 3-methoxy-4-hydroxymandelic acid in the urine. Pheochromocytomas display various appearances at the computed tomography imaging (Blake et al. 2004). Patients with pheochromocytoma experience skin sensation, flank pain, hypertension, anxiety, diaphoresis, headaches, weight loss, and elevated concentrations of free fatty acids and glucose (due to increases in lipolysis, glycogenolysis, and gluconeogenesis). The primary treatment is the surgical removal of the tumor. In addition, a phenylalanine- and tyrosine-restricted diet may be beneficial for affected individuals.

12.2.14 PROLINE AND 4-HYDROXYPROLINE

12.2.14.1 Hyperhydroxyprolinemia

Proline and 4-hydroxyproline are the major AAs in fibrillary collagen. Hyperhydroxyprolinemia, an autosomal recessive disorder, results from a deficiency of 4-hydroxyproline oxidase, which oxidizes 4-hydroxyproline to Δ^1-pyrroline-3-hydroxy-5-carboxylate (Phang et al. 2001). This condition leads to mental retardation. Affected individuals have high concentrations of 4-hydroxyproline in their plasma (up to 0.5 mM) and urine (up to 270 mg/day), but normal levels of other AAs (including proline) in both physiological fluids. No abnormality is found for collagen metabolism in persons with hydroxyprolinemia. Ingestion of a hydroxyproline-free diet or dietary supplementation with proline does not affect concentrations of 4-hydroxyproline in the plasma or urine, possibly due to the following two reasons. First, dietary arginine, glutamate, and glutamine are converted into proline and then 4-hydroxyproline in animals (Wu et al. 2011). Second, dietary 4-hydroxyproline may have different metabolic patterns than endogenously generated 4-hydroxyproline due to substrate channeling in the cells and the body.

12.2.14.2 Hyperprolinemia

This autosomal recessive disorder occurs due to a deficiency of either proline oxidase (also known as PRODH; the enzyme which oxidizes proline to P5C; type I) or P5C dehydrogenase (the enzyme which converts P5C to glutamate; type II) (Phang et al. 2001; Willis et al. 2008). Patients have high

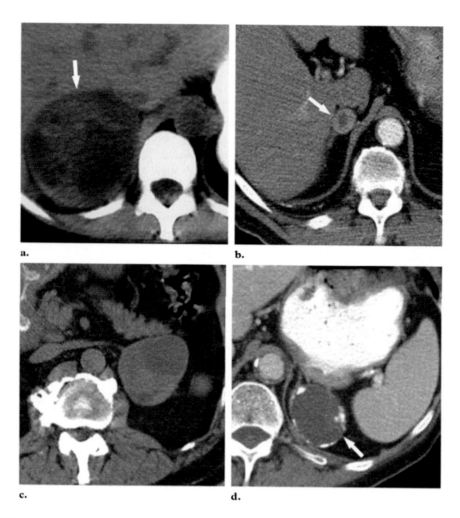

FIGURE 12.9 Spectrum of complex pheochromocytomas in humans. Pheochromocytomas display various appearances at the computed tomography (CT) imaging. (a) a heterogeneously reduced mass in the right adrenal gland (arrow) of a 72-year-old woman, as shown by unenhanced CT; (b) a mass of the right adrenal gland (arrow) with peripheral enhancement and a reduced central area in an 80-year-old man, as revealed by contrast-enhanced CT scan; (c) a mass with cystic and solid components in the left adrenal gland of a 41-year-old man, as demonstrated by unenhanced CT scan; (d) a cystic adrenal lesion with a calcified rim (arrow) in a 59-year-old woman, as identified by contrast-enhanced CT scan. (Reproduced from a photo freely available in the public domain from Blake, M.A. et al. 2004. *RadioGraphics* 24 (Suppl. 1):S87–S99. https://pubs.rsna.org/doi/10.1148/rg.24si045506.)

concentrations of proline in their plasma (0.5–2.6 mM in type I and 0.5–3.7 mM in type II) and excrete large amounts of free and peptide-bound proline (up to 3 g/day), hydroxyproline, and glycine (up to 0.7 g/day) when concentrations of proline in the plasma exceed 0.8 mM. The high levels of proline (up to 42 mM), hydroxyproline (up to 3 mM), and glycine (up to 20 mM) in the urine are likely caused by increased glomerular filtration and impaired renal reabsorption because proline, hydroxyproline, and glycine share the same transport system (Chapter 2). Affected individuals have convulsions, mental retardation, and renal disease. Results of recent genetic and clinical studies also indicate a close association between a deficiency of proline oxidase and schizophrenia in humans. Treatment involves a protein-restricted diet. Affected individuals can benefit from dietary supplementation with antioxidants, such as vitamin E, vitamin C, and glutathione (Mitsubuchi et al. 2014).

12.2.14.3 Iminoglycinuria

This is an autosomal recessive abnormality of the renal transport and reabsorption of imino acids (proline and hydroxyproline) and glycine (Rosenberg et al. 1968). This disorder is characterized by increased excretion of these three AAs in the urine. A defect in the proton-coupled AA transporter gene *SLC36A2* (PAT2) is the major factor responsible for iminoglycinuria (Bröer et al. 2008). Additional mutations occur in the genes encoding the imino acid transporter (SLC6A20; IMINO), a putative glycine transporter SLC6A18 (XT2), and a neutral AA transporter (SLC6A19; B⁰AT1) in families with either iminoglycinuria or hyperglycinuria (Bröer et al. 2008). Symptoms in affected patients include hypertension, glycosuria, nephrolithiasis, mental retardation, atypical gyrate atrophy, deafness, and blindness. Treatment involves: (1) a protein-restricted diet and (2) oral rehydration therapy.

12.2.14.4 Prolidase (Imidodipeptidase) Deficiency

Prolidase deficiency is an autosomal recessive disorder associated with imidodipeptiduria (Figure 12.10). Prolidase (a cytosolic enzyme) is particularly important in the hydrolysis of imidodipeptides that contain a C-terminal proline or hydroxyproline (Chapter 5). These dipeptides are generated from the breakdown of collagens (a family of proteins that are rich in proline and hydroxyproline) that are abundant in the extracellular matrix to support connective tissue, such as the skin, bone, tendons, and cartilage. Molecular analysis of prolidase deficiency cases identified 13 different mutations in the prolidase gene (*PEPD*): six missense and four exon-skipping mutations, two AA deletions, and a large genomic deletion (Hechtman 2001). A deficiency of prolidase

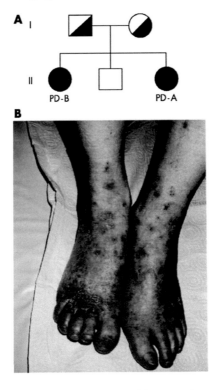

FIGURE 12.10 Prolidase deficiency in humans. Panel a illustrates the pedigree of a family carrying the 1234GRA mutant allele, causing the E412K substitution in the prolidase gene. Parents are heterozygotic for this mutation. Two sisters are homozygotic. Patient A (PD-A) is symptomatic, patient B (PD-B) is essentially asymptomatic, and their healthy brother does not carry the mutant allele. Panel b depicts severe skin ulcers at the lower legs and feet of patient A. (Reproduced from a photo freely available in the public domain from Lupi, A. et al. 2006. *J. Med. Genet.* 43:e58. https://pubmed.ncbi.nlm.nih.gov/17142620/.)

results in the urinary excretion of excessive dipeptides (up to 15 mmol/day) that include glycyl-proline, glutamyl-proline, and hydroxyproline dipeptides. Affected patients are unable to remodel their extracellular matrix, resulting in severe skin ulcers (particularly on their hands and feet) (Figure 12.4), mild-to-severe mental retardation, impaired wound healing, and increased susceptibility to infections. Treatment is aimed at controlling symptoms, particularly the skin lesions and ulceration, as well as local and systemic infections.

12.2.15 PURINES

12.2.15.1 Adenine Phosphoribosyltransferase Deficiency

This is an autosomal recessive disorder resulting from mutations of the adenine phosphoribosyltransferase (APRT) gene (Hidaka et al. 1987). The APRT protein catalyzes the synthesis of adenosine monophosphate from adenine and 5-phosphoribosyl-1-pyrophosphate. Patients with APRT deficiency have an impaired ability to degrade dietary or endogenous adenine, which is subsequently oxidized by xanthine dehydrogenase via the 8-hydroxy intermediate to 2,8-dihydroxyadenine. This results in the excessive production and urinary excretion of 2,8-dihydroxyadenine. Because 2,8-dihydroxyadenine is poorly soluble in the urine, its accumulation leads to urinary tract infections, as well as to the formation of kidney stones, kidney injury, and even kidney failure. Interestingly, up to 70% of affected patients have red hair or relatives with this hair color. Treatment involves: (1) a protein-restricted diet to reduce purine synthesis from AAs and a low-purine diet and (2) oral administration of allopurinol (an inhibitor of xanthine oxidase) to reduce the production of uric acid.

12.2.15.2 Adenosine Deaminase Deficiency

Adenosine deaminase (ADA) deficiency (an autosomal recessive disorder) is an immunodeficiency caused by the reduced conversion of adenosine to inosine (Flinn and Gennery 2018). ADA catalyzes the conversion of adenosine to inosine. ADA activity is particularly high in lymphocytes. A lack of ADA results in the accumulation of adenosine, deoxyadenosine, deoxy-ATP, and S-adenosylhomocysteine in the plasma as well as their elevated excretion in the urine. Adenosine is an activator of regulatory T-cells. Deoxyadenosine and deoxy-ATP inhibit ribonucleotide reductase and thus impair DNA synthesis, thereby leading to reduced proliferation and development of cells, particularly immature T and B lymphocytes and natural killer cells. Additionally, S-adenosylhomocysteine is cytotoxic to these immunocytes. Therefore, affected individuals have a small, underdeveloped thymus, lymphopenia, immunodeficiency, and increased risk for infectious diseases. Treatment involves: (1) a protein-restricted diet to reduce purine synthesis from AAs and a low-purine diet; (2) prevention and management of bacterial, viral, and fungal infections; and (3) intravenous administration of immunoglobulin to enhance whole-body immunity.

12.2.15.3 Adenylosuccinate Lyase Deficiency

This disorder (also known as adenylosuccinase deficiency) is an autosomal recessive disorder (Jurecka et al. 2015). This enzyme catalyzes several reactions in the *de novo* purine biosynthetic pathway (Chapter 5). In the first reaction, succinylaminoimidazolecarboxamide is converted to 5-aminoimidazole-4-carboxamide ribotide and fumarate. 5-Aminoimidazole-4-carboxamide ribotide proceeds through three more reactions to become adenylosuccinate (also called succinyladenosine monophosphate). Adenylosuccinate lyase (ADSL) cleaves adenylosuccinate to adenosine monophosphate and fumarate. Thus, this enzyme plays an important role in purine synthesis and also regulates metabolic processes by controlling the levels of AMP and fumarate in cells. ADSL deficiency is characterized by the appearance of succinylaminoimidazolecarboxamide and succinyladenosine in the plasma, cerebrospinal fluid, and urine. Affected individuals may have a range of symptoms that involve psychomotor retardation, epileptic seizures, and autistic features. To date, there is no specific and effective therapy for ADSL deficiency. Beneficial treatment may involve: (1) a protein-restricted diet to reduce purine synthesis from AAs and a low-purine diet, and (2) a ketogenic diet and with anticonvulsive drugs for the management of epilepsy.

12.2.15.4 Gout

Gout is caused by the excess deposition of monosodium urate crystals (the salts of uric acid, a metabolite of glutamine as well as ammonia and glutamate) within joints after chronic hyperuricemia. A deficiency of arginine also results in gout due to the impairment of the hepatic urea cycle. Inherited gout is a single joint arthritis, usually involving a toe, less often ankle or knee. Inherited gout mainly affects middle-aged and older men in the X-linked recessive manner (Jurecka 2009). At a physiological pH of 7.4, 98% of uric acid (the end product of purine catabolism) in the plasma is in the ionized form of urate, which is largely present as monosodium urate with a low solubility limit of about 380 μM. When plasma urate concentrations exceed 380 μmol/L, the risk of monosodium urate crystal formation and precipitation increases. Abnormal activity of two enzymes results in uric acid overproduction: superactivity of phosphoribosyl pyrophosphate synthetase (PRPS) and deficiency of hypoxanthine–guanine phosphoribosyltransferase (HGPRT) (Jurecka 2009). PRPS converts ribose-5-phopshate and ATP into phosphoribosyl pyrophosphate. HGPRT catalyzes the reaction of hypoxanthine and guanine with 5-phosphoribosyl 1-pyrophosphate to form inosine monophosphate and guanosine monophosphate, respectively, thereby playing a role in the generation of purine nucleotides through the purine salvage pathway (Chapter 5). A deficiency of HGPRT results in increased oxidation of hypoxanthine and guanine to uric acid. Symptoms of gout include red, tender, hot, and swollen joints, as well as neurological dysfunction (e.g., dystonia, mild-to-moderate mental retardation, and self-mutilation), and uric acid nephrolithiasis. Mutations in both PRPS and HGPRT are X-linked recessive traits. Treatment involves: (1) a protein-restricted diet to reduce purine synthesis from AAs and a low-purine diet; (2) the oral administration of allopurinol (an inhibitor of xanthine oxidase) to decrease the production of uric acid; and (3) the use of nonsteroidal anti-inflammatory drugs to reduce pain and inflammation.

12.2.15.5 Lesch–Nyhan Syndrome

This is an X-linked recessive disease caused by almost a complete deficiency of HGPRT due to mutations in the *HPRT* gene, which are usually carried by the mother and passed on to her son (Jurecka 2009). As noted previously, the HGPRT deficiency causes a buildup of uric acid in all body fluids, resulting in hyperuricemia and hyperuricosuria, as well as severe gout and kidney problems. Neurological symptoms include poor muscle control and mental retardation, which usually appear during the first year of life. Beginning in the second year of life, affected patients often exhibit self-mutilating behaviors, characterized by lip and finger biting. These patients generally have severe mental and physical problems throughout life. Treatment involves: (1) a protein-restricted diet to reduce purine synthesis from AAs and a low-purine diet; (2) the oral administration of allopurinol (an inhibitor of xanthine oxidase) to decrease the production of uric acid; and (3) supportive care, such as muscle relaxants for movement disorders and physical restraints to prevent self-injury.

12.2.15.6 Myoadenylate Deaminase Deficiency

This is an autosomal recessive disorder of purine metabolism in skeletal muscle (also known as type-1 AMP deaminase deficiency) (Sinkeller et al. 1988). AMP deaminase converts AMP into inosine monophosphate and ammonia and, therefore, plays an important role in the purine nucleoside cycle with physiological significance. A deficiency of AMP causes the accumulation of AMP in the exercising muscle and reduces the production of AMP metabolites, such as D-ribose. Affected individuals experience early fatigue, as well as pain, cramping, and weakness of skeletal muscle during exercise. Treatment involves: (1) a protein-restricted diet to reduce purine synthesis from AAs and a low-purine diet; (2) the oral administration of allopurinol (an inhibitor of xanthine oxidase) to decrease the production of uric acid; (3) a high oral dose of D-ribose (e.g., 4 g at the beginning of exercise; Zöllner et al. 1986); and (4) the avoidance of intense exercise.

12.2.15.7 Purine Nucleoside Phosphorylase Deficiency

This is an autosomal recessive disorder due to a deficiency of purine nucleoside phosphorylase (PNP), which catalyzes the conversion of inosine (a product of adenosine) and guanosine to hypoxanthine (Sasaki et al. 1988). PNP activity is particularly high in lymphocytes. Lack of PNP results in the accumulation of inosine, guanosine, and deoxy-GTP in the plasma, as well as elevated excretion in the urine. Deoxy-GTP inhibits ribonucleotide reductase and thus DNA synthesis, thereby leading to reduced proliferation of cells, particularly immature T-lymphocytes. Additionally, inosine, guanosine, and deoxy-GTP are cytotoxic to T-lymphocytes. Therefore, affected individuals have a small, underdeveloped thymus, reduced number of T-lymphocytes, immunodeficiency, and increased risk for infectious disease. Patients may also have neurological dysfunction (e.g., mental retardation) and are prone to the development of autoimmune disorders, including lupus erythematosus, hemolytic anemia, and idiopathic thrombocytopenic purpura. Treatment involves: (1) a protein-restricted diet to reduce purine synthesis from AAs and a low-purine diet and (2) the prevention and management of infections.

12.2.15.8 Xanthinuria

This disorder (an autosomal recessive trait) results from a deficiency of xanthine oxidase (also known as xanthine dehydrogenase or xanthine oxidoreductase) due to gene mutations (Ichida et al. 1997). This enzyme catalyzes the oxidation of hypoxanthine to xanthine and then to uric acid, the last two steps in the catabolism of purines (Chapter 6). The deficiency of xanthine oxidase, coupled with the continuous formation of xanthine from guanine by guanase, results in the accumulation of xanthine (a substance with low water solubility) in the plasma and urine. Hypoxanthine does not accumulate to an appreciable degree because this purine is recycled through a salvage pathway by HGPRT. Patients with xanthinuria experience arthropathy, myopathy, urinary tract infections, crystal nephropathy, urolithiasis, and renal failure. Treatment involves a protein-restricted diet to reduce purine synthesis from AAs and a low-purine diet.

12.2.16 PYRIMIDINES

12.2.16.1 β-Aminoisobutyric Aciduria

This is an autosomal recessive disorder (van Gennip et al. 1997). It is characterized by the high urinary excretion of β-aminoisobutyrate (up to 250 mg/day compared to a normal value of <10 mg/day for healthy individuals). This disorder is due to a defect in β-aminoisobutyrate-glutamate transaminase in the pathway of thymine (a pyrimidine) catabolism (Chapter 5). There is a large variation in the urinary excretion of β-aminoisobutyrate among individuals. So far, no clinical symptoms have been described for β-aminoisobutyric aciduria. However, high concentrations of β-aminoisobutyrate occur in the urine of fasted individuals and in patients with cancer, tuberculosis, liver disease, and lead poisoning (in each case likely due to increased degradation of pyrimidine). Treatment involves a protein-restricted diet to reduce purine synthesis from AAs and a low-pyrimidine diet.

12.2.16.2 Familial Pyrimidinemia

This autosomal recessive disorder results from a deficiency of dihydropyrimidine dehydrogenase (Diasio et al. 1988). This enzyme (also known as uracil reductase or thymine reductase) catalyzes the reduction of uracil and thymine to dihydrouracil and dihydrothymine, respectively (the first step in pyrimidine catabolism, Chapter 5). Thus, a deficiency of dihydropyrimidine dehydrogenase results in the accumulation of uracil and thymine in the plasma and urine but impaired synthesis of β-alanine and R-β-aminoisobutyrate. Clinical symptoms include convulsions, seizures, psychomotor retardation, hypertonicity, microcephaly, autism, and growth retardation. Affected individuals may be vulnerable to lethal toxicities after exposure to some pyrimidine-related chemotherapy drugs, such as 5-fluorouracil. Treatment involves a protein-restricted diet to reduce purine synthesis from AAs and a low-pyrimidine diet.

12.2.16.3 Hyper-β-Alaninemia

This autosomal recessive disorder results from a deficiency of β-alanine:α-ketoglutarate transaminase (Chapter 5) and the inhibition of renal reabsorption of β-AAs (including β-alanine, β-aminoisobutyrate, and taurine) (Gibson and Jacobs 2001). β-Alanine:α-ketoglutarate transaminase is responsible for the degradation of β-alanine (a product of pyrimidine catabolism) and, to some extent, GABA. Thus, affected individuals exhibit elevated levels of β-AAs and GABA in the plasma, cerebrospinal fluid, and urine, as well as elevated concentrations of carnosine in the skeletal muscle and urine. Excessive β-alanine and GABA are neurotoxic to the body. Clinical symptoms of hyper-β-alaninemia include neonatal respiratory distress, seizures, drowsiness, convulsions, mental retardation, hypotonia, and, if there is no liver transplantation, death. Treatment involves a protein-restricted diet to reduce purine synthesis from AAs, as well as a low-pyrimidine and low-β-alanine diet.

12.2.16.4 Orotic Aciduria

This is an autosomal recessive disorder that results from a deficiency of uridine monophosphate synthase (Suchi et al. 1997) or defects in urea cycle enzymes (Chapter 6). Uridine monophosphate synthase is a bifunctional enzyme catalyzing the last two steps of *de novo* pyrimidine biosynthesis and contains activities of orotate phosphoribosyltransferase and orotidine-5'-monophosphate decarboxylase (Chapter 5). A deficiency of this enzyme will lead to the accumulation of orotic acid in the plasma and urine. Orotic aciduria can also arise secondary to a blockage of the urea cycle (particularly in OCT deficiency) because ammonia is channeled to the synthesis of glutamine and then orotic acid. Patients with orotic aciduria exhibit anemia, abnormal changes in bone marrow, leukopenia, and retarded growth. Treatment involves: (1) a protein-restricted diet to reduce purine synthesis from AAs; (2) a low-pyrimidine diet; and (3) removal of ammonia in the blood.

12.2.17 SERINE

12.2.17.1 Hypophosphatasia

This autosomal recessive disorder is caused by reduced activity of tissue-nonspecific alkaline phosphatase (Whyte 2001). The enzyme catalyzes the catabolism of phosphoaminoethanol (a metabolite of serine and phosphocholine; Chapter 4) and plays a role in bone mineralization. Thus, a deficiency of alkaline phosphatase results in elevated concentrations of phosphoaminoethanol in the plasma and urine while impairing skeletal growth and development. Affected patients experience reduced food intake and inadequate weight gain, as well as clinical manifestations of rickets, bone lesions, teeth, central nervous system disease, and anemia. Asfotase alfa is approved for the treatment of hypophosphatasia to improve skeletal mineralization and motor capabilities.

12.2.17.2 Phosphoglycerate Dehydrogenase Deficiency

This is an autosomal recessive disorder and is also known as Neu–Laxova syndrome (Shaheen et al. 2014; Tabatabaie et al. 2011). It is a severe but potentially treatable inborn error of metabolism in humans due to mutations and a deficiency of phosphoglycerate dehydrogenase. The enzyme catalyzes the conversion of 3-phosphoglycerate to phosphohydroxypyruvate in the pathway of serine biosynthesis (Chapter 3). Patients with phosphoglycerate dehydrogenase deficiency have markedly low concentrations of serine (e.g., $50\,\mu M$ in the blood) and, to a relatively lesser extent, glycine (e.g., $105\,\mu M$ in the blood), in the plasma and cerebrospinal fluid. Affected individuals develop congenital microcephaly, profound psychomotor retardation, hypertonia, epilepsy, dysmyelination in the brain, growth restriction (including intrauterine growth restriction), and hypogonadism. Congenital bilateral cataracts may also occur in individuals with phosphoglycerate dehydrogenase deficiency. Dietary supplementation with L-serine (e.g., 0.6 g/kg BW/day in adults) or for those children with an insufficient response to L-serine alone, both L-serine and glycine (e.g., 0.25 g/kg BW/day) can ameliorate the symptoms of this disease (de Koning et al. 1998). Findings from this inborn error of metabolism indicate that: (1) endogenous synthesis of serine plays an essential role in maintaining serine homeostasis in neonates and (2) the intake of dietary serine from milk or the current milk formula is insufficient for optimal growth, development, and health.

12.2.18 SULFUR-CONTAINING AMINO ACIDS

12.2.18.1 Cystathioninuria

This autosomal recessive disorder is caused by a severe deficiency of cystathionase (also known as cystathionine γ-lyase) (Wang and Hegele 2003). The enzyme hydrolyzes cystathionine to cysteine and NH_4^+ (Chapter 6). Persons with cystathioninuria have high concentrations of cystathionine in their plasma (up to $20\,\mu M$), and a large amount of this metabolite is excreted in the urine (up to 1 g/day). Patients also suffer from mental retardation. Note that a deficiency of vitamin B_6 independent of a deficiency of cystathionase also results in cystathioninuria. Thus, both genetic and environmental (including nutritional) factors should be carefully considered in the interpretation of metabolite concentrations in the plasma and urine. Treatment includes: (1) a methionine-restricted diet and (2) an adequate intake of dietary cysteine (Finkelstein 2006).

12.2.18.2 Cystinosis

This disorder is an autosomal recessive lysosomal storage disorder due to mutations in the *CTNS* gene that codes for cystinosin, the lysosomal membrane-specific transporter for cystine in tissues and cells, including kidneys and polymorphonuclear leukocytes (Gahl et al. 2002). It is not to be confused with cystinuria (see below). As a result of the lysosomal transport defect, the cystine generated from intralysosomal protein degradation is not transported from the lysosomes into the cytosol for further catabolism. Instead, cystine is accumulated within the lysosomes at concentrations that are 10–100 times normal values. This eventually leads to intracellular crystal formation in the body. As indicated previously, cystinosis is the most common cause of Fanconi syndrome in infants and children. Individuals with mutations in the gene for cystine transport are normal at birth but develop renal abnormalities between 6 and 12 months of age. Clinical symptoms include dehydration, acidosis, vomiting, electrolyte imbalance, hypophosphatemic rickets, hypothyroidism, growth retardation, photophobia, renal glomerular damage, and retinal damage. Cystinosis is almost always treated with renal transplantation. This disorder is treated with cysteamine, which binds to cystine within the lysosome to facilitate the exit of cystine from the lysosome through a different transporter, thereby preventing the formation of cystine crystal in tissues. A methionine- and cysteine-restricted diet may also be beneficial for affected individuals.

12.2.18.3 Cystinuria

This transport disorder, which was the first aminoaciduria to be reported, is an autosomal recessive defect, with an overall incidence of approximately 1 in 7,000 newborn babies (Eggermann et al. 2012). The disease results from mutations in transporters of cystine and basic AAs, which are expressed at the apical surface of the small intestine and the renal tubular lumen; therefore, the absorption of dietary cysteine and basic AAs (arginine, lysine, and ornithine) from the lumen of the small intestine and the reabsorptive transport of these AAs from the luminal fluid of the renal proximal tubule into the blood are impaired. To date, two genes responsible for cystinuria in humans have been identified: (1) *SLC3A1* encoding the heavy subunit rBAT of a renal $b^{0,+}$ transporter and (2) *SLC7A9* encoding its interacting light subunit $b^{0,+}AT$. Cystinuria is characterized by the abnormally high urinary excretion of cystine, arginine, lysine, and ornithine and is a cause of persistent kidney stones in humans (Figure 12.11) and other animals such as dogs (Henthorn et al. 2009). In Newfoundland dogs exhibiting cystinuria in association with a nonsense mutation, R198X, in the *SLC7A9* gene encoding for the rBAT transporter, urinary excretion of cystine and lysine (but not arginine and ornithine) is high (Bannasch and Henthorn 2009). The major clinical

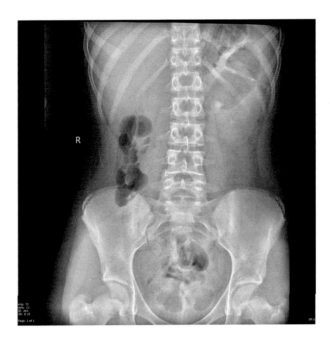

FIGURE 12.11 Abdominal radiograph in human with cystinuria. Cystine stones are present in the kidneys and frequently coalesce to form large branching staghorn calculi. (Reproduced from a photo freely available in the public domain from Knipe, H. and M.A. Morgan. 2020; https://radiopaedia.org/articles/cystinuria?lang=us.)

finding in cystinuria is renal calculi. Not all patients with cystinuria require renal transplantation. Penicillamine, a degradation product of penicillin, is used to treat patients with cystinuria because penicillamine reacts with cystine to form a mixed disulfide, penicillamine cysteine, for excretion. Nutritional management involving a methionine- and cysteine-restricted diet, drinking sufficient water, and restricting salt intake may also be beneficial for affected individuals.

12.2.18.4 Homocyst(e)inuria

This autosomal recessive disorder is caused by a deficiency of cystathionine β-synthase (Mudd et al. 2001). The enzyme converts homocysteine and serine into cystathionine (Chapter 4). Persons with this disease have high concentrations of homocyst(e)ine in their plasma (up to 50 μM) and urine (up to 100 mg/day), as well as high levels of methionine in their plasma. Patients with homocyst(e)inuria suffer from convulsions, mental retardation, cardiovascular disease, fatty liver, mottled red skin, lens dislocation, and fine sparse hair. In this disease, cysteine becomes a nutritionally essential AA. The incidence of the inherited homocyst(e)inuria is about 1:200,000 to 1:335,000 in the United States and can be much higher in some countries (e.g., 1:1,800 in Qatar and 1:6,400 in Norway) (Kožich and Stabler 2020). Note that a severe deficiency of either dietary folate plus vitamin B_6 or methylene-tetrahydrofolate reductase (MTHFR) also results in homocyst(e)inuria. Treatment of cystathionine β-synthase deficiency involves: (1) a methionine-restricted diet; (2) adequate intake of dietary cysteine; and (3) removal of homocysteine through the actions of methionine synthase and betaine–homocysteine methyltransferase.

12.2.18.5 Hypermethioninemia

Furujo et al. (2012) reported a case of hypermethioninemia in a female patient. It is an autosomal recessive disorder. The subject has a severe deficiency of methionine adenosyltransferase (MAT; also known as SAM synthetase) I/III and elevated concentrations of methionine in her plasma (10–15 times the normal value). This was found to result from two compound heterozygous missense mutations (R292C and R356L) in the gene, encoding the human MAT1A protein. Hypermethioninemia and mental retardation persisted until the age of 4 years and 8 months when dietary supplementation with SAM (a metabolite produced from methionine by MAT) was initiated [400–800 mg SAM disulfate tosylate (tosylate disulfate salt of SAM) twice daily]. This treatment improved the neurological development of the affected patient, although the concentration of methionine in the plasma remained substantially elevated. Other strategies of nutritional management include: (1) a methionine-restricted diet and (2) an adequate intake of dietary cysteine.

12.2.18.6   Glycine N-Methyltransferase Deficiency

This is an autosomal recessive disorder caused by a deficiency of glycine N-methyltransferase (GNMT) (Augoustides-Savvopoulou et al. 2003). This enzyme catalyzes the conversion of SAM and glycine into S-adenosylhomocysteine and sarcosine (Chapter 4). Symptoms of GNMT deficiency include elevations of serum liver transaminases, hepatic concentrations of methionine and SAM, and mild hepatomegaly. Similar observations have been reported for GNMT-knockout mice (Kožich and Stabler 2020). Treatment involves a methionine-restricted diet.

12.2.18.7   S-Adenosylhomocysteine Hydrolase Deficiency

This is an autosomal recessive disorder caused by a deficiency of S-adenosylhomocysteine hydrolase (SAHH) (Baric et al. 2004; Buist et al. 2006). This enzyme hydrolyzes S-adenosylhomocysteine into adenosine and homocysteine (Chapter 11). Affected individuals exhibit elevations of methionine, SAM, and creatine kinase (an indicator of tissue injury), as well as liver disease, neurologic abnormalities, and white matter abnormalities. Patients with SAHH show some improvement in response to the dietary restriction of methionine and supplementation with phosphatidylcholine and creatine.

12.2.19   Tryptophan

12.2.19.1   Carcinoid Syndrome

Carcinoid, which refers to tumors derived from the enterochromaffin (a type of enteroendocrine cells or argentaffin cells) or enterochromaffin-like cells in the gastric mucosa, is an autosomal recessive disorder (Schnirer et al. 2003). It results from the excessive formation of 5-hydroxytryptophan from tryptophan and the enhanced decarboxylation of 5-hydroxytryptophan to yield serotonin. Persons with this disease have elevated levels of serotonin and increased urinary excretion of serotonin and 5-hydroxyindoleacetate. Patients exhibit remarkable carcinoids (e.g., gastric carcinoids), cutaneous flushing, and pellagra-like skin lesions (Figure 12.12) and experience chronic

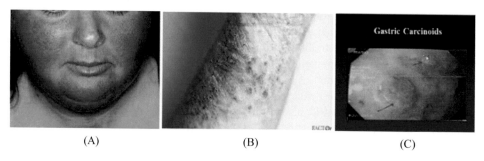

(A)　　　　　(B)　　　　　(C)

FIGURE 12.12 Abnormalities of the skin and stomach in patients with carcinoid syndrome gastric carcinoids). Panels a: Cutaneous flushing in a 32-year-old woman with carcinoid syndrome (Reproduced from a photo freely available in the public domain from Liu, L. 2020. https://step1.medbullets.com/endocrine/109033/carcinoid-syndrome.); Panel b: Pellagra-like skin lesions in a 42-year-old man with carcinoid syndrome (Reproduced from a photo freely available in the public domain from Liu, L. 2020. https://step2.medbullets.com/oncology/120477/carcinoid-syndrome.); Panel c: Gastric carcinoids in a 67-year-old man (Reproduced from a photo freely available in the public domain from Aaron Vinik et al. 2018. *Carcinoid Tumors.* https://www.ncbi.nlm.nih.gov/books/NBK279162/.)

diarrhea, abdominal cramps, heart disease, respiratory distress, and weight loss. Treatment is the surgical removal of the generally benign tumor. A tryptophan-restricted diet may be beneficial for affected individuals.

12.2.19.2 Hartnup Disease

This autosomal recessive disease occurs in persons with defects in intestinal transport and renal reabsorption of neutral AAs, particularly tryptophan, due to mutations of the SLC6A19 gene that encodes B°AT1 (Kleta et al. 2004). Thus, the production of nicotinamide or niacin from tryptophan in the liver is reduced. In addition, a relatively large amount of dietary tryptophan enters the large intestine for microbial fermentation and some of its metabolites are absorbed into the blood. Furthermore, the tryptophan filtered by the glomerulus into the lumen of the proximal renal tubules is not reabsorbed into the blood, thereby exacerbating tryptophan deficiency. The incidence of Hartnup disease is approximately one in 30,000 newborn infants in the United States. Affected individuals exhibit increases in the urinary excretion of indole compounds, histidine, and many neutral AAs (except for glycine, proline, and hydroxyproline), including alanine, asparagine, glutamine, BCAAs, phenylalanine, tyrosine, and tryptophan. Persons with this disease suffer from pellagra-like skin rashes (likely due to niacin deficiency; Figure 12.13), aberrations of the central nervous system, psychiatric disturbances, and mental retardation. Treatment includes: (1) a tryptophan-adequate and AA-balanced diet; and (2) dietary supplementation with nicotinamide or niacin; and (3) oral administration of L-tryptophan ethyl ester (0.2 g/kg BW/day; Jonas and Butler 1989).

12.2.19.3 Aromatic L-Amino Acid Decarboxylase Deficiency

This metabolic disorder affects the metabolism of aromatic AAs via decarboxylation, including phenylalanine, tyrosine, and tryptophan. See the "Phenylalanine and Tyrosine" section for a detailed discussion.

12.2.20 THE UREA CYCLE DEFECTS

Excess ammonia in the blood is highly toxic to the central nervous system in humans and other animals (Chapter 6). In mammals, the hepatic urea cycle plays a central role in the removal of ammonia by converting it into urea. Inherited disorders of the urea cycle have been reported for humans (Figure 12.14). Many of these defects are curable with liver transplantation early in life. Treatment generally includes: (1) a protein-restricted diet to reduce nitrogen loads and (2) intravenous or oral administration of sodium benzoate and sodium phenylacetate to remove ammonia (Singh et al. 2005). Additional therapies are indicated for specific disorders.

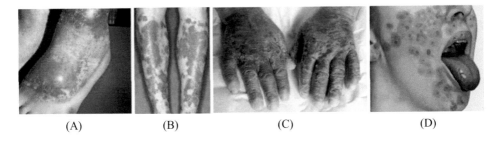

(A) (B) (C) (D)

FIGURE 12.13 Abnormalities of the skin in the feet (panel a), legs (panel b), hands (panel c), and face (panel d) of patients with Hartnup disease. (Reproduced from photos freely available in the public domain from Hartnup disease. http://medpics011.blogspot.com/2013/12/hartnup-disease.html.)

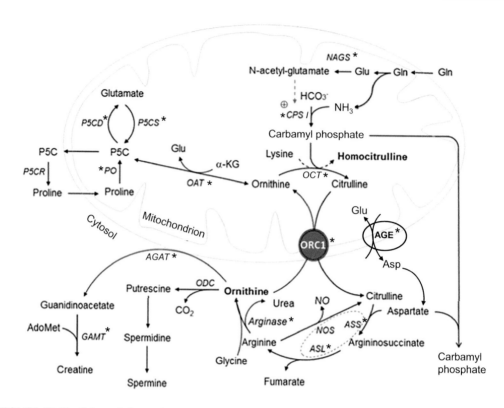

FIGURE 12.14 Inborn defects of urea cycle enzymes and related enzymes/transport proteins in humans. The hepatic urea cycle plays a major role in detoxifying ammonia as urea in humans. Defects in all enzymes of this metabolic cycle and related mitochondrial transporter proteins have been reported in individuals. AGAT, arginine;glycine amidinotransferase; AGE, aspartate-glutamate exchanger; ASL, argininosuccinate lyase; ASS, argininosuccinate synthetase; CPS I, carbamoyl phosphate synthetase-I; GAMT, guanidinoacetate *N*-methyltransferase; NAGS, *N*-acetylglutamate synthase; OAT, ornithine aminotransferase; OCT, ornithine carbamoyltransferase; NOS, nitric oxide synthase: ODC ornithine decarboxylase; ORC1, ornithine carrier 1; P5CD Δ^1-pyrroline-5-carboxylate dehydrogenase; P5CS, Δ^1-pyrroline-5-carboxylate synthase; P5CR, Δ^1-pyrroline-5-carboxylate reductase; PO, proline oxidase. * enzymes with inborn defects. (Adapted from a freely available article by Martinelli, D. et al. 2015. *Orphanet J. Rare Dis.* 10:29. https://ojrd.biomedcentral.com/articles/10.1186/s13023-015-0242-9.)

12.2.20.1 *N*-Acetylglutamate Synthase Deficiency

This is an autosomal recessive disorder (Caldovic et al. 2007). This mitochondrial enzyme catalyzes the conversion of glutamate and acetyl-CoA to *N*-acetylglutamate (NAG), which is an allosteric activator of CPS-I (a urea cycle enzyme; Chapter 6). Thus, a deficiency of NAG synthase results in elevated levels of alanine, glutamine, and ammonia in the plasma, spinal fluid, and urine but reduced concentrations of citrulline, arginine, and urea in these physiological fluids. Individuals with NAG synthase deficiency may experience growth retardation, lethargy, vomiting, mental retardation, deep coma, and death. Treatment involves oral administration of *N*-carbamoylglutamate (30–100 mg/kg BW/day for infants; Chapel-Crespo et al. 2016).

12.2.20.2 Argininosuccinic Aciduria

This autosomal recessive disorder results from the deficiency of argininosuccinate lyase in the liver and small intestine (Kleijer et al. 2002). The enzyme converts argininosuccinate to arginine and fumarate. This disease is associated with elevated concentrations of argininosuccinate in the plasma (up to 0.3 mM) and the excretion of relatively large amounts of argininosuccinate (up to 10 g/day) in the urine. Patients develop mental retardation, epilepsy, ataxia, and hepatomegaly within the first few years of life and may also exhibit hair defect (i.e., coarse brittle hair that breaks easily). Treatment includes dietary supplementation with arginine (e.g., 5 g/day for a 70-kg adult).

12.2.20.3 Carbamoyl Phosphate Synthetase I Deficiency

This disorder is an autosomal recessive disorder (Finckh et al. 1998). This mitochondrial enzyme converts NH_3 and HCO_3^- to carbamoyl phosphate, which then condenses with ornithine to form citrulline (Chapter 6). Thus, a deficiency of carbamoyl phosphate synthetase(CPS)-I impairs the urea cycle for ammonia detoxification in the liver and citrulline/arginine synthesis from glutamine in the small intestine, resulting in elevated concentrations of glutamine and ammonia in the plasma, spinal fluid, and urine but reduced concentrations of citrulline, arginine, and urea in these physiological fluids. Infants with CPS-I deficiency may experience growth restriction, developmental delay, lethargy, vomiting, mental retardation, deep coma, and even death. In some affected individuals, symptoms of CPS-I deficiency may be less severe and may not manifest until later in life. Treatment includes dietary supplementation with L-citrulline (e.g., 5 g/day for a 70-kg adult).

12.2.20.4 Hyperargininemia

This autosomal recessive disorder results from a deficiency of cytosolic arginase, which hydrolyzes arginine to urea plus ornithine (the last step of the urea cycle) (Scaglia and Lee 2006). Thus, affected individuals exhibit elevated levels of arginine and ammonia in their plasma, spinal fluid, and urine, but reduced concentrations of proline, urea, and ornithine in these fluids. Patients suffer from stiffness (especially in the legs) caused by the abnormal tensing of skeletal muscle, reduced growth, developmental delay, seizures, mental retardation, tremor, and ataxia (difficulty with balance and coordination). In response to high protein intake, a rapid increase in ammonia leads to episodes of irritability, nausea, and vomiting. Treatment includes an arginine- and citrulline-restricted diet.

12.2.20.5 Hypercitrullinemia

This autosomal recessive disorder results from the impairment of conversion of citrulline into arginine due to a deficiency of either enzymes or substrates (Endo et al. 2004). There are two forms of hypercitrullinemia, depending on its molecular basis, and both of them are characterized by elevated concentrations of citrulline and ammonia in the plasma and urine. Treatment for both type-I and type-II hypercitrullinemia includes dietary supplementation with L-arginine (e.g., 5 g/day for a 70-kg adult).

Type-I hypercitrullinemia (also known as type-I citrullinuria) occurs due to a deficiency of argininosuccinate synthase, which catalyzes the formation of argininosuccinate from citrulline and aspartate (Chapter 6). The concentrations of citrulline are greatly elevated in the plasma (up to 2 mM) and cerebrospinal fluid (up to 0.35 mM), as well as increased excretion in the urine (up to 0.5 to 2 g/day). Patients exhibit high circulating levels of ammonia (up to 170 µM), convulsion, alkalotic coma, and severe mental retardation.

Type-II hypercitrullinemia (also known as type-II citrullinuria) occurs due to a deficiency of citrin, a mitochondrial aspartate/glutamate exchanger that transports aspartate out of the mitochondria in exchange for the entry of glutamate from the cytosol into the mitochondria in the liver and small intestine. Aspartate is required by argininosuccinate synthase to convert citrulline into argininosuccinate in the cytosol. When citrin is deficient, this reaction is impaired, causing the accumulation of citrulline in the blood and urine, as well as the impairment of the urea cycle for ammonia detoxification. Type-II hypercitrullinemia is characterized by neonatal intrahepatic cholestasis. In adults, this disorder is often triggered by certain medications, infections, and alcohol consumption.

12.2.20.6 Hyperornithinemia

This is an X-linked recessive disease (also known as OCT deficiency) and the most common defect in the urea cycle (Wraith 2001). OCT catalyzes the formation of citrulline from ornithine and carbamoyl phosphate in the mitochondria of the liver and small intestine (Chapter 6). Thus, persons with OCT deficiency have elevated levels of ornithine, ammonia, orotic acid, glutamate, and glutamine in their plasma, spinal fluid, and urine but reduced concentrations of citrulline, arginine, and urea in these physiological fluids. Affected individuals develop severe episodes of nausea and vomiting, growth retardation, neurological dysfunction, seizures, mood swings, liver damage, skin lesions, and brittle hair. Treatment includes dietary supplementation with L-citrulline (e.g., 5 g/day for a 70-kg adult).

12.2.20.7 Hyperornithinemia–Hyperammonemia–Homocitrullinuria Syndrome

This disorder is an autosomal recessive disorder caused by mutations in the *SLC25A15* gene that encodes ORNT1 (mitochondrial ornithine transporter 1) (Camacho et al. 1999). Thus, the cytosolic ornithine cannot enter the mitochondria of the liver and small intestine, resulting in: (1) the accumulation of ornithine in the cytoplasm and its deficiency in the mitochondria and (2) an increase in the condensation of carbamoyl phosphate with lysine rather than ornithine by OCT to form homocitrulline. The HHH syndrome is diagnosed by persistent hyperornithinemia, episodic or postprandial hyperammonemia, and an increase in the urinary excretion of homocitrulline. Clinical symptoms are similar to those in other urea cycle defects but rarely develop in infancy. In the cases of neonatal onset (~12% of affected individuals), patients exhibit, on day 1 or 2 after birth, hyperammonemia-related problems, such as poor feeding, vomiting, lethargy, low body temperature, and rapid breathing. When the disease occurs in infancy, childhood, and adults (~88% of affected individuals), clinical manifestations include neurocognitive deficits, acute encephalopathy secondary to hyperammonemia, and liver dysfunction. These patients also excrete elevated amounts of polyamines in the urine that are about six times the normal values (Shimizu et al. 1990), possibly due to an enhanced conversion of ornithine into polyamines in cells. Treatment includes dietary supplementation with L-citrulline (e.g., 5 g/day for a 70-kg adult).

12.2.21 Other Organic Acidurias

12.2.21.1 Glutaric Acidemia

This autosomal recessive disorder occurs because glutaryl-CoA cannot be converted to crotonyl-CoA due to a deficiency of glutaryl-CoA dehydrogenase (Christensen et al. 2004). Glutaryl-CoA then undergoes hydrolysis to form glutaric acid. Thus, this disorder is associated with elevated levels of glutaric acid, glutaryl-CoA, 3-hydroxyglutaric acid, and glutaconic acid in the plasma and urine. Affected individuals may have difficulty moving and may experience spasms, jerking, rigidity, or decreased muscle tone. Some individuals with glutaric acidemia have developed bleeding in the brain or eyes. A lysine-restricted diet supplemented with carnitine can limit the progression of metabolic disorders to neurological damage in affected individuals.

12.2.21.2 Hyperoxaluria

This autosomal recessive disorder occurs because of the impaired oxidation of glycine- and hydroxyproline-derived glyoxylate to CO_2 (Hoppe 2012). Glyoxylate is then channeled to the formation of oxalate and glycolate. Hyperoxaluria is characterized by the excessive urinary excretion of both oxalate and glycolate, as well as the progressive deposition of calcium oxalate in the kidneys and other tissues. Individuals with hyperoxaluria have genitourinary tract disease and calculi. This disease may result in early death. Treatment includes: (1) a protein- and glycine-restricted diet; (2) dietary supplementation with vitamin B_6 (pyridoxine); and (3) sufficient water consumption.

12.2.21.3 α-Ketoadipic Acidemia

This autosomal recessive disorder occurs because α-ketoadipate (an intermediate in the catabolism of lysine, hydroxylysine, and tryptophan) cannot be converted to glutaryl-CoA due to a deficiency of the α-ketoadipate dehydrogenase complex (Danhauser et al. 2012). This disorder is characterized by the accumulation of α-keto, α-amino, and 2-hydroxy derivatives of adipic acid in the plasma (e.g., up to 120 μM α-aminoadipate) and their excessive excretion in the urine (e.g., up to 328 mmol α-aminoadipate, 970 mmol α-ketoadipate, and 40 mmol α-hydroxyadipate per mol creatinine). Clinical symptoms are varied and may include hypertonia, psychomotor abnormality, delayed development, seizures, and mental retardation. Treatment includes a lysine- and tryptophan-restricted diet.

12.2.21.4 Methylmalonic Acidemia

This autosomal recessive disorder is caused by a deficiency of methylmalonyl-CoA mutase, which converts methylmalonyl-CoA (a product of the propionyl-CoA carboxylation) into succinyl-CoA (Dionisi-Vici et al. 2006). Propionyl-CoA is generated from the catabolism of some AAs (including isoleucine, methionine, threonine, and valine). Adenosylcobalamin, a metabolite of vitamin B_{12}, is a cofactor for methylmalonyl-CoA mutase. Persons with a deficiency of methylmalonyl-CoA mutase have elevated levels of methylmalonic acid in their plasma and urine. Patients experience neurological, cardiac, and skeletal muscle dysfunction; episodic attacks of severe vomiting, leading to dehydration; severe metabolic acidosis; seizures and coma; and possibly death. Treatment includes a protein-restricted diet supplemented with biotin and vitamin B_{12}.

Combined methylmalonic aciduria and homocystinuria results from the impaired conversion of dietary cobalamin to methylcobalamin and adenosylcobalamin in the liver due to decreases in the activities of both methylmalonyl-CoA mutase and methionine synthase (Rossi et al. 2001). Patients with the early-onset variety develop symptoms within 12 months of age, which include poor feeding, failure to thrive, and hypotonia, as well as severe neurologic, hematologic, and gastrointestinal abnormalities. Magnetic resonance imaging typically shows diffuse supratentorial white matter edema and dysmyelination at the initial presentation but a bulk loss of white matter at the later stages of disease (Figure 12.15). These abnormalities may be caused by the reduced availability of the methyl group for methylation reactions and the homocysteine-induced damage to the endothelium. Treatment includes a protein-restricted diet supplemented with biotin and vitamin B_{12}.

12.2.21.5 Propionic Acidemia

This autosomal recessive disorder is caused by a deficiency of propionyl-CoA carboxylase, which converts propionyl-CoA [a product of the catabolism of some AAs (including isoleucine, methionine, threonine, and valine)] to D-methylmalonyl-CoA in a biotin-dependent mechanism (Dionisi-Vici et al. 2006; Scholl-Bürgi et al. 2012). Thus, this disease is associated with marked elevations of glycine in the plasma and urine, as well as the increased urinary excretion of propionate. The initial symptoms of propionic acidemia include poor feeding, vomiting, loss of appetite, weak muscle tone, and fatigue; many of these symptoms are related to metabolic acidosis. Children with this disease may experience intellectual disability or delayed development. As the disease progresses, affected individuals may have more serious medical problems, including heart abnormalities, seizures, coma, and possibly death. Treatment includes a protein-restricted diet supplemented with biotin and vitamin B_{12}.

12.2.22 POLYAMINES

Polyamines are synthesized from AAs, including arginine, proline, ornithine, and methionine. Defects in polyamine metabolism are closely linked with abnormal AA synthesis and catabolism in cells and, therefore, are discussed in this chapter.

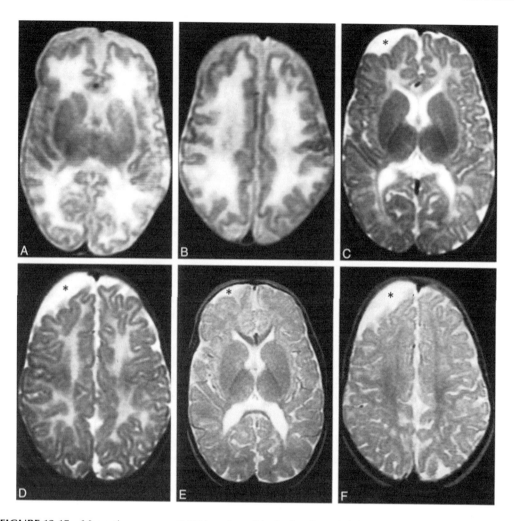

FIGURE 12.15 Magnetic resonance (MR) imaging of the brain of a male infant with combined methylmalonic aciduria and homocystinuria at the different stages of disease. The onset of this disorder occurred at 3 days of age and was diagnosed at 1 month of age. Panels a and b: Axial T2-weighted MR images at 2 months of age, showing that the supratentorial white matter was markedly edematous and hyperintense, the U fibers were diffusely organized, and the basal ganglia were spared, but the ventricular size was normal. Panels c and d: Axial T2-weighted MR images at 10 months of age, revealing the disappearance of edema, abnormally hyperintense supratentorial white matter, a loss of white matter particularly around the trigones of the lateral ventricles and in the parietal lobes, and the presence of an arachnoid cyst (asterisk) near the right frontal lobe. Panels e and f: Axial T2-weighted MR images at 24 months of age, indicating a severe loss of the white matter in the paratrigonal areas, the disorganization of the cortex on the ventricular surface and in the parietal lobes, bulk loss throughout the whole supratentorial white matter, and no change in the size of the right frontal arachnoid cyst (asterisk). (Reproduced from photos freely available in the public domain from Rossi, A. et al. 2001. *Am. J. Neuroradiol* 22:554–563. http://www.ajnr.org/content/ajnr/22/3/554.full.pdf.)

12.2.22.1 Spermine Synthase Deficiency

This is an X-linked recessive disorder caused by loss-of-function mutations in the spermine synthase (*SMS*) gene (Becerra-Solano et al. 2009). The SMS protein (an enzyme) catalyzes the conversion of spermidine (a product of putrescine) into spermine in all cell types (Chapter 5). A deficiency of SMS results in increases in the intracellular concentrations of putrescine and spermidine but decreases in the intracellular spermine concentrations and cognitive function, resulting in Snyder–Robinson syndrome in humans. Affected individuals exhibit mental retardation, skeletal defects, hypotonia, and movement disorders. Mechanistic studies with Drosophila have shown that a deficiency of SMS leads to the excessive catabolism of spermidine to generate toxic metabolites (e.g., acrolein and H_2O_2) that cause lysosomal defects and oxidative stress (Li et al. 2017). Consequently, autophagy-mediated lysosomal proteolysis and mitochondrial function are impaired in the nervous system and other cell types. Interestingly, oxidative stress induced by the deficiency of *SMS* can be alleviated by enhancing antioxidant activity through genetic or pharmacological therapies. A protein-restricted diet supplemented with spermine may be beneficial for affected individuals.

12.2.22.2 Elevation of Spermine in the Mucopolysaccharidoses

Mucopolysaccharidoses are a group of autosomal recessive disorders caused by the absence or reduced ability of lysosomal enzymes (e.g., α-L-iduronidase) to degrade glycosaminoglycans (glutamine-derived macromolecules), causing damage to tissues in the body, including the bone, cartilage, tendons, corneas, skin, and connective tissue (Hinderer et al. 2017). Humans with neuropathic subtypes of mucopolysaccharidoses (types I, II, IIIA, IIIB) exhibit severe somatic and neurological symptoms, as well as an elevated concentration of spermine in the cerebrospinal fluid (Hinderer et al. 2017). Interestingly, an elevation of spermine in the cerebrospinal fluid is closely associated with central nervous disorders and is normalized to the control value following the transplantation of hematopoietic stem cells. Similar findings have been reported for a canine model of type-I mucopolysaccharidose regarding a marked elevation of spermine in the cerebrospinal fluid of affected animals, as well as the normalization of the polyamine concentration to the value for normal dogs and the correction of brain lesions following the gene therapy (Hinderer et al. 2017). Of note, the pathway for spermine synthesis is not altered in humans and dogs with mucopolysaccharidoses. Thus, it is possible that the catabolism of spermine in cells is impaired in these mammals with mucopolysaccharidoses and is enhanced after the function of the lysosomes is improved. Although the underlying mechanisms remain unclear, spermine is a new useful biomarker to facilitate the development of therapeutics for the diseases. A protein- and spermine-restricted diet may be beneficial for affected individuals.

12.3 GENERAL CONSIDERATIONS FOR THE TREATMENT OF INBORN ERRORS OF AMINO ACID METABOLISM

Besides clinical management of symptoms and complications, traditional treatment for the inborn errors of AA metabolism varies with affected enzymes (Table 12.3). Management of diets is the mainstay for the treatment of many inborn errors of AA metabolism (Aliu et al. 2018; Endo et al. 2004; Kožich and Stabler 2020; Rumping et al. 2020). It should be borne in mind that such daily therapy is a lifelong process. Other means include: (1) restriction of specific AAs in the diet; (2) a reduction in the endogenous substrates of a defected enzyme; (3) dietary supplementation with a deficient product; (4) dietary replacement with an immediate precursor of a deficient AA; (5) stimulation of residual enzyme activity; (6) the administration of intermediary metabolites, compounds, or drugs that facilitate or inhibit specific metabolic pathway; (7) removal of ammonia from the systemic circulation; and (8) liver transplantation to correct the enzymatic defect. These approaches are designed for the daily management of affected patients to reduce ammonia production, remove toxic molecules (including ammonia) from tissues, and provide deficient AAs or metabolites.

Let us provide examples to illustrate the mechanism-based development of drugs to treat disorders resulting from inborn errors of AA metabolism (Scriver et al. 2001). First, allopurinol (a structural isomer of hypoxanthine) is an inhibitor of xanthine oxidase, the enzyme that is responsible for the successive oxidation of hypoxanthine and xanthine to produce uric acid (Chapter 6). Thus, this drug is used to treat hyperuricemia and its complications, including chronic gout and Lesch-Nyhan syndrome. Second, sodium phenylbutyrate (trade name Buphenyl) is the primary medication to treat urea cycle disorders. Phenylbutyrate is metabolized by β-oxidation to produce phenylacetate, which

TABLE 12.3

Traditional Means to Treat Inborn Errors of Amino Acid Metabolism in Humans[a]

Therapy	Example
Reduction of dietary protein and provision of high-quality protein	The mainstay of treatment for PKU and many other disorders of AA metabolism (maple syrup urine disease, homocystinuria, tyrosinemia, and defects of urea cycle enzymes)
Restriction of specific AAs in diets	Lysine and tryptophan in type I aciduria due to the deficiency of glutaryl-CoA dehydrogenase
	Isoleucine, valine, methionine, and threonine in propionic or methylmalonic aciduria due to propionyl-CoA carboxylase or methylmalonyl-CoA carboxylase deficiency
	Phenylalanine and tyrosine in PKU
	Arginine in the deficiency of ornithine carbamoyltransferase
Reduction of endogenous substrates of a defected enzyme	Use of 2-(2-nitro-4-trifluoromethylbenzoyl)-1,3-cyclohexanedione, an inhibitor of 4-hydroxyphenylpyruvate dioxygenase, to decrease the production of fumarylacetoacetate in patients with the deficiency of fumarylacetoacetase, a downstream enzyme in the pathway of tyrosine catabolism
Dietary supplementation with a deficient product of AA synthesis or catabolism	Oral or intravenous administration of arginine to patients with P5C synthase deficiency
	Use of creatine for individuals with guanidinoacetate methyltransferase deficiency
	Use of BH4 for patients with the defect of GTP cyclohydrolase I gene
Dietary replacement with an immediate precursor of a deficient AA	Use of citrulline to replace arginine in patients who lack arginine transporters
	Use of serine for patients with a defect in glycine synthesis
Stimulation of residual enzyme activity	Use of pyridoxine (vitamin B_6) to treat homocystinuria due to cystathionine β-synthase deficiency
Administration of intermediary metabolites, compounds, or drugs that facilitate or retard specific metabolic pathways	Use of ornithine or arginine to stimulate the hepatic urea cycle in infants with ornithine aminotransferase deficiency
	Use of NCG for individuals who do not express NAG synthase
	Inhibition of glutamine synthesis in urea cycle defects
Removal of ammonia from the systemic circulation	Dialysis (e.g., hemodialysis, hemofiltration, or peritoneal dialysis) to remove excessive amounts of ammonia and other toxic molecules
	Use of sodium benzoate, phenylacetate, or sodium phenylbutyrate to remove ammonia from the circulation in individuals with urea cycle defects

[a] These methods have also been used to treat inborn errors of amino acid metabolism in animal models.

Note: AA, amino acid; BH4, tetrahydrobiopterin; NAG, *N*-acetyl-glutamate; NCG, *N*-carbamoyl-glutamate; PKU, phenyl-ketonuria; P5C, pyrroline-5-carboxylate

then conjugates with glutamine (an ammonia sink) to form phenylacetylglutamine for elimination via the urine (Chapter 5). Third, BH4, an essential cofactor of AA hydroxylases, has been used to treat PKU due to a deficiency of GTP cyclohydrolase I (Werner et al. 2011). Because of its chemical instability, BH4 is often mixed with vitamin C either as a powder or in a deoxygenated solution before oral or intravenous administration to affected patients. Fourth, creatine is supplemented to patients with a deficiency of arginine:glycine amidinotransferase or guanidinoacetate methyltransferase to improve their neurological and muscular growth, development, and function.

With advanced biomedical research over the past 25 years, therapeutic means for inborn errors of AA metabolism now include new molecular biology and stem cell techniques (Table 12.4). A significant advance in this area is enzyme replacement through gene transfer or cell/organ transplantation (e.g., transplants of stem cells, liver, bone marrow, kidneys, or their combinations), which may be a promising permanent solution for affected individuals (Batshaw et al. 1999; Li et al. 2020; Malm

TABLE 12.4

Gene- and Transplantation-Based Means to Treat Inborn Errors of Amino Acid Metabolism in Humans and Animal Models

Therapy	Example
Gene transfer	T-lymphocyte-directed transfer of the ADA gene in humans and mice
	Hepatocyte-directed recombinant adenoviral gene delivery of the methylmalonyl-CoA mutase gene to mice with a severe form of methylmalonic acidemia (a deletion of exon 3 of the gene)
	Hepatocyte-directed recombinant adenoviral gene delivery of the OCT gene to sparse fur mice
	Hepatocyte-directed recombinant adenoviral gene delivery of the ASS gene in mice and bovine models
Stem cell transplantation	Correction for the deficiency of α-L-iduronidase in humans, a lysosomal enzyme that degrades the complex macromolecular glycosaminoglycans of heparan and dermatan sulfate
	Transplantation of human amnion epithelial stem cells to the liver of transgenic mice with BCKA dehydrogenase deficiency
	Treatment of PKU in mice with phenylalanine hydroxylase deficiency using hematopoietic stem cells
Bone marrow transplantation	Treatment for patients with aspartylglucosaminuria due to a deficiency of aspartylglucosaminidase[a]
	Treatment of PKU in mice with phenylalanine hydroxylase deficiency using bone marrow
Liver or hepatocyte transplantation	Treatment for patients with OCT deficiency using liver and hepatocytes from healthy individuals
	Transplant of liver to patients and mice with PKU
	Transplant of liver to patients with maple syrup urine disease
	Transplant of liver to patients with ASS deficiency
	Transplant of kidneys to patients with methylmalonic acidemia
Transplantation with a combination of two or more organs	Treatment of methylmalonic aciduria in humans using both the liver and kidneys from normal individuals
	Treatment of tyrosinemia in humans using both the liver and kidneys from normal individuals
CRISPR/Cas9 genome editing	Hemophilia B, PKU, hereditary tyrosinemia type I, OCT deficiency, aromatic L-amino acid decarboxylase deficiency, lysosomal storage disorders, and glycogen storage disorder

[a] This enzyme catalyzes the degradation of glycoproteins in the lysosomes.

Note: AA, amino acid; ADA, adenosine deaminase; ASS, argininosuccinate synthase; BCKA, branched-chain α-ketoacid; OCT, ornithine carbamoyltransferase; PKU, phenylketonuria.

et al. 2004; Wynn 2011). All of these modern methods for treating inborn errors of AA metabolism require interdisciplinary team's work, spanning clinical medicine, biochemistry, cell biology, and nutrition. Of particular note, the choice of a vehicle for carrying the gene of interest is vital to the safety and success of gene transfer for humans and other animals.

There is growing interest in the use of genome-editing techniques to correct gene mutations and deletions in humans and other animals with inborn errors of metabolism, including AA metabolism (Li et al. 2020; Schneller et al. 2017). Figure 12.16 illustrates the principle of this new gene therapy method, with clustered regularly interspaced short palindromic repeats-associated nuclease-9 (CRISPR/Cas9) as the editor. Specifically, a designer nuclease (e.g., CRISPR/Cas9, zinc finger nuclease, or transcription activator-like effector nuclease) cleaves a DNA molecule to generate a double-strand

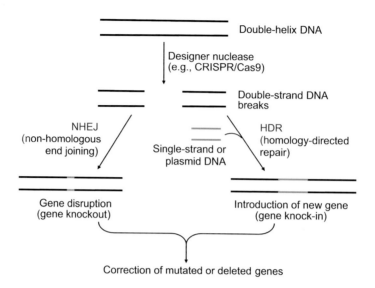

FIGURE 12.16 Genome editing of humans and other animals with inborn errors of metabolism using CRISPR/Cas9 (clustered regularly interspaced short palindromic repeats-associated nuclease-9) as the editor. CRISPR/Cas9 (a designer nuclease) cleaves a DNA molecule to generate a double-strand break (DSB) at a desired genomic locus. Thereafter, one of two endogenous repair mechanisms may repair the DSB DNA: the non-homologous end joining and the homology-directed repair. In the non-homologous end joining, the two ends of the DSB DNA are brought together and ligated without a homologous template for repair, which often inserts or deletes nucleotides (indels) to cause gene disruption (knockout). The homology-directed repair pathway requires the provision of an exogenous DNA template along with a site-specific genome editing nuclease to repair the DSB DNA, thereby causing the knock-in of a desired sequence of DNA into the genome of an embryo or animal cells. Because of its more precise targeting of genes, CRISPR/Cas9 is the preferred tool for genome editing. This gene editing system consists of a guide RNA and the Cas9 endonuclease, as well as a repair DNA template. The guide RNA provides sequence specificity to target the Cas9 endonuclease to a complementary site in the genome of an organism for creating a DSB.

break (DSB) at a desired genomic locus. Thereafter, one of two endogenous repair mechanisms may repair the DSB DNA molecule: the non-homologous end joining and the homology-directed repair. In the non-homologous end-joining pathway, the two ends of the DSB DNA are brought together and ligated without a homologous template for repair, which often inserts or deletes nucleotides (called indels) to cause gene disruption (knockout). The homology-directed repair pathway requires the provision of an exogenous DNA template along with a site-specific genome editing nuclease to repair the DSB DNA molecule, thereby causing the knock-in of a desired sequence of DNA into the genome of an organism. Compared with other gene editors, CRISPR/Cas9 (which was discovered in 2007 in bacteria and archaea as a defensive system against invading viruses) is simpler, faster, cheaper, and more accurate and, therefore, is the preferred tool for editing genomes in humans and other animals. The CRISPR/Cas9 technology has been used in preclinical trials as a therapy for the treatment of human inborn errors of metabolism, including hemophilia B, PKU, hereditary tyrosinemia type I, OCT deficiency, aromatic L-amino acid decarboxylase deficiency, lysosomal storage disorders, and glycogen storage disorder (Schneller et al. 2017; Yilmaz et al. 2020).

12.4 SUMMARY

Over the past 50 years, extensive research has determined the biochemical and genetic bases of abnormal AA metabolism in humans and other animals. Many of these inherited diseases are autosomal recessive disorders as two copies (one from each parent) of the same recessive, abnormal gene are present on the autosomal chromosomes of affected individuals. The availability of metabolic screening tests has led to the ability to accurately diagnose the diseases. Depending on affected enzymes in metabolic pathways, inborn errors of AA metabolism can result in: (1) little or no endogenous synthesis of AAs (e.g., arginine in infants without P5C synthase; glutamine in newborns with a severe deficiency of glutamine synthetase; and tyrosine in patients lacking phenylalanine hydroxylase) and their deficiencies; (2) complete or impaired blockage of the degradation of AAs (e.g., BCAAs in patients with BCKA dehydrogenase deficiency and phenylalanine in PKU) and substantial increases in their circulating levels; (3) the lack of or the impaired production of biologically active molecules (e.g., NO and serotonin in individuals with GTP cyclohydrolase I deficiency); (4) hyperammonemia (e.g., a deficiency of an enzyme in the urea cycle); or (5) disturbances in protein, lipid, and carbohydrate metabolism. Consequently, multiorgan dysfunction occurs, which severely compromises whole-body homeostasis, causes the abnormal development of organs (including the brain) and mental retardation, and even results in death. Thus, the treatment of disorders varies with their causes, but in most cases, affected individuals receive administration of sodium phenylbutyrate to remove excess ammonia from the circulation and are advised to adopt a lifelong reduction in dietary protein intake. Advances in gene therapy, stem cell biology, organ transplantation, and genome editing have led to the development of new, long-term treatments for inherited disorders of AA metabolism. Appropriate animal models for the study of inborn errors of AA metabolism (for example, humans and sparse fur mice with OCT deficiency) are needed to understand the underlying mechanisms and to develop effective therapies.

REFERENCES

Adams, D.R., S. Menezes, R. Jauregui, Z.M. Valivullah, B. Power, M. Abraham et al. 2019. One-year pilot study on the effects of nitisinone on melanin in patients with OCA-1B. *JCI Insight* 4:e124387.

Afink, G., W. Kulik, H. Overmars, J. de Randamie, T. Veenboer, A. van Cruchten et al. 2008. Molecular characterization of iodotyrosine dehalogenase deficiency in patients with hypothyroidism. *J. Clin. Endocrinol. Metab.* 93:4894–4901.

Aliu, E., S. Kanungo, and G.L. Arnold. 2018. Amino acid disorders. *Ann. Transl. Med.* 6:471.

Almaghlouth, I.A., J.Y. Mohamed, M. Al-Amoudi, L. Al-Ahaidib, A. Al-Odaib, and F.S. Alkuraya. 2011. 5-Oxoprolinase deficiency: report of the first human OPLAH mutation. *Clin. Genet.* 29:82:193–196.

Augoustides-Savvopoulou, P., Z. Luka, S. Karyda, S.P. Stabler, R.H. Allen, K. Patsiaoura et al. 2003. Glycine N-methyltransferase deficiency: a new patient with a novel mutation. *J. Inherit. Metab. Dis.* 26:745–759.

Bailey, C.G., R.M. Ryan, A.D. Thoeng, C. Ng, K. King, J.M. Vanslambrouck et al. 2011. Loss-of-function mutations in the glutamate transporter SLC1A1 cause human dicarboxylic aminoaciduria. *J. Clin. Invest.* 121:446–453.

Bandmann, O., K.H. Weiss, and S.G. Kaler. 2015. Wilson's disease and other neurological copper disorders. *Lancet Neurol.* 14:103–113.

Bannasch, D. and P.S. Henthorn. 2009. Changing paradigms in diagnosis of inherited defects associated with uroliths. *Vet. Clin. North Am. Small Anim. Prac.* 39:111–125.

Baric, I., K. Fumic, B. Glenn, M. Cuk, A. Schulze, J.D. Finkelstein et al. 2004. S-Adenosylhomocysteine hydrolase deficiency in a human: a genetic disorder of methionine metabolism. *Proc. Natl. Acad. Sci. USA* 101:4234–4239.

Batshaw, M.L., M.B. Robinson, X. Ye, C. Pabin, Y. Daikhin, B.K. Burton et al. 1999. Correction of ureagenesis after gene transfer in an animal model and after liver transplantation in humans with ornithine transcarbamylase deficiency. *Pediatr. Res.* 46:588–593.

Baumgartner, M.R., D. Rabier, M.C. Nassogne, J.-P. Padovani, P. Kamoun, D. Valle, and J.-M. Saudubray. 2005. Delta1-pyrroline-5-carboxylate synthase deficiency: neurodegeneration, cataracts and connective tissue manifestations combined with hyperammonaemia and reduced ornithine, citrulline, arginine and proline. *Eur. J. Pediatr.* 164:31–36.

Becerra-Solano, L.E., J. Butler, G. Castañeda-Cisneros, D.E. McCloskey, X. Wang, A.E. Pegg et al. 2009. A missense mutation, p.V132G, in the X-linked spermine synthase gene (SMS) causes Snyder-Robinson syndrome. *Am. J. Med. Genet. A* 149:328–335.

Blake, M.A., M.K. Kalra, M.M. Maher, D.V. Sahani, A.T. Sweeney, P.R. Mueller et al. 2004. Pheochromocytoma: an imaging chameleon. *RadioGraphics* 24(Suppl. 1):S87–S99.

Braissant, O., H. Henry, E. Béard, and J. Uldry. 2011. Creatine deficiency syndromes and the importance of creatine synthesis in the brain. *Amino Acids* 40:1315–1324.

Bröer, S. and M. Palacín. 2011. The role of amino acid transporters in inherited and acquired diseases. *Biochem. J.* 436:193–211.

Bröer, S., C.G. Bailey, S. Kowalczuk, C. Ng, J.M. Vanslambrouck, H. Rodgers et al. 2008. Iminoglycinuria and hyperglycinuria are discrete human phenotypes resulting from complex mutations in proline and glycine transporters. *J. Clin. Invest.* 118:3881–3892.

Buist, N.R., B. Glenn, O. Vugrek, C. Wagner, S. Stabler, R.H. Allen et al. 2006. S-Adenosylhomocysteine hydrolase deficiency in a 26-year-old man. *J. Inherit. Metab. Dis.* 29:538–545.

Caldovic, L., H. Morizono, and M. Tuchman. 2007. Mutations and polymorphisms in the human N-acetylglutamate synthase (*NAGS*) gene. *Hum. Mutat.* 28:754–759.

Camacho, J.A., C. Obie, B. Biery, B.K. Goodman, C.A. Hu, S. Almashanu et al. 1999. Hyperornithinaemia-hyperammonaemia-homocitrullinuria syndrome is caused by mutations in a gene encoding a mitochondrial ornithine transporter. *Nat. Genet.* 22:151–158.

Camargo, S.M.R., V. Makrides, R. Kleta, and F. Verrey. 2013. Kidney transport of amino acids and oligopeptides, and aminoacidurias. In: *Seldin and Giebisch's The Kidney: Physiology and Pathophysiology* (Alpern, R.J., M.J. Caplan, and O.W. Moe, eds). Elsevier, New York. pp. 2405–2423.

Centerwall, S.A. and W.R. Centerwall. 2000. The discovery of phenylketonuria: the story of a young couple, two retarded children, and a scientist. *Pediatrics* 105:89–103.

Chapel-Crespo, C.C., G.A. Diaz, and K. Oishi. 2016. Efficacy of N-carbamoyl-L-glutamic acid for the treatment of inherited metabolic disorders. *Expert Rev. Endocrinol. Metab.* 11:467–473.

Chinsky, J.M., R. Singh, C. Ficicioglu, C.D.M. van Karnebeek, M. Grompe, G. Mitchell et al. 2017. Diagnosis and treatment of tyrosinemia type I: a US and Canadian consensus group review and recommendations. *Genet. Med.* 19:1380.

Christensen, E., A. Ribes, B. Merinero, and J. Zschocke. 2004. Correlation of genotype and phenotype in glutaryl-CoA dehydrogenase deficiency. *J. Inherit. Metab. Dis.* 27:861–868.

Chuang, D.T. and V.E. Shih. 2001. Maple syrup urine disease (branched-chain ketoaciduria). In: *The Metabolic and Molecular Bases of Inherited Disease* (Scriver, C.R., A.L. Beaudet, W.S. Sly, and D. Valle, eds). McGraw Hill, New York. pp. 1971–2006.

Cohn, R.M., M. Yudkoff, R. Rothman, and S. Segal. 1978. Isovaleric acidemia: use of glycine therapy in neonates. *N. Engl. J. Med.* 299:996–999.

Coman, D.J., D.W. Murray, J.C. Byrne, P.M. Rudd, P.M. Bagaglia, P.D. Doran, and E.P. Treacy. 2010. Galactosemia, a single gene disorder with epigenetic consequences. *Pediatr. Res.* 67:286–292.

Crona, J., D. Taïeb, and K. Pacak. 2017. New perspectives on pheochromocytoma and paraganglioma: toward a molecular classification. *Endocr. Rev.* 38:489–515.

Danhauser, K., S.W. Sauer, T.B. Haack, T. Wieland, C. Staufner, E. Graf et al. 2012. DHTKD1 mutations cause 2-aminoadipic and 2-oxoadipic aciduria. *Am. J. Hum. Genet.* 91:1082–1087.

de Koning, T.J., M. Duran, L. Dorland, R. Gooskens, E. Van Schaftingen, J. Jaeken et al. 1998. Beneficial effects of L-serine and glycine in the management of seizures in 3-phosphoglycerate dehydrogenase deficiency. *Ann Neurol.* 44:261–265.

Diasio, R.B., T.L. Beavers, and J.T. Carpenter. 1988. Familial deficiency of dihydropyrimidine dehydrogenase. Biochemical basis for familial pyrimidinemia and severe 5-fluorouracil-induced toxicity. *J. Clin. Invest.* 81:47–51.

Dionisi-Vici, C., F. Deodato, W. Raschinger, W. Rhead, and B. Wilcken. 2006. Classical organic acidurias, propionic aciduria, methylmalonic aciduria, and isovaleric aciduria: long-term outcome and effects of expanded newborn screening using tandem mass spectrometry. *J. Inherit. Metab. Dis.* 29:383–389.

Eggermann, T., A. Venghaus, and K. Zerres. 2012. Cystinuria: an inborn cause of urolithiasis. *Orphanet J. Rare Dis.* 7:19.

El-Hattab, A.W. and F. Scaglia. 2015. Disorders of carnitine biosynthesis and transport. *Mol. Genet. Metab.* 116:107–112.

Endo, F., T. Matsuura, K. Yanagita, and I. Matsuda. 2004. Clinical manifestations of inborn errors of the urea cycle and related metabolic disorders during childhood. *J. Nutr.* 134:1605S–1609S.

Espinós, C., M. Pineda, D. Martínez-Rubio, V. Lupo, A. Ormazabal, M.A. Vilaseca et al. 2009. Mutations in the urocanase gene UROC1 are associated with urocanic aciduria. *J. Med. Genet.* 46:407–411.

Filho, J.A.F. and B.E. Shapiro. 2004. Tay-Sachs disease. *Arch. Neurol.* 61:1466–1468.

Finckh, U., A. Kohlschütter, H. Schäfer, K. Sperhake, J.P. Colombo, and A. Gal. 1998. Prenatal diagnosis of carbamoyl phosphate synthetase I deficiency by identification of a missense mutation in CPS1. *Hum. Mutat.* 12:206–211.

Finkelstein, J.D. 2006. Inborn errors of sulfur-containing amino acid metabolism. *J. Nutr.* 136:1750S–1754S.

Flinn, A.M. and A.R. Gennery. 2018. Adenosine deaminase deficiency: a review. *Orphanet J. Rare Dis.* 13:65.

Foreman, J.W. 2019. Fanconi syndrome. *Pediatr. Clin. North Am.* 66:159–167.

Fretzayas, A., M. Moustaki, O. Liapi, and T. Karpathios. 2012. Gilbert syndrome. *Eur. J. Pediatr.* 171:11–15.

Furujo, M., M. Kinoshita, M. Nagao, and T. Kubo. 2012. S-Adenosylmethionine treatment in methionine adenosyltransferase deficiency, a case report. *Mol. Genet. Metab.* 105:516–518.

Gahl, W.A., J.G. Thoene, and J.A. Schneider. 2002. Cystinosis. *N. Engl. J. Med.* 347:111–121.

Gibson, A.M. and C. Jacobs. 2001. Disorders of beta- and gamma-amino acids in free and peptide-linked forms. In: *The Metabolic and Molecular Basis of Inherited Disease* (Scriver, C.R., A.L. Beaudet, W.S. Sly, and D. Valle, eds). McGraw Hill, New York. pp. 2079–2210.

Guernsey, D.L., H. Jiang, D.R. Campagna, C.C. Evans, M. Ferguson, M.D. Kellog et al. 2009. Mutations in mitochondrial carrier family gene slc25a38 cause nonsyndromic autosomal recessive congenital sideroblastic anemia. *Nat. Genet.* 41:651–653.

Häberle, J., B. Görg, A. Toutain, F. Rutsch, J.F. Benoist, A. Gelot et al. 2006. Inborn error of amino acid synthesis: human glutamine synthetase deficiency. *J. Inherit. Metab. Dis.* 29:352–358.

Hechtman, P. 2001. Prolidase deficiency. In: *The Metabolic and Molecular Basis of Inherited Disease* (Scriver, C.R., A.L. Beaudet, W.S. Sly, and D. Valle, eds). McGraw Hill, New York. pp. 1839–1856.

Henthorn, P.S., J. Liu, T. Gidalevich, J. Fang, M.L. Casal, D.F. Patterson, and U. Giger. 2000. Canine cystinuria: polymorphism in the canine SLC3A1 gene and identification of a nonsense mutation in cystinuric Newfoundland dogs. *Hum. Genet.* 107:295–303.

Hidaka, Y., T.D. Palella, T.E. O'Toole, S.A. Tarle, and W.N. Kelley. 1987. Human adenine phosphoribosyltransferase. Identification of allelic mutations at the nucleotide level as a cause of complete deficiency of the enzyme. *J. Clin. Invest.* 80:1409–1415.

Hinderer, C., N. Katz, J.-P. Louboutin, P. Bell, J. Tolar, and P.J. Orchard. 2017. Abnormal polyamine metabolism is unique to the neuropathic forms of MPS: potential for biomarker development and insight into pathogenesis. *Hum. Mol. Genet.* 26:3837–3849.

Hoppe, B. 2012. An update on primary hyperoxaluria. *Nat. Rev. Nephrol.* 8:467.

Hou, Y.Q., Y.L. Yin, and G. Wu. 2015. Dietary essentiality of "nutritionally nonessential amino acids" for animals and humans. *Exp. Biol. Med.* 240:997–1007.

Hou, Y.Q., K. Yao, Y.L. Yin, and G. Wu. 2016. Endogenous synthesis of amino acids limits growth, lactation and reproduction of animals. *Adv. Nutr.* 7:331–342.

Ichida, K., Y. Amaya, N. Kamatani, T. Nishino, T. Hosoya, and O. Sakai. 1997. Identification of two mutations in human xanthine dehydrogenase gene responsible for classical type I xanthinuria. *J. Clin. Invest.* 99:2391–2397.

Isabella, V.M., B.N. Ha, M.J. Castillo, D.J. Lubkowicz, S.E. Rowe, Y.A. Millet et al. 2018. Development of a synthetic live bacterial therapeutic for the human metabolic disease phenylketonuria. *Nat. Biotechnol.* 36:857–864.

Item, C., S. Stöckler-Ipsiroglu, C. Stromberger, A. Mühl, M.G. Alessandri, M.C. Bianchi et al. 2001. Arginine:glycine amidinotransferase deficiency: the third inborn error of creatine metabolism in humans. *Am. J. Hum. Genet.* 69:1127–1133.

Jaeken, J.C.P., P. de Cock, L. Corbeel, R. Eeckels, and E. Eggermont. 1984. Gamma-aminobutyric acid-transaminase deficiency: a newly recognized inborn error of neurotransmitter metabolism. *Neuropediatrics* 15:165–169.

Jonas, A.J. and I.J. Butler. 1989. Circumvention of defective neutral amino acid transport in Hartnup disease using tryptophan ethyl ester. *J. Clin. Invest.* 84:200–204.

Jurecka, A. 2009. Inborn errors of purine and pyrimidine metabolism. *J. Inher. Metab. Dis.* 32:247–263.

Jurecka, A., M. Zikanova, S. Kmoch, and A. Tylki-Szymańska. 2015. Adenylosuccinate lyase deficiency. *J. Inherit. Metab. Dis.* 38:231–242.

Kleijer, W.J., V.H. Garritsen, M. Linnebank, P. Mooyer, J.G. Huijmans, A. Mustonen et al. 2002. Clinical, enzymatic, and molecular genetic characterization of a biochemical variant type of argininosuccinic aciduria: prenatal and postnatal diagnosis in five unrelated families. *J. Inherit. Metab. Dis.* 25:399–410.

Kleta, R., E. Romeo, Z. Ristic, T. Ohura, C. Stuart, M. Arcos-Burgos et al. 2004. Mutations in SLC6A19, encoding B0AT1, cause Hartnup disorder. *Nat. Genet.* 36:999–1002.

Koenig, M.K., R. Hodgeman, J.J. Riviello, W. Chung, J. Bain, C.A. Chiriboga et al. 2017. Phenotype of GABA-transaminase deficiency. *Neurology* 88:1919–1924.

Kogut, M.D., K.N. Shaw, and G.N. Donnell. 1967. Tyrosinosis. *Am. J. Dis. Child.* 113:47–53.

Korman, S.H. 2006. Inborn errors of isoleucine degradation: a review. *Mol. Genet. Metab.* 89:289–299.

Kožich, V. and S. Stabler. 2020. Lessons learned from inherited metabolic disorders of sulfur-containing amino acids metabolism. *J. Nutr.* 150:2506S–2517S.

Lecha, M., H. Puy, and J.C. Deybach. 2009. Erythropoietic protoporphyria. *Orphanet J. Rare Dis.* 4:19.

Li, C., J.M. Brazill, S. Liu, C. Bello, Y. Zhu, M. Morimoto et al. 2017. Spermine synthase deficiency causes lysosomal dysfunction and oxidative stress in models of Snyder-Robinson syndrome. *Nat. Commun.* 8:1257.

Li, H., Y. Yang, W. Hong, M. Huang, M. Wu, and X. Zhao. 2020. Applications of genome editing technology in the targeted therapy of human diseases: mechanisms, advances and prospects. *Sig. Transduct. Target. Ther.* 5:1.

Lupi, A., A. Rossi, E. Campari, F. Pecora, A.M. Lund, N.H. Elcioglu et al. 2006. Molecular characterisation of six patients with prolidase deficiency: identification of the first small duplication in the prolidase gene and of a mutation generating symptomatic and asymptomatic outcomes within the same family. *J. Med. Genet.* 43:e58.

Malm, G., J.E. Månsson, J. Winiarski, M. Mosskin, and O. Ringdén. 2004. Five-year follow-up of two siblings with aspartylglucosaminuria undergoing allogeneic stem-cell transplantation from unrelated donors. *Transplantation* 78:415–419.

Malmquist, J. and B. Hetter. 1970. Leucocyte glutaminase in familial protein intolerance. *Lancet* 296:129–130.

McAndrew, R.P., J. Vockley, and J. Kim. 2008. Molecular basis of dimethylglycine dehydrogenase deficiency associated with pathogenic variant H109R. *J. Inherit. Metab. Dis.* 31:761–768.

Mitchell, G., M. Grompe, M. Lambert, and R. Tanguay. 2001. Hypertyrosinemia. In: *The Metabolic and Molecular Basis of Inherited Disease* (Scriver, C.R., A.L. Beaudet, W.S. Sly, and D. Valle, eds). McGraw Hill, New York. pp. 1777–1806.

Mitsubuchi, H., K. Nakamura, S. Matsumoto, and F. Endo. 2014. Biochemical and clinical features of hereditary hyperprolinemia. *Pediatr. Int.* 56:492–496.

Montioli, R., M. Dindo, A. Giorgetti, S. Piccoli, B. Cellini, and C.B. Voltattorni. 2014. A comprehensive picture of the mutations associated with aromatic amino acid decarboxylase deficiency: from molecular mechanisms to therapy implications. *Hum. Mol. Genet.* 23:5429–5440.

Morii, K. and T. Yamamoto. 2016. Dubin–Johnson syndrome. *N. Engl. J. Med.* 375:e1.

Mudd, S.H., H.L. Levy, and J.P. Kraus. 2001. Disorders of transulfuration. In: *The Metabolic and Molecular Basis of Inherited Disease* (Scriver, C.R., A.L. Beaudet, W.S. Sly, and D. Valle, eds). McGraw Hill, New York. pp. 2007–2056.

Njålsson, R., E. Ristoff, K. Carlsson, A. Winkler, A. Larsson, and S. Norgren. 2005. Genotype, enzyme activity, glutathione level, and clinical phenotype in patients with glutathione synthetase deficiency. *Hum. Genet.* 116:384–389.

Noguchi, A. and T. Takahashi. 2019. Overview of symptoms and treatment for lysinuric protein intolerance. *J. Hum. Genet.* 64:849–858.

Oberiter, V., Z. Puretić, and V. Fabečić-Sabadi. 1978. Hyperglycinuria with nephrolithiasis. *Eur. J. Pediatr.* 127:279–285.

Oetting, W.S. 2002. New insights into ocular albinism type 1 (OA1): Mutations and polymorphisms of the OA1 gene. *Hum. Mutat.* 19:85–92.

Opitz, S., B. Käsmann-Kellner, M. Kaufmann, E. Schwinger, and C. Zühlke. 2004. Detection of 53 novel DNA variations within the tyrosinase gene and accumulation of mutations in 17 patients with albinism. *Hum. Mutat.* 23:630–631.

Orfao, A., A.C. Garcia-Montero, L. Sanchez, and L. Escribano. 2007. Recent advances in the understanding of mastocytosis: the role of KIT mutations. *Br. J. Haematol.* 138:12–30.

Phang, J.M., C.A. Hu, and D. Valle. 2001. Disorders of proline and hydroxyproline metabolism. In: *The Metabolic and Molecular Basis of Inherited Disease* (Scriver, C.R., A.L. Beaudet, W.S. Sly, and D. Valle, eds). McGraw Hill, New York. pp. 1821–1838.

Phornphutkul, C., W.J. Introne, M.B. Perry, I. Bernardini, M.D. Murphey, D.L. Fitzpatrick et al. 2002. Natural history of alkaptonuria. *N. Engl. J. Med.* 347:211–221.

Pinney, SE; C. MacMullen, S. Becker, Y.W. Lin, C. Hanna, P. Thornton et al. 2008. Clinical characteristics and biochemical mechanisms of congenital hyperinsulinism associated with dominant KATP channel mutations. *J. Clin. Invest.* 118:2877–2886.

Ristoff, E. and A. Larsson. 2007. Inborn errors in the metabolism of glutathione. *Orphanet J. Rare Dis.* 2:16.

Ristoff, E., C. Augustson, J. Geissler, T. de Rijk, K. Carlsson, J.L. Luo et al. 2000. A missense mutation in the heavy subunit of gamma-glutamylcysteine synthetase gene causes hemolytic anemia. *Blood* 95:2193–2196.

Rosenberg, L.E., J.L. Durant, and L.J. Elsas. 1968. Familial iminoglycinuria. An inborn error of renal tubular transport. *N. Engl. J. Med.* 278:1407–1413.

Rossi, A., R. Cerone, R. Biancheri, R. Gatti, M.C. Schiaffino, C. Fonda et al. 2001. Early-onset combined methylmalonic aciduria and homocystinuria: neuroradiologic findings. *Am. J. Neuroradiol* 22:554–563.

Rumping, L., B. Büttner, O. Maier, H. Rehmann, M. Lequin, J.-U. Schlump et al. 2019. Identification of a loss-of-function mutation in the context of glutaminase deficiency and neonatal epileptic encephalopathy. *JAMA Neurol.* 76:342–350.

Rumping, L., E. Vringer, R.H.J. Houwen, P.M. van Hasselt, J.J.M. Jans, and N.M. Verhoeven-Duif. 2020. Inborn errors of enzymes in glutamate metabolism. *J. Inherit. Metab. Dis.* 43:200–215.

Ruzzo, E.K., J.M. Capo-Chichi, B. Ben-Zeev, D. Chitayat, H. Mao, A.L. Pappas et al. 2013. Deficiency of asparagine synthetase causes congenital microcephaly and a progressive form of encephalopathy. *Neuron* 80:429–441

Salomons, G.S., S. Dooren, J.M. Van, N.M. Verhoeven, D. Marsden, C. Schwartz et al. 2003. X-linked creatine transporter defect: An overview. *J. Inher. Metab. Dis.* 26:309–318.

Sasaki, Y., M. Iseki, S. Yamaguchi, Y. Kurosawa, T. Yamamoto, Y. Moriwaki et al. 1998. Direct evidence of autosomal recessive inheritance of Arg24 to termination codon in purine nucleoside phosphorylase gene in a family with a severe combined immunodeficiency patient. *Hum. Genet.* 103:81–85.

Sauer, A.V., H. Morbach, I. Brigida, Y.S. Ng, A. Aiuti, and E. Meffre. 2012. Defective B cell tolerance in adenosine deaminase deficiency is corrected by gene therapy. *J. Clin. Invest.* 122:2141–2152.

Scaglia, F. and B. Lee. 2006. Clinical, biochemical, and molecular spectrum of hyperargininemia due to arginase I deficiency. *Am. J. Med. Genet.* 142C:113–120.

Schneller, J.L., C.M. Lee, G. Bao, and C.P. Venditti. 2017. Genome editing for inborn errors of metabolism: advancing towards the clinic. *BMC Med.* 15:43.

Schnirer, I.I., J.C. Yao, and J.A. Ajani. 2003. Carcinoid a comprehensive review. *Acta Oncol.* 42:672–692.

Scholl-Bürgi, S., J.O. Sass, J. Zschocke, and D. Karall. 2012. Amino acid metabolism in patients with propionic acidaemia. *J. Inherit. Metab. Dis.* 35:65–70.

Schulze, A. 2003. Creatine deficiency syndromes. *Mol. Cell. Biochem.* 244:143–150.

Scott, C.R. 2001. Sacrosinemia. In: *The Metabolic and Molecular Basis of Inherited Disease* (Scriver, C.R., A.L. Beaudet, W.S. Sly, and D. Valle, eds). McGraw Hill, New York. pp. 2057–2063.

Scriver, C.R., A.L. Beaudet, W.S. Sly, and D. Valle. 2001. *The Molecular and Metabolic Basis of Inherited Disease.* McGraw-Hill, New York.

Shaheen, R., Z. Rahbeeni, A. Alhashem, E. Faqeih, Q. Zhao, Y. Xiong et al. 2014. Neu-Laxova syndrome, an inborn error of serine metabolism, is caused by mutations in PHGDH. *Am. J. Hum. Genet.* 94:898–904.

Shimizu, H., K. Maekawa, and Y. Eto. 1990. Abnormal urinary excretion of polyamines in HHH syndrome (hyperornithinemia associated with hyperammonemia and homocitrullinuria). *Brain Dev.* 12:533–535.

Singh, R.H., W.J. Rhead, W. Smith, B. Lee, K.L. Sniderman, and M. Summar. 2005. Nutritional management of urea cycle disorders. *Crit. Care Clin.* 21:S27–S35.

Sinkeller, S.P.T., M.G. Joosten, R.A. Wevers, T.L. Oei, A.E.M. Jacobs, J.H. Veerkamp, and B.C.J. Hamel. 1988. Myoadenylate deaminase deficiency: a clinical, genetic and biochemical study in nine families. *Muscle Nerve* 11:312–317.

Soriano, J.R., L.S. Taitz, L. Finberg, and C.M. Edelmann. 1967. Hyperglycemia with ketoacidosis and leukopenia. *Pediatrics* 39:818–828.

Spodenkiewicz, M., C. Diez-Fernandez, V. Rufenacht, C. Gemeperle-Britschgi, and J. Haberle. 2016. Minireview on glutamine synthetase deficiency, an ultra-rare error of amino acid biosynthesis. *Biology* 5:50.

Sprute, R., D. Ardicli, K.K. Oguz, A. Malenica-Mandel, H.-S. Daimagüler, A. Koy et al. 2019. Clinical outcomes of two patients with a novel pathogenic variant in *ASNS*: response to asparagine supplementation and review of the literature. *Hum. Genome Var.* 6:24.

Sreelatha, O.K., E. Al-Harthy, P. Vanrijen-Cooymans, S. Al-Zuhaibi, and A. Ganesh. 2009. Albinism: images in ophthalmology. *Oman J. Ophthalmol.* 2:43–45.

Strassburg, C.P. 2010. Hyperbilirubinemia syndromes (Gilbert-Meulengracht, Crigler-Najjar, Dubin-Johnson, and Rotor syndrome). *Best Pract. Res. Clin. Gastroenterol.* 24:555–571.

Suchi, M., H. Mizuno, Y. Kawai, T. Tsuboi, S. Sumi, K. Okajima et al. 1997. Molecular cloning of the human UMP synthase gene and characterization of point mutations in two hereditary orotic aciduria families. *Am. J. Hum. Genet.* 60:525–539.

Tabatabaie, L., L.W.J. Klomp, M.E. Rubio-Gozalbo, L.J.M. Spaapen, A.A.M. Haagen, L. Dorland, and T.J. de Koning. 2011. Expanding the clinical spectrum of 3-phosphoglycerate dehydrogenase deficiency. *J. Inherit. Metab. Dis.* 34:181–184.

Tada, K. and S. Kure. 1993. Non-ketotic hyperglycinaemia: molecular lesion, diagnosis and pathophysiology. *J. Inherit. Metab. Dis.* 16:691–703.

Taylor, R.G., H.L. Levy, and R.R. McInnes. 1991. Histidase and histidinemia. Clinical and molecular considerations. *Mol. Biol. Med.* 8:101–116.

Teijema, H.L., H.H. van Gelderen, M.A. Giesberts, and M.S.L. de Angulo. 1974. Dicarboxylic aminoaciduria: an inborn error of glutamate and aspartate transport with metabolic implications, in combination with a hyperprolinemia. *Metabolism* 23:115–123.

Valle, D. and O. Simell. 2001. The hyperornithinemias. In: *The Metabolic and Molecular Basis of Inherited Disease* (Scriver, C.R., A.L. Beaudet, W.S. Sly, and D. Valle, eds). McGraw Hill, New York. pp. 857–96.

van Gennip, A.H., N.G.G.M. Abeling, P. Vreken, and A.B.P. van Kuilenburg. 1997. Inborn errors of pyrimidine degradation: clinical, biochemical and molecular aspects. *J. Inherit. Metab. Dis.* 20:203–213.

van Kuilenburg, A.B.P., M. Tarailo-Graovac, P.A. Richmond, B.I. Drögemöller, M.A. Pouladi, R. Leen et al. 2019. Glutaminase deficiency caused by short tandem repeat expansion in GLS. *N. Engl. J. Med.* 380:1434–1441.

Wang, J. and R. Hegele. 2003. Genomic basis of cystathioninuria (MIM 219500) revealed by multiple mutations in cystathionine gamma-lyase (CTH). *Hum. Genet.* 112:404–408.

Werner, E.R., N. Blau, and B. Thöny. 2011. Tetrahydrobiopterin: biochemistry and pathophysiology. *Biochem. J.* 438:397–414.

Whyte, M.P. 2001. Hypophosphatasia. In: *The Metabolic and Molecular Basis of Inherited Disease* (Scriver, C.R., A.L. Beaudet, W.S. Sly, and D. Valle, eds). McGraw Hill, New York. pp. 5313–5329.

Williams, R.A., C.D.S. Mamotte, and J.R. Burnett. 2008. Phenylketonuria: an inborn error of phenylalanine metabolism. *Clin. Biochem. Rev.* 29:31–41.

Willis, A., H.U. Bender, G. Steel, and D. Valle. 2008. *PRODH* variants and risk for schizophrenia. *Amino Acids* 35:673–679.

Wraith, J. E. 2001. Ornithine carbamoyltransferase deficiency. *Arch. Dis Child.* 84:84–88.

Wu, G. 2018. *Principles of Animal Nutrition.* CRC Press, Boca Raton, FL.

Wu, G., F.W. Bazer, R.C. Burghardt, G.A. Johnson, S.W. Kim, D.A. Knabe et al. 2011. Proline and hydroxyproline metabolism: implications for animal and human nutrition. *Amino Acids* 40:1053–1063.

Wynn, R. 2011. Stem cell transplantation in inherited metabolic disorders. *Hematology Am. Soc. Hematol. Educ. Program* 2011:285–291.

Yilmaz, B.S., S. Gurung, D. Perocheau, J. Counsell, and J. Baruteau. 2020. Gene therapy for inherited metabolic diseases. *J Mother Child* 24:1–12.

Zatkova, A. 2011. An update on molecular genetics of alkaptonuria (AKU). *J. Inherit. Metab. Dis.* 34:1127–1136.

Ziats, M.N., M.S. Comeaux, Y. Yang, F. Scaglia, S.H. Elsea, Q. Sun et al. 2015. Improvement of regressive autism symptoms in a child with TMLHE deficiency following carnitine supplementation. *Am. J Med. Genet. A* 167:2162–2167.

Zlotogora, J. 2015. *Mendelian disorders among Jews.* Department of Community Genetics, Public Health Services, Ministry of Health, Israel. https://www.health.gov.il/Subjects/Genetics/Documents/book_jews.pdf.

Zöllner, N., S. Reiter, M. Gross, D. Pongratz, C.D. Reimers, K. Gerbitz et al. 1986. Myoadenylate deaminase deficiency: successful symptomatic therapy by high dose oral administration of ribose. *Klinische Wochenschrift* 64:1281–1290.

13 Dietary Requirements of Amino Acids

Dietary protein is generally the primary source of amino acids (AAs) in healthy individuals under normal feeding conditions. According to the principles of nutrition, humans and other animals have requirements for dietary AAs but not protein (Fuller and Garlick 1994; Reeds 2020; Wu et al. 2010). AAs include those that are not synthesized or inadequately synthesized by the organisms [i.e., AAs that had traditionally been classified as nutritionally essential AAs (EAAs)], as well as the AAs that are synthesizable *de novo* in animal cells (AASAs) [i.e., AAs that had traditionally been classified as nutritionally nonessential AAs (NEAAs)]. In total parenteral nutrition (the provision of nutrients via intravenous administration), free AAs or their small peptides are used to support patients who cannot eat or have a dysfunctional small intestine. In enteral nutrition (eating via the mouth or feeding via a gastric tube), protein is generally part of the diet to provide AAs. The term "dietary protein requirement" is used in some sections of this chapter and some official publications as a proxy for dietary AA requirements for the following reasons. First, dietary protein is quantitatively the major source of AAs in the body under normal feeding conditions. Second, due to a lack of sufficient knowledge about AA nutrition and metabolism, FAO (2007), IOM (2005), and NRC (2012) have not recommended the requirements of humans and other animals for about half of the 20 canonical proteinogenic AAs. Third, the analysis of crude protein ($N\% \times 6.25$), rather than AAs, has become a routine procedure in global food/feed industries since the 1960s. Fourth, the content of most EAAs is generally correlated with that of proteins in common foodstuffs/feedstuffs. Fifth, some countries, such as Canada and the United States, require that the content of protein, but not AAs, in prepared foods/feeds be indicated on product labels.

Dietary proteins must be enzymatically hydrolyzed in the lumen of the gastrointestinal tract and their degradation products are absorbed by the small intestine to exert their nutritional value (Chapter 2). Adequate provision of AAs in the diet is essential to the health, growth, development, and survival of all organisms (Davis et al. 1993; Dillon 2013; Hoffer and Bistrian 2012; Millward 1998; Reeds et al. 2000). This is graphically illustrated by two human metabolic disorders resulting from protein malnutrition: (1) kwashiorkor (coined by the Jamaican pediatrician C. Williams in 1935; primarily resulting from a severe deficiency of dietary protein); and (2) marasmus ("wasting away" in Greek; the term first used by Soranio in 1656; primarily caused by severe deficiencies of both protein and energy in the diet) (Munro 1964). Kwashiorkor is a common nutritional problem in both children and adults in underdeveloped nations and also occurs in subpopulations (e.g., hospitalized trauma, cancer patients, and some elderly persons) in developed countries. Less severe forms of AA or protein deficiency are frequently observed in the elderly (e.g., the home-bound elderly) in the industrialized world, as well as children and adults in developing nations, thereby compromising their nutritional status, increasing their susceptibility to metabolic and infectious diseases, and reducing their physical strength and longevity. Thus, there has been growing recognition that the elderly have a higher requirement for dietary AAs than the currently recommended value [i.e., 0.8 g/kg body weight (BW)/day] (Fukagawa 2013; Kurpad and Vaz 2000).

In humans and other animals, the sources of AAs include (1) dietary proteins, peptides, and free AAs; (2) the degradation of whole-body proteins and peptides; and (3) in the case of AASAs, *de novo* endogenous synthesis. AAs are the building blocks of tissue proteins in all organisms (Table 13.1) and participate in vital metabolic processes in the body (Chapter 11). For carnivorous mammals (Wester et al. 2015), fish (Li et al. 2021a), and crustaceans (Li et al. 2021b) that ingest a small amount of carbohydrates, most of the dietary AAs are utilized for ATP and glucose production in

TABLE 13.1

Composition of Amino Acids in the Bodies of Humans and Other Animals[a]

Amino Acid (AA)	Rat[b]	Human[c]	Cattle[c]	Sheep[d]	Chick[e]	Pig[f] Intact AA	Pig[f] AA[g] Residues	HSB[h]	LMB[i]	Shrimp[j]
					mg AA/g Protein					
Ala	66.0	72	76	66.5	66.3	65.7	61.6	68.8	68.6	60.3
Arg	68.2	77	75	68.0	68.5	67.7	71.4	69.6	69.9	65.1
Asn	36.5	---	---	35.8	36.5	36.0	36.5	36.6	35.7	43.5
Asp	43.4	---	---	43.7	43.1	42.8	43.6	45.9	45.0	52.3
Asp+Asn	79.9	90	87	79.5	79.6	78.8	80.1	82.5	80.7	95.8
Cys	14.5	---	---	14.6	15.0	13.2	13.2	14.0	14.0	16.1
Gln	51.0	---	---	50.9	50.5	51.2	52.8	56.6	56.1	56.3
Glu	83.8	---	---	83.2	82.9	84.6	87.0	90.5	90.6	91.3
Glu+Gln	135	130	138	134	133	136	140	147.1	146.7	147.6
Gly	114	118	121	113	115	117	105	91.0	91.3	77.1
His	21.0	26	27	21.2	21.1	20.8	21.6	23.8	22.6	20.8
Ile	35.7	35	30	36.0	35.9	35.3	35.9	39.4	39.9	41.3
Leu	69.0	75	74	69.4	69.2	68.3	69.3	69.3	69.4	69.0
Lys	61.8	72	69	61.0	61.5	60.3	62.2	61.7	62.0	70.0
Met	19.2	20	18	19.0	18.9	18.7	19.3	28.5	29.0	21.2
Phe	34.1	41	39	34.6	34.8	34.3	35.9	40.5	40.6	45.9
Pro	85.7	84	87	85.5	85.3	86.1	85.3	66.2	66.3	68.2
OH-Pro	34.6	---	---	34.8	34.8	37.9	38.5	21.5	21.2	12.3
Pro+OH-Pro	120	---	---	120	120	124	124	87.7	87.5	80.5
Ser	44.8	44	47	45.2	45.0	44.3	43.1	49.0	49.2	52.4
Thr	36.0	41	43	36.8	36.3	35.1	35.0	40.6	41.0	40.7
Trp	12.0			11.4	11.6	11.1	11.9	11.4	11.6	12.2
Tyr	26.8	29	27	27.0	26.6	27.2	28.6	29.2	29.3	37.6
Val	42.0	47	42	42.6	41.8	42.2	42.0	46.0	46.9	46.6

Source: Wu et al. 2013. *Amino Acids* 44:1107–1113; Li et al. 2021a. *Adv. Exp. Med. Biol.* 1285:133–168; Li et al. 2021b. *Adv. Exp. Med. Biol.* 1285:169–197.

[a] Unless indicated otherwise, calculations were based on the molecular weights of intact AAs.

[b] Adult rats (60-day-old).

[c] Data for human fetuses (160–280 days of gestation) and cattle (12-week-old). It was not reported whether calculations were based on the molecular weights of intact AAs or AA residues.

[d] Adult sheep (12-month-old).

[e] Chickens (10-day-old).

[f] Pigs (30-day-old).

[g] Calculations were based on the molecular weights of AA residues (molecular weights of an intact AA: 18).

[h] Juvenile hybrid striped bass (HSB; 50 g of body weight).

[i] Juvenile largemouth bass (LMB; 50 g of body weight).

[j] Whole body of the whiteleg shrimp (*Litopenaeus vannamei*; 15 g of body weight).

their bodies. Thus, knowledge about AA biochemistry and functions provides the necessary foundation for determining the dietary requirements of AAs by humans and other animals. Requirements of dietary AAs can be classified as qualitative and quantitative. Qualitative requirements are related to the question of "*what* is required for maintenance, optimum performance (e.g., growth, lactation, reproduction, and physical activity), and optimum health (e.g., prevention of chronic metabolic disorders, resistance to infectious disease, and recovery from illness)?". Quantitative requirements refer to the question of *"how much* is required for maintenance, optimum performance, optimum health, and recovery from illness?". The major objectives of this chapter are to highlight (1) the classic and modern methods for determining dietary AA requirements and assessing the quality of dietary proteins in nutrition, and (2) the impacts of dietary protein and AA intake on the health of humans and other animals.

13.1 HISTORICAL PERSPECTIVES OF DIETARY AA REQUIREMENTS

13.1.1 An Overall View

Feeding experiments have traditionally been employed to determine both qualitative and quantitative requirements of dietary AAs by animals. Minimal requirements of AAs can also be estimated using the so-called factorial analysis, that is, measurements of the loss of nitrogen (as AAs and their metabolites) by animals fed a protein-free diet via urine, feces, gas, and other routes (maintenance) + AAs deposited in animals + AAs excreted as animal products (e.g., milk, egg, wool, and fetus) (Wu et al. 2014a). Over the past three decades, studies involving radioactive and stable isotope AA tracers have been used along with the nitrogen balance technique to determine dietary requirements of humans and farm animals for nutritionally essential (indispensable) AAs (EAAs). To date, advanced research methods include metabolomics, proteomics, and genomics. While much effort has been directed at EAA nutrition, little is known about dietary requirements of mammals, birds, fish, crustaceans, reptiles, amphibians, and insects for so-called "nutritionally nonessential (indispensable) AAs (NEAAs)".

In practice, a useful concept in protein nutrition is "limiting AA", which is defined as an AA that is in the shortest supply from the diet relative to its requirements by an animal for maintenance, growth, and health. Limiting AAs are usually EAAs, depending on diets. The first limiting AA is often an EAA that is present in the diet in the least amount, as compared to the animal's daily requirement. For example, lysine and methionine are often the first limiting AAs for corn- and soybean meal-based swine and poultry diets, respectively, and they are the most limiting AAs for ruminants fed corn- and forage-based diets. Results from nutritional studies indicate that (1) in corn- and soybean meal-based swine diets for growth, the second, third, fourth, fifth, and sixth limiting AAs are usually threonine, methionine, tryptophan, valine, and isoleucine, respectively (Baker 1996; Le Bellego et al. 2001); (2) in corn- and soybean meal-based poultry diets for growth, the second, third, fourth, fifth, and sixth limiting AAs are threonine, lysine, valine, arginine, and tryptophan, respectively (Fernandez et al. 1994). The concept of limiting AAs also applies to human nutrition. On the other hand, excess intakes of AAs must be avoided in both humans and other animals. This is particularly important for the economically important livestock, poultry, fish, and crustaceans to reduce the costs of feedstuffs and mitigate environmental pollution (Li et al. 2021a, b; Selle et al. 2020; Wu et al. 2014b).

13.1.2 Studies of Laboratory Animals

In 1816, F. Magendie reported that dogs fed a nitrogen-free diet died in a short period and that the death could be prevented by feeding a diet containing proteins. These results indicate that animals depend on preformed protein in their diets for survival. The question of "what" and "how much" AAs should be supplied in animal diets puzzled pioneers in the field. To quantify dietary intake of protein, J.B. Boussingault analyzed the nitrogen (N) content of foodstuffs in 1836. This work showed that dietary nitrogen content differed markedly between the foodstuffs of animal and plant origins, and among plant proteins. In 1872, H. Ritthausen speculated that various proportions of AAs among animal and plant proteins might be the cause of the differences in their nutritive value. Forty years later, this idea was supported by O. Abderhalden, who further proposed that the proportions of specific AAs in dietary protein were more important than their absolute amounts.

Research on qualitative requirements of individual AAs by animals began in 1904 when O. Abderhalden and P. Rona reported that mice fed either trypsin-digested casein hydrolysates or intact casein had the same rates of growth and survival, but the animals suffered from severe malnutrition, sickness, and even death when fed the neutralized acid hydrolysates of casein. One year later, these authors found that dogs exhibited a positive nitrogen balance when fed trypsin-digested casein but a negative nitrogen balance almost immediately after consuming the neutralized acid hydrolysates of casein. Similar results were obtained from rat studies by V. Henriques and C. Hansen in the same year. The reason for these intriguing observations was not known until 1906 when E.G. Willcock and F. Gowland Hopkins discovered that tryptophan, which is completely destroyed by acid hydrolysis, is essential for the growth and survival of rats. Based on nitrogen balance in dogs fed a tryptophan- or a proline-free basal diet that was supplemented either with or without the missing AA, E. Abderhalden proposed in 1912 that AAs could be classified as nutritionally essential (indispensable) or nonessential (dispensable). EAAs, not NEAAs, must be provided by diets to support protein accretion in growing animals and nitrogen balance in adults. After the seminal finding of the dietary essentiality of tryptophan for animals was presented, the importance of lysine in nutrition was demonstrated by T.B. Osborne and L.B. Mendel in 1914 when they noted that young rats did not grow when fed a gliadin-based diet that was severely deficient in lysine. However, when small, graded amounts of lysine were added to the basal diet, the young rats exhibited growth in a dose-dependent manner. In their original 1914 publication, T.B. Osborne and L.B. Mendel defined EAAs as those AAs that "cannot be manufactured *de novo* in the animal organism" and NEAAs as those AAs that can be formed adequately from other AAs *de novo* in the body. In 1916, H. Ackroyd and F. Gowland Hopkins reported that histidine is also an EAA for rats. Encouraged by these ground-breaking discoveries, many experiments were conducted between 1916 and 1926 to identify the dietary requirements of rats for other EAAs, but they were all unsuccessful and in most instances were discontinued because the animals rejected the food. Unfortunately, low food intake was not interpreted to indicate a dietary deficiency of an AA but rather was believed to be caused by the bad taste of the ration. Thus, by 1930, only three AAs (tryptophan, lysine, and histidine) had been unequivocally shown to be EAAs for rats.

In 1931, R.W. Jackson and R.J. Block reported that methionine or cystine was a dietary essential AA for the growth of rats fed a diet containing gelatin and a low level of whole milk powder. It was not until 1935 when W.C. Rose isolated threonine from casein that it became possible to prepare nutritionally complete crystalline AA-based diets for animals. Between 1937 and 1948, using rats fed various mixtures of AAs, W.C. Rose discovered that the lack of isoleucine, methionine, phenylalanine, threonine, or valine in the diet resulted in a loss of BW, diminished appetite, and eventual death. Of particular interest, this biochemist noted that animals grew at a low rate when arginine was missing from the diet but at a much higher rate when the diet contained adequate arginine. Recognizing a nutritional role for certain AAs that can be synthesized in the body but whose synthesis is insufficient for maximal growth, W.C. Rose and coworkers defined in 1946 an EAA as "one which cannot be synthesized by the animal organism out of materials ordinarily available to the cells *at a speed* commensurate with the demands for normal growth". According to this definition, EAAs vary with species, developmental stage, physiological status, and pathological conditions. For example, arginine, which is synthesized at a rate inadequate to support maximal growth of young mammals, can be considered to be an EAA. Therefore, by 1950, nine EAAs and one "nutritionally semi-essential" AA (i.e., arginine) had been identified for rats. Note that the major criterion used to assess whether an AA is nutritionally essential or nonessential was nitrogen balance or growth rates of animals. These simple methods, although imperfect, have played an important role in studies of AA metabolism and nutrition over the past century (Rose 1968; Wu 2018). The discovery of EAAs is a great example of testifying that creative ideas are a key element in advancing nutritional sciences.

13.1.3 HUMAN STUDIES

Based on the amounts of protein consumed by a group of German workmen doing moderate physical work, J. von Liebig estimated in 1840 that the average adult would require a dietary intake of 120 g protein per day. Extrapolating results from canine studies without consideration of a human equivalent dose, Liebig's student C. von Voit suggested a dietary intake of 118 g protein/day for the average adult in 1881. Influenced by the German school of nutritionists, in 1902, the American scientist W.O. Atwater (a former student of Voit) recommended the dietary intake of 125 g protein/day for the average adult, as he found that the U.S. workmen generally worked harder, ate more, and were wealthier than the Germans. However, in 1904, R.H. Chittenden (Professor of Physiological Chemistry at Yale University) challenged these high values of protein intake because they were not derived from human metabolic needs and were not consistent with his observations. In his experiments, Chittenden noted that (1) fifteen adults remained healthy and in nitrogen balance for 6 months on daily diets containing 61–62 g protein; and (2) seven college student-athletes consuming 64 g protein/day maintained their levels of athletic performance and well-being. Despite this advance in protein nutrition, little was known then about dietary requirements of individual AAs by humans.

Guided by results from his and others' animal studies, W.C. Rose undertook extensive research on dietary requirements of EAAs by adult humans at the University of Illinois between 1942 and 1955. This timely work arose partly from the urgent need to understand dietary AA requirements by soldiers who were fighting in World War II when food protein resources were scarce. To successfully complete his experiments, Rose cleverly designed the basal diet to contain nitrogen-free food ingredients, including cornstarch, sucrose, protein-free butterfat, corn oil, inorganic salts, and a vitamin mixture. The study participants consumed, for 8 days, an AA mixture lacking an AA under study, and N balance was the criterion for adequacy or inadequacy of the rations. In 1950, he identified methionine and valine as EAAs for young adults. One year later, Rose reported that threonine, but not histidine, was an EAA for adult humans. Specifically, the absence of dietary histidine did not affect nitrogen balance during a week-long experimental period. This finding was previously taken to suggest that histidine could be synthesized by humans. However, despite much effort by many biochemists worldwide, no pathway could be identified for histidine synthesis in animal cells. This discrepancy highlights a major weakness of nitrogen balance as the sole criterion to classify AAs as EAAs or NEAAs. Nonetheless, luck favored Rose in his subsequent studies during which he correctly identified isoleucine, leucine, lysine, phenylalanine, and tryptophan as EAAs for humans.

In all of these landmark experiments by W.C. Rose, the removal of isoleucine, leucine, lysine, methionine, phenylalanine, threonine, tryptophan, or valine from the diet resulted in a strongly negative nitrogen balance, low appetite, extreme fatigue, and nervous irritability. Conversely, these symptoms disappeared promptly after the addition of the missing AA to the ration. By contrast, Rose found that healthy young men fed a diet lacking one of the following AAs could maintain nitrogen balance: alanine, arginine, aspartate, cysteine, glutamate, glycine, proline, serine, and tyrosine. Note that he did not mention asparagine or glutamine in his work, possibly because he did not have the necessary methods for their analysis. In 1957, Rose defined an NEAA as "an amino acid which can be produced in sufficient quantities to fully meet the requirements of animals". Over the past five decades, studies involving stable isotope tracers have been undertaken by several groups of scientists in Canada, the United Kingdom, and the United States (including R.O. Ball, D.M. Bier, E.B. Marliss, P.B. Pencharz, P.J. Reeds, M.J. Rennie, J.C. Waterlow, R.R. Wolfe, and V.R. Young) to determine quantitative requirements of infants, children, and adults for dietary EAAs. Consistent with postnatal changes in the fractional rates of tissue protein synthesis, dietary EAA requirements (expressed as mg/kg BW) by humans generally decrease with age between birth and adulthood (FAO 2007, 2013).

13.1.4 STUDIES OF FARM ANIMALS

Farm animals grow faster than humans and, therefore, are useful biological models for sensitively detecting their responses to EAAs and defining their requirements for these nutrients (Baker 1996). Thus, along with the advent of AA nutrition research on rats and humans between the 1930s and the 1950s, there was much interest in studying the dietary requirements of poultry, swine, and cattle for EAAs during this period. Specifically, in 1938, A.A. Klose, E.L.R. Stokstad, and H.J. Almquist reported that arginine is an EAA for chickens. Subsequently, a series of elegant studies by E.T. Mertz and colleagues indicated the nutritional essentiality of tryptophan (1948), lysine (1949), threonine (1950), and methionine (1951), as well as arginine, leucine, phenylalanine, and valine (1952) in young pigs. Meanwhile, L.A. Maynard and coworkers demonstrated in 1951 that isoleucine is another EAA in swine. The Maynard group also used purified diets to determine the AA requirements of young ruminants in 1948. This seminal work was followed by extensive studies of AA requirements by lactating cows, growing beef, and growing sheep in the 1950s to 1980s. To bypass the microbial actions of the rumen in ruminants, these investigations involved direct infusion of individual AAs, casein, or other proteins into the abomasum, and generated unique concepts and terminologies in ruminant protein nutrition, which included (1) rumen-degradable protein (the protein that can be hydrolyzed in the rumen), (2) rumen-undegradable protein (the protein that cannot be hydrolyzed in the rumen), (3) microbial protein (protein synthesized by rumen bacteria), (4) metabolizable protein (true protein that is digested in the abomasum and the small intestine), and (5) nonprotein nitrogen (Schwab and Broderick 2017). Although ruminal bacteria can synthesize all AAs from ammonia, sulfur, and carbohydrate, the microbial source of protein and AAs is inadequate for supporting maximal growth of postweaning ruminants or maximum milk production by lactating cows when the animals are fed roughage diets.

Beginning in the late 1950s, H.H. Mitchell and H.M. Scott at the University of Illinois developed the ideal protein concept (optimal proportions and amounts of EAAs) for chicken diets. Early attempts were based on the EAA composition of eggs and casein but were largely unsuccessful because of the excess of many EAAs. In 1960, H.M. Scott's group simulated the profile of EAAs in the fat-free chick carcass to design a revised pattern of dietary EAAs for improving chick growth performance. An improvement was indeed achieved using this approach but remained unsatisfactory due to the lack of NEAAs in the diet. Subsequently, a mixture of several AAs (cystine, glycine, proline, and glutamate), which are synthesized by birds and had previously been thought to be NEAAs in chicken nutrition, was used in dietary formulations to yield better results on growth performance. This extensive research during the 1960s and the 1970s culminated in several versions of the "chick AA requirement standard" for the first three weeks post-hatching. Reference values were given in the Dean and Scott Standard (1965), the Huston and Scott (1968) Reference Standard, and the modified Sasse and Baker (1973) Reference Standard. The common features shared by these different recommended standards of dietary AA requirements by chickens are that the diets included (1) all protein EAAs that are not synthesized by chickens; (2) several AAs (cystine, glutamate, glycine, proline, and tyrosine) that are synthesized by animals to a various extent; and (3) no data on alanine, aspartate, asparagine, glutamine, or serine. Because the content of proline plus hydroxyproline in the body of chickens was not known at that time, the relatively small amount of proline in the recommended ideal protein was only arbitrarily set and was thought to limit their responses to dietary EAAs and their maximal growth. Thus, the lysine:proline ratio ranged from 4.75:1.00 in the Huston and Scott Reference Standard (1968) to 2.28:1.00 in the modified Sasse and Baker Reference Standard (1973). By contrast, very large amounts of glutamate (e.g., 13 times the lysine value in the modified Sasse and Baker Reference Standard) were used to presumably provide the entire need for "nonspecific AA nitrogen". However, key questions regarding whether glutamate fulfilled this role and whether excess glutamate might interfere with the transport, metabolism, and utilization of other AAs in chickens were not addressed by the Illinois investigators.

In 1980, the British nutritionist D.J.A. Cole suggested that swine diets could be formulated to contain ideal ratios of EAAs (with lysine as the reference AA) based on their concentrations in the pig carcass (almost exclusively tissue proteins). This idea was first adopted by the British Agricultural Research Council (ARC) in 1981 and then by the U.S. National Research Council (NRC) in 1988. Unfortunately, histidine, arginine, and all NEAAs were not included in the ARC's concept of "ideal protein". The absence of histidine, which is not synthesized by animal cells, from such a protein has no biochemical basis and, therefore, does not make any sense. Also, its conceptual foundation based solely on the EAA composition of the carcass was flawed, because the pattern of AAs in the diet does not necessarily reflect the composition of AAs in the body (Chapter 2). This mismatch arises from the fact that (1) individual AAs in the diet undergo extensive catabolism and transformations at different rates in the small intestine; (2) the pattern of AA concentrations in the circulation differs markedly from the AA composition in the diet; (3) individual AAs in the plasma have different metabolic fates in different animal tissues; and (4) the pattern of AAs in tissue proteins differs greatly from that in the diet (Chapter 3). Additionally, the "ideal protein" concept ignores all NEAAs, as well as the nutritional and physiological needs of the small intestine and immunocytes for NEAAs, which are not only major energy sources for enterocytes but also key regulators of gut integrity, immunity, health, and function (Wu et al. 2014a). These major shortcomings limit the usefulness of the early versions of the "ideal protein" in formulating swine diets for maximal growth performance.

Dietary AAs are required by humans and other animals primarily for maintenance (including the synthesis of nonprotein metabolites) and protein accretion (Cole 1980). However, the ARC's ideal protein concept did not take into consideration the relative contribution of maintenance to the total AA needs of the pig. This was due, in part, to technical challenges to accurately determine maintenance requirements for AAs, because their components include (1) protein synthesis, (2) the obligatory use of AAs as precursors for essential metabolites (including conventional neurotransmitters, NO, CO, and H_2S), (3) the obligatory oxidation of AAs (as major energy substrates for specific tissues, as the sole source of ammonia to link glucose and nitrogen metabolism, and as a source of CO_2 for acid–base balance and carboxylation reactions), (4) losses of AAs from gastrointestinal epithelia and blood via intestinal secretions, (5) losses of AAs from integument (hair and skin) and epidermal structures, and (6) the urinary excretion of unmodified AAs. In attempts to improve the original ideal protein concept, between 1989 and 1990, T.C. Wang and M.F. Fuller used gilts in the weight range of 25–50 kg to estimate an ideal AA pattern that included both maintenance and tissue protein accretion. However, these authors still did not consider arginine, histidine, or any so-called NEAAs in the ideal protein although they used glutamate at 826% of the lysine value to provide nonspecific AA nitrogen (Wang and Fuller 1989). Like the chicken studies in the 1960s and 1970s, there were also concerns over the assumptions for inclusion of this high level of glutamate in the swine diet that lack all other NEAAs.

Having recognized the need to modify the ideal protein concept for formulating swine diets, D.H. Baker (2000) took great efforts, between 1990 and 2000, to evaluate the dietary requirements of 10–20 kg swine for EAAs. In their original study, Baker and Chung (1992) added arginine (42% of lysine), glycine (100% of lysine), histidine (32% of lysine), and proline (33% of lysine) to the basal diet containing 1.2% true digestible lysine and using glutamate at 878% of the lysine value to provide nonspecific AA nitrogen. However, other NEAAs (including alanine, aspartate, asparagine, cysteine, glutamine, serine, and tyrosine) were not considered in the revised version of the ideal protein and the rationale for the use of arginine, glycine, histidine, and proline at different proportions to lysine was not explained. Furthermore, it was unknown (1) whether glutamate is an effective precursor for the synthesis of all other AAs (including aspartate, glutamine, and serine) in specific tissues (e.g., the small intestine, spleen, and lymph nodes) and the whole body, or (2) whether the high content of glutamate in the diet may affect the transport, metabolism, and utilization of other AAs in the diet. Disappointingly, after the 10th edition of the NRC Swine Nutrient Requirements was published in 1998 that did not recognize the needs of pigs for dietary proline or glycine, D.H. Baker omitted glycine and proline from the last version of his "ideal protein" for swine diet formulations in 2000. Over the past two decades, there have been successful approaches to refine the patterns of AAs in diets for lactating, suckling, weanling, finishing, or gestating pigs through the addition of arginine, glutamine, glutamate, or glycine improved neonatal and postweaning growth, lactation performance, and litter size in the swine (e.g., Hou and Wu 2018; Kim et al. 2005; Wang et al. 2014).

Based on an extensive review of the literature in 2009, G. Wu defined EAAs as either those AAs whose carbon skeletons cannot be synthesized or those that are insufficiently synthesized *de novo* by animals relative to their needs for optimal maintenance, growth, development, and health. EAAs must be provided in the diet to achieve optimal function in individuals. According to this definition, glutamine and glutamate have been classified as nutritionally EAAs for intestinal–mucosal integrity, function, and health in piglets within two weeks after weaning (Rezaei et al. 2013; Wu et al. 2011). Similarly, arginine is now considered to be an EAA for the maximum growth of neonatal pigs and for female reproduction (Wu et al. 2018). Furthermore, tyrosine, which is derived from phenylalanine hydroxylation but whose carbon skeleton cannot be synthesized *de novo*, should be classified as an EAA. In humans and other animals with a deficiency of tetrahydrobiopterin (BH4) or phenylalanine hydroxylase, diets must contain tyrosine to prevent a negative nitrogen balance and metabolic disorders. Likewise, cysteine, which is synthesized from methionine, should be considered to be an EAA, because the carbon skeleton of cysteine or methionine cannot be made *de novo* in animal cells. In birds, the carbon skeleton (P5C) of proline and arginine cannot be synthesized *de novo* (Wu et al. 1995) and the rate of glycine synthesis is normally lower than the rate of glycine utilization, and, therefore, these three AAs are classified as EAAs by definition.

In 2009, G. Wu defined NEAAs as those AAs that can be synthesized *de novo* in adequate amounts by animals to meet their requirements for maintenance, growth, development, and health and, therefore, need not be provided in the diet. According to this definition, the classification of AAs as NEAAs will depend on species, developmental stage, physiological state, environmental factors (e.g., heat stress and low temperature), and disease (Table 13.2). Disappointingly, to date, there is no compelling experimental evidence for the sufficient synthesis of NEAAs by animals under these conditions (Hou et al. 2015; 2016). Simply grouping, as NEAAs, all AAs that are synthesized *de novo* in animal cells without full consideration of the above factors have both conceptual and practical limitations. The list of AAs in the NEAA (now reclassified as AASA) category must be revised as new experimental data become available.

13.1.5 Dietary Requirements of Humans and Other Animals for AASAs (NEAAs plus CEAAs)

A key element of the historical classification of NEAAs is that all NEAAs were tactically assumed to be adequately synthesized in the animal to meet the needs for tissue protein synthesis. However, as recognized by V.R. Young (1994) and P.J. Reeds (2000), no such experimental data were ever obtained from all the previous studies involving humans and other animals. In agreement with W.C. Rose's 1946 definition of NEAAs and EAAs for rats, H.H. Mitchell stated in 1962 that "an amino acid may be a dietary essential nutrient even if an animal is capable of synthesizing it". Over the past decades, no studies have been performed systematically to provide quantitative data on dietary requirements of NEAAs by humans, livestock species, birds, or aquatic animals. Note that any data from short-term (e.g., up to 12 h) studies showing no difference in either the rates of skeletal muscle and whole-body protein synthesis or whole-body creatine synthesis between the control participants fed a diet providing EAAs and the participants fed a diet providing only EAAs but little or no NEAAs should not be taken to indicate whether the synthesis of NEAAs from EAAs meets their long-term (e.g., a prolonged period of days, months, and years) metabolic needs. This is because the amounts of preexisting plus newly synthesized NEAAs may be adequate only for a short period and may not be sufficient to meet physiological requirements during a longer period at the different stages of the life cycle. Official publications related to AA requirements by higher organisms (e.g., the Institute

TABLE 13.2

Classification of Amino Acids (AAs) as EAAs, NEAAs, and CEAAs in Animals[a]

Mammals[b]			Poultry			Fish		
EAA	AASA		EAA	AASA		EAA	AASA	
	NEAA	CEAA[c]		NEAA	CEAA[c]		NEAA	CEAA[c]
Arg[d]	Ala	Gln	Arg	Ala	Gln	Arg	Ala	Gln
Cys	Asn	Glu	Cys	Asn	Glu	Cys	Asn	Glu
His	Asp	Gly	Gly	Asp	Taurine	His	Asp	Gly
Ile	Ser	Pro	His	Ser		Ile	Ser	Taurine[f]
Leu		Taurine[e]	Ile			Leu		
Lys			Leu			Lys		
Met			Lys			Met		
Phe			Met			Phe		
Thr			Phe			Pro		
Trp			Pro			Thr		
Tyr			Thr			Trp		
Val			Trp			Tyr		
			Tyr			Val		
			Val					

Source: Wu, G. 2009. *Amino Acids* 37:1–17.

[a] Classification of AAs as EAAs, NEAAs, or CEAAs depends on species, developmental stage, physiological status, environmental factors, and disease. Based on recent advances in amino acid nutrition and metabolism, NEAAs and CEAAs should be considered as AASAs (amino acids that are synthesizable *de novo* in animal cells; Hou and Wu 2017).

[b] Preweaning ruminants have qualitatively similar requirements for dietary AAs to those for nonruminants. In postweaning ruminants, the microbial source of protein and AAs is inadequate for supporting their maximal growth or milk production when the animals are fed roughage diets.

[c] For neonates (including human infants and piglets), adults under stress conditions (e.g., heat stress, burns, and infection), and breeding stocks (both males and females). Taurine is an EAA for cats, human infants, and carnivorous fish.

[d] Arginine is synthesized *de novo* in most mammals except for cats, ferrets, mink, tigers, and possibly horses (Chapter 3). Although arginine synthesis occurs in the mammals (e.g., humans, swine, cattle, sheep, and rats) that express all the necessary enzymes, the rates of its synthesis do not meet requirements for growth or physiological functions (e.g., spermatogenesis in males, lactation and embryonic survival in females, as well as blood flow and ammonia detoxification via the urea cycle in both males and females). Aging is associated with a reduction in arginine synthesis.

[e] There is little synthesis of taurine in cats, tigers and cheetahs. Taurine synthesis is inadequate in human infants.

[f] Taurine synthesis may not occur in some carnivorous fish. Herbivorous fish synthesize taurine but the rates of its synthesis may be inadequate under stress conditions or when fed a low-protein diet.

AASA, an amino acid that is synthesizable *de novo* in animal cells; CEAA, conditionally essential AA; EAA, nutritionally essential AA (traditionally classified); NEAA, nutritionally nonessential AA (traditionally classified).

of Medicine-recommended dietary allowance for humans in 2005 and the NRC-recommended AA requirements for swine in 2012) do not provide data on dietary requirements of any NEAAs. Some of the explanations offered by the authors are not supported by our current understanding of AA metabolism and nutrition. For example, the Institute of Medicine stated in 2005 that dietary arginine was not required by healthy adults because arginine is synthesized via the hepatic urea cycle. However, there is no *net* synthesis of arginine in the mammalian liver via the hepatic urea cycle (Chapter 3). In addition, NRC (2012) indicated that typically, swine have sufficient capacity for the synthesis of all those AAs that are not classified as EAAs. However, ample evidence from recent studies is inconsistent with this notion (Hou et al. 2015, 2016). Furthermore, the synthesis of NEAAs in animals critically depends on the availability of EAAs that are usually provided from protein in expensive ingredients (Chapter 4), and *sufficient capacity* does not necessarily translate into *sufficient synthesis* of NEAAs in pigs fed an ordinary diet to minimize production costs and excretion of nitrogenous metabolites. This demonstrates the importance of ensuring that recommendations for dietary AA requirements be based on up-to-date knowledge of new developments in the field of AA metabolism. In humans and other animals, dependence on dietary EAAs to provide NEAAs via synthetic pathways not only wastes EAAs, but these metabolic pathways also produce a large amount of ammonia (a substance that is particularly toxic to the central nervous system at high concentrations and adversely increases the workloads of the liver and kidneys) and are energetically inefficient (Wu 2009). Humans and all other animals *do* have dietary requirements for NEAAs for optimal health and growth (Hou et al. 2016; Rasmussen et al. 2020; Wu et al. 2013).

The fact that some AAs can be synthesized in the body at the expense of considerable amounts of energy speaks highly of their physiological importance. Therefore, pathways for their *de novo* syntheses have evolved or have been highly conserved in the body. Likewise, all NEAAs undergo metabolic transformations and have crucial physiological functions (see Chapter 11). For example, the unusually high concentration (~1 mM) of glycine in the plasma of postnatal pigs has an important role in stimulating rapid growth, and the abundance of arginine (up to 6 mM) in porcine allantoic fluid during early gestation promotes placental growth and fetal development. Thus, there is compelling evidence that an inadequate supply of an NEAA in the diet may cause a severe metabolic disorder in animals. For example, the administration of a glutamine-free total parenteral nutrition (TPN) solution to postsurgical patients results in both reduced intestinal mass and a loss of skeletal muscle protein. Based on this finding, glutamine was classified by Lacey and Wilmore (1990) as a conditionally essential AA (CEAA), which is defined as an AA that can normally be synthesized in adequate amounts by animals but which must be provided in the diet to meet optimal needs under certain conditions wherein rates of utilization are greater than rates of synthesis. Furthermore, the results of recent studies indicate that (1) diets must contain sufficient amounts of arginine and glutamine to support optimal fetal, neonatal, and postweaning growth in swine; (2) dietary supplementation with proline enhances the growth performance of early-weaned pigs and young rats; and (3) whole-body protein synthesis in burn patients is enhanced by dietary supplementation with arginine, proline, and glycine (Hou et al. 2015, 2016; Wu et al. 2013). Based on the definitions of EAAs, NEAAs, and CEAAs, a revised classification of AAs in the nutrition of mammals, fish, and birds is summarized in Table 13.2.

Although EAAs must be included in diets to support the survival, growth, and development of all nonruminants (including humans, cats, dogs, swine, poultry, and fish), all the 20 canonical proteinogenic (protein-creating) AAs must be adequate to meet the needs of these organisms for physiologically essential metabolic processes (Wu 2009). In addition, individuals with inborn errors of AA synthesis must be provided with the affected AA for their survival (Chapter 12). Furthermore, as indicated previously, there is no compelling evidence for sufficient syntheses of NEAAs in normal animals (including humans, pigs, and rodents) that consume diets providing only EAAs. Of particular note, the ratio of NEAAs to EAAs in animals is 60:40 (Hou and Wu 2016), indicating that NEAAs are 50% more abundant than EAAs in the body. In rapidly growing swine, about 55% and 45% of the total dietary NEAAs entering the portal vein are used for protein accretion and other metabolic pathways, respectively, and about 40%–50% of the total NEAAs deposited in tissue proteins is derived from *de novo* synthesis from EAAs. These results indicate that dietary NEAA intake is substantially insufficient for protein synthesis when the animals are fed conventional diets. In adult humans, about 45% and 55% of the total dietary NEAAs are used for tissue protein replenishment and other metabolic pathways, respectively (Tessari 2019). Based on the results of both experimental and clinical studies over the past three decades, the century-old term "NEAA" has now been recognized to be a misnomer in nutritional sciences (Hou and Wu 2017). Thus, to avoid further confusion over AA nutrition, both NEAAs and CEAAs should be referred to as AAs that are synthesizable *de novo* in animal cells (AASAs). Criteria for assessing the dietary requirements of AASAs include embryonic survival and litter size, fetal growth, milk production, postnatal growth, skeletal muscle gain, absolute and proportional reductions of white adipose tissue (WAT), digestive function and intestinal integrity, immunity and health status, feed efficiency, and meat quality (Wu et al. 2013, 2014a, b, c). An AASA may be an EAA. For example, arginine is synthesized *de novo* in humans and pigs and, therefore, is an AASA in their nutrition. Much evidence shows that arginine is an EAA for the maximum growth, lactation, and reproduction of humans and pigs, as well as their optimum immunity and health, including cardiovascular health (Wu et al. 2013).

13.1.6 FUNCTIONAL AAs IN NUTRITION

The preceding discussion leads to the conclusion that whether an AA is called an EAA, CEAA, or NEAA is purely a matter of definition. Unfortunately, its conceptual limitation has hindered the development and practice of protein nutrition in humans and other animals. For example, traditionally, there was a lack of interest in conducting experiments to determine whether or not mammals, birds, fish, and crustaceans can sufficiently synthesize all of the AAs that are not classified as EAAs (Hou et al. 2015, 2016). Also, information on the composition of AAs in foodstuffs and the animal body was incomplete in previously published studies, resulting in inadequate knowledge about AA nutrition. Furthermore, the original classification of AA as EAAs or NEAAs in 1912 was based on nitrogen balance or animal growth but failed to consider regulatory roles for AAs in nutrition and metabolism. Therefore, historically, dietary AA requirements for whole-body growth and nitrogen balance in animals were the primary focus of protein nutrition research (Wu 2009). Since the 1990s, such shortcomings have become evident when the results of recent studies have indicated that (1) glutamate, glutamine, and aspartate are the major metabolic fuels for the small intestine of mammals, birds, fish, and crustaceans, as well as the liver, kidneys, and skeletal muscle of fish and crustaceans; (2) dietary glutamine is necessary for intestinal mucosal immunity; (3) dietary glutamine and glutamate ameliorates intestinal atrophy in early-weaned pigs fed a corn- and soybean meal-based diet and prevents intestinal dysfunction in rats receiving repetitive intragastric tube feeding of a protein-rich liquid diet; (4) dietary glycine modulates an animal's responses to inflammatory cytokines, thereby reducing mortality and morbidity in sepsis; (5) dietary arginine is required for maximum embryonic survival, as well as for the prevention and treatment of obesity and other metabolic syndromes (including hypertension); and (6) dietary proline and glycine are essential for skin health (Durante 2020; Le Floc'h et al. 2018; Li et al. 2021a, b; McNeal et al. 2018; Solano 2020; Wang et al. 2013; Wu 2009; Wu et al. 2011).

As a nonproteinogenic AA, taurine deserves special attention from nutritionists (Wright et al. 1986). Compared with other animal species (e.g., cattle, chickens, pigs, rats, and sheep), humans have a low ability to synthesize taurine at any stage during development. Thus, infants and children cannot produce a sufficient amount of taurine to meet their physiological needs and, therefore, must depend on a dietary source of taurine for optimal health, growth, and development. Depending on dietary protein intake, nutritional status, concentrations of hormones in the blood, and hepatic activity, a healthy adult synthesizes 50–125 mg taurine per day and excretes taurine primarily via the urine (95%) and, to a much lesser extent, the bile entering the feces (5%) (Jacobsen and Smith 1968; Sturman et al. 1975). Under stress or diseased conditions (e.g., heat stress, infection, obesity, diabetes, and cancer), taurine synthesis in the body may be impaired due to the suboptimal function of the liver and the reduced availability of its precursors. Notably, vegans generally have lower concentrations of taurine in their plasma and red blood cells than do their nonvegan counterparts (Laidlaw et al. 1988; Rana and Sanders 1986), likely due to its insufficient synthesis *de novo*. Additionally, there were reports that infants, children, and adults fed on taurine-free parenteral nutrition were deficient in taurine and greatly benefit from supplementation with taurine (Geggel et al. 1985; Stapleton et al. 1997). Taken together, these results suggest an inadequate synthesis of taurine by humans. However, the dietary requirements of taurine have not been established for nonfeline animals, including humans and most fish. Based on the urinary excretion of taurine (72 mg/day) by healthy adult humans, taurine requirement may be 75 mg/day (Wu 2020). Although swine, cattle, sheep, horses, poultry, and herbivorous fish can synthesize sufficient taurine from methionine or cysteine and generally do not require dietary taurine under healthy and adequately fed conditions, these animals may need dietary taurine for optimum health, well-being, growth, productivity, and physical performance under adverse environmental conditions (e.g., heat stress, weaning, long-distance transportation, infection, and other illnesses).

Some AASAs (e.g., arginine, glutamine, glutamate, glycine, and proline) play important roles in regulating gene expression, cell signaling, antioxidative responses, and immunity (Wu 2009). Additionally, glutamate, glutamine, and aspartate are major metabolic fuels for enterocytes (Beaumont and Blachier 2020) and they, along with glycine, D-aspartate, and D-serine, also regulate neurological development and function (Baccari et al. 2020). Furthermore, compelling evidence shows that (1) leucine activates MTOR to stimulate protein synthesis and inhibits proteolysis, and also enhances insulin secretion by pancreatic β-cells; (2) tryptophan modulates neurological and immunological functions by serving as a ligand for AhR receptors and as a precursor for the synthesis of numerous metabolites (including serotonin and melatonin); (3) S-adenosylmethionine (SAM, a metabolite of methionine) participates in protein and DNA methylation, and, therefore genetic and epigenetic regulation of cell growth and development; and (4) glutamine is essential for the synthesis of nucleotides and beneficially modulates the expression of anti-oxidative genes and redox signaling in enterocytes and immunocytes (Columbus et al. 2015; Fernstrom 2013; Strasser et al. 2016; Suryawan and Davis 2011; Wu et al. 2011). In addition, glutamine is a major metabolic fuel for the small intestine of mammals (Wu 2018) and the gut of aquatic animals (Li et al. 2021a,b). Of note, some AAs are required by an animal beyond protein synthesis and their inadequate provision has severe health consequences. For example, juvenile largemouth bass fed a low fishmeal diet (≤15% fishmeal CP) containing a large amount of proteins from soybean meal developed black skin syndrome characterized by skin darkening and retinal degeneration, as well as intestinal and liver atrophies and structural abnormalities, despite no change in BW gain (Li et al. 2020c). This metabolic disease resulted primarily from a deficiency of dietary methionine, as supplementing the diet with 0.5% methionine reduced the incidence of black skin syndrome by ~75% (Li et al. 2020d). Clearly, these findings indicate that methionine is a functional AA in animal nutrition.

Therefore, primarily based on a large body of published literature in the 1990s and 2000s, G. Wu proposed in 2010 the concept of functional AAs, which are defined as those AAs that participate in and regulate key metabolic pathways to improve health, survival, growth, development, lactation, and reproduction of the animal. Metabolic pathways include (1) AA synthesis and catabolism, (2) the generation of physiologically important low-molecular-weight peptides and nitrogenous substances, (3) intracellular protein turnover, (4) urea cycle and uric acid synthesis, (5) lipid and glucose metabolism, (6) immune responses, and (7) anti-oxidative reactions. Functional AAs can be EAAs (e.g., Cys, Leu, Met, and Trp in humans) and AASAs (e.g., Arg, Asp, Gln, Glu, Gly, Pro, and taurine in humans). Important roles of these AAs in physiology are not necessarily reflected by their relative or absolute concentrations in the plasma and cells, as tryptophan is among the least abundant AA in both free and peptide-bound pools (Hou et al. 2019). The concept of functional AAs takes into consideration the animal's metabolic needs for dietary AAs beyond tissue protein synthesis and unifies EAAs and AASAs in nutrition (Wu 2010). Humans and other animals have dietary requirements for functional AAs in health and under stress conditions (e.g., heat stress, gestation, lactation, weaning, intense exercise, and illness). The new nutritional concepts of functional AAs and dietary requirements for all proteinogenic AASAs have now been well accepted worldwide and are transforming the global practices of the nutrition of humans and other animals (including swine, poultry, sheep, cattle, fish, and shrimp) to (1) formulate balanced diets to maximize growth performance and feed efficiency in farm animals and to optimize the growth and development of neonatal mammals; (2) prevent or ameliorate intrauterine (mammals) or prehatching (poultry) growth restriction; (3) reduce risks for the postnatal development of chronic metabolic diseases (e.g., obesity, type-2 diabetes, and cardiovascular diseases); (4) optimize immune responses in all species to reduce risks for infectious diseases; and (5) enhance spermatogenesis and embryonic survival to prevent or treat infertility and pregnancy loss (Rasmussen et al 2020; Wu et al. 2013; Hou et al. 2016).

13.1.7 MOVING BEYOND THE "IDEAL PROTEIN" CONCEPT

The "ideal protein" concept had greatly advanced the field of swine and poultry protein nutrition over the last four and six decades, respectively (Baker 2009; van Milgen and Dourmad 2015; Kim et al. 2005) and had also been highlighted in the literature concerning the nutrition of other animals [including humans (FAO 2007), as well as fish and crustaceans (NRC 2011)]. However, the concept of "ideal protein" in animal nutrition, which was based solely on EAAs and ignored the more abundant AASAs, has major conceptual limitations due to the insufficient knowledge of AA biochemistry and nutrition, as well as inadequate research tools between the 1950s and the 1990s. Thus, the "ideal protein" is not ideal for the optimum nutrition and health of humans and other animals. Continuing to formulate diets based on the "ideal protein" concept is not an optimum practice in nutrition. Any ideal diet must provide all physiologically and nutritionally essential AAs (including EAAs, AASAs, and, in the cases of carnivores, also taurine). Thus, the "ideal protein" concept should be replaced with "optimum ratios of all proteinogenic AAs" for animals (Wu 2014). In the different stages of the life cycle, the requirements of humans and other animals for the amounts and ratios of all AAs, particularly AASAs whose synthesis depends on not only enzymes but also substrates and cofactors, are influenced by a plethora of factors, including genotypes, the environment, and diseases (Wu 2014). This means that dietary requirements for *all* proteinogenic AAs are dynamic and are not constant under all practical conditions. Optimal ratios of AAs in diets change with different physiological factors (e.g., exercise, gestation, lactation, and weanling of individuals, diseases, and other stressors (e.g., heat stress).

13.1.8 FORMULATING LOW-PROTEIN DIETS BASED ON OPTIMUM RATIOS OF ALL PROTEINOGENIC AAs

Both EAAs and AASAs limit the maximum growth and feed efficiency of animals (Hou et al. 2015, 2016). Reducing dietary protein intake by the inclusion of limiting AAs or animal-sourced feedstuffs that provide high-quality protein is an effective means to minimize feed cost and nitrogen excretion by farm animals (Hilliar and Swick 2019; Selle et al. 2020; Wu et al. 2014a). In addition, animal-sourced feedstuffs usually contain functional compounds, including taurine, creatine, carnosine, and anserine (Chapter 5) that are absent from plants. Those unique nutrients are critical and irreplaceable in the diets of carnivores and many omnivorous species. For example, animal plasma from bovine, porcine and even poultry sources provides immunoglobulins to young mammals (e. g. piglets, calves, kittens, and puppies) for boosting their feed intake, immunity, gastrointestinal health, and overall growth performance. In the face of diminishing resources of protein foodstuffs, it is necessary to formulate low-protein diets based on updated scientific knowledge. To date, this goal has been partially achieved due to dietary supplementation with limiting EAAs [e.g., methionine (or its α-ketoacid), lysine, threonine, and tryptophan]. However, a further reduction in dietary protein is constrained likely by the availability of AASAs. The optimum ratios of all proteinogenic AAs in the diets of humans and other animals are highlighted in Section 13.3 and must be considered to successfully develop low-protein and adequate AA diets for all animal species.

AASAs account for 60% of total AAs in the body (Chapter 3). Without dietary supplementation with AASAs, there is a limit to the minimum level of dietary protein because animals have the minimum requirements for *all* AAs to meet their needs for protein synthesis and other metabolic pathways but cannot synthesize adequate AASAs from low-protein diets. A minimum content of dietary CP with adequate EAAs varies with species, developmental stage, specific production (e.g., lactation or egg-laying), health status, and the environment, and may be, for example, 14% for 30–60 kg BW, 16% for 1- to 21-day-old broilers, and 30% for juvenile largemouth bass. For comparison, the optimum dietary CP levels with adequate amounts of all AAs to meet current growth and production expectations are 17%, 22%, and 40%, respectively, for these different animals. Optimum nutrition of AAs depends on their balances (ratios) and amounts in diets. As noted previously, the traditional "ideal protein" concept ignored the abundant AASAs that animals have a potential to form *de novo* but cannot synthesize adequately under normal feeding conditions due to insufficient substrates and/or relatively low enzymatic activities, as noted previously (Hou et al. 2016).

In the feeding of farm animals (e.g., pigs, poultry, fish, and shrimp) with a focus on reducing their AA intake and their excretion of nitrogenous and sulfurous wastes to the environment, low-protein diets must be fortified with (1) sufficient AASAs (including glutamate, glutamine, glycine, and proline), as well as possibly taurine and 4-hydroxyproline (a source of glycine to spare its synthesis from threonine and serine) in a species-dependent manner, or (2) the alternative low-cost sources of these AAs (e.g., animal byproducts) (Li and Wu 2020; Wu 2018). The inclusion of optimum ratios and amounts of all physiologically important AAs (including all AASAs) in the diets of livestock, poultry, fish, and crustaceans will help to improve the growth, feed efficiency, and health of animals while sustaining the global agriculture to provide humans with high-quality animal protein.

In support of the above notion, Kirchgessner et al. (1993) reported that, compared with the positive control [17% crude protein (CP) in the grower period (30–60 kg BW) and 14% CP in the finisher period (60 to 90 kg BW)], daily weight gain and feed conversion were reduced by up to 13% with the low protein diet with the same amount of EAAs during the grower (12% CP) and finisher (10% CP) periods despite similar feed intake. With dietary supplementation with 1%–4% glutamate, the weight gains and feed conversion of pigs fed a low CP diet were improved in a dose-dependent manner. However, pigs fed the low-protein diet supplemented with 4% glutamate still exhibited a lower weight gain and a lower feed efficiency, compared with the positive control group. This result suggests that pigs need AASAs other than glutamate for achieving maximal growth when fed a low-protein diet. In addition to swine feeding, glutamate, glutamine, glycine, and proline may be effectively used to replace a portion of fishmeal protein in the diets for fish (Li et al. 2021a), as well as shrimp and crabs (Li et al. 2021b). Furthermore, supplementing a mixture of AASAs (1.21% glutamate, 0.8% glycine, 0.43% proline, 0.33% alanine, and 0.99% aspartate) to a low (16.2%) CP diet for 1- to 21-d-old broilers improved their weight gain by 14% and feed efficiency by 10% (Awad et al. 2014). Animal byproducts are excellent sources of these and other AASAs, as well as all EAAs (including methionine, lysine, threonine, and tryptophan), taurine, and 4-hydroxyproline to prepare cost-effective, healthy, and environmentally sustainable low-protein diets for farm animals (Li and Wu 2020). The concept of a low-protein but adequate AA diet also applies to human nutrition, such as AA supplementation to women during pregnancy (Rasmussen et al. 2020; Weckman et al. 2019), recovery from illness, and the attenuation of lean tissue loss with aging.

13.2 METHODS FOR THE DETERMINATION OF DIETARY AA REQUIREMENTS

An inadequate or excess intake of AAs impairs the growth, development, and health of humans and other animals (Wu 2016) and can be detrimental under certain metabolic conditions (Herring et al. 2018). For example, a low maternal intake of dietary protein can cause oxidative stress, embryonic loss, and intrauterine growth restriction (IUGR) and reduce the postnatal growth of offspring due to a deficiency in specific AAs that are important for cell metabolism and function (Herring et al. 2018). Likewise, a high maternal intake of dietary protein can also result in IUGR and embryonic death in both humans and other mammals (e.g., cows, pigs, and rats) due to AA excesses, the elevation of homocysteine (an oxidant), and the toxicity of ammonia generated from AA catabolism (Herring et al. 2018). Of particular note, feeding a milk formula containing 50% more protein than that in porcine milk is fatal to neonatal piglets with a low birth weight (Jamin et al. 2010). In the production of farm animals, a major goal of nutritionists is to minimize dietary protein levels and feed costs without negatively affecting their growth performance, feed efficiency, and productivity. For example, in growing pigs (Kerr 2003) and growing broilers (Belloir et al. 2017), nitrogen excretion is reduced by approximately 8% and 10%, respectively, for every 1% unit reduction in dietary CP (Kerr 2003). Thus, it is imperative to determine the optimum requirements of mammals, birds, fish, and crustaceans for dietary AAs.

Over the past century, many methods have been developed to determine the dietary requirements of humans and other animals for EAAs and protein (Munro 1964; Pencharz and Ball 2003). Each method has its own strengths and weaknesses. The selection of a method will vary with species, developmental age, and the availability of research funding and facilities. Dietary requirements are affected by (1) dietary factors (e.g., AA composition and amounts, meal pattern, proportions of proteins consumed in daily meals, the content of other nutrients, energy intake, the presence or absence of anti-nutritional substances, the quality of drinking water, and food processing); (2) physiological characteristics of animals (e.g., age, sex, genetic backgrounds, circadian clock, hormones, pregnancy, and lactation); (3) pathological states (e.g., infection, trauma, neoplasia, diabetes, obesity, cardiovascular disease, and fetal growth restriction); and (4) environmental factors (e.g., temperatures, toxic agents, air pollution, physical activity, dietary habits, sanitation, and personal hygiene). These factors should be taken into consideration in estimating an animal's dynamic requirements for dietary AAs. Note that (1) different methods for assessing dietary AA requirements by animals may yield different results in the same animal; (2) the requirement of an individual AA in different tissues varies considerably; and (3) the type of food can affect the number and function of microbes in the gastrointestinal tract and, therefore, the bioavailability of dietary AAs.

13.2.1 Nitrogen Balance Studies

13.2.1.1 Measurement of Nitrogen Balances under Various Nutritional and Physiological Conditions

The nitrogen (N) atom is neither degraded nor synthesized in animals. In tissues or the whole body, nitrogen is present almost exclusively in proteins and AAs. Thus, when there is no nitrogen accumulation in the body, nitrogen intake from in the diet (nitrogen input) should be equal to nitrogen excretion by the animal in various forms, including urea, creatinine, uric acid, ammonia, nitrite, nitrate, and AAs in urine; NO gas; and fecal nitrogenous substances (nitrogen output) (Wu et al. 2014a; Young and Borgonha 2000). Nitrogen balance can be determined for the whole body or a specific tissue and is the classic approach for measuring the dietary requirements of protein (Table 13.3) and

TABLE 13.3
Dietary Protein Requirements of Humans of Different Age Groups

Age Group	Age (years)	Dietary Requirement of Protein (g/kg body weight/day)		
		IOM[a]	FAO/WHO/ UNU[b]	
			1985	2007
Infants	0.3–0.5	1.52	1.75	1.31
	0.75–1.0	1.50	1.57	1.14
Children	1–3	1.10	1.18	1.02
	4–8	0.95	1.05	0.92
Adolescents	9–13	0.95	0.99	0.90
	14–18 (boys)	0.85	0.97	0.87
	14–18 (girls)	0.85	0.94	0.85
Adults	≥19	0.80	0.75	0.83

[a] Recommended dietary allowance (RDA) published by the Institute of Medicine (IOM 2005).

[b] FAO/WHO/UNU (World Health Organization/Food and Agriculture Organization/United Nations University; 1985 and 2007).

TABLE 13.4

Dietary Requirements of Healthy Human Adults for Nutritionally Essential Amino Acids (EAAs)

EAA	Estimates from Nitrogen Balance Experiments[a]		MIT Values[a] (Tracer Studies) (2000)	IOM[b] (2005)	FAO/WHO/UNU[c] (2007)
	Men[d]	Women[e]			
			mg/kg body weight/day		
His	---	---	---	14	10
Ile	10	9.17	23	19	20
Leu	15.7	12.1	40	42	39
Lys	11.4	9.07	30	38	30
Met	2.36	3.23	---	---	---
Met+Cys	15.7	11.7	13	19	15
Phe	4.29	4.30	---	---	---
Phe+Tyr	15.7	---	39	33	25
Thr	7.14	6.25	15	20	15
Trp	3.57	2.80	6	5	4
Val	11.4	10.4	20	24	26
Total	90.6	65.8	186	214	184

Source: Young, V.R. and S. Borgonha. 2000. *J. Nutr.* 130:1841S–1849S.

[a] Recommended values of MIT, Massachusetts Institute of Technology.

[b] Recommended dietary allowance (RDA) published by the Institute of Medicine (IOM, 2005).

[c] FAO/WHO/UNU (World Health Organization/Food and Agriculture Organization/United Nations University, 2007).

[d] Body weight = 70 kg.

[e] Body weight = 60 kg.

EAAs (Table 13.4) by humans of all ages. For example, young adult humans exhibited a negative nitrogen balance on day 1 after consuming an EAA-complete diet except for no lysine (Rose et al. 1954a), no tryptophan (Rose et al. 1954a), no threonine (Rose et al. 1951), or an inadequate amount of L-tryptophan (0.10 g/day) (Rose et al. 1954b). This method is also applicable to both laboratory and farm animals, as shown in classical studies with young rats fed a diet containing zein or gliadin as the sole protein source (Osborne and Mendel 1914) and weanling pigs fed a purified diet containing no arginine or no leucine (Mertz et al. 1952). In nitrogen-balance studies, complete 24-h urine and fecal collections should be made. A glass-type urine container should contain a final concentration of 1% (v/v) H_2SO_4 to preserve ammonia and inhibit bacterial activity. Fecal samples should be immediately stored at $-20°C$ and freeze-dried. Care should be taken to avoid the evaporation of ammonia and urea hydrolysis. The loss of nitrogen via the skin, sweat, and other routes, which is sizable (e.g., 8 mg N/kg BW/day in human adults), should also be determined (FAO 2007).

$$\text{Whole-body N balance} = \text{Dietary N intake} - (\text{Urinary N} + \text{Fecal N} + \text{Other routes})$$

Growth in young animals results from protein deposition, namely a positive nitrogen balance (N intake > N excretion). It is often assumed that protein contains 16% nitrogen. Thus, to convert nitrogen to protein, a factor of 6.25 is used. It should be pointed out that this is based on the average molecular weight of AA residues found in protein. For proteins containing less or more than 16% nitrogen, the nitrogen-to-protein conversion factor of 6.25 should not be used to calculate protein content. Likewise, not all nitrogen in food is contained in protein (Hou et al. 2019). For example, conversion factors used to estimate the content of true protein plus peptides in different foods are

5.46, corn grains; 5.59, peanuts; 5.66, pistachio nuts; 3.27, potatoes; 6.22, soybeans; 4.08, sweet potatoes; 5.69, wheat flour; and 5.49, white rice (Hou et al. 2019). Thus, for highly digestible foods, the total content of individual AAs, rather than protein content, is most relevant to the nutrition of humans and other animals. To maintain a positive nitrogen balance, animals must be provided with AAs in diets and AAs from endogenous sources in appropriate ratios, because a deficiency of one AA can limit protein synthesis while increasing overall AA oxidation (Reeds 2000). The usefulness of growth and nitrogen balance studies has been instrumental in estimating the dietary requirements of farm animals (Baker 2009) and humans (Rose 1968) for AAs and proteins. Recommended values for growing and gestating swine of different BWs are summarized in Tables 13.5 and 13.6, respectively.

Diseased states are usually associated with a negative nitrogen balance, namely N intake<N excretion. This is due to an increase in AA oxidation and a decrease in the intake of dietary AAs. In patients with AIDS, burns, cancer, poorly-controlled diabetes, injury, metabolic acidosis, or sepsis, a negative nitrogen balance usually occurs primarily due to net protein degradation in skeletal muscle. This catabolic process provides the body with AAs to serve functional roles. However, the loss of 50% body protein is not compatible with survival in humans and other animals (Chapter 9). Affected individuals also exhibit a negative energy balance. Thus, treatment strategies for these patients may include the stimulation of protein synthesis, as well as the inhibition of intracellular protein degradation and whole-body AA oxidation to improve their nitrogen balance and survival, while assuring adequate energy intake.

TABLE 13.5

Dietary Requirements of Growing Swine at Different Body Weights for Nutritionally Essential Amino Acids (EAAs)[a]

Variable	Body Weight of Growing Swine (kg)						
	5–7	7–11	11–25	25–50	50–75	75–100	100–135
ME content of diet (kcal/kg)	3,400	3,400	3,350	3,300	3,300	3,300	3,300
ME intake (kcal/day)	904	1,592	3,033	4,959	6,989	8,265	9,196
Feed intake+wastage (g/day)	280	493	953	1,582	2,229	2,636	2,933
Content of total nitrogen in diet (%)	3.63	3.29	3.02	2.51	2.20	1.94	1.67
Content of crude protein in diet (%)	22.7	20.6	18.9	15.7	13.8	12.1	10.4
	Content of EAAs in Diet (%)						
Arginine	0.75	0.68	0.62	0.50	0.44	0.38	0.32
Histidine	0.58	0.53	0.48	0.39	0.34	0.30	0.25
Isoleucine	0.88	0.79	0.73	0.59	0.52	0.45	0.39
Leucine	1.71	1.54	1.41	1.13	0.98	0.85	0.71
Lysine	1.70	1.53	1.40	1.12	0.97	0.84	0.71
Methionine	0.49	0.44	0.40	0.32	0.28	0.25	0.21
Methionine+Cysteine	0.96	0.87	0.79	0.65	0.57	0.50	0.43
Phenylalanine	1.01	0.91	0.83	0.68	0.59	0.51	0.43
Phenylalanine+Tyrosine	1.60	1.44	1.32	1.08	0.94	0.82	0.70
Threonine	1.05	0.95	0.87	0.72	0.64	0.56	0.49
Tryptophan	0.28	0.25	0.23	0.19	0.17	0.15	0.13
Valine	1.10	1.00	0.91	0.75	0.65	0.57	0.49

*ME = metabolizable energy. The recommended arginine:*lysine ratios in diets for swine at various stages of growth and development may be underestimated.

[a] Values (as-fed basis) are adapted from NRC (2012) for swine fed typical corn- and soybean meal-based diets. Dry matter content in the diet is 90%.

TABLE 13.6

Dietary Requirements of Gestating Swine at Different Parities for Nutritionally Essential Amino Acids (EAAs)[a]

Variable		Gestating Sows							
	Parity	**1**		**2**		**3**		**4**	
	BW at Breeding (kg)	140		165		185		205	
	Litter Size	12.5		13.5		13.5		13.5	
	Days of Gestation	**<90**	**>90**	**<90**	**>90**	**<90**	**>90**	**<90**	**>90**
ME content of diet (kcal/kg)		3,300	3,300	3,300	3,300	3,300	3,300	3,300	3,300
ME intake (kcal/day)		6,678	7,932	6,928	8,182	6,928	8,182	6,897	8,151
Feed intake + wastage (g/day)		2,130	2,530	2,210	2,610	2,210	2,610	2,200	2,600
Content of total nitrogen in diet (%)		1.62	2.15	1.42	1.95	1.26	1.77	1.14	1.62
		Content of EAAs in Diet (%)							
Arginine		0.32	0.42	0.27	0.37	0.23	0.32	0.20	0.29
Histidine		0.22	0.27	0.19	0.23	0.16	0.20	0.14	0.18
Isoleucine		0.36	0.43	0.31	0.38	0.27	0.33	0.24	0.29
Leucine		0.55	0.75	0.47	0.66	0.41	0.59	0.36	0.53
Lysine		0.61	0.80	0.52	0.71	0.45	0.62	0.39	0.55
Methionine		0.18	0.23	0.15	0.20	0.13	0.18	0.11	0.16
Methionine + Cysteine		0.41	0.54	0.36	0.48	0.32	0.44	0.29	0.40
Phenylalanine		0.34	0.44	0.29	0.40	0.25	0.35	0.23	0.31
Phenylalanine + Tyrosine		0.61	0.79	0.53	0.70	0.46	0.62	0.41	0.56
Threonine		0.46	0.58	0.41	0.53	0.37	0.48	0.34	0.44
Tryptophan		0.11	0.15	0.10	0.14	0.09	0.13	0.08	0.12
Valine		0.45	0.58	0.39	0.52	0.34	0.46	0.31	0.42

BW = body weight; ME = metabolizable energy.

[a] Values (as-fed basis) are adapted from NRC (2012) for swine fed typical corn- and soybean meal-based diets. Dry matter content in the diet is 90%. The normal length of gestation in swine is 114 days.

Let us use, as an example, the loss of body protein in obese persons consuming a low-calorie, extremely low-carbohydrate, weight-reducing diet with the recommended protein intake maintained. These individuals develop metabolic acidosis because the mobilization of fat from white adipose tissue produces large amounts of free fatty acids, which are oxidized in the liver to form ketone bodies (acidic substances) (Gougeon-Reyburn and Marliss 1989; Hannaford et al. 1982). A concurrent loss of protein occurs to provide AA substrates for gluconeogenesis that yields glucose for tissues, especially the brain. These processes occur until blood ketone bodies increase considerably to serve as alternate metabolic fuels. The kidneys concurrently utilize glutamine to counter the acidosis (whose α-amino group is derived from branched-chain AAs and thus protein primarily in skeletal muscle) to generate ammonia to convert H^+ into NH_4^+. Thus, ketoacidosis in the hypocaloric state drives the loss of muscle protein and, therefore, a negative N balance in the

TABLE 13.7
Nitrogen Sparing by Bicarbonate Supplementation in Obese Persons on a Hypocaloric Protein Diet (400 kcal/day) for 21 Days[a]

	Group 1 (NaCl)	Group 2 (NaHCO₃)	Net Change due to HCO₃⁻ Feeding
Urine NH_4^+ nitrogen (mmol/day)	80.0	25.7	−54.3
Urine β-hydroxybutyrate (mmol/day)	34.4	8.9	−25.5
Glutamine utilization (mmol/day)	---	---	−27.15
β-hydroxybutyrate utilization (mmol/day)	---	---	+25.5
ATP from glutamine (mmol/day)[b]	---	---	−733
ATP from β-hydroxybutyrate (mmol/day)[b]	---	---	+689

Source: Wu, G. and E.B. Marliss. 1992. In: *Biology of Feast and Famine* (Anderson, G.H. and S.H. Kennedy, eds). Academic Press, San Diego. pp. 219–244.

[a] Healthy obese female persons (body mass index = 38.4±1.5 kg/m²; body weight = 100±4 kg) were given a 1.72 MJ (412 kcal), all protein (16.8 g N; partially hydrolyzed gelatin fortified with 0.41% L-tryptophan and 0.42% DL-methionine) liquid formula, 16 mmol KCl and a multivitamin–mineral supplement daily for 4 weeks. In addition, study participants in Group 1 (n = 5) received 60 mmol Na⁺ daily as sodium chloride (NaCl) for 3 weeks. Study participants in Group 2 (n = 5) were given 40 mmol/day NaHCO₃ during the first week, and 60 mmol/day during weeks 2 and 3. Urine excretion was collected every 24 h during the 3-week experimental period for biochemical analysis.

[b] It is assumed that the complete oxidation of 1 mole of glutamine or 1 mole of β-hydroxybutyrate potentially yields 27 moles of ATP in the kidneys.

whole body, despite keeping protein intake constant. By correcting for ketoacidosis and sparing renal ammoniagenesis from glutamine, which ultimately conserves AAs and muscle protein, the oral administration of NaHCO₃ to the obese individuals consuming this diet decreased the loss of body protein (Table 13.7). A variant of these metabolic responses became the theoretic basis for the current widely-promoted "keto-diet". The blood ketone-body levels reached with weight-reducing "keto-diets" are much lower than those in the studies described above. To date, in-depth studies of whole-body protein metabolism under such feeding conditions are scant.

The nitrogen balance across the placenta of a gestating mother illustrates unique patterns of nitrogen and AA utilization by the fetus (Wu et al. 2014a). Studies of AA uptake by the ovine fetus, calculated based on umbilical venous-arterial differences, indicate that most AAs, except lysine and histidine, are taken up by the fetus in 20%–30% excess above the amounts required for protein deposition. In pregnant sheep, uterine uptake of glutamine is the greatest among all of the measured AAs to support the needs of the growing fetus. Similar studies have shown the synthesis of urea from AA nitrogen by the fetus. In gestating swine, the accretion of nitrogen and AAs (particularly glycine, proline, glutamine, and arginine) in fetal pigs increases more rapidly during pregnancy than in non-nitrogen dry matter. AA nitrogen represents 83%–88% of total nitrogen, and arginine is the most abundant nitrogen carrier in the fetus at all gestational ages (Wu et al. 1999a). Such an abundance of arginine nitrogen in the fetus often goes unrecognized, but it reflects the important role for arginine in fetal nutrition, metabolism, survival, and growth.

13.2.1.2 Advantages and Limitations of Nitrogen Balance Studies

Nitrogen balance measurement is a relatively simple and relatively inexpensive approach to estimating the quantitative and qualitative requirements of humans and other animals for individual AAs and proteins (Munro 1964). However, this method has the following inherent limitations: (1)

failure to account for all the losses of nitrogen from the body (e.g., 0.5 g N/day or ~7.1% of daily nitrogen intake in the healthy adult humans consuming ~7.0 g N/day (FAO 2007); and in young pigs, 6.7% of dietary alanine nitrogen could not be recovered in the urine and feces), resulting in an underestimation of dietary AA requirements (Rasch and Benevenga 2004); (2) high variability in daily nitrogen balance, as small changes in nitrogen deposition may not be detected; (3) failure to detect functional changes in cells and organs (namely functional needs for AAs) or to fully evaluate the dietary requirements of individual AAs; (4) not being sufficiently sensitive to dietary intake of certain AAs particularly within a short experimental period; (5) an inability to provide information about the cellular processes of intermediary metabolism of AAs or protein; (6) difficulty in interpreting the experimental data either when dietary protein intake is high or when dietary protein intake is low because enzyme systems can adapt to low or high dietary AA intakes and the rates of AA catabolism can be altered; (7) nitrogen balance being strongly influenced by dietary energy intake, environmental conditions, and changes in endocrine status; (8) requirement of a relatively long period of adaptation to an experimental diet (e.g., 5–7 days for rats and pigs, and 7–10 days for adult humans); (9) possible inconsistency between animal growth and nitrogen balance, as an animal can lose weight (e.g., fat) and still be in a positive nitrogen balance; and (10) like all bioassays, the response per increment of intake declines as the maximum attainable response is approached.

Let us use histidine and arginine as examples to illustrate some shortcomings of nitrogen balance measurement for estimating dietary AA requirements. As mentioned previously, results of the nitrogen balance studies by W.C. Rose (1968) did not reveal dietary requirements of either histidine or arginine by healthy adults. Explanations for the failure to identify histidine as an EAA are that (1) hemoglobin contains a relatively large amount of histidine and the breakdown of this protein releases histidine; and (2) skeletal muscle contains millimolar concentrations of histidine in the form of dipeptides (e.g., carnosine) and the hydrolysis of these dipeptides provides histidine (Chapter 5). Extending the experimental period of feeding a histidine-free diet from 8 to 28 days or longer can substantially reduce the endogenous release of histidine from the catabolism of hemoglobin and intramuscular small peptides, thereby resulting in a negative nitrogen balance in normal and chronically uremic adult humans (Kopple and Swendseid 1975, 1981).

Based on nitrogen balance, arginine was traditionally not considered to be an EAA for healthy adult humans or livestock species. However, this notion is not consistent with the needs of both males and females for arginine to support their fertility. For example, L.E. Holt and A.A. Albanese (1944) notably reported that feeding an arginine-deficient diet to adult men for 9 days decreased both the number and motility of sperm cells by 90% despite nitrogen balance at equilibrium. This striking observation underlines a critical role for arginine in spermatogenesis. In addition, feeding an arginine-free diet to pregnant rats has been reported to increase fetal resorption, intrauterine growth retardation, and perinatal mortality, while decreasing the number of live fetuses. Such adverse effects can be prevented by adding arginine to the basal diet. These findings strongly argue that the functional needs beyond tissue protein synthesis and nitrogen balance should be important criteria for the classification of AAs as EAAs, NEAAs, or CEAAs. Thus, whether arginine is an EAA or NEAA for adults is only a matter of definition. The physiological functions of an AA must be fully considered when assessing its dietary requirements of animals. However, despite its shortcomings, the nitrogen balance study remains an invaluable procedure for determining the dietary requirements of AAs and protein for animals, until a new method is firmly established.

13.2.2 THE FACTORIAL METHOD

Dietary requirements for EAAs, NEAAs, and CEAAs by the whole body or tissues of interest (e.g., the small intestine) can be estimated according to factorial analysis, namely, the sum of fecal and urinary nitrogen in response to a protein-free diet (maintenance), AA deposited in the body, and AAs excreted as animal products (e.g., milk, egg, wool, and fetus growth) (Wu et al. 2014a). For certain AAs, the factorial method can also be based on the sum of the needs for the AAs for metabolic pathways and obligatory losses of the AAs via secretions from the body, including hair, sweat, nasal secretions, menstrual losses (women and the females of other primates), and seminal fluid (men). The obligatory losses of AAs occur when the animal is fed an essentially nitrogen-free diet that still meets energy requirements. The factorial method can be used only when data on AA oxidation in the whole body or tissues of interest are available. Recommended dietary requirements for AAs should be based on true digestible AAs. However, percentages of AAs in common food/feed ingredients with known true AA digestibilities may also be used to express the requirements of humans and other animals for dietary AAs.

$$\text{Dietary requirement of an AA} = \left(MN_{SI} + MN_{EIT} + LS_{ob} - ES_{IT} - ES_{EIT}\right)/RE$$

where

MN_{SI} and MN_{EIT} are the metabolic needs for the AA by the small intestine and extraintestinal tissues, respectively;

LS_{ob} is the obligatory loss of the AA by secretions from the body;

ES_{IT} is the endogenous synthesis of the AA in the small-intestinal tissues;

ES_{EIT} is the endogenous synthesis of the AA in extraintestinal tissues; and

RE is the true digestibility of the protein-bound AA (the release of the dietary protein-bound AA into the lumen of the small intestine).

For an AA that is not synthesized by animals or whose synthesis by intestinal microbes is negligible, the factorial method can be simplified because $ES_{EIT} = 0$.

Let us use, as examples, the requirements of young swine for glutamine and glutamate (Table 13.8). The metabolic needs of glutamine by a tissue include (1) oxidation as a metabolic fuel; (2) protein synthesis; (3) the generation of biologically active substances, and (4) the formation of tissue- or sex-specific products (e.g., mucins, embryo or fetus, and milk). In young pigs, major glutamine-utilizing tissues are the small intestine, skeletal muscle, lymphoid organs, vascular endothelia, kidneys, and nonsmall intestine portal-drained viscera (including the stomach, spleen, and pancreas) (Wu et al. 2011). The physiological requirement for glutamine in the whole body of young pigs and the rate of

---

TABLE 13.8

Physiological and Dietary Requirements of Young Pigs for Glutamine and Glutamate[a]

Variables	Glutamine Needs (mg/kg BW/day)	Glutamate Needs (mg/kg BW/day)
Physiological needs of the whole body	≥1,949	≥1,232
Small intestine	965	773
Skeletal muscle	310	236
Lymphoid organs	212	20
Vascular endothelia	163	15
Kidneys	151	184
Nonsmall intestine PDV tissue[b]	148	3.4
Endogenous synthesis in the whole body	1,149	746
Provision from diet[c]	≥889 [i.e., (1,949 − 1,149)/0.9]	≥ 540 [i.e., (1,232 − 746)/0.9]

Source: Wu et al. 2011 *J. Anim. Sci.* 89:2017–2030 for data on glutamine requirements; and Hou, Y.Q. and G. Wu. 2018. *Amino Acids* 50:1497–1510 for data on glutamate requirements.

Note: PDV, portal-drained viscera.

[a] Based on young pig weighing 7.92 kg and gaining 293 g body weight/day, while consuming a diet containing 21% crude protein.

[b] Including stomach, spleen, and pancreas.

[c] Assuming that the digestibility of glutamine and glutamate in dietary protein is 90%.

their endogenous synthesis of glutamine are ≥1,949 and 1,149 mg/kg BW/day, respectively, whereas glutamine synthesis in the small intestine is negligible or nondetectable. The obligatory losses of glutamine via hair, sweat, and nasal secretions from piglets are negligible. Thus, assuming that the digestibility of glutamine in dietary protein is 90% in pigs, glutamine provision from the diet must be ≥889 mg/kg BW/day. Similar estimations have also been made for glutamate metabolism and requirements in pigs (Hou and Wu 2018). Calculated values of dietary AA requirements should be verified by feeding trials, N-balance experiments, or studies of functional outcome (e.g., fertility, health, lactation, growth, athletic performance, or survival).

13.2.3   DOSE–RESPONSE FEEDING TRIALS

Protein accretion in growing animals is increased as the dietary intake of AAs is gradually augmented until the requirement is met (Ball et al. 1986). The physiological response does not change as the dietary intake of AAs is elevated beyond the requirement but below the upper limit level. Then, the intake of AAs greater than the upper limit level gradually becomes toxic due to AA imbalances or antagonisms or the excess accumulation of AA metabolites. The rationale for the use of dose–response feeding trials to determine dietary AA requirements is illustrated in Figure 13.1. Similarly, in adult animals gaining little or no nitrogen under adequate nutritional conditions, whole-body nitrogen balance becomes negative when the amount of a dietary AA is decreased from an adequate to an inadequate level. This principle has applied well to the assessments of the dietary requirements of adult humans for most EAAs (Rose 1968), but it is best with conceptual and practical limitations as noted above. Purified, semipurified, or whole-food-based diets can be used for the conduct of experiments involving the graded (ideally 6 or more) dietary levels of a test AA. The test AA intake should span both below and above a putative requirement based on published studies or fundamental nutritional knowledge. The measured variables may include growth rate, nitrogen balance, milk yield, embryonic/fetal survival, plasma AA concentration, intestinal integrity, or immune responses (Wu et al. 2014a). One or more of these variables can be used to

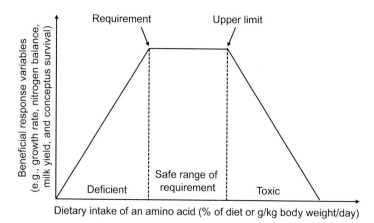

FIGURE 13.1   Determination of the requirements of animals for dietary amino acids (AAs) through dose–response feeding trials. Measured variables, which may include lean tissue growth, nitrogen balance, milk yield, conceptus (embryo/fetus and associated membranes) survival, plasma amino acid concentration, intestinal integrity, and immune responses, improve as the dietary AA intake increases towards the requirement. Then, a breakpoint in the response occurs once the dietary requirement is met. Until the upper limit of the dietary requirement is reached for a given response variable, a dietary intake greater than the nutritional requirement does not result in adverse effects. Above the upper limit of the dietary requirement, the test AA is toxic to animals because of AA imbalance or antagonism or the excess accumulation of harmful AA metabolites. One or more measured variables may be used to determine the requirements of animals for dietary AAs. Note that the requirements of animals for dietary AAs may vary substantially among individuals.

determine the requirements of humans and other animals for dietary AAs. Note that the requirements of the animal organisms for dietary AAs may vary substantially among individuals between species and within the same species, and in response to alterations in physiological, pathological, and environmental conditions (Le Floc'h et al. 2018; Waterlow et al. 1978).

13.2.4 Tracer Methods

13.2.4.1 General Considerations of AA Oxidation Methods for Estimating Dietary AA Requirements

The rate of oxidation of an AA depends on its concentration in the free pools (e.g., the plasma and intracellular fluids), the nutritional status, and the physiological needs of the animal (Chapter 4). When in excess, most AAs (possibly except for glutamine) cannot be stored in the body. Thus, an excessive amount of an AA will be disposed of primarily via biological oxidation and urea synthesis in mammals (or uric acid synthesis in avian species) (Figure 13.2). An increase in the oxidation of an AA is usually an indicator of its excessive availability in the body, provided that there are no significant changes in the concentrations of regulatory hormones or metabolites. In other words, if the supply of an AA exceeds its needs by the animal, this AA is oxidized to CO_2, water, ammonia, and urea. Note that an increase in the availability of an AA in the circulation does not necessarily indicate that its supply exceeds its needs by the animal. For example, a decrease in the rate of protein synthesis due to a deficiency of one essential AA in a diet may increase the availability of other AAs in the plasma for catabolism. Thus, the oxidation of an indicator AA can be used to estimate the requirement of dietary AAs and protein by humans and other animals.

In defining the dietary requirement of animals for an AA, it is important to consider the following general factors: (1) a requirement for the nitrogen of "nonessential AAs" from which other nitrogenous compounds can be synthesized; (2) a specific pattern of EAAs, CEAAs, and NEAAs within the digestible protein supply to allow the optimal utilization of dietary AAs or protein for maintenance and production (e.g., growth and reproduction); (3) a supply of AAs or digestible protein to replace basal losses due to the oxidation of AAs; and (4) an appropriate balance of protein and energy within the diet because excessive amounts of AAs can be oxidized for ATP production when the dietary supply of energy is inadequate. Furthermore, when using a tracer in the AA oxidation methods, one

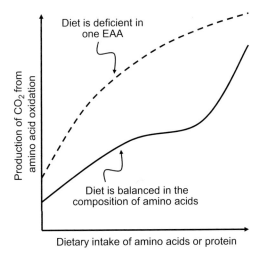

FIGURE 13.2 The interrelationships between amino acid (AA) oxidation and dietary intake of AAs in animals. In an animal fed a protein-adequate diet, an excess of a specific AA results in an increase in its oxidation but not necessarily the oxidation of other AA. By contrast, when an essential AA is deficient in a diet, the oxidation of other AA is increased progressively with increasing dietary intake of AA or protein.

should be aware that the rate of production of $^{14}CO_2$ (or $^{13}CO_2$) from a ^{14}C- or ^{13}C-labeled AA *in vivo* depends on the free pool size of the tracee AA (Chapter 7), the distribution of the enzymes involved in AA oxidation, and the activities of the enzymes in specific cell types and tissues (Chapter 11).

Now, let us consider the following situations relevant to the discussion of AA oxidation in the body when dietary energy intake is adequate. First, regardless of AA balance in the diet, when the dietary intake of AAs or protein is increased, the oxidation of AAs is also increased, because excessive AAs (possibly except for glutamine) must be oxidized to CO_2, water, and urea (Chapter 4). Second, when the dietary intake of AAs or protein is at the optimal amount for protein synthesis, the oxidation of the AAs is at a minimum level. Third, when the dietary intake of AAs or protein is below the animal's requirements, the oxidation of AAs is reduced to spare AAs for protein synthesis. This is partly because the enzymes involved in protein synthesis (e.g., tRNA-AA synthases) have much lower K_m values for AA substrates than the enzymes that degrade AAs. This means that AAs are preferentially channeled to the pathway of protein synthesis rather than AA catabolism. Therefore, only a small fraction of dietary AAs is available for oxidation in animals fed an AA-balanced diet. Fourth, in a protein-adequate diet, any excess of a specific AA (usually an EAA) would increase its oxidation, but not necessarily the oxidation of other AAs. By contrast, when an EAA is deficient in a diet, the oxidation of other AAs is increased progressively with increasing dietary intake of AA or protein. This is because the short supply of this AA limits the utilization of other AA for protein synthesis and all the excess AA are degraded in a tissue-specific manner. The interrelationships between AA oxidation and dietary intake of AAs or protein with or without a deficiency of one EAA are illustrated in Figure 13.2.

13.2.4.2 The Direct AA Oxidation Method

13.2.4.2.1 *Principle of the Direct AA Oxidation Method to Estimate Dietary AA Requirements*

When dietary intake of a test AA is below its physiological requirement by the animal, the rate of its oxidation in the whole body is relatively low. By contrast, when the dietary intake of a test AA

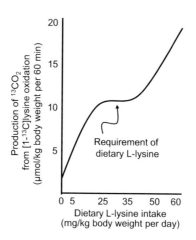

FIGURE 13.3 Oxidation of lysine to estimate dietary lysine requirement by adult humans (the direct AA oxidation method). Healthy adults consumed a diet providing adequate energy, 0.8 g protein/kg body weight (BW)/day, and a total amount of lysine at 5–60 mg/kg BW/day. At the end of each dietary period while subjects were in the fed state, the study participants received an intravenous bolus (priming dose) of L-[1-^{13}C]lysine (5.1 µmol/kg BW) and then 3-h intravenous infusions of L-[1-^{13}C]lysine at a constant rate of approximately 0.060 µmol/kg BW/min. Measurement of expired $^{13}CO_2$ for 60 min was made during the isotopic steady state of L-[1-^{13}C]lysine in the plasma to calculate the rate of CO_2 production from the oxidation of carbon-1 of lysine. The rate of oxidation of lysine was low at low dietary lysine intake, remained in a steady state at lysine intake of 25–35 mg/kg BW/day, and markedly increased at a lysine intake above 35 mg/kg BW/day. These results indicate that the requirement of healthy adults for dietary lysine may be between 25 and 35 mg/kg BW/day. (Adapted from Meredith et al. 1986.)

is above its physiological requirement by the animal, the rate of its oxidation is increased. At the optimal requirement, the rate of oxidation of a test AA is maintained at an optimal level and varies little within a narrow range of AA content in the diet (Figure 13.3). The word "direct" is used before "AA oxidation" because the oxidation of a test AA (e.g., lysine) is determined to estimate its dietary requirement (i.e., dietary lysine requirement).

13.2.4.2.2 Examples of the Direct AA Oxidation Method

In the early 1980s, V.R. Young and his colleagues introduced the direct AA oxidation technique to determine the dietary requirements of humans for AAs. Let's use lysine oxidation as an example to illustrate how this method can be used to estimate the dietary requirement of healthy adults for lysine (Meredith et al. 1986). The study participants consumed a diet providing adequate energy, 0.8 g protein/kg BW/day, and a total amount of lysine at 5–100 mg/kg BW/day (with a 7-day interval for each dose of lysine), and received continuous intravenous infusions of L-[l-^{13}C]lysine. The measurement of expired $^{13}CO_2$ for 60 min was made during the isotopic steady state of L-[l-^{13}C] lysine in the plasma. Results indicated that the oxidation of lysine was low at low dietary lysine intake, remained at a relatively constant rate at lysine intake of 25–35 mg/kg BW/day, and then it was markedly increased at lysine intake above 35 mg/kg BW/day (Figure 13.3). Based on these data, the dietary lysine requirement was estimated to be between 25 and 35 mg/kg BW/day. The precise dietary requirement of lysine could not be provided unless other variables could be available, including N balance, lysine balance, and concentrations of proteins and metabolites in the plasma (Young 1987). The direct AA oxidation method has been satisfactorily applied to determine dietary requirements of farm animals (e.g., young pigs) for EAA (e.g., phenylalanine).

13.2.4.3 The Indicator AA Oxidation Method

13.2.4.3.1 Principle of the Indicator AA Oxidation Method to Estimate Dietary AA Requirements

The indicator AA oxidation method (also known as the indirect AA oxidation method) is based on the hypothesis that the partition of any EAA between oxidation and protein synthesis is sensitive to the level of the most limiting AA in the diet (Elango et al. 2012). When an EAA, CEAA, or NEAA is limited for protein synthesis, all other AAs will become in excess and, therefore, must be oxidized. This means that increasing the dietary level of the limiting AA in graded amounts will increase the utilization of all dietary AAs for protein synthesis, resulting in a decrease in their oxidation until the requirement point is reached. Once the requirement point is reached, further increments of the test AA in the diet may not have any effect on the utilization of other AAs for oxidation or protein synthesis unless the test AA is capable of regulating these pathways. This method can also be used to estimate the requirements of humans and other animals for dietary protein. The word "indicator" is used before "AA oxidation" because the oxidation of a different AA (e.g., phenylalanine) than the test AA (e.g., proline) is determined to estimate the dietary requirement of the test AA. In essence, the indicator AA oxidation method for estimating AA requirements involves the oxidation of an indicator AA in response to the feeding of graded levels of a test AA. The oxidation of the indicator AA will decrease as the intakes of the test AA are increased until the animal's requirement of the test AA is met. Both at and above requirement, there is no further decrease in the oxidation of the indicator AA. The inflection (breakpoint) in the oxidation curve has been suggested to represent the physiological requirement for the test AA.

13.2.4.3.2 Examples of the Indicator AA Oxidation Method

The indicator AA oxidation method originated from a 1983 study by K.I. Kim, I. McMillan, and H.S. Bayley regarding the dietary requirements of neonatal pigs for lysine and histidine. In these animals, protein synthesis is very sensitive to a deficiency of dietary EAA (Kim et al. 1983). This technique was further refined by R.O. Ball and H.S. Bayley in the mid-1980s to estimate the dietary requirements of piglets for proline, arginine, and protein. The indicator AA oxidation method has

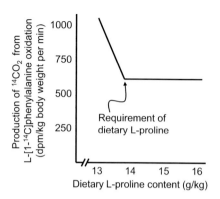

FIGURE 13.4 Oxidation of phenylalanine to estimate the requirement of neonatal pigs for dietary proline (the indicator amino acid oxidation method). Young pigs (2.5 kg body weight) were fed two meals that contained 20% crude protein, the total content of 1.31%, 1.35%, 1.38%, 1.44%, or 1.57% proline, and 10 μCi L-[1-^{14}C]phenylalanine, at 4 h and 2 h before a 60-min collection of expired $^{14}CO_2$. Production of $^{14}CO_2$ from L-[1-^{14}C]phenylalanine by the pigs decreased markedly as dietary proline content increased from 1.31% to 1.44% and then leveled off when dietary proline content increased from 1.44% to 1.57%. The break point for phenylalanine oxidation was 1.39% proline in the diet. Therefore, the dietary requirement of proline (expressed as g/100 food) by the neonatal pig is approximately 1.40%. (Adapted from Ball et al. 1986.)

also been successfully applied to humans (Kurpad and Thomas 2011; Zello et al. 2013) and horses (Mok et al. 2018). Let's use the determination of dietary proline requirement as an example to illustrate this technique. In the studies of R.O. Ball et al. (1986), 2.5-kg young pigs were fed meals containing 20% CP, total content of 1.31%–1.57% proline, and 10 μCi L-[1-^{14}C]phenylalanine. Expired $^{14}CO_2$ was measured for 1 h after feeding. Production of $^{14}CO_2$ from L-[1-^{14}C]phenylalanine by the piglets was decreased markedly due to enhanced whole-body protein synthesis as dietary proline content was increased from 1.31% to 1.44% and was then leveled off when dietary proline content was further increased from 1.44% to 1.57% (Figure 13.4). The break point for phenylalanine oxidation was 1.39% proline in the diet. When the experiment was repeated with piglets fed a diet containing 26% CP and the total content of 1.22%–1.82% proline, the break point for phenylalanine oxidation was at 1.42% proline in the diet. Based on these two experiments, the dietary requirement of the neonatal pig for proline (expressed as g/100 g food) is approximately 1.40%.

The indicator AA oxidation method can also be used to estimate the dietary requirements of animals for protein. For example, 2.5-kg young pigs were fed meals containing 12%, 16%, 20%, 24%, 28%, or 32% CP, the total content of 0.88% phenylalanine and 0.85% tyrosine, and 10 μCi L-[1-^{14}C]phenylalanine (Ball and Bayley 1986). The basal diet contained 29.6% skim milk, providing 10% CP. Various amounts of a mixture of NEAA (alanine, aspartic acid, asparagine, glutamate, glutamine, glycine, and proline) were added to the basal diet to provide 12%, 16%, 20%, 24%, 28%, and 32% CP (which is calculated from nitrogen content and does not necessarily reflect the amount of true protein or available AAs). Expired $^{14}CO_2$ was measured for 1 h after feeding. Production of $^{14}CO_2$ from L-[1-^{14}C]phenylalanine by the pigs decreased markedly as dietary protein content was increased from 12% to 24% and was then leveled off when dietary protein content increased from 24% to 32% diet (Figure 13.5). The break point for phenylalanine oxidation was 24% CP in the diet. When the experiment was repeated with piglets fed a diet containing an 11.18% mixture of NEAA and various amounts of skim milk to provide 16%, 20%, 24%, 26%, and 28% CP, the break point for phenylalanine oxidation was at 25.8% CP in the diet. The higher estimate of the dietary protein requirement of young piglets fed the 16%–28% CP diet may reflect the increasing proportions of AAs from intact protein and lower efficiency for the utilization of free crystalline AAs than intact protein. On average, the dietary requirement of CP (expressed as g/100 g food) by the neonatal pig

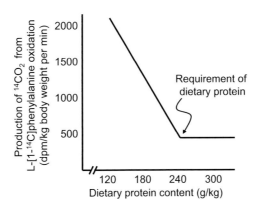

FIGURE 13.5 Oxidation of phenylalanine to estimate the requirement of neonatal pigs for dietary protein (the indicator AA oxidation method). Young pigs (2.5-kg body weight) were fed two meals that contained 12%, 16%, 20%, 24%, 28%, or 32% crude protein (CP), total content of 0.88% phenylalanine and 0.85% tyrosine, and 10 μCi L-[1-^{14}C]phenylalanine, at 4 h and 2 h before a 60-min collection of expired $^{14}CO_2$. The basal diet contained 29.6% skim milk providing 10% CP. Various amounts of a mixture of NEAAs (alanine, aspartic acid, asparagine, glutamate, glutamine, glycine, and proline) were added to the basal diet to provide 12%, 16%, 20%, 24%, 28%, and 32% CP. Production of $^{14}CO_2$ from L-[1-^{14}C]phenylalanine by the pigs decreased markedly as dietary protein content increased from 12% to 24% and was then leveled off when dietary protein content increased from 24% to 32%. The break point for phenylalanine oxidation was 24% CP in the diet. Therefore, the dietary requirement of CP (expressed as g/100 g diet) by the neonatal pig is approximately 25%. (Adapted from Ball and Bayley 1986.)

is approximately 25%, which is similar to the values of dietary CP levels ranging from 24% to 25% based on growth studies of piglets fed milk-based diets.

13.2.4.4 Advantages and Disadvantages of Tracer Studies for Estimating Dietary AA Requirements

The common advantages of both the direct and the indicator AA oxidation methods over the N balance technique are that (1) dietary requirements for AAs can be estimated within a short period after several days for adaptation to experimental diets, without a need for a long, expensive stay (e.g., one week or longer) in a metabolic facility before each measurement; and (2) more sensitive techniques than the nitrogen balance method are provided to evaluate changes in whole-body AA catabolism in response to different intakes of dietary AA or protein. In addition, the direct AA oxidation method can directly determine the rate of oxidation of the dietary AA of interest, making it possible to evaluate both the pattern of changes in the oxidation rate and the whole-body balance of the AA. Of note, the direct AA oxidation method does not result in substantial alterations in the pool size of AAs other than the test AA, potentially limiting the conceptual and technical problems associated with the metabolic compartmentation of the test AA and with estimates of the turnover of the indicator AA. Compared with the direct AA oxidation method, the indicator AA oxidation technique offers several unique advantages. First, the test AA and the tracer are separate. Therefore, there is no problem with giving various nutritionally significant quantities of the stable isotope tracer, because it is different from the test AA. Second, the indicator AA oxidation method is practically simpler and can be performed without the need for a long stay (e.g., one week or longer) in a metabolic facility before each measurement, as noted previously. Third, the break point is an operational indicator of the adequacy of dietary intake of the test AA. Therefore, no source of error varies systematically with the intake of the test AA. This helps eliminate the need for high precision and tedious measurement of CO_2 recovery for individuals. Fourth, one indicator AA (e.g., [1-^{14}C]- or [1-^{13}]-phenylalanine) can be used in theory to estimate the dietary requirements of all other AAs (including both EAAs and AASAs) by humans and other animals.

The common disadvantages of the direct and indicator AA oxidation methods are that (1) they can be used only in the fed state because food deprivation greatly affects the oxidation of all AAs in the body; (2) dietary intakes of both protein and energy critically influence the oxidation of the indicator AA, the test AA, and other AAs in a cell- and tissue-specific manner; (3) a break point in the oxidation of the labeled AA may not be easily identified in adults who have a relatively low rate of whole-body protein synthesis and in individuals who may not be sensitive to changes in the test AA (e.g., threonine, methionine, and tryptophan) in diets within a short period of time because of the complex metabolic pathways for AAs; (4) the production of labeled CO_2 from a [14]C- or ^{13}C-labeled AA may be influenced by the dilution of the precursor labeled AA and its intracellular SR or IE at the site of oxidation and, therefore, may not reflect the true oxidation of the labeled AA in specific cells and tissues; and (5) measurements of the oxidation of labeled AA within a short period of time may not reflect diurnal changes in the catabolism of the indicator AA, test AA, or other AAs over a 24-h period or days. In addition, the direct AA oxidation method has the following potential limitations. First, this technique can be used only if the carboxyl group of the test AA (e.g., lysine, phenylalanine, and a BCAA) is quantitatively released as CO_2 to the body bicarbonate pool when the test AA is oxidized. This poses a problem with AAs (e.g., arginine, glutamine, threonine, and tryptophan) with complex metabolic pathways. However, such a shortcoming can be eliminated by the indicator AA oxidation method. Second, an appropriately labeled AA may not always be available for use in determining their oxidation using the direct AA oxidation method. Third, in stable isotope studies, the indicator AA oxidation method requires experiments at low intakes of the test, unlabeled AA relative to the infused labeled AA, possibly leading to errors in the estimation of AA oxidation based on the production of labeled CO_2.

13.2.5 Substantial Differences in Current Estimated Dietary EAA and Protein Requirements by Humans or Other Animals

Short (e.g., 8 days)- and long (e.g., 24–89 days)-term nitrogen balance data on the obligatory losses of nitrogen via the urine, feces, and sweat from humans fed nitrogen-free or protein-graded diets, along with unaccounted losses of nitrogen via the skin, sweat, and respiration, led to the currently recommended requirement of humans for dietary protein (IOM 2005). This is indicated by the recommended daily allowance (RDA) for dietary protein (e.g., 800 mg/kg BW/day for adults), which is defined as an estimated amount that is considered necessary for satisfactory growth and/or the maintenance of good health in 97.5% of the human population. Likewise, short-term nitrogen balance studies in humans fed purified diets containing different levels (including zero) of a test EAA yielded an estimated dietary requirement for the EAA, with the currently recommended requirements for total EAAs being 90.6 and 65.8 mg/kg BW/day for adult men and women, respectively (Young and Borgonha 2000). Similarly, data on growth performance are commonly used to estimate the requirements of farm animals for dietary AAs and protein (NRC 2012).

Studies over the past three decades have shown that the nitrogen balance-based estimates of dietary EAA requirements by humans or other animals are considerably lower than the values obtained by the AA oxidation methods (Elango et al. 2012; Millward 1997). The differences can be up to 2- to 3-fold for many EAAs (Table 13.4). In addition, the recommended requirements of humans for dietary EAAs as based on nitrogen balance and isotopic studies are <15% and <30% of those for dietary protein, respectively (FAO 2007; IOM 2005). Likewise, the recommended requirement of growing pigs for dietary EAAs is <50% of that for dietary protein (NRC 2012). Furthermore, the sum of dietary requirements of hybrid striped bass for digestible EAAs is 10% of dietary dry matter, which is only 28% of the NRC-recommended requirement of 36% digestible protein (NRC 2011).

These discrepancies may result, in part, from both methodological differences and physiological factors. As indicated previously, the nitrogen balance or growth-performance experiments have inherent problems. In addition, the use of tracers in metabolic research is beset with potential issues associated with label dilution, isotope exchange, the sites of AA catabolism, the determination of intracellular specific activities of immediate precursors, and isotopic steady states (Chapter 7). The currently recommended requirements of humans for dietary EAAs may be substantially underestimated. The large disparities in the dietary requirements of humans, swine, and fish for EAAs vs protein are consistent with the very truth that these organisms have dietary requirements for large amounts of AASAs (Hou et al. 2015; Li et al. 2021a, b; Wu 2014; Wu et al. 2013, 2014a). Unfortunately, requirements of humans for dietary AASAs have long been ignored (e.g., IOM 2005; Katsanos et al. 2008). New knowledge about AA biochemistry and nutrition, as well as improved methodologies for studying whole-body AA metabolism, will be necessary to resolve the current disputes on the dietary requirements of humans and other animals for AAs or proteins.

13.2.6 POTENTIAL USE OF "-OMICS" TECHNOLOGIES TO ESTIMATE DIETARY AA REQUIREMENTS

The traditional approaches to studying dietary AA requirements have played a historically important role in advancing the field of protein and AA nutrition and remain irreplaceable today. However, these methods have limitations. With the completion of human and other mammalian genome projects, revolutionary technologies in life sciences characterized by high throughput, high efficiency, and rapid computation have been developed (Lin et al. 2011; Manjarín et al. 2020; Wang et al. 2009; Zhang et al. 2019). These advanced tools, such as genomics, proteomics, and metabolomics, are now available to determine optimal requirements of individuals for AAs because these nutrients can affect both the expression levels and biological activities of DNA, RNA, protein, and low-molecular-weight metabolites. In other words, changes in cell- and tissue-specific expression of genes, as well as in concentrations of proteins and metabolites in the plasma, urine, and tissues may serve as useful biomarkers for the adequacy or inadequacy of dietary requirements of AAs and proteins. These methods are particularly important to identify the responses of specific proteins in tissues to dietary AA intake and to explain interspecies or intraspecies individual variation in dietary AA requirements. This will provide a foundation for understanding and optimizing precision nutrition (also known as personalized nutrition) in humans and other animals.

13.2.6.1 Nutrigenomics

Different individuals respond differently to the same diet, as indicated by differences in their susceptibility to disease, as well as the efficiency of nutrient absorption and utilization for the synthesis of body constituents (including AAs and proteins). Genetic variability is most likely to be largely responsible for the diversity of biological outcomes in the animal kingdom. Among genomic variety, single-nucleotide polymorphisms (SNPs) are considered to be the major genetic source of phenotypic variability that differentiates individuals within a given species (Auton et al. 2015). An SNP refers to a substitution of a single nucleotide at a specific position in the genome to generate a modified DNA molecule that encodes for a different protein. For example, sickle-cell anemia (an abnormality in hemoglobin) and cystic fibrosis (a genetic mutation of the chloride transport channel) result from SNPs. In addition, other types of genetic variability (e.g., insertions or deletions of nucleotides and variability in copy number of repeated sequences) also make some contributions to phenotypic changes. To address this important issue, the term "nutrigenetics" has been coined, which can be defined as the relationship between diet and genotype as well as its impact on health and disease. A large body of data shows that mRNA levels in cells and tissues are affected by dietary adequacy or inadequacy of AAs (including arginine, glutamine, lysine, and tryptophan) (Wang et al. 2008), as well as the dietary intake of fats (Jobgen et al. 2009). Identifying key SNPs that may influence the nutritional response and health of an individual has been a primary driving force in the development of most nutrigenetic approaches to date. High-throughput genotyping methods for large-scale association studies include TaqMan SNP Genotyping Assay[R], single-base extension-based assays, mass spectrometry-based methods (e.g., the Sequenom MassARRAY genotyping system), the Invader assay, Pyrosequencing, gene chip methods (e.g., the new Affymetrix 500 K SNPChip Array), and next-generation sequencing technology (White and Cantsilieris 2017). Gene copy number variants, which may be an important source of changes in gene expression responsible for much of the variability in an organism's response to diets, have been recognized. Thus, future studies will be conducted beyond the consideration of the only variability between SNPs and will also take into account the other types of genetic variability. Genome-wide copy number detection using microarray technologies is one of the recent research topics on large-scale variations in genomes. Affymetrix GeneChip and Copy Number Analyzer for Affymetrix GeneChip v2.0 allow for not only accurate and high-resolution copy number estimations but also the analyses of allelic imbalances, thereby providing a powerful platform to explore the complexities of genomes.

13.2.6.2 Proteomics

Proteins are the final products of gene expression and have important structural and regulatory functions in cells and body fluids. Thus, proteomics technology has emerged as a revolutionary discovery tool to study how dietary AAs can alter the proteomes of organisms (Timp and Timp 2020; Wang et al. 2006). The workflow of this technology is illustrated in Figure 13.6. Using proteomics, researchers can simultaneously display and determine thousands of proteins in a study sample and identify their changes in response to physiological, pathological, and nutritional alterations. Currently, the most commonly used proteomics technologies are based on either the specific digestion of proteins by a protease (usually trypsin) or the direct analysis of intact proteins. The protein hydrolysis method, also known as the bottom-up approach, involves two-dimensional polyacrylamide gel electrophoresis and multidimensional protein identification. By contrast, the

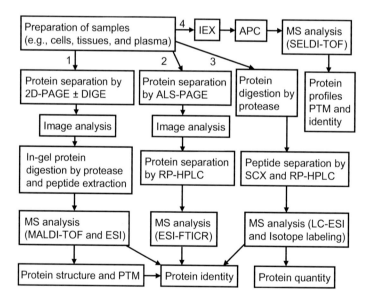

FIGURE 13.6 Workflows of commonly used proteomics technologies. The most commonly used proteomics technologies involve either specific digestion of proteins (the bottom-up approach using two-dimensional polyacrylamide gel electrophoresis and multidimensional protein identification technology) or direct analysis of intact proteins after their chromatographic separation (the top-down approach and surface-enhanced laser desorption ionization). This technology can be used to simultaneously analyze thousands of proteins in a tissue or cells. 1, 2D-PAGE MS; 2, top-down approach; 3, MudIPT; 4, SELDI. Abbreviations used: ALD, acid-labile detergent; APC, affinity protein capture; FTICR, Fourier transform ion cyclotron resonance; IEX, ion-exchange chromatography; PTM, posttranslational modifications; RP-HPLC, reversed-phase HPLC; SCX, strong cation exchange. (Reproduced from Wang, J.J. et al. 2006. *J. Nutr.* 136:1759–1762. With permission.)

analysis of intact proteins requires their chromatographic separation and their subsequent identification by mass spectrometry (MS), such as surface-enhanced laser desorption ionization. Recently, several quantitative proteomic techniques have been developed, such as 2D DIGE (difference gel electrophoresis), ICAT (isotope-coded affinity tag), iTRAQ (isobaric tags for relative and absolute quantification), and proteolytic O-18-labeling strategies. Finally, a promising approach for proteomics is protein microarray technology, which can be used to detect changes in the expression and posttranslational modifications of hundreds or even thousands of proteins in a parallel way. Identification of different phosphoproteins and their phosphorylation sites can be accomplished by combining proteomics with radioactive labeling, phospho-specific staining, immunoprecipitation, or immunoblotting, as well as metal affinity chromatography. This approach provides informational insights into the proteomes and their signaling pathways affected by the availability of dietary nutrients, including AAs and protein.

13.2.6.3 Metabolomics

Gene expression or protein concentration may indicate the potential for physiological or metabolic changes in cells, tissues, and organs but may not represent real endpoints of the complex regulatory processes in organisms. Nutrimetabolomics, defined as the analysis of the effects of diet on the metabolome (a complete set of small-molecule metabolites in a biological sample), is in its infancy in nutrition research. However, this technology has already provided novel and important insights into understanding the metabolic responses of humans or other animals to dietary interventions. Currently, the widely used methods for metabolomics studies involve proton nuclear magnetic resonance (NMR) technology and MS (Johnson et al. 2016). Liquid chromatography-MS, which is complementary to NMR, offers superb sensitivity but is limited by the essentially nonquantitative nature of the method and the requirement for internal standardization.

Let us use the piglet as an animal model to illustrate how metabolomics can be used to assess the dietary adequacy of arginine (He et al. 2009). Using ^{1}H-NMR spectroscopy, Q. He and colleagues determined changes in serum metabolome in growing pigs brought about by different levels of dietary arginine. Principal component analysis indicated that the concentrations of low-density lipoprotein, very low-density lipoprotein, and urea in the serum were lower, but the concentrations of creatinine, tricarboxylic acid cycle metabolites, ornithine, lysine, and tyrosine in the serum were greater in arginine-adequate as compared to arginine-inadequate pigs. Additionally, the concentrations of nitrogenous and lipid-signaling molecules (e.g., creatine ↑, glutamine ↑, glycerophosphorylcholine ↓, myo-inositol ↑) in the serum and of intestinal bacterial metabolites (ethanol ↓, methylamine ↑, dimethylamine ↓, and trimethylamine-N-oxide ↓) were all affected by dietary arginine supplementation in a way that depends on individual metabolites (He et al. 2009).

The metabolomics has also been used to assess differences in serum metabolic profiles between lean and obese pigs (He et al. 2012a). Specifically, with the NMR-based metabolomic technology, orthogonal projection to the latent structure with the discriminant analysis revealed that compared with lean pigs, high-density lipoproteins, very low-density lipoproteins, lipids, unsaturated lipids, glycoprotein, myo-inositol, pyruvate, threonine, tyrosine, and creatine were elevated in the serum of obese pigs, whereas opposite results were observed for serum glucose and urea. In addition, gut microbiota-related metabolites, including trimethylamine-N-oxide (reduced concentration) and choline (increased concentration), were altered in the serum of obese pigs relative to lean pigs. These findings indicate that the patterns of AA, lipid, and carbohydrate metabolism in the gastrointestinal microbes and their hosts in obese pigs are very different from those in lean pigs.

13.3 OPTIMUM RATIOS OF AASAs IN DIETS FOR HUMANS AND OTHER ANIMALS

The composition of AAs in the whole bodies of terrestrial animals (e.g., cattle, chickens, pigs, and rats) is generally similar (Wu et al. 2013). The content of many AAs does not differ appreciably between terrestrial animals and fish or shrimp (Li et al. 2021a, b). However, glycine, proline, and 4-hydroxyproline are more abundant in body proteins but aspartate, cysteine, glutamate, glutamine, isoleucine, lysine, methionine, phenylalanine, serine, threonine, tyrosine, and valine are less abundant in body proteins to various extents in young mammals and birds than in juvenile fish and shrimp (Li et al. 2021a, b). This is because of a much lower content of collagen in juvenile fish and shrimp than in young mammals and birds. The content of alanine in body proteins is similar between terrestrial animals and fish but is greater than that in shrimp. By contrast, histidine is less abundant in body proteins in terrestrial animals than in fish, whereas arginine and asparagine are less abundant in body proteins in terrestrial animals than in shrimp. Thus, the patterns of dietary AA requirements for protein deposition likely differ between terrestrial and aquatic animals (He et al. 2021; Li et al. 2021a, b; Zhang et al. 2021). Knowledge about the dietary requirements of animals for AASAs is crucial for reducing the dietary content of total protein for livestock, poultry, fish, and crustaceans, and for the identification of new feedstuffs or AA sources to replace the use of fishmeal in aquaculture. This will help to sustain the global animal agriculture to supply high-quality protein for human consumption and health.

TABLE 13.9
Recommended Requirements of Healthy Humans for AASAs[a]

Age Group	EAA[b]		Amino Acids that Are Synthesizable *de novo* in Animal Cells (AASAs)											
	Total	Lys	Total	Ala	Arg	Asn	Asp	Cys	Glu	Gln	Gly	Pro	Ser	Tyr
						mg/kg of body weight/day								
Infants[c] (0.3–1 y)	402	71.3	750	69.2	71.3	48.6	69.2	21.6	121	108	76.7	82.1	42.2	39.9
Children[d] (1–3 y)	295	52.3	550	50.7	52.3	35.6	50.7	15.8	88.7	79.2	56.2	60.2	30.9	29.3
Adult men and women (>18 y)														
Minimal PA	268	47.5	500	46.1	47.5	32.4	46.1	14.4	80.6	72.0	51.1	54.7	28.1	26.6
Moderate PA	348	61.8	650	60.0	61.8	42.1	60.0	18.7	105	93.6	66.4	71.1	36.5	34.6
Intense PA	429	76.0	799	73.8	76.0	51.8	73.8	23.0	129	115	81.8	87.5	45.0	42.6
						mg/kg of lean body mass/day								
Adult men (> 18 y)[e]														
Minimal PA	315	55.9	588	54.2	55.9	38.1	54.2	16.9	94.8	84.7	60.1	64.4	33.1	31.3
Moderate PA	409	72.7	765	70.6	72.7	49.5	70.6	22.0	124	110	78.1	83.6	42.9	40.7
Intense PA	505	89.4	940	86.8	89.4	60.9	86.8	27.1	152	135	96.2	103	52.9	50.1
Adult women (> 18 y)[f]														
Minimal PA	367	65.1	685	63.2	65.1	44.4	63.2	19.7	110	98.6	70.0	74.9	38.5	36.4
Moderate PA	477	84.7	890	82.2	84.7	57.7	82.2	25.6	144	128	91.0	97.4	50.0	47.4
Intense PA	588	104	1095	101	104	71.0	101	31.5	177	158	112	120	61.6	58.4

Source: Adapted from Wu, G. 2016. *Food Funct.* 7:1251–1265.

Note: PA, physical activity; y, year(s).

[a] Values are expressed as mg/kg body weight/day and refer to true digestible amounts. Except for glycine, all amino acids are L-isomers. Note that expressed as mg/kg of lean body mass/day, adult women have higher requirements for amino acids that are formed *de novo* than adult men. This is because adult women generally have a lower lean body mass than adult men.

[b] Values for adults with minimal physical activity are calculated as the IOM (2005) value×1.25. Nutritionally essential amino acids (EAAs) include His, Ile, Leu, Lys, Met, Phe, Thr, Trp, and Val, as defined by IOM.

[c] Values are calculated as 1.5×adult value (minimal PA).

[d] Values are calculated as 1.1×adult value (minimal PA).

[e] Calculated on the basis of 85% lean body mass in normal, nonobese adult men.

[f] Calculated on the basis of 73% lean body mass in normal, nonobese adult women.

Based on the composition, metabolism, and nutrition of AASAs in humans and other animals, Wu (2016) recommended for the first time the dietary requirements of infants, children, and adult humans for these AAs (Table 13.9). In addition, there has been great progress in our understanding of AA metabolism in farm animals over the past 30 years (He et al. 2021; Li et al. 2021a, b; Zhang et al. 2021). These recent advances in AA nutrition and metabolism led to the proposal of the optimal ratios of true digestible AAs in diets for (1) swine (Table 13.10) and chickens (broilers and laying hens; Table 13.11) during different phases of growth and production; (2) zoo carnivores and herbivores (young and adults; Table 13.12); (3) zoo mammalian and avian omnivores (young and adults; Table 13.13); and (4) cats (young and adults; Table 13.14). Furthermore, like chicks (He et al. 2021), pigs (Zhang et al. 2021), and rats (Hou et al. 2015), rainbow trout have dietary requirements for AASAs (Green et al. 2002), but no data are available regarding any specific AASA requirement. Of particular note, aquatic animals require much higher levels of dietary AAs (e.g., as 30% to 50% dietary protein; dry matter basis) than chickens, swine, and ruminants (18%–23%, 13%–23%, and 11%–20% dietary protein, respectively; dry matter basis) (Li et al. 2021a, b; Wu 2018). Most of the

TABLE 13.10

Optimal Ratios of True Digestible Amino Acids in Diets for Swine[a]

Amino Acid	Growing Pigs (kg)[b]				Gestating Pigs[c]		Lactating Sows[b]
	5–10	10–20	20–50	50–110	d 0–90	d 90–114	
	% of Diet (As-Fed Basis)						
Alanine	1.14	0.97	0.80	0.64	0.69	0.69	0.83
Arginine	1.19	1.01	0.83	0.66	1.03	1.03	1.37
Asparagine	0.80	0.68	0.56	0.45	0.50	0.50	0.66
Aspartate	1.14	0.97	0.80	0.64	0.61	0.61	0.94
Cysteine	0.32	0.28	0.24	0.20	0.19	0.19	0.26
Glutamate	2.00	1.70	1.39	1.12	0.89	0.89	1.81
Glutamine	1.80	1.53	1.25	1.00	1.00	1.60	1.38
Glycine	1.27	1.08	0.89	0.71	0.48	0.48	0.75
Histidine	0.46	0.39	0.32	0.26	0.29	0.29	0.39
Isoleucine	0.78	0.66	0.54	0.43	0.45	0.45	0.66
Leucine	1.57	1.33	1.09	0.87	1.03	1.03	1.41
Lysine	1.19	1.01	0.83	0.66	0.51	0.51	0.80
Methionine	0.32	0.28	0.24	0.20	0.16	0.16	0.25
Phenylalanine	0.86	0.73	0.60	0.48	0.54	0.54	0.77
Proline	1.36	1.16	0.95	0.76	0.89	0.89	1.24
Serine	0.70	0.60	0.49	0.39	0.45	0.45	0.74
Threonine	0.74	0.65	0.55	0.46	0.41	0.41	0.56
Tryptophan	0.22	0.19	0.17	0.14	0.11	0.11	0.18
Tyrosine	0.67	0.57	0.46	0.37	0.40	0.40	0.62
Valine	0.85	0.72	0.59	0.47	0.55	0.55	0.72

Source: Wu, G. 2014. *J. Anim. Sci. Biotechnol.* 5:34.

Note: d, day(s).

[a] Except for glycine, all amino acids are L-isomers. Values are based on true ileal digestible amino acids. Crystalline amino acids (e.g., feed-grade arginine, glutamate, glutamine, and glycine), whose true ileal digestibility is 100%, can be added to a diet to obtain their optimal ratios. The molecular weights of intact amino acids were used for all the calculations. The content of dry matter in all the diets was 90%. The content of metabolizable energy in the diets of growing pigs, gestating pigs, and lactating pigs is 3,330, 3,122, and 3,310 kcal/kg diet, respectively.

[b] Fed ad libitum (90% dry matter).

[c] Fed 2 kg/day on d 0–90, and 2.3 kg/day on d 90–114 (90% dry matter).

TABLE 13.11

Optimal Ratios of True Digestible Amino Acids in Diets for Broiler Chickens and Laying Hens[a]

Amino Acid	Age of Broiler Chickens			Laying Hens[e]	
	0–21 Days[b]	21–42 Days[c]	42–56 Days[d]	Content of Digestible AAs in Diet (%, As-Fed Basis)	Percentage of Digestible Lysine in Diet (%)
	(% of Digestible Lysine in Diet)				
Alanine	102	102	102	0.90	110
Arginine	105	108	108	1.03	126
Asparagine	56	56	56	0.72	88
Aspartate	66	66	66	1.03	126
Cysteine	32	33	33	0.29	35
Glutamate	178	178	178	1.45	177
Glutamine	128	128	128	1.58	193
Glycine	176	176	176	1.00	120
Histidine	35	35	35	0.41	50
Isoleucine	67	69	69	0.70	85
Leucine	109	109	109	1.52	185
Lysine	100	100	100	0.82	100
Methionine	40	42	42	0.38	46
Phenylalanine	60	60	60	0.53	65
Proline	184	184	184	1.31	160
Serine	69	69	69	0.80	98
Threonine	67	70	70	0.61	74
Tryptophan	16	17	17	0.19	23
Tyrosine	45	45	45	0.41	50
Valine	77	80	80	0.78	95

Source: He, W.L. et al. 2021. *Adv. Exp. Med. Biol.* 1285:109–131.

[a] Except for glycine, all amino acids are L-isomers. Values are based on true ileal digestible amino acids.

[b] Patterns of amino acid composition in the ideal protein are the same for male and female chickens. The amounts of digestible lysine in diet (as-fed basis; 90% dry matter) are 1.12% and 1.02% for male and female chickens, respectively.

[c] Patterns of amino acid composition in the ideal protein are the same for male and female chickens. The amounts of digestible lysine in diets (as-fed basis; 90% dry matter) are 0.89% and 0.84% for male and female chickens, respectively.

[d] Patterns of amino acid composition in the ideal protein are the same for male and female chickens. The amounts of digestible lysine in diets (as-fed basis; 90% dry matter) are 0.76% and 0.73% for male and female chickens, respectively.

[e] A diet that consists of 60% corn grain (containing 9.3% crude protein) and 24% soybean meal (43.5% crude protein) and is supplemented with 0.2% glycine and 0.1% L-methionine can meet the requirements of laying hens for all amino acids.

dietary AASAs are utilized by fish and crustaceans as metabolic fuels in their tissues, including the intestine, liver, kidneys, and skeletal muscle.

Data for nonprimate mammals can be useful references when developing the optimum requirements of humans for dietary AAs, particularly gestating and lactating women with whom it is challenging to perform experiments. Note that: (1) the requirements for AASAs by humans and other animals of all the age groups are much greater than those for EAAs; and (2) humans and other animals have particularly high requirements for dietary glutamate, glutamine, glycine, and proline that

TABLE 13.12

Recommended Requirements of Zoo Carnivores and Herbivores for Dietary Amino Acids[a]

Amino acid (AA)	Carnivores		Herbivores (Adult)		Herbivores (Young)[b]	
	AA Content in Diet (% of DM)	% of Lysine in Diet (g/100 g)	AA Content in Diet (% of DM)	% of Lysine in Diet (g/100 g)	AA Content in Diet (% of DM)	% of Lysine in Diet (g/100 g)
Ala	3.00	109	0.93	131	1.30	131
Arg	3.09	112	0.84	119	1.18	119
Asn	1.64	59.7	0.73	103	1.02	103
Asp	1.95	71.0	0.83	117	1.16	117
Cys	0.60	21.9	0.27	37.5	0.37	37.5
Gln	2.34	84.9	1.29	181	1.80	181
Glu	3.86	140	1.12	158	1.57	158
Gly	5.36	195	0.70	98.4	0.98	98.4
His	0.95	34.4	0.31	43.8	0.43	43.8
Hyp	1.73	62.9	---	---	---	---
Ile	1.61	58.6	0.60	84.4	0.84	84.4
Leu	3.12	113	1.19	167	1.66	167
Lys	2.75	100	0.71	100	0.99	100
Met	0.85	31.0	0.23	32.8	0.33	32.8
Phe	1.56	56.8	0.70	98.4	0.98	98.4
Pro	3.93	143	1.13	159	1.58	159
Ser	2.02	73.5	0.72	102	1.01	102
Thr	1.60	58.1	0.54	76.6	0.76	76.6
Trp	0.51	18.4	0.18	25.0	0.25	25.0
Tyr	1.24	45.0	0.53	75.0	0.75	75.0
Val	1.93	69.9	0.71	100	0.99	100
TPAA	45.7	---	14.3	---	20.0	---
Taurine	0.10	---	0.00	---	0.02	---

Source: Herring, C.M. et al. 2021. *Adv. Exp. Med. Biol.* 1285:233–253.

Note: DM, dry matter; Hyp, 4-hydroxyproline; TPAA, total proteinogenic amino acids.

[a] Values are AA content in diets for zoo carnivores and herbivores in general as references. Within carnivores or herbivores, various species may have moderately different requirements for dietary AAs. The molecular weights of intact amino acids are used for the calculation of AA content in the diet. Intakes of dry matter by zoo animals range from 1% to 5% of their body weight, depending on species, age, and physiological state.

[b] Before the normal weaning age. Within the first 1 month after weaning, the dietary content of all amino acids is reduced by 10%. A high intake of dietary protein in postweaning mammals increases risks for intestinal dysfunction.

are very abundant in rendered animal sources of feedstuffs, such as blood meal, feather meal, meat and bone meal, and poultry byproducts (Li et al. 2011). AASAs have now been included in swine (Hou and Wu 2018; Le Floc'h et al. 2018; Wu et al. 2018) and poultry (Belloir et al. 2017, 2019) diets worldwide to enhance the efficiency of their lean tissue growth and productivity. The recommended optimal ratios of dietary AAs for animals are expected to beneficially reduce dietary protein content and nitrogen excretion while improving the efficiency of nutrient utilization, growth, and production performance, thereby potentially sustaining global animal agriculture. It should be borne in mind that the recommended values of dietary AA requirements for farm, zoo, and companion animals may not be optimum, and are expected to serve as helpful guidelines for feeding practices and

TABLE 13.13

Recommended Requirements of Zoo Mammalian and Avian Omnivores for Dietary Amino Acids[a]

Amino Acid (AA)	Mammalian Omnivores						Avian Omnivores			
	Mammals (Adults)		Mammals (Young)[b]		Mammals (Lactating)		Birds (Adults)		Birds (Young)	
	AA Content in Diet[c]	% of Lysine in Diet	AA Content in Diet[d]	% of Lysine in Diet	AA Content in Diet[c]	% of Lysine in Diet	AA Content in Diet[c]	% of Lysine in Diet	AA Content in Diet[3]	% of Lysine in Diet
	(% of DM)	(g/g)	(% of DM)	(g/g)	(% of DM)	(g/g)	(% of DM)	(g/g)	(% of DM)	(g/g)
Ala	0.81	97.4	1.38	95.6	1.05	104	0.90	102	1.36	102
Arg	0.83	100	1.44	99.8	1.73	171	0.95	109	1.41	105
Asn	0.57	68.5	0.97	67.1	0.83	82.5	0.49	56.2	0.75	56.1
Asp	0.81	97.4	1.38	95.6	1.19	118	0.58	66.3	0.89	66.2
Cys	0.25	30.4	0.39	26.8	0.33	32.5	0.32	36.4	0.43	32.1
Gln	1.26	152	2.17	151	1.74	173	1.13	129	1.72	128
Glu	1.41	170	2.42	168	2.29	226	1.57	179	2.38	178
Gly	0.90	108	1.53	107	0.95	93.8	1.56	177	2.35	175
His	0.33	39.6	0.56	38.6	0.49	48.8	0.31	35.2	0.47	35.1
Ile	0.54	65.4	0.94	65.4	0.83	82.5	0.61	69.3	0.92	68.7
Leu	1.10	132	1.90	132	1.78	176	0.96	110	1.46	109
Lys	0.83	100	1.44	100	1.01	100	0.88	100	1.34	100
Met	0.25	30.4	0.39	26.8	0.32	31.3	0.37	42.2	0.54	40.1
Phe	0.61	73.0	1.04	72.1	0.97	96.3	0.53	60.3	0.81	60.2
Pro	0.96	116	1.64	114	1.57	155	1.63	185	2.46	184
Ser	0.49	59.3	0.85	58.7	0.93	92.5	0.61	69.3	0.93	69.2
Thr	0.58	70.0	0.89	62.1	0.71	70.0	0.62	70.3	0.90	67.2

(Continued)

TABLE 13.13 (Continued)
Recommended Requirements of Zoo Mammalian and Avian Omnivores for Dietary Amino Acids[a]

	Mammalian Omnivores						Avian Omnivores			
	Mammals (Adults)		Mammals (Young)[b]		Mammals (Lactating)		Birds (Adults)		Birds (Young)[3]	
Amino Acid (AA)	AA Content in Diet[c]	% of Lysine in Diet	AA Content in Diet[d]	% of Lysine in Diet	AA Content in Diet[c]	% of Lysine in Diet	AA Content in Diet[c]	% of Lysine in Diet	AA Content in Diet[3]	% of Lysine in Diet
	(% of DM)	(g/g)	(% of DM)	(g/g)	(% of DM)	(g/g)	(% of DM)	(g/g)	(% of DM)	(g/g)
Trp	0.18	21.3	0.27	18.5	0.23	22.5	0.15	17.0	0.22	16.0
Tyr	0.47	56.3	0.81	56.2	0.78	77.5	0.40	45.2	0.60	45.1
Val	0.59	71.5	1.03	71.3	0.91	90.0	0.71	80.3	1.07	79.9
TPAA	13.8	---	23.4	---	20.6	---	15.3	---	23.0	---
Taurine	0.00	---	0.05	---	0.00	---	0.00	---	0.00	---

Source: Herring, C.M. et al. 2021. *Adv. Exp. Med. Biol.* 1285:233–253.

Note: DM, dry matter; TPAA, total proteinogenic amino acids.

[a] Values are AA content in diets for zoo mammalian and avian omnivores in general as references. Within mammalian or avian omnivores, various species may have moderately different requirements for dietary AAs. The molecular weights of intact amino acids are used for the calculation of AA content in the diet. Intakes of dry matter by zoo animals range from 1% to 5% of their body weight, depending on species, age, and physiological state.

[b] Before weaning. Within the first month after weaning, the dietary content of all amino acids is reduced by 10%. A high intake of dietary protein in postweaning mammals increases risks for intestinal dysfunction.

[c] The true digestibility of amino acids in dietary protein and the content of dry matter in the diet are assumed to be 88% and 90%, respectively.

[d] The true digestibility of amino acids in dietary protein and the content of dry matter in the diet are assumed to be 92% and 90%, respectively.

TABLE 13.14

Recommended Requirements of Cats for Dietary Amino Acids[a]

Crude Protein and Amino Acid	Minimum Dietary Requirements of Cats For Amino Acids			Maximum Dietary Requirements of Young, Adult, and Elderly Adult Cats for Amino Acids
	Young Cats	Young Adult Cats	Elderly Adult Cats	
Crude protein	30	26	30	73.4
Taurine	0.2	0.2	0.2	0.29
Proteinogenic Amino Acids that Are Not Synthesized *de novo* by Cats				
Arg	2.14	1.86	2.33	5.24
Cys	0.50	0.50	0.50	1.12
His	1.30	1.12	1.12	3.17
Ile	1.68	1.46	1.46	4.11
Leu	2.73	2.36	2.36	6.67
Lys	2.94	2.55	2.56	7.20
Met	1.03	0.90	0.90	2.53
Phe	1.37	1.19	1.19	3.35
Thr	1.51	1.31	1.31	3.70
Trp	0.41	0.35	0.44	1.00
Tyr	1.23	1.07	1.07	3.01
Val	1.94	1.68	1.68	4.74
Proteinogenic Amino Acids that Are Synthesized *de novo* by Cats				
Ala	1.86	1.61	1.61	4.54
Asn	1.37	1.18	1.18	3.34
Asp	1.68	1.46	1.46	4.11
Glu	3.07	2.66	3.33	7.51
Gln	2.04	1.77	1.77	4.99
Gly	1.38	1.19	1.49	3.37
Pro[b]	1.42	1.23	1.23	3.47
Ser	1.45	1.25	1.25	3.54

Source: Che, D.S. et al. 2021. *Adv. Exp. Med. Biol.* 1285:217–231.

[a] Values are % of dry matter in the diet.

[b] Proline+4-hydroxyproline (the ratio of proline to 4-hydroxyproline = 18.6:1.0; g/g).

future research. Because the metabolism of animals is affected by physiological, environmental, and pathological factors (Waterlow et al. 1978), their optimum requirements for dietary AAs are not one set of fixed data, and likely undergo dynamic changes with changing conditions. This calls for a range of the recommended requirement values, which need to be modified under practical feeding conditions.

13.4 ASSESSMENT OF DIETARY PROTEIN QUALITY

While crystalline AAs can be used to prepare purified diets for consumption by humans and other animals, it is intact proteins in food that are the major sources of EAAs and AASAs in regular diets due to both tastes and costs. Thus, it is important that dietary protein quality be assessed so that the organisms will receive the balanced and adequate provision of all AAs (Harper and Yoshimura 1993). This should be done for any new sources of foodstuffs. The quality of any dietary protein depends on the following factors: (1) the amounts and profile of its AAs, particularly EAAs and functional AAs; and (2) the digestibility and availability of its AAs to the animal relative to require-ments for all AAs. Note, however, that a protein with the balanced composition of all AAs may not be a high-quality protein for animals if it cannot be hydrolyzed by proteases in the gastrointestinal tract. Thus, although the analysis of the AA content in foodstuffs is necessary to predict which AA is deficient or excessive in the diet, this chemical method should not be used as the sole means of evaluating the nutritive quality of food proteins. Therefore, biological studies to determine protein digestibility *in vivo* and the animal's growth performance must be carried out concurrently with the determination of dietary AA composition (Evans and Witty 1978). Fortunately, most common food-stuffs have been analyzed for their AA and protein content, as well as their digestibilities in vari-ous animal species (Chapter 2). However, both chemical analyses and biological experiments are needed to eliminate fake raw materials (e.g., melamine in pet foods) as sources of dietary protein. Taken together, the quality and adequacy of a dietary protein depend on its capability to provide *all* AAs in appropriate amounts and proportions.

Studies with farm animals have shown that the inclusion of animal protein (e.g., ruminant meat & bone meal, porcine mucosal hydrolysate, and chicken visceral digest) in plant-based diets can improve overall dietary protein quality and, therefore, the growth performance, feed efficiency, and health (including intestinal health and whole-body immune response) of swine, poultry, fish, and crustaceans (Wu 2018). In assessing dietary protein quality, taurine (a nonproteinogenic AA) must be determined in the diets of carnivores (including cats, dogs, tigers, and largemouth bass). Any plant-based diets for these animals must contain animal-sourced feedstuffs or be supplemented with taurine to protect their organs (particularly the small intestine and eyes) from damage (Che et al. 2021; Herring et al. 2021; Li et al. 2021a; Oberbauer and Larsen 2021).

13.4.1 CHEMICAL METHODS

13.4.1.1 AA Analysis

Dietary proteins must be hydrolyzed to individual AAs before AA analysis. This is usually done by acid hydrolysis (Chapter 1). Unfortunately, this process results in (1) the complete destruction of tryptophan, (2) the losses of methionine (20%), serine (10%), proline (6%), tyrosine (5%), aspar-tate (3%), and threonine (3%), and (3) the conversion of glutamine and asparagine to glutamate and aspartate, respectively (Chapter 1). Thus, correction for recovery rates of AAs from protein hydrolysis should be made. Alkaline hydrolysis of feedstuff is performed for the analysis of tryp-tophan (Chapter 1). Theoretically, food protein can be hydrolyzed with known proteases; however, this turns out to be practically difficult for the analysis of all AAs because they are released from protein at various rates. Alternatively, food can be incubated with fluids obtained from the stomach and small intestine of post-absorptive animals to mimic the *in vivo* digestion process. Although this latter process is promising, whether proteins can be completely hydrolyzed to free AAs may pose a serious problem. Separate acid and base hydrolyses of the same foodstuff provide a solution to this problem.

Free AAs can be measured by high-performance liquid chromatography (HPLC), gas chroma-tography, or enzymatic methods (Dai et al. 2014). HPLC is by far the most powerful technique for AA analysis. Whether the amounts of AAs in the hydrolysates of foodstuff proteins are calculated according to the molecular weights of intact AAs or AA residues must be stated in data presentation to avoid any confusion or an overestimation of true proteins. Values from AA analysis can tell us which AA in dietary proteins might be deficient, adequate, or excessive, but give little information on their availability to the animal. A good quality protein contains a high percentage of all EAAs and functional AAs. Data on their content in some foodstuffs for humans and other animals are shown in Tables 13.15–13.18. These data serve as useful references for the nutrition of humans and other animals, because there exist wide variabilities in the literature regarding the content of AAs (particularly methionine, cysteine, and tryptophan) within ingredients between laboratories (Hou et al. 2019; Li and Wu 2020). Note that glutamate, glutamine, asparagine, aspartate, proline, and

TABLE 13.15

Content of Total Amino Acids (Peptide-Bound Plus Free Amino Acids) in Human Foods[a]

Amino Acid (AA)	Corn Grain	Peanut	Pistachio Nut	Potato	Soybean	Sweet Potato	Wheat Flour	White Rice	Algae SM	Soy PC	Beef Cut Chuck	Beef Cut Round	Beef Cut Loin

Amino Acid (AA)	Corn Grain	Peanut	Pistachio Nut	Potato	Soybean	Sweet Potato	Wheat Flour	White Rice	Algae SM	Soy PC	Chuck	Round	Loin
Dry Matter (DM) Content (% of foodstuff) and Crude Protein (CP) Content (% of DM)													
DM	18.3	96.9	96.2	21.0	96.2	22.9	95.1	90.7	96.5	95.4	29.7	29.0	30.8
CP	10.1	27.7	21.5	9.84	44.6	6.91	13.4	8.25	68.8	67.5	68.0	72.1	73.4
Individual AAs (mg/g of Dry Matter)													
Ala	7.97	12.4	11.3	2.82	22.9	4.80	5.42	4.58	60.6	36.1	42.2	44.5	45.4
Arg	4.34	35.5	23.8	5.15	37.2	3.08	7.20	7.28	53.7	60.8	47.9	51.0	52.4
Asp	4.74	14.2	9.89	4.05	37.3	3.34	3.58	4.27	44.4	58.7	37.7	40.3	41.1
Asn	3.88	19.7	10.2	19.2	24.6	12.0	4.47	4.60	34.6	37.8	30.3	32.9	33.4
Cys	2.17	4.15	3.56	1.14	7.67	1.63	3.04	1.66	9.13	14.3	10.1	10.8	11.2
Glu	7.13	28.6	18.4	1.01	52.6	5.46	2.80	7.38	70.6	87.6	68.9	73.8	75.1
Gln	11.8	29.0	26.9	16.3	43.0	2.20	45.5	7.96	44.0	72.6	46.8	48.5	49.9
Gly	4.43	19.0	11.7	2.74	24.0	3.52	6.31	3.95	43.4	37.6	31.0	33.3	33.7
His	2.68	6.98	5.30	1.70	12.7	1.18	3.54	2.20	13.4	21.8	29.4	31.0	31.7
Hyp	0.04	0.79	0.59	0.08	0.78	0.05	0.43	0.04	0.15	0.14	1.73	1.74	1.77
Ile	3.85	10.8	10.2	3.19	23.9	3.31	4.92	3.74	42.3	39.6	38.4	40.5	41.1
Leu	12.8	18.1	16.9	4.72	40.0	4.88	10.0	7.26	65.5	60.7	61.8	65.1	66.7
Lys	2.85	9.98	11.9	5.13	32.6	3.61	3.64	2.33	43.3	52.9	66.6	70.4	72.0
Met	2.26	3.43	3.80	1.53	6.43	1.22	2.48	2.02	22.4	12.3	23.7	24.8	25.3
Phe	5.18	14.8	11.5	3.92	25.6	4.83	7.53	4.39	40.2	42.4	30.9	33.1	33.5
Pro	11.3	16.5	12.9	3.02	28.4	2.64	23.2	5.41	32.3	36.5	30.0	31.5	32.9
Ser	5.05	14.4	14.0	3.55	30.2	4.54	6.90	4.09	45.1	50.7	32.0	34.2	35.4
Thr	3.58	8.12	7.14	3.19	20.9	3.74	4.09	3.02	42.8	34.3	34.3	35.8	37.0
Trp	0.75	2.72	2.62	1.01	7.02	0.48	1.70	1.12	10.6	12.7	9.34	9.77	10.0
Tyr	4.80	11.0	5.32	2.34	18.4	2.99	3.86	2.37	39.3	30.1	27.1	28.9	30.1
Val	5.07	12.7	13.2	4.98	24.6	4.46	6.24	5.19	45.2	40.1	44.8	46.9	47.4
Total	107	293	231	90.8	521	73.9	157	84.9	803	840	745	789	807

Source: Hou, Y.Q. et al. 2019. *Amino Acids* 51:1153–1165; Li, P. and G. Wu. 2020. *Amino Acids* 52:523–542; Wu, G. et al. 2016. *J. Anim. Sci.* 94:2603–2613.

Note: CP, crude protein ($N\% \times 6.25$); Hyp, 4-hydroxyproline; PC, protein concentrate; SM, spirulina meal.

[a] Peptide-bound amino acids refer to amino acids in both proteins and non-protein peptides. The molecular weights of intact amino acids were used to calculate the amount of peptide-bound plus free amino acids in the acid or alkaline hydrolysates of foods. This calculation always overestimates the true content of protein and peptides in foods.

BCAAs represent most of the AA content in both plant and animal proteins. Certain plant (e.g., peanut meal and cottonseed meal) and animal (e.g., fish meal and gelatin) products provide high levels of arginine. However, foodstuffs of plant origin usually contain lower percentages of lysine, tryptophan, threonine, methionine, and cysteine than feedstuffs of animal origin. Unlike other animal products, the isoleucine content is relatively low in red blood cells or blood meal (only 22% of leucine). Overall, foodstuffs of animal origin (except for gelatin) are excellent sources of all AAs for livestock, avian, and aquatic species.

Animal products (e.g., meats and eggs) are abundant sources of EAAs and AASAs (including taurine) in human diets while providing polyamines, glutathione, and agmatine (Table 13.19). Meats also contain relatively large amounts of creatine, carnosine, and anserine (Table 13.19). For example, there are reports that the concentrations of taurine in beef, pork, lamb, and chicken meats

TABLE 13.16

Content of Amino Acids in Bovine Casein and Whey Protein, as well as Chicken Eggs as Human Foods

Amino Acid	Bovine Casein[a] (% of Protein)	Bovine Whey Protein[b] (% of Protein)	Whole-Egg Protein[c] (% of Protein)	Amino Acid Score[d]	
				Bovine Casein	Bovine Whey Protein
Ala	2.79	2.61	5.58	49.3	46.8
Arg	3.42	2.71	6.33	56.3	42.8
Asp	3.90	3.96[e]	5.97[g]	56.3	66.3
Asn	2.57	2.30[e]	4.33[g]	75.3	66.3
Asp+Asn	6.47	6.26	10.3	64.3	60.8
Cys	0.43	2.52	2.21	14.0	114
Glu	9.43	13.7[f]	8.55[h]	110	160
Gln	11.3	9.10[f]	4.65[h]	254	196
Glu+Gln	20.7	22.8	13.2	161	173
Gly	1.87	1.56	3.35	51.6	46.6
His	2.80	2.40	2.48	111	96.8
Ile	4.94	4.07	5.02	93.4	81.1
Leu	8.87	11.6	8.55	106	136
Lys	7.53	6.26	6.88	108	91.0
Met	2.65	2.50	3.08	89.3	81.2
Phe	4.90	4.59	5.22	93.7	87.9
Pro	10.9	10.6	3.78	272	280
Ser	5.11	3.86	7.78	65.6	49.6
Thr	4.12	3.44	4.39	92.9	78.4
Trp	1.25	1.85	1.60	95.6	116
Tyr	5.09	4.80	4.08	130	118
Val	6.06	5.53	6.17	99.2	89.6

[a] Li et al. (2011). All values were calculated on the basis of the molecular weights of intact amino acids in protein hydrolysates.

[b] Dangin, M. et al. (2001) for all amino acids, except for aspartate, asparagine, glutamate, and glutamine. Calculated on the basis of the molecular weights of intact amino acids in protein hydrolysates.

[c] USDA (2016; https://ndb.nal.usda.gov/ndb) for all amino acids, except for aspartate, asparagine, glutamate, and glutamine. Calculated on the basis of the molecular weights of intact amino acids in protein hydrolysates.

[d] Calculated as the (the amount of an amino acid in the bovine casein or whey protein × 100)/the amount of the same amino acid in whole-egg proteins.

[e] Calculated on the basis of the ratio of aspartate to asparagine (1.72:1.00) in bovine whey protein, as analyzed by an enzymatic method (Hou et al. 2019).

[f] Calculated on the basis of the ratio of glutamate to glutamine (1.50:1.00) in bovine whey protein, as analyzed by an enzymatic method (Hou et al. 2019).

[g] Calculated on the basis of the ratio of aspartate to asparagine (1.38:1.00) in whole-egg protein, as analyzed by an enzymatic method (Hou et al. 2019).

[h] Calculated on the basis of the ratio of glutamate to glutamine (1.84:1.00) in whole-egg protein, as analyzed by an enzymatic method (Hou et al. 2019).

range from 300 to 1,000, 400 to 1,200, 350 to 1,200, and 300 to 4,000 mg/kg wet weight, respectively (Purchas et al. 2004). These values correspond to 3.4 to 11.4, 4.5 to 13.5, 4.0 to 13.5, and 3.4 to 45 mM taurine in beef, pork, lamb, and chicken meats, respectively. A 3-ounce (84 g) beef steak would provide 67 mg taurine, which may meet approximately 89% of the daily taurine requirement of healthy adults (Wu 2020). Because plants contain no taurine, creatine, carnosine, or anserine, and

TABLE 13.17

Content of Total Amino Acids (Peptide-Bound Plus Free Amino Acids) in Feed Ingredients for Farm Animals[a]

AA	Blood Meal	Cookie Meal	Corn Grain	CSM	Feather Meal	Gelatin	MBM	Peanut Meal	PBM	SBM	SBM (P)	SGH Grain
General Nutrients (% of Foodstuff, As-Fed Basis)												
DM	91.8	90.8	89.0	90.0	95.1	88.9	96.1	91.8	96.5	89.0	96.4	89.1
CP	89.6	12.3	9.3	40.3	82.1	100.1	52.0	43.9	64.3	43.6	51.8	10.1
TP	88.0	10.5	8.2	32.3	81.0	97.4	50.7	35.1	60.4	38.2	41.6	8.8
EA	41.9	3.3	3.0	10.7	24.9	14.4	15.4	10.7	18.4	14.5	15.5	3.2
NA	46.1	7.2	5.2	21.6	56.1	83.0	35.3	24.3	42.0	23.7	26.1	5.6
Individual AAs (% of Foodstuff, As-Fed Basis)												
Ala	7.82	0.52	0.71	1.42	4.18	9.01	4.78	1.86	4.91	1.95	2.08	0.96
Arg	4.91	0.58	0.38	4.32	5.74	7.68	3.67	5.68	4.63	3.18	3.12	0.41
Asn	4.67	0.40	0.35	1.57	1.67	1.42	2.21	1.80	2.73	2.10	2.41	0.31
Asp	6.20	0.45	0.43	1.94	2.92	2.86	3.08	2.52	4.10	3.14	3.40	0.36
Cys	1.92	0.18	0.20	0.70	4.16	0.05	0.49	0.65	1.05	0.70	0.69	0.19
Gln	4.32	1.44	1.02	3.60	2.86	3.03	2.81	2.66	3.54	3.80	4.11	0.85
Glu	6.38	1.92	0.64	4.59	4.81	5.26	4.05	4.18	4.89	4.17	4.53	1.18
Gly	3.86	0.78	0.40	2.12	8.95	33.6	8.67	3.17	9.42	2.30	2.72	0.39
His	5.57	0.22	0.23	1.08	0.88	0.74	1.19	0.95	1.30	1.13	1.15	0.23
Hyp	0.20	0.00	0.00	0.05	4.95	12.8	2.88	0.07	3.31	0.09	0.07	0.00
Ile	2.54	0.51	0.34	1.19	3.79	1.17	1.92	1.41	2.32	2.03	2.10	0.38
Leu	11.4	0.88	1.13	2.26	6.75	2.61	3.56	2.48	4.21	3.44	3.70	1.21
Lys	8.25	0.41	0.25	1.66	2.16	3.75	3.13	1.37	3.44	2.80	2.87	0.21
Met	1.16	0.19	0.21	0.66	0.75	1.03	1.10	0.47	1.39	0.60	0.64	0.20
Phe	5.83	0.50	0.46	2.02	3.95	1.67	1.85	1.93	2.36	2.21	2.44	0.51
Pro	6.29	0.98	1.06	1.89	11.7	20.6	5.86	2.29	6.72	2.40	3.18	0.96
Ser	4.49	0.56	0.45	1.72	8.80	3.44	2.08	2.03	2.67	2.12	2.35	0.46
Trp	1.30	0.15	0.07	0.44	0.79	0.22	0.39	0.38	0.49	0.62	0.63	0.10
Thr	3.95	0.42	0.31	1.25	3.97	3.45	2.42	1.67	2.85	1.76	2.03	0.32
Tyr	2.86	0.55	0.43	1.10	2.04	0.93	1.45	1.39	1.84	1.66	1.72	0.45
Val	8.21	0.53	0.44	1.69	5.76	1.96	2.23	1.69	2.89	2.09	2.25	0.50
Total	102	12.2	9.51	37.3	91.6	117	59.8	40.7	71.1	44.3	48.2	10.2

Sources: Li, X.L. et al. 2011. *Amino Acids* 40:1159–1168.

Note: CP, crude protein (N%×6.25); CSM, cottonseed meal; DM, dry matter; EA, total amounts of essential AAs; MBM, meat and bone meal; NA, total amounts of nonessential AAs; P, processed; PBM, poultry byproduct meal; SBM, soybean meal; SGH, sorghum; TP, true protein, which was calculated on the basis of molecular weights of AA residues in protein.

[a] Peptide-bound amino acids refer to amino acids in both proteins and non-protein peptides. Molecular weights of intact amino acids (AAs) were used to calculate the content of AAs in feed ingredients.

abundant provision of these nutrients from all kinds of meats further underscores the importance of animal agriculture for improving human health and well-being worldwide.

13.4.1.2 AA Score (Chemical Score)

Because of the difficulty in comparing the quality of proteins with different AA compositions, H.H. Mitchell and R.J. Block proposed using chemical scores to rank proteins in 1946. The chemical scores are now known as AA scores (FAO 1991). The rationale behind this method is that a

TABLE 13.18

Content of Total Amino Acids (Peptide-Bound Plus Free Amino Acids) in Additional Feed Ingredients for Farm Animals[a]

AA	BSFM	CBPM	CVD	FM-M	FM-P	FM-SE	SDPM	PBM (PFG)	SDPP	SDEP	Algae SM	Bermuda grass hay	DDGS
				Dry Matter (DM) and Crude Protein (CP) Content (% of Foodstuff, As-Fed Basis)									
DM	95.3	98.0	93.2	92.8	91.6	92.1	88.7	96.8	95.4	95.1	96.5	87.2	90.3
CP	42.0	68.1	67.2	62.4	68.8	64.7	55.2	70.2	69.8	48.9	68.8	12.5	30.1
				Individual AAs (% of Foodstuff, As-Fed Basis)									
Ala	3.14	4.54	4.12	3.63	4.74	4.59	3.51	3.98	4.98	3.43	5.85	0.89	1.90
Arg	2.64	4.75	4.02	3.67	3.58	4.15	3.59	4.15	4.94	3.82	5.18	0.58	1.19
Asn	1.93	2.61	2.50	2.26	2.28	2.60	1.52	2.56	2.57	2.69	3.34	0.52	1.11
Asp	3.04	3.93	3.66	3.33	3.41	3.87	3.72	3.86	5.17	3.60	4.29	0.73	1.49
Cys	0.69	1.07	1.22	0.67	0.72	0.69	0.99	1.04	2.65	1.37	0.88	0.17	0.52
Gln	2.51	3.88	3.73	3.60	3.39	3.96	2.78	3.41	4.49	2.90	4.25	0.63	2.33
Glu	3.44	5.34	6.34	5.32	5.13	5.97	5.77	4.75	6.77	5.48	6.81	1.18	3.04
Gly	2.91	5.94	8.25	4.26	5.09	5.87	4.95	6.86	3.40	2.45	4.19	0.55	1.08
His	1.71	1.36	0.75	1.41	1.43	1.46	1.29	1.31	3.66	1.45	1.29	0.24	0.78
Hyp	1.27	1.85	1.73	1.57	1.82	1.98	0.79	2.25	0.021	0.023	0.014	0.010	0.035
Ile	2.02	2.72	3.84	2.42	2.75	2.79	2.44	2.38	2.77	2.97	4.09	0.50	1.01
Leu	3.25	5.28	6.10	4.50	5.27	4.59	4.30	4.33	7.56	4.61	6.32	0.92	3.14
Lys	3.21	4.52	5.02	4.46	5.25	4.57	4.07	3.54	6.85	4.09	4.18	0.52	0.92
Met	1.20	1.43	1.58	1.97	2.16	2.03	1.20	1.38	1.97	2.01	2.17	0.19	0.63
Phe	2.18	2.70	3.70	2.31	2.31	2.65	2.33	2.32	4.74	3.04	3.88	0.59	1.36
Pro	2.92	4.30	5.53	3.72	4.27	4.80	3.16	5.07	4.32	3.39	3.12	0.52	2.01
Ser	2.34	3.05	6.45	2.52	2.91	3.28	3.37	2.62	4.99	5.39	4.35	0.50	1.33
Thr	2.55	2.77	1.99	2.50	2.85	3.14	2.85	2.56	4.45	3.10	4.13	0.53	1.08
Trp	0.71	0.76	1.03	0.70	0.68	0.70	0.63	0.63	1.36	0.97	1.02	0.18	0.24
Tyr	3.85	2.29	2.56	1.89	2.01	2.36	2.24	1.88	3.51	2.61	3.79	0.38	0.95
Val	2.87	3.32	5.57	3.02	3.65	3.25	3.05	2.91	4.96	3.57	4.36	0.66	1.45
Total	50.4	68.4	79.7	59.7	65.7	69.3	58.6	63.8	86.1	63.0	77.5	11.0	27.6

Source: Gilbreath, K.R. et al. 2021. *J. Anim. Sci.* 98:skz370; Li, P. and G. Wu. 2020. *Amino Acids* 52:523–542.

Note: BSFM, black soldier fly larvae meal; CBPM, chicken byproduct meal; CP (crude protein, *N*%×6.25); CVD, chicken visceral digest; DDGS, dried distillers' grains with solubles; FM-M, fishmeal (United States Menhaden); FM-P, fishmeal (Peruvian anchovy); FM-SE, fishmeal (Southeast Asian miscellaneous marine fishes); Hyp, 4-hydroxyproline; PBM (PFG), poultry byproduct meal (pet-food grade); SDEP, spray-dried egg product; SDPM, spray-dried peptone from enzymes-treated porcine mucosal tissues; SDPP, spray-dried poultry plasma; SM, spirulina meal.

[a] Molecular weights of intact amino acids (AAs) were used to calculate the content of AAs in feed ingredients.

deficiency of an EAA would limit the rate of protein synthesis from other AAs. A chemical score for a protein is obtained by the following steps: (1) calculating the ratio of each EAA in the diet to that in a reference standard (whole egg), i.e., Lys/Lys$_{egg}$ and Met/Met$_{egg}$; and (2) assigning the lowest ratio as the AA score. The major disadvantages of this method are that: (1) besides the availability of an EAA, balances among all EAAs and the dietary intakes of other nutrients (e.g., magnesium and zinc) also affect tissue protein synthesis in humans and other animals (Harper and Yoshimura 1993; Young 1987); and (2) the AA score ignores the digestibility and balance of dietary AAs.

13.4.1.3 EAA Index

B.L. Oser (1951) proposed the EAA index method to assess protein quality. This approach was based on the assumption that each EAA must make some contribution to the nutritive value of a

TABLE 13.19

Content of Nonproteinogenic Substances (Including Amino Acids) in Feed Ingredients

Feedstuff	Cr	CrT	CrP	Car	Ans	GSH	Agm	Spd	Spm	Put	β-Ala	Cit	Orn	Tau
					Animal-Sourced Feedstuffs (mg/kg Feed, As-Fed Basis)									
BSFM	3.5	178	226	127	0.00	154	615	127	33.7	20.2	25.6	9.4	3.8	90.0
CBPM	4.6	1,447	90	5,506	7,966	113	225	494	504	174	51.0	1.1	109	2,096
CVD	3.4	1,056	601	136	48.2	19.8	1,727	384	330	161	120	13.6	93.0	1,317
Feather meal	1.0	134	7.5	2.0	6.7	0.71	118	775	310	32.4	84.0	1.1	14.7	142
FM-M	59.2	3,575	1,751	125	0.00	35.0	220	21.1	133	97.6	26.9	64.7	223	4,089
FM-P	127	5,412	6,150	665	0.00	23.8	908	232	1,587	171	118	213	218	7,486
FM-SE	14.0	4,161	2,403	35.9	0.00	225	1,649	351	210	1,074	142	327	177	9,864
SDPM	42.1	2,716	1,430	955	66.7	175	7,027	1,361	1,431	530	81.2	1,400	1,539	1,638
PBM (PFG)	3.5	1,768	233	545	1,146	73.2	310	556	802	66.2	53.5	1.3	27.3	3,884
SDPP	3.3	44.0	92.0	1,407	382	48.0	0.00	17.1	16.1	57.6	16.0	3.1	5.5	2,455
SDEP	7.0	102	87.8	1.8	6.5	34.2	0.00	29.1	18.0	143	59.6	1.8	2.8	326
					Plant-Sourced Feedstuffs (mg/kg Feed, As-Fed Basis)									
Algae SM	0.00	0.00	0.00	0.00	0.00	33.9	32.3	294	26.4	3.4	3.6	4.7	3.8	0.00
SBM	0.00	0.00	0.00	0.00	0.00	174	303	1,130	385	18.8	8.2	22.7	18.0	0.00
SPC	0.00	0.00	0.00	0.00	0.00	172	61.2	57.3	13.7	8.8	6.3	21.1	1.6	0.00

Source: Li, P. and G. Wu. 2020. *Amino Acids* 52:523–542.

Note: Agm, agmatine; β-Ala, β-alanine; Ans, anserine; Car, carnosine; Cit, citrulline; Cr, Creatine; CrT, creatinine; CrP, creatine phosphate; GSH, total glutathione; Orn, ornithine; Put, putrescine; Spd, spermidine; Spm, spermine; Tau, taurine.

$$\text{EAA Index} = \sqrt[n]{\frac{100\,a}{a_e} \times \frac{100\,b}{b_e} \times \frac{100\,c}{c_e}}$$

FIGURE 13.7 Essential amino acid (EAA) index. The geometric mean of the ratios of EAA in a test protein to those in a reference protein (usually egg protein) is defined as the EAA index. a, b, and c represent EAAs 1, 2, and 3 in a test protein, respectively, whereas a_e, b_e, and c_e represent EAAs 1, 2, and 3 in a reference protein, respectively. Depending on animal species and developmental stage, the number of traditionally classified EAAs ranges from 9 (e.g., adult humans) to 12 (e.g., chickens).

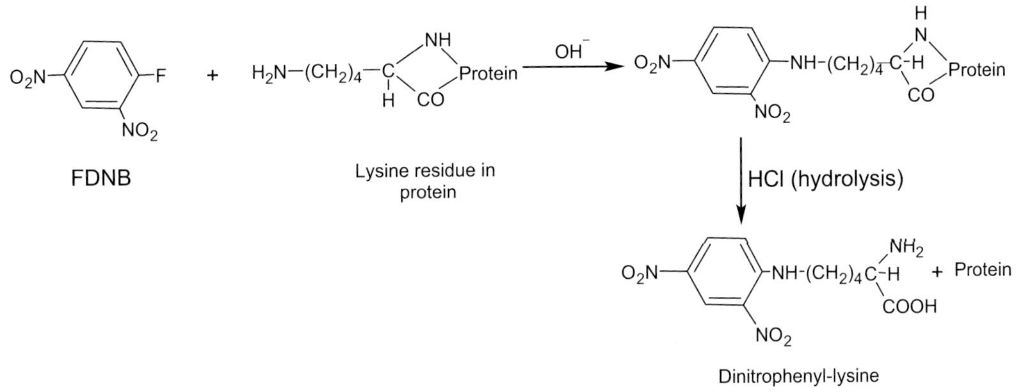

FIGURE 13.8 Dye-binding technique for the analysis of lysine involving the reaction between protein-bound lysine ε-NH$_2$ groups and 1-fluoro-2,4-dinitrobenzene (FDNB) to form a FDNB-protein derivative. After acid hydrolysis, dinitrophenyl-lysine is released for colorimetric determination. F, fluoride.

protein. The geometric mean of the ratios of EAAs in a test protein to those in a reference protein (usually egg protein) is called the EAA index. The mathematical equation describing the calculation of the EAA index is given in Figure 13.7.

13.4.1.4 Dye-Binding Techniques

A dye-binding technique involves assays of the reactive lysine content in a food measured by the difference between its dye-binding capacity before and after treatment with a reagent (usually propionic anhydride) to specifically block the basic ε-NH$_2$ group of lysine residues in peptide chains (Walker 1979). This is a very quick method to assess lysine content as a proxy for protein quality that assumes lysine is often the most limiting AA in a feedstuff. Orange G dye (trade name) interacts primarily with lysine and, to a lesser extent, other basic AA residues (e.g., Arg and His) of a protein at low pH. The amount of the unreacted dye is measured spectrophotometrically, and the amount of the reacted dye is determined by difference. As lysine is an EAA, its deficiency in the diet is expected to decrease the quality of the protein.

Another dye-binding technique involves the use of 1-fluoro-2,4-dinitrobenzene (FDNB; Figure 13.8). The lysine ε-NH$_2$ groups in an intact protein react with FDNB to form a covalently-bonded FDNB-protein derivative. After acid hydrolysis, dinitrophenyl-lysine is released and measured colorimetrically. This method is not highly specific for lysine but can be used to roughly estimate the lysine content of foodstuffs.

13.4.1.5 Mutual AA Ratios

This method was originally proposed by L.L.K. Morup and E.S. Olesen in 1976. It was based on the assumption that the optimum EAA ratios are of paramount importance. In this method, ratios of

EAAs in the test protein to those in a reference protein are calculated. EAAs in the test proteins are discounted if they are present in concentrations higher or lower than those in the reference pattern. The nutritive value of the test protein is predicted according to the ratios of lysine, threonine, tryptophan, sulfur-containing AAs, and aromatic AAs (Morup and Olesen 1976). Like all other chemical methods, the mutual AA ratio method fails to take into consideration the important contributions of NEAAs or CEAAs to protein nutrition in animals.

13.4.2 Animal Feeding Experiments

13.4.2.1 Overall Considerations

The quality of dietary protein is best evaluated by determining its bioavailability to organisms in a bioassay (Moughan 2003). Ideally, this is performed using multiple levels of a test protein in the diet that provides adequate caloric intake. Traditional concepts concerning protein utilization include (1) protein digestibility, which is a measure of the dietary protein-bound AAs that are made available to the animal after digestion and absorption; (2) biological value, which is a measure of how efficiently the absorbed AAs are utilized to synthesize proteins in the animal (namely, anabolic efficiency); and (3) overall protein utilization, as indicated by net protein utilization, which reflects both protein digestibility and biological value; this method has been most widely used in animal growth studies involving the utilization of dietary protein which can be either at a fixed amount or varying levels in the diet. Assessment of the quality or bioavailability of dietary protein can be made directly in human studies, however, with varying degrees of difficulty and high costs. Thus, feeding experiments can give meaningful information on the availability of dietary AAs to animals. Such studies normally involve small animals such as rats and chicks because of both practical convenience and low costs. These methods are summarized with appropriate equations in Table 13.20. In general, the overall efficiency of protein utilization by humans is lower than that in growing rodents, chickens, and piglets. Therefore, protein quality evaluation in nutrition should be performed to determine the relative efficiency of utilization of different protein sources and the absolute values. This further underscores the importance of using laboratory animals to assess dietary protein quality. A disadvantage of animal feeding experiments is that (1) bioassays are most specific to the animal being used in the assay, and (2) protein quality as measured in one animal may not be equivalent to that in another animal due to individual differences in requirements for AAs.

13.4.2.2 Biological Value

The "biological value" of a dietary protein was originally defined by K. Thomas in 1909 as the fraction of absorbed nitrogen retained in the body for the maintenance and growth of the animal. This method, modified by H.H. Mitchell in 1924, is a widely used procedure for the determination of dietary protein quality. A protein-free diet is used to measure metabolic fecal nitrogen and endogenous urinary nitrogen. This is because there is an excretion of nitrogen in the feces and urine in animals even when there is no dietary intake of AAs or protein. The biological value method is essentially a nitrogen balance technique. Major criticisms of this method are that the metabolic fecal nitrogen and the endogenous urinary nitrogen in animals fed a protein-free diet may not reflect their values under normal feeding conditions. This is partly because animals fed protein-free diets have mechanisms to spare nitrogen and, therefore, the endogenous urinary nitrogen and fecal nitrogen may be underestimated.

13.4.2.3 Protein Efficiency Ratio

In 1919, T.B. Osborne, L.B. Mendel, and E.L. Ferry introduced the protein efficiency ratio as a measure of the nutritive value of dietary protein for rats. This ratio is defined by the gain in BW per gram of dietary protein or nitrogen consumed. A standardized procedure for measuring the protein efficiency ratio was adopted first in Canada (1959) and then in the U.S. (1960). Subsequently, every new technique for assessing protein quality has been compared with the protein efficiency ratio method, which is the most widely used procedure for determining dietary protein quality and is

TABLE 13.20
Evaluation of Dietary Protein Quality for Humans and Other Animals

Method	Equation
(1) Chemical Analyses	
Chemical score	e.g., Lys/Lys_{egg} or Met/Met_{egg}, with the lowest ratio being the chemical score
EAA index	Geometric mean of ratios of EAAs in a test protein to those in a reference protein
Dye-binding	Reaction of Lys ε-NH_2 in protein with fluoro-2,4-dinitrobenzene
Mutual AA ratios	Ratios of EAAs in test protein to those in reference protein after discounting the EAAs that are present in concentrations higher or lower than those in the reference pattern
(2) Animal Feeding	
Biological value	$= [NI - (FN - MFN) - (UN - EUN)] \div [NI - (FN - MFN)] \times 100$
Protein efficiency ratio	$=$ weight gain/total protein intake
Net protein ratio	$= [\text{weight gain (test diet)} + \text{weight loss (N-free diet)}] \div \text{total protein intake (test diet)}$
Relative N utilization	$= [\text{weight gain (test diet)} + 0.1 (\text{initial} + \text{final weight})] \div \text{total N intake}$
Net protein utilization	$= [NI - (FN - MFN) - (UN - EUN)] \div NI \times 100$
Nitrogen growth index	$=$ slope of the regression of weight gain (Y-axis) on N intake (X-axis)
WBC-LTG	$=$ differences in whole-body composition and lean tissue gain within an experimental period
PDCAAS	$=$ lowest ratio for an EAA in test protein $\times$ true fecal AA digestibility/same EAA in a reference protein
DIAAS	$=$ lowest ratio for an EAA in test protein $\times$ true ileal AA digestibility/same EAA in a reference protein
(3) Metabolic indicators	
Concentrations of protein and free AAs in the plasma or serum; concentrations of ammonia and urea in the plasma or serum and urine; enzyme activities; whole-body protein turnover; flux of EAAs and certain AASAs in the plasma	
(4) MLA	
Utilization of protein hydrolysates by microorganisms and lower animals	

Note: AASA, an amino acid that is synthesizable *de novo* in animal cells; DIAAS, digestible indispensable amino acid score; EAA, nutritional essential amino acid; EUN, endogenous urinary nitrogen; FN, fecal nitrogen; MFN, metabolic fecal nitrogen; MLA, methods involving microorganisms and lower animals; NI, dietary nitrogen intake; FN − MFN, the amount of nitrogen from the diet that is excreted in the feces; UN — EUN, the amount of nitrogen from the diet that is excreted in the urine; NI − (FN − MFN) − (UN − EUN), the amount of dietary nitrogen retained by a test animal; NI − (FN − MFN), the amount of dietary nitrogen that is absorbed by a test animal; PDCAAS, protein digestibility corrected amino acid score; WBC-LTG, whole-body composition and lean tissue gain.

the official method in the U.S. The protein efficiency ratio assay requires that the protein source of interest is fed at a level of 10% protein in the diet. An advantage of the protein efficiency ratio is that there is no need to do a nitrogen balance experiment and only weight gains of a test animal are measured. A major criticism of this method is that weight gain depends on the amounts of food intake and may not necessarily be influenced by the quality of dietary protein. For example, an animal fed a diet containing a high percentage of fat but a low-quality protein may gain a substantial amount of weight mainly in the form of fat.

13.4.2.4 Net Protein Ratio

The net protein ratio method was proposed by A.E. Bender and B.H. Doell in 1957 to evaluate dietary protein quality. This technique is similar to the protein efficiency ratio, except that the consideration of maintenance required by the animal is included. Thus, weight gain, weight loss (on the protein-free diet), and protein intake by the test animal are usually determined. In addition, the original net protein ratio method requires that the protein source of interest is fed at a level of 10%

protein in the diet. This technique also assumes that the weight gain is directly proportional to high-quality dietary protein. This assumption may be misleading and invalid under some circumstances, as discussed previously. In addition, the percentage of BW gained as fat vs lean tissue in animals may vary with their intakes of energy and nutrients other than AAs, as well as their age and sex.

13.4.2.5 Net Protein Utilization

The net protein utilization method was originally developed by A.E. Bender and D.S. Miller in 1953 to accurately estimate nitrogen retention by animals. This bioassay is similar to the biological value technique, except that dietary nitrogen absorbed by a test animal is used in the net protein utilization method to replace total nitrogen intake in the biological value measurement. Calculation of values for net protein utilization is based on dietary nitrogen retained and total nitrogen intake by the test animal. Thus, this method is equivalent to Biological Value×Digestibility of Dietary N. Therefore, factors that affect the functions of the gastrointestinal tract will influence net protein utilization by animals independent of dietary protein quality.

13.4.2.6 Nitrogen Growth Index

The relationship between dietary nitrogen intake and BW gain in rats is usually curvilinear and can be considered essentially linear at the lower part of the curve. Thus, based on the finding that nitrogen retention is almost linear at points slightly above and below the protein maintenance requirement, J.B. Allison and H.W. Anderson proposed the nitrogen growth index technique (also called the slope ratio method) in 1945. The slope of the regression of weight gain (Y-axis) on dietary nitrogen intake (X-axis) is used to compare protein quality. An advantage of this method is that the slope of the line is affected by the utilization of dietary protein for weight gain in animals and is not independent of dietary nitrogen intake. However, a major criticism of the technique is that nitrogen gain can occur in animals fed lysine-deficient proteins (Bender 1982). In addition, the percentage of BW gained as fat vs lean tissue in animals may vary with their intakes of energy and nutrients other than AAs, as well as their age, and sex.

13.4.2.7 Relative Nitrogen Utilization

The relative nitrogen utilization method for assessing dietary protein quality was proposed by J.M. McLaughlan and M.O. Keith in 1975. This method includes a factor for the protein utilized for the maintenance and the value is expressed as a percent of that for the reference protein (lactalbumin). The authors assumed that 10% of the mean of the initial plus final BWs of an animal fed a protein-free diet reflects the maintenance requirement. In this assay, no additional animals are required to be on a protein-free diet. However, dietary nitrogen intake and weight gain of the test animal must be determined. A major weakness of this technique is that the components of weight gain in animals are not known and, therefore, may not be a valid indicator of dietary protein quality.

13.4.2.8 Whole-Body Composition and Lean Tissue Mass

The growth of lean tissue (mainly due to the accretion of protein) and whole-body composition in young animals (e.g., rats and pigs) are very sensitive to the amount and quality of dietary protein (Hu et al. 2015; Yang et al. 2015). The animals will gain more lean tissue but less WAT, when fed a diet containing adequate energy and high-quality protein during an experimental period (e.g., 2 months). Conversely, the animals will gain less lean tissue but more WAT when fed a diet containing adequate energy but low-quality protein during an experimental period (e.g., 2 months). Thus, the quality of dietary protein for young pigs or young rats can be assessed through: (1) the measurement of their initial and final BWs, as well as the analysis of their whole-body composition [i.e., water, CP (including true protein, AAs, and nitrogenous metabolites), crude lipids, carbohydrates, and minerals] at the end of the feeding trial. This can be accomplished through either the use of dual-energy X-ray absorptiometry (noninvasive) or the euthanasia of the research animals (e.g., rats, pigs, sheep, chickens, and fish). The proposed whole-body composition method is simple, rapid, and inexpensive (Hu et al. 2015; Yang et al. 2015), and the dual-energy X-ray absorptiometry technique can be readily applicable to humans of all age groups (McNeal et al. 2018).

TABLE 13.21

Suggested Patterns of Amino Acid Requirements for Humans for the Calculation of PDCAAS in Comparison with Amino Acid Patterns in Eggs and Cow's Milk

Amino Acid	Suggested Patterns of Amino Acid Requirements				Composition of Amino Acids in Food		
	Infant	Preschool Children (2–5 Years)	School Children (10–12 Years)	Adults	Eggs	Cows's Milk	Beef
			mg/g Crude Protein				
His	26	19	19	16	22	27	34
Ile	46	28	28	13	54	47	48
Leu	93	66	44	19	86	95	81
Lys	66	58	44	16	70	78	89
Met+Cystine	42	25	22	17	57	33	40
Phe+Tyr	72	63	22	19	93	102	80
Thr	43	34	28	9	47	44	46
Trp	17	11	9	5	17	14	12
Val	55	35	25	13	66	64	50
Total	460	339	241	127	512	504	479

Source: FAO. 1991. *Protein Quality Evaluation Report of Joint FAO/WHO Expert Consultation.* Rome, Italy.

Note: PDCAAS, protein digestibility-corrected amino acid score.

13.4.2.9 PDCAAS

The FAO (1991) recommended the protein digestibility corrected AA score (PDCAAS) to evaluate the quality of dietary proteins for human consumption. This approach can also be used in animal nutrition. In the PDCAAS method, a single value of apparent ("true fecal") CP digestibility is used as the digestibility of each EAA in the dietary protein. The ratio of the amount (mg) of an apparently digestible EAA in 1 g of the dietary protein to the amount (mg) of the same EAA in 1 g of the reference protein (the pattern of AA requirements) for preschool children is calculated for each EAA, and the lowest value (usually for the most limiting EAA) is designated as the PDCAAS. The pattern of AA requirements for preschool children is shown in Table 13.21. The equation for PDCAAS calculation is given below, with any value greater than 1.00 being truncated to 1.00.

$$PDCAAS = \frac{\text{Amount (mg) of the first limiting nutritionally essential amino acid (EAA) in 1 g of the dietary crude protein} \times \text{True fecal digestibility of the dietary crude protein}}{\text{Amount (mg) of the same EAA in 1 g of the reference crude protein for infants or preschool children (for other age groups of humans)}}$$

The rapidly growing rat (50–70 g) is the standard test animal used to assess the quality of dietary protein, as adopted by the FAO (1991). PDCAAS values for some common foods are provided in Table 13.22. Note that the FAO (1991) conferred the PDCAAS value of 1.00 to casein and egg white. With the rat model, Gilani and Sepehr (2003) and Rutherfurd et al. (2015) have determined that the PDCAAS score is 1.00 for whey protein. The PDCAAS values for milk, egg, and meat proteins are much greater than those of plant-sourced foods. Since 1993, the Food and Drug Administration of the United States (FDA; 1993, 2013, 2017) has adopted the PDCAAS of the FAO (1991) as the indicator of food protein quality. The FDA (2013, 2017) has also required that PDCAAS be used in calculating the percent daily value of protein in product labeling. The daily reference value of food protein requirement for a healthy adult human is 50 g/day (FDA 2013).

TABLE 13.22

Crude Protein (CP) Content, True Fecal CP Digestibilities, Amino Acid Scores, and Protein Digestibility-Corrected Amino Acid Scores (PDCAAS) for Foods[a]

Food	Crude Protein ($N\% \times 6.25$), %	True Fecal CP Digestibility (%)	Amino Acid Score	PDCAAS
Animal-Sourced Foods				
Beef	95.2	98	0.94	0.92
Casein	94.7	99	1.19	1.00
Egg white	87.0	100	1.19	1.00
Whey protein concentrate[b]	83.3	100	---	1.00
Whey protein hydrolysate[b]	84.4	100	---	1.00
Whey protein isolate[b]	---	100	---	1.00
Plant-Sourced Foods				
Black beans (autoclaved)	21.7	72	0.74	0.53
Chickpeas (canned)	21.2–21.4	88–89	0.74–0.81	0.66–0.71
Fababeans (autoclaved)	27.9	86	0.55	0.47
Kidney beans (canned)	18.9	81	0.84	0.68
Lentils (canned)	28.0	84	0.62	0.52
Lentils (autoclaved)	21.9	85	0.60	0.51
Peas (century, autoclaved)	13.9	83	0.82	0.68
Pea flour	30.8	88	0.79	0.69
Peas (trapper, autoclaved)	15.7	84	0.73	0.61
Pea protein concentrate	57.0	92	0.79	0.73
Peanut meal	61.2	94	0.55	0.52
Pinto beans (canned)	23.6–23.7	73–79	0.78–0.80	0.57–0.63
Pinto beans (autoclaved)	19.9	80	0.77	0.62
Rapeseed protein concentrate	68.3	95	0.98	0.93
Rapeseed protein isolate	87.3	95	0.87	0.83
Rice-wheat-gluten	20.3	95	0.27	0.26
Rolled oats	18.4	91	0.63	0.57
Seafarer bean (canned)	23.3	84	0.84	0.70
Soybean protein concentrate	70.2	95	1.04	0.99
Soybean protein isolate	92.2	98	0.94	0.92
Soy assay protein	93.0	95	0.97	0.92
Sunflower protein isolate	92.7	94	0.39	0.37
Wheat gluten	87.0	96	0.26	0.25
Whole wheat	16.2	91	0.44	0.40

Source: FAO. 1991. *Protein Quality Evaluation Report of Joint FAO/WHO Expert Consultation.* Rome, Italy.

Note: "---", values were not provided.

[a] Data were obtained from FAO (1991) for all foods except for whey protein concentrate and isolate.

[b] Data were obtained from Rutherfurd, SM. et al. 2015. *J. Nutr.* 145:372–379; and Gilani, G.S. and E. Sepehr. 2003. *J. Nutr.* 133:220–225.

The FAO (1991) has recognized that protein quality varies with the age of the individual consuming it. Because the pattern of AA requirements for preschool children differs from that for adults (Table 13.21), the pattern of AA requirements for adults should be used to calculate the PDCAAS values of foods to be consumed by adults. Thus, the current values of the PDCAAS for foods calculated according to the pattern of AA requirements for preschool children must be clarified as such. In addition, the PDCAAS method: (1) ignores co-limiting AAs and the balances of AAs (including AASAs) in dietary protein, (2) does not adequately account for the bioavailabilities of AAs in dietary protein, (3) does not credit high-quality proteins (due to the truncation of PDCAAS values > 1.00 to 1.00), (4) is also unfortunately based on the apparent (true fecal) protein digestibility that does not necessarily reflect true protein digestibility measured at the terminal ileum, (5) uses CP (which includes nonprotein and non-AA components) as protein in all components of the PDCAAS calculation; and (6) overestimates the protein quality of plant products containing anti-nutritional factors (e.g., protease inhibitors, amylase inhibitor, fiber, saponins, tannins, phytate, gossypol, lectins, and goitrogens) and the quality of poorly digestible proteins in diets supplemented with limiting AAs (FAO 2013).

13.4.2.10 DIAAS

In 2013, the FAO recommended the digestible indispensable AA score (DIAAS) method to evaluate protein quality in human nutrition. This approach can also be used in animal nutrition. The DIAAS is an improvement over the PDCAAS method because the new method is based on dietary protein (calculated as the sum of individual AA residues plus free AAs) and the true digestibility of the dietary protein (Wolfe et al. 2016). The FAO (2013) suggested that protein digestibility should be based on the true ileal digestibility of each AA preferably determined in humans, and in the case of no human data, in growing pigs (the most suitable animal model) or growing rats in that order. The AA scoring patterns of the reference protein to be used for the DIAAS calculation are those for (1) infants (birth to 6 months); (2) young children (6 months to 3 years); and (3) older children, adolescents and adults (Table 13.23).

In the DIAAS method, the true ileal digestibilities of individual AAs are used. The ratio of the amount (mg) of a truly digestible EAA in 1 g of the dietary protein to the amount (mg) of the same EAA in 1 g of the reference protein (the AA scoring pattern) for infants, young children, or other age groups of humans (Table 13.23) is calculated for each EAA, and the lowest value (usually for

TABLE 13.23

Recommended Amino Acid Scoring Patterns for Infants, Children, Adolescents, and Adults for the Calculation of Digestible Indispensable Amino Acid Score (DIAAS) in Human Nutrition

Amino Acid	Suggested Patterns of Amino Acid Requirements		
	Infant (Birth to 6 Months)	Children (6 Months to 3 Years)	Older Children, Adolescents, and Adults
	mg/g Protein Requirement		
His	21	20	16
Ile	55	32	30
Leu	96	66	61
Lys	69	57	48
Met + Cystine	33	27	23
Phe + Tyr	94	52	41
Thr	44	31	25
Trp	17	8.5	6.6
Val	55	43	40
Total	484.0	336.5	290.6

Source: FAO. 2013. *Protein Quality Evaluation Report of Joint FAO/WHO Expert Consultation.* Rome, Italy.

the first limiting EAA) is designated as the DIAAS. The equation for DIAAS calculation is given below, without the truncation of any values greater than 100% to 100%.

$$\text{DIAAS } (\%) = \frac{\substack{\text{Amount (mg) of the first limiting nutritionally essential} \\ \text{amino acid (EAA) in 1 g of the dietary protein}} \times \substack{\text{True ileal digestibility} \\ \text{of the dietary protein}}}{\substack{\text{Amount (mg) of the same EAA in 1 g of the reference protein for infants,} \\ \text{young children (0.5 to 3 years), or other age groups of humans}}} \times 100$$

There are still concerns over the recommended DIAAS method. First, the pattern of AA requirements for adolescents or adults is not used to calculate the DIAAS values of foods to be consumed by these individuals. Thus, the current values of the DIAAS for foods calculated according to the pattern of AA requirements for 3- to 10-year-old children must be clarified as such. In addition, like the PDCAAS method, the DIAAS method ignores co-limiting AAs and the balances of AAs (including AASAs) in dietary protein and does not adequately account for the bioavailabilities of AAs in dietary protein. Finally, like the PDCAAS method, the DIAAS may also overestimate the protein quality of products containing anti-nutritional factors that interfere with AA absorption and/or stimulate the utilization of AAs by microbes in the small intestine. To date, the DIAAS method has not been adopted by the FDA.

13.4.3 Metabolic Indicators in Animals

13.4.3.1 Concentrations of Free AAs in the Plasma or Serum

Concentrations of free AAs in the plasma or serum reflect their provision from the diet, rates of their synthesis and utilization, and rates of whole-body protein turnover to affect the release of AAs from proteins into the blood, and, therefore, are of important value in assessing dietary protein quality (Liao et al. 2018). Changes in plasma or serum AA concentrations are useful in identifying dietary deficiencies of some EAAs in nonruminants such as rats (McLaughlan 1974). However, the data should be interpreted with caution and evaluated according to the updated knowledge of AA metabolism in animals. For example, an increase in the plasma or serum concentrations of some AAs (e.g., leucine and glycine) may be an indicator of an inadequate intake of dietary protein resulting in increased degradation of intracellular proteins, rather than an excessive intake of dietary protein that is abundant in these AAs. On the other hand, the intake of excessive protein from the diet causes a decrease in concentrations of some plasma or serum AAs (e.g., threonine). This phenomenon has been referred to as the "dietary protein paradox" (Moundras et al. 1993). Nonetheless, reduced concentrations of arginine, proline, and glutamine in the plasma or serum of neonatal pigs are sensitive and useful indicators of their low dietary intake (Wu et al. 2014a).

13.4.3.2 Concentrations of Proteins in the Plasma or Serum

The liver of a 70-kg healthy human produces about 15 g albumin per day (Hou et al. 2020). Protein deficiency usually results in a decreased synthesis of proteins, including those exported by the liver (Evans and Witty 1978). In clinical medicine, the concentrations of some proteins (e.g., albumin, the most abundant protein) in the plasma or serum are often measured as a noninvasive indicator of dietary protein quality (Bender 1982). For example, during the period of recovery from protein malnutrition, patients fed a milk protein-based diet exhibit a faster rise in serum albumin concentrations than those fed an isonitrogenous, vegetable protein-based diet (Semba 2016; Waterlow et al. 1978). However, because the composition of AAs in albumin is not representative of other proteins in the body, the concentration of albumin in the plasma or serum alone may not reflect overall dietary protein quality. In addition, the concentration of albumin in the plasma or serum depends on the clearance of the protein from the circulation. Furthermore, hypoalbuminemia can be caused by some acute and chronic medical conditions such as nephrotic syndrome, hepatic cirrhosis, and inflammatory responses, independent of dietary protein quality. Nonetheless, low concentrations of serum albumin correlate with an increased risk of morbidity and mortality in humans and other animals, and, therefore, are a useful prognostic indicator (Waterlow et al. 1978).

13.4.3.3 Concentrations of Urea and Ammonia in the Plasma or Serum and Urine

As end products of AA oxidation, urea and ammonia concentrations in the plasma or serum and urine may be useful indicators of dietary protein quality. The circulating levels of urea and ammonia are generally reduced in response to the feeding of high-quality protein or a better profile of AAs but are elevated following the intake of low-quality protein. This notion gains support from studies involving animals, such as rats (Bassily et al. 1982), young pigs (Liao et al. 2018), and growing sheep (Wang and Lu 2002). However, it should be recognized that concentrations of urea and ammonia in the plasma or serum and urine may be influenced by the amount and quality of the dietary protein consumed, and by the activity of the hepatic urea cycle. Feeding large amounts of low-quality protein to animals is often associated with increased levels of urea and ammonia in the blood circulation because the oxidation of excess dietary AAs in the body is enhanced substantially due to their imbalance (Tojioka et al. 2011). Conversely, animals fed an adequate amount of high-quality protein diet exhibit relatively low concentrations of both urea and ammonia in the plasma or serum and urine but elevated levels of glutamine in the plasma or serum. However, metabolic acidosis is often associated with the increased urinary excretion of NH_4^+ independent of dietary protein quality. Furthermore, a deficiency of manganese (a cofactor of arginase) can also result in decreased concentrations of urea in the plasma or serum and urine, as well as increased concentrations of glutamine in the plasma due to the increased synthesis of glutamine from ammonia and glutamate, but these changes may not necessarily be caused by a low-quality dietary protein (Wu 2018). Thus, like concentrations of AAs, caution should be exercised in interpreting concentrations of urea and ammonia in the plasma or serum and urine. The urine volume over a defined period of time should be determined to calculate the total amounts of urinary urea and ammonia excretion in individuals.

13.4.3.4 Enzyme Activities

The enzymes which have been used as indicators of dietary protein quality include xanthine oxidase, catalase, arginase, aspartate transaminase, and glutamate transaminase in the plasma, liver, and/or other tissues (Harper and Yoshimura. 1993; Iwalokun et al. 2006). This is based on the assumptions that: (1) increased expression of certain enzymes is required to degrade excessive AAs in the body and (2) protein malnutrition compromises the integrity of cells (particularly hepatocytes), therefore releasing enzymes to the circulation. These methods have the potential to be good indicators of protein quality, especially when samples are obtained from the blood for analyses, but more work is required to establish their validity in practice. In this regard, it is noteworthy that cofactors are required for the catalytic activity of many enzymes. For example, hepatic arginase activity is decreased either when an animal is fed a diet with high-quality protein or when the diet is deficient in manganese (Wu 2018). Because there are diurnal changes in plasma or tissue activities of some enzymes (e.g., alanine transaminase and aspartate transaminase) within reference ranges possibly due to meal protein intakes and the effect of the biological clock, blood and other tissues should be collected from test animals in the same fed state (e.g., the same time after food ingestion).

13.4.3.5 Whole-Body Protein Turnover

Whole-body protein synthesis is maximized and whole-body protein degradation is minimized when the intake of high-quality dietary protein is optimized (Chapter 8). In addition, the skeletal muscle of healthy individuals responds positively to the increased intakes of high-quality protein, as assessed by increases in muscle protein accretion and mass (Chapter 8). Thus, the rates of protein synthesis and degradation in the whole body or skeletal muscle can be used to assess the quality of dietary protein (Tomé 2012). This method is most sensitive in rapidly growing animals (e.g., rats, piglets, and chicks) but can be applied to adults, and its disadvantages are high costs in chemical analysis and shortcomings associated with *in vivo* tracer studies (Chapter 7).

13.4.3.6 Flux of EAAs and Certain AASAs in the Plasma

Measuring the flux of EAAs (e.g., lysine and tryptophan; Young 1987) and certain AASAs (e.g., glutamine, glycine, and proline; Hou et al. 2016) in the plasma may be a potentially noninvasive method for assessing dietary protein quality. The assumption of this method is that the flux of an EAA in the plasma reflects the availability of the AA in the diet if the digestive and absorptive functions of the gastrointestinal tract are normal. However, determination of the flux of only one EAA or AASA will not reflect the amounts and balances of all AAs in the diet, and simultaneous measurements of the fluxes of many EAAs and AASAs are time-consuming, labor- and resource-intensive, and expensive. In addition, the flux of an EAA in the plasma is also influenced by its release from intracellular protein degradation in tissues, particularly skeletal muscle, and the flux of an AASA in the plasma may also depend on the rate of its endogenous synthesis. Furthermore, in humans and other animals, the flux of AAs in plasma is affected by both insulin secretion and the sensitivity of tissues to insulin, and the concentrations of BCAAs and aromatic AAs in serum are more responsive than other AAs to insulin levels and sensitivity. Thus, the flux of EAAs or AASAs in the plasma with respect to dietary protein quality should be carefully interpreted. Nonetheless, the use of this method, coupled with the direct measurement of protein synthesis in specific tissues or the whole body, will be a powerful approach to assess dietary protein quality. Disadvantages of this technique are that it is highly complex and expensive.

13.4.4 METHODS USING MICROORGANISMS AND LOWER ANIMALS

The principle of these methods is that good quality protein would better support the growth of the microorganisms that have the patterns of AA requirements for protein synthesis similar to those of higher animals (Evans and Witty 1978). Sample proteins are hydrolyzed by proteases or acid/base and the AA hydrolysates are included in the culture medium. Microorganisms and lower animals used for assessing dietary protein quality include the following: (1) *Tetrahymena pyriformis* (protozoa); (2) *Streptococcus fecalis* (bacteria); (3) *Streptococcus zymogenes* (bacteria); (4) *Leuconostoc mesenteroides* (bacteria); (5) *E. coli.* (a bacterium); and (6) mealworm (an insect). The advantages of these microbial methods are that only small amounts of sample proteins are required for an experiment and that many different feedstuffs can be easily and quickly tested at one time. The technique may also be useful for evaluating dietary protein for ruminants. However, the microorganisms-based methods cannot directly provide data on AA composition in dietary proteins or their digestibilities in the small intestine of all animals. Additionally, microbes commonly used to evaluate protein quality differ substantially from nonruminant animals in protein digestion, from the mixed ruminal microbes of ruminants in protein fermentation, and from all animals in peptide/AA metabolism. Furthermore, a heat-treated protein may not be utilized by ruminal microbes, but may still be digested by the small intestine. Therefore, the microbial methods are of limited value for evaluating the quality of proteins in feedstuffs fed to ruminants and nonruminants.

13.5 IMPACTS OF AA NUTRITION ON HUMAN HEALTH

13.5.1 GENERAL CONSIDERATIONS

Metabolism of AAs in humans occurs via multiple pathways (Figure 13.9) and is closely related to energy homeostasis. This is because intestinal AA absorption, AA uptake by extra-intestinal tissues, intracellular protein turnover, ammonia detoxification, purine and pyrimidine formation,

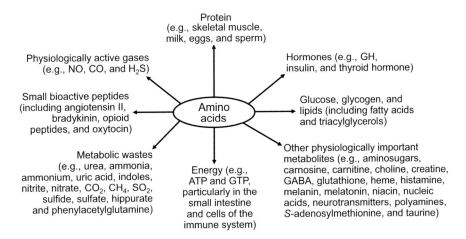

FIGURE 13.9 Utilization of amino acids (AAs) via multiple metabolic pathways in humans and other animals. Rates of the utilization of AAs for protein synthesis in tissues and, therefore, protein deposition in the whole body (particularly skeletal muscle), export of proteins by tissues (e.g., ~15 g albumin from the liver of a 70-kg fed adult person per day), as well as milk and egg production (in females), affect the rates of production of metabolic wastes (e.g., ammonia, urea, and gases) by the organisms. AAs are also used for the generation of bioactive peptides, small signaling molecules, and other physiologically important substances (e.g., creatine, carnosine, and polyamines). Depending on nutritional and physiological states, excess AAs can be either oxidized to CO_2 and water or converted into glucose, glycogen, and lipids. Of note, the small intestine utilizes certain AAs (glutamate, glutamine, and aspartate) as the primary energy sources in mammals, birds, fish, and crustaceans, whereas cells of the immune system (e.g., lymphocytes and macrophages) depend on glutamine as a major metabolic fuel. Thus, dietary AAs are particularly important for intestinal health. CH_4, methane; CO, carbon monoxide; GABA, γ-aminobutyrate; GH, growth hormone; H_2S, hydrogen sulfide; NO, nitric oxide; SO_2, sulfur dioxide.

renal AA reabsorption, and the excretion of nitrogenous metabolites require energy. In addition, the metabolism of many AAs requires NADPH for both biosynthetic and anti-oxidative reactions, with NADPH being generated from $NADP^+$ primarily via glucose metabolism through the pentose cycle. Physiological energy substrates in foods are fatty acids, glucose, and AAs; these nutrients exist primarily in the forms of triacylglycerols, starch, and protein, respectively. Therefore, ingestion of AAs must be considered in the context of the intake of other energy substrates and micronutrients (aiding in AA metabolism). The use of AAs as major metabolic fuels for tissues other than the small intestine and immune cells is not desirable because of their lower energetic efficiency, as compared with fatty acids and glucose. As discussed in Chapter 4, the extensive degradation of glutamate, glutamine, and aspartate (which are highly abundant in all animal- and plant-sourced proteins but neurotoxic at elevated concentrations) by enterocytes provides these cells with the most energy, while preventing the central nervous system from potential injury. Similarly, glutamine is utilized by lymphocytes, macrophages, and other cells of the immune system to produce a large amount of ATP; glutamine, glutamate, and aspartate stimulate DNA and protein syntheses in response to immunological challenges. Ideally, dietary AAs are balanced in each meal to support physiological processes, such as the syntheses of proteins and neurotransmitters that undergo continuous turnover in the body. A deficiency of an AA at any time will impair whole-body protein synthesis and increase the tissue-specific oxidation of all other AAs to ammonia and urea. Animal models can be used to develop mechanism-based methods for resolving significant issues over impacts of dietary AA intake on human health and disease.

The gross calories of fat, protein, and starch, as determined in bomb combustion, are 9.4, 5.4, and 4.1 kcal/g, respectively. The amounts of energy released from the oxidation of fat, protein, and starch to water and CO_2 *in vivo* are 9.4, 4.1, and 4.1 kcal/g, respectively. Because not all dietary fat, protein, and starch are digested in the stomach and small intestine, and because protein oxidation in the body is incomplete, the physiological values of energy in dietary fat, protein, and starch for humans are generally considered to be 9, 4, and 4 kcal/g, respectively. The resting metabolic rate of healthy humans, expressed as kcal/kg BW/day, decreases with age, ranging from 55 kcal/kg BW/day in the 5-year-old to 25 kcal/kg BW/day in the 45-year-old (Elia 1992). Because of energy requirements for physical activity (e.g., walking, lifting, and doing home chores) beyond rest, free-living individuals should have dietary energy intake above their resting metabolic rate. For example, a 45-year-old adult with minimum physical activity would need 30 kcal energy/kg BW/day (1.2×resting metabolic rate). Data on the impacts of dietary AA intake on human physical performance and health have important implications for livestock, birds, fish, crustaceans, horses, and other companion animals (e.g., cats and dogs).

13.5.2 Sarcopenia in Humans during Aging

During the aging process, sedentary adults exhibit sarcopenia that is characterized by a gradual decline in skeletal muscle mass and physical function (Lonnie et al. 2018; Tessier et al. 2019). For example, adults experience a 0.5–1% loss in skeletal muscle mass per year from the age of 50 years when receiving no nutritional intervention (Lonnie et al. 2018). This is due, in part, to a 20–30% decrease in muscle protein synthesis in the elderly (Chapter 8). Generally, sarcopenia affects people in their 30s and beyond (e.g., a 30%–50% decrease between the ages of 40 and 80 years). Sarcopenia increases the risks of falls, fractures, dependent living, morbidity, and mortality, as well as health care expenditure. With an increase in life expectancy due to improvements in living conditions and health management, the global aging population is increasing. It has been estimated, for example, that by the year 2050, 20% of the U.S. population will be aged >65 years (Mather et al. 2015). This will be associated with a dramatic increase in the incidence of sarcopenia, which will reduce longevity. Adequate protein intake (both quality and quantity) can play an important role in mitigating the progression of skeletal muscle loss and alleviating a significant public health concern worldwide.

It has been recognized that a mild loss of skeletal muscle mass occurs between 26 and 30 years of age in men and women (Silva et al. 2010). In both sexes, the age of 27 years is the cut-off after which skeletal muscle starts to show a negative association with age. Likewise, Lindle et al. (1997) have reported significant age-related reductions in concentric and eccentric peak torque in both men and women between 20 and 93 years of age. Furthermore, in 22- to 65-year-old men, the percentage of type-1 fibers (oxidative) in skeletal muscle increases but the percentage of its type-II fibers (glycolytic) decreases linearly with increasing age (Larsson et al. 1978), indicating a structural change of the muscle. Thus, it would be prudent to prevent skeletal muscle loss at an early age in adults through a combination of improved protein nutrition and regular exercise.

Sarcopenia also occurs in nonprimates during aging. For example, in Fisher 344×Brown Norway rats, the mass, fiber number, and cross-sectional area of skeletal muscle (*vastus lateralis*) are decreased by about 60%, 40%, and 60%, respectively, between 12 and 36 months of age, while the content of collagen in skeletal muscle is increased by ~610% during this 24-month period (Lushaj et al. 2010). In addition, aging cats lost 34% of their lean body mass over an 8-year period at an average rate of 4.3%/year (Cupp et al. 2007). Furthermore, aging dogs lose lean body mass over a 4-year period at an average rate of 2.4%/year (Adams et al. 2015). Finally, horses also lose a substantial amount of skeletal muscle mass and muscle function during aging (e.g., between 5 and 25 years of age) (Ochoa 2020). These animals are useful models to elucidate the underlying complex and multifactorial mechanisms responsible for sarcopenia in humans and develop AA-based strategies to mitigate this health problem. Although exercise can help to mitigate sarcopenia by enhancing the mass and function of skeletal muscle, such a means is unsuitable for the frail elderly who are not capable of physical exercise. Thus, adequate AA intake, hormonal intervention, or their combination is required to support healthy aging in humans (Sun 2020).

13.5.3   HEALTHY HUMANS WITH MINIMUM PHYSICAL ACTIVITY

13.5.3.1   The Current RDA of Protein

A sedentary lifestyle has a profound negative effect on skeletal muscle. For example, a 7-day bed rest in young healthy males can decrease leg muscle mass by 3% and muscle O_2 consumption by 4% (Ringholm et al. 2011). Thus, healthy humans must be physically active to prevent muscle loss. Based on the meta-analysis of short-term nitrogen balance studies in humans, the RDA of protein for the healthy adult with minimal physical activity represents only the minimum daily average dietary intake that meets the nutrient requirements of nearly all (97.5%) healthy individuals in a particular life stage and is currently 0.8 g protein/kg BW/day (Table 13.3). Dietary protein is assumed to be of high quality (a proper mixture of animal- and plant-sourced proteins) with a biological value of at least 75%, contributing to 10.7% of the total dietary energy (i.e., 120 kJ/kg BW/day for 31- to 50-year-old healthy men with minimal physical activity).

13.5.3.2   Functional Needs of Humans for Dietary AAs to Maximize Muscle Protein Synthesis and Mass

Cellular protein concentration depends on the balance between protein synthesis and proteolysis and is beneficially influenced by adequate intakes of dietary AAs. Gaining muscle is essential for the growth of infants and children, whereas maintaining muscle protein mass is critical for preventing sarcopenia in aging people. As indicated previously, functional needs (e.g., support of spermatogenesis, fetal survival and growth, blood circulation, resistance to infectious disease, as well as skeletal muscle mass and health) should also be an important criterion for recommending dietary AA requirements for humans. The consumption of a single meal providing 25–30 g of high-quality protein (0.333–0.40 g/kg BW) and adequate energy maximally stimulates skeletal muscle protein synthesis in the resting 75-kg young adult man (Phillips et al. 2012; Volpi et al. 2013). This translates to a daily intake of 75–90 g protein when 25–30 g of protein is consumed per meal for 3 meals daily (1.0–1.2 g/kg BW/day). An increase in skeletal-muscle protein synthesis occurs within 1–2 h after the ingestion of dietary protein or AA and is sustained for 3 h thereafter (Bohe et al. 2001; Rasmussen et al. 2000). The underlying mechanism involves primarily increases in AA availability and insulin secretion, as well as the activation of the MTOR cell signaling pathway to protein synthesis and inhibit proteolysis in skeletal muscle (Adegoke et al. 2009; Kimball 2014). Thus, concurrently-improved insulin sensitivity in response to AAs can help to mitigate sarcopenia in humans and other animals.

13.5.3.3   Suboptimal Values of the Current Protein RDA for Humans and the Nutritional Significance of a Higher RDA for Adult Humans

Estimates of dietary AA requirements by humans based on nitrogen balance studies are considerably lower than those obtained by AA oxidation methods. The differences can be up to 2- to 3-fold for many EAAs. These discrepancies likely result from both methodological and physiological factors. In all the various versions of recommended AA requirements, only EAAs are considered and represent 8%–27% of the RDA for protein requirement. This is a limitation in protein nutrition because AASAs are more abundant than EAAs in tissues and can also limit protein synthesis in tissues, including skeletal muscles (Hou et al. 2015, 2016; Wu et al. 2011). The current RDA of protein for humans is recommended to meet nitrogen balance without consideration of other physiological needs and, therefore, must not be regarded as the optimal amount for the maintenance, health, or functions of specific organs or the whole body. Deutz et al. (2014) have suggested that dietary protein intake be at least 1.0–1.2 g/kg BW/day for healthy elderly adults and 1.2–1.5 g/kg BW/day for malnourished elderly adults. The additional AAs required by humans are mainly AASAs.

13.5.3.4   Higher Recommended Protein Requirements for Adult Humans

Research findings over the past two decades indicate that the current RDA of protein is even insufficient for adult humans with minimum physical activity. First, elderly adults who consumed diets providing 0.8 g protein/kg BW/day for 14 weeks lost skeletal muscle mass (Campbell et al. 2001). Second, men and women (70–79 years of age) lost the most amount of skeletal muscle during a 3-year period when they consumed the lowest amount of dietary protein (≤0.8 g protein/kg BW/day) (Campbell et al. 2002). Third, increasing dietary protein intake moderately above the RDA by 25%–35% enhanced muscle protein anabolism and reduced the progressive loss of muscle mass in adults with advanced age (Campbell et al. 2001, 2002). Fourth, older community-dwelling adults (70–79 years) consuming 1.2 g protein/kg BW/day (as 18.6% of dietary energy) lost 40% less lean body mass over a 3-year period than those ingesting 0.8 g protein/kg BW/day (as 10.9% of dietary energy) (Houston et al. 2008). Thus, adequate protein intake is highly beneficial for healthy aging, and the optimum requirement of adult humans with minimal physical activity for dietary protein (high quality) is 1.0 g/kg BW/day and can be increased to 1.1 or 1.2 g/kg BW/day for the elderly (Morais et al. 2006). This is particularly important for the elderly with minimal physical activity, as they have a reduced ability to digest dietary protein and absorb peptides/AAs, have a lowered sensitivity to insulin, and experience progressive muscle loss if receiving no nutritional intervention (Lonnie et al. 2018). Finally, there are reports that frailty in the elderly can exacerbate the catabolic effects of aging on protein metabolism through a combined effect of increasing muscle protein degradation and reducing muscle protein synthesis (Morais et al. 1997, 2000; Chevalier et al. 2003). Long-term adequate consumption of high-quality protein is necessary to counteract sarcopenia in humans while improving their health and well-being.

13.5.4   Healthy Humans with Moderate or Intense Physical Activity

13.5.4.1   Benefits of Dietary Protein Plus Adequate Exercise on the Protein Synthesis and Mass of Skeletal Muscle

Moderate exercise is beneficial for improving skeletal muscle mass and strength, as well as whole-body health while reducing the risk for metabolic syndrome in humans consuming adequate AAs (Wolfe 2006). In addition, improvement in the sensitivity of myofibrillar protein synthesis to AA supply can persist for up to 24 h after resistance exercise (Burd et al. 2011). Furthermore, in the elderly, resistance exercise (e.g., weight lifting) can enhance skeletal muscle mass and strength (Layman et al. 2015). Of note, dietary protein and moderate exercise have synergistic effects on skeletal-muscle protein synthesis. Thus, the American College of Sports Medicine (ACSM 2009) has recommended strength training for the elderly to sustain muscle mass and function.

13.5.4.2   Negative Protein Balance during Moderate or Intense Exercise

During exercise, there is a negative balance between the rates of protein synthesis and breakdown in the whole body, as well as an increase in the rate of whole-body AA oxidation, resulting in a transient catabolic state (Rennie et al. 1981, Young and Torún 1981). The underlying mechanisms differ with the intensity of exercise. For example, exhaustive endurance exercise reduces the rate of protein synthesis without affecting protein breakdown in the whole body (including skeletal muscle), whereas a prolonged bout of resistance exercise results in an increase in the rate of protein breakdown in the whole body (including skeletal muscle) being greater than an increase in the rate of protein synthesis (Norton and Layman 2006). The magnitudes of these changes also depend on the type of exercise. Even moderate exercise (e.g., 1-h treadmill exercise at 55% of VO_2 max) enhances whole-body protein catabolism by 25% in healthy adults (Lemon et al. 1997). This translates into a dietary protein requirement of ≥1 g/kg BW/day.

13.5.4.3 Importance of Adequate Protein Intake to Prevent Muscle Loss after Exercise

During the recovery period after a single bout of moderate or intense exercise, unless sufficient dietary protein is consumed to increase muscle protein synthesis, protein degradation will exceed protein synthesis, resulting in a net loss of skeletal muscle mass and a negative whole-body nitrogen balance. In support of this view, healthy adults who performed intense exercise daily (9.9 kcal/min for six 20-min periods) for 3 weeks and consumed 1 g protein/kg BW/day exhibited negative nitrogen balance during each day of the training program (Young and Torún 1981). Furthermore, healthy human adults performing endurance exercise require 88% more dietary protein to maintain nitrogen balance than sedentary persons (1.37 versus 0.73 g protein/kg BW/day) (Tarnopolsky et al. (1988). Likewise, healthy human adults performing strength training exercise require 104% more dietary protein to maintain nitrogen balance than sedentary persons (1.41 versus 0.69 g protein/kg BW/day) (Tarnopolsky et al. 1992).

When the dietary intake of AAs and energy is sufficient during a post-exercise period of recovery, a positive protein balance occurs in the whole body (including skeletal muscle) (Biolo et al. 1997; McGlory and Phillips 2016). For example, compared with the placebo group (20 g dextrose), consumption of 14 g of high-quality protein (primarily whey) plus 6 g free AAs for 10 weeks at one hour before and after resistance training and one-morning bolus on rest days resulted in greater increases in fat-free mass (+2.92 kg), thigh mass (+0.32 kg), and muscle strength (+21% in bench press and +28% in leg press)] in previously untrained young men (Willoughby et al. 2007). In addition, compared with the placebo (flavored water), the acute ingestion of either 20 g whey protein or 20 g casein after exercise augmented the rate of muscle protein synthesis and the net balance of muscle protein (Tipton et al. 2004). Likewise, when supplemental whey protein (0.15 g protein/kg BW/day) was consumed for 24 weeks by postmenopausal women immediately after weight training, skeletal-muscle strength was consistently improved by 9%, compared with the placebo supplement group (Holm et al. 2008). Similarly, compared with the rest state, the fractional synthetic rates of mixed, myofibrillar, mitochondrial, and sarcoplasmic proteins in the skeletal muscles of humans were 30%–160% greater at 4 h following resistance or endurance exercise, depending on the types of protein and exercise (Table 13.24). Also, acute unilateral resistance exercise (leg press and knee extension exercise) augments cumulative myofibrillar protein synthesis by 25% in adequately fed humans over the 16 h following the exercise, when compared to the contralateral leg without exercise (Gasier et al. 2012). Furthermore, in adequately fed people, rates of muscle protein synthesis were increased by 112%, 65%, and 34% at 3, 24, and 48 h postexercise respectively, whereas rates of muscle protein breakdown were increased by 31% and 18% at 3 and 24 h after exercise, respectively and returned to resting levels by 48 h (Phillips et al. 1997). At each time point following

TABLE 13.24
Fractional Synthetic Rates (FSRs) of Proteins in the Skeletal Muscles of Adult Humans at 4 h Following Resistance or Endurance Exercise

Type of Proteins	FSRs of Proteins (%/h)			Increase Over the Rest State (%)	
	Rest	4 h Following Resistance Exercise	4 h Following ER Endurance Exercise	4 h Following Resistance Exercise	4 h Following Endurance Exercise
Mixed	0.04–0.06	0.10–0.16	0.10–0.12	160	120
Myofibrillar	0.02–0.05	0.05–0.11	0.03–0.06	129	29
Mitochondrial	0.05–0.10	0.10–0.15	0.12–0.15	73	80
Sarcoplasmic	0.04–0.06	0.08–0.10	0.08–0.10	80	80

Source: McGlory, C. and S.M. Phillips. 2016. In: *The Molecular Nutrition of Amino Acids and Proteins* (Dardevet, D., ed). Academic Press, San Diego. pp. 67–78.

exercise, the rates of protein synthesis were greater than those of protein breakdown, resulting in net protein accretion. The effective period for anabolism can last for up to 48 h after a single workout (Rasmussen and Phillips 2003).

13.5.4.4 Amount and Timing of Dietary Protein to Maximally Enhance Skeletal Muscle Protein Synthesis after Exercise

The consumption of 20 g high-quality protein after exercise maximally enhances muscle protein synthesis in healthy adult humans. For example, in adult participants (with ≥4 months of previous recreational weight-lifting experience) who consumed drinks containing 0, 5, 10, 20, or 40 g of egg protein after resistance exercise, muscle protein synthesis exhibited a dose-dependent increase in response from 0 to 20 g of oral protein and was maximally stimulated at the dose of 20 g (Moore et al. 2009). Instead of further stimulating muscle protein synthesis, 40 g of oral protein resulted in a marked increase in whole-body leucine oxidation rates (Moore et al. 2009). Similarly, in healthy adults (with ≥6 months of previous recreational weight-lifting experience) who consumed drinks containing 0, 10, 20, or 40 g of whey protein at both rest and after resistance exercise, muscle myofibrillar protein synthesis exhibited a dose-dependent increase in response from 0 to 20 g of oral protein intake and was maximally stimulated at the dose of 20 g (Witard et al. 2014). Ingestion of 40 g whey protein did not further stimulate muscle myofibrillar protein synthesis but markedly increased whole-body AA oxidation (Witard et al. 2014). Likewise, the ingestion of 20 g of whey protein in a meal every 3 h within a 12-h period was a superior strategy for stimulating muscle myofibrillar protein synthesis in healthy adults after resistance exercise (Areta et al. 2013). Furthermore, compared with a protein intake of <0.91 g/day in physically inactive adults (walking<0.8 km/day), higher protein intake (>1.11 g/day) in physically active adults (walking>3.2 km/day) is associated with beneficial improvements in body composition and cardiometabolic health in adults (Brown et al. 2019). Collectively, these findings indicate that consumption of 20 g high-quality protein (e.g., whey protein) in a meal is sufficient to maximize muscle protein synthesis in humans with experiences of active physical exercise at both rest and after exercise. A combination of adequate AA intake and regular exercise is an effective method to minimize sarcopenia and improve health in aging adults (Bauer et al. 2013) and in patients with type 2 diabetes mellitus (Campbell and Rains 2015). In these individuals, exercise will increase energy expenditure to reduce body WAT.

The underlying molecular mechanisms for the beneficial effect of protein intake on muscle mass and function involve: (1) the improved sensitivity of tissues (particularly skeletal muscle) to insulin and the activation of the MTOR signaling pathway to stimulate protein synthesis (Moore et al. 2011); (2) increased uptakes of glucose and fatty acids by skeletal muscle; and (3) activated autophagy to promote proteolysis for the provision of AAs as gluconeogenic substrates and regulators of metabolic responses (He et al. 2012b). In healthy adult men with moderate physical activity (90 min on a cycle ergometer at 45%–50% of maximal O_2 uptake two times daily), the frequent consumption of small meals providing 2.5 g protein/kg BW/day resulted in a positive whole-body protein balance, compared with a protein intake of 1 g/kg BW/day (Forslund et al. 1999). Thus, the net effect of exercise on muscle protein accretion critically depends on the sufficient provision of dietary AAs and energy. In adequately fed persons, the overall chronic responses of protein metabolism to regular exercise are anabolic and beneficial for inducing skeletal muscle hypertrophy, improving muscle protein mass and function, and preventing muscle wasting (Layman et al. 2005).

It is important to note that the timing of protein or AA consumption is crucial for muscle recovery after exercise. Skeletal muscle takes up nutrients (e.g., AAs, glucose, and fatty acids) from the blood circulation most efficiently within the first 30–60 min after an exercise program is completed, followed by great reductions several hours later (Wolfe 2006). Thus, the response of muscle protein synthesis to exercise-induced anabolism is much greater when AA intake is initiated immediately following exercise, as compared to 3 h after the end of exercise (Levenhagen et al. 2001). As noted previously, the proportions and amounts of all AAs in diets should be considered when specific

EAAs are supplemented to persons after exercise. For example, consuming individual BCAAs alone cannot enhance muscle protein synthesis when the availability of other AAs is limited (Leenders et al. 2011). This is because protein synthesis requires all 20 different AAs as synergistic building blocks.

13.5.4.5 New Recommended Requirements for Dietary Protein in Humans with Moderate or Intense Exercise

Based on the results of published studies, ACSM, the American Dietetic Association, and Dietitians of Canada recommend that endurance-training (moderate exercise) athletes and strength-training (intense exercise) athletes consume 1.2–1.4 and 1.4–1.7 g high-quality protein/kg BW/day, respectively, depending on the type of physical activity (ACSM 2009). For example, recommendations for dietary protein intake by adult humans are 1.2 and 1.4 g protein/kg BW/day for aerobic moderate and intense exercise, respectively; 1.4 and 1.7 g protein/kg BW/day for resistance moderate and intense exercise, respectively (ACSM 2009). Dietary intake of 1.5 g protein/kg BW/day has also been recommended for aerobic intense exercise (Geliebter et al. 1997). Due to the current obesity pandemic, future refined recommendations should be based on lean tissue mass or ideal BW appropriate for height (Simmons et al. 2016). A combination of whey protein (a rapidly digested protein) with casein (a protein that is digested at a slower rate than whey protein) seems to be an effective formula for skeletal-muscle protein synthesis after exercise. The inclusion of high-quality animal protein or combinations of high-quality plant-based proteins can stimulate muscle anabolism (van Vliet et al. 2015). As noted previously, the consumption of 20 g protein by adult humans at 30–60 min after exercise can maximize protein synthesis in skeletal muscle. Recent data also indicate that the adequate intake of protein at each meal of the day has an advantage over a large amount of protein in a single meal to support skeletal-muscle mass and function in individuals at rest and performing exercise (Layman et al. 2015).

13.5.5 OBESE HUMANS ON A WEIGHT-REDUCING PROGRAM

An effective weight-reducing diet for obese persons is to provide protein intake that meets their physiological needs while adjusting the content of digestible carbohydrates and lipids to create a calorie deficit. In addition, a combination of physical activity and increased intake of high-quality protein provides an effective strategy to enhance fat loss and improve metabolic profiles in obese persons. In a study by Layman et al. (2005), obese women in a 16-week weight-loss program were assigned to various intensities of exercise and protein intake levels. The authors found that the study participants in the high protein-exercise group lost 3 kg body fat without a loss of lean body mass, whereas those in the low protein plus exercise group lost both white fat and skeletal muscle. Similarly, combining exercise training with a higher protein intake (mainly derived from dairy foods) results in the loss of body fat and the preservation of muscle mass in obese people (Trouwborst et al. 2018). Augmenting the dietary provision of protein can increase the circulating levels of arginine, which enhances insulin sensitivity, stimulates the oxidation of fatty acids and glucose in skeletal muscle, promotes whole-body energy expenditure, and reduces white fat mass in obese humans (McKnight et al. 2010). Furthermore, in free-living subjects, adequate consumption of dietary protein can have a satiety effect and, therefore, reduce food or energy intake by inhibiting the release of ghrelin (an appetite-promoting polypeptide) and stimulating the release of peptide YY and glucagon-like peptide 1 (appetite-suppressing polypeptides) (Leidy et al. 2015). These changes in the endocrine status help to control white fat gains and preserve skeletal muscle mass in a long-term, sustainable manner.

On top of habitual protein intake (e.g., 1.07 g/kg BW/day in U.S. adults), additional consumption of 0.31 protein/kg BW/day to achieve an intake of 1.38 g protein/kg BW/day is beneficial for the long-term management of BW to minimize WAT and maximize skeletal muscle mass (Leidy et al.

2015). In healthy adults consuming adequate amounts of energy, as well as protein, carbohydrates, and lipids, dietary AAs are used to primarily support the intracellular synthesis of proteins and polypeptides, as well as low-molecular-weight bioactive substances. Interestingly, within 8 hours after healthy young adults consumed eggs (providing 23 g protein, 19 g fat, and a negligible amount of carbohydrate), only 8% of the dietary protein is used for gluconeogenesis and the remainder for the maintenance of whole-body protein turnover and tissue-specific AA oxidation (Fromentin et al. 2013). However, if the period with oral carbohydrate just sufficient to inhibit hepatic ketogenesis is prolonged, a much larger proportion of the ingested AAs must be converted into glucose to meet the obligate requirements of the brain for glucose (~125 g/day in a 70-kg adult). This compromises the above essential roles of dietary protein in the body.

There are reports that the dietary intake of high-quality protein required to optimize fat loss and improve metabolic profiles in overweight or obese persons is 1.2–1.5 g/kg BW/day (Kim et al. 2016; Krieger et al. 2006; Wycherley et al. 2012), is 50–87.5% higher than the currently recommended value of 0.8 g/kg BW/day. With these beneficial changes, adequate protein consumption can ameliorate metabolic syndrome and may extend lifespan in these individuals.

13.5.6 Distribution of Daily Protein Intake or the Frequency of Meals

AAs undergo continuous catabolism in mammals (e.g., humans, pigs, and rats), with half-lives ranging from 0.5 to 2 h, depending on AA and physiological state (Chapter 4). After the ingestion of a meal containing protein or AAs, the concentrations of AAs in their plasma increase gradually to peak values and then decline thereafter to baseline values within 4–6 h. Thus, in addition to the daily intake of total protein, the quantity of protein in each meal and the temporal pattern of protein ingestion are also crucial factors in influencing the balance of muscle protein synthesis and catabolism, and, therefore, skeletal muscle mass. The consumption of three meals a day, with each meal providing ~25–30 g of high-quality protein, can maximally stimulate muscle protein synthesis over 24 h in healthy young and older adults (Mamerow et al. 2014; Symons et al. 2009). The rate of skeletal muscle protein synthesis in healthy adults is 25% higher when protein intake is evenly distributed across breakfast, lunch, and dinner, compared with a pattern where most protein is consumed at the evening meal despite the same daily intake of total protein (Mamerow et al. 2014). In addition, spreading protein intake equally among three daily meals can improve muscle mass and strength in the elderly (Farsijani et al. 2016). These findings have important implications for improving skeletal-muscle mass, strength, and function in older, physically active adults who generally have resistance to stimuli of muscle protein synthesis and have a higher threshold of dietary protein intake to promote muscle protein synthesis (McGlory and Phillips 2016). Because humans usually eat breakfast, lunch, and dinner at regular times of the day (e.g., 7:00 AM, 12:00 noon, and 7:00 PM), the recommended values of their requirements for dietary proteins are intended for three meals in a day (~25–30 g of high-quality protein per meal). This should apply to both athletic and nonathletic adults, as well as growing children.

13.5.7 Sources of Dietary AAs

13.5.7.1 Plant- vs Animal-Sourced Proteins

Both animal and plant products are excellent sources of select vitamins (e.g., vitamin B_{12} from meat and folate from green leafy vegetables) and select minerals (e.g., iron from meat and magnesium from whole grains), whereas animal products generally provide more biologically available minerals than plant products (Wu et al. 2014b). Animal-sourced foods [e.g., meat, dairy products, egg, poultry, seafood (including fish and shellfish), and other products] contain higher quantities and more balanced proportions of AAs relative to human tissues, than plant-sourced foods (e.g., rice, wheat, corn, potato, vegetables, cereals, beans, peas, processed soy products, nuts, and seeds) (Hou et al. 2019; Moughan and Rutherfurd 2012; Wu et al. 2016). For example, beef contains 63%–68% protein on the dry matter basis (Wu et al. 2016), but most staple foods of plant origin (except for legumes) have a protein content <12% (dry matter basis) and are deficient in most AAs, including lysine, methionine, cysteine, tryptophan, threonine, and glycine (Hou et al. 2019). Additionally, proteins isolated from animal products or present in whole animal-sourced foods generally have a higher digestibility (~95%–100%) than proteins isolated from plant-sourced foods (~85%–92%) or present in whole plant foods (~80%–85%) which usually contain anti-nutritional factors (FAO 1991, 2007; Moughan and Rutherfurd 2012). To meet the Institute of Medicine-recommended dietary allowance of methionine plus cysteine by the 70-kg adult human, the daily intake of meat, corn grain, potato, sweet potato, wheat flour, or white rice would be 38.4, 371, 560, 897, 262, or 402 g dry matter, respectively (Table 13.25). A large amount of ingested starch can be converted into glucose and fat in the body, thereby possibly contributing to the development of hyperglycemia, obesity, and dyslipidemia, particularly in persons who are sensitive to high starch intake and have elevations of plasma cholesterol and low-density lipoproteins. A 38.4 g dry beef provides only 7.7 g lipids (Wu et al. 2016), which provide only 3.5% of the daily energy (2000 kcal) needed by a 70-kg adult. Note that lipids are an important source of energy and essential components in humans, and some fatty acids (e.g., oleic acid and conjugated fatty acids) in beef can increase high-density lipoproteins (HDL; "good cholesterol") and decrease low-density lipoproteins (LDL; "bad cholesterol") in the blood of men and women (Smith et al. 2020). Thus, an appropriate amount of meat can contribute to an AA-balanced, healthy diet for humans without inducing metabolic syndrome.

Several research findings indicate that animal-sourced protein has a greater nutritional value than plant-sourced protein to build and sustain skeletal muscle mass. First, dietary supplementation of 17.5 g milk protein per day during a 12-week resistance exercise program increased lean body mass more than an isonitrogenous amount of soy protein (3.9 vs. 2.8 kg; Hartman et al. 2007).

TABLE 13.25

Provision of L-Methionine (Met) Plus L-Cysteine (Cys) from Meat or Plant-Sourced Foods to Meet Requirements by a 70-kg Healthy Adult[a]

Variable	Meat (Beef)[b]	Corn Grain	Peanut	Pistachio Nut	Potato	Soybean	Sweet Potato	White Flour	White Rice
Content of Met plus Cys, mg/g[c]	36.5	4.43	7.58	7.36	2.67	14.1	2.85	5.52	3.68
True digestibility of food protein, %[d]	95[e]	81	91	80[f]	89	80	52	92	90
Needed intake of food[g], g/day	38.4	371	193	226	560	118	897	262	402
Content of Dig carb in food, mg/g[c]	31.4	834	174	280	840	316	881	844	910
Intake of Dig carb in food, g/day	1.2	309	33.6	63.3	470	37.3	790	221	366

Source: Hou, Y.Q. et al. 2019. *Amino Acids* 51:1153–1165; Wu, G. et al. 2016. *J. Anim. Sci.* 94:2603–2613.

Note: Dig carb, digestible carbohydrate (glycogen or starch).

[a] The recommended dietary allowance of L-methionine plus L-cysteine for a 70-kg healthy adult is 1.33 g/day (IOM 2005).

[b] Loin cut of beef.

[c] Values are expressed on the dry matter basis.

[d] Moughan and Rutherfurd (2012). The true digestibility of protein in soybean (cooked) was calculated as the average value for its constituent amino acids.

[e] The true digestibility of protein in beef (cooked) is 95% (Bax et al. 2013).

[f] The standardized ileal digestibility of L-methionine plus L-cysteine in roasted pistachio nuts is 80% (Bailey and Stein 2020).

[g] Food intake (dry matter basis) needed to meet the requirement for digestible dietary L-methionine plus L-cysteine.

Second, compared with an equal amount of soy protein, dietary supplementation with 24 g whey per day to young men enhanced their lean tissue gains after 36 weeks of resistance exercise training (3.3 vs. 1.8 kg; Volek et al. 2013). Third, the ingestion of animal-sourced protein by healthy adults ranging from 17.5 to 40 g from whey, skimmed milk, or beef stimulated skeletal-muscle protein synthesis to a greater extent than the same amount of soy protein under resting and post-exercise conditions (van Vliet et al. 2015). Fourth, long-term vegetarianism resulted in reduced skeletal-muscle mass in older women, compared with the consumption of an omnivorous diet (18.2 vs. 22.6 kg lean body mass) (Aubertin-Leheudre and Adlercreutz 2009). Fifth, the consumption of a meat-containing omnivorous diet contributed to greater gains in skeletal muscle mass and fat-free body mass in older men (51-69 years of age) with 12-week of resistance training, compared with a lactoovovegetarian (meat-free) diet (Campbell et al. 1999). Thus, as a nutritional strategy, the adequate ingestion of AAs from animal-sourced protein (e.g., nutrient-dense lean meat) can reverse a current decline in protein intake by adults in the age groups of ≥51 years. This simple means is vitally important for sustaining skeletal-muscle mass and improving health in aging adults.

An ideal human diet would consist of both animal- and plant-sourced foods in appropriate amounts and proportions to ensure the intake of sufficient quantity and quality of protein while consuming adequate dietary fiber. As noted previously, plant- and animal-based foods contribute ~65% and 35% of protein, respectively, in human diets worldwide, and the opposite is true in North America. While proper combinations of large amounts of legumes with cereals could sufficiently provide most AAs, the global availability of legumes as a staple food is increasingly limited and in many parts of the world, these foods are not produced (Akibode and Maredia 2011). At best, such combinations may meet protein requirements (0.8 g/kg BW/day) for adults with minimal physical activity to maintain a short-term nitrogen balance but not for optimal growth or development in children when a variety of plant-sourced foods is carefully chosen. In the home-bound elderly, consuming <65% of total protein from animal-sourced foods results in the deficiency of at least one EAA, leading to protein undernutrition (Dasgupta et al. 2005). Similarly, results of a recent study indicated that in the community-dwelling older adults of Canada, United States, and Europe, the prevalence of protein intake below the current recommendation of 0.8 g/kg BW/day is substantial (14%–30%) and increases to 65%–76% according to a proposed cut-off value of 1.2 g/kg BW/day (Hengeveld et al. 2020; Houston et al. 2008; Morais et al. 2006). In any case, the assessment of dietary protein quality solely based on ratios of EAAs to lysine without the consideration of the total amount of protein and its true digestibility is potentially misleading. Appropriate proportions of animal- vs. plant-sourced proteins in the diet (e.g., 65% vs. 35% for the elderly; Dasgupta et al. 2005) should provide sufficient EAAs and AASAs, as well as their optimal ratios relative to lysine. However, as noted previously, the consumption of a combination of different plant-based foods may result in a complementary effect to raise dietary protein quality and quantity, but greater care must be taken to achieve desirable EAA and AASA intakes than a diet consisting of adequate animal protein (Hou and Wu 2018). Recent advances in AA biochemistry and nutrition can guide the development of plant-based foods for human consumption and optimum human health. To prevent AA deficiency and stunting, children should consume sufficient animal protein.

13.5.7.2 Diets Based Solely or Primarily on Plant-Sourced Foods

Legumes and nuts contain relatively high amounts of lysine, methionine, threonine, and tryptophan, but these AAs, glycine, and proline are generally deficient in grains and vegetables (Hou et al. 2019; Mariotti and Gardner 2019). In addition, glutamate, glutamine, aspartate, asparagine, and the three BCAAs are abundant in all plant proteins (Hou et al. 2019), whereas proline can be synthesized from arginine (abundant AA in legumes and nuts), and glycine from other AAs (including proline, glutamate, and serine) (Li and Wu 2018). Thus, it is possible for adult humans to obtain adequate AAs from a carefully prepared mixture of plant-sourced foods with different protein quality and quantity. However, plant-protein diversity is crucial to ensure proper AA provision in individuals consuming diets based solely on plant-sourced foods (Salomé et al. 2020). This can be achieved through either advanced training to learn about the principles of AA nutrition and metabolism or professional advice from protein-nutrition experts.

There is epidemiological evidence that vegetarian diets consisting of whole-grain cereals, legumes, nuts, seeds, a variety of vegetables, and fruits may provide adults with many health benefits, such as reductions in risks for metabolic syndrome (including obesity, type-2 diabetes, hypertension, and other cardiovascular diseases) and various types of cancer (Fresán and Sabaté 2019; Kim et al. 2019). Such findings are highly significant in both nutrition and medicine. However, this kind of diet may include dairy products and eggs, and, therefore, animal protein and related nutrients that are absent from plants (i.e., taurine). Furthermore, nonstrict vegetarian diets (e.g., lacto-ovo, pesco-, and semi-vegetarian diets) typically contain dairy products and eggs. There is evidence that strict vegetarian diets do not provide taurine (an AA essential for cardiovascular, muscular, and retinal functions) and can cause taurine deficiency in children and adults (Chapter 5).

Debate exists about whether a certain amount of all-plant-derived protein (e.g., 55–70 g/day for a 70-kg BW) is adequate for the long-term health of adults, particularly the elderly (Mariotti and Gardner 2019). Nutritional adequacy of all plant-sourced diet foods in individuals should be assessed according to not only the concentrations of total protein (or albumin) and micronutrients in the plasma but also those of taurine, other AAs (e.g., methionine, histidine, and tryptophan), and hemoglobin, as well as functional variables (e.g., skeletal-muscle protein concentrations and strength). Given a limited intake of total protein by many elderly people, they have a high risk for protein deficiency when their diets contain no animal-sourced foods or <65% of their dietary protein is derived from animal products (Dasgupta et al. 2005). Because children usually eat foods prepared by their parents, all-plant-based foods may result in a high risk for AA deficiency and, therefore, stunting and impaired physical development. This is clearly illustrated by the finding that in China, as the consumption of animal-source foods was increased by 115% and that of grain foods was decreased by 43% between 1990 and 2010, the prevalence of growth stunting in children under 5 years of age decreased from 33% in 1990 to 9.5% in 2010 (Wu et al. 2014c). Thus, children and adolescents should be encouraged to consume both plant- and animal-sourced foods providing adequate AAs to prevent growth restriction and optimize health.

13.5.7.3 Differential Effects of Different Animal Proteins on Protein Accretion in the Body

The speed of the digestion of various animal-sourced proteins and their AA composition can differ substantially. For example, individual AAs are released more rapidly from whey protein (a "fast-release" protein digested within 1 h) than casein (a "slow-release" protein) in the small intestine to elevate plasma AA concentrations and support muscle protein synthesis in the resting state or after exercise (Dangin et al. 2003). In addition, the nutritional quality of animal-sourced proteins is not equal even though they are all highly digestible in the human gastrointestinal tract. Furthermore, there are age-dependent differential nutritional values of animal-sourced proteins in humans. For example, in young men, the ingestion of 30 g bovine casein induced a higher rate of protein accretion in the whole body due to a longer period of elevated AA concentration in the plasma, when compared with the ingestion of 30 g bovine whey protein (Dangin et al. 2001). It is also possible that young men can effectively generate cysteine from methionine to compensate for the severe deficiency of cysteine in casein. By contrast, the consumption of whey protein (0.48 g/kg BW) is more effective than the same amount of casein protein for protein gains in healthy elderly men with minimal physical activity (Dangin et al. 2003). Likewise, the consumption of whey protein stimulated postprandial muscle protein synthesis and accretion more effectively than casein or casein hydrolysate in elderly men (Pennings et al. 2011). The underlying mechanisms may be complex, and one of them may be that whey protein provides an abundant amount of cysteine for protein synthesis and other metabolic pathways in aging adults, and the elderly have a reduced ability to convert methionine into cysteine.

13.5.8 Protein Intake and AA Deficiency in Humans

13.5.8.1 Global Protein Intake by Adult Humans

Protein sources of human diets include animal- (e.g., dairy products, eggs, fish, and meats) and plant- (e.g., cereals, legumes, potatoes, cassava, vegetables, and fruits) based agricultural products. The mean protein intake per adult person varies greatly among different regions [for example, from <0.66 g/kg BW/day in some developing nations (Schönfeldt and Hall 2012) to ~1.2 g/kg BW/day in North America (Berryman et al. 2018)]. Plant- and animal-based foods contribute ~65% and ~35%, respectively, of protein in human diets on a worldwide basis, and ~32% and ~68% of protein in human diets, respectively, in North America (Wu et al. 2014b). Note that these are population mean values, with either lower or higher values for some individuals. Adequate AA intake is essential for: (1) optimizing the growth and development of fetuses and children; (2) preserving skeletal muscle mass during adulthood, inactivity (e.g., bed rest, spaceflight, or microgravity), or the experience of certain metabolic dysfunction (e.g., hypertension and other cardiometabolic syndromes, obesity, and type 2 diabetes); (3) improving anti-oxidative and immune responses; and (4) maintaining the health and well-being of people in all age groups, including the elderly (Phillips et al. 2020; Wu 2016).

13.5.8.2 Global Scope and Consequences of Protein Deficiencies

AA deficiency affects about one billion people worldwide, including (1) 165 million children under 5 years of age; (2) more than 50% of the home-bound elderly receiving home-delivered meals in the United States; and (3) 25%–85% of patients with a plethora of diseases and disorders (e.g., cancers, renal failure, cardiometabolic diseases, dementia, and burns) in long-term care facilities (Wu 2016). Dietary AA deficiency not only contributes to compromised pregnancies (e.g., reductions in the survival and growth of conceptuses), stunting, cardiovascular dysfunction, impaired immunity, and high risk for infectious disease (e.g., recurrent viral or bacterial infections) but also exacerbates the deficiencies of other nutrients (including vitamin A and iron) and worsens metabolic profiles (e.g., dyslipidemia and hyperglycemia) in humans and other animals (Chauhan et al. 1965; Herring et al. 2018; Langley-Evans 2007; Li et al. 2007; Smythe et al. 1962; Wharton et al. 1967). Other clinical symptoms for protein deficiency (hypoproteinemia) include low concentrations of total proteins (particularly albumin), trace minerals, and lipid-soluble vitamins in the plasma; fatigue and weakness; the loss of hair, brittle nails and dry skin, liver abnormality, and edema; mood changes and irritability; and cardiac failure (Wharton et al. 1967; Wu 2016). These disorders occur because an insufficient provision of dietary AAs impairs their roles in: (1) the digestion and absorption of dietary nutrients by the small intestine; (2) antioxidative and immune responses; (3) the synthesis of protein carriers that transport nutrients (including long-chain fatty acids, vitamin A, and iron) and other molecules (e.g., cholesterol and triacylglycerols) in the blood; (4) the biological oxidation of fatty acids and glucose to water and CO_2 for ATP production and fuel homeostasis; and (5) the syntheses of NO, hormones, neurotransmitters, and other bioactive molecules that are essential to life (Chapter 11). A severe deficiency of an AA can cause death, as indicated by an inadequate provision of arginine and the resultant hyperammonemia in infants (Heird et al. 1972).

Inadequate AA intake during gestation and postnatal periods has far-reaching adverse consequences in humans and other animals through mechanisms involving fetal and neonatal programming (Herring et al. 2018; Wang et al. 2012). This nutritional problem causes not only impairments in the growth and development of fetuses and live-born offspring but also a high risk for metabolic syndrome (including hypertension, obesity, and diabetes) and a low quality of life as adults. Of particular interest, stunting in boys and girls has serious negative effects on society and human physical strength, as well as the health (including reproductive health) of affected individuals and their generations of offspring (Langley-Evans 2007). In the elderly population, protein undernutrition exacerbates sarcopenia and further compromises skeletal muscle function (Wolfe 2006), leading to dynapenia (the loss of muscle strength; Tessier et al. 2019).

13.5.8.3   Means to Prevent AA Deficiency in Humans

In regular feeding practice, protein from food is the major source of AAs for humans. As noted previously, the quantity and quality of dietary protein are determinants of the adequacy of AA nutrition in organisms, including humans as well farm and companion animals. Consumption of animal-based foods (e.g., lean beef, fish, pork, and poultry) with high protein content and quality (Wu et al. 2014; Wu 2016), or dietary supplementation with specific AAs (Dillon 2013; Fukagawa 2013; Smriga et al. 2004), is a simple and effective means to ameliorate the impairment of growth and development in millions of children and aging elderly worldwide. For example, in 7-year-old children in Kenya who consumed basal diets (7,300 kJ/day) consisting of almost exclusively staple crops (corn and beans) that met energy requirement, isocaloric supplementation (1,050–1,255 kJ/day) with meat improved growth and cognitive development (Grillenberger et al. 2003). Of particular note, supplementation with animal protein increased upper arm muscle area by 80% in Kenyan children, compared with the control group. Similarly, in China, as the consumption of animal-sourced foods increased by 115% between 1990 and 2010, the prevalence of growth stunting in children under 5 years of age decreased from 33% in 1990 to 9.5% in 2010 (Wu et al. 2014b). Likewise, in low-income countries, consumption of milk and other animal-sourced foods by undernourished children improved anthropometric indices, while reducing morbidity and mortality (Dror and Allen 2011). In addition, ingestion of animal protein as ≥65% of total dietary protein can prevent protein deficiency in the elderly (Dasgupta et al. 2005). Furthermore, in diabetic patients, the insulin resistance of tissues (e.g., skeletal muscle) in the regulation of protein synthesis and catabolism makes the utilization of ingested protein and the restraint of protein breakdown inefficient (Marliss and Gougeon 2002). In support of this view, postprandial hyperaminoacidaemia can overcome the insulin resistance of protein anabolism (Bassil et al. 2011a) and adequate AA intake is necessary to mitigate muscle loss in patients with type 2 diabetes (Campbell and Rains 2015). These findings indicate that plant proteins alone may not be adequate to support maximal growth and development in infants and children or optimize health and well-being in adults.

13.5.8.4   Restriction of Dietary AAs or Protein for Medical Therapy and Longevity

13.5.8.4.1   Cancers

AAs are major energy and protein substrates in tumors. Thus, there is an interesting hypothesis that restricting dietary AAs or protein may starve cancer cells, thereby inhibiting their growth (Kang 2020). For example, feeding a purified diet containing no serine or glycine beginning at the age of 60–80 days after birth impeded tumor growth in autochthonous tumors in genetically engineered mouse models of intestinal cancer or lymphoma, while enhancing their survival (Maddocks et al. 2017). However, in the serine- and glycine-free diet, all other AAs increased proportionally to achieve the same total AA content as that in the control diet. Thus, the control and therapy diets were not isonitrogenous and differed in the content of not only serine and glycine but also all other AAs. This experimental design seriously confounded data interpretation to preclude a definite conclusion from the study. It is possible that the increase in the combination of all AAs but serine and glycine or some of them, rather than the simultaneous absence of serine plus glycine, contributes to the benefit of the serine-and glycine-free diet. Further complicating this picture is that the authors did not provide data on food intake by the two groups of mice. Of particular note, Weber et al. (1983) reported that dietary protein deficiency reduced the growth of primary and metastatic hepatoma in rats, but substantially increased their mortality. Thus, adequate AA nutrition must be considered in cancer prevention and therapy. Taken together, it can be surmised that an increase in the intake of certain AAs, rather than a deficiency of a few or all AAs, may be beneficial for the survival of animals with cancers. Limiting dietary AA intake below physiological needs will promote negative nitrogen balance and, therefore, will not likely improve the health or survival of cancer patients.

13.5.8.4.2 Obesity and Type 2 Diabetes Mellitus

Another recent provocative suggestion regarding the role of AA deficiency in medical therapy is the use of leucine deprivation to treat obesity or type 2 diabetes. Specifically, feeding a leucine-free diet to mice for 7 days was found to reduce their white adipose, lean tissue, and whole-body weight (Cheng et al. 2010). Thus, these authors proposed that the short-term deprivation or restriction of dietary leucine could be used to treat obesity and associated metabolic diseases. Similarly, in a study involving diet-induced obese mice, feeding an AA-adequate diet for 14 weeks decreased body weight (by ~30%) and lean tissue mass (by ~25%) but enhanced insulin sensitivity, when compared to a diet containing insufficient amounts of either all EAAs or three BCAAs that were only 23% of either all EAAs or the BCAAs in the adequate diet (Cummings et al. 2017). Such a severe dietary deficiency of either all EAAs or only three BCAAs can result in a great decrease in the whole-body synthesis of proteins (including enzymes responsible for lipogenesis) and a negative nitrogen balance and is harmful to the health and survival of humans and other animals. It should also be borne in mind that leucine, isoleucine, and valine are not formed *de novo* in all animals (including humans) and must be sufficiently included in the diet for their protein synthesis, maintenance, and survival. A dietary intervention based on a severe deficiency of any EAA, if used for a long term, will cause tremendous health problems and even deaths in patients with obesity or type 2 diabetes and, therefore, should not be touted as scientifically sound therapy. To avoid this concern, Wei et al. (2018) fed db/db mice (a type 2 diabetic model) a leucine-free diet every other day for 8 weeks. Although the intermittent leucine-free diet attenuated hyperglycemia in the animals, their fasting blood glucose concentration (11 mM) remained very high within the range of severe diabetes. The lack of dietary leucine will cause AA imbalances, inhibit whole-body protein synthesis, impair neurological function, result in metabolic burdens on the liver (producing excess amounts of both ammonia and urea) and the kidneys (excreting the wastes in the urine), and increase the risk for ammonia toxicity. Therefore, such nutritional management will have adverse effects on vital organs (particularly the liver, kidneys, and brain) and, therefore, should not be adopted to treat patients with type 2 diabetes.

13.5.8.4.3 Longevity

As humans and other animals continue to age, their rates of energy expenditure are gradually decreased. Results of an early study indicated that restricting energy intake by up to 65% (albeit too severe for humans) retarded the aging process and increased lifespan in mice (Weindruch et al. 1986). These authors did not report whether restricting AA or protein intake *per se* could result in the same outcome. Subsequent studies with male (Fischer 344) rats showed that reducing the dietary content of methionine from 0.86% to 0.17% beginning at 6 weeks of age completely abolished their growth but resulted in a 30% increase in their life-span (Orentreich et al. 1993). Stunting is a severe adverse effect of nutritional treatment and should not be recommended for humans. A careful examination of this study revealed that the content of methionine in the control diet (containing 0.86% methionine) was 33% higher than that in a normal diet for young rats (Wu et al 1999b) and substantially exceeded normal methionine requirement for adult rats (Jobgen et al. 2009). Because the excess production of some metabolites (e.g., H_2S, methanethiol, and sulfate) of methionine is toxic, the high intake of methionine in the control diet may have adverse effects on animals. Thus, the higher longevity of rats fed the 0.17%-methionine diet (Orentreich et al. 1993) occurred possibly because of a shortened lifespan of animals in the control group but not necessarily a beneficial response to dietary methionine restriction.

Similarly, a study with female mice showed that reducing the dietary content of methionine from 0.43% to 0.11%, 0.12%, and 0.15% at 6 weeks, 4 months, and 6 months of age, respectively, substantially impaired their growth but moderately increased life-span (Miller et al. 2005). Unfortunately, the basal diet used in the study lacked cysteine or cystine, tyrosine, and most AASAs and, therefore, was neither balanced in AAs nor representative of a normal diet consumed by humans. Such an imbalanced diet could be used in scientific experiments but should not be fed to any individuals as a nutritionally desirable means for improving their health and longevity. Using the same breed of rats and the same diets as those previously reported by Orentreich et al. (1993), Hasek et al. (2010) found that dietary methionine restriction appeared to enhance both food/energy intake per kg BW and whole-body energy expenditure per kg fat-free body mass. However, because rats fed the high- and low-methionine diets possessed different masses of WAT (which has a much lower metabolic rate than lean tissues), interpretation of the data is confounded because they were expressed in different units of measurement. As indicated previously, there are concerns over the content of methionine in both diets.

To date, there is no compelling evidence for supporting the use of protein- or AA-restricted diets as the optimum nutritional means for enhancing longevity in humans or other animals. Any diets designed for increasing the lifespan of individuals should not compromise their growth or health (including immune and anti-oxidative responses). Future experiments with scientifically sound design and rationale are warranted to determine whether a reduction in the ingestion of a specific AA, a group of AAs, or all AAs within physiological ranges can result in long-term benefits on physical strength, health, longevity, and life quality.

13.5.9 Safe (Tolerable) Upper Limits of Dietary Protein Intake by Humans

The tolerable upper intake level of a nutrient is defined as the highest level of daily nutrient intake that is likely to pose no risk of adverse health effects to almost all individuals in the general population (IOM 2005). An adverse effect is defined as any significant alteration in the structure of humans or any impairment of a physiologically important function. An intake above the upper intake limit will increase the risk of adverse effects. Safe (tolerable) upper limits for dietary protein intake (maximum safe intake) by young and adult humans have not been established and can differ among individuals and metabolic conditions. Like any nutrient, divided protein intake at different meals of the day is preferred to reduce a sudden excess of any AAs in the gastrointestinal tract, liver, brain, heart, kidneys, and other tissues. The IOM (2005) recommended an acceptable macronutrient distribution range for protein intake at 10%–35% of total energy for adults. Note that dietary intake of energy should not exceed requirements and that the safety of protein intake is influenced by the ingestion of carbohydrates and lipids (Wu 2016). In view of large variations among people in any age population, caution must be exercised not to adopt "one shoe fits all" guidelines when establishing safe upper limits of dietary protein intake by humans.

13.5.9.1 Healthy Infants and Children

Results of dietary surveys indicate that protein intake by infants during the complementary feeding (a combination of breast- and formula feeding) period in industrialized countries is generally 2–3 times the RDA value. For example, in the 1997 Copenhagen Cohort Study, the median protein intake of healthy 12-month-old weaned infants in Denmark was 3.2 g/kg BW/day (14% of energy intake) and the 90th percentile was 4.7 g/kg BW/day (18% of energy intake) (Michaelsen 1997). The mean protein intake of healthy 9–12 month-old infants in other industrialized European countries was even higher than that from the Copenhagen Cohort Study, with the highest value being in Italy where the mean intake of protein was 5.1 g/kg BW/day (19.5% of energy intake) (Rolland-Cachera et al. 1999). In healthy older (2.5-year-old) Danish children, the 10th, 50th, and 90th percentiles of dietary protein intake were 2.4, 2.9, and 4.0 g/kg BW/day, respectively, with 63% of the dietary protein being derived from animal-sourced foods (Hoppe et al. 2004). These data indicate that healthy 1- to 3-year-old children can tolerate a dietary intake of 5 g protein/kg BW/day (Table 13.26). For comparison, young pigs and preweaning ruminants can well tolerate 20% protein in their diets (on the as-fed basis; 90% DM; Bergen 2021; Cao et al. 2021; Gilbreath et al. 2021).

TABLE 13.26

Safe Upper Limits and Recommended Values of Dietary Protein Intakes by Healthy Humans

Group (Age)	Safe Upper Limits of Dietary Protein Intake		Recommended Values of Dietary Protein Intake	
	Value[a]	Reference	Value[a]	Reference
Infants (0.3–1 year)	4.7	Michaelsen (1997)	1.5	IOM (2005)
Children (1–3 years)	5.1	Hoppe et al. (2004)	1.1	IOM (2005)
Adults (>18 years)	3.5	Macdermid and Stannard (2006)	1.0–1.6	ACSM (2009)
		Bilsborough and Mann (2006)	1.0–1.5	Deutz et al. (2014)
Minimal physical activity	---	---	1.0	Volpi et al. 2013
Moderate physical activity	---	---	1.2 – 1.4	ACSM (2009)
Intense physical activity	---	---	1.5 –1.7	ACSM (2009); Geliebter et al. (1997)

[a] Expressed as g/kg body weight/day, depending on the type of physical activity. The body weight of an individual should be the ideal body weight appropriate for height.

13.5.9.2 Healthy Adult Humans

Healthy adults can tolerate the long-term consumption of 2 g dietary protein/kg BW/day (Wolfe 2006) or even higher amounts (Wu 2016). For example, the consumption of 3 g dietary protein/kg BW/day (the highest amount tested in the study) for 3 weeks (duration of the study) did not cause any side effects in elite cyclists (Witard et al. 2011). In addition, cyclists could well tolerate 3.3 g dietary protein/kg BW/day (the highest amount tested in the study) for 7 days (duration of the study) (Macdermid and Stannard 2006). Furthermore, based on the capacity of urea synthesis, healthy adults can tolerate a dietary intake of 3.5 g protein/kg BW/day without side effects (Bilsborough and Mann 2006). This is equivalent to 280 g protein/day for an 80-kg subject. Interestingly, the Greenland Inuit, who have lived on an almost exclusive meat diet for generations, consume daily 280 g protein, 135 g fat, and 54 g carbohydrate per person without renal or hepatic abnormality (McClelland and DuBois 1930). However, a higher intake of protein may present a problem for some adults, as shown in a study involving forty healthy resistance-trained individuals who were assigned to ingest 4.4 g protein/kg BW/day (Antonio et al. 2014). The protein was derived from a regular diet plus a mixture of whey and casein powder. Among the ten subjects who dropped out, three stated an inability to consume the required amount of protein and one person complained about gastrointestinal distress. By contrast, thirty persons (including men and women with an average age of 24 years) could consume 4.4 g protein/kg BW/day for 8 weeks without side effects. Based on these studies, well-adapted healthy adults can tolerate a dietary intake of 3.5 g protein/kg BW/day for a prolonged period. There are reports that hospitalized adult humans with burns can tolerate well the ingestion of 2.5 g protein/kg BW/day (Jaksic et al. 1991).

The average protein intake (e.g., 1.07 g/kg BW/day for young adults) being 15% of dietary energy in the United States is well within the acceptable macronutrient distribution range (IOM 2005), but well below the recommended intake for most athletes (ACSM 2009). Even the 95th percentile of protein intake for United States adults is still far below the highest acceptable macronutrient distribution range for protein (i.e., 35% of dietary calories). Dietary intake of protein (up to 1.7 g protein/kg BW/

day) recommended for athletes is well within the acceptable macronutrient distribution range. Based on an extensive review of the literature, Bilsborough and Mann (2006) suggested the maximum intake of 2–2.5 g protein/kg BW/day for healthy people, totaling 160–200 g protein/day for an 80-kg adult consuming 2,900 kcal daily. This is equivalent to 25% of dietary energy from protein. For comparison, adult swine (nonpregnant), growing poultry, and carnivores (e.g., cats, tigers, and largemouth bass) well tolerate at least 20%, 23%, and 50% dietary protein (on the as-fed basis; 90% DM), respectively (He et al. 2021; Herring et al. 2021; Li et al. 2021a; Zhang et al. 2021), and lactating ruminants (e.g., cows, goats, and sheep) have maximum milk yields when fed diets containing 18% protein (on the as-fed basis; 90% DM; Bergen 2021; Cao et al. 2021; Gilbreath et al. 2021).

13.5.10 CONCERNS OVER ADVERSE EFFECTS OF HIGH PROTEIN INTAKE ON HUMAN HEALTH

13.5.10.1 General Considerations

Dietary protein intake must meet the physiological needs of infants, children, and adolescents, as well as young and elderly adults for AAs, and must not be harmful to their health. The terms "low and high intakes of dietary protein" should be defined quantitatively for constructive discussions on any adverse effects of high protein intake on the health of humans. At present, protein intake less than the currently recommended value for a given population (Table 13.3) is considered to be low (FAO 2013), and high protein intake may be defined as at least 25% of dietary energy intake in the form of protein (i.e., at least 125 g protein/day for a 70-kg adult consuming 2,000 kcal of energy per day; Westerterp-Plantenga et al. 2012).

There is active debate over the effects of high protein intake on human health due to different results from either epidemiological or clinical studies, as well as the conflicting opinions of experts working in the field (e.g., Bilsborough and Mann 2006; Phillips et al. 2020; Van Elswyk et al. 2018). These confusions result, in part, from the different expression of dietary protein intakes, such as g/day, g/kg BW/day, and the percent of energy consumption, especially BW-based units in increasingly obese populations (Hruby and Jacques 2020). The bodyweight of adult persons of the same sex may differ by more than 2-fold and the content of their adipose tissue may vary by more than 4-fold. Thus, the unit of protein consumption by humans in g/day or g/kg BW/day has a severe limitation. In addition, depending on the amount of caloric intake, the unit of protein consumption by humans in the percent of energy consumption cannot be used to compare their actual ingestion of protein per day. It would be desirable to express dietary protein intake per (1) kg of nonfat lean tissue, (2) kg of nonfat lean tissue plus the normal amount of fat (namely, a standardized BW), or (3) kg BW of a normal (nonoverweight, nonobese) person. Furthermore, the recommended values may not be the true requirements of humans for dietary AAs due to the methodological difficulties and conceptual limitations of clinical studies (Fuller and Garlick 1994), and have undergone continuous revisions over the past three decades as more accurate data are available (FAO 1991, 2007, 2013).

Healthy individuals have a relatively high capacity to oxidize dietary AAs to water-soluble metabolites, including ammonia, NO, homocysteine, and sulfate (Chapter 4). In addition, bacteria in the intestine can produce both beneficial (e.g., short-chain fatty acids) and potentially deleterious (e.g., p-cresol, skatole, and sulfide) metabolites from AAs. In mammals (including humans) with adequate availabilities of arginine and glutamine, AA-derived ammonia can be readily detoxified as urea in hepatocytes and enterocytes (Chapter 6), whereas the kidneys remove H^+ through the production of ammonia to form NH_4^+ (Chapter 4). Urea and NH_4^+ are then excreted in the urine, which is facilitated by NO via renal blood flow and glomerular filtration. When vitamins B_6, B_{12}, and folate are adequate, homocysteine (an oxidant) is effectively recycled into methionine in the liver.

13.5.10.2 Definition of and General Concern over High Protein Intake

High protein intake may be defined as at least 25% of the adequate dietary energy intake in the form of protein (i.e., at least 125 g protein/day for a 70-kg adult consuming 2000 kcal of energy per day;

Westerterp-Plantenga et al. 2012), and is a common method for weight management for overweight or obese persons by stimulating the oxidation of fatty acids and increasing energy expenditure in the whole body (Oliveira et al. 2020). Elevated ingestion of AAs increases the loads of nitrogen to the gastrointestinal tract, liver, kidneys, heart, blood vessels, brain, and other organs. Thus, there are legitimate concerns that the long-term consumption of large amounts of dietary protein may have adverse effects on human health (Blachier et al. 2010; Bonjour 2011; Rosenvinge et al. 1999). Protein intake greater than its safe upper limits in different age groups can exceed the ability of the liver, intestine, and kidneys to detoxify ammonia and should be avoided. Adverse effects of high protein intake include intestinal discomfort, hyperaminoacidemia, hyperammonemia, hyperinsulinemia, dehydration, irritation, nausea, diarrhea, liver and kidney injuries, fatigue, headache, seizures, high risk for cardiovascular disease, or even death (Santesso et al. 2012). Problems of high protein intake can be exacerbated by low intake of carbohydrates because of additional burdens on the liver and kidney to produce large amounts of glucose from AAs besides the roles of these two organs in disposing of excessive ammonia and urea. Under this nutritional condition, the synthesis of glucose from AAs is crucial for survival because glucose is essential for meeting the energy requirements of the brain (that uses 125 g glucose/day in a 70-kg person), red blood cells, renal medulla, and retinal cells, and for the production of NADPH to support numerous biochemical (including anti-oxidative) reactions in all cell types (Wu and Marliss 1992).

Pregnant mammals (e.g., humans, swine, and cattle) are more sensitive to high dietary protein intake than their non-pregnant counterparts, because ammonia is particularly toxic to conceptuses and decreases placental-fetal blood flow (Herring et al. 2018). For example, in 1040 healthy women (a median body weight of 57 kg at the beginning of pregnancy) who consumed daily 70 to 350 g protein during the third trimester of pregnancy, an increase in 10 g of protein intake/day was associated with a reduction in the birth weight of offspring by 17.8 g (Andreasyan et al. 2007). Likewise, pregnant gilts fed a high-protein diet (30% CP) produced piglets with intrauterine growth restriction (IUGR) in comparison to gilts fed the normal diet (12.1% CP; Herring et al. 2018). Furthermore, increasing the CP level of diets for gilts from 12% to 16% increases the concentration of ammonia in the maternal plasma and reduces the number of live-born piglets at birth in a dose-dependent manner (Ji et al. 2017). Thus, the physiological state of individuals should be considered when assessing the safety of protein intake.

Dietary proteins are generally consumed by humans as part of complex food matrices, which contain not only proteins and AAs but also other nutrients and substances, such as digestible and nondigestible carbohydrates (e.g., starch, fibers, and oligosaccharides), lipids (fats, as well as saturated, unsaturated, cis-, and *trans* fatty acids), vitamins, minerals, and anti-nutritional factors (Richter et al. 2015). All these nutrients and nonnutritive compounds can affect whole-body metabolism and health both independently and in concerted actions. Thus, caution must be exercised when interpreting results from inadequately controlled studies, in which precise intakes of nutrients and anti-nutritional substances are unknown or are beset with a plethora of other possible confounding factors (such as lifestyles, emotional stress, and living environments). The following paragraphs highlight findings from clinical studies to address major-specific concerns over the potential adverse effects of high protein intake on human health.

13.5.10.3 Digestive, Cardiovascular, and Renal Functions

Dietary protein may influence the population, numbers, and activities of the intestinal microbiota and health, as well as heart rates, and glomerular blood flow (Diether and Willing 2019). There are concerns that excessive AAs and their metabolites are harmful to the gastrointestinal, circulatory, and urinary tract systems (Santesso et al. 2012). However, comprehensive reviews of Blachier et al. (2019) and Pedersen et al. (2013) indicate that protein intake of ≤2 g/kg BW/day does not negatively affect intestinal, hepatic, renal, or cardiovascular function in healthy people. For example, the ingestion of protein up to 34% of dietary energy intake as an effective method of weight management for overweight or obese persons does not change their intestinal microbiota or induce colonic inflammation (Blachier et al. 2019). In addition, results of epidemiologic studies indicate a significant relationship between increased protein intake and lower risks for hypertension and coronary heart disease in humans (Hu 2005). Similarly, in well-controlled clinical trials, increasing dietary protein intake can improve cardiovascular health in overweight or obese persons through weight loss and lean tissue maintenance, ameliorating dyslipidemia, and reducing blood pressure (Leidy et al. 2015). Current data supports the notion that risk for cardiovascular disease can be reduced by a dietary pattern that provides adequate protein with balanced AAs (Richter et al. 2015).

A recent comprehensive review indicates that: (1) most ($n = 8$), but not all ($n = 5$), studies with healthy adult humans showed higher glomerular filtration rates in response to high protein intake ($\geq 20\%$ but $<35\%$ of energy consumption); (2) all the glomerular filtration rates were within the physiological ranges for healthy adults; and (3) high protein intake does not increase the risk of kidney stones or renal dysfunction and has no adverse effect on blood pressure (Van Elswyk et al. 2018). Furthermore, a diet providing 130–140 g protein per day as 25% of total energy intake for 6 months does not adversely influence renal function in overweight and obese persons with no preexisting kidney disease (Skov et al. 1999). Likewise, consumption of a weight-loss diet containing 90–120 g of protein/day did not affect renal function in overweight persons or in obese adults with type 2 diabetes, compared with those consuming 55–70 g protein/day (Jesudason et al. 2013). There is epidemiological evidence that: (1) in patients with reduced kidney function, dietary protein intake at ~0.8 g/kg ideal BW/day can limit renal function decline without affecting the functions of cardiovascular and other systems; and (2) long-term lower protein intake increases mortality in these patients (Bilancio et al. 2019). These results do not support the view that low protein diets are beneficial for preventing kidney failure progression. Patients with renal dysfunction or gout are advised to consume an adequate amount of high-quality protein but not an excessive amount of protein (Santesso et al. 2012). In addition, individuals who have consumed a low-protein diet for a prolonged period should not suddenly ingest large amounts of protein due to the preexisting reductions in the expression of hepatic urea-cycle enzymes for ammonia detoxification, as well as the rates of glomerular filtration and the transport of ammonia and urea from the blood into the proximal renal tubules.

13.5.10.4 Bone Mass and Integrity

Efficient absorption of dietary minerals (particularly calcium and phosphorus), biomineralization, and the cross-linkage of collagen molecules in bone depends on protein, which makes up about 50% of the volume of bone and about one-third of its mass (Heaney and Layman 2008). For example, there are positive associations between the amount of ingested proteins and bone mass gain in children and adolescents of both sexes (Bonjour et al. 2011). Furthermore, dietary supplementation with 20 g protein per day for 1 year attenuated the reduction of proximal bone mineral density by 50% in persons with hip fracture (Schürch et al. 1998). Thus, adequate intake of protein, particularly from calcium- and phosphorus-rich milk products, is essential to support bone growth in infants and children and to sustain the mass and health of the skeleton in adults. There is a concern that high protein intake may stimulate the urinary excretion of calcium, which may contribute to bone loss and subsequent development of osteopenia and osteoporosis (Bonjour 2011). However, in free-living individuals, high protein intake is likely associated with high calcium intake, and, therefore, may compensate for a moderate increase, if any, in urinary excretion of calcium. In addition, whether dietary protein intake affects bone health will depend on a variety of other dietary factors (e.g., calcium, phosphorus, vitamins, fats, and acid-base balance), physiological status (e.g., hormones and renal function), and physical activity. Based on extensive and systematic reviews of the literature, Sahni et al. (2013) and Wallace (2019) concluded that: (1) dietary protein provides a significant benefit to bone health in humans; and (2) adequate protein intake [for example, up to 35% of total calories (2000 kcal) per day or up to 175 g protein per day for the 70-kg adult] is safe, increases bone mass and mineral density in both young and older adults, and reduces bone fracture in older adults. Thus, consumption of high-quality protein (e.g., meat, milk, and fish) plays a key role in improving skeletal health to reduce the risk for osteopenia and osteoporosis, which are estimated to affect 53.6 million U.S. adults of ≥ 50 years of age (Wright et al. 2014).

13.5.10.5 Cancers

Patients with cancers exhibit a great loss of skeletal muscle proteins due to diminished protein synthesis and increased proteolysis (Prado et al. 2020). The muscle is the major reservoir of protein and free AAs in the body and is essential for respiration, physical movement, and balance, as well as physical strength and power generation in humans. Thus, rapidly losing muscle mass impairs physical motility, shortens the survival time of cancer patients (particularly those with pancreatic cancers), compromises anti-inflammatory responses to the cancers, and reduces the whole-body metabolism of both glucose and protein, especially in persons with diabetes. For example, a review of 150 studies has indicated that cancer patients with less muscle mass experience more surgical and post-operative complications, longer hospital stays, lower physical capacity and function, poorer quality of life, shorter survival, and higher mortality rates, in comparison to those with more muscle mass (Prado et al. 2018). In support of this view, the consumption of red meat was positively associated with a 7-year survival rate among 992 individuals with stage III colon cancer (Van Blarigan et al. 2018), indicating that higher protein intake is beneficial for these patients. To sustain life, these patients have greater requirements for dietary protein (e.g., ≥1.5 g/kg BW/day) than people without cancers (Prado et al. 2020). Arends et al. (2017) recommended a protein intake of 1.2–1.5 g/kg BW/day for patients with various types of cancers to minimize the negative nitrogen balance in the whole body.

Some epidemiological studies showed that the consumption of large quantities of protein (particularly animal protein) could be linked to an increase in risks for the development of cancers (e.g., Chow et al. 1994; Levine et al. 2014). Although the results of those investigations revealed a correlation between the ingestion of animal-based protein (e.g., red meats) and certain diseases [e.g., colon cancer and hyperglycemia (see below)], it should be noted that: (1) there is a clear difference between correlation and causation; and (2) findings of the epidemiological studies do not establish a role for the adequate intake of animal-sourced protein (e.g., lean meat) in causing chronic diseases in humans. There are no rigorous long-term clinical trials to determine the effects of animal-sourced protein on the incidence of cancer in adults or children because such studies are unethical. Likewise, there is little evidence in human beings for the carcinogenicity of an adequate intake of animal protein (Alexander et al. 2015). Lean meat and fish are a major source of high-quality protein for human consumption. Recent studies from large cohorts such as the Nurse's Health Study, the Health Professional Follow-up Study, and the Multiethnic Cohort showed nonsignificant associations and even beneficially inverse associations between consumption of unprocessed red meat and colorectal cancer (Bernstein et al. 2015; Ollberding et al. 2012). Of note, findings from the intervention studies on diet and cancer, such as the Women's Health Initiative and the Polyp Prevention Trial, indicated that a decrease in dietary intake of animal protein (e.g., red meat and processed meat) did not reduce the risk of colorectal cancer and/or had no effect on adenoma recurrence in the large bowel (Beresford et al. 2006; Lanza et al. 2001; Schatzkin et al. 2000).

13.5.10.6 Type 1 and Type 2 Diabetes Mellitus

In acute studies, patients with diabetes (type 1 and type 2) are characterized by a negative balance of protein in the whole body (particularly skeletal muscle) due to decreased protein synthesis and increased proteolysis (Hebert and Nair 2010; Marliss and Gougeon 2002). In addition, type 2 diabetes is associated with the insulin resistance of both glucose and protein metabolism (Pereira et al. 2008). Importantly, acute hyperaminoacidemia (excessive AAs in the blood) overcomes insulin resistance to result in protein anabolism and does not worsen the already attenuated glucose disposal in hyperglycemic type 2 diabetic patients (Bassil et al. 2011a,b). Similarly, raising AAs and insulin to postprandial levels in normal people increases protein synthesis and induces protein anabolism in their skeletal muscle (Sheffield-Moore et al. 2000), without causing insulin resistance or impeding insulin-mediated glucose synthesis and catabolism in the whole body (Burgos et al. 2021). These results are important because of the major public health issue due to the current global epidemic of type 2 diabetes.

Epidemiological reports regarding a role of protein intake in causing diabetes have been inconsistent. Some studies found that the consumption of large quantities of dairy protein could be linked to an increased risk for the development of type 1 diabetes in children (Lamb et al. 2015) and type 2 diabetes mellitus in adults (Shang et al. 2016; van Nielen et al. 2014). By contrast, other longitudinal studies have shown that persons consuming higher amounts of dairy products have a lesser incidence of type 2 diabetes (Bhavadharini et al. 2020; Drehmer et al. 2015; Talaei et al. 2018). However, it is unknown whether animal protein *per se* or other dietary factors (e.g., fats, carbohydrates, vitamins, and minerals) may potentially contribute to the putative disorders of glucose metabolism in humans. As noted previously, an association does not mean a causal effect. To date, there is no direct evidence that the ingestion of cow's milk or other animal proteins causes type 1 diabetes (an autoimmune disease targeting pancreatic β-cells) in humans or other animals. By contrast, the results of studies with the BB rat (a spontaneous animal model of type 1 diabetes) indicate that all the animals develop diabetes when fed a plant-based diet but hyperglycemia occurs in only about 5% of them when fed a casein-based semi-purified diet (Scott and Marliss 1991; Wu 1995). Interestingly, wheat gluten in plant-based rodent diets (containing wheat as a major component) has been identified to be a potent protein to cause the autoimmune attack in the pancreas and induce type 1 diabetes in the BB rat (MacFarlane et al. 2003). Likewise, given the important functions of AAs (Chapter 11), it is unlikely that the consumption of animal protein *per se* increases insulin resistance in humans or other animals and is associated with an increased risk for the development of type 2 diabetes. However, diets must be balanced in the composition and amounts of all nutrients, including AAs, lipids, starch, fibers, vitamins, and minerals, to maintain health and well-being.

Much evidence shows that adequate protein intake is important for preventing or alleviating protein loss in patients with type 1 or type 2 diabetes (Hebert and Nair 2010; Marliss and Gougeon 2002; Pfeiffer et al. 2020). There are suggestions that the daily intake of high-quality protein for type 1 diabetic adult patients with minimal physical activity be 70–80 g/day, with the amount being divided into 6 meals (14–16 g each for breakfast and lunch, 21–24 g for dinner, and 7–8 g in each of three snacks; Marković-Jovanovic 2013). In addition, regular exercise is important for the health, fitness, and longevity of persons with type 1 or type 2 diabetes (ADA 2021a,b; Marliss and Vranic 2002; Wu et al. 2019), and many of them train and compete in sports, such as swimming (Riddell et al. 2020). Patients with type 1 diabetes must receive treatment with insulin to prevent hyperglycemia and ketoacidosis for their survival. Of note, insulin deficiency for as short as 8 h promotes protein catabolism (Riddell et al. 2017). Thus, in an exercise program with integrated insulin therapy, type 1 diabetic patients should be frequently monitored for blood glucose concentrations and advised to consume high-quality protein (20% of energy consumption each for breakfast and lunch, 30% of energy consumption for dinner, and 10% of energy consumption in each of three snacks) to support whole-body protein synthesis and muscle mass (Marković-Jovanovic 2013). Other recommendations for the nutritional management of people with type 1 diabetes include: (1) the daily consumption of protein along with other nutrients in foods be divided into six meals: breakfast, lunch, and dinner (20%, 30%, and 20% of the daily intake, respectively), as well as two snacks and one bedtime meal (with each accounting for 10% of the daily intake); (2) the regular ingestion of the same amount of carbohydrates in each meal (Marković-Jovanovic 2013).

Marliss and Gougeon (2002) presented a strong argument for increasing the recommended intake of high-quality dietary protein (e.g., the proportions of animal- and plant-sourced proteins being 60% and 40%, respectively) for patients with type 2 diabetes) from <0.8 to 1.2 g/kg BW/day. In support of this view, a review of 18 randomized control trials (ranging from 4 to 56 weeks) involving 1099 adults with type 2 diabetes revealed that high protein intake (e.g., the ratio of protein to carbohydrates and lipids being 32:47:18) is beneficial for ameliorating dyslipidemia and weight management in these patients (Zhao et al. 2018). In addition, the consumption of a high-protein/low-carbohydrate, weight-maintaining, nonketogenic diet (the ratio of protein to carbohydrates and lipids being 30:20:50) by persons with untreated type 2 diabetes for 5 weeks reduced serum glucose concentrations by 36% (from 11 to 7 mM) and the percentage of total glycohemoglobin in the blood by 22%, when compared with a control diet (the ratio of protein to carbohydrates and lipids being 15:55:30) (Gannon and Nuttall 2004). Thus, high dietary protein of at least 27% of restricted but nutritionally adequate energy intake is safe and beneficial for type 2 diabetic patients with normal renal function. Successful management of type 2 diabetes may include the dietary intake of high-quality protein at 20–30% of energy intake (ADA 2021a).

13.6 SUMMARY

The proportions and amounts of dietary AAs have a profound impact on the food intake, growth, development, and health of mammals, birds, and aquatic animals. Thus, dietary AA intake by the organisms must meet their physiological needs. To provide scientifically sound nutritional guidelines for the public and agricultural industries, considerable efforts have been made over the past century to determine dietary requirements of AAs and proteins by humans and other animals. Nitrogen balance studies and growth trials have traditionally been used to accomplish this goal. Minimal requirements for dietary AAs or protein can also be estimated by factorial analysis; namely, the sum of fecal and urinary nitrogen in response to a protein-free diet (maintenance), AAs deposited in the body, and AAs excreted as animal products. Direct and indirect AA oxidation methods have also been used to estimate AA requirements by humans and other animals. Based on protein accretion in growing animals and nitrogen balance in adults, AAs have been traditionally classified as EAAs, NEAAs, or CEAAs. To avoid further confusion over their nutritional and physiological significance, both NEAAs and CEAAs can be considered together as AASAs that are needed in the diets of both humans and other animals. Dietary requirements of humans and other animals for AAs should be based on the metabolic needs of *all* canonical proteinogenic AAs (including AASAs) for maintenance, tissue protein synthesis, the generation of physiologically essential nonprotein metabolites (e.g., NO, taurine, β-alanine, creatine, and polyamines), and their regulatory functions. Dietary optimum ratios of all proteinogenic AAs must replace the long-standing "ideal protein" concept to formulate animal diets and guide the practice of human nutrition. Because dietary protein is the ultimate source of all AAs in the body, its quality must be evaluated by reliable methods involving both chemical analyses and animal feeding experiments (e.g., AA score, biological value, PDCAAS, DIAAS, and lean tissue gain), metabolic indicators, and the utilization of protein hydrolysates by microorganisms. In addition, physiologically important nonproteinogenic AAs (e.g., taurine) should be included in diets for infants and individuals with limited or no ability to synthesize them. Animal protein can contribute to healthy diets for maximum growth and good health (including skeletal muscle, reproductive, and and immune-system health) in both humans and other animals while preventing the excessive accretion of WAT in the body, reducing the excretion of nitrogenous wastes, delaying aging, and mitigating sarcopenia, while meeting the high demands of exercising individuals for high-quality protein.

Much work is needed to define optimum requirements of humans and other animals for dietary AAs under various physiological and pathological conditions. Physically active humans must consume adequate AAs to maintain or promote the strength, function, and mass of their skeletal muscles, mitigate sarcopenia, and maintain their well-being. This notion applies to other animals (e.g., cats, dogs, horses, and breeding stocks). To meet the functional needs, the daily dietary intake of 1.0, 1.2 to 1.4, and 1.5 to 1.7 g protein/kg BW/day is recommended for adult humans with minimal, moderate, and intense physical activity, whereas the daily dietary intake of 1.2 g high-quality protein per kg BW is recommended for elderly persons and type 2 diabetic patients. The tolerable upper limit of protein intake is 3.5 g/kg BW/day for well-adapted adult humans and is greater for younger persons (e.g., 5.1 g/kg BW/day for 1- to 3-year-old children). Long-term consumption of 2 g protein/kg BW/day is safe for healthy adults and children and does not negatively affect their digestive, renal, cardiovascular, endocrine, or immune function or increase risks for bone loss, obesity, diabetes, cardiovascular disease, or cancer. Likewise, adult swine (nonpregnant), growing poultry, lactating cows, and carnivores (e.g., cats, tigers, and largemouth bass) tolerate at least 20%, 23%, 18%, and 50% dietary protein (on the as-fed basis; 90% DM), respectively. Protein intakes of humans and other animals should be adjusted according to physiological, pathological, and environmental alterations to avoid excess consumption. Adequate AA nutrition is essential for the optimum growth, development, and health of people, as well as companion and farm animals.

REFERENCES

ACSM. 2009. American College of Sports Medicine, American Dietetic Association, and Dietitians of Canada. Joint Position Statement: nutrition and athletic performance. *Med. Sci. Sports Exerc.* 41:709–731.

ADA (American Diabetes Association). 2021a. Facilitating behavior change and well-being to improve health outcomes: Standards of medical care in diabetes—2021. *Diabetes Care* 44 (Suppl. 1):S53–72.

ADA (American Diabetes Association). 2021b. Obesity Management for the Treatment of Type 2 Diabetes: Standards of Medical Care in Diabetes—2021. *Diabetes Care* 44 (Suppl. 1):S100–110.

Adams, V.J., P. Watson, S. Carmichael, S. Gerry, J. Penell, and D.M. Morgan. 2015. Exceptional longevity and potential determinants of successful ageing in a cohort of Labrador retrievers: results of a prospective longitudinal study. *Acta Vet. Scand.* 58:29.

Adegoke, O.A., S. Chevalier, J.A. Morais, R. Gougeon, S.R. Kimball, L.S. Jefferson et al. 2009. Fed-state clamp stimulates cellular mechanisms of muscle protein anabolism and modulates glucose disposal in normal men. *Am. J. Physiol.* 296:E105–E113.

Akibode, S. and M. Maredia. 2011. *Global and Regional Trends in Production, Trade and Consumption of Food Legume Crops.* Michigan State University, East Lansing, MI.

Alexander, D.D., D.L. Weed, P.E. Miller, and M.A. Mohamed. 2015. Red meat and colorectal cancer: a quantitative update on the state of the epidemiologic science. *J. Am. Coll. Nutr.* 34:521–543.

Andreasyan, K., A.-L. Ponsonby, T. Dwyer, R. Morley, M. Riley, K. Dear, and J. Cochrane. 2007. Higher maternal dietary protein intake in late pregnancy is associated with a lower infant ponderal index at birth. *Eur. J. Clin. Nutr.* 61:498–508.

Antonio, J., C.A. Peacock, A. Ellerbroek, B. Fromhoff, and T. Silver. 2014. The effects of consuming a high protein diet (4.4 g/kg/d) on body composition in resistance-trained individuals. *J. Int. Soc. Sports Nutr.* 11:19.

ARC (Agricultural Research Council). 1981. *The Nutrient Requirements of Pigs: Technical review.* Commonwealth Agricultural Bureaux, Slough, UK.

Arends, J., V. Baracos, H. Bertz, F. Bozzetti, P.C. Calder, N.E.P. Deutz et al. 2017. ESPEN expert group recommendations for action against cancer-related malnutrition. *Clin Nutr* 36:1187–1196.

Areta, J.L., L.M. Burke, M.L. Ross, D.M. Camera, D.W. West, E.M. Broad et al. 2013. Timing and distribution of protein ingestion during prolonged recovery from resistance exercise alters myofibrillar protein synthesis. *J. Physiol.* 591:2319–2331.

Atwater, W.O. 1902. Principles of nutrition and nutritive value of food. *USDA Farmers' Bull*, no. 142.

Aubertin-Leheudre, M. and H. Adlercreutz. 2009. Relationship between animal protein intake and muscle mass index in healthy women. *Br. J. Nutr.* 102:1803–10.

Auton, A., L.D. Brooks, R.M. Durbin, E.P. Garrison, H.M. Kang, J.O. Korbel et al. 2015. A global reference for human genetic variation. *Nature* 526:68–74.

Awad, E.A., I. Zulkifli, A.S. Farjam, and L.T. Chwen. 2014. Amino acids fortification of low-protein diet for broilers under tropical climate. 2. Nonessential amino acids and increasing essential amino acids. *Italian J. Anim. Sci.* 13:3297.

Baccari, G.C., S. Falvo, A. Santillo, F.D.G. Russo, and M.M. Di Fiore. 2020. D-Amino acids in mammalian endocrine tissues. *Amino Acids* 52:1263–1273.

Bailey, H.M. and H.H. Stein. 2020. Raw and roasted pistachio nuts (Pistacia vera L.) are 'good' sources of protein based on their digestible indispensable amino acid score as determined in pigs. *J. Sci. Food Agric.* 100:3878–3885.

Baker, D.H. 1996. Advances in amino acid nutrition and metabolism of swine and poultry. In: *Nutrient Management of Food Animals to Enhance and Protect the Environment* (Kornegay, E.T. ed). CRC Press, Boca Raton, FL. pp. 41–53.

Baker, D.H. 2000. Recent advances in use of the ideal protein concept for swine feed formulation. *Asian-Aust. J. Anim. Sci.* 13:294–301.

Baker, D.H. 2009. Advances in protein-amino acid nutrition of poultry. *Amino Acids* 37:29–41.

Ball, R. and H.S. Bayley. 1986. Influence of dietary protein concentration on the oxidation of phenylalanine by the young pig. *Br. J. Nutr.* 55:651–658.

Ball, R.O., J.L. Atkinson, and H.S. Bayley. 1986. Proline as an essential amino acid for the young pig. *Br. J. Nutr.* 55:659–668.

Bassil, M., E.B. Marliss, J.A. Morais, S. Pereira, S. Chevalier, and R. Gougeon. 2011a. Postprandial hype-raminoacidaemia overcomes insulin resistance of protein anabolism in men with type 2 diabetes. *Diabetologia* 54:648–656.

Bassil, M., S. Burgos, E.B. Marliss, J.A. Morais, S. Chevalier, and R. Gougeon. 2011b. Hyperaminoacidemia at postprandial levels does not modulate glucose metabolism in type 2 diabetes mellitus. *Diabetologia* 54:1810–1818.

Bassily, N.S., K.G. Michael, and A.K. Said. 1982. Blood urea content for evaluating dietary protein quality. *Food* 26:759–764.

Bauer, J., G. Biolo, T. Cederholm, M. Cesari, A.J. Cruz-Jentoft, and J.E. Morley. 2013. Evidence-based recom-mendations for optimal dietary protein intake in older people: a position paper from the PROT-AGE Study Group. *J. Am. Med. Dir. Assoc.* 14:542–559.

Bax, M., C. Buffière, N. Hafnaoui, C. Gaudichon, I. Savary-Auzeloux, D. Dardevet et al. 2013. Effects of meat cooking, and of ingested amount, on protein digestion speed and entry of residual proteins into the colon: a study in minipigs. *PLoS One* 8:e61252.

Beaumont, M. and F. Blachier. 2020. Amino acids in intestinal physiology and health. *Adv. Exp. Med. Biol.* 1265:1–20.

Belloir, P., B. Méda, W. Lambert, E. Corrent, H. Juin, M. Lessire, and S. Tesseraud. 2017. Reducing the CP content in broiler feeds: impact on animal performance, meat quality and nitrogen utilization. *Animal* 11:1881–1889.

Belloir, P., M. Lessire, W. Lambert, E. Corrent, C. Berri, and S. Tesseraud. 2019. Changes in body com-position and meat quality in response to dietary amino acid provision in finishing broilers. *Animal* 13:1094–1102.

Bender, A.E. 1982. Evaluation of protein quality: methodological considerations. *Proc. Nutr. Soc.* 41:267–276.

Beresford, S.A., K.C. Johnson, C. Ritenbaugh, N.L. Lasser, L.G. Snetselaar, H.R. Black et al. 2006. Low-fat dietary pattern and risk of colorectal cancer: the women's health initiative randomized controlled dietary modification trial. *JAMA* 295:643–654.

Bergen, W.G. 2021. Amino acids in beef cattle nutrition and production. *Adv. Exp. Med. Biol.* 1285:29–42.

Bernstein, A.M., M. Song, X. Zhang, A. Pan, M. Wang, C.S. Fuchs et al. 2015. Processed and unprocessed red meat and risk of colorectal cancer: analysis by tumor location and modification by time. *PLoS One* 10(8):e0135959.

Berryman, C.E., H.R. Lieberman, V.L. Fulgoni, and S.M. Pasiakos. 2018. Protein intake trends and con-formity with the Dietary Reference Intakes in the United States: analysis of the National Health and Nutrition Examination Survey, 2001–2014. *Am. J. Clin. Nutr.* 108:405–413.

Bhavadharini, B., M. Dehghan, A. Mente, S. Rangarajan, P. Sheridan, V. Mohan et al. 2020. Association of dairy consumption with metabolic syndrome, hypertension and diabetes in 147 812 individuals from 21 countries. *BMJ Open Diab Res Care* 8:e000826.

Bilancio, G., P. Cavallo, C. Ciacci, and M. Cirillo. 2019. Dietary protein, kidney function and mortality: review of the evidence from epidemiological studies. *Nutrients* 11:196.

Biolo, G., K.D. Tipton, S. Klein, and R.R. Wolfe. 1997. An abundant supply of amino acids enhances the metabolic effect of exercise on muscle protein. *Am. J. Physiol.* 273:E122–E129.

Bilsborough, S. and N. Mann. 2006. A review of issues of dietary protein intake in humans. *Int. J. Sport Nutr. Exerc. Metab.* 16:129–152.

Blachier, F., A.M. Davila, S. Mimoun, P.H. Benetti, C. Atanasiu, M. Andriamihaja et al. 2010. Luminal sulfide and large intestine mucosa: friend or foe? *Amino Acids* 39:335–347.

Blachier, F., M. Beaumont, K.J. Portune, N. Steuer, A. Lan, M. Audebert et al. 2019. High-protein diets for weight management: interactions with the intestinal microbiota and consequences for gut health. A posi-tion paper by the my new gut study group. *Clin. Nutr.* 38:1012–1022.

Bohe, J., J.F. Low, R.R. Wolfe, and M.J. Rennie. 2001. Latency and duration of stimulation of human muscle protein synthesis during continuous infusion of amino acids. *J. Physiol.* 532:575–579.

Bonjour, J.P., P. Ammann, T. Chevalley, and R. Rizzoli. 2011. Protein intake and bone growth. *Can. J. Appl. Physiol.* 26:S153–S166.

Brown, A.F., C.M. Prado, S. Ghosh, S.M. Leonard, P.J. Arciero, K.L. Tucker, and M.J. Ormsbee. 2019. Higher-protein intake and physical activity are associated with healthier body composition and cardiometabolic health in Hispanic adults. *Clin. Nutr. ESPEN* 30:145–151.

Burd, N.A., D.W. West, D.R. Moore, P.J. Atherton, A.W. Staples, T. Prior et al. 2011. Enhanced amino acid sensitivity of myofibrillar protein synthesis persists for up to 24 h after resistance exercise in young men. *J. Nutr.* 141:568–573.

Burgos, S.A., S. Chevalier, J.A. Morais, M. Lamarche, S. Kellett, and E.B. Marliss. 2021. Acute hyperaminoacidemia does not suppress insulin-mediated glucose turnover in healthy young men. *Appl. Physiol. Nutr. Metab.* 46:397–403.

Campbell, A.P. and T.M. Rains. 2015. Dietary protein is important in the practical management of prediabetes and type 2 diabetes. *J. Nutr.* 145:164S–169S.

Campbell, W.W., M.L. Barton, Jr., D. Cyr-Campbell, S.L. Davey, J.L. Beard, G. Parise, and W.J. Evans. 1999. Effects of an omnivorous diet compared with a lactoovovegetarian diet on resistance-training-induced changes in body composition and skeletal muscle in older men. *Am. J. Clin. Nutr.* 70:1032–1039.

Campbell, W.W., T.A. Trappe, R.R. Wolfe, and W.J. Evans. 2001. The recommended dietary allowance for protein may not be adequate for older people to maintain skeletal muscle. *J. Gerontol. A* 56:M373–M380.

Campbell, W.W., T.A. Trappe, A.C. Jozsi, L.J. Kruskall, R.R. Wolfe, and W.J. Evans. 2002. Dietary protein adequacy and lower body versus whole body resistive training in older humans. *J. Physiol.* 542:631–642.

Cao, Y., J. Yao, X. Sun, S. Liu, and G.B. Martin. 2021. Amino acids in the nutrition and production of sheep and goats. *Adv. Exp. Med. Biol.* 1285:63–79.

Chauhan, S., N.C. Nayak, and V. Ramalingaswami. 1965. The heart and skeletal muscle in experimental protein malnutrition in rhesus monkeys. *J. Pathol. Bacteriol.* 90:301–309.

Che, D.S., P.S. Nyingwa, K.M. Ralinala, G.M.T. Maswanganye, and G. Wu. 2021. Amino acids in the nutrition, metabolism, and health of domestic cats. *Adv. Exp. Med. Biol.* 1285:217–231.

Cheng, Y., Q. Meng, C. Wang, H. Li, Z. Huang, S. Chen et al. 2010. Leucine deprivation decreases fat mass by stimulation of lipolysis in white adipose tissue and upregulation of uncoupling protein 1 (UCP1) in brown adipose tissue. *Diabetes* 59:17–25.

Chevalier, S., R. Gougeon, K. Nayar, and J.A. Morais. 2003. Frailty amplifies the effects of aging on protein metabolism: role of protein intake. *Am. J. Clin. Nutr.* 78:422–429.

Chow, W., G. Gridley, J.K. McLaughlin, J.S. Mandel, S. Wacholder, W.J. Blot et al. 1994. Protein intake and risk of renal cell cancer. *J. Natl. Cancer Institute* 86:1131–1139.

Chung, T.K. and D.H. Baker. 1992. Ideal amino acid pattern for 10-kilogram pigs. *J. Anim. Sci.* 70:3102–3111.

Cole, D.J.A. 1980. The amino acid requirements of pigs: the concept of an ideal protein. *Pig News Info.* 1:201–205.

Columbus, D.A., M.L. Fiorott, and T.A. Davis. 2015. Leucine is a major regulator of muscle protein synthesis in neonates. *Amino Acids* 47:259–270.

Cummings, N.E., E.M. Williams, I. Kasza, E.N. Konon, M.D. Schaid, B.A. Schmidt. 2017. Restoration of metabolic health by decreased consumption of branched-chain amino acids. *J. Physiol.* 596:623–645.

Cupp, C.J., C. Jean-Philippe, W.W. Kerr, A.R. Patil, and G. Perez-Camargo. 2007. Effect of Nutritional Interventions on Longevity of Senior Cats. *Int. J. Appl. Res. Vet. Med.* 5:133–149.

Dai, Z.L., Z.L. Wu, S.C. Jia, and G. Wu. 2014. Analysis of amino acid composition in proteins of animal tissues and foods as pre-column *o*-phthaldialdehyde derivatives by HPLC with fluorescence detection. *J. Chromatogr. B.* 964:116–127.

Dangin, M., Y. Boirie, C. Garcia-Rodenas, P. Gachon, J. Fauquant, P. Callier, O. Ballèvre, and B. Beaufrère. 2001. The digestion rate of protein is an independent regulating factor of postprandial protein retention. *Am. J. Physiol.* 280:E340–E348.

Dangin, M., C. Guillet, C. Garcia-Rodenas, P. Gachon, C. Bouteloup-Demange, K. Reiffers-Magnani et al. 2003. The rate of protein digestion affects protein gain differently during aging in humans. *J. Physiol.* 549:635–644.

Dasgupta, M., J.R. Sharkey, and G. Wu. 2005. Inadequate intakes of indispensable amino acids among homebound older adults. *J. Nutr. Elderly* 24:85–99.

Davis, T.A., M.L. Fiorotto, and P.J. Reeds. 1993. Amino acid compositions of body and milk protein change during the suckling period in rats. *J. Nutr.* 123:947–956.

Deutz, N., J. Bauer, R. Barazzoni, G. Biolo, Y. Boirie, and A. Bosy-Westphal et al. 2014. Protein intake and exercise for optimal muscle function with aging: recommendations from the ESPEN Expert Group. *Clin Nutr.* 33:929–936.

Diether, N.E. and B.P. Willing. 2019. Microbial fermentation of dietary protein: an important factor in diet–microbe–host interaction. *Microorganisms* 7:19.

Dillon, E.L. 2013. Nutritionally essential amino acids and metabolic signaling in aging. *Amino Acids* 45:431–441.

Drehmer, M., M.A. Pereira, M.I. Schmidt, M.D.C.B. Molina, S. Alvim, P.A. Lotufo, and B.B. Duncan. 2015. Associations of dairy intake with glycemia and insulinemia, independent of obesity, in Brazilian adults: the Brazilian Longitudinal Study of Adult Health (ELSA-Brasil). *Am. J. Clin. Nutr.* 101:775–782.

Dror, D.K. and L.H. Allen. 2011. The Importance of milk and other animal-source foods for children in low-income countries. *Food Nutr. Bull.* 32:227–243.

Durante, W. 2020. Amino acids in circulatory function and health. *Adv. Exp. Med. Biol.* 1265:39–56.

Elango, R., R.O. Ball, and P.B. Pencharz. 2012. Recent advances in determining protein and amino acid requirements in humans. *Br. J. Nutr.* 108 (Suppl 2):S22–S30.

Elia, M. 1992. Organ and tissue contribution to metabolic rate. In: *Energy Metabolism: Tissue Determinants and Cellular Corollaries* (Kinney, J.M. and H.N. Tucker, ed). Raven Press, New York. pp. 61–79.

Evans, E. and R. Witty. 1978. An assessment of methods used to determine protein quality. *World Rev. Nutr. Diet.* 32:1–26.

FAO (Food and Agriculture Organization of the United Nations). 1991. *Protein quality evaluation Report of Joint FAO/WHO Expert Consultation.* Rome, Italy.

FAO (Food and Agriculture Organization of the United Nations). 2007. *Protein and amino acid requirements in human nutrition. Report of a Joint WHO/FAO/UNU Expert Consultation.* Rome, Italy.

FAO (Food and Agriculture Organization of the United Nations). 2013. *Dietary protein quality evaluation in human nutrition. Report of an FAO Expert Consultation.* Rome, Italy.

FDA (U.S. Food and Drug Administration). 1993. Federal Register. 58(3):2301–2426.

FDA (U.S. Food and Drug Administration). 2013. A Food Labeling Guide: Guidance for Industry. www.fda.gov/FoodLabelingGuide. Accessed on April 18, 2021.

FDA (U.S. Food and Drug Administration). 2017. CFR - Code of Federal Regulations Title 21. The information is available online and is current as of April 1, 2017. https://www.accessdata.fda.gov/scripts/cdrh/cfdocs/cfcfr/cfrsearch.cfm. Accessed on April 18, 2021.

Farsijani, S., J.A. Morais, H. Payette, P. Gaudreau, B. Shatenstein, K. Gray-Donald, and S. Chevalier. 2016. Relation between mealtime distribution of protein intake and lean mass loss in free-living older adults of the NuAge study. *Am. J. Clin. Nutr.* 104:694–703.

Fernandez, S.R., S. Aoyagi, Y. Han, C.M. Parsons, and D.H. Baker. 1994. Limiting order of amino acids in corn and soybean meal for growth of the chick. *Poult. Sci.* 73:1887–1896.

Fernstrom, J.D. 2013. Large neutral amino acids: dietary effects on brain neurochemistry and function. *Amino Acids* 45:419–430.

Forslund, A.H., A.E. El-Khoury, R.M. Olsson, A.M. Sjodin, L. Hambraeus, and V.R. Young. 1999. Effect of protein intake and physical activity on 24-h pattern and rate of macronutrient utilization. *Am. J. Physiol.* 276:E964–E976.

Fresán, U. and J. Sabaté. 2019. Vegetarian diets: planetary health and its alignment with human health. *Adv. Nutr.* 10:S380–S388.

Fromentin, C., D. Tomé, F. Nau, L. Flet, C. Luengo, D. Azzout-Marniche et al. 2013. Dietary proteins contribute little to glucose production, even under optimal gluconeogenic conditions in healthy humans. *Diabetes* 62:1435–1442.

Fukagawa, N.K. 2013. Protein and amino acid supplementation in older humans. *Amino Acids* 44:1493–1509.

Fuller, M.F. and P.J. Garlick. 1994. Human amino acid requirements: can the controversy be resolved? *Annu. Rev. Nutr.* 14:217–241.

Gannon, M.C. and F.Q. Nuttall. 2004. Effect of a high-protein, low-carbohydrate diet on blood glucose control in people with type 2 diabetes. *Diabetes* 53:2375–2382.

Gasier, H.G., J.D. Fluckey, S.F. Previs, M.P. Wiggs, and S.E. Riechman. 2012. Acute resistance exercise augments integrative myofibrillar protein synthesis. *Metabolism* 61:153–156.

Geggel, H., M. Ament, and J. Heckenlively. 1985. Nutritional requirement for taurine in patients receiving long-term, parenteral nutrition. *N. Engl. J. Med.* 312:142–146.

Geliebter, A., M.M. Maher, L. Gerace, B. Gutin, S.B. Heymsfield, and S.A. Hashim. 1997. Effects of strength or aerobic training on body composition, resting metabolic rate, and peak oxygen consumption in obese dieting subjects. *Am. J. Clin Nutr.* 66:557–563.

Gilani, G.S. and E. Sepehr. 2003. Protein digestibility and quality in products containing antinutritional factors are adversely affected by old age in rats. *J. Nutr.* 133:220–225.

Gilbreath, K.R., G.I. Nawaratna, T.A. Wickersham, M.C. Satterfield, F.W. Bazer, and G. Wu. 2020. Metabolic studies reveal that ruminal microbes of adult steers do not degrade rumen-protected or unprotected L-citrulline. *J. Anim. Sci.* 98:skz370.

Gilbreath, K.R., F.W. Bazer, M.C. Satterfield, and G. Wu. 2021. Amino acid nutrition and reproductive performance in ruminants. *Adv. Exp. Med. Biol.* 1285:43–61.

Gougeon-Reyburn, R. and E.B. Marliss. 1989. Effects of sodium bicarbonate on nitrogen metabolism and ketone bodies during very low energy protein diets in obese subjects. *Metabolism* 38:1222–1230.

Green, J.A., R.W. Hardy, and E.L. Brannon. 2002. The optimum dietary essential: nonessential amino acid ratio for rainbow trout (*Oncorhynchus mykiss*), which maximizes nitrogen retention and minimizes nitrogen excretion. *Fish. Physiol. Biochem.* 27:109–115.

Grillenberger, M., C.G. Neumann, S.P. Murphy, N.O. Bwibo, P. van't Veer, J.G. Hautvast, and C.E. West. 2003. Food supplements have a positive impact on weight gain and the addition of animal source foods increases lean body mass of Kenyan schoolchildren. *J. Nutr.* 133:3957S–3964S.

Hannaford, M.C., L.A. Leiter, R.G. Josse, M.B. Goldstein, E.B. Marliss, and M.L. Halperin. 1982. Protein wasting due to acidosis of prolonged fasting. *Am. J. Physiol.* 243:E251–256.

Harper, A.E. and N.N. Yoshimura. 1993. Protein quality, amino acid balance, utilization, and evaluation of diets containing amino acids as therapeutic agents. *Nutrition* 9:460–469.

Hartman, J.W., J.E. Tang, S.B. Wilkinson, M.A. Tarnopolsky, R.L. Lawrence, A.V. Fullerton, and S.M. Phillips. 2007. Consumption of fat-free fluid milk after resistance exercise promotes greater lean mass accretion than does consumption of soy or carbohydrate in young, novice, male weightlifters. *Am. J. Clin. Nutr.* 86:373–381.

Hasek, B.E., L.K. Stewart, T.M. Henagan, A. Boudreau, N.R. Lenard, C. Black et al. 2010. Dietary methionine restriction enhances metabolic flexibility and increases uncoupled respiration in both fed and fasted states. *Am. J. Physiol.* 299:R728–R739.

He, Q.H., X.F. Kong, G. Wu, P.P. Ren, H.R. Tang, F.H. Hao et al. 2009. Metabolomic analysis of the response of growing pigs to dietary L-arginine supplementation. *Amino Acids* 37:199–208.

He, Q.H., P.P. Ren, X.F. Kong, Y.N. Wu, G. Wu, P. Li et al. 2012a. Comparison of serum metabolite compositions between obese and lean growing pigs using an NMR-based metabonomic approach. *J. Nutr. Biochem.* 23:133–139.

He, C., R. Sumpter, Jr., and B. Levine. 2012b. Exercise induces autophagy in peripheral tissues and in the brain. *Autophagy* 8:1548–1551.

He, W.L., P. Li, and G. Wu. 2021. Amino acid nutrition and metabolism in chickens. *Adv. Exp. Med. Biol.* 1285:109–131.

Heaney, R.P. and D.K. Layman. 2008. Amount and type of protein influences bone health. *Am. J. Clin. Nutr.* 87:1567S–1570S.

Hebert, S.L. and K.S. Nair. 2010. Protein and energy metabolism in type 1 diabetes. *Clin. Nutr.* 29:13–17.

Heird, W.C., J.F. Nicholson, J.M. Driscoll, J.N. Schullinger, and R.W. Winters. 1972. Hyperammonemia resulting from intravenous alimentation using a mixture of synthetic L-amino acids: a preliminary report. *J. Pediatr.* 81:162–165.

Hengeveld, L.M., J.M.A. Boer, P. Gaudreau, M.W. Heymans, C. Jagger, N. Mendonca et al. 2020. Prevalence of protein intake below recommended in community-dwelling older adults: a meta-analysis across cohorts from the PROMISS consortium. *J Cachexia Sarcopenia Muscle* 11:1212–1222.

Herring, C.M., F.W. Bazer, G.A. Johnson, and G. Wu. 2018. Impacts of maternal dietary protein intake on fetal survival, growth and development. *Exp. Biol. Med.* 243:525–533.

Herring, C.M., F.W. Bazer, and G. Wu. 2021. Amino acid nutrition for optimum growth, development, reproduction, and health of zoo animals. *Adv. Exp. Med. Biol.* 1285:233–253.

Hilliar, M. and R.A. Swick. 2019. Nutritional implications of feeding reduced-protein diets to meat chickens. *Anim. Prod. Sci.* 59:2069–2081.

Hoffer, L.J. and B.R. Bistrian. 2012. Appropriate protein provision in critical illness: a systematic and narrative review. *Am. J. Clin. Nutr.* 96:591–600.

Holm, L., J.L. Olesen, K. Matsumoto, T. Doi, M. Mizuno, T.J. Alsted et al. 2008. Protein-containing nutrient supplementation following strength training enhances the effect on muscle mass, strength, and bone formation in postmenopausal women. *J. Appl. Physiol.* 105:274–281.

Holt, L.E. Jr. and A.A. Albanese. 1944. Observations on amino acid deficiencies in man. *Trans. Assoc. Am. Physicians* 58:143–56.

Hoppe, C., T.R. Udam, L. Lauritzen, C. Mølgaard, A. Juul, and K.F. Michaelsen. 2004. Animal protein intake, serum insulin-like growth factor I, and growth in healthy 2.5-y-old Danish children. *Am. J. Clin. Nutr.* 80:447–452.

Hou, Y.Q. and G. Wu. 2017. Nutritionally nonessential amino acids: a misnomer in nutritional sciences. *Adv. Nutr.* 8:137–139.

Hou, Y.Q. and G. Wu. 2018. L-Glutamate nutrition and metabolism in swine. *Amino Acids* 50:1497–1510.

Hou, Y.Q., Y.L. Yin, and G. Wu. 2015. Dietary essentiality of "nutritionally nonessential amino acids" for animals and humans. *Exp. Biol. Med.* 240:997–1007.

Hou, Y.Q., K. Yao, Y.L. Yin, and G. Wu. 2016. Endogenous synthesis of amino acids limits growth, lactation and reproduction of animals. *Adv. Nutr.* 7:331–342.

Hou, Y.Q., W.L. He, S.D. Hu, and G. Wu. 2019. Composition of polyamines and amino acids in plant-source foods for human consumption. *Amino Acids* 51:1153–1165.

Hou, Y.Q., S.D. Hu, X.Y. Li, W.L. He, and G. Wu. 2020. Amino acid metabolism in the liver: nutritional and physiological significance. *Adv. Exp. Med. Biol.* 1265:21–37.

Houston, D.K., B.J. Nicklas, J. Ding, T.B. Harris, F.A. Tylavsky, A.B. Newman et al. 2008. Health ABC Study. Dietary protein intake is associated with lean mass change in older, community-dwelling adults: the Health, Ageing, and Body Composition (Health ABC) Study. *Am. J. Clin. Nutr.* 87:150–155.

Hruby, A. and P.F. Jacques. 2020. Protein intake and human health: implications of units of protein intake. *Adv. Nutr.* 12:71–88.

Hu, F.B. 2005. Protein, body weight, and cardiovascular health. *Am. J. Clin. Nutr.* 82:242S–247S.

Hu, S.D., X.L. Li, R. Rezaei, C.J. Meininger, C.J. McNeal, and G. Wu. 2015. Safety of long-term dietary supplementation with L-arginine in pigs. *Amino Acids* 47:925–936.

Huston, R.L. and H.M. Scott. 1968. Effect of varying the composition of crystalline amino acid mixture on weight gain and pattern of free amino acids in chick tissue. *Fed. Proc.* 27:1204–1209.

IOM (Institute of Medicine). 2005. *Dietary Reference Intakes for Energy, Carbohydrates, Fiber, Fat, Fatty Acids, Cholesterol, Proteins, and Amino Acids.* The National Academies Press, Washington, D.C.

Iwalokun, B.A., S.B. Bamiro, and A. Ogunledun. 2006. Levels and interactions of plasma xanthine oxidase, catalase and liver function parameters in Nigerian children with Plasmodium falciparum infection. *APMIS.* 114:842–850.

Jacobsen, J.G. and L.H. Smith. 1968. Biochemistry and physiology of taurine and taurine derivatives. *Physiol. Rev.* 48:424–511.

Jaksic, T., D.A. Wagner, J.F. Burke, and V.R. Young. 1991. Proline metabolism in adult male burned patients and healthy control subjects. *Am. J. Clin. Nutr.* 54:408–413.

Jamin, A., R. D'Inca, N. Le Floc'h, A. Kuster, J. Orsonneau, D. Darmaun et al. 2010. Fatal effects of a neonatal high-protein diet in low-birth-weight piglets used as a model of intrauterine growth restriction. *Neonatology* 97:321–328.

Jesudason, D.R., E. Pedersen, and M. Clifton. 2013. Weight-loss diets in people with type 2 diabetes and renal disease: a randomized controlled trial of the effect of different dietary protein amounts. *Am. J. Clin. Nutr.* 98:494–501.

Ji, Y., Z.L. Wu, Z.L. Dai, X.L. Wang, J. Li, B.G. Wang, and G. Wu. 2017. Fetal and neonatal programming of postnatal growth and feed efficiency in swine. *J. Anim. Sci. Biotechnol.* 8:42.

Jobgen, W., W.J. Fu, H. Gao, P. Li, C.J. Meininger, S.B. Smith et al. 2009. High fat feeding and dietary L-arginine supplementation differentially regulate gene expression in rat white adipose tissue. *Amino Acids* 37:187–198.

Johnson, C.H., J. Ivanisevic, and G. Siuzdak. 2016. Metabolomics: beyond biomarkers and towards mechanisms. *Nat. Rev. Mol. Cell Biol.* 17:451–459.

Kang, J.S. 2020. Dietary restriction of amino acids for cancer therapy. *Nutr. Metab.* 17:20.

Katsanos, C.S., D.L. Chinkes, D. Paddon-Jones, X.J. Zhang, A. Aarsland, and R.R. Wolfe. 2008. Whey protein ingestion in elderly persons results in greater muscle protein accrual than ingestion of its constituent essential amino acid content. *Nutr. Res.* 28:651–658.

Kerr, B.J. 2003. Dietary manipulation to reduce environmental impact. In: *9th International Symposium on Digestive Physiology in Pigs* (Ball, R.O., ed). Banff, Alberta, Canada. pp. 139–158.

Kim, K.I., I. McMillan, and H.S. Bayley. 1983. Determination of amino acid requirements of young pigs using an indicator amino acid. *Br. J. Nutr.* 50:369–382.

Kim, S.W., G. Wu, and D.H. Baker. 2005. Ideal protein and amino acid requirements by gestating and lactating sows. *Pig News Inform.* 26:89N–99N.

Kim, J., L. O'Connor, L. Sands, M. Slebodnik, and W. Campbell. 2016. Effects of dietary protein intake on body composition changes after weight loss in older adults: a systematic review and meta-analysis. *Nutr. Rev.* 74:210–224.

Kim, H., L.E. Caulfield, V. Garcia-Larsen, L.M. Steffen, J. Coresh, and C.M. Rebholz. 2019. Plant-based diets are associated with a lower risk of incident cardiovascular disease, cardiovascular disease mortality, and all-cause mortality in a general population of middle-aged adults. *J. Am. Heart Assoc.* 8:e012865.

Kimball, S.R. 2014. Integration of signals generated by nutrients, hormones, and exercise in skeletal muscle. *Am. J. Clin. Nutr.* 99:237S–242S.

Kirchgessner, M., F.X. Roth, and B.R. Paulicks. 1993. Effects of adding glutamic acid to low protein diets for fattening pigs on criteria of growth and carcass composition. *Agribiol. Res.* 46:346–358.

Kopple, J.D. and M.E. Swendseid. 1975. Evidence that histidine is an essential amino acid in normal and chronically uremic man. *J. Clin. Invest.* 55:881–891.

Kopple, J.D. and M.E. Swendseid. 1981. Effect of histidine intake of plasma and urine histidine levels, nitrogen balance and N-tau-methylhistidine excretion in normal and chronically uremic men. *J. Nutr.* 111:931–942.

Krieger, J., H. Sitren, M. Daniels, and B. Langkamp-Henken. 2006. Effects of variation in protein and carbohydrate intake on body mass and composition during energy restriction: a meta-regression. *Am. J. Clin. Nutr.* 83:260–274.

Kurpad, A.V. and T. Thomas. 2011. Methods to assess amino acid requirements in humans. *Curr. Opin. Clin. Nutr. Metab. Care* 14:434–439.

Kurpad, A.V. and M. Vaz. 2000. Protein and amino acid requirements in the elderly. *Eur. J. Clin. Nutr.* 54 (Suppl 3):S131–S142.

Laidlaw, S.A., T.D. Shultz, J.T. Cecchino, and J.D. Kopple. 1988. Plasma and urine taurine levels in vegans. *Am. J. Clin. Nutr.* 47:660–663.

Lacey, J.M. and D.W. Wilmore. 1990. Is glutamine a conditionally essential amino acid? *Nutr. Rev.* 48:297–309.

Lamb, M.M., M. Miller, J.A. Seifert, B. Frederiksen, M. Kroehl, M. Rewers, and J.M. Norris. 2015. The effect of childhood cow's milk intake and HLA-DR genotype on risk of islet autoimmunity and type 1 diabetes: the Diabetes Autoimmunity Study in the Young (DAISY). *Pediatr Diabetes* 16:31–38.

Langley-Evans, S.C. 2007. Developmental programming of health and disease. *Proc. Nutr. Soc.* 65:97–105.

Lanza, E., A. Schatzkin, C. Daston, D. Corle, L. Freedman, R. Ballard-Barbash et al. 2001. Implementation of a 4-y, high-fiber, high-fruit-and-vegetable, low-fat dietary intervention: results of dietary changes in the polyp prevention trial. *Am. J. Clin. Nutr.* 74:387–401.

Larsson, L., B. Sjödin, and J. Karlsson. 1978. Histochemical and biochemical changes in human skeletal muscle with age in sedentary males, age 22–65 years. *Acta. Physiol. Scand.* 103:31–39.

Layman, D.K., E. Evans, J.I. Baum, J. Seyler, D.J. Erickson, and R.A. Boileau. 2005. Dietary protein and exercise have additive effects on body composition during weight loss in adult women. *J. Nutr.* 135:1903–1910.

Layman, D.K., T.G. Anthony, B.B. Rasmussen, S.H. Adams, C.J. Lynch, G.D. Brinkworth, and T.A. Davis. 2015. Defining meal requirements for protein to optimize metabolic roles of amino acids. *Am. J. Clin. Nutr.* 101:1330S–1338S.

Le Bellego, L., J. Van Milgen, S. Dubois, and J. Noblet. 2001. Energy utilization of low-protein diets in growing pigs. *J. Anim. Sci.* 79:1259–1271.

Le Floc'h, N., A. Wessels, E. Corrent, G. Wu, and P. Bosi. 2018. The relevance of functional amino acids to support the health of growing pigs. *Anim. Feed Sci. Technol.* 245:104–116.

Leidy, H.J., P.M. Clifton, A. Astrup, T.P. Wycherley, M.S. Westerterp-Plantenga, N.D. Luscombe-Marsh et al. 2015. The role of protein in weight loss and maintenance. *Am. J. Clin. Nutr.* 101:1320S–1329S.

Leenders, M., L.B. Verdijk, L. van der Hoeven, J. van Kranenburg, F. Hartgens, W.K. Wodzig et al. 2011. Prolonged leucine supplementation does not augment muscle mass or affect glycemic control in elderly type 2 diabetic men. *J. Nutr.* 141:1070–1076.

Levenhagen, D.K., J.D. Gresham, M.G. Carlson, D.J. Maron, M.J. Borel, and P.J. Flakoll. 2001. Postexercise nutrient intake timing in humans is critical to recovery of leg glucose and protein homeostasis. *Am. J. Physiol.* 280:E982–E993.

Lemon, P.W., D.G. Dolny, and K.E. Yarasheski. 1997. Moderate physical activity can increase dietary protein needs. *Can. J. Appl. Physiol.* 22:494–503.

Levine, M.E., J.A. Suarez, S. Brandhorst, P. Balasubramanian, C.W. Cheng, F. Madia et al. 2014. Low protein intake is associated with a major reduction in IGF-1, cancer, and overall mortality in the 65 and younger but not older population. *Cell Metab.* 19:407–417.

Li, P. and G. Wu. 2018. Roles of dietary glycine, proline and hydroxyproline in collagen synthesis and animal growth. *Amino Acids* 50:29–38.

Li, P., and G. Wu. 2020. Composition of amino acids and related nitrogenous nutrients in feedstuffs for animal diets. *Amino Acids* 52:523–542.

Li, P., Y.L. Yin, D.F. Li, S.W. Kim, and G. Wu. 2007. Amino acids and immune function. *Br. J. Nutr.* 98:237–252.

Li, X.L., R. Rezaei, P. Li, and G. Wu. 2011. Composition of amino acids in feed ingredients for animal diets. *Amino Acids* 40:1159–1168.

Li, X.Y., S.X. Zheng, and G. Wu. 2021a. Nutrition and functions of amino acids in fish. *Adv. Exp. Med. Biol.* 1285:133–168.

Li, X.Y., T. Han, S.X. Zheng, and G. Wu. 2021b. Nutrition and functions of amino acids in aquatic crustaceans. *Adv. Exp. Med. Biol.* 1285:169–197.

Li, X.Y., S.X. Zheng, X.K. Ma, K.M. Cheng, and G. Wu. 2021c. Use of alternative protein sources for fishmeal replacement in the diet of largemouth bass (*Micropterus salmoides*). Part I: effects of poultry by-product meal and soybean meal on growth, feed utilization, and health. *Amino Acids* 53:33–47.

Li, X.Y., S.X. Zheng, K.M. Cheng, X.K. Ma, and G. Wu. 2021d. Use of alternative protein sources for fishmeal replacement in the diet of largemouth bass (*Micropterus salmoides*). Part II: effects of supplementation with methionine or taurine on growth, feed utilization, and health. *Amino Acids* 53:49–62.

Liao, S.F., N. Regmi, and G. Wu. 2018. Homeostatic regulation of plasma amino acid concentrations. *Front. Biosci.* 23:640–655.

Lin, G., C. Liu, T.J. Wang, G. Wu, S.Y. Qiao, D.F. Li, and J.J. Wang. 2011. Biomarkers for optimal requirements of amino acids by animals and humans. *Front. Biosci.* S3:1298–1307.

Lindle, R.S., E.J. Metter, N.A. Lynch, J.L. Fleg, J.L. Fozard, J. Tobin et al. 1997. Age and gender comparisons of muscle strength in 654 women and men aged 20–93 yr. *J. Appl. Physiol.* 83:1581–1587.

Lonnie, M., E. Hooker, J.M. Brunstrom, B.M. Corfe, M.A. Green, A.W. Watson et al. 2018. Protein for life: review of optimal protein intake, sustainable dietary sources and the effect on appetite in ageing adults. *Nutrition* 10:360.

Lushaj, E.B., J.K. Johnson, D. McKenzie, and J.M. Aiken. 2010. Sarcopenia accelerates at advanced ages in Fisher 344×Brown Norway rats. *J. Gerontol. A* 63:921–927.

Macdermid, P.W. and S.R. Stannard. 2006. A whey-supplemented, high-protein diet versus a high-carbohydrate diet: effects on endurance cycling performance. *Int. J. Sport. Nutr. Exerc. Metab.* 16:65–77.

MacFarlane, A.J., K.M. Burghardt, J. Kelly, T. Simell, O. Simell, I. Altosaar, and F.W. Scott. 2003. A type 1 diabetes-related protein from wheat (*Triticum aestivum*). *J. Biol. Chem.* 278:54–63.

Maddocks, O.D.K., D. Athineos, E.C. Cheung, P. Lee, T. Zhang, N.J.F. van den Broek et al. 2017. Modulating the therapeutic response of tumours to dietary serine and glycine starvation. *Nature* 544:372–376.

Mamerow, M.M., J.A. Mettler, K.L. English, S.L. Casperson, E. Arentson-Lantz, M. Sheffield-Moore et al. 2014. Dietary protein distribution positively influences 24-h muscle protein synthesis in healthy adults. *J. Nutr.* 144:876–880.

Manjarín, R., C. Boutry-Regard, A. Suryawan, A. Canovas, B.D. Piccolo, M. Maj et al. 2020. Intermittent leucine pulses during continuous feeding alters novel components involved in skeletal muscle growth of neonatal pigs. *Amino Acids* 52:1319–1335.

Mariotti, F. and C.D. Gardner. 2019. Dietary protein and amino acids in vegetarian diets-A Review. *Nutrients* 11:2661.

Marković-Jovanovic, S. 2013. Nutritional management in type 1 diabetes mellitus. In: *Type 1 Diabetes* (Escher, A.P. and A. Li, ed). IntechOpen doi:10.5772/52465.

Marliss, E.B. and R. Gougeon. 2002. Diabetes mellitus, lipidus Et... proteinus! *Diabetes Care* 25:1474–1476.

Marliss, E.B. and M. Vranic. 2002. Intense exercise has unique effects on both insulin release and its roles in glucoregulation: implications for diabetes. *Diabetes* 51(Suppl 1):S271–S283.

Mather, M., L.A. Jacobsen, and K.M. Pollard. 2015. Aging in the United States. *Population Bulletin* 70:1–18.

McClelland, W. and E. DuBois. 1930. Prolonged meat diets with a study of kidney function and ketosis. *J. Biol. Chem.* 87:651–680.

McGlory, C. and S.M. Phillips. 2016. Amino acids and exercise: molecular and cellular aspects. In: *The Molecular Nutrition of Amino Acids and Proteins* (Dardevet, D., ed). Academic Press, San Diego, CA. pp. 67–78.

McKnight, J.R., M.C. Satterfield, W.S. Jobgen, S.B. Smith, T.E. Spencer, C.J. Meininger et al. 2010. Beneficial effects of L-arginine on reducing obesity: potential mechanisms and important implications for human health. *Amino Acids* 39:349–357.

McLaughlin, J.M. 1974. Nutritional significance of alterations in plasma amino acids and serum proteins. In: *Committee on Amino Acids, Food and Nutrition.* National Academy of Sciences, Washington, DC. pp. 89–108.

McNeal, C.J., C.J. Meininger, C.D. Wilborn, C.D. Tekwe, and G. Wu. 2018. Safety of dietary supplementation with arginine in adult humans. *Amino Acids* 50:1215–1229.

Meredith, C.N., Z.M. Wen, D.M. Bier, D.E. Matthews, and V.R. Young. 1986. Lysine kinetics at graded lysine intakes in young men. *Am. J. Clin. Nutr.* 43:787–794.

Mertz, E.T., W.M. Beeson, and H.D. Jackson. 1952. Classification of essential amino acids for the weanling pig. *Arch. Biochem. Biophys.* 38:121–128.

Michaelsen, K.F. 1997. Nutrition and growth during infancy. The Copenhagen Cohort Study. *Acta Paediatr.* 86:1–36.

Miller, R.A., G. Buehner, Y. Chang, J.M. Harper, R. Sigler, and M. Smith-Wheelock. 2005. Methionine-deficient diet extends mouse lifespan, slows immune and lens aging, alters glucose, T4, IGF-I and insulin levels, and increases hepatocyte MIF levels and stress resistance. *Aging Cell* 4:119–125.

Millward, D.J. 1997. Human amino acid requirements. *J. Nutr.* 127:1842–1846.

Millward, D.J. 1998. Metabolic demands for amino acids and the human dietary requirement: Millward and Rivers (1988) revisited. *J. Nutr.* 128:2563S–2576S.

Mok, C.H., C.L. Levesque, and K.L. Urschel. 2018. Using the indicator amino acid oxidation technique to study threonine requirements in horses receiving a predominantly forage diet. *J. Anim. Physiol. Anim. Nutr. (Berl)* 102:1366–1381.

Moore, D.R., M.J. Robinson, J.L. Fry, J.E. Tang, E.I. Glover, S.B. Wilkinson et al. 2009. Ingested protein dose response of muscle and albumin protein synthesis after resistance exercise in young men. *Am. J. Clin. Nutr.* 89:161–168.

Moore, D.R., P.J. Atherton, M.J. Rennie, M.A. Tarnopolsky, and S.M. Phillips. 2011. Resistance exercise enhances mTOR and MAPK signalling in human muscle over that seen at rest after bolus protein ingestion. *Acta Physiol.* 201:365–372.

Morais, J.A., R. Gougeon, P.B. Pencharz, P.J. Jones, R. Ross, and E.B. Marliss. 1997. Whole-body protein turnover in the healthy elderly. *Am. J. Clin. Nutr.* 66:880–889.

Morais, J.A., R. Ross, R. Gougeon, P.B. Pencharz, P.J. Jones, and E.B. Marliss. 2000. Distribution of protein turnover changes with age in humans as assessed by whole-body magnetic resonance image analysis to quantify tissue volumes. *J. Nutr.* 130:784–791.

Morais, J.A., S. Chevalier, and R. Gougeon. 2006. Protein turnover and requirements in the healthy and frail elderly. *J. Nutr. Health Aging* 10:272–283.

Morup, I.K. and E.S. Olesen. 1976. New method for prediction of protein value from essential amino acid pattern. *Nutr. Rep. Int.* 13:355–365.

Moughan, P.J. 2003. Amino acid availability – aspects of chemical analysis and bioassay methodology. *Nutr. Res. Rev.* 16:127–141.

Moughan, P.J. and S.M. Rutherfurd. 2012. True ileal amino acid and protein digestibility (%) for selected human foods. In: *Report of a Sub-Committee of the 2011 FAO Consultation on "Protein Quality Evaluation in Human Nutrition"*. FAO, Rome.

Moundras, C., C. Remesy, and C. Demigne. 1993. Dietary protein paradox: decrease of amino acid availability induced by high-protein diets. *Am. J. Physiol.* 264:G1057–G1065.

Munro, H.N. 1964. Historical introduction: the origin and growth of our present concepts of protein metabolism. In: *Mammalian Protein Metabolism* (Munro, H.N. and J.B. Allison, eds). Academic Press, New York.

Norton, L.E. and D.K. Layman. 2006. Leucine regulates translation initiation of protein synthesis in skeletal muscle after exercise. *J. Nutr.* 136:533S–S537.

NRC (National Research Council). 2011. *Nutrient Requirements of Fish and Shrimp*. National Academies Press, Washington DC.

NRC (National Research Council). 2012. *Nutrient Requirements of Swine*. National Academy Press, Washington, D.C.

Oberbauer, A.M. and J.A. Larsen. 2021. Amino acids in dog nutrition and health. *Adv. Exp. Med. Biol.* 1285:199–216.

Ochoa, S. 2020. Muscle atrophy in horses. https://www.innovetpet.com/blogs/horses/muscle-atrophy. Accessed, December 21, 2020

Oliveira, C.L.P., N.G. Boulé, A.M. Sharma, S.A. Elliott, M. Siervo, S. Ghosh et al. 2020. A high-protein total diet replacement increases energy expenditure and leads to negative fat balance in healthy, normal-weight adults. *Am. J. Clin. Nutr.* doi:10.1093/ajcn/nqaa283.

Ollberding, N.J., L.R. Wilkens, B.E. Henderson, L.N. Kolonel, and L. Le Marchand. 2012. Meat consumption, heterocyclic amines and colorectal cancer risk: the Multiethnic Cohort Study. *Int. J. Cancer* 131:E1125–E1133.

Orentreich, N., J.R. Matias, A. DeFelice, and J.A. Zimmerman. 1993. Low methionine ingestion by rats extends life span. *J. Nutr.* 123:269–274.

Osborne, T.B. and L.B. Mendel. 1914. Amino acids in nutrition and growth. *J. Biol. Chem.* 17:325–350.

Oser, B. L., 1951. Method for integrating essential amino acid contents in the nutritional evaluation of protein. *J. Am Dietet. Assoc.* 27:396–402.

Pedersen, A.N., J. Kondrup, and E. Børsheim. 2013. Health effects of protein intake in healthy adults: a systematic literature review. *Food Nutr. Res.* 57:21245.

Pencharz, P.B. and R.O. Ball. 2003. Different approaches to define individual amino acid requirements. *Annu. Rev. Nutr.* 23:101–116.

Pennings, B., Y. Boirie, J.M. Senden, A.P. Gijsen, H. Kuipers, and L.J. van Loon. 2011. Whey protein stimulates postprandial muscle protein accretion more effectively than do casein and casein hydrolysate in older men. *Am. J. Clin. Nutr.* 93:997–1005.

Pereira, S., E.B. Marliss, J.A. Morais, S. Chevalier, and R. Gougeon. 2008. Insulin resistance of protein metabolism in type 2 diabetes. *Diabetes* 57:56–63.

Pfeiffer, A.F.H., E. Pedersen, U. Schwab, U. Risérus, A. Aas, M. Uusitupa et al. 2020. The effects of different quantities and qualities of protein intake in people with diabetes mellitus. *Nutrients* 12:365.

Phillips, S.M., K.D. Tipton, A. Aarsland, S.E. Wolf, and R.R. Wolfe. 1997. Mixed muscle protein synthesis and breakdown after resistance exercise in humans. *Am. J. Physiol.* 273:E99–E107.

Phillips, B.E., Hill, D.S., and Atherton, P.J. 2012. Regulation of muscle protein synthesis in humans. *Curr. Opin. Clin. Nutr. Metab. Care* 15:58–63.

Phillips, S.M., D. Paddon-Jones, and D.K. Layman. 2020. Optimizing adult protein intake during catabolic health conditions. *Adv. Nutr.* 11:S1058–S1069.

Prado, C.M., S.A. Purcell, C. Alish, S.L. Pereira, N.E. Deutz, D.K. Heyland et al. 2018. Implications of low muscle mass across the continuum of care: a narrative review. *Ann. Med.* 50:675–693.

Prado, C.M., S.A. Purcell, and A. Laviano. 2020. Nutrition interventions to treat low muscle mass in cancer. *J Cachexia Sarcopenia Muscle* 11:366–380.

Purchas, R.W., S.M. Rutherfurd, P.D. Pearce, R. Vather, and B.H.P. Wilkinson. 2004. Concentrations in beef and lamb of taurine, carnosine, coenzyme Q_{10}, and creatine. *Meat Sci.* 66:629–637.

Rasch, T.W., and N.J. Benevenga. 2004. Recovery of ^{15}N in the body, urine, and gas phase of piglets infused intravenously with ^{15}N L-alanine from 12–72 hours of age. *J. Nutr.* 134:847–854.

Rana, S.K. and T.A. Sanders. 1986. Taurine concentrations in the diet, plasma, urine and breast milk of vegans compared with omnivores. *Br. J. Nutr.* 56:17–27.

Rasmussen, B.B. and S.M. Phillips. 2003. Contractile and nutritional regulation of human muscle growth. *Exerc. Sport Sci. Rev.* 31:127–131.

Rasmussen, B.B., K.D. Tipton, S.L. Miller, S.E. Wolf, and R.R. Wolfe. 2000. An oral amino acid-carbohydrate supplement enhances muscle protein anabolism after resistance exercise. *J. Appl. Physiol.* 88:386–392.

Rasmussen, B.F., M.A. Ennis, R.A. Dyer, K. Lim, and R. Elango. 2020. Glycine, a dispensable amino acid, is conditionally indispensable in late stages of human pregnancy. *J. Nutr.* 151:361–369.

Reeds, P.J. 2000. Dispensable and indispensable amino acids for humans. *J. Nutr.* 130:1835S–1840S.

Reeds, P.J., D.G. Burrin, B. Stoll, and J.B. van Goudoever. 2000. Role of the gut in the amino acid economy of the host. *Nestle Nutr. Workshop Ser. Clin. Perform. Programme* 3:25–40.

Rennie, M.J., R.H. Edwards, S. Krywawych, C.T. Davies, D. Halliday, J.C. Waterlow, and D.J. Millward. 1981. Effect of exercise on protein turnover in man. *Clin. Sci. (Lond)* 61:627–639.

Rezaei, R., D.A. Knabe, C.D. Tekwe, S. Dahanayaka, M.D. Ficken, S.E. Fielder et al. 2013. Dietary supplementation with monosodium glutamate is safe and improves growth performance in postweaning pigs. *Amino Acids* 44:911–923.

Richter, C.K., A.C. Skulas-Ray, C.M. Champagne, and P.M. Kris-Etherton. 2015. Plant protein and animal proteins: do they differentially affect cardiovascular disease risk? *Adv. Nutr.* 6:712–728.

Riddell, M.C., I.W. Gallen, C.E. Smart, C.E. Taplin, P. Adolfsson, A.N. Lumb et al. 2017. Exercise management in type 1 diabetes: a consensus statement. *Lancet Diabetes Endocrinol.* 5:377–390.

Riddell, M.C., S.N. Scott, P.A. Fournier, S.R. Colberg, I.W. Gallen, O. Moser et al. 2020. The competitive athlete with type 1 diabetes. *Diabetologia* 63:1475–1490.

Ringholm, S., R.S. Bienso, K. Kiilerish, A. Guadalupe-Grau, N.J. Aachmann-Andersen, B. Saltin et al. 2011. Bed rest reduces metabolic protein content and abolishes exercise-induced mRNA responses in human skeletal muscle. *Am. J. Physiol.* 301:E649–E658.

Rolland-Cachera, M.F., M. Deheeger, and F. Bellisle. 1999. Increasing prevalence of obesity among 18-year-old males in Sweden: evidence for early determinants. *Acta Paediatr.* 88:365–367.

Rosenvinge, S.A., A. Toubro, J. Bülow, K. Krabbe, H. Parving, and A. Astrup. 1999. Changes in renal function during weight loss induced by high vs low-protein low-fat diets in overweight subjects. *Int. J. Obes.* 23:1170–1177.

Rose, W.C. 1968. The sequence of events leading to the establishment of the amino acid needs of man. *Am. J. Public Health* 58:2020–2027.

Rose, W.C., W.J. Haines, D.T. Warner, and J.E. Johnson. 1951. The amino acid requirements of man: II. The role of threonine and histidine. *J. Biol. Chem.* 188:49–58.

Rose, W.C., W.J. Haines, and D.T. Warner. 1954a. The amino acid requirements of man: V. The role of lysine, arginine, and tryptophan. *J. Biol. Chem.* 206:421–430.

Rose, W.C., G.F. Lambert, and M.J. Coon. 1954b. The amino acid requirements of man. VII. General procedures; the tryptophan requirement. *J. Biol. Chem.* 211:815–827.

Rutherfurd, S.M., A.C. Fanning, B.J. Miller, and P.J. Moughan. 2015. Protein digestibility-corrected amino acid scores and digestible indispensable amino acid scores differentially describe protein quality in growing male rats. *J. Nutr.* 145:372–379.

Sahni, S., K.E. Broe, K.L. Tucker, R.R. McLean, D.P. Kiel, L.A. Cupples, and M.T. Hannan. 2013. Association of total protein intake with bone mineral density and bone loss in men and women from the Framingham Offspring Study. *Public Health Nutr.* 29:1–7.

Salomé, M., E. de Gavelle, A. Dufour, C. Dubuisson, J. Volatier, H. Fouillet et al. 2020. Plant-protein diversity is critical to ensuring the nutritional adequacy of diets when replacing animal with plant protein: observed and modeled diets of French adults (INCA3). *J. Nutr.* 150:536–545.

Santesso, N., E.A. Akl, M. Bianchi, A. Mente, R. Mustafa, D. Heels-Ansdell, and H.J. Schünemann. 2012. Effects of higher- versus lower-protein diets on health outcomes: a systematic review and meta-analysis. *Eur. J. Clin. Nutr.* 66:780–788.

Sasse, C.E. and D.H. Baker. 1973. Modification of the Illinois reference standard amino acid mixture. *Poult. Sci.* 52:1970–1972.

Schatzkin, A., E. Lanza, D. Corle, P. Lance, F. Iber, B. Caan et al. 2000. Polyp Prevention Trial Study Group. Lack of effect of a low-fat, high-fiber diet on the recurrence of colorectal adenomas. *N. Engl. J. Med.* 342:1149–1155.

Schönfeldt, H.C. and N.G. Hall. 2012. Dietary protein quality and malnutrition in Africa. *Br. J. Nutr.* 108:S69–S76.

Schürch, M.A., R. Rizzoli, D. Slosman, L. Vadas, P. Vergnaud, and J.P. Bonjour. 1998. Protein supplements increase serum insulin-like growth factor-I levels and attenuate proximal femur bone loss in patients with recent hip fracture. A randomized, double-blind, placebo-controlled trial. *Ann. Intern. Med.* 28:801–809.

Schwab, C.G. and G.A. Broderick. 2017. A 100-year review: protein and amino acid nutrition in dairy cows. *J. Dairy Sci.* 100:10094–10112.

Scott, F.W. and E.B. Marliss. 1991. Diet as an environmental factor in development of insulin-dependent diabetes mellitus. *Can. J. Physiol. Pharmacol.* 69:311–319.

Sheffield-Moore, M., R.R. Wolfe, D.C. Gore, S.E. Wolf, D.M. Ferrer, and A.A. Ferrando. 2000. Combined effects of hyperaminoacidemia and oxandrolone on skeletal muscle protein synthesis". *Am. J. Physiol.* 278:E273–279.

Selle, O.H., J.C.D.P. Dorigam, A. Lemme, P.V. Chrystal, and S.Y. Liu. 2020. Synthetic and crystalline amino acids: alternatives to soybean meal in chicken-meat production. *Animals* 10:729.

Semba, R.D. 2016. The rise and fall of protein malnutrition in global health. *Ann. Nutr. Metab.* 69:79–88.

Shang, X., D. Scott, A.M. Hodge, D.R. English, G.G. Giles, P.R. Ebeling, K.M. Sanders. 2016. Dietary protein intake and risk of type 2 diabetes: results from the Melbourne Collaborative Cohort Study and a meta-analysis of prospective studies. *Am. J. Clin. Nutr.* 104:1352–1365.

Silva, A.M., W. Shen, M. Heo, D. Gallagher, Z. Wang, L.B. Sardinha, and S.B. Heymsfield. 2010. Ethnicity-related skeletal muscle differences across the lifespan. *Am. J. Hum. Biol.* 22:76–82.

Simmons, E.E., J.D. Fluckey, and S.E. Riechman. 2016. Cumulative muscle protein synthesis and protein intake requirements. *Annu. Rev. Nutr.* 36:17–43.

Skov, A.R., S. Toubro, B. Ronn, L. Holm, and A. Astrup. 1999. Randomized trial on protein vs carbohydrate in ad libitum fat reduced diet for the treatment of obesity. *Int. J. Obes. Relat. Metab. Disord.* 23:528–536.

Smith, S.B., D.K. Lunt, D.R. Smith, and R.L. Walzem. 2020. Producing high-oleic acid beef and the impact of ground beef consumption on risk factors for cardiovascular disease: A review. *Meat Sci.* 163:108076.

Smriga, M., S. Ghosh, Y. Mouneimne, P.L. Pellett, and N.S. Scrimshaw. 2004. Lysine fortification reduces anxiety and lessens stress in family members in economically weak communities in Northwest Syria. *Proc. Natl. Acad. Sci. USA* 101:8285–8288.

Smythe, P.M., A. Swanepoel, and J.A.H. Campbell. 1962. The heart in kwashiorkor. *Br. Med. J.* 1:67–73.

Solano, F. 2020. Metabolism and functions of amino acids in the skin. *Adv. Exp. Med. Biol.* 1265:187–199.

Stapleton, P.P., R.P. Charles, H.P. Redmond, and D.J. Bouchier-Hayes. 1997. Taurine and human nutrition. *Clin. Nutr.* 16:103–108.

Strasser, B., J.M. Gostner, and D. Fuchs. 2016. Mood, food, and cognition: role of tryptophan and serotonin. *Curr. Opin. Clin. Nutr. Metab. Care* 19:55–61.

Sturman, J.A., G.W. Hepner, A.F. Hofmann, and P.J. Thomas. 1975. Metabolism of [^{35}S]taurine in man. *J. Nutr.* 105:1206–1214.

Sun, Y. 2020. Thrifty hormone ghrelin: the secret of aging muscularly. *J. Aging Sci.* 8:S3.005.

Suryawan, A. and T.A. Davis. 2011. Regulation of protein synthesis by amino acids in muscle of neonates. *Front. Biosci.* 16:1445–1460.

Symons, T.B., M. Sheffield-Moore, R.R. Wolfe, and D. Paddon-Jones. 2009. A moderate serving of high-quality protein maximally stimulates skeletal muscle protein synthesis in young and elderly subjects. *J. Am. Diet. Assoc.* 109:1582–1586.

Talaei, M., A. Pan, J.M. Yuan, and W.P. Koh. 2018. Dairy intake and risk of type 2 diabetes. *Clin. Nutr.* 37:712–718.

Tarnopolsky, M.A., J.D. MacDougall, and S.A. Atkinson. 1988. Influence of protein intake and training status on nitrogen balance and lean body mass. *J. Appl. Physiol.* 64:187–193.

Tarnopolsky, M.A., S.A. Atkinson, J.D. MacDougall, A. Chesley, S. Phillips, and H.P. Schwarcz. 1992. Evaluation of protein requirements for trained strength athletes. *J. Appl. Physiol.* 73:1986–1995.

Tessari, P. 2019. Nonessential amino acid usage for protein replenishment in humans: a method of estimation. *Am. J. Clin. Nutr.* 110:255–264.

Tessier, A.-J., S.S. Wing, E. Rahme, J.A. Morais, and S. Chevalier. 2019. Physical function-derived cut-points for the diagnosis of sarcopenia and dynapenia from the Canadian longitudinal study on aging. *J. Cachexia Sarcopenia Muscle* 10:985–999.

Timp, W. and G. Timp. 2020. Beyond mass spectrometry, the next step in proteomics. *Sci. Adv.* 6:eaax8978.

Tipton, K.D., T.A. Elliott, M.G. Cree, S.E. Wolf, A.P. Sanford, and R.R. Wolfe. 2004. Ingestion of casein and whey proteins result in muscle anabolism after resistance exercise. *Med. Sci. Sports Exerc.* 36:2073–2081.

Tomé, D. 2012. Criteria and markers for protein quality assessment - A review. *Br. J. Nutr.* 108 (Suppl. 2):S222–S229.

Trouwborst, I., A. Verreijen, R. Memelink, P. Massanet, Y. Boirie, P. Weijs, and M. Tieland. 2018. Exercise and nutrition strategies to counteract sarcopenic obesity. *Nutrients* 10:605.

Tujioka, K., M. Ohsumi, K. Hayase, and H. Yokogoshi. 2011. Effect of the quality of dietary amino acids composition on the urea synthesis in rats. *J. Nutr. Sci. Vitaminol.* 57:48–55.

Van Blarigan, E.L., C.S. Fuchs, D. Niedzwiecki, S. Zhang, L.B. Saltz, R.J. Mayer et al. 2018. Association of survival with adherence to the American Cancer Society Nutrition and Physical Activity Guidelines for cancer survivors after colon cancer diagnosis: the CALGB 89803/Alliance TrialAssociation of colon cancer survival with ACS Guideline Adher. *JAMA Oncol.* 4:783–790.

Van Elswyk, M.E., C.A. Weatherford, and S.H. McNeill. 2018. A systematic review of renal health in healthy individuals associated with protein intake above the US recommended daily allowance in randomized controlled trials and observational studies. *Adv. Nutr.* 9:404–418.

van Milgen, J. and J.-Y. Dourmad. 2015. Concept and application of ideal protein for pigs. *J. Anim. Sci. Biotechnol.* 6:15.

van Nielen, M., E.J.M. Feskens, M. Mensink, I. Sluijs, E. Molina, P. Amiano et al. 2014. Dietary protein intake and incidence of type 2 diabetes in Europe: the EPIC-InterAct Case-Cohort Study. *Diabetes Care* 37:1854–1862.

van Vliet, S., N.A. Burd, and L.J.C. van Loon. 2015. The skeletal muscle anabolic response to plant- versus animal-based protein consumption. *J. Nutr.* 145:1981–1991.

Volek, J.S., B.M. Volk, A.L. Gomez, L.J. Kunces, B.R. Kupchak, D.J. Freidenreich et al. 2013. Whey protein supplementation during resistance training augments lean body mass. *J. Am. Coll. Nutr.* 32:122–135.

Volpi, E., W.W. Campbell, J.T. Dwyer, M.A. Johnson, G.L. Jensen, J.E. Morley, and R.R. Wolfe. 2013. Is the optimal level of protein intake for older adults greater than the recommended dietary allowance? *J. Gerontol. A* 68:677–681.

Walker, A.F. 1979. A comparison of the dye-binding and fluorodinitrobenzene methods for determining reactive lysine in leaf protein concentrates. *Br. J. Nutr.* 42:455–465.

Wallace, T.C. 2019. Optimizing dietary protein for lifelong bone health: a paradox unraveled. *Nutr. Today.* 54:107–115.

Wang, T.C. and M.F. Fuller. 1989. The optimum dietary amino acid patterns for growing pigs. 1. Experiments by amino acid deletion. *Br. J. Nutr.* 62:77–89.

Wang, H.R. and D.X. Lu. 2002. A study on the optimal amino acid pattern at the proximal duodenum in growing sheep. *Asian-Austral. J Anim. Sci.* 15:38–44.

Wang, J.J., D.F. Li, L.J. Dangott, and G. Wu. 2006. Proteomics and its role in nutrition research. *J. Nutr.* 136:1759–1762.

Wang, J.J., L.X. Chen, P. Li, X.L. Li, H.J. Zhou, F.L. Wang et al. 2008. Gene expression is altered in piglet small intestine by weaning and dietary glutamine supplementation. *J. Nutr.* 138:1025–1032.

Wang, J.J., G. Wu, H.J. Zhou, and F.L. Wang. 2009. Emerging technologies for amino acid nutrition research in the post-genome era. *Amino Acids* 37:177–186.

Wang, J.J., Z.L. Wu, D.F. Li, N. Li, S.V. Dindot, M.C. Satterfield et al. 2012. Nutrition, epigenetics, and metabolic syndrome. *Antioxid. Redox Signal.* 17:282–301.

Wang, W.W., Z.L. Wu, Z.L. Dai, Y. Yang, J.J. Wang, and G. Wu. 2013. Glycine metabolism in animals and humans: implications for nutrition and health. *Amino Acids* 45:463–477

Wang, W.W., Z.L. Dai, Z.L. Wu, G. Lin, S.C. Jia, S.D. Hu et al. 2014. Glycine is a nutritionally essential amino acid for maximal growth of milk-fed young pigs. *Amino Acids* 46:2037–2045.

Waterlow, J.C., P.J. Garlick, and D.J. Millward. 1978. *Protein Turnover in Mammalian Tissues and in the Whole Body*. North Holland Publishing Company, Amsterdam.

Weber, T.R., M.C. Dalsing, A. Sawchuck, P. Sieber, and J.L. Grosfeld. 1983. The effect of protein deficiency on growth and response of primary and metastatic hepatoma. *J. Surg. Res.* 34:395–403.

Weckman, A.M., C.R. McDonald, J.B. Baxter, W.W. Fawzi, A.L. Conroy, and K.C. Kain. 2019. Perspective: L-arginine and L-citrulline supplementation in pregnancy: a potential strategy to improve birth outcomes in low-resource settings. *Adv. Nutr.* 10:765–777.

Wei, S., J. Zhao, S. Wang, M. Huang, Y. Wang, and Y. Chen. 2018. Intermittent administration of a leucine-deprived diet is able to intervene in type 2 diabetes in db/db mice. *Heliyon* 4:e00830.

Weindruch, R., R.L. Walford, S. Fligiel, and D. Guthrie. 1986. The retardation of aging in mice by dietary restriction: longevity, cancer, immunity and lifetime energy intake. *J. Nutr.* 116:641–654.

Wester, T.J., K. Weidgraaf, M. Hekman, C.E. Ugarte, S.F. Forsyth, and M.H. Tavendale. 2015. Amino acid oxidation increases with dietary protein content in adult neutered male cats as measured using $[1-^{13}C]$ leucine and $[^{15}N_2]$urea. *J. Nutr.* 145:2471–2478.

Westerterp-Plantenga, M.S., S.G. Lemmens, and K.R. Westerterp. 2012. Dietary protein - its role in satiety, energetics, weight loss and health. *Br. J. Nutr.* 108 (Suppl. 2):S105–S112.

Wharton, B.A., G.R. Howells, and R.A. McCance. 1967. Cardiac failure in kwashiorkor. *Lancet* 2(7512):384–387.

White, S.J. and S. Cantsilieris. 2017. *Genotyping: Methods and Protocols*. Springer, New York.

Willoughby, D.S., J.R. Stout, and C.D. Wilborn. 2007. Effects of resistance training and protein plus amino acid supplementation on muscle anabolism, mass, and strength. *Amino Acids* 32:467–477.

Witard, O.C., S.R. Jackman, A.K. Kies, A.E. Jeukendrup, and K.D. Tipton. 2011. Effect of increased dietary protein on tolerance to intensified training. *Med. Sci. Sports Exerc.* 43:598–607.

Witard, O.C., S.R. Jackman, L. Breen, K. Smith, A. Selby, and K.D. Tipton. 2014. Myofibrillar muscle protein synthesis rates subsequent to a meal in response to increasing doses of whey protein at rest and after resistance exercise. *Am. J. Clin. Nutr.* 99:86–95.

Wolfe, R.R. 2006. The underappreciated role of muscle in health and disease. *Am. J. Clin. Nutr.* 84:475–482.

Wolfe, R.R., S.M. Rutherfurd, I.Y. Kim, and P.J. Moughan. 2016. Protein quality as determined by the digestible indispensable amino acid score: evaluation of factors underlying the calculation. *Nutr. Rev.* 74:584–599.

Wright, C.E., H.H. Tallan, Y.Y. Lin, and G.E. Gaull. 1986. Taurine: biological update. *Annu. Rev. Biochem.* 55:427–453.

Wright, N.C., A.C. Looker, and K.G. Saag. 2014. The recent prevalence of osteoporosis and low bone mass in the United States based on bone mineral density at the femoral neck or lumbar spine. *J. Bone Miner. Res.* 29:2520–2526.

Wu, G. 1995. Nitric oxide synthesis and the effect of aminoguanidine and N^G-monomethyl-L-arginine on the onset of diabetes in the spontaneously diabetic BB rat. *Diabetes* 44:360–364.

Wu, G. 2009. Amino acids: metabolism, functions, and nutrition. *Amino Acids* 37:1–17.

Wu, G. 2010. Functional amino acids in growth, reproduction and health. *Adv. Nutr.* 1:31–37.

Wu, G. 2014. Dietary requirements of synthesizable amino acids by animals: a paradigm shift in protein nutrition. *J. Anim. Sci. Biotechnol.* 5:34.

Wu, G. 2016. Dietary protein intake and human health. *Food Funct.* 7:1251–1265.

Wu, G. 2018. *Principles of Animal Nutrition*. CRC Press, Boca Raton, FL.

Wu, G. 2020. Important roles of dietary taurine, creatine, carnosine, anserine and 4-hydroxyproline in human nutrition and health. *Amino Acids* 52:329–360.

Wu, G., and E.B. Marliss. 1992. Interorgan metabolic coordination during fasting and underfeeding: an adaptation for mobilizing fat and sparing protein in man. In: *Biology of Feast and Famine* (Anderson, G.H. and S.H. Kennedy, eds). Academic Press, San Diego, CA. pp. 219–244.

Wu, G., N.E. Flynn, W. Yan, and D.G. Barstow, Jr. 1995. Glutamine metabolism in chick enterocytes: absence of pyrroline-5-carboxylate synthase and citrulline synthesis. *Biochem. J.* 306:717–721.

Wu, G., T.L. Ott, D.A. Knabe, and F.W. Bazer. 1999a. Amino acid composition of the fetal pig. *J. Nutr.* 129:1031–1038.

Wu, G., N.E. Flynn, S.P. Flynn, C.A. Jolly, and P.K. Davis. 1999b. Dietary protein or arginine deficiency impairs constitutive and inducible nitric oxide synthesis by young rats. *J. Nutr.* 129:1347–1354.

Wu, G., F.W. Bazer, R.C. Burghardt, G.A. Johnson, S.W. Kim, X.L. Li et al. 2010. Impacts of amino acid nutrition on pregnancy outcome in pigs: mechanisms and implications for swine production. *J. Anim. Sci.* 88:E195–E204.

Wu, G., F.W. Bazer, G.A. Johnson, D.A. Knabe, R.C. Burghardt, T.E. Spencer et al. 2011. Important roles for L-glutamine in swine nutrition and production. *J. Anim. Sci.* 89:2017–2030.

Wu, G., Z.L. Wu, Z.L. Dai, Y. Yang, W.W. Wang, C. Liu et al. 2013. Dietary requirements of "nutritionally nonessential amino acids" by animals and humans. *Amino Acids* 44:1107–1113.

Wu, G., F.W. Bazer, Z.L. Dai, D.F. Li, J.J. Wang, and Z.L. Wu. 2014a. Amino acid nutrition in animals: protein synthesis and beyond. *Annu. Rev. Anim. Biosci.* 2:387–417.

Wu, G., J. Fanzo, D.D. Miller, P. Pingali, M. Post, J.L. Steiner, and A.E. Thalacker-Mercer. 2014b. Production and supply of high-quality food protein for human consumption: sustainability, challenges and innovations. *Ann. N.Y. Acad. Sci.* 1321:1–19.

Wu, G., F.W. Bazer, and H.R. Cross. 2014c. Land-based production of animal protein: impacts, efficiency, and sustainability. *Ann. N.Y. Acad. Sci.* 1328:18–28.

Wu, G., H.R. Cross, K.B. Gehring, J.W. Savell, A.N. Arnold, and S. H. McNeill. 2016. Composition of free and peptide-bound amino acids in beef chuck, loin, and round cuts. *J. Anim. Sci.* 94:2603–2613.

Wu, G., F.W. Bazer, G.A. Johnson, and Y.Q. Hou. 2018. Arginine nutrition and metabolism in growing, gestating and lactating swine. *J. Anim. Sci.* 96:5035–5051.

Wu, N., S.S.D. Bredin, Y. Guan, K. Dickinson, D.D. Kim, Z. Chua et al. 2019. Cardiovascular health benefits of exercise training in persons living with type 1 diabetes: a systematic review and meta-analysis. *J. Clin. Med.* 8:253.

Wycherley, T., L. Moran, P. Clifton, M. Noakes, and G. Brinkworth. 2012. Effects of energy-restricted high-protein, low-fat compared with standard-protein, low-fat diets: a meta-analysis of randomized controlled trials. *Am. J. Clin. Nutr.* 96:1281–1298.

Yang, Y., Z.L. Wu, S.C. Jia, S. Dahanayaka, S. Feng, C.J. Meininger et al. 2015. Safety of long-term dietary supplementation with L-arginine in rats. *Amino Acids* 47:1907–1920.

Young, V.R. 1987. Kinetics of human amino acid metabolism: nutritional implications and some lessons. *Am. J. Clin. Nutr.* 46:709–725.

Young, V.R. 1994. Adult amino acid requirements: The case for a major revision in current recommendations. *J. Nutr.* 124:1517S–1523S.

Young, V.R. and S. Borgonha. 2000. Nitrogen and amino acid requirements: the Massachusetts Institute of Technology amino acid requirement pattern. *J. Nutr.* 130:1841S–1849S.

Young, V.R. and B. Torún. 1981. Physical activity: impact on protein and amino acid metabolism and implications for nutritional requirements. *FAO/WHO/UNU. Report No. EPR/81/28A.* Rome, Italy.

Zello, G.A., P.B. Pencharz, and R.O. Ball. 1993. Dietary lysine requirement of young adult males determined by oxidation of L-[1–^{13}C]phenylalanine. *Am. J. Physiol.* 264:E677–E685.

Zhang, J.M., D. Zhao, D. Yi, M.J. Wu, H.B. Chen, T. Wu et al. 2019. Microarray analysis reveals the inhibition of intestinal expression of nutrient transporters in piglets infected with porcine epidemic diarrhea virus. *Sci. Rep.* 9:19798.

Zhang, Q., Y.Q. Hou, F.W. Bazer, W.L. He, E.A. Posey, and G. Wu. 2021. Amino acids in swine nutrition and production. *Adv. Exp. Med. Biol.* 1285:81–107.

Zhao, W., Y. Luo, Y. Zhang, Y. Zhou, and T. Zhao. 2018. High protein diet is of benefit for patients with type 2 diabetes. *Medicine (Baltimore)* 97:e13149.

Index

Note: **Bold** page numbers refer to tables and *italic* page numbers refer to figures.

A *see* adenine (A)
AA *see* amino acids (AAs)
D-AA *see* D-amino acid (D-AA)
L-AA *see* L-amino acids (L-AA)
AA-tRNA *see* aminoacyl-tRNA (AA-tRNA)
Abderhalden, E. 76, 117
Abderhalden, O. 76
Abel, J. J. 276, 306
AbPC *see* Antibody-producing cells (AbPC)
Abs *see* Antibodies (Abs)
absorption
    definitions of 74–76
    developmental changes in intestine 79–81
    free AA and small peptides 75
    intact immunoglobulins 67
    portal vein-drained system *75*
    routes 75
AcAc *see* Acetoacetate (AcAc)
Acacia angustissima 33, 109
acceptor site *see* aminoacyl site (A site)
3-acetamidopropanal *278, 281*
acetoacetate (AcAc) **393**, 511
acetylcholinesterase 242, 507, 508
acetyl-CoA (Ac-CoA) 153, 161, 181, 183, 244
N-acetyl-cysteine 37
N-acetyl-5-methoxytryptamine *see* Melatonin
        (*N*-acetyl-5-methoxytryptamine)
acid hydrolysis
    for AA analysis 709
    in dye-binding technique 715, *715*
    of tryptophan 674
Ackermann, D. 258
acrylamide 35, 48
acryl-CoA dehydrogenation 215
actinomycin D 577
activators 513
active proteases and peptidases *78*
acute respiratory syndrome coronavirus 2 478
acyl-carnitine 285; *see also* L-carnitine
ADA *see* adenosine deaminase (ADA)
ADC *see* arginine decarboxylase (ADC)
adenine (A) 103, 291, 648
adenine phosphoribosyltransferase (APRT) 292, **629,** 648
    deficiency 648 (*see also* amino acid metabolism errors)
adenosine deaminase (ADA) 648
    deficiency 648 (*see also* amino acid metabolism errors)
adenosine monophosphate (AMP) 291, 648; *see also* myoadenylate deaminase deficiency
adenosine monophosphate succinate (AMPS) *134*
adenylosuccinase *see* adenylosuccinate lyase (ADSL)
adenylosuccinate lyase (ADSL) **629** *see* amino acid metabolism errors
    deficiency 648–649
adenylyl transferase 158
ADMA *see* asymmetrical dimethylarginine (ADMA)
adrenaline 304; *see also* epinephrine

ADSL *see* adenylosuccinate lyase (ADSL)
African Sleeping Sickness 277
AGA *see* agmatinase (AGA)
AGAT *see* arginine:glycine amidinotransferase (AGAT)
Agelenopsis aperta 30
agmatinase (AGA) 206, 211, 559
agmatine 278, 538
AgPC *see* antigen-presenting cells (AgPC)
Ags *see* antigens (Ags)
AhR *see* aryl hydrocarbon receptor (AhR)
AIB *see* aminoisobutyrate (AIB)
Ala *see* alanine (Ala)
ALA *see* δ-aminolevulinic acid (ALA)
alanine (Ala) 3
    catabolism 198–205
    glyoxylate transaminase *218*
    ketone bodies effect on synthesis of *513*
    L-Alanine 16
    synthesis 126–127, 133–136
    transaminase 199
ALAS *see* δ-aminolevulinic acid synthase (ALAS)
albinism 640; *see also* amino acid metabolism errors
alkaline hydrolysis 21, 43
alkaptonuria 26, 641, 642
allantoicase 364, 365
allantoinase 364, 365, 366
Allison, J.B. 198
allo-form 6
allopurinol 648, 649, 661
allosteric activators 510, 518
allosteric inhibitors 510
allosteric regulation 509, 510
α-acetylamino-γ-phenylbutyric acid 133
α-amino acids **44, 45**; *see also* amino acids (AAs)
    amino and carboxyl groups
        condensation 50–52
        metals, AAs chelates 49
        N^α-dehydrogenation 49
        oxidative deamination 50
        peptide synthesis 52
    amino group in α-AAs **44–45**
        amino–imino tautomerization 48
        deamination 47
        keto–enol tautomerization 48
        o-phthalaldehyde, conjugation **45–47**
        oxymethylation 47
        transamination 47
    chemical reactions
        amino and carboxyl groups 49–52
        amino group in α-AAs 44–48
        carboxyl group in α-AAs 48
        proteins 52–59
        side chain in α-AAs 48
    oxidation rate *693,* 693–694
α-aminoadipate-6-semialdehyde 221
α-aminoisovaleric acid 26

α-carbon 3, 6
α-decay 378
α-dicarbonyls 47
α-difluoromethylornithine (DFMO) 277, 508
α-hydrogen 3
α-hydroxy-γ-phenylbutyric acid 133
α-ketoacids 47, 103, 169–170
α-ketoadipate (α-keto-hexanedioic acid) 659
α-ketoadipic acidemia 659; *see also* amino acid
    metabolism errors
α-ketobutyrate 160
α-ketoglutarate (α-KG) 103, 104, 127, 128, 133, 338
α-keto-hexanedioic acid *see* α-ketoadipate
    (α-keto-hexanedioic acid)
α-ketoisocaproate (KIC) 156, 169, 213, 214
α-keto-β-hydroxy-butyric acid 133
α-keto-γ-methylthiobutyrate 170
α-keto-γ-phenylbutyric acid 133
α-KG *see* α-ketoglutarate (α-KG)
α-*N*-Oxalyl-α,β-diamino propionic acid (α-ODAP) 33–34
α-particle 378
α-sulfonic acid group (–SO3H) 27
αβT *see* αβ T cell (αβT)
αβ T cell (αβT) *525*
α,δ-dibromopropylmalonic ester 25
Alzheimer's disease 33
Amanita mushrooms (fungi) 34
amidophosphoribosyltransferase (APRT) 292
aminoacetic acid *see* glycine
amino acid degradation *see* degradation
amino acid epimerases 167
amino acid functions 537, 606; *see also* amino acid
    degradation; amino acid metabolism errors
    AA-derived gas chemical properties 543–544
    AA nitrogenous product roles 557
    arginine 548, **548–549**
    carnosine 568–569
    CO functions 546–547
    creatine 559–561, *560*
    D-AA 572
    gaseous signaling 543–548, *544*
    glucosamine 570–571
    glutamate 552, **553,** 554
    glutamine 550–552
    glutathione *561,* 561–564, *562,* **563**
    glycine *554,* 554–555
    histamine 565, 568
    H$_2$S functions 547–548
    4-hydroxyproline 569–570
    immune response 583–592
    as ligands and activators 571
    melanin 568
    melatonin 568
    NO functions *544,* 544–546
    nonpeptide molecule synthesis 542–543
    in nutrition, therapy, and health 592–599, *593, 598*
    peptide synthesis 537, 542
    polyamine functions 557–559
    proline 555–556
    protein synthesis 537, 542
    purine and pyrimidine 564
    regulatory roles 573–583
    small peptide synthesis 542
    supplementation efficacy and safety 600–606, **601**

    taurine functions 564–565
    tryptophan 556–557
amino acid-induced sensing 596–599
    AA sensing in tongue 597–598
    in gastrointestinal tract 598–599
    glutamate receptors 597–598
    taste cells 596–597
    taste signaling mechanisms *598*
amino acid metabolism 517, 527–530; *see also* amino acid
    degradation; amino acid synthesis; metabolism
    concepts
    AA catabolism 520–522
    intracellular protein turnover 522–528
    nutritional and physiological factors effect on 518
amino acid metabolism errors 623–665
    basic AA 631
    branched-chain AA 632
    carnitine 632–633
    clinical diagnosis 623
    creatine 633
    Fanconi syndrome 626, 630
    galactosemia 630
    glutamate 633–634
    glutamine 634–635
    glutathione 635–636
    glycine 636–637
    heme 637–639
    histidine 639–640
    hyperornithinemia 631
    inherited diseases 625–626
    lysinuric protein intolerance 631
    organic acidurias 658–659
    phenylalanine and tyrosine 640–645
    proline and 4-hydroxyproline 645–648
    purines 648–650
    pyrimidines 650–651
    serine 651–652
    sulfur-containing AA 652–654
    treatment 661–664
    tryptophan 654–655
    urea cycle 655–658
    Wilson's disease 630
amino acid racemases 166–167
amino acid regulatory roles 573
    AA imbalances and disorders 574
    cell signaling 581–583, *583*
    DNA methylation and histone modifications *580*
    in epigenetics 579–580
    in food intake 573–574
    in gene expression 577, *579*
    interorgan metabolism *578*
    in nutrient metabolism 574–577, *575, 576*
    one-carbon unit metabolism *576*
amino acids (AAs) 1, 592; *see also* conditionally essential
    amino acid (CEAA); dietary protein quality
    assessment; essential amino acid (EAA);
    nonessential amino acid (NEAA); sulfur-
    containing AA
    amino and carboxyl groups
        condensation 50–52
        metals, AAs chelates 49
        N$^\alpha$-dehydrogenation 49
        oxidative deamination 50
        peptide synthesis 52

amino group in α-AAs **44–45**
   amino–imino tautomerization 48
   deamination 47
   keto–enol tautomerization 48
   o-phthalaldehyde, conjugation **45–47**
   oxymethylation 47
   transamination 47
in animal bodies **672, 679**
in animal kingdom 31–33
in aqueous solution **41**
arginine 681
by birds 676
cell culture 599
chemical properties **4–5**
   solubility, water and organic solvents 37–38
   tastes of crystalline AAs 35–36
   zwitterionic form 38–42
chemical reactions
   amino and carboxyl groups 49–52
   amino group in α-AAs 44–48
   carboxyl group in α-AAs 48
   proteins 52–59
   side chain in α-AAs 48
chemical stability 42–44
in cosmetic and toiletry products 599
definition of 3–5
degradation and catabolism
   age-dependent changes 192–194
   blood plasma 194–197
   catabolic pathways 182–186
   cell -, tissue-, and species-specific 190–192
   energetic efficiencies 186–190
   overall view of 181–182
   rates and patterns 197–198
discovery **2–3**
   D-AAs 28–30
   L-Alanine (α-aminopropionic acid) 16–26
   β-Alanine (β-aminopropionic acid) 27–28
in food 596–599, **712**
free and peptide (protein)-bound 12–16
functional 682
glutamine 681
glycine 681
hydrochloric acid **10**
imbalances 600–602
immune response 583–592
induced sensing 596–599
isomers
   cis- and *trans*-AAs 11
   L- and D-AAs 5–9
   R- and *S*-AAs 9–11
isotopes **377**
in medical and pharmaceutical therapy 592–594
metabolites 537, **538–541**
in microbes 34–35
mother to fetus 529
mutual AA ratios 715–716
nomenclature 6
nutritionally semi-essential AA 674
in nutrition and metabolism **543**
optimum ratios 701–707, **702–708**
oxidation rate of *693*, 693–694
in plants 33–34
in plasma 722

in processed foods 35
proteinogenic and non-proteinogenic 12
proteins 585
in spoiled animal products 33
taurine 681
L-amino acids (L-AA); *see also* amino acids (AAs)
   catabolism
      in microbes 239–241
      nitrogenous metabolites 241–242
   deaminase 47
amino acid synthesis 518–519
   arginine 518–519
   D-AAs conversion *168*
      humans and other animals 167–168
      microorganisms 168–169
   D-AAS synthesis
      human and other animals 164–166
      microorganisms 166–167
   general pathways, in animal cells
      amino acid transamination 133
      animal cells 132–133
   glutamine 519–520
   microorganisms
      amino acid epimerases 167
      amino acid racemases 166–167
      2-aminoethylphosphonate 163–164
      arginine 158–159
      aspartate and asparagine 159
      cysteine and tyrosine 159–160
      2,6-diaminopimelic acid 163–164
      essential amino acids 160–161
      glutamate and glutamine 156–158
      N-acetylated amino acids 161–163
      overall pathways 155–156
      phosphoryl amino acids 164
   overall view of 118
   specific pathways, in humans and other animals
      alanine, glutamine, and glutamate 133–136
      arginine and lysine 140
      arginine, citrulline, and ornithine 136–138
      aspartate and asparagine 138
      cysteine and taurine 138–140
      glycine and serine 140–146
      homoarginine 140
      methylarginines 146–147
      N-acetyl-aspartate 153
      phosphoryl amino acids 154
      proline and hydroxyproline 148–150
      sulfur-containing AAs 151–153
      tyrosine 150
      β-alanine 150–151
   tissues and cells 118
      cell -, tissue-, and species-specific 118
      disease, AA rates 131
      in endothelial cells 127
      in heart, brain, lungs 125–127
      homeostasis 128–131
      in liver 125
      in macrophages and lymphocytes 127
      in ovaries, testes 128
      in placentae, mammary glands 128
      in sense organs 128
      in skeletal muscle 125–127
      in small intestine 127

amino acid synthesis (*cont.*)
       in smooth muscle cells 127
       in white adipose tissue 125–127
       α-ketoacids into L-AAS 169–170
amino acid transamination 133
aminoacylation 416
aminoacyl site (A site) 415
aminoacyl-tRNA (AA-tRNA) 29, 416–417
2-aminoethanethiol dioxygenase 140
2-aminoethylphosphonate 163–164
amino–imino tautomerization 48
aminoisobutyrate (AIB) **629**
aminomalonic acid 17, 19, 21, 43
aminopeptidases 272, *463,* 464; *see also* exopeptidases
ammonia 105, 136
    biochemical mechanisms responsible 338–339
    concentrations in plasma and tissues 499
    conversion 358
    detoxification *350*
    historical observations 333–334
    hyperammonemia treatment 339
    microbial assimilation 103
    nitrogen 103
    normal and abnormal concentrations 335–337
    production and toxicity 333–334, 337–338
    production and utilization *102*
    removal, physiological conditions 334–335
    utilization of 157
AMP *see* adenosine monophosphate (AMP)
AMP-activated protein kinase (AMPK) *523,* **549,** 581
AMPK *see* AMP-activated protein kinase (AMPK)
AMPS *see* adenosine monophosphate succinate (AMPS)
Angelini, C. 286
angiotensin-converting enzyme 275
animals
    animal products 60
    animal tissues 255
    immune function assessments 586, *586*
    intestinal immunity and health 586
    proteinogenic amino acids *7–8*
    proteinogenic L-AAs and glycine 6
anserine 258, 260, 262, *263; see also* carnosine
antagonism 600–602
antibodies (Abs) *525*
antibody-producing cells (AbPC) *525*
anticodon 414, 415, 418
antigenic peptides 474
antigen-presenting cells (AgPC) *525*
antigens (Ags) *525*
antihypertensive peptides 273
anti-inflammatory macrophages (M2) *525*
antimicrobial peptides **275**
antioxidative peptides **274**
antipain 465
antizyme 1 279
APF1 *see* ATP-dependent proteolysis factor 1 (APF1)
apparent digestibility 81
APRT *see* adenine phosphoribosyltransferase (APRT);
        amidophosphoribosyltransferase (APRT)
aquaporins 517
ARC *see* British Agricultural Research Council (ARC)
arcamine 19
Archaea methylamine methyltransferase 1
Arg *see* arginine (Arg)

arginase expression 207
arginine (Arg) 21, 99, 136; *see also* amino acids (AAs)
    AA supplementation safety 602–603
    as allosteric activator 575
    catabolism 520–522
    functions 548, **548–549**
    in growth, health, and disease **548–549**
    interorgan metabolism *578*
    NO-dependent and NO-independent actions **550**
    precursors 519
    substrate oxidation enhancement and adiposity
        reduction *575*
    synthesis 518–519
arginine catabolism 205, *206*
    arginase expression 207
    arginine decarboxylase 211
    arginine paradox 209–210
    multiple enzymes 205–206
    NO synthases 207–209
    polyamines syntheses 211
arginine decarboxylase (ADC) *206,* 211
arginine:glycine amidinotransferase (AGAT) **629**
    deficiency 633 (*see also* amino acid metabolism errors)
arginine metabolism 192
arginine paradox 209–210
arginine-proline cycle 227
arginine synthesis 22, 33, 136–138, *137,* 140, *158,*
        158–159
argininosuccinate (AS) *206,* 341
argininosuccinate lyase (ASL) 125, 656, *656*
argininosuccinate synthase (ASS) 125, 341, 657
argininosuccinic aciduria 656–657; *see also* amino acid
        metabolism errors
aromatic L-amino acid decarboxylase deficiency 641, 655
aryl hydrocarbon receptor (AhR) 571
AS *see* argininosuccinate (AS)
A site *see* aminoacyl site (A site)
ASL *see* argininosuccinate lyase (ASL)
Asn *see* asparagine (Asn)
Asp *see* aspartate (Asp)
asparaginase 203–205
asparagine (Asn) 3, 48; *see also* amino acids (AAs)
    catabolism 198–205
    L-asparagine 21
    synthesis 138, 159
    synthetase deficiency 630–631
aspartate (Asp) 21
    catabolism 198–205
    L-aspartate 21
    peptidases 464
    synthesis 138, 159
ASS *see* argininosuccinate synthase (ASS)
astigmatism 640
asymmetrical dimethylarginine (ADMA) 521
atomic number 375, 376
atom percent enrichment *see* isotope enrichment (IE)
ATP 501
    arginine kinase 25
    carnosine synthetase 258
    consuming pathways 281
    producing pathways 281
ATP-binding cassette (ABC) 288–289
ATP-dependent glutamine synthetase 125
ATP-dependent proteolysis factor 1 (APF1) 462

ATP-dependent proteolytic system 470–471, *473*
autolysosome 468, *469*
5-aza-CdR *see* 5-aza-2′-deoxycytidine (5-aza-CdR)

B *see* B lymphocytes (B)
Bacillus anthracis 168
Bacillus–Lactobacillus–Streptococcus group 96
Bacillus subtilis 168
Bacillus subtilis in vivo 164
Bacteroides fragilis 157
Baeyer, A. 17
Baldes, K. 223
balenine 265
Ball, R.O. 136
Barbieri, A. 24
Barbieri, J. 24
Barger, G. 24, 303
Barrett, A.J. 467
basal cells 597; *see also* taste cells
BAT *see* brown adipose tissue (BAT)
Baudrimont, A.E. 22
Baumann, E. 22
Baumann, L. 23, 256
BCA *see* bicinchoninic acid (BCA)
BCAAs *see* branched chain amino acids (BCAA)
BCKA *see* branched-chain α-ketoacid (BCKA)
BCKD *see* branched-chain α-ketoacid dehydrogenase
        (BCKD)
Beccari, G.B. 71
Becker, C.E. 311
Becquerel (Bq) 379
Becquerel, Henri 375
Bell, E.A. 23
Benda, C. 425
Benevenga, N.J. 230
benzoylornithine 21
Bequette, B.J. 345
Bergmann, M. 22
Bertholet, P.E.M. 71
Berthollet, C.L. 334
Bertin-Sans, H. 296
Berzelius, J.J. 22, 419
Best, C. 317
betaine (trimethylglycine) 290
betaine/choline/carnitine transporter (BCCT) 289
β-alanine 3, 27, 37, 261–262
        synthesis 150–151
        α-ketoglutarate transaminase 651
        β-aminopropionic acid 27–28
β-alanyl-L-histamine *see* carcinine
β-alanyl-L-histidine 256, 258 *see* carnosine
β-aminoethylimidazole *see* histamine
β-aminoisobutyrate 295
β-aminoisobutyric acid 27
β-aminoisobutyric aciduria 650; *see also* amino acid
        metabolism errors
β-aminopropionic acid *see* β-alanine
β-casomorphins 272
β-elimination 280
β-Hydroxybutyrate (BHB) 511
β-hydroxy-trimethyllysine 287
β-hydroxy-β-methylbutyrate (HMB) 214, **541**
β-iminazolylethylamine *see* histamine
β-indolealdehyde 26

β-methylthiolpropaldehyde 24
β-*N*-acetyl-D-hexosaminidase 317
β-*N*-oxalyl-α,β-diamino propionic acid (β-ODAP)
        33–34
β-(1–4)-poly-*N*-acetyl-d-glucosamine *see* chitin
β-sulfinylpyruvate 139
β-γ-carbon configuration 6
Beyer, K.H. Jr 354
BHB *see* β-hydroxybutyrate (BHB)
BH4-dependent tryptophan hydroxylase (TPH) 236
bicinchoninic acid (BCA) 54
Bieber, L.L. 215
bilirubin 296
biliverdin reductase 301, 302
bioactive peptides in protein hydrolysates
        animal nutrition and health 275–276
        human nutrition and health 271–275
bioavailability 72, 73
biochemical pathways, protein synthesis 408
biological value 716
birds, immune system *584,* 584–585
Biuret Assay (Piotrowski' Test) 53–54
Blachier, F. 136, 345
blank radioactivity values (dpm) 382
Bloch, K. 215
Bloch, W. 303
blood ammonia 337
blood plasma proteins 489–490
B lymphocytes (B) *525,* 584
Bödeker, C. 26
body weight (BW) 13, 28, 171, 269, 438, 687
Boerhaave, H. 339
Bopp, F. 26
Borsook, H. 221, 227
Bosch, C. 334
Bosshard, E. 22
Bourgeois, A. 16
Boutron-Charlard, A.F. 21
Bouveault, L. 23
Brachet, J. 407
Braconnot, H. 1, 22, 23
branched-chain AAs catabolism
        BCKA dehydrogenase 214
        BCKAs degradation 215–216
        KIC dioxygenase 214–215
        nutritional regulation 216–217
        physiological regulation 216–217
        transaminase 212–214
branched-chain amino acids (BCAA) 23, 24, 26, *160, 212,*
        212–213, **541**
        interorgan metabolism *578*
        isovaleric acidemia 632
        ketone bodies effect on synthesis of *513*
        maple syrup urine disease 632
        methylbutyric acidemia 632
branched-chain α-ketoacid (BCKA) 134, **629** *see* maple
        syrup urine disease
        degradation 215–216
        dehydrogenase 214
        ketone effect on oxidative decarboxylation *513*
branched-chain α-ketoacid dehydrogenase (BCKD) *212,*
        403, *521*
Braunstein, A.E. 133, 231
Brieger, Ludwig 276

British Agricultural Research Council (ARC) 677
Brosnan, J.T. 136, 281
brown adipose tissue (BAT) **549**
brush cells 597
B⁰ system transporter 238
Buchanan, J.M. 358
Buck, P.S. 24
buphenyl *see* sodium phenylbutyrate
Burger, A. 281
Buston, H.W. 26
BW *see* body weight (BW)¹⁴

C-acetoacetate 398
Ca²⁺-dependent protease 462, 470
Ca²⁺-dependent proteolytic system 470
Cahours, A.T. 22
calpain system 470; *see also* Ca²⁺-dependent proteolytic system
canavanine 17, 34
cancers 737, 743–744
Cantoni, G.L. 227
Cara, F. 260
carbamoyl phosphate (CP) 136, 352
carbamoylphosphate synthetase-I (CPS-I) 657; *see also* amino acid metabolism errors
carbobenzoxy-L-glutamic acid anhydride 22
carbon monoxide (CO) functions 546–547
    cytoprotective effects 546
    in immune system 546
carboxypeptidases 78, 464; *see also* exopeptidases
carcinine 259, 260
carcinoid 654, 654–655; *see also* amino acid metabolism errors
Cardini, C.E. 311
cardiovascular risk factors (CVRF) **549**
Cargill, R.W. 260
Carisano, A. 260
carnitine
    primary carnitine deficiency 632–633
    TML dioxygenase deficiency 633
carnosine 255, 256, 262, 263
    dipeptidase 263
    functions 568–569
carnosine catabolism
    anserinase 263
    carnosinase 263
    species-specific tissue distribution 263
carnosine synthesis 258, 260, 262
    age, sex, muscle fiber type 262
    physical activity 262
    substrates availability 261–262
Carter, H.E. 26
caspases 470
Caspersson, T. 407
catalytic site 464–467
catecholamines, synthesis and catabolism 304–306
catechol-O-methyltransferase 305
caveolin-1-dependent endocytosis 279
CD8 *see* cytotoxic T cells carrying CD8 marker (CD8)
CEAA *see* conditionally essential amino acid (CEAA)
cell signaling pathways 583
certain teleost fish 356–357
chemical reactions of AAs
    amino and carboxyl groups

condensation 50–52
metals, AAs chelates 49
Nᵅ-dehydrogenation 49
oxidative deamination 50
peptide synthesis 52
amino group in α-AAs **44–45**
    amino–imino tautomerization 48
    deamination 47
    keto–enol tautomerization 48
    o-phthalaldehyde, conjugation **45–47**
    oxymethylation 47
    transamination 47
carboxyl group in α-AAs **44–45**, 48
side chain in α-AAs 48
chemical stability of AAs
    crystalline forms 42
    strong acid and alkaline solutions 43–44
    water and buffered solutions 42–43
    water at high temperatures 43
    water, high-pressure and high-temperature 43
chickens, amino acids, endogenous ileal flows **83–84**
chitin synthesis 315
choline
    choline catabolism
        humans and other animals 318–319
        in microbes 319
    choline synthesis
        in farm and laboratory animals 318
        in humans 317–318
    history of 317
chromatographic method 53
chymotrypsin activity 80, 508
Ciechanover, A. 462
cinnamycin 50
cis-4-Hydroxy-L-proline 34
cis/*trans* nomenclature 11, *11*
citric acid cycle 333; *see also* Krebs cycle
citrulline 136
    catabolism 205
    synthesis 119, 125, 136–138
citrullinuria *see* hypercitrullinemia
c-Jun NH(2)-terminal kinase (JNK) 581
CK *see* creatine kinase (CK)
cl cells (Mast) *525*
Clementi, A. 340
Clifford, W.M. 258
Clostridium clusters 96
Coghill, R.D. 26
Cohnheim, O. 76
Cole, S.W. 26
Colson, A. 45
Comb, D.G. 312
condensation 50–52
Conditionally essential amino acid (CEAA) 680, 746
    in animals **679**
conventional method 379
Coomassie Brilliant Blue dye 53
copper-containing enzyme 364
copper–glycine complex 49
copper–leucine chelate 49
Corynebacterium glutamicum 157
cottonseed meal (CSM) **712**
covalent modifications 516
Coyne, F.P. 24

CP *see* carbamoyl phosphate (CP); crude protein (CP)
CPS-I *see* carbamoylphosphate synthetase-I (CPS-I)
Craig, L.C. 28
Cramer, E. 26
creatine
    AGAT deficiency 633
    creatine synthesis
        interorgan cooperation 281–283
        metabolism of 284–285
        regulation of 283
        tissue distribution of 285
    functions 559–561
    guanidinoacetate methyltransferase deficiency 633
    history of 281
    kinase 559
    X-linked creatine transporter deficiency 633
creatine kinase (CK) *206*, 281, 285, 559
creatine-phosphate (Cr-P) *206*
creatine-synthetic enzymes 283
Crick, F. 408
Crigler–Najjar syndrome *see* Gilbert's syndrome
Cr-P *see* creatine-phosphate (Cr-P)
crude protein (CP) 71–72, 106, **712**
Crumpler, H.R. 27
crustaceans, immune system 585
crystalline forms of AAs 42
crystalline lysine 24
CSM *see* cottonseed meal (CSM)
CVRF *see* cardiovascular risk factors (CVRF)
cyanobacterium 158
cyanohydrin 26
cyclic metabolic pathways concept 333
cyclization 42
Cys *see* cysteine (Cys)
cystamine (2,2′-dithiobisethanamine) 140
cystathionase 652
cystathionine β-synthase 652
cystathionine γ-lyase 228
cystathioninuria 652; *see also* amino acid
        metabolism errors
cysteine (Cys) 39; *see also* amino acids (AAs)
    catabolism 229
    L-cysteine 22
    synthesis 138–140, *139, 159,* 159–160
cystine 22
cystinosis 652; *see also* amino acid metabolism errors
cystinuria *652,* 652–653; *see also* amino acid metabolism
        errors
cytochromes 296, 545
cytokines 520, 521, *525*
cytoplasm 340
cytosolic arginase 657
cytosolic protein synthesis 408–409
cytotoxic T cells carrying CD8 marker (CD8) *525*

Daft, Floyd S. 26
Dakin, H.D. 199, 205, 225
D-alanine 28, 29, 167
Dale, H. 303, 317
D-Amino acid (D-AA) 166–167; *see also* amino
        acids (AAs)
    amino acid synthesis
        human and other animals 164–166
        microorganisms 166–167

    in animal kingdom 29–30
    catabolism
        bacteria and animals 242–244
        D-AA transporters 238
        enzymatic activity 238–239
        in microbes 241
        nitrogenous metabolites 241–242
    conversion, amino acid synthesis 168–169
        humans and other animals 167–168
        microorganisms 168–169
    D-alanine 572
    D-aspartate 573
    deaminase 47
    D-serine functions 573
    functions 572
    in microbes 30
    in plant- and animal-sourced foods 28–29
    racemase (*see* amino acids (AAs))
    transporters 238
Damodaran, M. 21, 22
D-amyl alcohol 23
D'Aniello, A. 29
DAPA *see* 2,6-diaminopimelic acid (DAPA)
D-arginine 28
D-aspartate 29, 30
D-aspartate racemase 166
data interpretation 394–395
Davis, T.A. 431
Davis, W.S. 306
Day, H.G. 311
DC *see* dendritic cell (DC)
DCAM *see* decarboxylated *S*-adenosylmethionine (DCAM)
3,4-DCI *see* 3,4-dichloroisocoumarin (3,4-DCI)
2D difference gel electrophoresis (2D DIGE) 701
deamination 47
decarboxylated *S*-adenosylmethionine (DCAM) *206*
decarboxylation 222–223
de Duve, C. 462
degradation
    AA catabolism
        age-dependent changes 192–194
        blood plasma 194–197
        catabolic pathways 182–186
        cell -, tissue-, and species-specific 190–192
        energetic efficiencies 186–190
        overall view of 181–182
        rates and patterns 197–198
    in animal cells
        alanine catabolism 198–205
        asparagine catabolism 198–205
        aspartate catabolism 198–205
        glutamate catabolism 198–205
        glutamine catabolism 198–205
        historical perspectives 198
    arginine catabolism 205, 520–522
        arginase expression 207
        arginine decarboxylase 211
        arginine paradox 209–210
        multiple enzymes 205–206
        NO synthases 207–209
        polyamines syntheses 211
    arginine-proline cycle 227
    asparaginase 203–205
    branched-chain AAs catabolism

degradation (*cont.*)
    BCKA dehydrogenase 214
    BCKAs degradation 215–216
    KIC dioxygenase 214–215
    nutritional regulation 216–217
    physiological regulation 216–217
    transaminase 212–214
  citrulline catabolism 205
  D-AAs catabolism
    bacteria and animals 242–244
    D-AA transporters 238
    enzymatic activity 238–239
    in microbes 241
    nitrogenous metabolites 241–242
  enzyme-catalyzed reactions 199–202
  glutamine 522
  glycine and serine catabolism
    glycine cleavage system 217
    glycine *N*-methyltransferase 219
    serine degradation 219
    serine hydroxymethyltransferase 217–219
  histidine catabolism 220–221
  3-hydroxyproline catabolism 225
  4-hydroxyproline catabolism 225
  3-hydroxyproline oxidase 226
  4-hydroxyproline oxidase 226
  kidney- and liver-type glutaminases 202–203
  L-AAs catabolism
    in microbes 239–241
    nitrogenous metabolites 241–242
  lysine catabolism
    decarboxylation 222–223
    via saccharopine and pipecolate pathways 221–222
  methionine catabolism
    transamination pathway 230–231
    transsulfuration pathway 228–229
  N-acetylated AAs catabolism 237–238
  ornithine catabolism 205
  P5C metabolism 226
  phenylalanine and tyrosine catabolism 223–225
  proline catabolism 225
  proline oxidase 226
  selenocysteine catabolism 237
  sulfur-containing AAs catabolism
    cysteine catabolism 229
    methionine catabolism 228–231
    taurine catabolism 231
  threonine catabolism 231–234
  tryptophan catabolism
    kynurenine pathway 234–236
    serotonin pathway 236
    transamination pathway 237
3-dehydrocarnitine 290
de La Rue, W. 26
Delluva, A.M. 304
δ-aminolevulinic acid (ALA) 298
δ-aminolevulinic acid synthase (ALAS) 298
Δ¹-pyrroline-5-carboxylate (P5C) 118, *132,* 136, 207
Demarcay, H. 27
dendritic cell (DC) *525*
de novo synthesis 117, 126, 135, 148, *155,* 266, *293*
  cysteine and tyrosine 159
Dent, C.E. 27
deoxyribonucleic acid (DNA) 291
  methylation 579

dermatan sulfates 314–315
Dessaignes, V. 21, 22, 321
deubiquitinating enzyme *see* ubiquitin-isopeptidase
dextrorotatory 6
DFP *see* di-isopropylfluorophosphate (DFP)
D-glucosamine 311
  historical perspectives 311
D-glucosamine 311; *see also* glycosaminoglycans
D-glutamate 29
D-glyceraldehyde 5, *6*
diamine oxidase 280
2,6-diaminopimelic acid (DAPA) 34, 163–164
dicarboxylic aminoaciduria 631
3,4-dichloroisocoumarin (3,4-DCI) 465
didehydroalanine 52
Diem, K. 354
dietary AA requirement 671–746; *see also* amino acids
    (AAs); dietary protein quality assessment
  classification 672
  determination (*see* dietary AA requirement
    determination; Dietary AA requirement
    determination)
  EAA requirement 686
  estimation 673
  factors to consider 693
  farm animal studies 676–678
  functional AA 681–682
  glutamine requirement **391**
  human studies 675
  ideal protein concept 676, 677
  Kwashiorkor 671
  laboratory animal studies 673–674
  limiting AA 673
  marasmus 671
  sparing nitrogen by bicarbonate supplementation
    689
  for tissue proteins 671
dietary AA requirement determination 684–685, 690,
    692; *see also* nitrogen balance measurement;
    "-omics" technologies; tracer method
  dose–response feeding trials 692, *692*
  factorial method 690–692, **691**
dietary AA supplementation 594–599
  AA imbalances 600–602
  advantages of 595–596
  animal nutrition and production 595–596
  antagonism 600–602
  arginine 602–603
  definition 594
  efficacy and safety 600
  glutamate 604–606
  glutamine 603–604
  human nutrition 594
dietary glutamate 203
dietary glycosaminoglycans 315–317
dietary N intake (NI) **717**
dietary nucleic acids 104
dietary protein 72, 76–79, 77, 81, 100
dietary protein quality assessment 708–724
  AA analysis 709–712
  AA in plasma 722
  biological value 716
  chemical score 712–713
  digestible indispensable AA score 721–722
  dye-binding techniques 715, *715*

EAA flux in plasma 724
EAA index 713, 715
enzyme activities 723
lean tissue mass 718
mutual AA ratios 715–716
net protein ratio 717–718
nitrogen growth index 718
protein digestibility corrected AA score 719–721, **719, 720**
protein efficiency ratio 716–717
proteins concentration in plasma 722–723
relative N utilization 718
urea and ammonia concentration in plasma and urine 723
using microorganisms 724
whole-body composition 718
whole-body protein turnover 723–724
dietary protein requirements **685**
digestibility 72, 73
digestible indispensable AA score (DIAAS) 721–722
digestion
    definitions of 72–74
    digestive system 67, **68**
    monogastric animals
        AAs across, net balance 94–96
        dietary protein digestion 76–79
        free AAs absorption 88–94
        historical perspective 76
        nitrogen, extensive recycling 96–99
        protein digestibility 81–88
        proteolytic digestive capacity 79–81
    proteases and peptidases **74**
    ruminants
        AA degradation inhibition 108–109
        chemical treatment 107
        free AAs absorption 105
        gastrointestinal tract 100–103
        heating 106–107
        high-quality protein 106–107
        nitrogen recycling 105–106
        nucleic acids digestion 103–105
        nutritional implications 105–106
        nutritional significance 99–100
        physical encapsulation 108
        polyphenolic phytochemicals 107–108
        rumen degradation 106–107
        small peptides 105
dihydropyrimidine dehydrogenase (DPD) 650
5,6-dihydroxyindole-2-carboxylic acid 309
di-isopropylfluorophosphate (DFP) **465**
dimethylglycine dehydrogenase (DMGDH) *141,* 156, 636; *see also* amino acid metabolism errors
2,4-dinitro-α-naphthol-7-sulfonic acid 21
dioxin receptor *see* aryl hydrocarbon receptor (AhR)
dipeptides 568–569
    production of 255
    synthesis 256–257, 261
Diphosphoglucuronateglucuronosyltransferase 1A1 (UGT1A1) **629**
dipolarion *see* zwitterionic form
direct AA oxidation method 694–695
disintegrations per minute (dpm) 379
disintegrations per second (dps) 379
D-isovaleraldehyde 23
DL-α-amino-γ-phenylbutyric acid 133

DL-β-hydroxybutyrate (HB) **393**
DM *see* dry matter (DM)
D-methylmalonyl-CoA dehydrogenation 216
DMGDH *see* dimethylglycine dehydrogenase (DMGDH)
DNA *see* deoxyribonucleic acid (DNA)
dose–response feeding trials 692, *692*
DPD *see* dihydropyrimidine dehydrogenase (DPD)
dpm *see* disintegrations per minute (dpm)
D-proline 28
dps *see* disintegrations per second (dps)
Drechsel, E. 24
Driscoll, J. 462
Drosophila melanogaster 277
Drury, A.N. 291
dry matter (DM) 71, **712**
D-serine 30, 166
    functions 573
    racemase 166–167 (*see also* amino acids (AAs))
Dubin–Johnson syndrome 637
Dumas, J.B. 27
Dunlop, D.S. 29
duramycin 50
du Vigneaud, V. 227
dye-binding techniques 715, *715*

E-64 *see* L-3-carboxy-*trans*-2,3-epoxypropylleucylamido(4-guanidino) butane (E-64)
EAA *see* essential amino acid (EAA)
EAA synthesis 160–161
EAAT1 *see* excitatory amino acid transporter 1 (EAAT1)
Eagles, B.A. 265
4E-BP1 *see* eIF4E-binding protein-1 (4E-BP1)
EC *see* endothelial cell (EC)
edestin 21
Edgar, G. 281
Edlbacher, S. 220
Edson, N.L. 211
eEF *see* eukaryotic elongation factors (eEF)
Eggleton, G. 281
Eggleton, P. 281
Ehrlich, F. 23
EIAA *see* small intestine, monogastric animals
eIF *see* eukaryotic initiation factors (eIF)
eIF5A modification 557
eIF4E-binding protein-1 (4E-BP1) 414, 524
elasmobranchs 356–357
Ellinger, A. 24, 26
Elsholz, A.K.W. 164
Embden, G. 26, 211, 223
ENaC *see* Epithelial sodium channels (ENaC)
endocytosis and autophagy 467–468
endogenous opioid peptides 270
endogenous urinary N (EUN) **717**
endoglycosidase *see* heparanases (endoglycosidase)
endopeptidases 464; *see also* peptidases
endoplasmic reticulum 467
endothelial cell (EC) *525,* **550**
endothelial nitric oxide synthesis *339*
endothelial NO synthase (eNOS) **208, 475**; *see also* nitric oxide synthase (NOS)
energy-dependent proteolysis 462
energy requirement, uric acid 361
    from ammonia via adenosine 361–362
    from ammonia via guanosine 362–363

energy requirement, uric acid (*cont.*)
    kidneys, arterial circulation 366–367
    nutritional and metabolic significance 364
    reactive nitrogen species 365–366
    reactive oxygen species 365–366
    species-specific degradation 364–365
    uric acid from ammonia 364
Engel, A.G. 286
Engel, L.L. 47
enkephalins 270
eNOS *see* endothelial NO synthase (eNOS)
enteramine 310; *see also* serotonin
enterocytes, anatomical relationships **68**
enteroendocrine L and K cells 597
enterokinase 78
enthalpy change 503
entropy 503
enzymatic activity 238–239
enzymatic hydrolysis **272**
enzyme 127, 166, 260, 263, 506
    activity regulation 509, *511*, 518
    induction 509
    irreversible inhibition of 508
    kinetics 506
    Michaelis–Menton equation 506
    reversible inhibition of 506–507
enzyme-catalyzed reactions 199–202
enzyme-catalyzed transamination 133
eosinophil (ESP) *525*
epichlorhydrin 23
epidermin 50
epigenetics 579
    regulation of gene expression *581*
epinephrine (EPN) 304, **541**; *see also* catecholamines
epithelial sodium channels (ENaC) 597
EPN *see* epinephrine (EPN)
Epps, H.M. 303
ε-*N*-L-lysine methyltransferase 286, 287
equilibrium 504
    constant 505
"erepsin" 76
eRF *see* eukaryotic protein release factors (eRF)
ERK 1 and 2 *see* extracellular signal-regulated kinases (ERK 1 and 2)
Erlenmeyer, E. 24, 26
Erspamer, V. 310
Escherichia coli 19–21, 157, 159, 167
E site *see* exit site (E site)
ESP *see* eosinophil (ESP)
essential amino acid (EAA) 160–161, 673–674, 675, 678; *see also* amino acids (AAs)
    in animals 678
    flux in plasma 724
    index 713, 715
    requirement **686, 687**
ethanolamine 154, *155*
eukaryotes *vs.* prokaryotes cytosol
    gene transcription 426–427
    mRNA translation initiation 427
    peptide elongation and termination 427–428
eukaryotic elongation factors (eEF) 412
eukaryotic initiation factors (eIF) *410*, 412, 414, 452
    4E-BP1 524
eukaryotic protein release factors (eRF) 418

eumelanin 568; *see also* melanin
EUN *see* endogenous urinary N (EUN)
evolutionary relationship 467
excitatory amino acid transporter 1 (EAAT1) **92**
exit site (E site) 414, 416
exopeptidases 464; *see also* peptidases
Exton, J.H. 135
extracellular glycosaminoglycans 316
extracellular matrix proteins 55–58, 487
extracellular proteins degradation
    blood plasma proteins 489–490
    extracellular matrix proteins 487
    interstitial space of tissues 490–491
    measurement 491
    via proteases and peptidases 487–489
extracellular signal-regulated kinases (ERK 1 and 2) 581

FA *see* fatty acid (FA)
factorial method 690–692, **691**; *see also* N balance measurement; "-omics" technologies; tracer method
FAD *see* flavin adenine dinucleotide (FAD)
familial pyrimidinemia 650; *see also* amino acid metabolism errors
fanconi syndrome 626, 630; *see also* amino acid metabolism errors
fatty acid (FA) **550**
fecal N (FN) **717**
felidae species 151
felinine synthesis *151, 152*
Fernstrom, J.D. 310
ferrochelatase 638
fetal fluids 60
fibrous proteins 69; *see also* protein
5-aza-2′-deoxycytidine (5-aza-CdR) 300
Fischer, E. 5, 22–26, 76, 291, 357–358, 407
Fisher, H. 296
fish, immune system 585
Fiske, C. 281
Flamand, C. 26
flavin adenine dinucleotide (FAD) *141*, 156
flooding dose technique 438–440
9-fluorenylmethyl chloroformate (FMOC-Cl) 52
fMet *see* *N*-Formylmethionine (fMet)
FMOC *see* 9-fluorenylmethyl chloroformate (FMOC)
FN *see* fecal N (FN)
Følling, I.A. 24
Foltz, C.M. 419
forkhead box protein O1 (FOXO1) 300
formic acid
    formate catabolism
        in humans and other animals 321
        in microbes 321
    formate synthesis
        in humans and other animals 320–321
        in microbes 321
    historic perspectives 319–320
Fourcroy, A.F. 53
FOXO1 *see* forkhead box protein O1 (FOXO1)
F6P synthesis *see* fructose-6-phosphate (F6P) synthesis
Frankel, S. 27
Frankia sp. 157
free amino acids (FAAs) **18–19**; *see also* amino acids (AAs)

absorption 88–94, 105
    concentrations 499, 500
Freeburgh, B. 260
free energy 503
Fricker, L.D. 78
Fritz, I.B. 285
fructose-6-phosphate (F6P) synthesis 201, *312*
4-fumuraylacetoacetate 224
functional amino acids 682
    formulating low-protein diets 683
    "ideal protein" concept 683
    in nutrition 681–682

G *see* guanine (G)
GA *see* guanidinoacetate (GA)
GABA *see* γ-aminobutyric acid (GABA)
galactosemia 630; *see also* amino acid metabolism errors
galactose-1-phosphate uridyltransferase (G1PUT) **629**
γ-aminobutyrate catabolism 37, *201*
γ-aminobutyric acid (GABA) 3, 27, 128
    transaminase deficiency 633–634 (*see also* amino acid metabolism errors)
γ-amino-β-hydroxybutyric and trimethylbetaine *see* carnitine
γ-butyrobetaine aldehyde 287
γ-butyrobetaine dioxygenase 288
γ-butyrobetaine hydroxylase *see* γ-butyrobetaine dioxygenase
γ-cyanopropylmalonic ester 24
γ-Glu-Cys-Gly 265
γ-glutamyl cycle 88, *93*
γ-glutamylcysteine synthetase 266, 268
    deficiency 635 (*see also* amino acid metabolism errors)
Gamow, G. 407
gaseous signaling 543–548, *544*
gastric pepsinogen C 80
gastric prorennin 78
gastrointestinal tract (GI tract) 100–103, 598–599
    active proteases and peptidases 78
    dietary protein digestion *77*
    proteases and peptidases 79
Gautier, H. 45
GC *see* guanylyl cyclase (GC)
GCN2 *see* general control nonderepressible protein 2 (GCN2)
GCS *see* glycine cleavage system (GCS)
GDH *see* glutamate dehydrogenase (GDH)
GEF *see* guanine nucleotide exchange factor (GEF)
Geiger-Mueller counter 378
Gelarden, R.T. 354
gelatin 23
gene mutations
    autosomal dominant/autosomal recessive inheritance 625
    X-linked dominant/recessive inheritance 625
general control nonderepressible protein 2 (GCN2) 577
gene transcription 409–410, 426–427; *see also* protein synthesis
Gerhardt, C. 24
gestation 21
GFAT *see* glutamine:fructose-6-phosphate transaminase (GFAT)
GH *see* growth hormone (GH)
Ghosh, S. 311

Gibbs free energy 503–504
Gilbert's syndrome 637–638; *see also* amino acid metabolism errors
GI tract *see* gastrointestinal tract (GI tract)
gizzerosine (toxic amino acid) *17*, 33
Gln *see* glutamine (Gln)
globular proteins 69; *see also* protein
Glu *see* glutamate (Glu)
glucagon 54
glucosamine 256
    functions 570–571
glucosamine-6-phosphate deaminase (GNPDA) 312
glucose–alanine cycle 135, *135*
glucose metabolism *391*
glucose-6-phosphate dehydrogenase (G6PDH) 338, *339*, **629**, 637
glutamate (Glu) 103; *see also* amino acids (AAs); glutamine
    catabolism 198–205
    decarboxylase 27
    dehydrogenase 334, 340
    dietary AA supplementation 604–606
    GABA transaminase deficiency 633–634
    HA syndrome 634
    P5C synthase deficiency 634
    peptidases 464–465
    receptors 597
    synthesis 133–136, 156–158, 160, *171*
glutamate dehydrogenase (GDH) 99, 133, 334, 340
glutamate oxaloacetate transaminase 127; *see also* aspartate (Asp)
glutamate-pyruvate transaminase 127; *see also* alanine (Ala)
glutamate γ-semialdehyde 225
glutamic acid 39
glutaminase *1*, 133, *158*, 199; *see also* glutamine (Gln)
glutamine (Gln) 3; *see also* amino acids (AAs); glutamate; glutaminase
    catabolism 198–205, *204*, 522
    cell signaling pathway regulation 551
    dietary AA supplementation 603–604
    functions 550–552
    GS deficiency 634–635
    interorgan metabolism *578*
    ketone bodies effect on synthesis of *513*
    metabolism 479
    phosphate-activated glutaminase deficiency 635
    regulatory enzymes 519
    requirement by young pigs **691**
    synthesis 126, 133–136, 156–158, 160, *172*
glutamine:fructose-6-phosphate transaminase (GFAT) 201
glutamine synthetase (GS) 99, *157*, 334
    deficiency 634–635 (*see also* amino acid metabolism errors)
glutaminolysis 203
glutaric acidemia 658; *see also* amino acid metabolism errors
glutathione (GSH) 265
    in animal metabolism and physiology **563**
    concentrations of 265–266
    de novo synthesis 266
    in formaldehyde removal and d-lactate synthesis *562*
    functions *560, 561*, 561–564, *562*, **563**
    GSH synthesis 266

glutathione (GSH) (cont.)
  history of 265
  in mercapturate formation *561*
  5-oxoprolinuria 635–636
  peroxidase 561
  physiological fluids 265–266
  regulation of 266–268
  synthetase 635
  in thiol and free radical homeostasis *562*
  transport and degradation 268, *269*
  γ-Glutamyl-cysteine synthetase deficiency 635
glutathione disulfide (GSSG) *209,* 265
glutathione-*S*-transferase 561
gluten (gliadin) hydrolysate 22, 71
gly *see* glycine (Gly)
glycine (Gly) 6, 15, 22, 36; *see also* amino acids (AAs)
  amidinotransferase 283
  concentrations of 268
  DMGDH deficiency 636
  encephalopathy 636
  functions 552, 554
  glycinemia 636
  glycinuria 636
  sarcosinemia 637
  sideroblastic anemia 637
glycine and serine catabolism
  glycine cleavage system 217
  glycine *N*-methyltransferase 219
  serine degradation 219
  serine hydroxymethyltransferase 217–219
glycine cleavage system (GCS) 217, *219*
glycine (Gly)-encephalopathy 636
glycinemia 636; *see also* amino acid metabolism errors
glycine *N*-methyltransferase (GNMT) 219, 654
glycine-proline-4-hydroxyproline 269
Glycine-Proline-X 55
glycine-related tripeptides **259**
glycine synthesis 131, 140–146, *141,* **142,** *143*
Glycine-X-hydroxyproline 55
glycinuria 636; *see also* amino acid metabolism errors
glycolic aldehyde 26
glycosaminoglycans 55–58; *see also* D-glucosamine
  catabolism of 312, 315–317
  historical perspectives 311
  synthesis of 311–312, *312*–315
glycosaminoglycans catabolism *314*
glycosaminoglycans synthesis *313*
gly-pro-4-hydroxyproline
  metabolism *270*
  in milk and plasma 268–269
  utilization, animals 269–270
GMAT *see* guanidinoacetate
GM-CSF *see* granulocyte/macrophage colonystimulating
  factor (GM-CSF)
Gmelin, L. 27
GMP *see* guanosine monophosphate (GMP)
GNPDA *see* glucosamine-6-phosphate deaminase
  (GNPDA)
Gobley, T. 317
Goldberg, A.L. 134, 462
Goldstein, G. 462
Gortner, R.A. 26
gout 649; *see also* amino acid metabolism errors
Gowland Hopkins, F. 265

GPCR *see* G-protein-coupled receptors (GPCR)
G6PDH *see* glucose-6-phosphate dehydrogenase
  (G6PDH)
G protein 515, 597
G protein beta subunit-like (GβL) 524
G-protein-coupled receptors (GPCR) 583
  cell-specific 597
G1PUT *see* galactose-1-phosphate uridyltransferase
  (G1PUT)
granulocyte/macrophage colony-stimulating factor
  (GM-CSF) *525*
GRAS (Generally Recognized as Safe) 15
Greenberg, D.M. 231, 232
growth hormone (GH) **550**
Grunberg-Manago, M. 407
GS *see* glutamine synthetase (GS)
GSH *see* glutathione (GSH)
GSH synthesis 266
GSSG *see* glutathione disulfide (GSSG)
GTP *see* guanosine triphosphate (GTP)
guanidinoacetate (GA)
  methyltransferase deficiency 633 (*see also* amino acid
    metabolism errors)
guanine (G) 35, 291, 360, 650
guanine nucleotide exchange factor (GEF) **412,** 415,
  419, 583
guanosine monophosphate (GMP) 292
guanosine triphosphate (GTP) *134*
guanylyl cyclase (GC) **550**
Guiditta, A. 29
Gulewitsch, W. 27, 255, 256, 285
Gunsalus, I.C. 167
Gurin, S. 304
Guroff, G. 462
György, P. 220
GβL *see* G protein beta subunit-like (GβL)

HA *see* homoarginine (HA); hyaluronan (HA);
    hyperammonemia (HA)
Haber, F. 334
Habermann, J. 22
Hamalainen, R. 277
Harington, C.R. 306
hartnup disease 655; *see also* amino acid metabolism
    errors
Hashimoto, A. 30
Haussinger, D. 203
Haworth, W. 311
healthy adult humans
  dietary amino acids and nitrogen **85**
heating 106–107
heat shock protein 551; *see also* heme oxygenase (HO)
Hediger, M.A. 354
Hedin, S.G. 21, 23
Heintz, W.H. 27
heme oxygenase (HO) 546
heme synthesis
  and catabolism 296–302
  containing pigments (*see* cytochromes)
  Dubin–Johnson syndrome 637
  Gilbert's syndrome 637–638
  history of 296–298
  pathways of 298
  protoporphyria 638–639

regulation 298
    in animal cells 301–302
    in erythroid cells 300–301
    in hepatocytes 298–300
  synthase (*see* ferrochelatase)
hemoglobin protein 23
Henderson–Hasselbalch equation 39
Henry, E.O. 21
Henseleit, K. 21, 333, 340
heparan and heparin synthesis 315
heparanases (endoglycosidase) 315–316
hepatic acute-phase proteins 450
hepatic urea cycle 340, *344*, 348
hepatolenticular degeneration *see* Wilson's disease
Herbst, R.M. 47
Herrmann, H. 303
Hershko, A. 462
de Hevesy, George 375
hexosamine-synthetic pathway 202, *312*
HGPRT *see* hypoxanthine-guanine
    phosphoribosyltransferase (HGPRT)
HHH syndrome *see* hyperornithinemia–
    hyperammonemia–homocitrullinuria syndrome
    (HHH syndrome)
HI *see* hyperinsulinsim (HI)
high-performance liquid chromatography (HPLC) 6, *16*,
    46, 434, 709
high-quality protein 106–107; *see also* protein
HI/HA syndrome *see* hyperinsulinism and
    hyperammonemia (HI/HA syndrome)
His *see* histidine (His)
histamine
    catabolism 303
    functions 565, 568
    synthesis 303
histidine (His); *see also* amino acids (AAs)
    catabolism *220*, 220–221
    mastocytosis 639
    Tay–Sachs disease 639
    urocanic aciduria 639–640
histidinemia 639; *see also* amino acid metabolism errors
histidine-related dipeptides **259**
histidine synthesis *161*
histidinoalanine 50, *51*
histone modifications
    regulation of gene expression *581*
Hlasiwetz, H. 22
HMB *see* β-Hydroxy-β-methylbutyrate (HMB)
HO *see* heme oxygenase (HO)
Hoagland, M.B. 407
Hoffmann, E. 357
Hoffmann, W.F. 26
Hofmeister, F. 76
Holden, J.T. 167
Holley, R.W. 408
homeostasis 499
  regulation of 499
homoanserine 260
homoarginine (HA) 140
homocarnosine 260
homocyst(e) inuria 653; *see also* amino acid metabolism
    errors
homogentisic acid 26
Hopkins, F.G. 26, 209

Hoppe-Seyler, E.F. 296
Horbaczewski, Ivan 357
Horsford, E.N. 22
HPLC *see* high-performance liquid chromatography
    (HPLC)
H₂S *see* hydrogen sulfide (H₂S)
human atherosclerotic plaque 21
human consumption 271
human health
    adverse effects 741–745
    aging process 726
    amino acids, endogenous ileal flows **83–84**
    animal proteins 735
    continuous catabolism 732
    general considerations 724–726, *725*
    global protein intake 736
    global scope and consequences 736
    healthy adult humans 740–741
    healthy infants and children 739
    intense physical activity 728–731, **729**
    major source 737
    medical therapy and longevity 737–739
    minimum physical activity 727–728
    plant-sourced foods 734–735
    plant- vs animal-sourced proteins 732–734, **733**
    proteinogenic amino acids *7–8*
    proteinogenic L-AAs and glycine 6
    tolerable upper intake level 739, **740**
    weight-reducing program 731–732
Hünefeld, F.L. 296
Hunter, G. 265
Hurtwitz, J. 408
hyaluronan (HA) 313–314
hyaluronic acid *see* hyaluronan (HA)
hyaluronidases 316
hydrochloric acid (HCl) **10**, 76, 77, 78
hydrochloride salts 38
hydrogen sulfide (H₂S)
    antiinflammatory effect 547
    Ca²⁺-dependent effect 547
    cell metabolism regulation 547–548
    functions 547
5-hydroxyindole-3-acetate 310
4-hydroxy-L-proline 23
5-hydroxylysine 33
hydroxyproline 25, 127, 149
3-hydroxyproline
    catabolism 225
    oxidase 226
4-hydroxyproline 5, 55, 56, 79, 483
    catabolism 225
    functions 569–570
    oxidase 226
hydroxyproline synthesis 148–150
5-hydroxytryptamine *see* serotonin
hyperammonemia (HA) 336, 631
    syndrome 634
hyperargininemia 657
hypercitrullinemia 657
hyperhydroxyprolinemia 645
hyperinsulinism and hyperammonemia (HI/HA
    syndrome) **629**; *see also* amino acid
    metabolism errors
hyperinsulinsim (HI) 524, 634

hypermethioninemia 653–654; *see also* amino acid
 metabolism errors
hyperornithinemia 631, 658; *see also* amino acid
 metabolism errors
hyperornithinemia–hyperammonemia–homocitrullinuria
 syndrome (HHH syndrome) 658; *see also*
 amino acid metabolism errors
hyperoxaluria 658; *see also* amino acid metabolism
 errors
hyperprolinemia 645–646, *646*; *see also* amino acid
 metabolism errors
hypersarcosinemia 637; *see also* sarcosinemia
hypertyrosinemia 641–643, *642, 643*; *see also* amino acid
 metabolism errors
hyper-β-alaninemia 651; *see also* amino acid metabolism
 errors
hypoalbuminemia 723
hypophosphatasia 651; *see also* amino acid metabolism
 errors
hypothyroidism 643–644; *see also* amino acid
 metabolism errors
hypoxanthine-guanine phosphoribosyltransferase
 (HGPRT) 649

ICAT *see* isotope-coded affinity tag (ICAT)
IDA *see* iodoacetate (IDA)
"ideal protein" concept 683
IDO *see* indoleamine 2,3-dioxygenase (IDO)
IE *see* isotope enrichment (IE)
IFN *see* interferon (IFN)
Ig *see* immunoglobulins (Ig)
IGF *see* insulin-like growth factor (IGF)
iGluRs *see* ionotropic glutamate receptors (iGluRs)
Ikeda, K. 22
IL *see* interleukin (IL)
Ile *see* isoleucine (Ile)
imidodipeptidase deficiency *see* prolidase deficiency
imino acids, definition 5; *see also* amino acids (AAs)
iminoglycinuria 647; *see also* amino acid
 metabolism errors
immune and circulatory systems 127
immune system 584
 acquired 585
 B-lymphocytes 584
 fish and crustaceans 585
 innate 584–585
 mammals and birds *584,* 584–585
 M1 and M2 cell balance *525*
immunoglobulins (Ig) 67, 109, 424, 490
IMP *see* inosine monophosphate (IMP)
inborn metabolic disorder 24
indandione-2-N-2'-indanone enolate 50
indicator AA oxidation method 695–697
indirect AA oxidation method *see* indicator AA oxidation
 method
indole-3-acetaldehyde 237
indoleamine 2,3-dioxygenase (IDO) 234, *235*
inducible NOS (iNOS) 551; *see also* nitric oxide synthase
 (NOS)
inflammatory macrophages (M1) *525*
Ingvaldsen, T. 23, 256
inhibitors 513
iNOS *see* inducible NOS (iNOS)
inosine monophosphate (IMP) 134, 292, 293, 596, 649

inositol trisphosphate (IP₃) 597
Insulin 349
insulin-like growth factor (IGF) **528**
intercellular glutamine-glutamate cycle 203, *205*
interferon (IFN) *525*
interleukin (IL) *525*
interorgan synthesis 128
interstitial space of tissues 490–491
intracellular glycosaminoglycans 317
intracellular labeled precursor pool
 decreased dilution 396
 increased dilution 395–396
intracellular protein degradation *493*
 biological half-lives 474–477
 historic perspectives 461–462
 intracellular protein turnover 477
 physiological significance 477–479
 proteases and peptidases 463
 catalytic site 464–467
 endopeptidases 464
 evolutionary relationship 467
 exopeptidases 464
 in vitro measurement
 general considerations 479–481
 tracer and nontracer methods 481–483
 in vivo measurement
 general considerations 483–484
 labeled AA single administration 484–485
 leucine oxidation method 485
 3-methylhistidine urinary excretion 485–487
intracellular protein synthesis 429
intracellular protein turnover 461, *461,* 477
intracellular proteolytic pathways
 lysosomal proteolytic pathway
 endocytosis and autophagy 467–468
 lysosomal proteolytic system 468–470
 proteases in lysosomes 468
 nonlysosomal proteolytic pathway
 ATP-dependent proteolytic system 470–471
 Ca²⁺-dependent proteolytic system 470
 caspases 470
 nonlysosomal proteolytic system 470, 474
 26S proteasome structure 471–472
 ubiquitin-dependent protein degradation 472–474
 ubiquitin-independent proteolytic system 470–471
 ubiquitin-proteasome system functions 474
in vitro measurement
 intracellular protein degradation
 general considerations 479–481
 tracer and nontracer methods 481–483
 protein synthesis
 AA tracers 433–434
 general considerations 432–433
 protein synthesis rate 434–435
 in vitro preparations 433
in vivo measurement
 intracellular protein degradation
 general considerations 483–484
 labeled AA single administration 484–485
 leucine oxidation method 485
 3-methylhistidine urinary excretion 485–487
 protein synthesis
 flooding dose technique 438–440
 general considerations 435–436

labeled AA single administration 437–438
leucine oxidation method 442–445
protein turnover 436–437
radioactive/stable tracers 436
tissues, ^2H_2O use 445–448
tracer AA continuous infusion 440–442
iodoacetate (IDA) 465, **465**
ion-exchange chromatography 42
ionizable groups in amino acids **39–40**
ionotropic glutamate receptors (iGluRs) 598
IP3 *see* inositol trisphosphate (IP3)
irreversible inhibitors 508
isobaric tags for relative and absolute quantification
        (iTRAQ) 701
isobuteine synthesis 151, *151, 153*
isoleucine (Ile) 6, 23, 134, 212, 501; *see also* amino
        acids (AAs)
isotope-coded affinity tag (ICAT) 701
isotope enrichment (IE), 381
    radioactive isotopes 382–383
    significance 385–392
    stable isotope enrichment 383–385
isotope experiments
    data interpretation 394–395
    exchange 397–398
    intracellular labeled precursor pool
        decreased dilution 396
        increased dilution 395–396
    isotopic non-steady state 400–401
    randomization 396–397
    recycling 398–400
isotopes; *see also* radioactive isotopes
    amino acid **377**
    definition of 375–377
    isotopic enrichment 381
    isotopic studies 401–403
    metabolic research
        radiotracer methods, high sensitivity 394
        tracing metabolic pathways 392–394
    radioactive expression 379–381
    radioisotopes 377–379
    specific radioactivity 381
        radioactive isotopes 382–383
        significance 385–392
        stable isotope enrichment 383–385
    tracer and tracee 381
isotopes randomization 396–397, *398*
isotopes recycling 398–400
isotopic enrichment 381
isotopic non-steady state 400–401
isovaleric acidemia 632; *see also* amino acid metabolism
        errors
isovaleric aciduria *see* isovaleric acidemia
isovalthine synthesis 151, *151, 153*
iTRAQ *see* isobaric tags for relative and absolute
        quantification (iTRAQ)

Jacobs, W.A. 28
Jaffé, M. 24, 220
JNK *see* c-Jun NH(2)-terminal kinase (JNK)
Johanson–Blizzard syndrome 476
Johnson, A.B. 225
Johnson, P. 211
Jones, M.E. 136

Jones, N.R. 263
Jungas, R.L. 182

KADH *see* 2-Ketoadipate dehydrogenase complex
        (KADH)
Karyagina, M.K. 133
Kaufman, S. 150, 224
k-casein 78
Kendall, E.C. 265, 306
3-ketoacid CoA-transferase 290
2-ketoadipate dehydrogenase complex (KADH) **649**
keto–enol tautomerization 48, 358
KIC *see* α-Ketoisocaproate (KIC)
KIC dioxygenase 214–215
kidney- and liver-type glutaminases 202–203
Kim, P.M. 166
Kjeldahl method 72
Klebsiella aerogenes 159
Knoop, F. 17, 133
Knopf, L. 199
Koeppe, R.E. 136
Kolbe, H. 27
Kornberg, A. 407
Kossel, A. 21, 23, 24, 205, 291, 407
Krebs bicarbonate buffer 94
Krebs cycle 106, 183, *183, 185,* 222, 338, 394
Krebs, H.A. 21, 22, 24, 47, 133, 148, 198, 199, 225, 333,
        334, 340, 358
Krebs–Henseleit bicarbonate buffer 53
Kreil, G. 30
Krimberg, R. 285
Kritzmann, M.G. 133
Kutscher, F. 303
Kwashiorkor 671
kynurenine pathway 234–236

labeled AA single administration 437–438, 484–485
Lactobacillus sakei LT-13 167
Ladenburg, A. 276
L-alanine (α-aminopropionic acid) 16–27
lanthionine 50, *51,* 52
L-arginine 21, 25, 36
    monohydrochloride 49
    phosphate 24
L-asparagine (α-aminosuccinamic acid) 21
L-aspartate (α-aminosuccinic acid) 21
Laurent, A. 22, 24
lauric arginate 49
Lavoisier, Antoine 76, 198
laws of thermodynamics *see* thermodynamics
L-3-carboxy-*trans*-2,3-epoxypropylleucylamido
        (4-guanidino) butane (E-64) 465
L-carnitine
    catabolism of 288–290
    diet, contribution of 287
    endogenous synthesis 287
    history of 285–286
    interorgan cooperation 286–287
    regulation of 288
L-Citrulline (α-amino-δ-carbamidovaleric acid) 21
LCT *see* lysosomal cystine transporter (LCT)
L-Cysteine (α-amino-β-mercaptopropionic acid) 22
L-DOPA [3,4-dihydroxy-L-phenylalanine (3-hydroxy-L-
        tyrosine) 31

Leavenworth, C.S. 24
Ledderhose, G. 311
Leder, P. 408
Leloir, L.F. 311
Lesch–Nyhan syndrome 649; *see also* amino acid
        metabolism errors
Leu *see* leucine (Leu)
Leucaena leucocephala 34, 109
Leuchs, F.H. 26
Leuchs, H. 23
leucine (Leu) 23–24, 37
    ketone and pyruvate on transamination of **512**
leucine oxidation method 442–445, 485
Levene, P.A. 26, 291
levorotatory 6
levulinic acid 22
L-glutamate (α-aminoglutaric acid) 22
L-glutamine (α-aminoglutaramic acid) 22
L-glutamyl-D-alanine 28
L-histidine (α-amino-β-imidazolepropionic acid) 23, *261*
L-histidine-HCl 36
L-homoarginine 23, 140
Liebreich, O. 317
ligand 515
limiting AA 673
lipid metabolism 136
Lipmann, F.A. 26, 30
lipolysis and palmitate recycling **386**
lipopolysaccharide (LPS) *525*
Lipp, A. 24, 26
liquid-phase peptide synthesis 52
Liquori, A.M. 277
L-isoleucine (α-amino-β-methylvaleric acid) 23
L. latifolius 33
L-leucine (α-aminoisocaproic acid) 23
L-leucyl-*asparagine* 42
L-lysine (α,ε-diaminocaproic acid) 23, 24, 25
L,L-α-ε-diaminopimelate (DAPA) 34
L-methionine (α-amino-γ-methylthiobutyric acid) 24
L-methionine sulfoximine 34
Locquin, R. 23
Loewi, O. 317, 407
Lohmann, K. 24, 281, 291
longevity 738–739
L-Ornithine (α,δ-diaminovaleric acid) 24
Lowry assay 54
L-phenylalanine (α-amino-β-phenylpropionic acid) 24, 379
L-phosphoarginine 24–25
L-proline (pyrrolidine-2-carboxylic acid) 25
LPS *see* lipopolysaccharide (LPS)
L-pyrrolysine 25, 428
L-selenocysteine *25*
    formation 419–420
    historical perspectives 419
    selenoproteins 419–420
L-serine (α-amino-β-hydroxypropionic acid) 26
L. sylvestris 33
L-threonine (α-amino-β-hydroxybutyric acid) 26
L-tryptophan (α-amino-β-3-indolepropionic acid) 26
L-tyrosine 26
Lusk, G. 199
L-valine (α-aminoisovaleric acid) 26, 27, 36
Lyons, P.J. 78
Lys *see* lysine (Lys)

lysine (Lys); *see also* amino acids (AAs)
    catabolism
        decarboxylation 222–223
            via saccharopine and pipecolate pathways 221–222
    lysinoalanine 50, *51*
    synthesis 140, *162*
lysinoalanine 50, *51*
lysinuric protein intolerance 631; *see also* amino acid
        metabolism errors
lysosomal cystine transporter (LCT) 91, 92
lysosomal proteolytic pathway
    endocytosis and autophagy 467–468
    lysosomal proteolytic system 468–470
    proteases in lysosomes 468
lysosomal proteolytic system 468–470
lysosome 467–468
L-α,γ-diaminobutyric acid 33

M1 *see* inflammatory macrophages (M1)
M2 *see* anti-inflammatory macrophages (M2)
MacMunn, C.A. 296
macroautophagy 468
macrophage (MΦ) *525*
macrophage colony-stimulating factor (M-CSF) *525*
Maillard reaction 106, *107*
Malaguti, F.J. 22
Mallette, L.E. 135
malonomycin 19
mammalian vacuolar protein sorting mutant 34
        (mVps34) 524
mammals 118, 127
    immune system *584*, 584–585
Mandelstam, J. 462
mannose-6-phosphate 467
MAPK *see* mitogen-activated protein kinase (MAPK)
maple syrup urine disease 632; *see also* amino acid
        metabolism errors
marasmus 671
Marliss, E.B. 133–134
Martinez, R.E. 137
mass spectrometry (MS) 701
mast *see* mast cells (mast)
mast cells (mast) 303, 313, 315, 639
mastocytosis 639; *see also* amino acid metabolism errors
MAT *see* methionine adenosyltransferase (MAT)
Matsuoka, Z. 234
Matthews, J.C. 93
MBM *see* meat and bone meal (MBM)
M-CSF *see* macrophage colony-stimulating factor
        (M-CSF)
ME *see* 2-mercaptoethanol (ME); metabolizable
        energy (ME)
Me-AIB *see* 2-methylaminoisobutyric acid (Me-AIB)
meat and bone meal (MBM) **712**
mechanistic target of rapamycin (MTOR) 24, 314, 407,
            541, 543
    cell signaling 522
    MTORC1 524
    MTORC2 524
Meijer, A.J. 349
Meister, A. 117
melamine 72, 709; *see also* protein
melatonin (*N*-acetyl-5-methoxytryptamine)
    elimination and catabolism of 309–310

functions 568
serotonin catabolism 310–311
serotonin synthesis 310
synthesis 308–309
synthesis of 306–309
Meltzer, H.L. 231
Menghini, V.A. 296
2-mercaptoethanol (ME) 42, 45, 237
MEROPS database 467
Merrifield, R.B. 52
messenger RNA (mRNA) 408
met *see* methionine (Met)
metabolic fecal N (MFN) **717**
metabolic pathways 394
metabolic research, isotopes
    radiotracer methods, high sensitivity 394
    tracing metabolic pathways 392–394
metabolism concepts 73, 501; *see also* amino acid
        metabolism
    activator and inhibitor concentrations 513–514
    allosteric regulation 510
    changes in cell volume 517
    chemical reactions 501
    enzyme activity regulation 518
    enzymes as biochemical reactions 506–508
    equilibrium concept 504–505
    metabolic design principles 508–509
    metabolic pathways 508
    metabolism regulation 509
    near-equilibrium and nonequilibrium reactions 505
    phosphorylation and dephosphorylation 510–511
    signal transduction 514–517
    substrate and cofactor concentrations 511–513
    thermodynamics 501–504
metabolizable energy (ME) **687, 688**
metabolizable protein 676
metabolomics 701
metabolon 509
metabotropic glutamate receptors (mGluRs) 597
metals, AAs chelates 49
Metcalf, B.W. 277
methionine (Met) 24, 33, 138; *see also* amino acids (AAs)
    catabolism 227, 228–231
        transamination pathway 230–231
        transsulfuration pathway 228–229
    sulfoximine 338
    synthesis *162,* 170
methionine adenosyltransferase (MAT) 653
5-methoxytryptamine 310
2-methylaminoisobutyric acid (Me-AIB) 92
methylarginines synthesis 146–147, *147*
methylated derivatives 255
methylbutyric acidemia 632; *see also* amino acid
        metabolism errors
1-methylhistidine 260
3-methylhistidine urinary excretion 485–487
methyllanthionine 52
3-methyl-lanthionine 50, *51*
3-methyl-lysinoalanine 50, *51*
methylmalonic acidemia 659; *see also* amino acid
        metabolism errors
methylmalonyl-CoA mutase 659
methylthioadenosine (MTA) 206, 278
Meyer, G.M. 76

Meyerhof, O. 24
MFN *see* metabolic fecal N (MFN)
mGluRs *see* metabotropic glutamate receptors (mGluRs)
Michaelis–Menton equation 506
microbes 30, 34
microbial metabolism 81
microbial protein 676
    fermentation 273
    synthesis *101,* 106
microorganisms, AAs synthesis 67, 99
    amino acid epimerases 167
    amino acid racemases 166–167
    2-aminoethylphosphonate 163–164
    arginine 158–159
    aspartate and asparagine 159
    cysteine and tyrosine 159–160
    D-AAs conversion 168–169
    D-AAs synthesis 166–167
    2,6-diaminopimelic acid 163–164
    essential amino acids 160–161
    glutamate and glutamine 156–158
    N-acetylated amino acids 161–163
    overall pathways 155–156
    phosphoryl amino acids 164
microRNA (miRNA) 580
    biogenesis *582*
Miescher, J.F. 291
Miller, G.L. 265
Miller, L.L. 221
miRNA *see* MicroRNA (miRNA)
mitochondrial arginine decarboxylase 279
mitochondrial basic AA carriers (BAC) 207
mitochondrial electron transport system 183
mitochondrial ornithine transporter 1 (ORNT1) 341, 658
mitochondrial proteins 424–426
mitochondrial β-hydroxyisobutyryl-CoA hydrolase 216
mitogen-activated protein kinase (MAPK) 552
    family 581
    induced cell signaling *583*
de Moitessier, J. 296
molar percent enrichment *see* isotope enrichment (IE)
molecular circuit 515; *see also* signal transduction
monoamine oxidase 305
monogastric animals digestion 96–97
    AAs across, net balance 94–96
    dietary protein digestion 76–79
    free AAs absorption 88–94
    historical perspective 76
    nitrogen, extensive recycling 96–99
    protein digestibility 81–88
    proteolytic digestive capacity 79–81
monosodium glutamate (MSG) 22
Mörner, K. 306
Morris, S.M. 207
mRNA *see* messenger RNA (mRNA)
mRNA translation 411–412
    active 80S initiation complex 415–416
    inactive free 80S ribosomes 412–414
    48S initiation complex 414–415
    43S preinitiation complex 414
    translation initiation 427
MS *see* mass spectrometry (MS)
MTA *see* methylthioadenosine (MTA)
MTHF *see* N^5-N^{10}-Methylenetetrahydrofolate (MTHF)

MTOR *see* mechanistic target of rapamycin (MTOR)
mucopolysaccharidoses 661
Mueller, J.H. 24
Mulder, G.J. 22, 23, 53, 296
"multicatalytic protease complex" 462
multidrug and toxin extrusion (MATE) 285
multiple enzymes 205–206
Munro, H. 198
mutual AA ratios 715–716
mVps34 *see* mammalian vacuolar protein sorting mutant
        34 (mVps34)
MWC model 510
myoadenylate deaminase deficiency 649; *see also* Amino
        acid metabolism errors
myofibrillar proteins 58–59, 526
myosin 58, 69
MΦ *see* macrophage (MΦ)

N-acetyl-AA synthetase 35
N-acetyl-aspartate synthesis 31, **32,** 33, 153
N-acetylated AAs catabolism 237–238
N-acetylated amino acids 161–163
N-acetylcysteine 139
N-acetylglutamate (NAG) 153, 513, 514, **549,** 656
N-acetylglutamate synthase (NAGS) 118, 334, 574
        deficiency 656 (*see also* amino acid metabolism errors)
N-acetyl-L-histidine 31, **32,** 153
N-acetyl-5-methoxytryptamine *see* Melatonin
        (*N*-acetyl-5-methoxytryptamine)
N-acetylornithine 159
N-acetyltransferases catalyze 35
N-acetyl-π-methylhistidine 31, **32**
Nachmansohn, D. 281
NAG *see* N-acetylglutamate (NAG)
NAGS *see* N-acetylglutamate synthase (NAGS)
natural amino acids discoveries **2–3**
natural killer cells (NK) *525*
N balance measurement **685–689,** 685–689; *see also*
        factorial method; "-omics" technologies; tracer
        method
        advantages and limitations 689–690
NBB *see* neutral brush border (NBB)
NCA *see* N-Carboxy amino acid anhydride (NCA)
N-carbamoylglutamate (NCG) 513, 514
N-carbobenzoxyglutamate-α-methyl ester 265
N-carboxy amino acid anhydride (NCA) 45, 49, 52
NCG *see* N-carbamoylglutamate (NCG)
ND *see* not detectable (ND); not determined (ND)
NEAA *see* nonessential amino acid (NEAA)
near-equilibrium reactions 505
Needham, D.M. 133
NEPN *see* norepinephrine (NEPN)
Neptune, E.M. 22
net protein ratio 717–718
net protein utilization 718
NETs *see* neutrophil excellular traps (NETs)
Neubauer, O. 117, 150, 223
neurolathyrism 34
neuromodulators 574
neuronal NO synthase (nNOS) 208; *see also* nitric oxide
        synthase (NOS)
Neurospora crassa 287, 311
neutral brush border (NBB) 92
neutrophil (NTP) *525*

neutrophil extracellular traps (NETs) *525*
Newey, H. 75, 92
newly synthesized proteins
        cytosol, extracellular space 424
        posttranslational modifications 420–424
Newsholme, E.A. 203
N-formiminoglutamate 221
N-formylmethionine (fMet) 426
N-glycosyl-L-asparagine 35
N^G-monomethyl-l-arginine (NMMA) 522
N^G*N*^G-dimethyl-L-arginine *see* asymmetrical
        dimethylarginine (ADMA)
N^G*N*^NG-dimethyl-L-arginine *see* symmetrical
        dimethylarginine (SDMA)
NI *see* dietary N intake (NI)
NIDDM *see* noninsulin-dependent diabetes mellitus
        (NIDDM)
ninhydrin 50
Nirenberg, M. 408
Nishikawa, T. 30
nisin 50
nitric oxide (NO) 21, 106, 127, 261, *525,* **529, 550**
        AMP-activated protein kinase phosphorylation 545
        in cardiovascular system 545
        facets 545–546
        functions of *544,* 544–546
nitric oxide synthase (NOS) 338, **541**
nitrogen 103
        balance measurement 689, 690
        extensive recycling 96–99
        growth index 718
        recycling 105–106
nitrogen growth index 718
nitrogenous metabolites 241–242, **335**
NK *see* natural killer cells (NK)
NKHG *see* nonketotic hyperglycinemia (NKHG)
N-leucine infusion technique 86
N-malonyl-D-alanine 28
NMDA *see* N-Methyl-d-aspartate (NMDA)
N-methylaminoisobutyrate (MeAIB) 88
N-methyl-d-aspartate (NMDA) 557
N-methyltransferase 282, 303
NMMA *see* NG-Monomethyl-l-arginine (NMMA); ω-
        NG-monomethyl-l-arginine (NMMA)
N^5-N^10-Methylenetetrahydrofolate (MTHF) 145–146
nNOS *see* neuronal NO synthase (nNOS)
NO *see* nitric oxide (NO)
non-canonical proteinogenic AAs 12
nonequilibrium reactions 505
nonessential amino acid (NEAA) 673–674, 675, 678;
        see also amino acids (AAs)
        in animals **679**
        of humans and animals 678–681, **679**
        roles of 682
nongenomic mechanisms 516
non-human monogastric mammals **68**
noninsulin-dependent diabetes mellitus (NIDDM)
        197–198
nonketotic hyperglycinemia (NKHG) 636; *see also* glycine
        (Gly)-encephalopathy
nonlysosomal proteolytic pathway
        ATP-dependent proteolytic system 470–471
        Ca^2+-dependent proteolytic system 470
        caspases 470

nonlysosomal proteolytic system 470, 474
26S proteasome structure 471–472
ubiquitin-dependent protein degradation 472–474
ubiquitin-independent proteolytic system 470–471
ubiquitin-proteasome system functions 474
nonlysosomal proteolytic system 470, 474
nonprimates, anserine 264–265
nonprotein AA see amino acids (AAs)
non-protein nitrogen (NPN) *100,* 103, 106, 676
non-proteinogenic amino acids 12, *15, 17,* 30, 33, 118
nonsense codon 418, 652
nontracer method 481–483
norepinephrine (NEPN) **541**
NOS see nitric oxide synthase (NOS); NO synthase (NOS)
NO synthase (NOS) 205, 207–209
not detectable (ND) 14, 20, 43
not determined (ND) 341, 386
N-phosphoarginine 154, 164
N-phosphohistidine synthesis 164
N-phosphorylation 154
NPN see nonprotein nitrogen (NPN)
NRC see U.S. National Research Council (NRC)
NRF-1 see nuclear respiratory factor 1 (NRF-1)
N-terminal amino acid 476, **476**
NTP see neutrophil (NTP)
nuclear respiratory factor 1 (NRF-1) 300
nucleic acids digestion 103–105
nuclein see nucleic acids
nucleotidases 103
nutrient sensing 598–599
nutrigenomics 699–700
nutritional implications 105–106
nutritional regulation 216–217
nutritional significance 99–100
nystagmus 640
N$^\alpha$-dehydrogenation 49

OAT see ornithine aminotransferase (OAT)
obesity 738
Ochoa, S. 407
ochronosis 641, *642; see also* amino acid metabolism errors
OCT see ornithine carbamoyltransferase (OCT)
ocular albinism, type 1 641
Odake, S. 24
ODC see ornithine decarboxylase (ODC)
'Official Methods of Analysis of the AOAC International' 71
Ohsumi, Yoshinori 468
oligopeptides 52, 79
ω-*N*G-monomethyl-L-arginine (NMMA) 146
"-omics" technologies 699
one-carbon unit metabolism *576*
o-phthaldialdehyde (OPA) *16,* 45–46, **45–47**
opioid peptides
bioactive peptides 271–275
endogenous synthesis of 270–271
enzymatic hydrolysis **272**
optic nerve hypoplasia 640
organic acidurias 658–659; *see also* amino acid metabolism errors
organic anion transporters (OAT) 366

ornithine 24
catabolism 205
cycle 340 (*see also* urea cycle)
synthesis 136–138, *158*
ornithine aminotransferase (OAT) 136
inborn deficiency of 504
ornithine carbamoyltransferase (OCT) 136, 334–335; *see also* hyperornithinemia
ornithine decarboxylase (ODC) 211, 277, 279, 551
ornithinoalanine 50, *51*
ORNT1 see mitochondrial ornithine transporter 1 (ORNT1)
orotic aciduria 651; *see also* amino acid metabolism errors
ovine allantoic fluid 21
oxaloacetate 133
oxidative deamination 50
oxidative stress 563
5-oxoprolinuria 635–636; *see also* amino acid metabolism errors
oxymethylation 47

PA see polyamines (PA)
Palade, G.E. 407
palmitate oxidation **388**
p-aminophenylalanine 26
Pan, A. 93
pancreatic protein hydrolysate 26
pancreatic trypsin 76
PAO see polyamine oxidase (PAO)
Paracolobactrum aerogenoides 103
Park, C.R. 135
Pasteur, L. 5
PAT see proton-coupled amino acid transporter (PAT)
Pauly, H. 23
PBM see Poultry by-product meal (PBM)
P5C see pyrroline-5-carboxylate (P5C)
P5CD see pyrroline-5-carboxylate dehydrogenase (P5CD)
P5C metabolism 226
P5CR see pyrroline-5-carboxylate reductase (P5CR)
P5CS see pyrroline-5-carboxylate synthase (P5CS)
P5C synthase deficiency 634; *see also* amino acid metabolism errors
PDV see Portal-drained viscera (PDV)
Pegg, A.E. 277
Pelouze, E. 27
Pelouze, T.J. 21
Pencharz, P.B. 136
penicillamine 653
PEPCK see phosphoenolpyruvate carboxykinase (PEPCK)
pepsins 76, 77
peptidases; *see also* protease
protein degradation 463
catalytic site 464–467
endopeptidases 464
evolutionary relationship 467
exopeptidases 464
peptide; *see also* peptidases
bond formation 417–418
chain elongation 418–419
small 542
peptide bond-linked AAs 12–13, *15*
peptide-bound amino acids (PAAs) **18–19**
peptide-bound asparagine 21
peptide-bound proline 148

peptide elongation; *see also* protein synthesis
    aminoacyl-tRNA 416–417
        peptide bond formation 417–418
        peptidyl-tRNA translocation 418
        tRNA-bound AA on 80S ribosome 416
peptide elongation and termination 427–428
peptides absorption
    monogastric animals
        AAs across, net balance 94–96
        dietary protein digestion 76–79
        free AAs absorption 88–94
        historical perspective 76
        nitrogen, extensive recycling 96–99
        protein digestibility 81–88
        proteolytic digestive capacity 79–81
    protein classification 69–71
    protein content 71–72
    ruminants
        AA degradation inhibition 108–109
        chemical treatment 107
        free AAs absorption 105
        gastrointestinal tract 100–103
        heating 106–107
        high-quality protein 106–107
        nitrogen recycling 105–106
        nucleic acids digestion 103–105
        nutritional implications 105–106
        nutritional significance 99–100
        physical encapsulation 108
        polyphenolic phytochemicals 107–108
        rumen degradation 106–107
        small peptides 105
    toxic AAs degradation 109
peptides separation 54
peptide synthesis 52
peptidyl site (P site) 416
peptidyl-tRNA translocation 418
perchloric acid 25
peroxisome proliferator-activated receptor-α (PPAR-α) 298
Perutz, M. 296
phagophore 468
Phe *see* phenylalanine (Phe)
phenolsulfotransferase 305
phenylacetylglutamine 322
phenylalanine (Phe) 35, 76, 117; *see also* amino
        acids (AAs)
    catabolism 24
    L-phenylalanine 24
    synthesis *163*
    and tyrosine catabolism 223–225
phenylethylaminoalanine 50, *51*
phenylketonuria (PKU) 24, *644,* 644–645; *see also* amino
        acid metabolism errors
phenylmethylsulfonylfluoride (PMSF) 465
phenylpyruvate 224
pheochromocytoma 645; *see also* amino acid
        metabolism errors
pheomelanin 568; *see also* melanin
philothion 265
phorbol myristate acetate (PMA) *525*
phosphagen 281
phosphate-activated glutaminase
    deficiency 635
phosphocreatine 559

3′, 5′-phosphodiester bridges 292
phosphoenolpyruvate carboxykinase (PEPCK) 184
phosphoethanolamine 154, *155*
phosphoglycerate dehydrogenase deficiency 651–652;
        see also amino acid metabolism errors
phosphoinositide 3 (PI3) 597
5-phosphoribosyl-1-pyrophosphate (PRPP) 292, 295
phosphoribosylpyrophosphate synthetase (PRPS) 649
5-phosphoribosyl-α- pyrophosphate 160
phosphoryl amino acids 154, 164
phosphorylation 510
    of BCKA dehydrogenase 511
    enzyme regulation by reversible *511*
    tyrosine hydroxylase 511
phosphoserine synthesis 164
phosphothreonine synthesis 164
phosphotyrosine synthesis 164
phosvitin 510
phthalimidopropylmalonic ester 24
p-hydroxyphenylpyruvate 224
physical encapsulation 108
physiological regulation 216–217
physiological significance, protein synthesis
    animal growth 430–431
    cells production and replacement 431
    immune responses and health 432
    injury, wound healing and recovery 431
    protein concentrations regulation 430–431
    proteins physiological functions 430
PI3 *see* phosphoinositide 3 (PI3)
pigs
    amino acids, endogenous ileal flows **83–84**
    amino acids utilization **119**
    dietary amino acids **120**
    gestating gilts, metabolism **121–122**
    lactating sows, metabolism **123–124**
    nitrogen absorption **98**
Pinhey, K.G. 265
Pinner, A. 291
Pinosch, H. 303
pipecolic acid pathways 221
Pirie, N.W. 265
Piwi RNA 580
PKU *see* phenylketonuria (PKU)
plasma 60
plasmalemmal and T-tubular caveolae (PTC) 208
plasma membrane caveolae (PMC) 208
Plisson, A. 21
PM *see* postsynaptic membrane (PM)
PMA *see* phorbol myristate acetate (PMA)
PMC *see* plasma membrane caveolae (PMC)
PMSF *see* phenylmethylsulfonylfluoride (PMSF)
PNP *see* purine nucleoside phosphorylase (PNP)
PO *see* proline oxidase (PO)
Polidori, C. 309
polyamine oxidase (PAO) 278–280
polyamines (PA) 528, **549**
    catabolism *280*
    eIF5A modification 557
    functions 557–559
    history of 276–277
    metabolism 277
    mucopolysaccharidoses 661
    polyamine degradation

diamine oxidase 279–281
N^1-acetylpolyamine oxidase 281
N^1-acetyltransferase 281
polyamine oxidase 279–281
polyamine synthesis
pathways of 277–279
regulation of 279
spermine synthase deficiency 660–661
synthesis 211, *278*
poly(A)-binding protein (PABP) 410
Polygonatum multiflorum 33
polypeptide synthesis 22, 54
polyphenolic phytochemicals 107–108
porcine placenta 134
porphyrin 296
portal-drained viscera (PDV) **691**
portal vein-drained system *75*
Porter, K. 407
positional isotopomers 381
postsynaptic membrane (PM) 208
posttranslational modifications 12, 25, 52, 58, 408, 420,
422; *see also* protein synthesis
potassium hydroxide 21
poultry by-product meal (PBM) **712**
PPAR-α *see* peroxisome proliferator-activated receptor-α
(PPAR-α)
Priestley, J. 333
primary carnitine deficiency 632–633; *see also* amino acid
metabolism errors
primary messenger *see* ligand
primed constant infusion 387
PRMT *see* protein arginine *N*-methyltransferases (PRMT)
Pro *see* proline (Pro)
PRODH *see* proline oxidase
prokaryotes cytosol 426
prolidase deficiency *647*, 647–648; *see also* amino acid
metabolism errors
proline (Pro) 5, 25, 117, 136, 148, **550**; *see also* amino
acids (AAs)
catabolism 225
chemical structures *148*
functions 555–556
hyperhydroxyprolinemia 645
hyperprolinemia 645–646, *646*
iminoglycinuria 647
oxidase 645
prolidase deficiency *647*, 647–648
synthesis 148–150
proline oxidase (PO) *132,* 225, 226
prolyl-4-hydroxyproline 79
propionic acidemia 659; *see also* amino acid
metabolism errors
propionyl-CoA carboxylase 659
proteases 463; *see also* peptidases
activities 80
catalytic site 464–467
endopeptidases 464
evolutionary relationship 467
exopeptidases 464
inhibitors *466*
in lysosomes 468
protein
animals, physiological roles in **71**
classification **69–70,** 69–71

content 71–72, *72*
determination
Biuret Assay (Piotrowski' Test) 53–54
Coomassie Brilliant Blue dye 53
Lowry assay 54
efficiency ratio 716–717
extracellular degradation 79
intracellular synthesis of 128
microarray technology 700–701
over-consumption 71
in plasma or serum 722–723
polypeptide aggregates 69
proteins *versus* peptides 54
extracellular matrix proteins 55–58
glycosaminoglycans 55–58
myofibrillar proteins 58–59
peptides separation 54
protein arginine *N*-methyltransferases (PRMTs) 146
proteinases *see* endopeptidases
protein biosynthesis 461
protein-bound lysine residues 47, 287
protein catabolism 364
protein degradation *see* intracellular protein degradation;
peptidases; tracer and nontracer methods
protein digestibility 81–88
protein digestibility corrected AA score (PDCAAS)
719–721, **719, 720**
protein digestion
monogastric animals
AAs across, net balance 94–96
dietary protein digestion 76–79
free AAs absorption 88–94
historical perspective 76
nitrogen, extensive recycling 96–99
protein digestibility 81–88
proteolytic digestive capacity 79–81
protein classification 69–71
protein content 71–72
ruminants
AA degradation inhibition 108–109
chemical treatment 107
free AAs absorption 105
gastrointestinal tract 100–103
heating 106–107
high-quality protein 106–107
nitrogen recycling 105–106
nucleic acids digestion 103–105
nutritional implications 105–106
nutritional significance 99–100
physical encapsulation 108
polyphenolic phytochemicals 107–108
rumen degradation 106–107
small peptides 105
toxic AAs degradation 109
protein hydrolysates 271
protein hydrolysis 76, 78
protein malnutrition
arginine 587–588
glutamate 589–590
glutamine 588–589
glycine 590
tryptophan 590–591
proteinogenic amino acids 1, *7,* 12, 118
proteinogenic L-AAs 6

protein synthesis (PS) 12, **549**
  biochemical characteristics
    energy requirement 429–430
    physiological significance 430–432
  biochemical pathways 408
  cytosolic protein synthesis 408–409
  eukaryotes *vs.* prokaryotes
    gene transcription 426–427
    mRNA translation initiation 427
    peptide elongation and termination 427–428
  gene transcription 409–410
  historical perspectives 407–408
  L-pyrrolysine 428
  L-selenocysteine
    formation 419–420
    historical perspectives 419
    selenoproteins 419–420
  mitochondrial proteins 424–426
  mRNA translation 411–412
    active 80S initiation complex 415–416
    inactive free 80S ribosomes 412–414
    48S initiation complex 414–415
    43S preinitiation complex 414
  newly synthesized proteins
    cytosol, extracellular space 424
    posttranslational modifications 420–424
  peptide chain elongation 418–419
  peptide elongation
    aminoacyl-tRNA 416–417
    peptide bond formation 417–418
    peptidyl-tRNA translocation 418
    tRNA-bound AA on 80S ribosome 416
  physiological significance
    animal growth 430–431
    cells production and replacement 431
    immune responses and health 432
    injury, wound healing and recovery 431
    protein concentrations regulation 430–431
    proteins physiological functions 430
  prokaryotes cytosol 426
  in vitro measurement
    AA tracers 433–434
    general considerations 432–433
    protein synthesis rate 434–435
    in vitro preparations 433
  in vivo measurement
    flooding dose technique 438–440
    general considerations 435–436
    labeled AA single administration 437–438
    leucine oxidation method 442–445
    protein turnover 436–437
    radioactive/stable tracers 436
    tissues, ^2H_2O use 445–448
    tracer AA continuous infusion 440–442
  whole-body and tissue-specific 448–451
protein turnover, intracellular 436–437, 522; *see also*
    intracellular protein degradation
  blood flow as AA metabolism regulator 527–528
  factors affecting 525–526
  MTOR cell signaling 522–524
  nutritional factors affecting **527**
  physiological factors affecting **528**
  stress and pathological factors affecting **529**
Proteobacteria 96

proteolysis *see* intracellular protein degradation
proteolytic digestive capacity 79–81
proteolytic enzymes **465**
proteolytic pathways *see* intracellular protein degradation
proteomics 700–701
proton-coupled amino acid transporter (PAT) 92
protoporphyria 638–639; *see also* amino acid metabolism
    errors
Proust, J.L. 23
Prout, W. 76, 339–340
PRPP *see* 5-phosphoribosyl-1-pyrophosphate (PRPP)
PRPS *see* phosphoribosylpyrophosphate synthetase
    (PRPS)
PS *see* protein synthesis (PS)
Pseudomonas aeruginosa 241
P site *see* peptidyl site (P site)
PTC *see* plasmalemmal and T-tubular caveolae (PTC)
purine 103
  ADA deficiency 648
  ADSL deficiency 648–649
  APRT deficiency 648
  catabolism of 295–296
  de novo synthesis 293
  gout 649
  history of 290–291
  Lesch–Nyhan syndrome 649
  myoadenylate deaminase deficiency 649
  in nucleotides 291–292
  PNP deficiency 650
  synthesis of 292–293
  xanthinuria 650
purine nucleoside phosphorylase (PNP) 650
purine nucleosides 358–360
  functions 564
purine nucleotide cycle *134*
PUT *see* putrescine (PUT)
putrescine (PUT) 211, 277, 278; *see also* polyamines
Pyman, F.L. 23
pyridoxal phosphate 167
pyridoxal phosphate-dependent enzyme 279
pyrimidine 290–291
  catabolism of 295–296
  de novo synthesis 294
  familial pyrimidinemia 650
  functions 564
  history of 290–291
  hyper-β-alaninemia 651
  in nucleotides 291–292
  nucleotide synthesis 295
  orotic aciduria 651
  synthesis of 293–295
  β-aminoisobutyric aciduria 650
pyrrolidine 25
pyrroline-5-carboxylate (P5C) **629,** 678
pyrroline-5-carboxylate dehydrogenase (P5CD) 206, 240,
    322, 656
pyrroline-5-carboxylate reductase (P5CR) 158, 206, 400,
    445, 656
pyrroline-5-carboxylate synthase (P5CS) 137,
    206, 656
pyrrolysine 1, 12
pyruvate 133, 160
pyruvate carboxylase 397
pyruvic acid 47

QH2 *see* reduced quinone (QH2)radioactive expression 379–381

radioactive isotopes 382–383; *see also* isotope
radioactive/stable tracers 436
radioisotopes 375, 377–379
    disintegration 377
    half-lives and types 377, **378**
    nutrient metabolism 386
    nutrients plasma fluxes calculations 387–388
    product formation calculations 386–387
    radioisotope decay *378*
    substrate oxidation calculations 386–387
radionuclides *see* radioactive isotopes
Raistrick, H. 220
Rapamycin-insensitive companion of TOR (rictor) 524
Rapport, M. 310
raptor *see* regulatory associated protein of TOR (raptor)
ras homolog enriched in brain (Rheb) 524
Rawling, N.D. 467
reactive nitrogen species (RNS) 364
reactive oxygen species (ROS) 364, **549**
Redtenbacher, J. 27
reduced quinone (QH2) 294
Reeds, P.J. 431
regulation 360–361
regulatory associated protein of TOR (raptor) 524
regulatory molecules *525*
relative N utilization 718
renal urea transporters 354–355, 354–356
rennin (chymosin) 77
respective aminoaldehydes (RCHO) 279
reversible enzyme inhibition 506; *see also* enzyme
    competitive inhibition 506–507
    double reciprocal plots 506, 507
    noncompetitive inhibition 507
    uncompetitive inhibition 507
de Rey-Paihade, J. 265
Rheb *see* ras homolog enriched in brain (Rheb)
Rhizobium leguminosarum 157–158
Rhizobium meliloti 157
ribonucleic acid (RNA) 291
    small noncoding 580
ribose-1-phosphate (R-1-P) 294
ribose-5-triphosphate (R-5-P-P-P) 294
ribosomal protein S6 (RPS6) 415
ribosomal RNA (rRNA) 408, 411
rictor *see* rapamycin-insensitive companion of TOR
    (rictor)
Ringer, A.I. 199, 211, 221
Rittenberg, D. 296
Ritthausen, K.H. 22
RNA *see* ribonucleic acid (RNA)
Roberts, E. 27
Robiquet, P.J. 1, 21
Roche, J. 221
Roentgen, Wilhelm Conrad 375
Rona, P. 76
ROS *see* reactive oxygen species (ROS)
Rose, Irwin 462
Roseman, S. 312
Rosenheim, O. 277
Rose, W.C. 1, 21, 26, 117, 136, 148, 150
Röthler, H. 220

Roth, M. 45
Rothstein, M. 221
Rouelle, H. 339
rough endoplasmic reticulum (RER) 423, *423*
R-1-P *see* ribose-1-phosphate (R-1-P)
R-5-P-P-P *see* ribose-5-triphosphate (R-5-P-P-P)
RPS6 *see* ribosomal protein S6 (RPS6)
rRNA *see* ribosomal RNA (rRNA)
Ruhemann, S. 50
rumen degradation 106–107
    AA degradation inhibition 108–109
    chemical treatment 107
    heating 106–107
    physical encapsulation 108
    polyphenolic phytochemicals 107–108
ruminal protein synthesis 101
ruminants, digestion
    AA degradation inhibition 108–109
    chemical treatment 107
    free AAs absorption 105
    gastrointestinal tract 100–103
    heating 106–107
    high-quality protein 106–107
    nitrogen recycling 105–106
    nucleic acids digestion 103–105
    nutritional implications 105–106
    nutritional significance 99–100
    physical encapsulation 108
    polyphenolic phytochemicals 107–108
    protein digestion 676
    rumen degradation 106–107
    small peptides 105
Russell, D.H. 277
Ryan, W.L. 23
R-β-aminoisobutyrate (D-β-aminoisobutyrate) 27

S *see* svedberg unit of flotation (S)Sabourin, P.J. 215
saccharopine acid pathways 221
S-adenosylhomocysteine (SAHC) 146, 219, 228, 229
S-adenosylhomocysteine hydrolase deficiency 654
S-adenosylmethionine (SAM) 255, 410, **541**
S-adenosylmethionine decarboxylase (SAMD) *206, 278*
SAHC *see* *S*-adenosylhomocysteine (SAHC)
Sallach, H.J. 136
Salmonella typhimurium 157
Salzmann, L. 22
SAM *see* *S*-adenosylmethionine (SAM)
SAMD *see* *S*-adenosylmethionine decarboxylase (SAMD)
SAM-dependent protein methyltransferase 287
sample radioactivity values (dpm) 382
SAM synthetase *see* methionine adenosyltransferase (MAT)
Sands, J.M. 354
sarcolemmal membrane (SM) 208
sarcoplasmic proteins 526
sarcosinemia 637; *see also* amino acid metabolism errors
S-benzylcysteinylglycine methyl ester 265
SBM soybean meal (SBM)
SCF *see* stem cell factor (SCF)
Schayer, R.W. 303
Schenker, S. 338
Scherer, H. 296
Schiff, H. 47
Schmidt-Nielsen, B. 354
Schoenheimer, R. 225, 375, 407, 461

Schotten, K. 27
Schreiner, P. 276
Schryver, S.B. 26
Schulze, E. 21, 22, 24
Schulz, H. 24
Schutzenberger, P. 16, 26
Schwann, T. 76
Schwarz, K. 419
Schwarze, W. 24
SDMA *see* symmetrical dimethylarginine (SDMA)
Sec *see* selenocysteine (Sec)
SECIS (selenocysteine inserting sequence) element 419
second messengers, intracellular 516
selenocysteine (Sec) 1, 12; *see also* Amino acids (AAs)
    catabolism 237
    identification 1
    L-selenocysteine 25
selenoproteins 419–420
Sendju, Y. 285
sensing
    AAs 571–572
Ser *see* serine (Ser)
Sera, Y. 220
serine (Ser); *see also* Amino acids (AAs)
    degradation 219
    hypophosphatasia 651
    phosphoglycerate dehydrogenase deficiency 651–652
    synthesis 140–146, *141*
serine hydroxymethyltransferase (SHMT) 140, 141, 144,
    217–219
serotonin pathway 236, 310
SGH *see* sorghum (SGH)
S-(iso-ethylcarboxymethyl)-glutathione 151
S-(iso-propylcarboxymethyl)-glutathione 151
Shemin, D. 140, 296
Sherwin, C.P. 322
Shiver, H.E. 281
SHMT *see* serine hydroxymethyl transferase (SHMT);
        serine hydroxymethyltransferase (SHMT)
sideroblastic anemia 637
Siegfried, M.A. 24
signaling proteins 583
signal transduction 514
    in cells *515*
    covalent modifications of target proteins 516
    extracellular ligand binding 515–516
    intracellular second messenger generation 516
    processes 515
    signaling cascade termination 516–517
silk protein 26
Simpson, M.V. 461
single-nucleotide polymorphisms (SNPs) 699
S6K1 *see* S6 kinase-1 (S6K1)
skeletal muscle 60
S6 kinase-1 (S6K1) 524
Skita, A. 26
SLC *see* solute carrier (SLC)
slope ratio method *see* nitrogen growth index
SM *see* sarcolemmal membrane (SM)
small intestine, monogastric animals
    nitrogen flows and recycling *97*
    transport
        AAs via the γ-glutamyl cycle 88–93
        free AAs via transmembrane transporters 88
        small peptides, by small intestine 93–94

small noncoding RNAs 580
small peptides 105
SMO *see* spermine oxidase (SMO)
Smyth, D.H. 75, 92
Snell, E.E. 167
SNPs *see* single-nucleotide polymorphisms (SNPs)
Snyder, S.H. 277
Soddy, Frederick 375
sodium
    malonic ester 23
    phenylbutyrate 661, 665
    transduction 597
solid-phase peptide synthesis 52
solid-state fermentation 274–275
solute carrier (SLC) 88
Sörensen, S.P.L. 47
sorghum (SGH) **712**
soybean meal (SBM) **712**
Spaeth, A.E. 21, 136, 199
SPDS *see* spermidine synthase (SPDS)
specific radioactivity, isotopes 381
    radioactive isotopes 382–383
    significance 385–392
    stable isotope enrichment 383–385
spermidine synthase (SPDS) 206, 211, 277, 575
spermine 276; *see also* polyamines
    concentrations 244
    synthase deficiency 660–661
spermine oxidase (SMO) 278, 279, 280
Sprinson, D.B. 231
26S proteasome structure 470, 471–472, *472*
S. ruminantium 103
stable isotopes; *see also* isotope
    application of 391
    nutrient metabolism 388
    nutrients plasma fluxes calculations 390–391
    product formation calculations 388–390
    product-precursor relationships 392
    substrate oxidation calculations 388–390
standard AA *see* protein
Steib, H. 23
Steiger, E. 21
stem cell factor (SCF) *525*
sterol regulatory element binding protein 1c
    (SREBP1c) 525
Stetten, M.R. 225
Steudel, H. 291
Steward, F.C. 27
Strecker, Adolph 16
Strecker, H.J. 225
Strecker method 1
Streptococcus faecalis 167
Streptomyces 34
Streptomyces coelicolor 157
Streptomyces viridochromogenes 157
strong acid and alkaline solutions 43–44
Subbarow, Y. 281
substrates availability 261–262
subtilin 52
suicide inhibition 508
sulfur-containing AA; *see also* amino acids (AAs)
    cystathioninuria 652
    cysteine catabolism 229
    cystinosis 652
    cystinuria *652*, 652–653

glycine *N*-methyltransferase deficiency 654
    homocyst(e)inuria 653
    hypermethioninemia 653–654
    methionine catabolism 228–231
    S-adenosylhomocysteine hydrolase deficiency 654
    synthesis 151–153
    taurine catabolism 231
sulfuric acid 1
Suzuki, U. 260
svedberg unit of flotation (S) 412, 413
symmetrical dimethylarginine (SDMA) 146, 147
synaptic cells 597; *see also* taste cells
Synechocystis PCC 6803 157
Szent-Gyorgyi, A. 291
S-β-aminoisobutyrate (L-β-aminoisobutyrate) 27

T3 *see* triiodothyronine (T3)
T4 *see* thyroxine (T4)
Tabor, H. 277, 303
Tachau, H. 26
Takamine, J. 304
tannin–alkaloid complex 108
taste cells 596–597
    brush cells 597
    ENaC 597
    enteroendocrine L and K cells 597
    types 596–597
taste signaling mechanisms *598*
taurine (2-aminoethanesulfonic acid) 15, 27, 28, **679**
    catabolism 231
    functions 564–565
    synthesis 138–140, 139, *139*
Tavares, C.D.J. 230
Tay–Sachs disease 639; *see also* Amino acid metabolism errors
t-BOC *see* t-butyloxy carbamate (t-BOC)
t-butyloxy carbamate (t-BOC) 52
TCA *see* trichloroacetic acid (TCA)
T cells carrying CD4 marker (Th0 CD4) *525*
TDO *see* tryptophan 2,3-dioxygenase (TDO)
Teichmann, L.K. 296
Temin, H.M. 408
teozein 26
terminating codon *see* nonsense codon
tetrahydrobiopterin (THF) *132, 141*
    metabolomics 701
    nutrigenomics 699–700
    proteomics 700–701
    synthesis *209*
Th1 *see* T helper cell 1 (Th1)
Th2 *see* T helper cell 2 (Th2)
Th0 CD4 *see* T cells carrying CD4 marker (Th0 CD4)
theanine 15, 17, 540; *see also* amino acids (AAs)
T helper cell 1(Th1) *525*
T helper cell 2 (Th2) *525*
thermodynamics 501
    enthalpy change 503
    entropy 503
    first law of 502–503
    Gibbs free energy 503–504
    second law of 503
THF *see* tetrahydrobiopterin (THF)
thiamine pyrophosphate (TPP) *160, 201,* 214
Thierfelder, H. 322
thionyl chloride (SOCl2)- 49

Thompson, J.F. 27
Thompson, J.R. 230
Thr *see* threonine (Thr)
threonine (Thr) 1
    aldolase 231
    catabolism 231–234
    synthesis *162*
thromboxane B2 (TXB2) **550**
Thudichum, J.L.W. 296
thymine reductase *see* dihydropyrimidine dehydrogenase (DPD)
thyroglobulin 306
thyroid hormones
    synthesis and catabolism of 306
thyroxine (T4) **541**
Tiedermann, F. 27
tissue-specific protein degradation 491–492
TLR *see* toll-like receptors (TLR)
TML *see* trimethyllysine (TML)
TNF-α *see* tumor necrosis factor-α(TNF-α)
Todd, Margaret 375
Tolkatschevskaya, N. 258
toll-like receptors (TLR) 546
Tomita, M. 285
Tomlinson, C. 136
total parenteral nutrition (TPN) 336, 592
toxic AAs degradation 109
TP *see* true protein (TP)
TPH *see* tryptophan hydroxylase (TPH)
TPN *see* total parenteral nutrition (TPN)
TPP *see* thiamine pyrophosphate (TPP)
tracer and nontracer methods 481–483
tracer method 481–483, 693–698; *see also* factorial method; N balance measurement; "-omics" technologies
    advantages and disadvantages 697–698
    direct AA oxidation method 694–695
    factors to consider 695
    indicator AA oxidation method 695–697
    obligatory losses 698–699
tracer/tracer ratio (TTR) 381, **384,** 390
transaminase 212–214
transamination pathway 47, 230–231, 237
transcription factors 577
transfer RNA (tRNA) 408
trans-4-Hydroxy-L-proline 23
transient receptor potential melastatin 5 (TRPM5) 595
trans-L-4-hydroxyproline 34
transport of AAs
    AAs via the γ-glutamyl cycle 88–93
    free AAs via transmembrane transporters 88
    small peptides, by small intestine 93–94
    substances in animal cells **89–92**
transsulfuration pathway 228–229
trichloroacetic acid (TCA) 25, 54, 60
triiodothyronine (T3) **541**
triiodothyronine synthesis *307*
trimethylglycine *see* betaine (Trimethylglycine)
trimethyllysine (TML) 633
    dioxygenase deficiency 633
tRNA *see* transfer RNA (tRNA)
tRNA-bound AA on 80S ribosome 416
Trp *see* tryptophan (Trp)
TRPM5 *see* transient receptor potential melastatin 5 (TRPM5)

"true ileal" digestibility coefficients 81–82
true protein (TP) **712**
Trypanosoma brucei 277
Trypanosoma cruzi 30
trypsin 78
tryptophan (Trp) 26, 35, 43, 556–557
    aromatic L-amino acid decarboxylase deficiency 655
    carcinoid *654*, 654–655
    Hartnup disease 655
    synthesis *163*
tryptophan catabolism 310
    kynurenine pathway 234–236
    serotonin pathway 236
    transamination pathway 237
tryptophan 2,3-dioxygenase (TDO) 234
tryptophan hydroxylase (TPH) 310
tumor necrosis factor-α (TNF-α) *525*, **529**
type 2 diabetes mellitus 738
tyrosinase (Tyrosine hydroxylase) 640
tyrosine (Tyr) 35, 39, 48, 76
    albinism 640, *640*
    alkaptonuria 641
    aromatic L-amino acid decarboxylase deficiency 641
    conversion *308*
    hypertyrosinemia 641–643, *642, 643*
    hypothyroidism 643–644
    ocular albinism, type 1 641
    phenylketonuria *644*, 644–645
    pheochromocytoma 645
    synthesis 127, 150, 159–160, *163*
tyrosine hydroxylase *see* tyrosinase (Tyrosine hydroxylase)
tyrosinosis 150, 643; *see also* Amino acid metabolism errors

U *see* uracil (U)
ubiquitin-activating enzyme (E1) 462
ubiquitin-conjugating enzyme (E2) 462
ubiquitin-dependent protein degradation 472–474
ubiquitin-independent proteolytic system 470–471
ubiquitin isopeptidase 472, *473*
ubiquitin-proteasome cascade 461
ubiquitin-proteasome system functions 474
ubiquitin-protein ligase (E3) 462
UDP *see* uridine diphosphate (UDP)
UDP-D-glucose dehydrogenation 313
UDP-*N*-acetylgalactosamine 315
UGT1A1 *see* diphosphoglucuronate
            glucuronosyltransferase 1A1 (UGT1A1)
ultraviolet (UV) 568, 639
UMP *see* uridine monophosphate (UMP)
5′- untranslated region (5′-UTR) 414
uracil (U) 291, 297, 650
uracil reductase *see* dihydropyrimidine dehydrogenase
            (DPD)
urate oxidase *see* uricase
urea 106
    certain teleost fish 356–357
    elasmobranchs 356–357
    excretion, urine 353–354
    extrahepatic cells of mammals 345–346
    hepatic urea cycle 340
    historical perspectives 339–340
    by kidneys 353
    nutritional and metabolic implications 347–348
    in plasma and urine 723

    production in mammals 339
    recycling in ruminants 352–353
    urea cycle
        characteristics of 340–344
        discovery of 340
        gluconeogenesis in liver 344–345
        regulation of 348–349
    ureagenesis 349–352
    urea production 346–347
urea cycle 21, 125, *343*
    argininosuccinic aciduria 656–657
    characteristics of 340–344
    CPS-I deficiency 657
    discovery of 340
    gluconeogenesis in liver 344–345
    HHH syndrome 658
    hyperargininemia 657
    hypercitrullinemia 657
    hyperornithinemia 658
    NAG synthase deficiency 656
    regulation of 348–349
urea excretion 353–354
ureagenesis 349–352; *see also* urea production
urea–nitrogen recycling **353**
urea production 346–347; *see also* urea cycle
urea resynthesis 98
urea transporter (UT) 340, 352, 354, *355*
uric acid synthesis
    ammonia conversion 358
    chemistry 358
    energy requirement 361
        from ammonia via adenosine 361–362
        from ammonia via guanosine 362–363
        kidneys, arterial circulation 366–367
        nutritional and metabolic significance 364
        reactive nitrogen species 365–366
        reactive oxygen species 365–366
        species-specific degradation 364–365
        uric acid from ammonia 364
    historical perspectives 357–358
    purine nucleosides 358–360
    regulation 360–361
    vs. urea syntheses 367–368
uricase 364
uridine diphosphate (UDP) 294, 350, 630
uridine diphosphoglucuronate glucuronosyltransferase
            1A1 (UGT1A1) 637
uridine monophosphate (UMP) **629**
    synthase 651
uridylyl-removing enzyme 158
urinary excretion
    conjugation products 321
    glycine utilization 321–322
    important roles 354–355
    phenylacetylglutamine 322–323
    phenylalanine and glutamine 322–323
    renal transporters 354–355
    urea excretion 353–354
urocanase 639
urocanic aciduria 639–640; *see also* amino acid
            metabolism errors
US Food and Drug Administration 71
U.S. Food and Drug Administration (FDA) 15
U.S. National Research Council (NRC) 677

UT *see* Urea transporter (UT)
UV *see* ultraviolet (UV)

Val *see* valine (Val)
valine (Val) 26; *see also* Amino acids (AAs)
    metabolism 403
    transamination of **512**
    α-ketoacids 134
van Caulaert, C. 334
Van Leeuwenhoek, A. 276
Van Slyke assay 47
Van Slyke, D.D. 47, 76, 334
vasopressin 356
Vauquelin, L.N. 1, 21, 71, 276
vesicular Glu transporter (VGT) **92**
vesicular Gly/GABA transporter (VGGT) **92**
VGGT *see* vesicular Gly/GABA transporter (VGGT)
VGT *see* vesicular Glu transporter (VGT)
Vickery, H.B. 24, 26
Vilenkina, G.Y. 231
vitamin B_6-dependent, D-AA **165**
vitamin B_6-dependent transamination 237
Vogt, W. 303
von Gorup-Besanez, E. 26
von Kninerem, W. 357
von Liebig, J. 21, 26, 50, 53, 71, 281, 321
Von Poehl, A. 277

Wada, M. 21
Wagner, H. 24
Wang, X.Q. 278
Warren, K.S. 338
water
    amino acids solubility **37**
    and buffered solutions 42–43
    free AAs stability 42–43
        high pressure and high temperatures 43
        at high temperatures 43
        strong acid and alkaline solutions 43–44
    high-pressure and high-temperature 43
    at high temperatures 43
water-insoluble proteins 71
water-soluble proteins 71
Watford, M. 185

Watson, J.D. 408
Weigert, F. 24
Weiss, S. 408
Wells, I.C. 23
Werle, E. 303
Weyl, T. 17
whole-body catabolism **197–198**
whole-body infusion system 383
whole-body phenylalanine (Phe) catabolism **390**
whole-body protein turnover *477,* 723–724
Wilheim Scheele, K. 357
Williams-Ashman, H.G. 277
Willstatter, R.M. 25
Wilson's disease 630; *see also* Amino acid
            metabolism errors
Windaus, A. 303
Windmueller, H.G. 21, 136, 199
Wohler, F. 340
Wolff, Ludwig 22
Wollaston, W.H. 22
Wolosker, H. 166, 312
Wood, W.A. 167
Work, E. 34
Wray, John 319
Wu, G. 21, 98, 136, 142, 203, 230, 345
Wurtman, R.J. 310

xanthine oxidase 359, 650
xanthinuria 650; *see also* Amino acid metabolism errors
xenobiotics 561, 562
Xenopus laevis oocytes 93
X-linked creatine transporter deficiency 633; *see also*
            Amino acid metabolism errors

Yada, S. 220
Yoshimatsu, N. 234

Zak, R. 436
Zeisel, S.H. 318
Zeller, E. 277
zero-order reaction 501
Zervas, L. 22
zwitterionic form 38–42

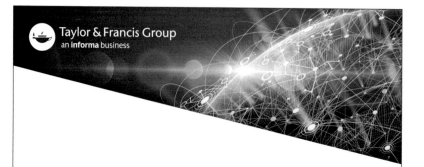